Recommended Dietary Allowances (RDA), 1980[a]

Age (years)	Weight (kg)	Weight (lbs)	Height (cm)	Height (in)	Protein (g)	(RE) Vitamin A	(µg) Vitamin D	(mg) Vitamin E	(mg) Vitamin C	(mg) Thiamin	(mg) Riboflavin	(mg equiv.) Niacin	(mg) Vitamin B₆	(µg) Folacin	(µg) Vitamin B₁₂	(mg) Calcium	(mg) Phosphorus	(mg) Magnesium	(mg) Iron	(mg) Zinc	(µg) Iodine
Infants																					
0.0-0.5	6	13	60	24	kg × 2.2	420	10	3	35	0.3	0.4	6	0.3	30	0.5	360	240	50	10	3	40
0.5-1.0	9	20	71	28	kg × 2.0	400	10	4	35	0.5	0.6	8	0.6	45	1.5	540	360	70	15	5	50
Children																					
1-3	13	29	90	35	23	400	10	5	45	0.7	0.8	9	0.9	100	2.0	800	800	150	15	10	70
4-6	20	44	112	44	30	500	10	6	45	0.9	1.0	11	1.3	200	2.5	800	800	200	10	10	90
7-10	28	62	132	52	34	700	10	7	45	1.2	1.4	16	1.6	300	3.0	800	800	250	10	10	120
Males																					
11-14	45	99	157	62	45	1,000	10	8	50	1.4	1.6	18	1.8	400	3.0	1,200	1,200	350	18	15	150
15-18	66	145	176	69	56	1,000	10	10	60	1.4	1.7	18	2.0	400	3.0	1,200	1,200	400	18	15	150
19-22	70	154	177	70	56	1,000	7.5	10	60	1.5	1.7	19	2.2	400	3.0	800	800	350	10	15	150
23-50	70	154	178	70	56	1,000	5	10	60	1.4	1.6	18	2.2	400	3.0	800	800	350	10	15	150
51+	70	154	178	70	56	1,000	5	10	60	1.2	1.4	16	2.2	400	3.0	800	800	350	10	15	150
Females																					
11-14	46	101	157	62	46	800	10	8	50	1.1	1.3	15	1.8	400	3.0	1,200	1,200	300	18	15	150
15-18	55	120	163	64	46	800	10	8	60	1.1	1.3	14	2.0	400	3.0	1,200	1,200	300	18	15	150
19-22	55	120	163	64	44	800	7.5	8	60	1.1	1.3	14	2.0	400	3.0	800	800	300	18	15	150
23-50	55	120	163	64	44	800	5	8	60	1.0	1.2	13	2.0	400	3.0	800	800	300	18	15	150
51+	55	120	163	64	44	800	5	8	60	1.0	1.2	13	2.0	400	3.0	800	800	300	10	15	150
Pregnant					+30	+200	+5	+2	+20	+0.4	+0.3	+2	+0.6	+400	+1.0	+400	+400	+150	[b]	+5	+25
Lactating					+20	+400	+5	+3	+40	+0.5	+0.5	+5	+0.5	+100	+1.0	+400	+400	+150	[b]	+10	+50

[a] The allowances are intended to provide for individual variations among most normal, healthy people in the United States under usual environmental stresses. They were designed for the maintenance of good nutrition. Diets should be based on a variety of common foods in order to provide other nutrients for which human requirements have been less well defined. See the text for a more detailed discussion of the RDA and of nutrients not tabulated.

The Committee on RDA has published a separate table showing energy allowances in ranges for each age-sex group and another table for vitamins and minerals not previously covered by the recommendations. These tables appear in Appendix O. The FDA has published a special table of selected RDA values for use on food labels: these, the U.S. RDA, appear on the inside back cover.

Reproduced from *Recommended Dietary Allowances*, 9th ed. (1980), with the permission of the National Academy of Sciences, Washington, D.C.

[b] Supplemental iron is recommended.

Understanding Nutrition

THIRD EDITION

Understanding Nutrition

THIRD EDITION

Eleanor Noss Whitney   Eva May Nunnelley Hamilton

Revised by
Eleanor Noss Whitney
with
Marie A. Boyle

West Publishing Company
St. Paul   New York   Los Angeles   San Francisco

Copyediting Beverly Peavler, Naples Editing Service
Composition K. F. Merrill Co.
Text Illustration Brenda Booth
Cartoons Barbara Clark
Cover Photomicrograph of pantothentic acid. Tore Johnson from Woodfin Camp &
Associates

PHOTO CREDITS

1, 49, 123, 155, 193, 231, 269, 321, 367, 409, 521, 547 From D. W. Fawcett,
The Cell 2nd ed., (Philadelphia: Saunders, 1981). **34** © Robert Gaylord. **85**
From D. W. Fawcett, *An Atlas of Fine Structure,* (Philadelphia: Saunders, 1966).
222 © Kent Reno, Jeroboam. **225** Lorraine Rorke/Icon. **322** Ron Alexander,
Stock, Boston, Inc. **327** David J. Farr. **385** Courtesy of Gjon Mili. **449** Reprinted
from *Food Technology*, Vol. 31, No. 10, p. 34, 1977. Copyright © by Institute of
Food Technologists. Courtesy of E. Varriano-Marston, Ph.D. **487** Courtesy of
Landrum B. Shettles, M.D. **493, 500** George Malave, Stock, Boston, Inc. **516**
Elizabeth Crews/Icon. **548** Frank Siteman, Stock, Boston, Inc.

Library of Congress Cataloging in Publication Data
Whitney, Eleanor Noss.
  Understanding nutrition.
  Includes bibliographical references and index.
  1. Nutrition. 2. Metabolism. I. Hamilton, Eva May Nunnelley. II. Title.
QP141.W46 1984 613.2 83-23568
ISBN 0-314-77862-4

To the world's children, born and unborn—
may they be nourished both with the
understanding of nutrition and with love.

Ellie Whitney
Marie Boyle

About the Authors

Eleanor Noss Whitney, Ph.D., R.D., received her B.A. in Biology from Radcliffe College in 1960 and her Ph.D. in Biology from Washington University, St. Louis, in 1970. Formerly on the faculty at the Florida State University, she now devotes full time to research, writing, and consulting in nutrition and health. She is president of The Nutrition Company of Tallahassee, Inc., a nutrition information resource center. Her previous publications include articles in *Science*, the *Journal of Nutrition*, *Genetics*, and other journals, and the textbooks *Nutrition: Concepts and Controversies* and *Understanding Normal and Clinical Nutrition*.

Marie Ann Boyle received her B.A. in Psychology from the University of Maine in 1975 and is presently completing her M.S. in Nutrition and the requirements for the R.D. at the Florida State University. She has worked in the outpatient and dietetics departments of the Maine Medical Center, Portland, in the operation of a health-oriented restaurant in New York, and as nutritionist for a children's weight-loss camp in Florida.

Contents

Appendixes

Preface

The wide acceptance of *Understanding Nutrition* since its first publication in 1977 has been gratifying. May Hamilton and I are happy to know that our efforts at communicating the excitement and fascination of nutrition have reached so many readers. At the same time, we have become keenly aware of the burden of responsibility we bear as a consequence, to make the text as accurate and complete as possible. This third edition represents a major undertaking, not unlike writing a whole new book. It has been a challenge to incorporate new, important information without making the book unmanageably large and without cramping the style that has made it interesting and fun to read. Marie Boyle and I hope we have successfully met this challenge.

This edition has two new chapters—Chapters 1 and 12—yet is shorter by two chapters than the second edition. A multitude of new insights and findings enrich its pages. Chapter 1 brings together into one place an introduction to the nutrients and kcalories; foods and food group plans; the nutrient density concept; exchange systems; the RDA and other standards; the scientific method; and dietary guidelines; it also introduces the basics of nutrition assessment (the details are reserved for Chapter 12). Chapters 2, 3, and 4 are devoted to the energy nutrients—carbohydrates, lipids, and protein; and Chapter 5 reveals the body's handling of them during digestion, absorption, and transport. Chapter 6 explains metabolism; Chapter 7 explores the causes of obesity and also includes approaches to weight control. Chapters 8, 9, 10, and 11 present the vitamins, minerals, and water. Chapter 12 presents nutrition assessment techniques in greater depth, shows their uses in nutrition surveys, presents results of the major recent U.S. and Canadian surveys, and concludes with recommendations for improved diet planning. Chapters 13, 14, and 15 then develop the themes important in nutrition throughout life, from conception to old age. A complete course in nutrition could logically stop after Chapter 11; a more comprehensive course would include Chapter 12 or all 15 chapters.

New Highlights

1A *Natural Foods*—puts into perspective their pros and cons and explains the meaning of the term *organic*

1B *Vitamin-Mineral Supplements*—shows how to decide rationally whether you need one.

2 *Sugar Stands Accused*—clears sugar of all charges except its contribution to dental caries—but look at Highlight 7 for more on sugar.

4 *Nutrition and the Brain*—shows the relationship of diet to the neurotransmitters, and their connections to pain and sleep.

6 *Nutrition for the Athlete*—explores the areas of nutrition important to peak athletic performance.

7 *Sugar Addiction*—explains why sugar is so attractive, describes binge eating, and discusses its relationship to puritanical attitudes about food.

9 *World Hunger*—makes vivid the problem of world hunger, reviews recent successful attempts at local solutions, identifies U.S. and multinational corporations' responsibilities for some of the problems, and concludes with suggestions for individual action.

11 *Contaminants in Foods*—uses mercury, lead poisoning, DDT, and PBB as examples to show how contaminants can affect the body, where they come from, how serious a concern they are.

Note on Self-Study 7: We have revised the energy portion of the Self-Study in accordance with current research. Students should find that their estimated energy expenditures agree well with the extent of their activity.

Alternating with the chapters are Highlights on topics of great interest to today's readers. A few of these are adapted from *Nutrition: Concepts and Controversies*; all but a few are new to *Understanding Nutrition* as of this edition, and the original ones have been completely revised. We have thoroughly enjoyed all the new learning involved in each area and have found it challenging to attempt to present a balance of viewpoints where controversy is rife.

As before, one of the main missions of the book is to assist the reader who wants not only to learn nutrition "facts," but also to become a discriminating consumer of newly emerging nutrition information. "How can I decide what to believe?" the reader wants to know. Portions of every chapter—the digressions—and most of the Highlights are devoted to constructing a sieve through which readers can filter new nutrition claims and separate the valid ones from the rest.

In the past, the book has attempted to reserve chapters for "solid information" and highlights and digressions for controversial items. Highlights and digressions were printed on shaded paper to remind the reader that they were tentative. This edition, too, shades digressions and Highlights, but the distinction is not as clear-cut in this edition. A few of the Highlights are quite factual (for example, the one on labeling) and here and there some information is presented in chapters that may well become "yesterday's news"—that is, out of date—five years from now. Selections from the original Note to the Student, written for the first edition, convey an important message about this problem, and are appended right after this Preface. In brief, the message is that there is no absolute certainty, even in science's "facts," and that human critical thinking and judgment must always be applied in assessing claims. Students often find this news difficult to accept, but we cannot make it otherwise.

In fact, if the book were to be utterly, rigidly true to the nature of nutrition science, it would present no statements without a "may," a "probably," or an "is thought to be." The only reason why these phrases don't appear throughout is because they would take up too much space. The reader should read them in. Nothing here is gospel.

Space has also been saved by reducing the number of footnotes to a minimum. Many statements that have appeared in the previous editions with footnotes now appear without them. The reader who has an older edition of *Understanding Nutrition* can easily find them there; the reader who is new to this edition should know that every statement is backed by evidence and that the authors will supply references on request. If all references were retained, however, this third edition would have more footnotes than text on many of its pages. The suggested readings, formerly at the ends of chapters, have been gathered into a continuous sequence in Appendix J, also to save space. The space saved by these means has been spent developing nutrition concepts in a complete and orderly fashion.

The Self-Studies are all in Appendix Q, where they form a coherent unit parallel to the chapters. Notes at the ends of the chapters alert you to the references and Self-Studies.

A new feature of this book is the photographs of cells at the start of each chapter, which add depth to the understanding of nutrition. Most of them were taken through an electron microscope, and they magnify their subjects some 10,000 to 100,000 times. In most cases, the original reference did not give the exact magnification, and no attempt was made to estimate it; it seems necessary only to know that the pictures reveal views of cellular activity so intimate that you can almost see the molecules at work.

An abundance of interesting information, related to the basics presented here, is available in the *Instructor's Manual*, which includes 14 optional lectures on topics of interest, and TH (transparency/handout) masters that expand on text topics. Figures and tables in this book that are marked with "TH" numbers indicate which ones are available for projection as transparencies; notes at the ends of the chapters inform you of additional TH masters in the *Manual*.

The explosion of new information since the last edition prompts a new thought. Nutrition science has enlarged its domain in the ten years since the first edition of *Understanding Nutrition* was in the early stages of preparation. It is not only that the authors have learned more (although that is certainly true), but that interest, support, and research in nutrition have greatly expanded nationwide. The time has come when nutrition could claim, with biology, chemistry, and the other sciences, to be worth a full year's attention at the college level for students who wish to say they really understand it, but until it is accorded that status, this text will remain usable for a one-term college course.

The expansion of nutrition knowledge is reflected in this book's revised Appendixes. New in this edition are (among others) Appendix E, which offers a dozen nutrition assessment standards and tools; Appendix H, which presents 71 new foods in addition to the 730 foods of the standard handbook; and, in addition to the three minerals and five vitamins in previous editions, the zinc and folacin contents of all foods for the first time; and Appendix P, which compares the composition of national-brand vitamin-mineral supplements and offers rational guidelines for selecting one. The reader who takes time to explore the appendixes will discover a broad and convenient array of information for reference.

A note on style: In writing, we sometimes split infinitives, sometimes start sentences with "And" or "But," now and then speak of ourselves as "we," and often address the reader as "you," not because we don't know any better, but because we think of the book as a conversation with students in which such practices are relaxed and comfortable. We hope the style is pleasing to readers and eases learning.

In other ways, however, we are conservative. We use the adjectival form *nutrition* to modify "status," "assessment," "education," and the like, reserving *nutritional* for its proper meaning: "conveying nutrients." We have been careful to use the recently agreed-upon nomenclature for the vitamins: "vitamin C" (not ascorbic acid), and "folacin" (not folic acid), for example. To avoid gender bias without going to vague uninteresting plural forms, we have alternated between "he" and "she" in examples; in doing so, we hope we have been fair to both genders.

Finally, to give credit where it is due, we have been assisted and supported by the finest group of associates any authors could ask for. We are especially grateful to Annette Franklin for her untiring, meticulous work on the word processor; Delores Truesdell for her monumental effort and skill in assembling the new food composition data; Sharon Rady Rolfes for her loving attention to the *Instructor's Manual*; Lorraine Bailey for the *Student Study Guide*; Frances Sizer for her creation of Appendix P and of the diet-rating table in Chapter 7 and for innumerable other contributions; and our wonderful, enthusiastic, patient, and long-suffering editors Gary Woodruff, Phyllis Cahoon, and Lenore Franzen. Our reviewers have also made many helpful contributions: Barbara Gilpin, Carol Bishop, William Lockhart, Fay Dong, Diane Wakat, J. DeWolfe, Susan Dougherty, Jeanne Mott, Carolyn Knutson, Kathy Timmons, Annamarie Herndon, Carolyn Lara-Braud, Constance Jordan, Merrill Christensen, and especially Kay B. Franz and Stan Winter. Most importantly, we want readers to know that, although this edition appears under our names, it is still May Hamilton's book, too. She participated in giving birth to the first edition and nurtured the second, and her loving care is apparent everywhere in this, the third edition.

Eleanor N. Whitney
Marie A. Boyle
January 1984

Note to the Student

You may have some questions in mind as you approach the study of nutrition. In getting to know students over the years, we have some idea of what your concerns may be.

I keep hearing exciting news about nutrition. How can I tell what to believe? This is the complaint we hear most often from students. Because of it, we have designed this book not to be just a book of facts but also a book of principles that you can use to assess the nutrition information you encounter elsewhere. Today's nutrition science stands firmly on the principles of chemistry and molecular biology. This book is based on those principles.

Even with the principles clearly in mind, however, it is sometimes hard to tell whether a statement made in the marketplace is a valid fact or a myth. Some major controversies currently raging in our field concern sugar, fiber, cholesterol, vitamin C and cancer, additives, and many other issues. It would not be fair to present these issues to you in textbook fashion as if they were settled, but it makes the study of our lively science needlessly dull to omit them. Our decision has been to reserve the **chapters** mostly for solid information, on which the experts in our field largely agree, and to present separate **highlights** on the current issues, for more speculative material. The highlights alternate with the chapters and are printed on colored pages to remind you that they convey more tentative information.

Even though we are scientists, in some cases we have no facts. Researchers in nutrition are earnestly endeavoring to learn more, but there are many areas where we are still in the dark. Students can be infuriated when a teacher seems to weasel: "I want the facts, and you are hedging. Give me the answer, straight and simple." It is frustrating to ask why and have a cautious scientist reply, "Well, we know this, and this, and . . ." but leave your question dangling. It is insulting to be told, "It's too complicated to understand," which sounds suspiciously like what mother used to say: "Wait until you are older, dear." But the truth of the matter is that there are a great many things we do not understand. One of the most exciting, as well as frustrating, experiences for students can be the dawning realization that they are approaching the outer bounds of human knowledge. The answers are simply not all in yet; no one knows what they all are; no one ever has. This is true in many areas of nutrition; it is a growing, young science. Although its questions are immensely important and fascinating, that is all they are—questions. We have tried to be honest in this respect: to show you what we do know (with a high probability) and to admit what we don't.

In attempting to present a fair picture of current nutrition research in the highlights, we have found ourselves at times confused, frustrated, angered, and amused. If you too respond this way in reading the maybes and probablys of today's nutrition issues, then be assured that you are close to the reality of our science. Any book that claims at this time to present absolute answers to all questions is actually only presenting one person's prejudices. The writer may be proved right in years to come, but some of the winners have not yet been declared. If you wish to be informed on the current issues, you will have to accept the ambiguities and contradictions in the evidence and the disagreements among the experts as an instrinsic part of scientific research in progress.

But then how can I choose what to believe? In the absence of all the facts, we still have to live and make decisions. Should you eat polyunsaturated fats? Avoid tuna? Beef? Sugar? It would not be fair to answer simply "We don't know" to all these questions. Where the answers are uncertain today, we owe it to you to help in developing the skill to evaluate new information as it appears tomorrow. Our field is beset with claims and appeals, and all of us as consumers need to be equipped to deal with them.

There are some guidelines that would help you discriminate between reliable information and false advertising. It seems to us that a separate chapter devoted to this subject would not serve the purpose. You need continuous, repeated exposure to the kinds of claims made to consumers, and you need practice in assessing them. We offer frequent opportunities, by way of **digressions** throughout the text, for you to examine such sources of nutrition information and to assess their reliability against the criteria of accurate scientific reporting. In these digressions we have identified the most common characteristics of fraudulent advertising and the most common misunderstandings that arise from reading about nutrition research.

The digressions are set off with color like this; if they prove too distracting you can skip them and possibly come back to them later. But they constitute a theme that runs throughout the book.

Caution

In some cases we have clear-cut evidence that a claim being made on the marketplace is fraudulent. We feel obligated to explain and elaborate on these cases. It is not enough to tell you these are myths and provide nothing to replace them. But there is another problem. It seems to us that it is also not enough to say "That is a myth, and this is a fact." After all, aren't "they" saying their myth is a fact? Confronted with a choice between what "they" say and what "we" (in a nutrition text) say, you are in the bind of having to choose whom to believe, with nothing further to go on. We hope, by providing relevant information, to show you that what we say is more probably true than the myth you might otherwise believe. You will understand why the low-carbohydrate diet is ill advised when you know that carbohydrate is needed to metabolize fat in the body and how the body may be damaged when carbohydrate is not available. You will understand why taking large doses of vitamin C may be harmful when you know what can happen to people who indulge in that practice.

In using some of our space to deal with current issues, consumer questions, and health food myths, we have elected not to present an encyclopedic book of all the knowledge that has been accumulated in our rapidly expanding field. Instead, we have stressed concepts, using selected facts to illustrate the principles on which they are based. Information in the chapters is, however, amplified by abundant additional information in the **appendixes**. We hope you will explore them and find them useful. We believe it is important to gain an acquaintance with the general principles of nutrition, as well as to develop the incentive and ability to identify reliable nutrition information on your own. Armed with this skill, you can continually gather and apply the information that is relevant to your own particular concerns.

Understanding Nutrition

THIRD EDITION

CHAPTER 1
Introduction to Nutrition

CONTENTS

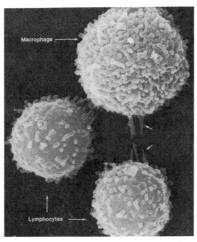

The body's cells are highly sensitive and energetic, and require many nutrients to sustain their activities. Shown here are three white blood cells—the body's defenders against disease.

You are what you eat.

UNKNOWN

You are a collection of molecules that move. All these moving parts are arranged into patterns of extraordinary complexity and order—cells, tissues, and organs. The arrangement is constant, but its parts are continuously being replaced by a process using nutrients, and using energy derived from nutrients. Your skin, which has reliably covered you from the time you were born, is not the same skin that covered you seven years ago; it is made entirely of new cells. The fat beneath your skin is not the same fat that was there a year ago. Your oldest red blood cell is only 120 days old, and the entire lining of your digestive tract is renewed every three days. To maintain your "self," you must continually replenish the energy you burn and replace the pieces you lose.

All these pieces have come from your food. You are made entirely of what you have eaten. Amazingly, though, whether you ate spaghetti or apple pie last night, the nutrients supplied by these foods are handled the same way by your body, so that in the end there is no way to know which food you ate. Only if the spaghetti and the apple pie, together with the other foods you choose to eat, do not contain the nutrients you need, do you fail to function as well as you might. For optimum health, you need not only adequate amounts of the essential nutrients

1

science of nutrition: the study of nutrients and of their ingestion, digestion, absorption, transport, metabolism, interaction, storage, and excretion. A broader definition includes the study of the environment and of human behavior as it relates to these processes.

nutrient: a substance obtained from food and used in the body to promote growth, maintenance, and/or repair. The **essential nutrients** are those the body cannot make for itself in sufficient quantity but has to obtain from food.

The six classes of nutrients are carbohydrate, fat, protein, vitamins, minerals, and water.

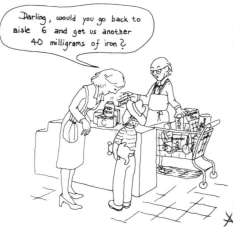

Darling, would you go back to aisle 6 and get us another 40 milligrams of iron?

Atoms, molecules, and compounds: Appendix B summarizes basic chemistry facts and provides definitions.

Intentional additives are the subject of Highlight 10. Incidental additives (pollutants and contaminants in foods) are treated in Highlight 11.

but, ideally, an assortment of nutrients in good proportion to each other. The science of nutrition is the study of the nutrients in food and the body's handling of these nutrients.

The Nutrients

Almost any food you eat is composed of dozens or even hundreds of different kinds of materials, atoms and molecules—tinier by far than the smallest things that can be seen with the most powerful microscope. The complete chemical analysis of a food such as spinach shows that it is composed mostly of water (95 percent) and that most of the solid materials are organic compounds: carbohydrate, fat, and protein. If you could remove these materials, you would find a tiny residue of minerals, vitamins, and other materials. Water, carbohydrate, fat, protein, vitamins, and some of the minerals are nutrients. Some of the other materials are not.

A complete chemical analysis of your body would show that it is made of similar materials. If you weigh 150 pounds, your body contains about 90 pounds of water and (if 150 pounds is the ideal weight for you) about 30 pounds of fat. The other 30 pounds are mostly protein, carbohydrate, related organic compounds made from them, and the major minerals of your bones: calcium and phosphorus. Vitamins, other minerals, and incidental extras constitute a fraction of a pound. Thus you, like spinach, are composed largely of nutrients (see Figure 1–1).

(This book is devoted mostly to the nutrients, but you should be aware that other constituents are found in foods and in your body—both intentional additives and incidental ones, such as pollutants. Some are beneficial, some are of no recognized positive value to humans, and some are harmful. Later sections of the book focus on these constituents and their significance.)

If you burn a food such as spinach in air, it disappears. The water evaporates, and all the organic compounds are oxidized to gas (carbon dioxide) and water vapor, leaving only a residue of ash (minerals). This leads us to a definition of the word *organic*.

An organic compound is one that contains carbon atoms. The first organic compounds known were natural products synthesized by plants or animals; indeed, it used to be thought that only living things contributed organic compounds to our world. The term has since been expanded to include all carbon compounds, whatever their origin. Actually, in a sense, all organic compounds are produced by living things. Some of them, like petroleum (which comes from the remains of microorganisms, plants, and animals that grew in prehistoric times), began and ended their lives millions of years ago. Others are produced by plants and animals alive today. Still others come from laboratories where chemists (who are also living things) produce them in the test tube.

Labels on food products sometimes make the claim that the product is "organic," implying that it is therefore somehow superior. By the definition given above, any carbon compound is organic, even a synthetic vitamin preparation from the laboratory of a pharmaceutical company. Is there any reason to believe that "organic" or "natural" foods or nutrient preparations sold in "health food" stores are superior to grocery store foods or synthetic vitamins? Highlight 1A investigates this question.

In any case, four of the six classes of nutrients—carbohydrate, fat, protein, and vitamins—are organic, while the other two (minerals and water) are not. On being oxidized during metabolism, three of these four (carbohydrate, fat, and protein) provide energy the body can use. In contrast, minerals and water are inorganic and are not oxidized in the human body to yield energy (they can oxidize, however, as iron does when it rusts).

At this point it is clear that molecules account both for your body's structure and for its activities. You are made of atoms taken from some of the molecules of food and rearranged into the molecules of your body. You are able to go about your various pursuits thanks to the energy released when other food molecules are taken apart.

FIGURE 1–1 Food and the human body are made of the same classes of chemicals. (Vitamins are not shown because the amount is too small to be seen in a picture this size.)

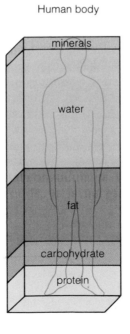

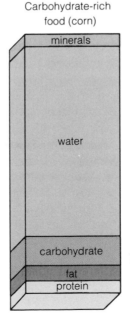

organic: containing carbon or, more strictly, containing carbon and hydrogen or carbon-carbon bonds. This definition excludes coal (which has no defined bonds); a few carbon-containing compounds such as carbon dioxide (which contains only a single carbon and no hydrogen); and salts such as calcium carbonate ($CaCO_3$), magnesium carbonate ($MgCO_3$), and sodium cyanide ($NaCN$). See also pp. 35–36.

The organic nutrients are carbohydrate, fat, protein, and vitamins. The first three yield energy for human use.

oxidation: often, a reaction in which atoms from a molecule are combined with oxygen, usually resulting in the release of energy. Chemical oxidation of nutrients differs from oxidative combustion (burning) in that the energy released is largely chemical and mechanical, rather than heat and light energy. A more complete and accurate explanation is given in Appendix B.

Metabolism, the set of processes by which nutrients are rearranged into body structures or broken down to yield energy, is defined and described in Chapter 6.

The energy nutrients are carbohydrate, fat, and protein.

calorie: a unit in which energy is measured. Technically, a calorie is the amount of heat necessary to raise the temperature of a gram of water one degree Centigrade. Food energy is measured in **kilocalories** (thousands of calories), abbreviated **kcalories** or **kcal**, or capitalized: **Calories**. Most people, even nutritionists, speak of these units simply as calories, but on paper they should be prefaced by a k. (The pronunciation of *kcalories* ignores the k, but some people when speaking pronounce it "KAY-calories" or "KAY-cal.") We will use *kcalories* and *kcal* throughout this book.

The Energy Nutrients

You can metabolize all four classes of organic nutrients, but derive energy from only three. These three are the energy nutrients. They are vital to life, for without continual replenishment of the energy you spend daily, you would soon die. When oxidized in the body, the energy nutrients break down; that is, their carbon and hydrogen atoms (and others) come apart and are combined with oxygen, yielding carbon dioxide and water, waste materials that must be excreted.

If you burn a potful of food on the range, the same kind of thing happens. Heat is released together with carbon dioxide and water vapor, and you are left with a ruined pot, blackened with the carbon and mineral residue from the food. But when you oxidize food in your body, the energy is not all released as heat. (You aren't left with a black carbon residue, either!) Some energy is transferred into other compounds (including fat) that compose the structures of your body cells, and some of the energy that holds the atoms of the energy nutrients together is used as fuel for your activities.

The amount of energy the energy nutrients release can be measured in calories (or more properly, kilocalories), which are familiar to everyone as those things that make foods "fattening."[1] The calorie content of a food thus depends on how much carbohydrate, fat, and protein it contains. If you don't use these nutrients immediately after you eat them, your body rearranges them (and the energy they contain) into storage compounds such as body fat and puts them away for later. Thus an excess intake of any of the three energy nutrients can lead to overweight. Too much meat (a protein-rich food) is just as fattening as too many potatoes (a carbohydrate-rich food).

It is important not to forget the organic compound found in some beverages: alcohol. Alcohol is not properly called a nutrient by the definition given earlier, because it doesn't promote growth, maintenance, or repair in the body. Still, people do consume it, and it shares several characteristics with the energy nutrients. Like them, it is metabolized in the body to yield energy. When taken in excess of energy need, it, too, is converted to body fat and stored. But when alcohol contributes a substantial portion of the energy in a person's diet, its effects are damaging. (Highlight 8A is devoted to alcohol and nutrition.)

Practically all foods contain mixtures of all three energy nutrients, although they are sometimes classified by the predominant nutrient. Thus it is not correct to speak of meat as a protein or of bread as a carbohydrate; they are *foods* rich in these nutrients. A protein-rich food like beef actually contains a lot of fat as well as protein; a carbohydrate-rich food like corn also contains fat and protein, as shown in Figure 1–1. Only a few foods are exceptions to this rule, the common ones being sugar (which is pure carbohydrate) and oil (which is almost pure fat).

---

1   Food energy can also be measured in kilojoules (kJ): A kilojoule is the amount of energy expended when a kilogram is moved one meter by a force of one newton. One kcalorie equals 4.2 kJ. The kilojoule is now the international unit of energy, and the United States and Canada will slowly be switching over to it in the next decades, but it is not in popular use yet. This book does not use the kilojoule.

Figure 1–2 outlines very simply the flow of the energy nutrients into and through the body. The next six chapters reveal the many services they render to you.

The energy nutrients are (by molecular standards) tremendous in size. A single molecule of carbohydrate may be composed of 300 sugar (glucose) units, each containing 24 atoms, for a total of some 7,000 atoms. Fats and proteins are similar in size. Even when they are broken down during digestion, they are absorbed as sizable units—and these are often reassembled back into macromolecules in the cells. Only if they are oxidized for fuel do they diminish in size to tiny molecules of carbon dioxide and water (three atoms each). When this occurs, they release tremendous quantities of energy for your use.

Furthermore, you eat (by molecular standards) tremendous quantities of the three energy nutrients. Some people eat a hundred or more grams a day of each. If you could purify the carbohydrate, fat, and protein in your daily diet, they would fill two or three measuring cups.

Carbohydrate, fat, and protein: large, organic molecules. Definitions appear in Chapters 2, 3, and 4, respectively.

macromolecule: a huge molecule, composed of hundreds or thousands of atoms. (A molecule of water, by contrast, is composed of only three atoms: 2 Hs and 1 O.)

A Note about Grams

Most people don't think of foods in terms of grams. It's easy to learn to do so, though, and a good idea for those who plan to work with foods in the future. The United States and Canada are both in the midst of a shift from the old British system of measurement to the metric system, so grams can be expected to become more and more a part of our lives. Food scientists already use 100 grams of foods as standard sizes for analysis, so 100 grams is a good size to learn to visualize. For a start, remember first that 100 grams is (very roughly) the weight of a normal serving (a half cup) of most vegetables or a half cup of milk or juice. Second, remember that a teaspoon of any dry powder such as sugar, salt, or flour weighs (very roughly) 5 grams. For accurate conversion factors, look on the inside back cover.

Normal vegetable servings (½ cup) are about 100 grams. A half cup of vegetables, juice, or milk is about 100 grams. 1 teaspoon any dry powder is about 5 grams.

The vitamins, the next class of nutrients, differ profoundly from the first three classes in almost every way: in their size and shape, in the roles they play in the body, and in the amounts you consume. Perhaps the only characteristics they share with the first three classes of nutrients are that they are vital to life, they are organic, and they are available in food.

The Vitamins

The vitamins are organic compounds generally much smaller than the energy nutrients. Their use in the body is not to be metabolized for energy; in fact, if they do happen to be broken down, they yield no usable energy. Their role is to serve as helpers, making possible the processes by which the other nutrients are digested, absorbed, and metabolized or built into body structures. There are 15 different vitamins, each with its own special roles to play (see Table 1–1).

vitamin: an organic compound, vital to life, indispensable to body function, needed in minute amounts; an essential nutrient.

vita = life

amine = containing nitrogen (the first vitamins discovered were amines)

FIGURE 1–2 **Metabolism of the energy nutrients**. The atoms in a molecule are held together by energy in the form of chemical bonds. When a large molecule, such as a carbohydrate molecule, is broken apart, some of the chemical bonds are broken and energy is released. The atoms themselves are never broken apart in chemical reactions, only regrouped.

Note: We will use the convention throughout this book that arrows pointing downward represent reactions in which molecules (groups of atoms) are being broken into smaller molecules and energy is being released. Arrows pointing upward represent reactions in which larger molecules are being built, with energy used for the bonding.

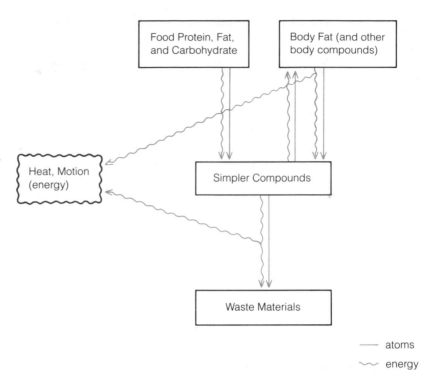

TABLE 1–1 **The Vitamins**[a]

The fat-soluble vitamins
    Vitamin A
    Vitamin D
    Vitamin E
    Vitamin K
The water-soluble vitamins
    B Vitamins
        Thiamin
        Riboflavin
        Niacin
        Vitamin B_6
        Vitamin B_{12}
        Folacin
        Biotin
        Pantothenic Acid
    Vitamin C

---

[a] The names given here for the vitamins are those agreed on by the American Institute of Nutrition and other scientific societies and published in Nomenclature policy: Generic descriptors and trivial names for vitamins and related compounds, *Journal of Nutrition* 112 (1982): 7-14.

The fact that vitamins are organic has several consequences. For one thing, vitamins are destructible. They can be broken down, oxidized, altered in shape. They must therefore be handled with care. The body makes special provisions to absorb and transport them, providing many of them with custom-made protein carriers. A vitamin may be useful in one form here and another there, so special metabolic equipment is provided that can subtly alter the characteristics of a vitamin to allow it to perform a particular task.

The destructibility of vitamins also has implications for food handlers and cooks. You are well advised, when working with food, to keep in mind that excessive acid, alkali, air, heat, or light can destroy them.

The vitamins are divided into two classes: some are soluble in water (the B vitamins and vitamin C) and others in fat (vitamins A, D, E, and K). This fact has many implications for the kinds of foods they are found in, and the ways the body absorbs, transports, stores, and excretes them. The vitamins are the subjects of Chapters 8 and 9.

The Minerals

The minerals are inorganic compounds, smaller than vitamins and found in even simpler forms in foods. Sodium, for example, can exist as a single charged atom (ion), tiny in comparison to starch, which may be composed of hundreds or thousands of atoms. Some minerals may be put together into orderly arrays in such structures as bones and teeth—but only with the help of the body's lively metabolic machinery, which itself is composed of protein and assisted by vitamins and some minerals. When minerals are withdrawn from bone and excreted, they yield no energy. When they float about in the fluids of the body, they give the fluids certain characteristics, but they are not metabolized—arranged and rearranged—in the complicated ways or to the same extent as the energy nutrients are. You consume small amounts of minerals daily, roughly similar to the amounts of vitamins in your diet. There are 21 different minerals important in nutrition (see Table 1–2).

The water-soluble vitamins are the B vitamins and vitamin C. The fat-soluble vitamins are vitamins A, D, E, K.

The minerals are elements, whereas the other nutrients are all compounds. This means the minerals cannot lose their identity; they exist "forever," like the carbon, hydrogen, and oxygen of which the energy nutrients are composed. When you cook a food containing vitamins and minerals, the vitamins can come apart or be altered in shape as their elements undergo rearrangement. Thus the vitamins can "disappear" (lose their chemical identity), but the minerals remain unchanged. Calcium, for example, enters the body as an ion with two positive charges. It may be combined with any of a number of negative ions (phosphate, sulfate, and the like) to form salts in foods, or it may become part of a large, organic molecule, but it never loses its identity as calcium. Iron may vary, in the sense that it may exist in two different ionic states, but it, too, retains its identity and cycles repeatedly within and through living things.

Element, compound, ion: see Appendix B.

Salts and their effects on water balance are discussed in Chapter 10.

Ionic states of iron: see Appendix B.

Because they are indestructible, minerals in food need not be handled with the very special care that vitamins need. You do need to make sure, however, not to soak them out of food or throw them away in cooking water. Chapters 10 and 11 are devoted to the minerals.

Water

Water, indispensable and abundant, forms the major part of every body tissue. It is often ignored—because, like air, it is everywhere and we take it for granted. Water is inorganic, a single molecule being composed of three atoms (H_2O).[2] The amounts you must consume relative to the other nutrients are enormous: two to three liters (about two to three quarts) a day. That's 2,000 to 3,000 grams, nearly ten times the amount of the energy nutrients you need. Of course, you need not drink water as such in these quantities; it comes abundantly in foods and beverages.

Water provides the medium in which nearly all the body's activities are conducted. It participates in many of the body's metabolic reactions, and supplies the medium for transporting vital materials to cells and waste products away from them.

In addition to the obvious dietary source—water itself—virtually all foods contain water (as a look at Figure 1–1 will remind you). In addition,

TABLE 1–2 **The Minerals**

THE MAJOR MINERALS
  Calcium
  Phosphorus
  Potassium
  Sodium
  Chloride
  Magnesium
  Sulfur
THE TRACE MINERALS
  Iron
  Iodine
  Zinc
  Chromium
  Selenium
  Fluoride
  Cobalt
  Molybdenum
  Copper
  Manganese
  Vanadium
  Tin
  Silicon
  Nickel

---

2 A more accurate way to describe how water is organized would be to say that, although we know that the ratio of hydrogen atoms to oxygen atoms is 2 to 1, we do not know that water exists as discrete molecules.

water is generated from the energy nutrients in foods (recall that the carbon and hydrogen in these nutrients combine with oxygen during metabolism to yield carbon dioxide and water). Daily water intake from these three sources, which amounts to about 2½ liters or quarts a day, normally balances perfectly with daily water excretion, which takes place by way of four routes—urination, evaporation from the lungs, losses in the feces, and evaporation from the skin. Water is further discussed in Chapter 10, but is mentioned in every chapter. If you watch for it, you cannot help but be impressed by its participation in all life processes.

Food Group Plans

Now that the individual nutrients have been introduced, the question can be asked, how the available foods can be juggled to create a diet that supplies all the needed nutrients in the appropriate amounts for good health. The principle is simple enough: just select a variety of foods that present the nutrients you need. But in practice, how does this work out? It is helpful to think in terms of adequacy, balance, kcalorie control, and variety. We named adequacy first, here, for alphabetical order, but let's begin by discussing dietary balance.

Diet-planning principles are ABCV—adequacy, balance, kcalorie control, and variety.

The minerals calcium and iron illustrate the importance of dietary balance. Iron is one of the essential nutrients. You can only get it into your body by eating foods that contain it. If you miss out on these foods you can develop iron-deficiency anemia. You feel weak, tired, and unenthusiastic, may have frequent headaches, and can do very little muscular work without disabling fatigue. If you make the needed correction and add iron-rich foods to your diet, you soon feel more energetic.

Some foods are rich in iron; others are notoriously poor. Meats, fish, poultry, and legumes are in the iron-rich category, and an easy way to obtain the needed iron is to include these foods in your diet regularly. Most food group plans recommend two or more servings a day.

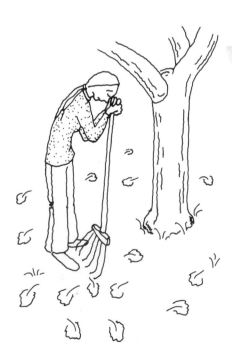

Calcium is another essential nutrient. A diet lacking calcium causes poor bone development during the growing years and a gradual bone loss in adults that can totally cripple a person in later life. The foods just named (meats and meat substitutes) are poor sources of calcium; you can get enough of this nutrient only by making frequent use of milk and milk products or carefully selected milk substitutes. Most food group plans recommend two or more cups of milk or the equivalent every day for adults and more for growing children, teenagers, and women who are either pregnant or breastfeeding their babies.

Most foods that are rich in iron are poor in calcium, and vice versa. In fact, milk (except breast milk) and milk products are so poor in iron that the overuse of these foods can actually cause iron-deficiency anemia if they displace iron-rich foods from the diet. The anemia even has a special name: milk anemia. And yet no one could accuse milk of not being a nutritious food. It is the single most nutritious food for children and is important in the diet of people of all ages.

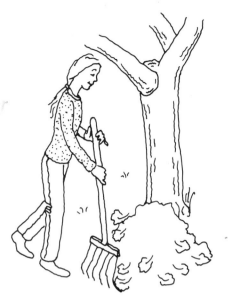

The concept to grasp from this illustration is that of dietary balance. Use enough—but not too much—meat or meat substitutes for iron; use enough —but not too much—milk and milk products for calcium. Save some space in the diet for other foods needed for other nutrients.

Iron and calcium are only two of some 40-odd essential nutrients. What foods provide the others? One of the most familiar systems of grouping foods in the United States fits the major foods into four groups, as shown in Table 1–3. Each of the four groups contains foods that are similar in origin and nutrient content. The nutrients named in the table are representative of all the nutrients, and the assumption is that once you have adequate amounts of these you'll probably have enough of the other two dozen or so essential nutrients as well, because they occur in the same groups of foods. This is not an entirely safe assumption; when fortified foods are involved, some eight or ten nutrients may be listed on the label, making the food appear nutritious, but they may be the only nutrients present. Still, with the precaution that primarily whole foods be used, the Four Food Group Plan provides a suitable foundation for diet planning.

The Four Food Group Plan specifies that a certain quantity of food must be consumed from each group. For the adult, the number of servings recommended is two, two, four, and four (see Table 1–4).

Many foods don't fit into any of the four food groups. Consider butter, margarine, cream, sour cream, salad dressing, mayonnaise, jam, jelly, broth, coffee, tea, alcoholic beverages, synthetic products, and others. These items are grouped together into a miscellaneous category. Some of them

TABLE 1–3 **The Four Food Groups[a]**

FOOD GROUP	SAMPLE FOODS	MAIN NUTRIENT CONTRIBUTIONS
Meat and meat substitutes	Beef, pork, lamb, fish, poultry, eggs, nuts, legumes	Protein, iron, riboflavin, niacin, zinc, vitamin B_{12},[b] thiamin
Milk and milk products	Milk, buttermilk, yogurt, cheese, cottage cheese, soy milk, ice cream	Calcium, protein, riboflavin, zinc, vitamin, B_{12},[b] thiamin
Fruits and vegetables	All fruits and vegetables	Vitamin A, vitamin C,[c] thiamin, additional iron and riboflavin; fiber, folacin
Grains (bread and cereal products)	All whole-grain[d] and enriched flours and products	Additional amounts of niacin, iron, thiamin;[e] zinc in whole grains; fiber

[a] This is a U.S. plan. A similar plan developed for Canada is presented in Appendix M.

[b] Vitamin B_{12} is contributed only by the animal food members of this group.

[c] Dark green and deep orange vegetables are especially reliable vitamin A sources; other fruits and vegetables are not. For vitamin C, citrus fruits, green leafy vegetables, and selected other fruits and vegetables are superior sources. See Chapters 8 and 9 for more details.

[d] Whole grains include wheat, oats, rice, barley, millet, rye, bulgur.

[e] One serving is not a significant source of any of these nutrients, but the recommended four or more servings contribute significant quantities to the diet. This group also contributes most of the complex carbohydrate of the diet. Whole-grain products are highly recommended in place of refined enriched products.

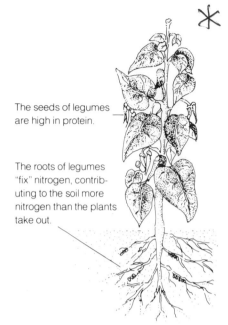

The seeds of legumes are high in protein.

The roots of legumes "fix" nitrogen, contributing to the soil more nitrogen than the plants take out.

Legumes are rich in protein and B vitamins like meat; but unlike meat, they are low in fat and high in healthful complex carbohydrates, both starch and fiber. Long scorned by the middle class as "beans" or "the poor man's meat," legumes are now coming into their own as an inexpensive, health-promoting, land-sparing, nutritious food. From them are made food products that are used in many kinds of cooking: Orientals' bean curd (tofu) and soy sauce, Americans' peanut butter and baked beans, vegetarians' bean sprouts, and Mexicans' bean paste, among others.

TABLE 1–4 **Servings in the Four Food Group Plan** TH1-1 KNOW!

FOOD GROUP	SERVINGS (ADULT)	SERVING SIZE
Meat and meat substitutes	2	2–3 oz cooked meat, fish, or chicken; ¼ cup tuna; 2 eggs; 4 tbsp peanut butter; 1 cup cooked legumes; ½ cup nuts
Milk and milk products	2[a]	1 cup (8 oz) milk; 1 cup yogurt; 1½ cup cottage cheese; 2 cups ice cream; 5 tbsp milk pudding; 1–2 oz cheese
Fruits and vegetables	4[b]	½ cup fruit, vegetable, or juice; 1 medium apple, orange, banana, or peach
Grains (bread and cereal products)	4[c]	1 slice bread; ½ cup cooked cereal or 1 cup (1 oz) ready-to-eat cereal; ½ hamburger or hot dog bun or English muffin; ½ cup cooked rice, grits, macaroni, or spaghetti; 2 tbsp flour; 6 saltines; 1 6-inch tortilla

[a] For children up to 9, 2–3 cups; for children 9 to 12, 3–4 cups; for teenagers and pregnant women, 3–4 cups; for nursing mothers, 4 cups or more.
[b] One should be rich in vitamin C; at least one every other day should be rich in vitamin A.
[c] Enriched or whole-grain products only.

do contribute some nutrients to the day's intake. However, either they are not foods, their nutrient content is not significant in enough of the nutrients characteristic of a food group, or their nutrient content has been greatly diluted by fat, sugar, or water.

The Four Food Group Plan appears quite rigid, but it can be used with great flexibility once its intent is understood. For example, cheese can be substituted for milk because it supplies protein, calcium, and riboflavin in about the same amounts. Legumes and nuts are alternative choices for meats. The plan can be adapted to casseroles and other mixed dishes and to different national and cultural cuisines.

The Four Food Group Plan was originally devised several decades ago. Despite much study and effort on its behalf, it has never worked perfectly. Very few people follow it to the letter, and of those who do, many overconsume kcalories, especially kcalories from fat. One of the problems, some critics say, is that half of the food classes identified (two of the four groups) are animal products: milk and meat. This leads many people to think that half of the foods they consume should be milk and meat. Actually, though, the plan recommends *two* milk, *two* meat, and *eight* food items from the plant food groups.[3]

Since the Four Food Group Plan was originally devised, many more nutrients have been identified and studied. A person can follow all its rules

3   S. Clapp, Chuck the basic four? *The Community Nutritionist* II, January–February 1983, p. 1.

and still fail to meet the day's needs for some nutrients—especially vitamin B_6, magnesium, zinc, and vitamin E. Iron has been a problem from the beginning.

A modification of the Four Food Group Plan designed to solve these problems was published in 1978. It recommends:

● Two servings milk/milk products (as before).
● Two servings meat, fish, or poultry (portion size 3 ounces, not 2 to 3 ounces).
● Two servings legumes and/or nuts (portion size ¾ cup), to provide more of the five nutrients just mentioned.
● Four servings fruits and vegetables (as before).
● Four servings whole-grain (not enriched) products, for more of those same nutrients.
● One serving fat or oil (for vitamin E).[4]

Most selections of food based on this plan would supply 100 percent of the recommended amounts of all nutrients for men and all except iron for women and would miss providing a woman's full recommended amount of iron by only 10 percent on the average. The average energy content of a diet selected according to this plan, however, is high—2,200 kcalories—and the authors of the plan acknowledge that this is a disadvantage. A person whose kcalorie allowance is 2,200 or less finds no leeway in this plan for free food choices. But the authors feel that this disadvantage is outweighed by the advantage of a virtual guarantee of diet adequacy. This book assumes an openminded willingness on the part of the reader to learn the Modified Plan's recommendations and see how they work out in practice. Demonstrations throughout Chapters 8 through 11 show repeatedly that the addition of legumes to the daily meal plan makes the needed difference between barely adequate intakes and ample intakes of many vitamins and minerals.

The vegetarian faces a special problem in diet planning—that of obtaining the needed nutrients from fewer food groups. There are two major classes of vegetarians (with many variations). The lacto-ovo vegetarian uses milk and eggs (animal products) but excludes meat, fish, and poultry (animal flesh) from the diet, while the pure vegetarian, or vegan, excludes all these foods and uses only plant foods. For both lifestyles it is necessary to know how to combine foods to obtain the nutrients nonvegetarians get from the meat and milk groups.

The lacto-ovo vegetarian can adapt the Four Food Group Plan by making a change in the meat group (see Table 1–5). The strict vegetarian, who doesn't use dairy products, should take a vitamin B_{12} supplement or use vitamin B_{12}–fortified soy milk. Additional guidelines are offered elsewhere (see note at end of chapter).

TABLE 1–5 **Four Food Group Plan for the Vegetarian**

2 servings milk or milk products (or soy milk fortified with vitamin B_{12})

2 servings protein-rich foods (include 2 cups legumes daily to help meet iron requirements for women; count 4 tbsp peanut butter as 1 serving)

4 servings whole-grain foods

4 servings fruits and vegetables (include 1 cup dark greens to help meet iron requirements for women)

Adapted from *Vegetarian Food Choices* (Gainesville: Shands Teaching Hospital and Clinics, Food and Nutrition Service, University of Florida, 1976).

---

4   J. C. King, S. H. Cohenour, C. G. Corrucini, and P. Schneeman, Evaluation and modification of the basic four food guide, *Journal of Nutrition Education* 10 (1978): 27–29.

nutrient density: a characteristic of a food. A nutrient-dense food provides a high quantity (relative to need) of one or (preferably) several essential nutrients, with a small quantity (relative to need) of kcalories. Self-Study 12 in Appendix Q permits you to compute the nutrient densities of foods you like to eat.

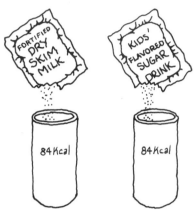

All the kcalories from protein and lactose—280 mg calcium, 180 RE vitamin A, 0.4 mg riboflavin, and more.

All the kcalories from sucrose—insignificant nutrients.

An example of nutrient density

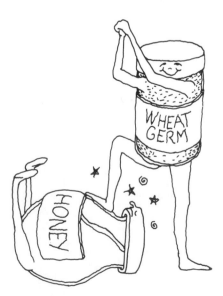

The preceding discussion has highlighted a problem that concerns many people today. Eating well seems to necessitate eating a lot. Some people don't even spend 2,200 kcalories in their daily activities. If they were to eat this many kcalories, they would get fat.

How can a person get all the essential nutrients without overeating? The answer lies in selecting the foods within each group that deliver the most nutrients at the lowest kcalorie cost: foods with high nutrient density. Take foods containing iron, for example: a 3-ounce portion of either sirloin steak or sardines provides 2.5 milligrams of iron; but the beef contains 330 kcalories and the sardines, only 175 kcalories.[5] The sardines, then, are more iron-dense (they have the same amount of iron for a smaller number of kcalories). If you asked a nutritionist whether beef or sardines were more nutritious, he or she would have to say both were nutritious, in the sense that both provide valuable, needed nutrients. But based on the amount of iron they offer for a given kcalorie amount, the sardines are more nutritious than the beef. This concept, the concept of nutrient density, may someday become the basis for a new kind of food labeling. Foods that provide more nutrients than kcalories, relative to a person's need, qualify to be labeled *nutritious foods.*

The concept that a nutritious food is one that delivers nutrients at a low kcalorie cost can help the weight-conscious consumer make informed choices. The food industry has enthusiastically endorsed the selling of the nutritional *adequacy* concept. The dairy people proclaim, "Drink milk—it's good for you." The meat people boast that meat is rich in protein and iron, as indeed it is. These foods can be advertised as loaded with nutrients, bursting with vitamins, high in health value. But the aware consumer realizes that whole milk and meat can also contribute many fat kcalories. Thus the advertisement of these and other products may benefit the milk and meat industries more than it benefits our bodies. This doesn't mean we should avoid them, but that we should use them in moderation.

Another case in point is honey, a much-beloved and much-advertised "health-food" product. Honey does provide a few B vitamins and trace minerals in very small amounts in contrast to white sugar, which does not supply them at all. But to say that honey is actually nutritious is to mislead the consumer. On the other hand, wheat germ, another favorite item in "health-food" stores, provides abundant B vitamins, iron, and other nutrients relative to its kcalories. If the two should enter a contest for the title of "nutritious food," the wheat germ would win, hands down. (Chapter 2 offers more about honey.)

No list of nutritious foods (by this definition) has been published yet, but systems already exist that are useful to the consumer who wants to eat well and control kcalories at the same time. These are known as exchange systems. Foods listed in the exchange system are considered protective foods.

5   These figures were taken from items 170 and 154 in Appendix H.

Exchange Systems

developed solely for calorie counting not nutrients

Unlike a food group system, which sorts foods by their protein, vitamin, and mineral contents only, the exchange systems presented here pay special attention to kcalories, proportions of carbohydrate, fat, and protein, and portion sizes. All the food portions on a list have approximately the same number of kcalories and the same amounts of energy nutrients (protein, fat, and carbohydrate). The U.S. exchange system will be presented here as an example; the Canadian system is in Appendix M. There are six lists of foods in the exchange system, and each has a typical member—with portion size specified—that you can remember it by. The lists, and their typical representatives, are:

- Milk—1 cup skim milk (80 kcalories).
- Vegetable—½ cup green beans (25 kcalories).
- Fruit—½ small banana (40 kcalories).
- Bread—1 slice bread (70 kcalories).
- Meat—1 ounce lean meat or low-fat cheese (55 kcalories).
- Fat—1 teaspoon butter (45 kcalories).

Table 1–6 shows the protein, fat, and carbohydrate values that pertain to each list, and Figure 1–3 shows the foods that belong together in this system. Notice that cheese is classed as a meat in this system, because its protein and fat contents are similar to those of meat (calcium is not being considered here).

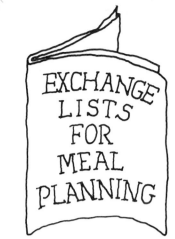

The exchange lists were originally developed for people with diabetes. They proved so useful, however, that they are now in general use for diet planning. The complete lists of all the foods in the U.S. and Canadian exchange systems appear in Appendix M. (Other kinds of exchange systems also exist. For example, foods can be grouped on the basis of their sodium content.)

---

kCalorie Values of Carbohydrate, Fat, and Protein

If you know the number of grams of carbohydrate, fat, and protein in a food, you can derive the number of kcalories. Simply multiply the carbohydrate grams times 4, the fat grams times 9, and the protein grams times 4, and add them all together.

The energy values for the exchange list items in Table 1–6 were derived this way. For example, a slice of bread contains 15 grams of carbohydrate (that's 60 kcalories) and 2 grams protein (that's another 8 kcalories), or 68 kcalories in all—rounded off to 70 kcalories for ease in calculating. A half-cup of vegetables (not including starchy vegetables) contains 5 grams of carbohydrate (20 kcalories) and 2 grams of protein (8 more) and has been rounded *down* to 25 kcalories. (This slight understatement of the energy value of vegetables is probably intended to encourage people to use them in abundance. At 25 kcalories a half cup, you could eat 4 cups of vegetables for less than the kcalorie cost of a single 3-ounce hamburger patty.)

1 g carbohydrate = 4 kcal
1 g fat = 9 kcal
1 g protein = 4 kcal

FIGURE 1–3 **Sets of similar foods, exchange system.**

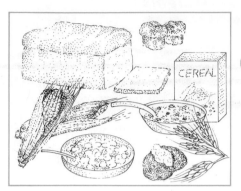

Breads

1 slice bread is like:

¾ cup ready-to-eat cereal
½ cup cooked beans
⅓ cup corn
1 small potato

(1 bread = 15 g carbohydrate, 2 g protein, and 70 kcal)

Milks

1 cup skim milk is like:

1 cup skim-milk yogurt, plain
1 cup buttermilk
½ cup evaporated skim milk

(1 milk = 12 g carbohydrate, 8 g protein, and 80 kcal)

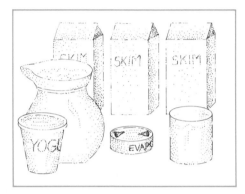

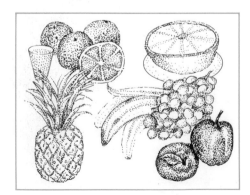

Vegetables

½ cup green beans is like:

½ cup greens
½ cup carrots
½ cup beets

(1 vegetable = 5 g carbohydrate, 2 g protein, and 25 kcal)

Fruits

½ small banana is like:

1 small apple
½ grapefruit
½ cup orange juice

(1 fruit = 10 g carbohydrate and 40 kcal)

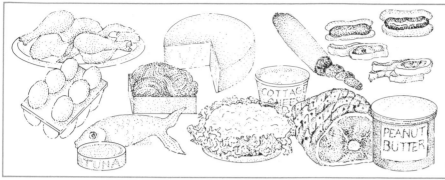

Meats (medium-fat)

1 oz medium-fat meat is like 1 oz lean meat in protein content, but is estimated to have an extra ''½ fat''—that is, to have the 3 g fat of a lean meat and 2½ g additional fat. Examples:

1 oz pork loin
1 egg
¼ cup creamed cottage cheese[a]

(1 medium-fat meat = 7 g protein, 5½ g fat, and about 80 kcal)

Peanut Butter

Peanut butter is like a meat in terms of its protein content but stands alone in being very high in fat. It is estimated as:

2 tbsp peanut butter = 1 lean meat + 2½ fat
(2 tbsp peanut butter = 7 g protein, 15½ g fat, and about 170 kcal)

(Don't stop reading now, and don't swear off peanut butter, necessarily. You'll need to read about the polyunsaturated character of its fat in Chapter 3, and the B-vitamin contributions it makes in Chapter 8, before deciding how much of a place it should have in your diet.)

[a] Cheeses are grouped with milk in food group plans because of their calcium content but with meats in this system because, like meat, they contribute kcalories from protein and fat and have negligible carbohydrate content.

Meats (lean)

1 oz lean meat is like:

1 oz chicken meat without the skin
1 oz any fish
¼ cup canned tuna
1 oz low-fat cheese[a]

(1 low-fat meat = 7 g protein, 3 g fat, and 55 kcal)

Meats (high-fat)

1 oz high-fat meat is like 1 oz lean meat in protein content but is estimated to have an extra ''1 fat''—that is, to have the 3 g fat of a lean meat and 5 g additional fat. Examples:

1 oz country-style ham
1 oz cheddar cheese[a]
1 small hot dog (frankfurter)

(1 high-fat meat = 7 g protein, 8 g fat, and 100 kcal)

Fats

1 tsp butter is like:

1 tsp margarine
1 tsp any oil
1 tbsp salad dressing
1 strip crisp bacon
5 small olives
10 whole Virginia peanuts

(1 fat = 5 g fat and 45 kcal)

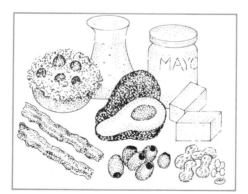

Legumes

Legumes are an odd kind of plant food. They are like meats because they are rich in protein and iron, but many are lower in fat than meat. Besides, they contain a lot of starch. They can be treated as:

½ cup legumes = 1 lean meat + 1 bread
(½ cup legumes = 15 g carbohydrate, 9 g protein, 3 g fat, and 125 kcal)

Legumes can also be considered similar to breads in being rich in complex carbohydrate, and the additional protein can be ignored, but this treatment underestimates their kcalorie value, especially that of the higher-fat legumes such as peanuts.

Whatever you do with legumes on paper, however, use them often in cooking. You will learn many more reasons why they are an inexpensive, nutritious, high-quality, and health-promoting food. The Modified Four Food Group Plan recommends the use of two ¾-cup servings of legumes a day. For calculating, this would amount to three ½-cup portions in the exchange system.

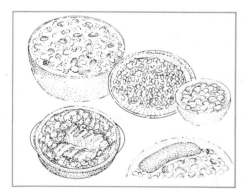

TABLE 1–6 **The Six Exchange Lists**[a] TH1-3

LIST	PORTION SIZE	CARBOHYDRATE (g)	PROTEIN (g)	FAT (g)	ENERGY (kcal)
Milk (skim)[b]	1 cup	12	8	0	80
Vegetable[c]	½ cup	5	2	0	25
Fruit	1 portion	10	0	0	40
Bread[d]	1 slice	15	2	0	70
Meat (lean)[e]	1 oz	0	7	3	55
Fat	1 tsp	0	0	5	45

[a] This is the U.S. exchange system. The complete details, and those of the Canadian system, are shown in Appendixes L and M.
[b] 1 cup low-fat milk = 1 skim milk + 1 fat; 1 cup whole milk = 1 skim milk + 2 fats.
[c] This list includes low-kcalorie vegetables only.
[d] This list includes starchy vegetables such as lima beans and corn, as well as cereal, bread, pasta, and other grain products. For portion sizes see Appendixes L and M.
[e] This list includes cheese and peanut butter as well as meat.

The user of the exchange system is encouraged to think of skim milk as milk and of whole milk as milk with added fat. A glass of whole milk is described, in fact, as "one milk plus two fats," and a glass of low-fat milk as "one milk plus one fat." The vegetable list includes only low-kcalorie vegetables, so that a half-cup of any of them will provide about 25 kcalories. The fruit list specifies "no added sugar or sugar syrup"—not necessarily to forbid you to eat fruits with sugar but to make you aware when you do and to help you keep track of sugar consumption. Portion sizes are adjusted so that fruit portions are equal in kcalories. One small banana counts as "two fruits." But a piece of cherry pie is *not* "a fruit." It *includes* a fruit if it contains ten large cherries, but it also includes bread and fat exchanges, and added sugar. (Thus it might be counted as "one fruit, two breads, and three fats, with 3 teaspoons added sugar.") The bread list also clearly specifies portion sizes and makes clear which grain products contain added fat. Corn, lima beans, and other starchy vegetables are listed with the breads, not the vegetables, because they are similar to breads in kcalorie and carbohydrate content.

Perhaps most important of all, meats and cheeses are separated into three categories—lean, medium-fat, and high-fat—and the fat list, by including items like bacon and olives, alerts the user to foods that are unexpectedly high in fat kcalories. More details of the exchange system will appear in later chapters.

If you are a diet planner who wants to choose foods that contain all the nutrients you need, you are well advised to follow a food group plan, because it promotes adequacy and provides for balance among the different kinds of foods to help you avoid overemphasis on any one. But if you want to control kcalories as well, you will find it convenient to use the exchange lists as lists of nutritious foods from which to make your selections. You need to be aware of only one additional principle of diet planning to do very well for yourself: variety. It is generally agreed that people should not eat the same foods day after day, for two reasons. One reason is that you can't keep track of all the nutrients individually, and some foods may be better sources of some of them than other foods are. The second reason is that a monotonous diet may deliver unwanted amounts of undesirable food constituents, such as contaminants. Each food's ingredients are diluted by the bulk of all the other foods eaten and even further diluted if several days are skipped before it is eaten again.

Suppose you want to use the Four Food Group Plan to make menus that are adequate but not excessive in kcalories. Most people (notably women) say, "I couldn't possibly eat all that food without getting fat!" The demonstration in Table 1–7 shows that it can be done; it may come as a surprise that it can be done extremely well by using the exchange system to choose the actual items. Table 1–7 shows that all 12 recommended items can total about 900 kcalories while providing adequacy for most of the major nutrients. An average adult would still have more than 1,000 kcalories to spend. A wise choice would be to invest many of those additional kcalories in additional fruits, vegetables, and whole-grain foods, or in the two large servings of legumes/nuts and the one serving of fat recommended by the Modified Four Food Group Plan. (Two ¾-cup portions of legumes at about 180 kcalories each and 1 teaspoon of margarine at 45 kcalories would add only about 400 kcalories to the total and still leave some room to spare.) Some of the extra kcalories could be spent adding more starch-containing foods like additional whole-grain bread or snacks like popcorn. Others could be invested in occasional sweet desserts, even alcohol. If these additions were made, they would be made by choice rather than through the unintentional use of high-kcalorie foods to begin with. Adequacy and balance would be achieved, not necessarily at each meal, but within each day.

With judicious selections, the diet can meet the need for all the nutrients and provide some luxury items as well. The final plan might be like that outlined in Table 1–8 (one of many possible examples). The planner then could achieve variety by selecting different foods each day from the exchange lists.

A last refinement that is useful to the conscientious diet planner is to learn to use different patterns of exchanges for different kcalorie levels. A person eating 3,000 kcalories per day could use considerably more bread exchanges, for example, than a person eating 1,500 kcalories per day. Table 1–9 shows diet plans for different kcalorie intakes.

An **adequate** diet is one that provides all the essential nutrients and kcalories necessary to maintain health and body weight. Ideally, a diet will be more than just adequate; it will be **optimal**, providing an assortment and balance of nutrients and kcalories that maintains ideal body weight and the best possible state of health.

protective or **foundation foods**: nutrient-dense foods around which a nutritious diet can be constructed. These foods are: milk, cheese, meat, fish, poultry, eggs, legumes, nuts, fruits, vegetables, and grains.

TABLE 1–8 **A Sample Diet Plan**[a]

EXCHANGES	ENERGY (kcal)
2 skim milk	160
2 vegetable	50
3 fruit	120
7 bread	490
6 medium-fat meat	465
4 fat	180
	1,465

[a] This diet derives about 20 percent of its kcalories from protein, about 30 percent from fat, and nearly 50 percent from carbohydrate. Self-Study 1 in Appendix Q shows how to do calculations like this.

TABLE 1–7 **How to Use a Food Group Plan and an Exchange System to Plan Diets** TH1-4

FOUR FOOD GROUP PLAN	USING THE EXCHANGE SYSTEM	EXAMPLE	ENERGY COST (kcal)
Milk—2 cups	Milk list—select 2 exchanges	2 cups skim milk	160
Meat—2 servings (2–3 oz each)	Meat list—select 6 exchanges[a]	6 oz lean meat	330
Fruits and vegetables —4 servings	Fruit and vegetable lists—select 4 exchanges	2 vegetable exchanges; 2 fruit exchanges	50 80
Grains (breads and cereals)—4 servings	Bread list—select 4 exchanges	4 bread exchanges	280
Total			900

[a] In the Four Food Group Plan, 1 serving is 2–3 oz. In the exchange system, 1 exchange is 1 oz.

TABLE 1–9 **Diet Patterns for Different kCalorie Levels**[a]

EXCHANGES	ENERGY LEVEL (kcal)					
	1,000	*1,200*	*1,500*	*1,800*	*2,000*	*2,200*
Skim milk	2	2	2	2	3	3
Vegetable	2	3	3	3	4	5
Fruit	3	4	4	5	5	6
Bread	4	5	8	10	10	11
Lean meat	4	5	5	6	7	7
Fat	4	5	6	7	8	9

[a] These patterns of exchanges supply about 30 percent of the kcalories as fat, in accordance with the view that a moderate fat intake is desirable.

Recommended Nutrient Intakes

RDA: Recommended Dietary Allowances. The RDA are daily recommended intakes of nutrients intended to provide for individual variations among most normal, healthy people in the United States under usual environmental stresses. RDA are set for:

Energy—a range.

Vitamins—A, D, E, C, folacin, niacin, riboflavin, thiamin, B₆, B₁₂.

Minerals—calcium, phosphorus, iodine, iron, magnesium, zinc.

"Estimated safe and adequate intakes" are set for:

Vitamins—K, biotin, pantothenic acid.

Minerals—sodium, potassium, chloride, copper, manganese, fluoride, chromium, selenium, molybdenum.

The RDA should not be confused with **MDR** (minimum daily requirements), a term used on the labels of nutrient supplements. (The MDR are not much used anymore because they often misled the public into thinking of them as absolute minimum requirements.)

Diet adequacy can be achieved through the use of a food group plan aided by the principles of nutrient density and kcalorie control. However, the science of nutrition is actually based on the study of how the body uses nutrients, and one of the most important aspects of that study is to ask how much of each nutrient the body needs and how we can tell if it is getting enough. This section shows how nutrition experts arrive at recommended nutrient intakes, and the next section shows how the adequacy of people's nutrient intakes is assessed.

Many countries have developed nutrient standards, and three sets are presented at the ends of the book (inside front cover, Appendix O): those of the United States, of Canada, and of the World Health Organization (WHO). They differ from one another in a variety of ways that will be explained for individual nutrients in the chapters to come. Here, the RDA are presented as an example of recommended intakes. (The U.S. RDA used on food labels are different from these RDA and are described later in this chapter.)

The RDA are recommendations published by the United States government. They are used and referred to so often that they are presented on the inside front cover of this book. The main RDA table includes recommendations for protein, 10 vitamins, and 6 minerals, while another table specifies energy needs for people of different ages and still another presents tentative recommendations for 12 more vitamins and minerals. About every five years, the Committee on RDA meets to re-examine and revise these recommendations on the basis of new evidence regarding people's nutrient needs.[6] It then publishes an updated set of RDA.[7]

The RDA have been much misunderstood. One person, on first learning of their existence, was outraged: "You mean Uncle Sam tells me that I must

6   The committee on RDA is a committee of the Food and Nutrition Board (FNB) of the National Academy of Sciences/National Research Council (NAS/NRC).

7   Food and Nutrition Board, Committee on Recommended Allowances, *Recommended Dietary Allowances*, 9th ed. (Washington, D.C.: National Academy of Sciences, 1980).

eat exactly 45 grams of protein every day?" This is not the government's intention, and the RDA are not commandments. The following facts will help put the RDA in perspective:

● They are published by the government, but the study group that determines them is composed of highly qualified scientists selected by the National Academy of Sciences.

● They are based on available scientific evidence to the greatest extent possible, and the committee reviews them about every five years in the light of new findings and revises them if necessary.

● They are recommendations, not requirements, and certainly not minimum requirements. They include a margin of safety so substantial that an intake of two-thirds of the RDA is often deemed adequate, except for energy.

● They take into account the differences among individuals and define a range within which most healthy persons' intakes of nutrients probably should fall. Individuals whose needs are higher than the average are included within this range.

● They are for healthy persons only. Medical problems alter nutrient needs.

Separate recommendations are made for different sets of people. Children aged 4 to 6 are distinguished from men aged 19 to 22, for example. Each individual can look up the recommendations for his or her own age and sex group.

How Do We Know What We Know?
The Scientific Method

Faced with the public's confusion over what to believe about nutrition, authorities often express the view that our country's young people should have at least a short course in epistemology—the study of knowledge, its limits and validity. If people realized that "knowledge" means different things as used by different people, and that it arises in different ways, they might be better equipped to decide what knowledge to accept as their own.

Consider the following statements:

● I just *know* the sun will rise at 6:00 tomorrow.
● I know the sun will rise at 7:00 tomorrow, because I have timed the sunrise every morning for 20 years and have fully described the changes in its timing from day to day. From the pattern I have identified, I can predict the timing of the sunrise repeatedly, without errors.

Both speakers claim to know when the sun will come up—but how do they know what they know?

The first speaker is speaking on faith: "I just *know*." Whether we accept or reject his statement depends on whether we share his faith. He has offered no proof of its validity.

The second speaker has based his statement on evidence gathered

epistemology (episs-tuh-MOLL-o-gee): the study of knowledge, its limits and validity.

Nutrition experts can be identified on the basis of their credentials. They have college and graduate degrees (**M.S., Ph.D.**) *in nutrition* from recognized universities. An **R.D.** (registered dietitian) is a trained professional with some 70 or so undergraduate hours in nutrition and food science, a year's internship or the equivalent, and a passing score on the R.D. exam, a four-hour qualifying exam administered over six competency areas by the American or Canadian Dietetic Association. A "nutritionist" is not necessarily a nutrition expert. Anyone can call himself a "nutritionist." Watch out for *self-styled* nutrition experts.

At many points in the following chapters, help is offered on how to distinguish a trustworthy nutrition authority from a quack. If you want to become competent in nutrition yourself, watch for these pointers and learn how to tell the difference.

validity: the quality of being supported by objective evidence.

and predictions made and tested in the past. He has used the scientific method:

1 He has made a series of observations (time of sunrise each day for 20 years).

2 He has perceived a pattern and developed a hypothesis (the sun will continue to rise at times consistent with this pattern).

3 He has made and tested predictions based on this hypothesis and has confirmed them by means of further observations (indeed, the sun does rise at the times predicted by the hypothesis).

4 He has made a further prediction based on the hypothesis (the sun will rise at 7:00 tomorrow morning). This prediction is testable by observation.

We may want to ask him some questions, of course, but assuming he answers them satisfactorily, this method would seem to provide a prediction we can rely on.

This book presents nutrition knowledge derived from use of the scientific method. Further refinements of its applications are presented throughout as digressions in the text. Questions are raised and answered about many different aspects of the use of science. In terms of our example, these questions have to do with:

● The method of making measurements. Did he just look at the sun, did he use an instrument, how did he determine the exact instant of the sunrise?

● The accuracy of the instrument that he used. Was it a clock? What kind of clock?

● The accuracy of the standard he used for reference. Did he use international time? Is that a suitable standard?

● The number of observations he made. Did he make enough observations to see all possible variations on the pattern?

● The agreement of his findings with those reported by other observers. How well do his findings fit into our established picture of the relationships of the sun, earth, and other heavenly bodies?

The method our observer used was the *descriptive method.* There are others. In nutrition, the *experimental method* is often used, in which the scientist not only observes, but also intervenes and manipulates his material or subjects. Still, whatever the details, the scientific method always approaches reality by means of this series of steps: making observations that others can repeat and confirm, developing hypotheses, making predictions from them, and testing the predictions. A piece of scientific knowledge (a scientific fact) is thus based on externally observable evidence and so has validity.

We who rely on scientists' observations as reported in various media (books, journals, newspapers, television, word of mouth) also have to ask questions about the media themselves. How far can we trust them to report accurately? How do we know where they get their information? These problems too are dealt with later in the book.

The Setting of Recommended Allowances

It is important to understand how the RDA and other such recommendations are set. Especially if you use them to evaluate the adequacy of your own diet, you need to be aware that individuals' nutrient needs vary widely, and that the allowances have been chosen so that they can be used for whole groups of people. A theoretical discussion based on the way the Committee on RDA made its recommendation for protein will illustrate the limitations and qualifications you must keep in mind when dealing with the RDA.

Suppose we were the Committee on RDA and we had the task of setting an RDA for nutrient X (any nutrient). Ideally, our first step would be to try to find out how much of that nutrient each person needs. We would review and select the most valid studies of deficiency states, of the body's nutrient stores and their depletion, and of many other relevant factors. We could also measure the body's intake and excretion of nutrient X (in the case of nutrients that aren't changed before they are excreted) and find out how much of an intake is required to achieve balance (this is called a balance study). For each individual subject, we could determine a *requirement* for nutrient X. Below the requirement, that person would slip into negative balance or experience declining stores.

We would find that different individuals have different requirements. Mr. A might need 40 units of the nutrient each day to maintain balance; Ms. B might need 35; Mr. C, 65. If we looked at enough individuals, we might find that their requirements fell into an even distribution—that most were near the midpoint, and only a few were at the extremes. Figure 1–4 depicts this situation.

Then we would have to decide what intake to recommend for everybody; that is, we would have to set the RDA. Should we set it at the mean (shown in Figure 1–4 at 45 units)? This is the average requirement for nutrient X; it is the closest to everyone's need. But if people took us literally and consumed exactly this amount of nutrient X each day, half of the population would develop deficiencies, Mr. C among them.

Perhaps we should set the RDA for nutrient X at or above the extreme—say, at 70 units a day—so that everyone would be covered. (Actually, we

balance study: a laboratory study in which a person is fed a controlled diet and the intake and excretion of a nutrient are measured. Balance studies are valid only for nutrients like calcium that don't change while they are in the body.

requirement: the amount of a nutrient that will just prevent the development of specific deficiency signs; distinguished from the RDA, which is a recommended allowance that includes a safety factor to provide for individual variability.

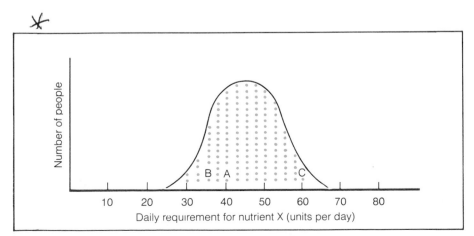

FIGURE 1–4 Each dot represents a person. A, B, and C are Mr. A, Ms. B, and Mr. C.

didn't study everyone, so we would have to worry that some individual we didn't happen to test would have a still higher requirement.) This might be a good idea in theory, but what if nutrient X is expensive or scarce? A person like Ms. B, who needs only 35 units a day, would then try to consume twice that, an unnecessary strain on her pocketbook. Or she might overeat as a consequence or overemphasize foods containing nutrient X to the exclusion of foods containing other valuable nutrients.

The choice we would finally make, with some reservations, would be to set the RDA at a reasonably high point so that the bulk of the population would be covered. In this example, a reasonable choice might be to set it at 63 units a day. By moving the RDA further toward the extreme we would pick up very few additional people but inflate the recommendation as it applies to most people (including Mr. A and Ms. B).

It is this kind of choice that the committee members make in setting the RDA for nutrients. They set it well above the mean requirement as best they can determine it from the available information. (Actually, they don't usually have enough data to be sure that the population's requirements are evenly distributed.) Relatively few people's requirements, then, are not covered by the RDA.

If you have followed this line of reasoning, you will see why the RDA cannot be taken literally by any individual. Remember, you can't know exactly what your own personal requirement may be. Moreover, the Committee on RDA makes several assumptions that do not apply to all real situations. It assumes, among other things, that you are eating a generally adequate diet including protein of good quality and that you are consuming adequate kcalories and nutrients. It assumes that you store and cook your foods with reasonable care and that large amounts of nutrients aren't lost in these processes. When you use the RDA for yourself and compare your nutrient intakes with them, you should keep two principles in mind:

● They are not absolute requirements. *R* stands for *recommended*, not for *required*. They are allowances, and they are generous. Even so, they do not necessarily cover every individual for every nutrient. In planning your own diet, it is probably wise to aim at getting 100 percent or more of the RDA for every nutrient.

● Beyond a certain point, though, it is unwise to consume large amounts of any nutrient. It is naive to think of the RDA as minimum amounts. A more accurate view is to see your nutrient needs as falling within a range, with danger zones both below and above it. Figure 1–5 illustrates this point. The 1980 RDA reflect this consideration especially clearly in the tables for the trace minerals, which are stated in terms of "safe and adequate" ranges of intakes.

It is also important to remember that the RDA and other such recommendations are for the maintenance, not the restoration, of health. Under the stress of illness or malnutrition, a person may require a much higher intake of certain nutrients. Separate recommendations are made for therapeutic diets; for use after surgery, burns, or fractures; or in the treatment of other illnesses.

Nutrient needs:

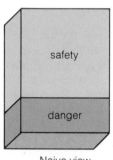

Naive view

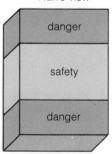

Accurate view

FIGURE 1–5 The RDA are not minimum amounts but represent the approximate midpoints of ranges within which nutrient intakes probably should fall. Nutrient intakes above or below these ranges might be equally harmful.

With the understanding that they are approximate, flexible, and generous, we can use the RDA as a yardstick, not to assess the adequacy of individual diets, but to measure the adequacy of diets in whole populations, like that of the United States. Diets of individuals cannot be meaningfully assessed by comparison to the RDA, because individuals' needs differ unpredictably, but the diets of groups can be assessed. For example, a diet providing at least two-thirds of the RDA for seven indicator nutrients may be deemed "good"; one providing less than two-thirds for one or more may be considered "poor." Standards like these have been applied in a number of surveys of the U.S. population to determine the people's nutrition status.

The RDA for Energy (kCalories)

In setting allowances for kcalorie intakes, the Committee on RDA took a different approach than for the nutrients. Its members had reasoned that it would be sensible to set generous allowances for protein, vitamins, and minerals. They felt that small amounts of a *nutrient* in excess of the minimum required to maintain freedom from deficiency symptoms would be less harmful than small deficits. However, *energy* intakes either above or below need are undesirable. Obesity is as much to be avoided as underweight. The Committee on RDA therefore set the energy RDA at the mean—halfway between the lowest and highest needs of the individuals it studied. The latest version of the RDA provides a wide range of suggested kcalorie intakes surrounding the mean for each age-sex group, showing how variable individual people's kcalorie needs are. Figure 1–6 illustrates the difference between the nutrient and kcalorie RDA set by the committee. As the figure shows, most people's energy needs fall close to the mean, but few fit the mean exactly. The best way to ensure that your kcalorie intake actually fits your own particular requirement is to monitor your weight over a period of time.

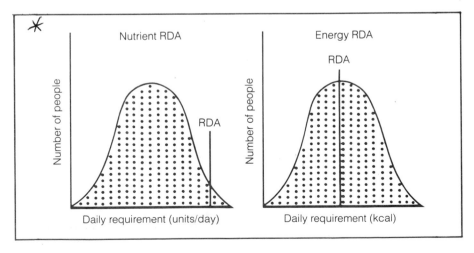

FIGURE 1–6 The nutrient RDA are set so that only a few people's requirements will exceed them. The energy RDA are set so that half the population's requirements will fall below and half above them. TH1-5

No RDA is set for carbohydrate or fat. The assumption is that you will first use a certain minimum number of kcalories for the protein you specifically need, and then will use the remaining kcalories for carbohydrate, fat, and possibly alcohol (according to your personal preference) to meet your energy RDA.

The U.S. RDA

The term *U.S. RDA* appears on food labels and so deserves an explanation. When you read a food label, you may want to have it express the food's nutrient contents as a percentage of your need. For example, it would be useful to see on the label of a cereal box that one serving of the cereal provides you with 25 percent of the iron you need for the day. Your RDA could be used to give you this information; but the trouble is, the makers of the label don't know who you are: a 10-year-old boy, a 70-year-old woman, or a pregnant teen-age girl. To standardize labels, four sets of U.S. RDA were developed for different groups of people. The most commonly used of these is the U.S. RDA for adults, and this is the one referred to here. The idea behind the U.S. RDA for adults was to develop a single set of standards for a sort of generalized adult human being whose nutrient needs are high —as high as people's needs generally go. So if you read on a label that a serving of cereal provides 25 percent of the U.S. RDA of iron, you can be sure that it will also provide at least 25 percent of *your* iron RDA. Your nutrient needs, in other words, are covered by the U.S. RDA.

The U.S. RDA are a set of figures chosen by the Food and Drug Administration (the FDA, which is responsible for nutrition labeling). For most nutrients, the U.S. RDA are the same as the RDA for an adult man. But for iron—because a woman's need is greater than a man's—the woman's RDA is used. The thing to remember about the U.S. RDA is that they are about equal to the highest numbers for each nutrient that you can find in the RDA table. The table on the inside back cover shows the U.S. RDA used on labels that make nutrition claims.

Highlight 12 explains nutrition labeling in detail. The U.S. RDA are on the inside back cover.

Other Recommendations

As mentioned, different nations and international groups have published different sets of standards similar to the RDA. The Canadian equivalent to the RDA is the Dietary Standard for Canada, a table of recommended daily nutrient intakes (shown in Appendix O). The Canadian recommendations differ from the RDA in some respects, partly because of differences in interpretation of the data they were derived from and partly because conditions in Canada differ somewhat from those in the United States. Some of the differences between the two sets of recommendations will be explained as the nutrients are discussed in the coming chapters.

Among the most widely used recommendations are a set developed by two international groups: the Food and Agriculture Organization (FAO) and the World Health Organization (WHO). The FAO/WHO recommendations are considered sufficient for the maintenance of health in "nearly all people."[8] They are sometimes higher, usually lower, than the RDA, not because the RDA are wrong, but because different judgment factors apply to each. FAO/WHO, for example, assumed a protein quality lower than that commonly available in the United States and so recommended a higher intake. The United States sets its calcium recommendation higher to keep it in balance with the higher phosphorus and protein intakes of its people. Nevertheless, the various recommending agencies have arrived at figures that are all within the same range.

Assessment of Nutrition Status

The RDA and other such standards for daily intakes of nutrients are based on determination of people's needs—and people's needs are determined by observation of what happens when they don't get enough of the nutrients. They get sick, one way or another, and they exhibit symptoms. A nutrient already used as an example is iron; iron can be used again here to illustrate the stages in development of an overt nutrient deficiency.

The overt, or outside, symptoms of an iron deficiency are pallor, weakness, tiredness, apathy, and headaches. These overt symptoms are the outward manifestations of an internal state of the blood—anemia—in which there is too little of the iron-containing protein hemoglobin to carry oxygen to the cells and enable them to get energy.

In reality, however, the appearance of overt iron deficiency is the last of a long sequence of events, as shown in Figure 1–7. First, there is a deficiency

overt (oh-VERT): out in the open. A condition can be **covert** (KOH-vert), or hidden, but when it has become obvious, it is said to be overt.

ouvrire = to open

co + operire = to hide thoroughly

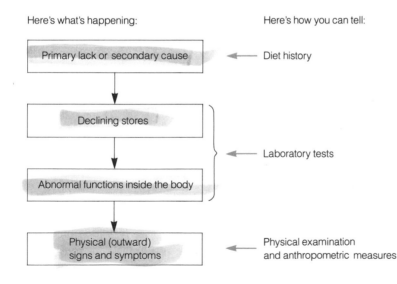

Here's what's happening:

Here's how you can tell:

Primary lack or secondary cause ← Diet history

Declining stores

Abnormal functions inside the body ← Laboratory tests

Physical (outward) signs and symptoms ← Physical examination and anthropometric measures

FIGURE 1–7 **Stages in the development of a nutritional deficiency**. Notice that attention to diet can prevent problems at the earliest possible time.

Source: Adapted from H. H. Sandstead and W. N. Pearson, Clinical evaluation of nutrition status, in *Modern Nutrition in Health and Disease*, ed. R. S. Goodhart and M. E. Shils (Philadelphia: Lea and Febiger, 1973), p. 585.

8   FAO Nutrition Meetings, *Requirements of Vitamin A, Thiamine, Riboflavin, and Niacin,* report series 41 (Rome: Food and Agriculture Organization, 1967).

A **primary deficiency** is a nutrient deficiency caused by inadequate dietary intake of a nutrient; a **secondary deficiency** is caused by something other than diet, such as a disease condition that reduces absorption, increases excretion, or causes destruction of the nutrient. Either of these can be a **subclinical** deficiency—that is, a deficiency in the early stages, before the signs have become obvious.

Methods Used in Nutrition Assessment

1 Diet history

2 Physical examination

3 Laboratory tests

4 Anthropometric measures

  anthropos = man

  metric = measuring

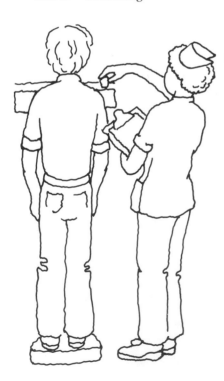

of iron getting into the body—either because there is not enough iron in the person's food (a primary deficiency) or because the person's body cannot absorb enough of the iron taken in or use it normally (a secondary deficiency). The body then begins to use up its own stores of iron; so there is a period of declining stores. At this point, a deficiency might be said to exist already, but there are no outward signs of it yet, and the person hasn't started to feel bad. Finally, the stores are used up, and not enough hemoglobin can be made to fill the developing, new red blood cells. At this point, the number of red blood cells declines, the new cells made are small and their color is pale, and every part of the body feels the effects of an oxygen lack. Weakness, fatigue, pallor, and headaches ensue.

As Figure 1–7 shows, there are ways to get at the problem of deficiencies before the end stage is reached. One way a deficient diet can be discovered is by means of a diet history. First a careful recording is made of all the foods a person eats over a period of time (say, three days or a week), with special attention to portion sizes. The foods are looked up in a table of food composition like Appendix H in this book, which shows the amounts of nutrients in each food. Then the nutrient intakes are compared with recommended intakes like the RDA. This kind of study is recommended for you, the reader, in the exercises in Appendix Q. The only cautions you have to exercise are to be aware that the Appendix H values are not absolute (different oranges vary in vitamin C contents, for example), and that the values presented assume reasonable care was taken in the preparation of foods (for example, they weren't so seriously overcooked that vitamins were lost). You are also assumed to be healthy, to be taking no medications that interfere with your body's use of nutrients, and to absorb and use the nutrients normally.

A second nutrition assessment technique is a physical examination that looks for cues to poor nutrition status. Every part of the body that can be inspected can offer such clues: the hair, eyes, skin, posture, tongue, fingernails, and others.

A third way to detect a developing deficiency is to take samples of body tissues (like blood or urine) and study them in the laboratory for the effects of a nutrient lack. If body changes are already occurring but are not yet obvious, such laboratory tests may reveal them. In the case of iron, for example, there are many tests to detect declining stores. A blood sample that shows a high level of the iron-carrier protein transferrin is an early indicator of a developing iron deficiency, because one of the body's first responses to such a deficiency is to increase its output of this protein in the effort to pick up more iron from the intestinal tract. (A less sensitive but much more widely used test of iron status is the red blood cell count, which detects overt iron-deficiency anemia.)

A fourth technique that may reveal nutrient deficiencies or other nutrition problems (although not useful for iron) is the taking of height, weight, and other body measurements. These anthropometric measures alert the clinician to such serious problems as growth failure in children and wasting or swelling of body tissue in adults, which may reflect severe nutrient or kcalorie deficiencies or imbalances. Many more details of nutrition assessment techniques are offered in Chapter 12 and Appendix E.

In reading further, you may want to keep this example of nutrition assessment in mind. It illustrates several nutrition principles. For one thing, inside-the-body changes precede the outward signs of deficiencies or excesses. As a corollary, we do not have to wait for the signs of sickness to appear before doing something about it. There are tests that can be used to show deficiencies in the early stages or to confirm that nutrient stores are adequate. These principles underlie several later chapters about the vitamins and minerals.

Dietary Guidelines

Since the mid-1960s, there has been increasing concern that overnutrition may be contributing to the illnesses many people suffer from today: heart disease, cancer, diabetes, liver disease, and others. These diseases may arise in part from excesses in fat, salt, sugar, even protein intake. Government authorities are now as much concerned to protect people from consuming too much of these substances as they once were about deficient intakes. In the last decade, the governments of several of the developed countries have published recommendations that people reduce their intakes of fat, salt, and sugar and turn back toward the more whole-food-based diets of their predecessors.

Among the new sets of recommendations have been the *Dietary Recommendations for Canadians* (1976), the *Dietary Goals for the United States* (1977), and the *Dietary Guidelines for Americans* (1980). These sets of guidelines differ somewhat from each other, but there is more agreement than disagreement. The emphasis in all of them is on prevention of overnutrition and disease.

overnutrition: overconsumption of energy or nutrients.

Many nutrition surveys in the United States and Canada have also revealed *undernutrition*, but a discussion of these survey findings is reserved for Chapter 12, after the chapters on vitamins and minerals, because it will then be more meaningful.

In the preface, we presented the view that science never possesses or conveys "the truth" or "reality." Rather, the progress of science is marked by the development of a continuously changing *picture* of reality. We can never get at reality itself. The picture that scientists continuously work on developing keeps changing because new observations keep coming to light that don't quite fit in the old picture. Therefore we cannot be dogmatic in stating nutrition facts. In fact, they aren't facts, they are only *findings* from which we keep trying to generalize—even though we sometimes seem to treat them as facts when we do not take the time to qualify them with wordy phrases like "The present view is," or "Some authorities believe," and the like.

Some people are fully aware that science is an evolving process, but many are uncomfortable on the shifting ground and resent having to adjust constantly to integrate new information. It is a task we need to become comfortable with, even to enjoy, if we are to adopt the scientific attitude toward nutrition.

A further level of sophistication is demanded of us when we listen to

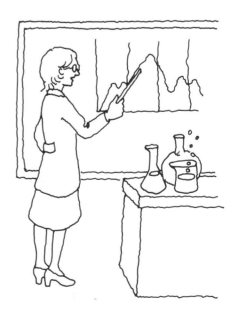

what scientists themselves have to say about applying "the facts" (the findings). No two scientists have quite the same picture of reality, even if they have access to the same set of findings; and to complicate the situation further, they may have different sets of values or philosophies.

These differences among scientists need not upset us, but we should be aware of them. We can then take what scientists say with the appropriate degree of openmindedness toward other possible points of view. This attitude is especially needed when we deal with recommendations scientists make about our behavior, as they do when they offer dietary guidelines.

Caution

Nutrition scientists are of divergent opinions about advising the public on diet. Some feel that no advice can reasonably be given at all; others feel justified in offering very concrete advice. Three points of view along the spectrum might be expressed as follows (we'll take dietary fat as an example):[9]

● Even though the facts are not all in, we know enough to recommend major and sweeping changes in the diet of the public. On fat consumption, the facts will eventually prove that dietary fat is the primary culprit in the development of heart disease; therefore every citizen should reduce fat intake to less than 30 percent of kcalories and preferably 20 percent right now.

● Not all the facts are in, but it is safe to suggest modest dietary changes, at least for some people. On fat consumption, it appears that the public eats too much fat and this fat is usually eaten at the expense of other food that contains important nutrients. Furthermore, no present evidence suggests that any harm would result from reducing fat consumption. Therefore most people should probably reduce their fat intakes to 35 percent of kcalories and consume more protective foods in place of fat.

● We don't know enough yet to make any recommendations to the public. On fat consumption, not enough information is yet available to prove that fat is the primary culprit in heart disease. If people were advised on this matter at the present time, and the advice were to turn out later to be wrong, public confidence in science would be shaken.

The *Dietary Goals* and other guidelines offered to the public represent a compromise between the two extremes, not a consensus opinion of all scientists. They are tentative, and they are offered here not because they represent the absolute truth on diet, but because students of nutrition need to know what they are.

The first U.S. *Dietary Goals* were seven in number.[10] One of them had to

9   We are indebted to Dr. Kay B. Franz, assistant professor of food science and nutrition, Brigham Young University, for expressing the distinctions that follow.

10   U.S. Senate, Select Committee on Nutrition and Human Needs, *Dietary Goals for the United States* (Washington, D.C.: Government Printing Office, 1977).

do with energy (kcalorie) consumption, two with carbohydrate, three with fat, and one with salt (see box). The recommended changes in diet are illustrated in Figure 1–8, which shows that the most dramatic change recommended was that we should increase our consumption of complex carbohydrate. Chapter 2 presents the reasons for this and the message, surprising to many consumers, that carbohydrate is not "bad" but "good" for you.

Dietary Goals for the United States

1 To avoid overweight, consume only as much energy (kcalories) as is expended; if overweight, decrease energy intake and increase energy expenditure.

2 Increase the consumption of complex carbohydrates and "naturally occurring" sugars from about 28 percent of energy intake to about 48 percent of energy intake.

3 Reduce the consumption of refined and other processed sugars by about 45 percent to account for about 10 percent of total energy intake.

4 Reduce overall fat consumption from approximately 40 percent to about 30 percent of energy intake.

5 Reduce saturated fat consumption to account for about 10 percent of total energy intake; and balance that with polyunsaturated and monoun-saturated fats, which should account for about 10 percent of energy intake each.

6 Reduce cholesterol consumption to about 300 milligrams a day.

7 Limit the intake of sodium by reducing the intake of salt (sodium chloride) to about 5 grams a day.

FIGURE 1–8   **The U.S. *Dietary Goals*.**

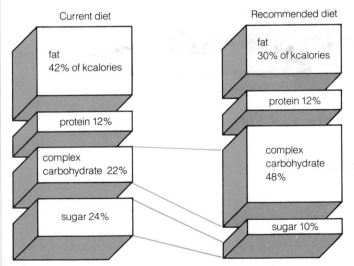

Source: *Dietary Goals for the United States*, 2nd ed., Select Committee on Nutrition and Human Needs, United States Senate (Washington, D. C. : Government Printing Office, 1977).

The publication of the *Dietary Goals* kicked up a whirlwind of conflicting opinions. Proponents hailed the *Goals* as long overdue and only regretted that they were understated and conservative. Opponents criticized them as premature, exaggerated, and inappropriate for distribution to the public. One of the objections to the *Goals* was that they had come out under the auspices of a political body—a powerful Senate committee—rather than a group of scientists. This criticism, among others, led to the disbanding of the Senate committee at the end of 1977, and the distribution of its responsibilities to two government departments whose charges include matters of nutrition and health: the Department of Agriculture (USDA) and the Department of Health and Human Services (USDHHS).

In 1979, after much more discussion and disagreement, representatives of these two departments produced *Dietary Guidelines for Americans*, which included seven guidelines similar to the *Goals* but less specific and less controversial (see box).

✳

Dietary Guidelines for Americans and Suggestions for Food Choices

1 *Eat a variety of foods daily.* Include these foods every day: fruits and vegetables; whole grain and enriched breads and cereals; milk and milk products; meats, fish, poultry, and eggs; dried peas and beans.

desireable — 2 *Maintain ideal weight.* Increase physical activity; reduce kcalories by eating fewer fatty foods and sweets and less sugar, and by avoiding too much alcohol; lose weight gradually.

3 *Avoid too much fat, saturated fat, and cholesterol.* Choose low-fat protein sources such as lean meats, fish, poultry, dried peas and beans; use eggs and organ meats in moderation; limit intake of fats on and in foods; trim fats from meats; broil, bake, or boil—don't fry; read food labels for fat contents.

4 *Eat foods with adequate starch and fiber.* Substitute starches for fats and sugars; select whole-grain breads and cereals, fruits and vegetables, dried beans and peas, and nuts to increase fiber and starch intake.

5 *Avoid too much sugar.* Use less sugar, syrup, and honey; reduce concentrated sweets like candy, soft drinks, cookies, and the like; select fresh fruits or fruits canned in light syrup or their own juices; read food labels—sucrose, glucose, dextrose, maltose, lactose, fructose, syrups, and honey are all sugars; eat sugar less often to reduce dental caries.

6 *Avoid too much sodium.* Reduce salt in cooking; add little or no salt at the table; limit salty foods like potato chips, pretzels, salted nuts, popcorn, condiments, cheese, pickled foods, and cured meats; read food labels for sodium or salt contents especially in processed and snack foods.

÷ don't drive 7 *If you drink alcohol, do so in moderation.* For individuals who drink —limit all alcoholic beverages (including wine, beer, liquors, and so on) to one or two drinks per day. NOTE: use of alcoholic beverages during pregnancy can result in the development of birth defects and mental retardation called Fetal Alcohol Syndrome.

Source: *Nutrition and Your Health, Dietary Guidelines for Americans* (Washington, D.C.: USDA, USDHHS, 1979).

The publication of these two sets of recommendations—the *Goals* and the *Guidelines*—so close together in time reveals the nation's intense interest in nutrition and especially its concern about overnutrition. Whichever document you look at, you see the same general principles stressed: the *Goals* state them in terms of nutrients; the *Guidelines* translate them into foods.

The United States is not alone in being concerned about its citizens' ways of eating. As we mentioned earlier, many other nations have studied the same issues and have presented their people with similar sets of recommendations. The Canadian government's recommendations are shown here for comparison; you can see that many of the concerns are the same (see box).

Dietary Recommendations for Canadians

These should not be considered a replacement for treatment of a particular disease. The recommendations are:

a) A reduction in kcalories from fat, to 30 to 35 percent of total kcalories, mainly as a decrease in saturated fat.
b) A partial substitution of polyunsaturated for saturated fat.
c) A reduction in dietary cholesterol intake to 400 milligrams daily or less.
d) A diet that contains less alcohol, salt, and refined sugars, and more whole grain products, fruits, and vegetables,
e) The prevention and control of obesity through reducing excess kcalories and increasing physical activity. Precautions should be taken that no deficiency of vitamins and minerals occurs when total kcalories are reduced.

The dietary recommendations for special groups are that:

a) Normal infants should be excluded from any dietary modifications recommended for cardiovascular disease.
b) In the diets of obese children, reduction of kcalories (except from foods like sugar that are devoid of essential nutrients) should be cautiously undertaken so as to maintain adequate growth rates. A preferable regimen for the obese child is a program of increased physical activity.
c) The elderly or infirm, or persons with additional requirements, such as pregnant women, nursing mothers, or growing persons, should be particularly careful that there be no deficiency of essential nutrients if total kcalories are reduced. In growing children, kcalorie intake should be sufficient to ensure adequate growth.

Source: *Report of the Committee on Diet and Cardiovascular Disease* (Canada: Department of Health and Welfare, 1976), pp. 81–82.

The sets of guidelines presented here are not the only ones that have appeared, and are certain not to be the last, but they suffice to illustrate the kinds of efforts being made to provide useful dietary advice to the public. Unlike the food group plans described earlier, these guidelines do not focus on "getting enough" but rather on "not getting too much." In truth, there may be a need for such advice; but in heeding it, we would be ill served if we forgot to try to make our diets adequate. Except for such recommendations as "Eat a variety of foods," the goals and guidelines have been phrased largely negatively: "Avoid. . . ." They don't deal fully with the need for dietary adequacy.

Recent surveys undertaken to assess the nutrition status of families in the United States have revealed that both concerns are still real. Described fully in Chapter 12, the surveys have shown both overnutrition and undernutrition to be problems in our population. There is a need, then, for all of us to choose our foods intelligently in the interest of our nutritional health.

This chapter has taken you a long way—from introduction of the nutrients and foods through a discussion of the assessment of people's nutrition status to a conclusion that for our health's sake we should perhaps, be eating differently, than we do now. Chapter 2 takes a closer look at the first of the energy nutrients, carbohydrate, and presents the reasons why this conclusion may, indeed, be valid.

Summing Up

To achieve optimum health, we need both adequacy and variety in the nutrients we ingest. The major classes of nutrients vital to health and found in our food supply are carbohydrate, fat, protein, vitamins, minerals, and water. The first four are organic nutrients; the last two are inorganic.

After ingestion, carbohydrate, fat, and protein are metabolized to simpler compounds which may become incorporated into body structures or be oxidized to yield energy. The energy released is measured in kcalories and supports body processes such as growth, maintenance, repair, and movement. The main excretory products of these oxidations are carbon dioxide and water; protein yields additional excretory products which will be discussed later.

There are at least five concepts to keep in mind when planning a nutritious diet: adequacy, balance, kcalorie control, variety, and nutrient density. Food group plans and exchange systems use these concepts.

The Four Food Group Plan divides foods into groups according to similarity of protein, vitamin, and mineral content. A specific number of daily food servings is recommended from each group. Exchange systems list foods according to the number of kcalories and amount of protein, carbohydrate, and fat each contains. Each list defines specific portion sizes for individual foods. Exchange systems are recommended to consumers who wish to eat well while monitoring their kcalorie intakes. Individuals may also find it helpful to use both systems simultaneously to ensure adequate nutrient intakes along with controlled kcalorie intakes.

The RDA (Recommended Dietary Allowances) represent suggested daily nutrient intakes for healthy people in the United States. Canada and other nations have their own similar standards. The RDA can be used as a yardstick against which the intakes of groups of people can be measured and as a guide for planning group diets; their use for individuals is limited.

The RDA were developed for different age and sex groups, but a single set of values has been drawn from them for use in nutrition labeling. Called the U.S. RDA, these standards are equal or close to the highest RDA values for any group for each nutrient. Nutrient contents of foods are then stated on labels as a percentage of the U.S. RDA.

A diet providing two-thirds of the RDA for a set of seven indicator nutrients is deemed good. This is one of the standards used in surveys of the U.S. population to determine its people's nutrition status. Other ways of evaluating nutrition status of individuals or groups of people include the use of clinical tests and physical examinations; these means are also used in nutrition status surveys.

Recent recommendations for diet planning emphasize preventive nutrition. These include the *Dietary Recommendations for Canadians* (1976), the *Dietary Goals for the United States* (1977), and the *Dietary Guidelines for Americans* (1980).

NOTE: References recommended for further reading are in Appendix J; see "Food Group Plans, Exchange Systems, Recommendations, and Dietary Guidelines." For more on the credentials of reliable nutrition authorities, and on ways of evaluating the validity of nutrition information, see "Misinformation" in Appendix J.

Self-Study exercises in Appendix Q show you how to:

● Record what you eat.
● Determine the percentage of kcalories you consume from protein, fat, and carbohydrate.
● Score your diet against the Four Food Goup Plan.

The *Instructor's Manual* that accompanies this text includes an extra transparency/handout master relating to the Four Food Group Plan: "Low Cost Foods for Survival." TH1-2 It also includes an entire supplementary lecture on "Diet Planning for the Vegetarian."

HIGHLIGHT 1A
Natural Foods

*The ingredients listed are mostly "whole" foods.
This "wholeness" means that the flour . . . or flakes
contain all the elements of the whole grain,
particularly the "germ," that part of the grain
kernel from which the grain would sprout if
planted. So this germ is the most life-containing,
life-giving part of the grain.*

EDWARD ESPE BROWN,
The Tassajara Bread Book

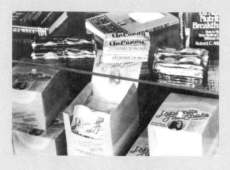

This Highlight introduces the first of many controversial subjects discussed in this book. It deals with something close to many people's hearts—the foods we choose to buy and eat. No one will be completely in agreement with all that is said here. If your own view is not the first to be presented, please be aware that it will probably receive fair treatment later on. If you love whole-grain bread, for example, be assured that some very favorable statements are made about it in the chapters to come. First the cons, then the pros of "natural" foods are given, before a balanced view is reached.[1]

Long ago, an experiment was performed in which six rats were fed a diet of white bread and water. Within 13 weeks, all of them were sick and their hair was falling out.[2] This experiment has been widely reported, and some people have taken it as "proof" that white bread is not nutritious, and in fact is even bad for health. Actually, however, the experiment only proved that white bread by itself does not provide all the nutrients animals need to grow and stay healthy. No other single food—not even hamburger—supports life much better. In fact, in that same experiment, six animals were fed hamburger and all developed paralysis; all but one were dead by the thirteenth week. Dr. D. M. Hegsted, professor of nutrition at the Harvard School of Public Health, in reporting the experiment, cautioned that any single food consumed in excess and in the absence of other foods may appear to be toxic.[3]

Rather than feeding single foods, it is possible to offer rats—or human

---

1   This Highlight is adapted from E. M. N. Hamilton and E. N. Whitney, Controversy 1: Natural foods, in *Nutrition: Concepts and Controversies*, 2nd ed. (St. Paul, Minn.: West, 1982), pp. 17–23.

2   D. M. Hegsted and L. M. Ausman, Sole foods and some not so scientific experiments, *Nutrition Today*, November/December 1973, pp. 22–25.

3   Hegsted and Ausman, 1973.

beings, for that matter—a mixed diet that includes members of all four food groups; they will then stay healthy and active and suffer no apparent ill effects. In such a diet, the bread group could be represented by the same white bread fed previously, and the meat group by hamburger as before, but two other food groups would also be represented: fruits and vegetables and milk and milk products. In this diet, the nutrient deficits of each food would be compensated for by the other foods.

Would this diet of white bread, hamburger, fruits and vegetables, and milk be a healthy diet? There are two schools of thought on the merits of ordinary foods bought in ordinary grocery stores.

An article in *The Miami Herald* is typical of the "No!" answer to this question. Its headline states "OUR FOOD IS KILLING US," and it refers to grocery-store foods as "denutrified, contaminated and deeply embalmed garbage."[4] The quoted writer subscribes to the view that our food has been subjected to all kinds of violence:

● It has been processed to the point where it no longer contains any nutrients worth mention ("denutrified").
● It has been sprayed or otherwise treated with poisons that can do us harm when we eat it ("contaminated").
● It has been pumped full of additives to change its texture, color, and flavor (more "contaminated"); and it has preservatives added to make it imperishable ("embalmed").
● Furthermore, it was grown on such poor soil that it had virtually no nutritive value to begin with ("garbage").

It is dangerous, according to this point of view, to eat such unnatural food. People who hold this view, and there are many of them, urge consumers to abandon the grocery store and shop instead at stores that sell foods described as "organic," "natural," or "health" foods.

There are actually several issues here, and all are complex. The accusations quoted have to be translated into more objective language before they can be dealt with at all, and discussion of some will be postponed to later places in the book. Regarding the "denutrification" of foods, an objective wording of the question might be "Does food processing cause such great nutrient losses that consumers should seek out unprocessed foods?" This question is further explored elsewhere.[5] Regarding "embalming" and "contamination," two whole highlights (Highlights 10 and 11) address the issues of additives and contaminants. Here, let us begin to deal with the merits of "natural" foods. It is necessary to start with some definitions.

Organic, Natural, and Health Foods

The term *organic* has two meanings. One meaning was made popular by J. I. Rodale, a Pennsylvania editor whose magazine *Prevention* has enjoyed

---

4   *Miami Herald,* January 9, 1979.

5   Nutrient losses incurred by food processing are described in "Foods in the Home," a supplementary lecture in the *Instructor's Manual* that accompanies this text.

The chemist's definition of **organic** is given on p. 3. There is also a popular definition: a food or nutrient produced without the use of chemical fertilizers, pesticides, or additives. As used on labels, this term may misleadingly imply unusual power to promote health. It has not been legally defined.

A natural food is one that has been altered as little as possible from the original farm-grown state. As used on labels, this term may misleadingly imply unusual power to promote health. Not legally defined as of 1983.

health food: a misleading term used on labels, usually of organic or natural foods, to imply unusual power to promote health. This term has no legal definition as of 1983.

a wide readership for several decades among people interested in health. According to Rodale, an organic food is a food fertilized with natural organic matter such as manure rather than chemical fertilizers, grown without application of pesticides, and processed without the use of food additives. However, as defined by chemists, the term *organic* merely means containing organic compounds, or molecules with carbon atoms in them. By this definition, all foods are organic.[6] Your body cannot tell whether the nutrients it receives come from an "organic" food or any other food.

When you read the word *organic* on a food label it usually conveys the Rodale meaning: free of chemical fertilizers, pesticides, and additives. The word *natural* has similar connotations but means more generally foods altered as little as possible from their original farm-grown state. *Health foods* encompass both organic and natural foods. They include "conventional foods which have been subjected to less processing than usual (such as unhydrogenated nut butters and whole-grain flours) and less conventional foods such as brewer's yeast, pumpkin seeds, wheat germ, and herb teas."[7] The latter items are supposed to have special power to promote health. None of these words has any legal meaning; so they may express different intents when used on different labels.

Cons of Health Foods

Does the consumer obtain any advantage by buying health foods? When the foods themselves have been studied, no evidence has ever been found to show that they confer any special physical benefit. But when the *users* are observed it is found that what they are trying to buy is peace of mind. They are described as people who long for purity, who distrust technology and especially "chemicals," and who are anxious about their health.[8] Health food store operators have been seen to play the role of doctors. They "diagnose" the ailments their customers complain of and "prescribe" foods or pills or powders to relieve the symptoms. For this service, customers may pay prices inflated 50 percent or more above the prices of comparable grocery-store items.

Mail-order houses also cater, often dishonestly, to people's anxiety and needs for reassurance. Herbal products available for order by mail are required by law to carry a special label that says, in part:

> The following information should not be used for the diagnosis, treatment or prevention of diseases . . . [and] should not be used to . . . replace the services of a physician. . . .

But the people selling these products correctly anticipate that buyers will overlook the label. Right below the disclaimer are promises that these

6   Position paper on food and nutrition misinformation on selected topics, *Journal of the American Dietetic Association* 66 (1975): 277–279.

7   L. A. Barness, Nutritional aspects of vegetarianism, health foods, and fad diets, *Nutrition Reviews* 35 (June 1977): 153–157.

8   R. T. Frankle and F. K. Heussenstamm, Food zealotry and youth: New dimensions for professionals, *American Journal of Public Health* 64 (January 1974): 11–18.

products will help "impotence, memory, kidney and bladder complaints, arthritis, cancer..." (the list goes on and on). They will correct "miscarriage even after hemorrhaging and pain have begun."[9] (Imagine a woman beginning to bleed, with an impending miscarriage, delaying her trip to the doctor or hospital in order to take an herbal preparation! And yet it is easy to see why a young woman fearful of doctors and hospitals and trusting "nature" would make such a choice, even against all reason and evidence.) Almost $100 million a year is spent on herbal products, much of it by mail.[10]

Taking herbal products is risky for several reasons. They cannot be monitored or held to defined standards by government agencies, as packaged, labeled foods can be. Many contain natural toxins and should be used with moderation if at all. Sassafras, for example, contains the liver toxin safrole.[11] The overuse of the herb ginseng produces a cluster of symptoms including high or low blood pressure, nervousness, sleeplessness, diarrhea, depression, confusion, and many others.[12] The popular herb chamomile can cause shock.[13] The *Journal of the American Medical Association* warns physicians that when they see food poisoning symptoms they should keep in mind the possibility that herbal teas from natural food stores may be involved:

> The American public is unaware of the potential dangers of certain of these products; they assume and are accustomed to the fact that foods purchased from retail stores generally have been tested and approved for human use. However, many...plant products have not been tested; their effects on the body are not fully understood, or their effects simply are unknown to the majority of casual purchasers.... Unfortunately the Food and Drug Administration [FDA] does not have the authority to require such labels except via a cumbersome product-by-product procedure.[14]

As of the fall of 1979, 700 different plants had been reported to cause deaths or serious illnesses in the Western hemisphere.[15] (At the same time, there had been—apparently—no cases of food-borne illness attributed to the consumption of legally permitted levels of artificial additives in processed foods.[16])

Among health foods, none is innocent of all charges, even honey. Honey has been found to contain spores which, in the human body, produce bacteria that synthesize the deadly botulism toxin. The small amounts normally involved may constitute no risk for most people, but infants under

sassafras (SASS-uh-frass), **ginseng** (JINN-seng), **chamomile** (CAM-oh-meel): plants whose leaves, flowers, or other parts are popularly used for the making of herbal teas. Hazards are associated with the overuse of these and many others.

shock: an emergency reaction of the body in which the blood pressure drops suddenly; a dangerous condition.

botulism (BOTT-you-lizm): poisoning by the toxin produced by a certain species of bacteria (*Clostridium botulinum*); this toxin is the most potent biological poison known.

9   B. McPherrin, Mail order health fraud, *ACSH News and Views* 1 (September/October 1980): 10.

10   McPherrin, 1980.

11   McPherrin, 1980.

12   Ginseng abuse syndrome, *Nutrition and the MD*, September 1979.

13   W. H. Lewis, Reporting adverse reactions to herbal ingestants (letter to the editor), *Journal of the American Medical Association* 240 (1978): 109–110.

14   Lewis, 1978.

15   A. Brynjolfsson, Food irradiation and nutrition, *Professional Nutritionist*, Fall 1979, pp. 7–10.

16   M. W. Pariza, Food safety from the eye of a hurricane, *Professional Nutritionist*, Fall 1979, pp. 11–14.

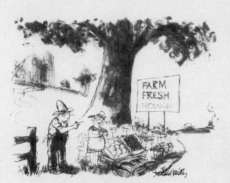

"Remember, now, the stuff is organic for those that want organic."

Drawing by Donald Reilly; © 1971 The New Yorker Magazine, Inc.

one year of age should probably never be fed honey.[17] (It can also be contaminated with environmental pollutants picked up by the producer bees.) Honey is believed to be implicated in several cases of sudden infant death.[18]

More dangerous by far than either herbal preparations or foods like honey are pills and supplements, especially of minerals. Highlight 1B deals with some of these.

From all this information it is apparent that products sold under the label "health" may not be so healthful after all. In fact, the term is considered so misleading that the Federal Trade Commission has proposed that the terms *health food*, *natural*, and *organic* be prohibited from use on labels.[19] The term *organic*—meaning pesticide-free—may sometimes be an outright lie. Many foods sold as organic contain pesticide residues at the same levels as conventional foods, in some cases because the farmers secretly spray them and in others because pesticide residues remain in the environment from previous uses. Moreover, organic foods in several experiments have been found not to differ chemically from conventional foods.[20] And it is not surprising—even if it is disappointing—that some sellers will label their products organic just to be able to sell them at twice the price they would get for the same foods without the label. Even though this is unethical, it is not illegal; nor is it false advertising, since *organic* has not been legally defined.

All this is not to say that all health-food operators are dishonest. Many are utterly sincere and are trying to sell their customers the purest and finest products. But many people who have turned to health foods sooner or later become disillusioned with most of them. One health-food store owner gave up the business because she couldn't square it with her conscience. "I just didn't believe it any more. It got to the point where I was almost hiding from my customers. I couldn't look them in the eye. After I stopped believing I just couldn't sell [health foods] any more."[21]

If health-food store products often are not what they appear to be and will not do for the consumer what he hopes they will do, some questions still remain about their merits. One question of great concern in this shrinking, pollution-threatened, energy-starved world relates to the methods of organic farming. Even if organic foods do not differ chemically from conventional foods, they are produced differently. Does the method of production make any difference—to anybody?

17   Corn syrup can also be contaminated with *C. botulinum* spores. D. A. Kautter, T. Lilly, H. M. Solomon, and R. K. Lynt, *Clostridium botulinum* spores in infant foods—a survey, *Journal of Food Protection* 45 (1982): 1028–1029.

18   I. B. Vyhmeister, What about honey? *Life and Health*, August 1980, pp. 5–7; R. W. Miller, Honey: Making sure it's pure, *FDA Consumer* 13 (September 1979): 12–13.

19   M. Stephenson, The confusing world of health foods, *FDA Consumer* 12 (July/August 1978): 18–22.

20   Stephenson, 1978.

21   Singing the health food blues, an interview with B. Cavanaugh, former owner of a health food store, *ACSH News and Views* 1 (February 1980): 10–11.

Pros of Organic Farming

Organic foods are grown in soil fertilized only with natural waste materials such as manure and compost (rotted vegetable matter and garbage). Like "chemical" fertilizers, these materials are composed of chemicals, and they support the growth and health of plants only to the extent that they provide the chemicals the plants need: potassium, nitrogen, phosphate, and others. There is nothing superior about organic fertilizer from that standpoint. Both organic and "chemical" fertilizers can be excellent for a plant if they provide it with a "balanced diet," and both types of fertilizer can be poor if they provide an imbalance of nutrients or are missing one or more nutrients.[22] The ultimate chemical composition achieved by a plant depends on the genetic program it has received in its seed. It makes protein or vitamins or fiber according to those inherited instructions and is not at the mercy of the quality of the soil—as long as the needed raw materials are there in a usable form. Plants grow normally if they grow at all. If the fertilizer is inadequate, then the crop yield will be less—but what plants there are will be of the usual composition. The only known exception to this relates to minerals. Plants grown in soil lacking iodine will produce iodine-poor fruits and vegetables, for example. But crop rotation, soil testing, soil enrichment, and crop analysis are all safeguards intended to ensure that plants don't lack minerals.[23]

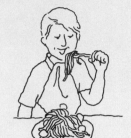

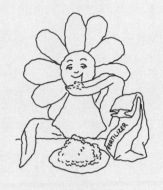

There may, however, be fringe benefits to the use of natural fertilizers like compost. For example, such fertilizers affect the structure (tilth) of the soil to give a mechanical advantage to the plant. Moreover, organic material returned to the soil is recycled in the natural way. It might otherwise be burned (polluting the air) or dumped to wash into the rivers, lakes, and oceans (polluting the water).

The recycling aspect may be one of the most significant differences between organic and conventional farming, and its chief advantage may be not to the nutrition of the individual consumer but to the ecology. Dr. Joan D. Gussow, professor of nutrition at Columbia University, points out that organic farming conserves energy and doesn't pollute. In contrast, conventional agriculture consumes vast amounts of energy and produces fully *half* of the more than four billion tons of solid waste the United States generates each year. Organic farming attempts to make use of its own waste. It is "ecologically sound agriculture." Besides, it breaks no laws, and it can produce foods as safe and as nutritious as conventional foods.[24]

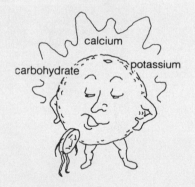

To sum up what has been said so far, foods carrying the labels *organic*, *health*, and *natural* have no proven nutritional advantage over conventional, comparable grocery-store foods. They are often considerably more expensive; they are often fraudulently advertised; and their use—especially that of herbal preparations—may be risky because they are not well

22   W. H. Allaway, *The Effect of Soils and Fertilizer on Human and Animal Nutrition*, Agriculture Information Bulletin no. 378 (Washington, D.C.: Government Printing Office, March 1975).

23   R. B. Alfin-Slater, Vitamin supplementation: An appraisal of values—and dangers, *Professional Nutritionist*, Winter 1980, pp. 8–11.

24   J. D. Gussow, The organic alternative, *Nutrition Today*, March/April 1974, pp. 31–32.

regulated or inspected. When health foods or herbal remedies are substituted for competent medical advice and treatment they may be tragically ill-chosen. Organic foods are not different chemically from their conventional counterparts, and often are not even pesticide-free. If any reason exists to recommend organic over conventional agriculture, it relates to the ecology, not to the food produced.

Does all this mean there is *no* advantage to natural foods? The questions of food processing and additives have been postponed to later parts of the book, and they need to be considered before a full answer can be given, but for the moment it might be appropriate to offer a few conclusions here. Generally speaking, the more a food resembles the original, farm-grown product, the more nutritious it is likely to be. During processing, nutrients are lost, and often nutrient-empty additions like sugar, salt, and fat are made. A potato contains 20 milligrams of vitamin C; the same number of kcalories in french fries contains only about 7 milligrams; and the same number of kcalories of potato chips contains only 2 milligrams of vitamin C. (By this standard, it isn't really fair to call potato chips "natural" even if they are organically grown!) An apple contains 50 IU of vitamin A, applesauce with the same number of kcalories contains about 30, and apple jelly contains less than 1. And so forth. Regardless of where these products were purchased—whether at the health food store or at the grocery store—there is something to be said for buying the potato and the apple. They don't have to be *labeled* natural, they only have to *be* natural.

(Incidentally, something funny about health-food stores is that they ignore the nutrient density principle. Among their most popular items are candy bars loaded with sugar and fat. Because the candy bars are made from sources labeled "natural," like fruit sugar, honey, and carob beans, rather than from cane sugar and chocolate, they are advertised as superior sources of nutrients.)

When you want to choose nutritious foods, a useful guideline is to choose whole, natural foods. But you don't have to do this all the time. Not every potato product you use must be recognizably potato. A principle that helps with making food choices is to ask, "What am I using this food for?" or "How big a part of my diet is this food?" The more you depend on a food as a staple item, the more important its wholesomeness. If bread, for example, is one of your staple foods, then whole-grain bread is certainly a better choice than refined, white bread.[25] In the same way, the less often or heavily you use a food, the less its quality matters. An example is the use of candy bars. If you eat them only on picnics and you picnic only once a year, they'll hardly detract from your nutrition on a year-round basis. But if you are eating nothing but candy bars for breakfast and lunch every day, then they are a staple item in your diet and a very poor choice indeed. You can no doubt think of many similar examples of harmless versus harmful uses of food items.

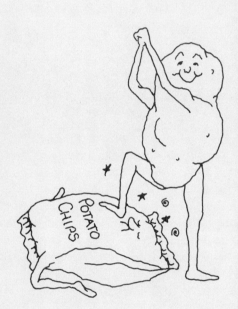

staple: with respect to food, one used frequently or daily in the diet —for example, potatoes (in Ireland) or rice (in the Far East).

---

25 The *Instructor's Manual* accompanying this text includes a detailed description of the many nutritional advantages of whole-grain bread in its optional lecture, "Foods in the Home."

Something else to keep in mind is that not all choices are necessarily positive or negative; some are simply neutral. If you happen to know an organic farmer locally and want to buy his produce, there is certainly no reason not to. His products may be more attractive, more flavorsome, more desirable to you as a consumer than the same kind of foods available elsewhere. You may want to support his "ecologically sound agriculture" even if it means paying a higher price to do so. And if you have taken a fancy to a particular product sold at the local health food store, whatever it may be, there is no reason why you should not buy it and use it. Some products sold as natural (such as the local baker's whole-grain bread, for example) are truly delicious, nourishing, and worth the extra price to consumers who have the money to spend.

But if you don't have the money, or don't have a personal preference for specific products in these special categories, there is no reason why you should make any effort in that direction. It is perfectly possible to obtain all the wholesome, nutritious foods you need for a balanced and adequate diet by making educated choices in the grocery store.

NOTE: References recommended for further reading are in Appendix J; see "Books," and also the special section on "Misinformation."

Vitamin, Mineral, and Other Supplements

All substances are poison. The right dose differentiates a poison and a remedy.

PARACELSUS (16th century)

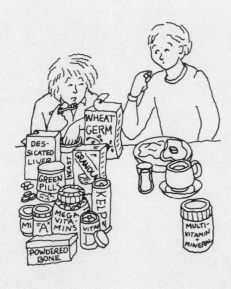

nutritional yeast: a preparation of yeast cells, often praised for its high nutrient content. Yeast is a concentrated source of B vitamins, as are many other foods. The type of yeast used is brewer's, not baker's, yeast; see items 729 and 730 in Appendix H and the end of this Highlight.

Billions of dollars are spent on vitamin pills in the United States each year. Two-thirds of our citizens use them. Some people buy them because their doctors have told them to, but most people decide independently that they need them.[1] One person takes a single pill every morning, expecting it to deliver all the vitamins she requires. Another puts together a veritable arsenal of pills and powders in a pattern tailored to what he sees as his own personal needs.

Who's right? Or is it necessary to take vitamin pills at all? The vitamins are not dealt with in detail until Chapter 8, but it seems only fair to introduce this question early because it is of such general concern.[2]

Many takers of the single, daily pill seem to view it as a kind of nutritional insurance. This attitude (to anticipate the conclusion of this discussion) is not an extreme practice and, although unnecessary, does little harm even to the pocketbook. However, most people can learn to adjust their diets and meet their nutrient needs much better from foods than from pills. All you need in order to feel secure doing this is an understanding of a plan like the Four Food Group Plan and of a standard such as the RDA (Chapter 1), along with an acquaintanceship with the vitamins and minerals (Chapters 8-11).

The person to worry about is the one with the huge stockpile of nutrient preparations. Before breakfast, this person takes, say, 500 milligrams of vitamin C, 1,000 units of vitamin E, several tablespoons of "nutritional yeast," some kelp tablets, a capsule of vitamins A and D, a spirulina tablet, some green pills, and assorted other pills containing trace minerals, and sprinkles dessicated liver, powdered bone, bone meal, and wheat germ on his granola, followed by powdered skim milk. Such practices reveal that the person wants pills and powders to play a role that is better entrusted to

1   H. G. Schutz and coauthors, Food supplement usage in seven Western states, *American Journal of Clinical Nutrition* 36 (1982): 897–901.

2   This Highlight is adapted from E. M. N. Hamilton and E. N. Whitney, Controversy 2: Vitamin supplements, in *Nutrition: Concepts and Controversies*, 2nd ed. (St. Paul, Minn.: West, 1982), pp. 45–49.

food. (Not all the choices just listed are equally questionable, however. The wheat germ, granola, and milk are nutritious foods.)

All that such a person is trying to do is to obtain all the nutrients he needs. He is persuaded that he can't do this using ordinary foods. Highlight 1A dealt with one aspect of this belief—the "magic" associated with health foods—but even if this person agreed with the conclusion reached there, he would still use his pills and powders. "I need them," he would say, "because I may have unusually high needs for vitamins and minerals, and besides, it can't hurt to take a little extra."

These beliefs are typical of nutritional faddism, which is born of inadequate knowledge applied with sincere interest. Our supplement-taker, then, is a faddist because he cares profoundly about his health and knows no better way to care for it. Let us take a close look at the first of his reasons: "I may have unusually high needs."

Nutritional Individuality

Biologically speaking, no two people are exactly alike except identical twins, and no two people have exactly the same nutrient needs. You may need a bit more vitamin C than your friend, and your friend a bit more protein than you, to maintain peak health. Not only are people different biologically, but their different lifestyles affect their nutrient needs. Even identical twins, if they live differently, may not have identical needs. If one of them has a highly stressful job, for example, she may need a bit more of certain nutrients than the other; but rarely (only once in 100 cases) is a person's need above the RDA. These differences between individuals— which are nothing more than normal variations—may make our nutrient requirements differ as much as twofold or threefold, one from another; that is, you may need up to twice or three times as much vitamin C as your friend does, if his requirement is near the bottom end of the range and yours is near the top.

One person may even need seven times as much of a nutrient as someone else—but to say this is to display the full range of needs from the very lowest to the very highest. That is, the comparison is between someone with extraordinarily small needs and someone with extraordinarily high ones.[3] Such a comparison can't be used as the basis for recommending that any normal person take doses of nutrients seven or so times higher than the *average requirement*.

In some instances, *very* large differences in nutrient needs are seen. Some people are born with rare genetic defects that keep them from using certain nutrients in the normal way. These people may have extraordinarily high or low nutrient requirements, differing tenfold or a hundredfold from the average. But these are rare defects indeed. Only one person in 10,000 may have such a defect, and it demands diagnosis if the person is to live a normal life.

kelp: a kind of seaweed used by the Japanese as a foodstuff. Kelp tablets are made from dehydrated kelp.

spirulina: a kind of algae ("blue-green manna") said to contain large amounts of vitamin B_{12} and to suppress appetite. It does neither.

green pills: pills containing dehydrated, crushed vegetable matter. One pill contains nutrients equal to those in one small forkful of fresh vegetable—minus losses incurred in processing. Sixty pills costing $15.00 deliver vegetable matter worth about $1.50.

dessicated liver: dehydrated liver, a powder sold in health food stores and supposed to contain in concentrated form all the nutrients found in liver. Possibly not dangerous, this supplement has no particular nutritional merit, and grocery-store liver is considerably less expensive. *Dessicated* means "totally dried."

powdered bone, **bone meal**: two among many nutrient supplements intended to supply calcium and other bone minerals.

wheat germ: a part of the wheat grain, rich in nutrients.

granola: a cereal made from mixed oats and other grains.

normal variation: the variation normally expected in a biological system. Nutrient needs, for example, normally vary over a twofold or threefold range from the mean, although individuals are much more likely to have needs falling near the mean than near the extreme. See Figure 1-4.

---

3   R. Dubos, The intellectual basis of nutrition science and practice, a paper presented at the NIH conference on the biomedical and behavioral basis of clinical nutrition, June 19, 1978, in Bethesda, Maryland, and reprinted in *Nutrition Today*, July/August 1979, pp. 31–34.

Illness also imposes differences in nutrient requirements. Under the stress of surgery or high fever or after suffering extensive burns, for example, a person's needs for protein are much greater than usual, up to perhaps five times normal, and the needs for vitamins and minerals may be increased even more. Some prescription and over-the-counter medicines also increase specific vitamin and mineral needs. These special needs are the subject of large volumes on diet therapy used by health professionals in hospital work.[4]

What we are concerned with here, however, are normal variations, and these don't justify the taking of large quantities of vitamins and minerals in concentrated form by the normal, healthy person. Foods contain enough vitamins and minerals so that a reasonably careful selection of them will supply all that most people need. The food group plans described in Chapter 1 provide a healthful balance of nutrients—enough to meet the needs of people at the top of the range of normal variation.

"But," the supplement-taker may say, "that argument is based on too many assumptions for my comfort. You assume that the foods you speak of have the nutrients in them—whereas they may be poor in nutrients. You assume that they haven't lost those nutrients in cooking—when in fact they could be cooked to pieces and have no nutritional value." The nutrient contents of ordinary grocery-store foods were defended in Highlight 1A. Losses in cooking are moderate if you are careful. The choice of a variety of foods from day to day minimizes the risk of suffering a lack of nutrients in case one item chosen should happen to be nutrient-poor. But the debate between the self-doser and the ordinary-food user goes on and on, and will pop up again often in the chapters to come.

One other aspect of the self-dosing practice should at least be mentioned here: the risks. It is a myth that the vitamins are nontoxic. All of them, not only the well-known vitamins A and D, but also the water-soluble B vitamins and vitamin C, have been shown to have toxic effects, at least in some people, when taken in large doses.

How Vitamins Are Promoted

"Three-fourths of the public believe that extra vitamins provide more pep and energy. Twenty-six percent [use] nutritional supplements expecting observable benefits—without a physician's advice," reports Dr. P. L. White, director of the Department of Foods and Nutrition of the American Medical Association.[5] If it isn't necessary to do this, why have so many people been bamboozled into believing that it is? Dr. White has identified one of the kinds of claims made by pill-pushers: "The idea of nutritional individuality promotes the notion that you should try it [a fad] even though it didn't work for me." Dr. V. Herbert, professor of medicine and pathology at Columbia College of Physicians and Surgeons, has noted many other earmarks of

4   One such text is E. N. Whitney and C. B. Cataldo, *Understanding Normal and Clinical Nutrition* (St. Paul, Minn.: West, 1983).

5   P. L. White, Food faddism, *Contemporary Nutrition* 4 (February 1979).

faddism. Dr. Herbert says you can tell it may be a quack talking if he tries to persuade you:

- That you should buy something you wouldn't otherwise buy.
- That your disease condition is due to a faulty diet.
- That you have a "subclinical" deficiency.
- That, in fact, you should take supplements of any kind.
- That you should take "natural" vitamins.[6]

The last of these notions, that "natural" vitamins are of more virtue than synthetic vitamins, resembles the now-familiar argument about fertilizers. The body cannot tell whether a vitamin in the bloodstream came from an organically grown cantaloupe melon or from a chemist's laboratory. Pills made from the melon and from some chemical in the lab may differ from one another in their *other* ingredients, but insofar as they contain a certain vitamin, they are identical. If either kind of pill has an advantage of any kind, it is as often the synthetic as the "natural" pill. In one instance, vitamin C from *synthetic* pills was found to be absorbed better than that from "natural" pills, because something in the "natural" pills was interfering with the absorption of the vitamin.[7] In another case, the "natural" pills were found to be so weak that synthetic vitamin C had to be added to them to bring the concentration up to acceptable levels.[8]

In any case, there is nothing natural about a pill, no matter what its source. If we define *natural* more carefully and insist that the word be used only to refer to foods, not pills, and only to foods in their original, farm-grown state, then we can make a statement that will hold up to critical inspection. The natural food (like a cantaloupe melon) may be better for you than any pill—not because it has better vitamin C in it but because it conveys "fringe benefits" along with the vitamin C: carbohydrate, fiber, and fluid with dissolved calcium, potassium, and many other nutrients:

> There is no advantage to eating a nutrient from one source as opposed to another, but there may be fringe benefits to eating that nutrient in a natural food as opposed to a purified nutrient preparation.[9]

Minerals: Even More Dangerous

Takers of self-prescribed pills need a warning about the risks of overdosing with vitamins, but if they also take minerals they need a more urgent warning. Minerals are often "prescribed" by people calling themselves homeopathic physicians. "Homeopathy is a therapeutic system based on

subclinical: a nutrient deficiency that has no visible or otherwise detectable (clinical) symptoms. It is possible for such a deficiency to develop (see the discussion of loss of iron from body stores in Chapter 1), but the term is often used as a scare tactic to persuade consumers to buy nutrient supplements they don't need.

homeopathy (home-ee-OPP-athee): a branch of medicine (supposedly) that focuses on preventing disease, promoting health, and restoring disturbed body balances by feeding needed nutrients. Homeopathic "physicians" may or may not have M.D. degrees.

6   V. Herbert, The health hustlers, in *The Health Robbers*, ed. S. Barrett and G. Knight (Philadelphia: George F. Stickley, 1976).

7   O. Pelletier and M. O. Keith, Bioavailability of synthetic and natural ascorbic acid, in *The Nutrition Crisis, a Reader*, ed. T. P. Labuza (St. Paul, Minn.: West, 1975), pp. 192–200.

8   A. Kamil, How natural are those "natural" vitamins? *Co-op News*, March 13, 1972, p.3, reprinted in *Nutrition Reviews/Supplement: Nutrition Misinformation and Food Faddism*, July 1974, p. 34.

9   Position paper on food and nutrition misinformation on selected topics, *Journal of the American Dietetic Association* 66 (1975): 277–279.

cell salts: a mineral preparation sold in health food stores supposed to have been prepared from living, healthy cells. It is not necessary to take such preparations, and it may be dangerous.

minute doses of various remedies, many of which are mineral salts.... These 'cell salts' are alleged to have therapeutic value in a wide range of diseases."[10] The reasons why ill-informed dosing with minerals is especially dangerous will become fully apparent in the chapters on minerals; Dr. White expresses his concern this way:

> The newer research on the trace minerals has been exploited by the health food set; one sees glowing claims for zinc, selenium and chromium, the last being promoted as GTF, or glucose tolerance factor. Laboratories that "evaluate" nutritional status by hair analysis flourish, as does their business in food supplements to "correct" the "metabolic imbalances" uncovered by such analysis. Admittedly useful for certain determinations, hair analysis has not yet been found appropriate for general nutritional evaluation. A most disturbing aspect is that some physicians and dentists are utilizing the "services" of hair analysis laboratories.[11]

With all there is to be said against the use of vitamin pills, is there anything to be said *for* them? Yes, when a doctor prescribes them, and yes, in at least two other instances:

● When your kcalorie intake is below about the 1,500 level, so that you can't eat enough total food to be sure of meeting your vitamin needs.
● When you know that—for whatever reason—you are going to be eating irregularly for a limited time.

For a listing and comparison of available vitamin-mineral supplements, turn to Appendix P.

On these occasions, a single, balanced vitamin-mineral pill should suffice. It is then important to remember that, if vitamins are needed, minerals will be needed too, and a "vitamin pill" is not enough. A vitamin-mineral supplement is called for.

A problem that remains for the reader who is persuaded of the view presented here is "How do I tell my friends about this?" Trying to persuade a pill-popping friend not to take pills and powders can easily turn into the unfortunate experience of losing the friend. As Dr. A. E. Harper, professor of nutritional sciences at the University of Wisconsin, has put it, "Isn't it amazing how when you explain to someone that what they have accepted as fact is not so, they become angry with you rather than with the person who gave them the inaccurate information in the first place?"[12] Yes, it is amazing—and painful. But the response is not surprising when you recall that the person who has paid his or her own money as the price for believing a bogus "fact" has a personal stake in having the fact be true.

To avoid alienating the people we are trying to reach with valid information we can adopt several strategies. For one thing, we can always acknowledge the validity of the feelings and values that underlie the faddist's practices. Then, we can distinguish between practices that are dangerous and those that are merely neutral. We can ignore the neutral ones and

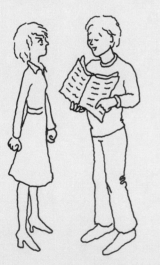

10   B. McPherrin, Mail order health fraud, *ACSH News and Views* 1 (September/October 1980): 10.

11   White, 1979.

12   A. E. Harper, Science and the consumer, *Journal of Nutrition Education* 11 (October–December 1979): 171.

confront only the dangerous ones. Finally, we can make ourselves responsible for learning the facts of the matter as thoroughly as we can, getting them all in perspective, and communicating them clearly.

In closing, it may be of interest to demonstrate how good judgment would rank the items selected by the pill-and-powder breakfaster described at the start. They can be sorted into groups as follows:

● *Most risky*: The A and D capsules and the minerals, because overdoses are a real possibility and have serious ill effects. Potassium chloride, for example, is sold in health-food stores, carries no warning label, and is known to have caused deaths of otherwise healthy individuals.[13]

● *Second*: The powdered bone (the calcium from such a source is very poorly absorbed, and some bone meal has been found to contain high levels of lead[14]) and the kelp tablets (the urine of people who use kelp tablets has been found to contain raised concentrations of arsenic, a poison and a possible cancer-causing agent[15]).

● *Third*: The vitamin C and the vitamin E. The doses (500 mg of vitamin C and 1,000 units of vitamin E) are not the highest doses people get away with taking, but they are high enough to be toxic in some individuals. (See Chapters 8 and 9 for more about vitamin C and E toxicity.)

● *Fourth*: The spirulina. It has little vitamin B_{12} itself, and some of the vitamin B_{12}-like compounds in it may actually compete with the vitamin B_{12} from other sources, rendering the vitamin less effective. Also, spirulina does not suppress appetite.[16]

● *Fifth*: The dessicated liver and the green pills. These are probably neutral items (although some risks could still come to light). It is easy to get the same nutrients delivered in ordinary foods, but there may be no harm in taking them in this form.

● *Sixth*: The nutritional yeast and the granola. Using them is probably a neutral practice. Live, baker's yeast cells, used to leaven bread, consume nutrients, but nonliving, brewer's yeast cells do not. Brewer's yeast is grown specially as a nutrient supplement, particularly for vegetarian diets; it is a good source of protein, B vitamins, and iron. Added to cereal, it improves the cereal's protein quality—important for the vegetarian whose total protein intake may be nearer the minimum needed than is the meat-eater's intake. Granola is a fairly nutritious cereal, although it contains more sugar than most people realize (see Appendix F), and is unpopular with dentists concerned about sugar and tooth decay.

13   One case was that of a baby whose mother had read the book *Let's Have Healthy Children* by Adelle Davis and had given the supplement to the infant, as the book suggested, for colic; M. Stephenson, The confusing world of health foods, *FDA Consumer* 12 (July/August 1978): 18–22.

14   FDA has requested that bone meal makers place a warning label on the product to protect infants, young children, and pregnant and lactating women; but as of early 1983, only 1 in 50 had complied. FDA request for lead warning rejected, *Nutrition Week*, June 9, 1983, p.6.

15   Stephenson, 1978.

16   V. Herbert and G. Drivas, *Spirulina* and vitamin B_{12}, *Journal of the American Medical Association* 248 (1982): 3096–3097; Spirulina discounted (Update), *FDA Consumer*, September 1981, p. 3.

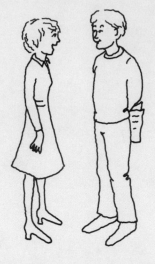

● *Last:* The wheat germ and the powdered skim milk. These are nutritious foods, they can be bought in the grocery store, and the skim milk in particular is a very economical source of valuable nutrients.

In counseling the user, you might praise the value system that puts such a high premium on health, and express support of the desire to take good care of the body. Then, you might reinforce the use of the last pair of items, agreeing that these foods are nutritious, reasonable in cost, and delicious. When you are sure of your listener's openness to whatever else you might have to say, you might offer a caution about the use of the potent supplements listed first, but keep your own counsel about the remaining ones unless you are asked. This way you probably won't lose a friend, and you may provide a substantial boost to exactly what he treasures most—his good health.

NOTE: References recommended for further reading are in Appendix J; see "Books," "Misinformation," and "Nutritional Individuality."

CHAPTER 2
The Carbohydrates: Sugar, Starch, and Fiber

CONTENTS

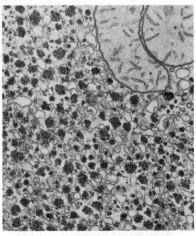

Within a single cell lie hundreds of coils of membranes enfolding materials the cell makes and uses. Shown here is part of a liver cell. The clusters of dark beads are glycogen—the form in which the cell stores carbohydrate energy.

The two bodies in the upper right-hand corner are mitochondria. Much of the cell's metabolic activity takes place inside these structures. Millions of enzymes are mounted on their internal membranes, in the order in which they perform their reactions.

French bread, biscuit, tortillas, pumpernickel, corn pone, scones, rice cakes . . . the very names conjure up old cultures that produced breads as characteristic as their makers.

IRMA S. ROMBAUER AND
M. R. BAKER
The Joy of Cooking

Most of us would like to feel good all the time. The enjoyment available in a day, no matter what the day may bring, can be tremendous if our bodies and minds are tuned for it. The feeling of well-being that comes with energy, alertness, clear thinking, and confidence is so rewarding that if you know how to produce it, you will probably make the necessary effort.

It would be an exaggeration to say that good eating habits alone produce this feeling of well-being. If you try to think of what makes you feel good, you can come up with several answers. Being in love, for example, is certainly one. Facing and solving a personal problem is another. Being well rested helps, and so does exercise. Being clean is still another help; a cold shower after heavy work or exercise can be bracing and exhilarating. Sparkling weather, clean air, beautiful scenery, pleasant company—all these play a part.

Even among the best of these pleasures, however, some limits are set by your nutritional state. You can feel really good only when your blood sugar (glucose) level is right. If that condition isn't met, neither the most beautiful mountaintop nor the most stimulating companion can compensate.

The health and functioning of every cell in your body depend on blood glucose to a greater or lesser extent. Ordinarily the cells of your brain and nervous system depend *solely* on this sugar for their energy. The brain cells are continually active, even while you're asleep, so they are continually drawing on the supply of glucose in the fluid surrounding them and it permits them to use other fuels as well. They oxidize glucose for the energy they need to perform their functions. To maintain the supply, a continuous flow of blood moves past these cells, replenishing the glucose as the cells use it up.

Glucose, a simple sugar, is often called blood sugar, because it is the principal carbohydrate found in mammalian blood (see also p. 53).

For the exception to this rule, ketosis, see Chapter 6.

Oxidation: see p. 3.

Because the brain and other nerves ordinarily cannot obtain energy without glucose, they are especially vulnerable to a temporary deficit in the blood glucose supply. When the brain is deprived of energy, mental processes are affected. The body's attempts to compensate may lead to other symptoms—weakness, trembling, anxiety, dizziness, nausea. Hypoglycemia—too little glucose in the blood—can cause these symptoms.

The symptoms of anxiety, dizziness, weakness, and the rest can be caused by a number of conditions other than hypoglycemia, however, such as oxygen deprivation to the brain. They may also be caused psychologically, by an anxiety state. Even such a serious condition as multiple sclerosis can be mistaken for hypoglycemia by the unwary diagnostician. Thus we laypersons, who are not trained in the diagnosis of conditions that present similar symptoms, are extremely unwise if we try to diagnose ourselves. The point of introducing blood glucose by talking about hypoglycemia is not to persuade you that you have the condition, but to show how indispensable glucose is to your feeling of well-being. A little knowledge is a dangerous thing. Don't self-diagnose.

hypoglycemia (HIGH-po-gligh-SEEM-ee-uh): a too-low blood glucose concentration. Hypoglycemia may arise briefly in any normal person or can be a symptom of a number of disease conditions.

hypo = too little

glyce = glucose

emia = in the blood

Caution

The maintenance of the body's temperature and blood glucose are examples of **homeostasis** (HOME-ee-oh-STAY-sis). Homeostasis is defined as the maintenance of relatively constant internal conditions in body systems by corrective responses to forces that, unopposed, would cause unacceptably large changes in those conditions. A homeostatic system is not static. It is constantly changing, but within tolerable limits.

homeo = the same

stasis = staying

The body has an amazing ability to adapt to changing conditions by altering its own chemistry to maintain an internal balance. It maintains your temperature within a degree, and your blood glucose level with equal precision. An awareness of how blood glucose is maintained can enable you to cooperate with your body in the best interest of both of you.

The Constancy of the Blood Glucose Level

When you wake up in the morning, your blood probably contains between 70 and 120 milligrams (mg) of glucose in each 100 milliliters (ml) of blood. This range, which is known as the fasting blood glucose concentration, is normal and is accompanied by a feeling of alertness and well-being (provided that nothing else is wrong, of course—that you don't have the flu, for example). If you don't eat, the blood glucose level gradually falls as the cells all over your body keep drawing on the diminishing supply. At 60 or 65 milligrams per 100 milliliters, the low end of the normal range, a feeling of hunger is often experienced. The normal response to this sensation is to eat; then the blood glucose level rises again.

It is important that the blood glucose level should not rise too high, and the body protects itself against this eventuality. The first organ to respond to raised blood glucose is the pancreas, which detects the excess and puts out a message about it; then liver and muscle cells receive the message, remove the glucose from the blood, and store it.

Special cells of the pancreas are sensitive to the blood glucose concentration.[1] When it rises, they respond by secreting more of the hormone insulin into the blood. As the circulating insulin bathes the body's other cells, they take up glucose from the blood. Most of the cells can only use the glucose for energy right away, but the liver and muscle cells have the ability to store it for later use; they assemble the small glucose units into long chains of glycogen. The liver cells also convert glucose to fat for export to other body cells. Fat cells can conserve the energy of glucose in this form (see Figure 2–1).

After you have eaten, then, your blood glucose concentration has returned to normal, and any excess glucose has been put in storage. During the hours that follow, before you eat again, the stored liver glycogen (but not the stored fat) can replenish the glucose supply as the brain and other body cells use it to meet their energy needs. Normally, only glycogen from the liver, not from the muscle, can return glucose units to the blood; muscle cells only use them internally.

One of the hormones that can call glucose out of the liver cells is the famous "fight-or-flight" hormone, epinephrine.[2] Epinephrine is produced quickly when you are under stress, ensuring that all your body cells have energy fuel in emergencies. At ordinary times other hormones guarantee that liver glycogen returns glucose to the blood whenever it is needed for maintenance.

Muscle glycogen, too, can be dismantled to glucose, but this glucose is used primarily within the muscle cells themselves, where it serves as an important fuel for muscle action. Long-distance runners know that adequate stores of muscle glycogen can make a crucial difference in their endurance toward the end of a race. Before an event, the athlete is well advised to eat meals high in carbohydrate (see Highlight 6). If there is an extraordinary need for blood glucose and the liver supply has run low, muscle glycogen can break down to an intermediate product, lactate, which enters the blood. The liver picks it up, converts it to glucose, and

A **milligram (mg)** is 1/1,000 of a gram; a **milliliter (ml)** is 1/1,000 of a liter. Blood concentrations of many substances are measured in milligrams per 100 milliliters (mg/100 ml.).

milli = 1,000

Chapter 5 describes the functions of the pancreas and liver. Their places in the digestive system are shown in Figure 1 in that chapter.

A **hormone** is a chemical messenger. Hormones are secreted in response to altered conditions by a variety of glands in the body. Each affects one or more specific target tissues or organs and elicits specific responses to restore normal conditions.

insulin (IN-suh-lin): a hormone secreted by the pancreas in response to (among other things) increased blood glucose concentration.

glycogen (GLIGH-co-gen): a storage form of glucose in liver and muscle.

glyco = glucose

gen = gives rise to

Epinephrine used to be called **adrenaline** (uh-DREN-uh-lin). Another hormone that brings glucose forth from storage is **glucagon** (GLOO-kuh-gon). Glucagon is produced by the alpha cells of the pancreas.

---

1 These special cells are the beta (BAY-tuh) cells, one of several types of cells in the pancreas. The beta cells secrete insulin in response to increased blood glucose concentration.

2 Epinephrine (epp-ih-NEF-rin) is a hormone secreted by the adrenal glands in response to stress. It is produced by the adrenal glands, which lie on top of the kidney.

Chapter 6 tells how protein yields glucose.

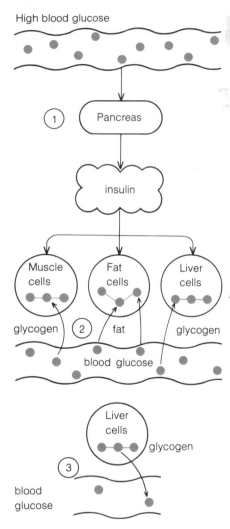

High blood glucose

FIGURE 2–1 **Regulation of blood glucose concentration.** TH2-1

1 High blood glucose stimulates pancreas to release insulin.
2 Insulin stimulates the uptake of glucose into cells. Liver and muscle cells store it as glycogen. Liver cells also convert it to fat, and fat cells store it in that form.
3 Later, low blood glucose is raised when liver glycogen is reconverted to glucose and released into the blood. (Other hormones are involved but not shown.)

releases it once again. Thus muscle glycogen can contribute indirectly to the blood glucose supply if necessary.[3]

The maintenance of a normal blood glucose level thus depends ordinarily on two processes. When the level gets too low, it can be replenished quickly either from liver glycogen stores or from food. When the level gets too high, insulin is secreted to siphon the excess into storage. (There is more to this story. Insulin performs other roles, too. This description is intended only to give you a sense of how the body maintains its blood glucose level.)

The way you eat can help your body keep a happy medium between the extremes. Two guidelines apply. First, when you are hungry, you should eat without waiting until you are famished. Second, when you do eat, you should eat a balanced meal, including some protein and fat as well as complex carbohydrate. The fat slows down the digestion and absorption of carbohydrate, so that it trickles gradually into the blood, providing a steady, ongoing supply. The protein elicits the secretion of glucagon, which is antagonistic to insulin and damps its effect. The protein also provides a more slowly digested, alternative source of blood glucose for use in case the glycogen reserves are used up.

A question people often wonder about in relation to blood glucose is, What is diabetes? Diabetes is a disease, most probably hereditary, characterized either by a deficiency of insulin in the circulating blood or by a surplus of ineffective insulin. Either the pancreas becomes unable to synthesize insulin (Type I diabetes) or the cells are not able to respond to the insulin that is supposed to stimulate them to take up glucose (Type II). In either case, blood glucose rises too high when the person with diabetes eats foods or drinks beverages containing carbohydrate.

When the blood glucose rises too high, and insulin fails to bring it back down to normal, the body brings a second control mechanism into play. The kidneys, through which blood flows each time it passes through the lower body, serve as a filter to remove unwanted materials from the blood and funnel them into the urinary bladder for excretion. Blood glucose levels above about 170 mg/100 ml trigger a compensatory action of the kidneys that causes the excess glucose to spill into the urine.

An early symptom of diabetes is excessive hunger (perhaps the brain cells don't get a prompt message when glucose is present in the body). Another is excessive thirst, because the kidneys excrete water to get rid of the excess blood glucose. The person with diabetes who learns to use nutrition knowledge to manage the disease may be able to live a nearly normal life in spite of this defect in carbohydrate metabolism. Because diabetes is present in about one out of every four families in the United States and Canada, this book offers information about it wherever it is relevant.

3   This cycle is known to biochemists as the Cori cycle. G. F. Cahill, T. T. Aoki, and A. A. Rossini, Metabolism in obesity and anorexia nervosa, in *Nutrition and the Brain*, vol. 3, Disorders of Eating and Nutrients in Treatment of Brain Diseases, Chap. 1, pp. 1–70.

The Chemist's View of Sugars

Those who work with atoms and molecules—chemists, physicists, and other scientists—are people whose curiosity has impelled them to ask questions about everything. The answers they seek are explanations of substances in terms of the next smaller units of which they are made. These scientists also explain *you* in this way; that is, you are a bundle of a great many atoms (perhaps 3,000,000,000,000,000,000,000,000,000,000, give or take 1,000,000,000,000,000,000,000,000,000,000), held together and moved about by virtue of their associated energy.

If your mind boggles at such a thought, don't be dismayed. It staggers anyone's imagination to contemplate the ultimate realities of our universe. If you willingly go along with the chemists, all the way down to the atoms of which the carbohydrates are made, you may feel that you are in unfamiliar territory at first, but you stand to gain much insight. An understanding of how energy is contained in glucose molecules and how it is released when these molecules are metabolized in the body will help you achieve some desirable ends—to acquire the energy you need from your food at a minimum dollar cost, for example, or to balance your food energy sources for maximum health and efficiency without weight gain.

Glucose

A chemist views a glucose molecule as a compound composed of 24 atoms: 6 carbons, 12 hydrogens, and 6 oxygens. These atoms are symbolized by the letters C, H, and O. Thus the chemical formula for glucose is $C_6H_{12}O_6$.

Each type of atom has a characteristic amount of energy available for forming chemical bonds with other atoms. A carbon atom can form four such bonds; a nitrogen atom three; an oxygen atom two; and a hydrogen atom only one. One way to represent the number of bonds associated with each type of atom is to use lines radiating from the letters. The bond of a hydrogen atom is represented by a single line radiating from the H; the bonds of an oxygen atom are represented by two such lines; those of a nitrogen atom by three; and those of a carbon atom by four (see margin).

Atoms may be put together in any way that satisfies their bonding requirements. The structure of the active ingredient of alcoholic beverages, shown here as an example, meets each atom's bonding needs. The carbons both have four lines (bonds), the oxygen has two, and the hydrogens each have one to connect them to other atoms. In any drawing of a chemical structure these conditions must be met, not because a fussy scientist made them up but because they represent what nature demands.

Glucose is a larger and more complicated molecule than alcohol, but it obeys the same rules—as do all chemical compounds. The complete structure of a glucose molecule is shown here. Again, each carbon atom has four bonds, each oxygen two, and each hydrogen one.

The diagram of a glucose molecule shows all the relationships between the parts and proves simple on examination. Since you will be viewing other complex structures (not necessarily to memorize them but rather to

diabetes (DYE-uh-BEET-eez): a disorder of blood glucose regulation, usually caused by insufficiency or relative ineffectiveness of insulin. Other, less common causes of diabetes are explained in Highlight 2.

A too-high blood glucose level is **hyperglycemia**. Glucose in the urine is **glycosuria** (GLIGH-cose-YOUR-ee-uh). There's more about the kidneys in Chapter 5.

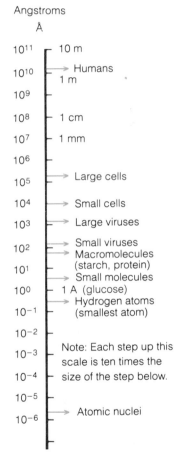

Relative sizes of atoms, cells, and organisms.

Compound, chemical formula: Appendix B presents basic chemistry.

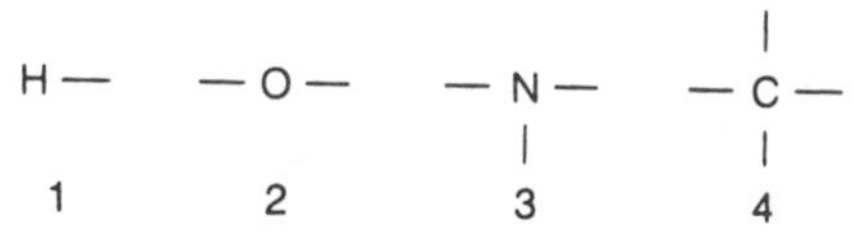

H—   —O—   —N—   —C—

1   2   3   4

Bonds of the four main types of atoms found in nutrients. (Nitrogen doesn't appear in glucose, but is important in protein; see Chapter 4.)

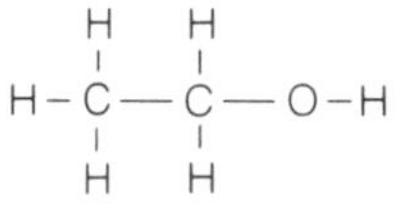

H—C—C—O-H

Chemical structure of ethyl alcohol.

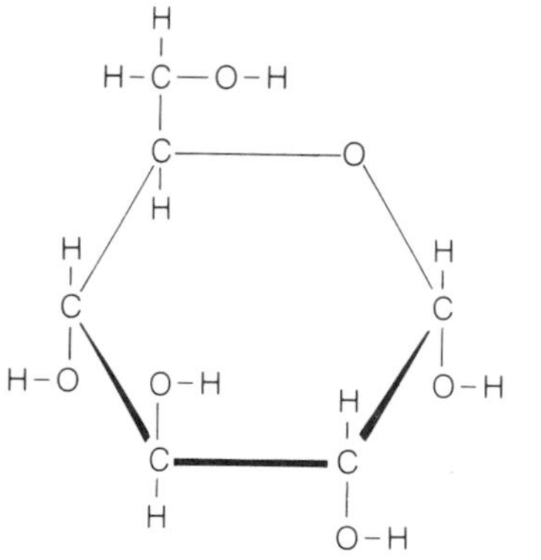

Chemical structure of glucose. On paper, it has to be drawn flat, but in nature the ring is on a plane and the attached structures extend above and below it.

Chemical reaction: See Appendix B.

FIGURE 2–2 **Simplified diagrams of glucose.** TH2-3

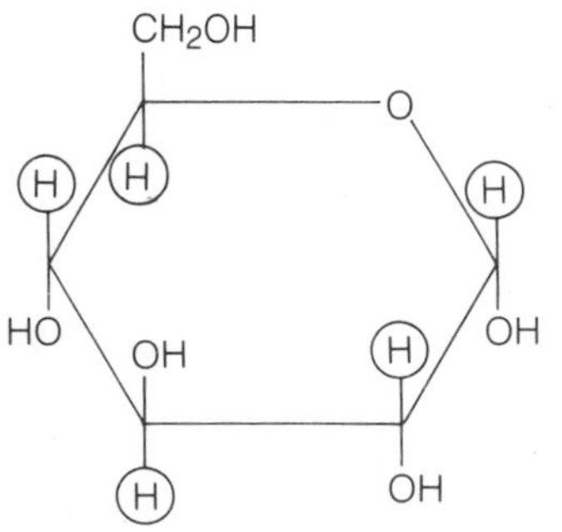

understand certain things about them), let us adopt a simpler way to depict them—one that shows fewer details. In the drawings of Figure 2–2, the corners where lines intersect represent carbon atoms; thus many of the bonds need not be shown. Wherever a carbon atom needs hydrogens (Hs) to complete its four bonds, the Hs are not shown but are simply assumed to be present. Knowing the rules of chemical drawings, we can reconstruct the complete structure, with all its details, from such a picture.

All carbohydrates are composed of glucose and other C-H-O compounds very much like glucose in structure. They come in three main sizes: single molecules, like glucose; pairs (for example, two glucose molecules bonded together); and chains (for example, 300 glucose molecules strung in a line). The chemist's terms for these three types of carbohydrates are monosaccharides, disaccharides, and polysaccharides.

Knowing about the chemist's terms for the carbohydrates will help you understand more precisely the common terms we use to describe them— sugars and starches. The sugars are the monosaccharides and disaccharides, also known as the simple carbohydrates; store-bought white sugar is one of the disaccharides. Starch, glycogen, and some fibers are the polysaccharides, also known as the complex carbohydrates.

Next, we'll examine how these units are put together and taken apart in the continuous flow of matter and energy through living things.

Making and Breaking Pairs: Chemical Reactions

When a disaccharide is formed from two monosaccharides, a chemical reaction known as a condensation reaction takes place (see Figure 2–3). In a condensation reaction, a hydrogen atom is removed from one monosaccharide and an oxygen-hydrogen (OH) group is removed from the other, leaving the two molecules bonded by a single O. The H and OH that were removed from the monosaccharides in this reaction also bond to form a molecule of water (H_2O).

When a disaccharide is taken apart to form two monosaccharides again, as during digestion in the human body, a molecule of water participates in the reaction. H is added to one monosaccharide and OH to the other to re-form the original structures. This reaction is a hydrolysis reaction (Figure

Future drawings of the glucose structure will be made simpler still, by omitting the circled Hs:

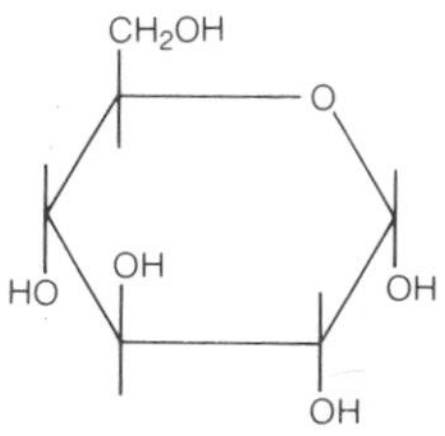

Another way to look at glucose is to notice that its six carbon atoms are all connected:

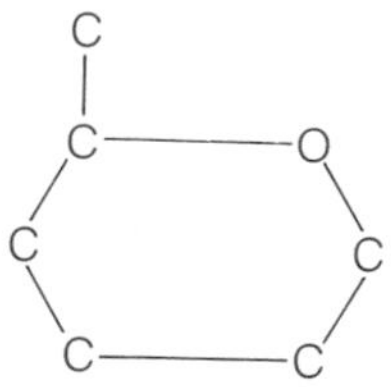

In the simplest diagrams of all, when the number of carbon atoms is the only concern, glucose is symbolized this way:

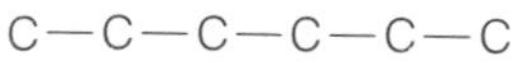

C—C—C—C—C—C

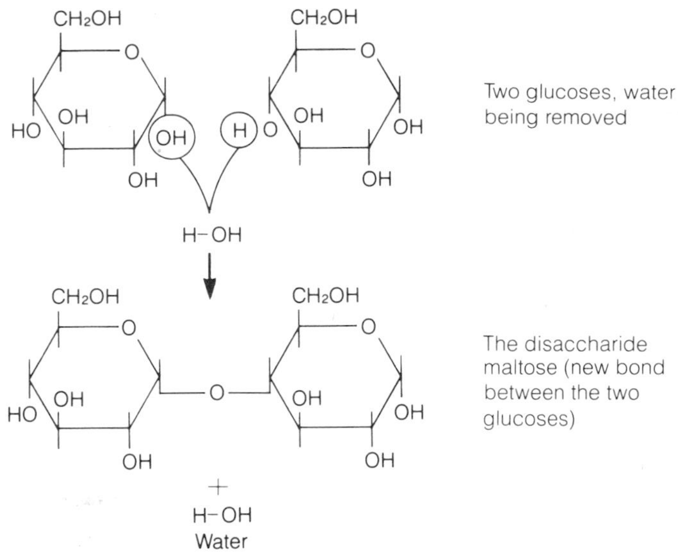

Two glucoses, water being removed

The disaccharide maltose (new bond between the two glucoses)

+

H–OH
Water

FIGURE 2–3 **Condensation.** TH2-4

2–4). It is by condensation and hydrolysis reactions that all the carbohydrates are put together and taken apart.

Condensation and hydrolysis reactions seldom take place spontaneously; they require enzymes to facilitate them. The enzymes are described fully in Chapter 4, but for the moment, let us adopt a simple definition. An enzyme is a giant protein molecule (about the size of 300 or more glucose molecules clumped together) that provides a surface on which other molecules may react with one another. Since the making and breaking of chemical bonds tells the whole story of growth, maintenance, and change in living creatures, the enzymes that facilitate these reactions are indispensable to life.

But enough about chemical bonds. You know now that glucose is the predominant energy source for all the body's cells and can appreciate the importance of having a constant energy supply if you are to feel well. So let's return to the more familiar chemical mixtures called foods, which are the sources of glucose in the diet.

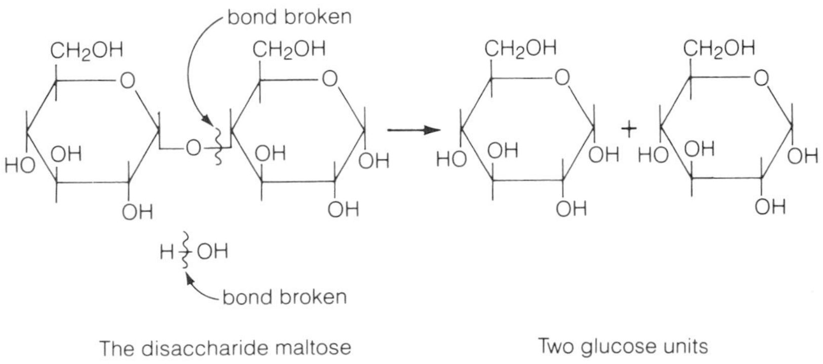

bond broken

H–OH

bond broken

The disaccharide maltose

Two glucose units

FIGURE 2–4 **Hydrolysis.** TH2-4

carbohydrate: a compound composed of carbon, hydrogen, and oxygen, arranged as monosaccharides or multiples of monosaccharides.

carbo = carbon (C)

hydrate = water (H_2O)

complex carbohydrates: the polysaccharides (starch, glycogen, and cellulose).

simple carbohydrates: the monosaccharides (glucose, fructose, and galactose) and the disaccharides (sucrose, lactose, and maltose); also called the sugars.

monosaccharide (mon-oh-SACK-uh-ride): a carbohydrate of the general formula $C_nH_{2n}O_n$; *n* may be any number, but the monosaccharides important in nutrition are all hexoses (n = 6) with the formula $C_6H_{12}O_6$).

mono = one

saccharide, ose = sugar

hex = six

disaccharide: a pair of monosaccharides bonded together.

di = two

polysaccharide: many monosaccharides bonded together.

poly = many

condensation: a chemical reaction in which two reactants combine to yield a major product, with the elimination of water or a similar small molecule.

hydrolysis (high-DROL-uh-sis): a chemical reaction in which a major reactant is split into two products, with the addition of H to one and OH to the other (from water).

hydro = water

lysis = breaking

An enzyme is not a hormone. Enzymes are large protein molecules; hormones are small or medium-sized molecules, usually made of protein or lipid. Enzymes facilitate specific chemical reactions; hormones act as master controllers, often regulating enzymes. Enzymes are fully described in Chapter 4.

glucose: a monosaccharide; sometimes known as blood sugar, sometimes as grape sugar; also called **dextrose**. Nearly all plant foods contain glucose.

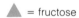 = glucose

fructose: a monosaccharide; sometimes known as fruit sugar. Most plants contain fructose, especially fruits and saps.

fruct = fruit

▲ = fructose

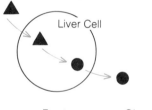

Fructose ⟶ Glucose

(Sometimes fructose breaks down to intermediates, which are used for other purposes.)

FIGURE 2–5 **Two monosaccharides**. Can you see the similarities? If you learned the rules on p. 54, you will be able to "see" 6 Cs, 12 Hs, and 6 Os in both these compounds. TH2-3

The Sugars

Practically all your energy comes from the food you eat, about half from carbohydrate and half from protein and fat. In fact, one of the principal roles of carbohydrate in the diet is to supply energy in the form of blood glucose. Starch is the most significant contributor of glucose to people's diets, but any of the sugars can supply it, too. There are actually six common sugars found in foods—glucose, fructose, galactose, sucrose, lactose, and maltose. A number of other sugars are familiar to the users of special dietary products, notably the sugar alcohols—maltitol, mannitol, sorbitol, and xylitol.

Glucose

Glucose is not especially sweet tasting; a pinch of the purified sugar on your tongue gives only the faintest taste sensation. However, it is absorbed with extraordinary rapidity into the bloodstream. If a diabetic person has become unconscious with extreme hypoglycemia (for example, from an overdose of insulin), a quick way to supply the needed blood glucose is to tip his head to one side and to drip a water solution of glucose into his cheek pocket. The glucose will be absorbed directly into his bloodstream.

Fructose

If you have ever sampled pure, powdered fructose, you will not be surprised to learn that it is the sweetest of the sugars. Curiously, fructose has exactly the same chemical formula as glucose—$C_6H_{12}O_6$—but its structure is quite different (see Figure 2–5). The different arrangements of the atoms in these two sugars stimulate the taste buds on your tongue in different ways.

Fructose can be absorbed directly into the bloodstream. When the blood circulates past the liver, the fructose is taken up into the liver cells, where enzymes rearrange the C, H, and O atoms to make compounds indistinguishable from those derived from glucose and sometimes to make glucose itself. Thus the effect of fructose on the body is very similar to the effect of glucose.

Food chemists have studied sweet-tasting substances, such as fructose, and have identified the exact arrangement of atoms that stimulates the

Glucose

Fructose

sweet-taste receptors in the tongue. All sweet-tasting substances share this structure, including the artificial sweeteners saccharin, cyclamate, and aspartame. A later section of this chapter deals with these.

Galactose

Glucose and fructose are the only monosaccharides of importance in foods. A third, galactose , is seldom found free in nature but occurs as part of the disaccharide lactose. Like glucose and fructose, galactose is a hexose with the formula $C_6H_{12}O_6$. It is shown in Figure 2–6 beside a molecule of glucose for comparison.

Sucrose

The other three common sugars are disaccharides—pairs of monosaccharides linked together. Glucose is found in all three; the second member of the pair is either fructose, galactose, or another glucose.

Sucrose, table sugar, is the most familiar of the three disaccharides. Sugar cane and sugar beets are two sources from which it is purified and granulated to various extents to provide the brown, white, and powdered sugars available in the supermarket. Because it contains fructose in an accessible position, it is a very sweet sugar.

When you eat a food containing sucrose, enzymes in your digestive tract hydrolyze the sucrose to yield glucose and fructose. These monosaccharides are absorbed, and the fructose may be converted to glucose in the liver. (Alternatively, the fructose may be broken down to smaller compounds identical to those derived from glucose.) Thus one molecule of sucrose can ultimately yield two of glucose.

You can see from this description that it ultimately makes no difference whether you eat these monosaccharides hitched together as table sugar or already broken apart. In either case they will end up as monosaccharides in the body. People who think that the "natural sugar" honey is chemically different from purified table sugar fail to understand this point.

It so happens that honey, like table sugar, contains glucose and fructose. The only difference is that in table sugar, they are hitched together

galactose: a monosaccharide; part of the disaccharide lactose.

■ = galactose

sucrose: a disaccharide composed of glucose and fructose; commonly known as table sugar, beet sugar, or cane sugar. Actually, sucrose occurs in many fruits and some vegetables and grains.

sucro = sugar

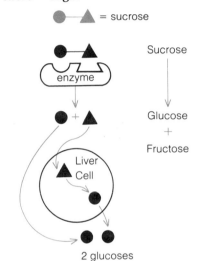

Digestion of sucrose. TH2-5

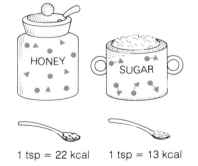

1 tsp = 22 kcal   1 tsp = 13 kcal

FIGURE 2–6 **Two monosaccharides.** Can you see the difference? TH2-3

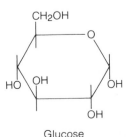

Glucose   Galactose

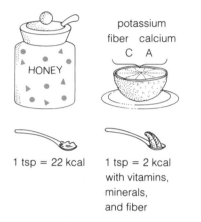

potassium
fiber   calcium
C   A

HONEY

1 tsp = 22 kcal

1 tsp = 2 kcal
with vitamins,
minerals,
and fiber

while in honey they are not. Like table sugar, honey is concentrated to the point where it contains very few impurities, even such desirable ones as vitamins and minerals. In fact, being a liquid, honey is more dense than its crystalline sister and so contains more kcalories per spoon. Table 2–1 shows that honey is not significantly more nutritious than sugar:

To say that honey is no more nutritious than sugar, however, is not to say that there are no differences among sugar sources. Consider a piece of fruit, like an orange. From the fruit you could receive the same monosaccharides and the same kcalories as from sugar or honey. But the packaging is different. The fruit's sugars are diluted in a large volume of water which contains valuable trace minerals and vitamins, and the flesh and skin of the fruit are supported by fibers that also offer health value.

From these two comparisons you can see that the really significant difference between sugar sources is not between "natural" and "purified" sugar but between concentrated sweets and the dilute, naturally occurring sugars that sweeten nutritious foods. You can suspect an exaggerated nutrition claim when you hear the assertion that a product is more nutritious because it contains honey.

A popular fad diet, the fructose diet, claims to be a wonderfully effective means of losing weight. Purified fructose, according to its proponents, is a "natural sugar" that gives you energy without accumulating as body fat. The diet plan requires that you buy packages of purified fructose and use this sugar in place of the "unnatural sugar" sucrose, which causes ugly weight gain. In light of what has just been said about honey versus oranges, it should be clear that there is nothing more natural about purified, crystalline fructose than about purified, crystalline sucrose. Be skeptical whenever you hear the assertion that purified fructose (or any other sugar, for that matter) is more natural than table sugar.

Caution

Sucrose is the principal energy-nutrient ingredient of carbonated beverages, candy, cakes, frostings, cookies, and other concentrated sweets.

TABLE 2–1   **Vitamins and Minerals Supplied by Some Sugar Sources**

	CALCIUM (mg)	IRON (mg)	VITAMIN A (IU)	THIAMIN (mg)	RIBOFLAVIN (mg)	VITAMIN C (mg)
1 tbsp sugar (white granulated)	0	trace[a]	0	0	0	0
1 tbsp honey (strained or extracted)	1	0.1	0	trace[a]	0.01	trace[a]
Possible daily nutrient need[b]	1,000	18	5,000	1.5	1.7	60

[a] A trace is an amount large enough to be detectable in chemical analysis but too small to be significant in comparison to the amounts recorded in these tables.

[b] These are amounts that an adult might typically need in a day. Not all the vitamins and minerals are listed.

Highlight 2 at the end of this chapter addresses the question whether sucrose is a useful, neutral, or harmful part of the diet.

Lactose

Lactose is the principal carbohydrate found in milk, comprising about 5 percent of its weight. A human baby is born with the digestive enzymes necessary to hydrolyze lactose into its two monosaccharide parts, glucose and galactose, so that they can be absorbed. The galactose is then converted to glucose in the liver, so each molecule of lactose yields two molecules of glucose to supply energy for the baby's growth and activity. Babies can digest lactose at birth, but they don't develop the ability to digest starch until they are several months old (see Chapter 14). This is one of the many reasons why milk is such a good food for babies; it provides a simple, easily digested carbohydrate in the right amount to supply energy to meet their needs.

Some individuals lose the ability to digest lactose and become lactose-intolerant. When such a person drinks milk, the unhydrolyzed lactose in the intestine becomes food for intestinal bacteria instead. The multiplying bacteria produce gas and irritate the intestine, making the person sick with nausea and diarrhea. Lactose intolerance arises predictably at around the age of four in certain races—in fact, in the majority of the world's people: Native American, Oriental, African, Mediterranean, and Middle Eastern peoples. It can also appear temporarily in anyone who is ill, making the person unable to tolerate milk for a while. Lactose intolerance is not the same as the commonly observed milk allergy, which is caused by an immune reaction to the protein in milk.

Maltose

The third disaccharide is found at only one stage in the life of a plant. When the seed is formed, it is packed with starch—glucose units strung together in long arrays—to be used as fuel for the germination process. When the seed begins to sprout, an enzyme cleaves the starch between pairs of glucose units, making maltose. Another enzyme then splits the maltose units into glucose units, and other enzymes degrade these still further, releasing energy for the sprouting of the plant's shoot and root. By the time the young plant has put forth leaves, all the starch in the seed has been used up, but the leaves can now capture the sun's light to garner additional energy for growth. Thus the sugar maltose is present briefly during the early germination process, as the starch is being broken down. The malt found in beer contains maltose formed as the starch in the grains breaks down. (The alcohol is produced by yeast in a process known as fermentation.)

As you might predict, when you eat or drink a food source of maltose, your digestive enzymes hydrolyze the maltose into two glucose units, which are then absorbed into the blood. Thus, maltose, like the other disaccharides, contributes glucose to the body.

In summary, then, the major simple carbohydrates, or sugars, are those

lactose: a disaccharide composed of glucose and galactose; commonly known as milk sugar.

lact = milk

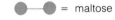

Digestion of lactose. TH2-5

lactose intolerance: inherited or acquired inability to digest lactose, due to failure to produce the enzyme lactase. Lactose intolerance is prevalent in the majority of adult human population groups.

maltose: a disaccharide composed of two glucose units; sometimes known as malt sugar.

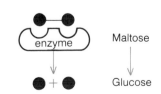

Digestion of maltose. TH2-5

TABLE 2–2 **The Major Simple Carbohydrates**

MONOSACCHARIDES		DISACCHARIDES	
Glucose	●	Maltose	●—●
Fructose	▲	Sucrose	●—▲
Galactose	■	Lactose	●—■
(found only in lactose)			

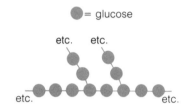

● = glucose

Portion of a starch molecule.

starch: a plant polysaccharide composed of glucose and digestible by humans.

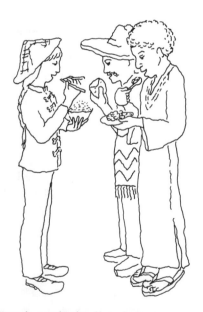

Starch can be broken down to shorter chains of glucose units known as **dextrins**. The word sometimes appears on food labels, because dextrins can be used as thickening agents in foods.

shown in Table 2–2. Glucose, fructose, maltose, and sucrose are from plants; lactose and its component galactose, from milk.

The Chemist's View of Complex Carbohydrates

While the sugars contain three monosaccharides in different combinations, the polysaccharides are composed almost entirely of only one—glucose. The differences between them have to do with the ways glucose is combined into the large molecules of starch, glycogen, and cellulose.

Starch

As the chemist sees it, starch is a branched chain of dozens of glucose units connected together. These units would have to be magnified more than 10 million times to appear at the size shown on this page. However, as molecules go, starches are rather large. A single starch molecule may contain from 300 to 1,000 or more glucose units linked together. These giant molecules are packed side by side in the rice grain or potato root—as many as a million in a cubic inch of food.

In the plant, starch serves a function similar to that served by the glycogen in your liver. It is a storage form of glucose needed for the plant's first growth. (When you eat the plant, of course, you get the glucose to use for your own purposes.)

All starchy foods are in fact plant foods. Seeds are the richest food source; 70 percent of their weight is starch. Many human societies have a staple grain from which 50 to 80 percent of their members' food energy is derived. Rice is the staple grain of the Orient. In Canada, the United States, and Europe the staple grain is wheat. If you consider all the food products made from wheat—bread (and other baked goods made from wheat flour), cereals, and pasta—you will realize how all-pervasive this grain is in the food supply. Corn is the staple grain of much of South America and of the southern United States; the Mexicans use corn in their tortillas. The staple grains of other peoples include millet, rye, barley, and oats. In each society a bread, meal, or flour is made from the grain, then used for many purposes. These staple foods are the major source of food energy for the world's people, supporting human life and activity.

A second important source of starch is the bean and pea family, including such dry beans found in the supermarket as butter beans, kidney beans, "baked" beans, black-eyed peas (cowpeas), chickpeas (garbanzo beans), and soybeans. These vegetables are about 40 percent starch by weight and also contain a significant amount of protein. A third major source of starch is the tubers, such as the potato, yam, and cassava. These serve as the primary starch sources in many non-Western societies.

When you eat any of these foods, the starch molecules are taken apart by enzymes in your mouth and intestine. The enzymes hydrolyze the starch molecules to yield glucose units, which are absorbed across the intestinal wall into the blood. One to four hours after a meal, all the starch has been digested and is circulating to the cells as glucose.

Glycogen

Glycogen is not found in plants and is stored in animal meats only to a limited extent. It is not, therefore, of major importance as a nutrient, although it performs an important role in the body, as already described. Glycogen is more complex and more highly branched than starch, a structure permitting rapid breakdown. When the hormonal message "Break down glycogen" arrives at a liver or muscle cell, enzymes can attack all the branches simultaneously, producing a surge of energy for emergency action. The photograph at the start of this chapter shows part of a single liver cell, in which a multitude of glycogen packages await such a call.

glycogen (GLIGH-co-gen): an animal polysaccharide composed of glucose, manufactured and stored in liver and muscle.

Cellulose

The third polysaccharide of importance in nutrition is cellulose. Cellulose, like starch, is found abundantly in plants and is composed of glucose units connected in long chains. However, the bonds holding its glucose units together are different. This difference is of major importance for humans, because each type of bond requires a different enzyme to hydrolyze it. The human digestive tract is supplied with abundant enzymes to hydrolyze the bonds in starch, but has none that can attack the bonds in cellulose. As a result, starch is digestible for humans and cellulose is not. Cellulose passes through the digestive tract largely unchanged, which explains the different roles of these two major plant polysaccharides. Starch is the most abundant energy source in the staple foods of the world, whereas cellulose provides no energy for humans at all.

cellulose (CELL-you-loce): a plant polysaccharide composed of glucose and indigestible by humans.

Cellulose is, however, one of the fibers, and the fibers are important to health in their own right. In recent years, cellulose and other plant fibers have received increasing attention as the public has learned of their value. Researchers are still actively trying to determine what they do and do not do, and there is much disagreement about their role, but clearly they are important. The last section of this chapter is devoted to the fibers.

The Carbohydrates in Foods

You need some carbohydrate daily as a source of glucose. If you don't eat carbohydrate, your body devours its own protein to generate glucose—and it needs its protein for other vital purposes. The "protein-sparing effect" of carbohydrate is important and will come up again (Chapters 4, 6). How much carbohydrate is enough?

Estimation of Carbohydrate Intake

Most authorities agree that you need considerably more than 50 grams— probably more than 100 grams—of carbohydrate a day.[4] To be safe, you should probably aim at at least 125 grams; and 300 grams might be an ideal intake for many people. At 4 kcalories per gram, that would be 1,200 kcalories from carbohydrate.

4   For example, *Recommended Dietary Allowances*, 9th ed. (Washington, D.C.: National Academy of Sciences, 1980), p. 33.

*Carbohydrate values are—
milk, 12; bread, 15; fruit, 10;
vegetable, 5; and sugar, 5. See
Figure 2–7.*

The exchange system described in Chapter 1 (pp. 13–18) provides a convenient way to estimate the amount of carbohydrate in your lunchbox or on your dinner plate. In exchange systems, foods are sorted into lists in such a way that the carbohydrate contents of foods on any one list are similar. To use such a system, all you need to know is the carbohydrate value for the list and the members of that list with their portion sizes (see Figure 2–7). Carbohydrate is found in only four of the six types of food listed in the exchange system; so you need only know four values and learn a value for sugar (which is not on exchange lists).

Sugar Intake

Exchange systems do not include sugary foods like candy, jam, and soft drinks, because they are not considered desirable in diet plans. But people

FIGURE 2–7 **Foods containing carbohydrate.**

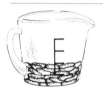

12 g in 1 c milk

1 c skim milk (or any other serving of food in the milk list) provides 12 g carbohydrate as lactose, a naturally occurring sugar. Cheeses have negligible carbohydrate and so are not included with milk in this system.

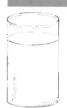

5 g in 1/2 c vegetables

½ c green beans (or any other serving of food on the vegetable list) provides 5 g carbohydrate, mostly as naturally occurring sugars. Starchy vegetables are not included on this list.

10 g in one fruit exchange

1 serving of fruit (serving sizes are shown on the fruit list) provides 10 g carbohydrate as naturally occurring sugars.

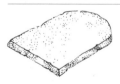

15 g in one slice bread

1 slice of bread (or any other serving of food on the bread list) provides 15 g carbohydrate, mostly in the form of starch. All grain foods, such as cereal and pasta, and such starchy vegetables as corn, lima beans, and potatoes are included on this list.

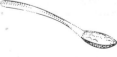

5 g in 1 tsp sugar

1 tsp white sugar (or any other concentrated sweet) provides 5 g carbohydrate.

do consume them, and they certainly contain carbohydrate. To estimate an accurate total of the carbohydrate you consume, you may need a "sugar list," and we have invented one for the purpose (Figure 2–7). Among the concentrated sweets treated as equivalent to 1 teaspoon of white sugar are:

- 1 teaspoon brown sugar.
- 1 teaspoon candy.
- 1 teaspoon corn sweeteners.
- 1 teaspoon corn syrup.
- 1 teaspoon honey.
- 1 teaspoon jam.
- 1 teaspoon jelly.
- 1 teaspoon maple sugar.
- 1 teaspoon maple syrup.
- 1 teaspoon molasses.

These sugars can all be assumed to provide about 20 kcalories per teaspoon. Some are closer to 10 kcalories (for example, 13 kcalories for sucrose), while some are over 20 (22 kcalories for honey); so an average figure of 20 kcalories is an acceptable rough approximation.

For a person who uses catsup (ketchup) liberally, it may help to remember that 1 tablespoon of catsup supplies about 1 teaspoon of sugar. A 12-ounce can of a sugary carbonated beverage contains about 9 teaspoons of sugar, or 45 grams of carbohydrate.

Finally, while we're still on the subject of sugar, you need to recognize its many aliases. The accompanying miniglossary presents the multitude of names that denote sugar on food labels.

All of the foods containing carbohydrate have now been identified in five categories. Some practice with estimating portion sizes and a familiarity with the gram amounts gives you a command of the total carbohydrate content of any diet. The example given in Figure 2–8 demonstrates the system's usefulness.

This kind of calculation provides only an estimate but is close enough for most purposes. A more accurate way to determine the carbohydrate composition of foods is to refer to Appendix H, which lists individual foods. Adding the individual carbohydrate amounts found in Appendix H yields 138 grams of carbohydrate for the meals shown in Figure 2–8.

1 tbsp catsup = 1 tsp sugar.
12 oz sugary carbonated beverage = 9 tsp sugar.

The difference between the 157-gram estimate and the 138-gram amount obtained by the more accurate calculation may be disconcerting. Rough estimates are often more valuable than close calculations, however, because of the time saved and because often only a "ballpark" figure is needed. In this example, we know that an intake of 50 grams of carbohydrate is far below the recommended minimum of 125 grams, but 138 and 157 grams are both comfortably above it and in the same range. The difference between them becomes insignificant from this perspective.

Most estimates of the nutrient contents of foods are rough but serviceable approximations. If we refer to a "90-kcalorie potato," you should

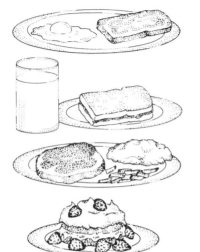

FIGURE 2–8 **How to estimate carbohydrate intake.**
Suppose that one day's meals consisted of the menus illustrated here. That day's meals contain the following carbohydrate exchanges (you'd have to look in Appendix L to discover the serving size units):

Breakfast:	1 bread
Lunch:	2 bread
	2 tsp sugar[a]
	1 milk
Dinner:	2 bread[b]
	1 vegetable[c]
Snack:[d]	1 bread
	1 fruit
	6 tsp sugar

Thus the total carbohydrate consumption for the day is:

6 bread	=	90 g carbohydrate
8 tsp sugar	=	40
1 milk	=	12
1 vegetable	=	5
1 fruit	=	10
Total		157 g carbohydrate

This is more than the minimum of 125 g and so is an adequate day's intake.

[a] The sandwich contains 2 tsp jelly; that would count as 2 sugars.
[b] This is a 1 c serving of mashed potato and would count as 2 breads.
[c] This is a ½ c serving of green beans; it would count as 1 vegetable.
[d] This is a 2-inch diameter biscuit with ¾ c strawberries, 1 tbsp heavy cream, and 6 tsp sugar added in preparation. The biscuit would count as 1 bread; the strawberries as 1 fruit; and the sugar as 6 tsp.

understand this to mean "90 plus-or-minus-about-20-percent," which makes it not significantly different from a 100-kcalorie potato. In general, for most purposes, a variation of about 20 percent is expected and is considered perfectly reasonable.

Caution

It takes only one or two calculations of this kind to give you a feel for the carbohydrate content of your diet. Once you are aware of the major carbohydrate-contributing foods you eat, you can return to thinking simply in terms of the foods, developing a sense of how much of each is enough.

This chapter began by showing you how important glucose is for the functioning of the brain and the body's other tissues. Then it went on to demonstrate how the body can derive glucose from all carbohydrates. Now it has shown where the carbohydrates are in foods. Armed with this information, you can explode some of the myths perpetrated by advertisers of carbohydrate-containing foods and beverages. Sugar is "quick energy"— right? When you need quick energy, you should reach for a candy bar and a cola beverage, right? Wrong. The best pick-me-ups are not concentrated sugars. True, sugars (monosaccharides) offer energy, and are indispensable to the body's best functioning—but you now can see that any food containing carbohydrate can offer them to you. How about a delicious lettuce-and-tomato-and-meat sandwich, a tall, cool glass of milk, and a fresh, juicy orange for your pick-me-up?

Miniglossary of kCaloric Sweeteners

brown sugar: sugar crystals contained in molasses syrup with natural flavor and color, 91 to 96 percent pure sucrose. (Some refiners add syrup to refined white sugar to make brown sugar.)

confectioner's sugar: finely powdered sucrose, 99.9 percent pure.

corn sweeteners: corn syrup and sugars derived from corn.

corn syrup: a syrup produced by the action of enzymes on cornstarch. High-fructose corn syrup (HFCS) may contain as little as 42 percent or as much as 90 percent fructose; dextrose makes up the balance.

dextrose, fructose, galactose, glucose: already defined (pp. 56–57).

granulated sugar: crystalline sucrose, 99.9 percent pure.

honey: invert sugar formed by an enzyme from nectar gathered by bees. Composition and flavor vary, but honey usually contains fructose, glucose, maltose, and sucrose.

invert sugar: a mixture of glucose and fructose formed by the splitting of sucrose in a chemical process. Sold only in liquid form, sweeter than sucrose, invert sugar is used as an additive to help preserve food freshness and prevent shrinkage.

lactose: already defined (p. 59).

levulose: the technical name for fructose.

maltitol, mannitol, sorbitol, xylitol: sugar alcohols, which can be derived from fruits or produced from dextrose; absorbed and metabolized differently from sugar in the human body, and not utilizable by ordinary mouth bacteria.

maltose: already defined (p. 59).

maple sugar: although once a common sweetener, this sugar is rarely added to foods and is commonly replaced by sucrose and artificial maple flavoring. The only source of true maple sugar is the concentrated sap of the sugar maple tree. Maple sugar is expensive, compared with other sweeteners.

molasses: a thick, brown syrup, which tastes bitter and sour as well as sweet, created during cane sugar production. Molasses contains a few minerals.

natural sweeteners: any of the sugars listed here.

raw sugar: the residue of evaporated sugar cane juice, tan or brown in color. Raw sugar can only be sold in the United States if the impurities (dirt, insect fragments, and the like) have been removed.

sucrose: already defined (p. 57).

Alternative Sweeteners

Among alternative sweeteners familiar to people who use special dietary products are the sugar alcohols—among them, mannitol, sorbitol, xylitol, and maltitol. These carbohydrates are either absorbed more slowly or metabolized differently than the sugars and so may be suitable for use by people who must restrict their intakes of ordinary sweets.

Mannitol is the least satisfactory of the alternative sweeteners just named. It is considerably less sweet than sucrose, so sizable amounts have to be used when it is substituted for sucrose. Because it lingers unabsorbed in the intestine for a long time, it is available to intestinal bacteria for their energy. As they use it, they multiply, attracting water, and produce irritating waste, causing diarrhea. It is therefore not much used as an alternative sweetener.

Sorbitol has been popular as a sweetener for sugar-free gums and candies, but it too, has drawbacks. It is only half as sweet as sucrose, so twice as many kcalories have to be used to deliver a given amount of sweetness. Also, like mannitol, it causes diarrhea. Advantages are that it is absorbed very slowly, so that it has little or no effect on blood glucose; and little or no insulin is needed to make it available to the body's cells. Thus people with diabetes, who have either no insulin or ineffective insulin, may benefit from using small amounts of sorbitol. Its threshold for causing diarrhea is higher than mannitol's; so of the two, sorbitol is preferred.

Xylitol has also been popular, especially in chewing gums, because it has been reported to help prevent dental caries. (It not only doesn't support caries-producing bacteria; it actually inhibits their growth.[5]) Like all the sugar alcohols, it has as many kcalories per gram as sucrose, but it is as sweet as fructose, so that less can be used. Xylitol occurs in foods, and some xylitol is produced in the body during normal metabolic processes; so it is not a foreign substance. Xylitol is widely used in many western European countries and in Canada; however, reports that it may cause tumors in animals have led to the voluntary curtailing of its use by U.S. food producers.

Maltitol has a sweetness equal to about 90 percent that of sucrose. It is used in some carbonated beverages and canned fruits, and in Japanese bakery products and other sweets intended not to cause tooth decay. At first thought not to be absorbed from the GI tract, maltitol was recommended for use in food products for dieters and people with diabetes. This claim is doubtful; the sugar probably does have kcalorie value. Manufacturing maltitol from maltose is expensive and limits its use; using maltose directly costs less.

> The person who wishes to cut kcalories should be aware that the sugar alcohols *do* contain kcalories, just as many per gram as sucrose. In spite of this fact, products that contain them are labeled "sugar-free." The reason they are suitable for people who must limit their intakes of ordinary sweets is because the body handles them differently, not because they are kcalorie-free. The person who is limiting kcalories must limit sugar alcohols just as carefully as sugars.

Another sweetener of possible usefulness to people with abnormal carbohydrate metabolism is fructose, already discussed. It is twice as sweet as sucrose, and it neither requires nor stimulates insulin secretion, so it has been advocated as an alternative sweetener for use by people with diabetes

---

5   Xylitol as a sucrose substitute—relation to dental caries, *Nutrition Reviews* 39 (1981): 368–371.

and hypoglycemia.[6] Many authorities oppose the use of fructose by people with diabetes, however, because it may tend to increase their already raised blood lipid levels.[7] Because fructose, like sucrose, contains 4 kcalories per gram, however, it is not useful as a weight-loss aid.

Artificial Sweeteners

The artificial sweeteners are compounds, developed or discovered by chemists, that "fool" the taste buds into conveying a sweet taste to the brain, but convey negligible or no kcalories the body can use. Foremost among those in present use in the United States and Canada are aspartame, cyclamate, and saccharin (see Miniglossary).

Cyclamate's use was banned some years ago in the United States because of a possible threat of cancer; but cyclamate is still used in Canada. The reverse is true of saccharin; it is no longer available over the counter in Canada because of a possible link to cancer, but is still in wide use in the United States, though it must carry a warning label. Aspartame ("Nutra Sweet" or "Equal") is a relative newcomer among the artificial sweeteners and has an unsullied reputation so far.

Artificial sweeteners whose use may become more common in the future are the so-called left-handed sugars, or L- sugars. A sugar is an asymmetrical molecule (as a hand is an asymmetrical body part), and so it can theoretically occur in two shapes that are mirror-images of each other (as the right and left hands are). Those found naturally in plants are the right-handed, or D-sugars, and the body's enzymes and absorptive machinery are equipped to handle these. L-sugars are just as sweet as D-sugars, and they mix well into baked goods, but they pass through the body unchanged, offering no kcalories. The most promising of the L-sugars appears to be L-fructose.[8]

L-sugar: a mirror-image of natural sugar, unutilizable by the body. The L version of glucose (D-glucose or dextrose) is L-glucose.

dextro = right

Miniglossary of Artificial Sweeteners

aspartame (aspartyl-phenylalanine methyl ester): a dipeptide (see p. 125) that tastes remarkably like sugar, but is 200 times sweeter than sucrose. Aspartame, also called "Nutra Sweet," is blended with lactose and with an anticaking agent and is sold commercially as "Equal." It turns sour when heated and so cannot be used for cooking or baking, but is effective in warm and cold beverages and in and on warm and cold foods. Unlike saccharin, it has no bitter aftertaste, and so may prove more acceptable to consumers.

cyclamate: a zero-kcalorie sweetener used in Canada but banned in the United States (see Highlight 10).

saccharin (sodium saccharine): discovered in 1879 and used in the United States since that time, a zero-kcalorie sweetener that is at least 200 times sweeter than sucrose; banned in Canada (see Highlight 10).

---

6   P. A. Crapo and J. M. Olefsky suggest allowing up to 75 grams per day of fructose in the diabetic diet: Fructose—its characteristics, physiology, and metabolism, *Nutrition Today*, July/August 1980, pp. 10–15.

7   Both fructose and sucrose are thought to have adverse effects on blood lipids in at least 20 percent of the population. Nutritionists say reevaluation of sucrose "appears to be warranted," *Food Chemical News*, February 21, 1983, pp. 1–3.

8   New sugar, new fat/new thoughts, *Health*, March 1982, p. 28.

The Fibers

Many of the fibers are carbohydrates. Besides cellulose, already mentioned, two other carbohydrates—pectin and hemicellulose—are classed
as fibers. Another material classified as fiber is lignin, a noncarbohydrate.
Still others are the gums and mucilages often used as thickening agents in
prepared foods.

Although cellulose and other fibers are not attacked by human enzymes,
some fibers, notably hemicellulose, can be digested by bacteria in the
human digestive tract, and can yield products similar to those the body
obtains from the so-called available carbohydrates. These products may be
absorbed by the body or excreted as waste. Food fibers are therefore not all
kcalorie-free.[9]

Beneficial Effects of Fiber

Based on the experience of researchers in Africa, the "fiber hypothesis"
suggests that consumption of unrefined, high-fiber carbohydrate foods
protects against many Western diseases.[10] Rural Africans naturally consume
a diet very high in fiber and show a low incidence of these chronic conditions. Some researchers, however, stress that it may be the higher Western
intake of salt, sugar, and animal fat rather than the absence of fiber that is
responsible for these conditions.

Fiber may also play a role in weight control. According to the "fiber
hypothesis," obesity is not seen in those parts of the world where large
amounts of fiber are eaten. Foods high in fiber tend to be low in fat and
simple sugars. High-fiber breads have fewer kcalories per pound than
refined breads. High-fiber foods, because of their water-holding capacity,
satisfy hunger readily. Many of the diet aids on the market today are composed of bulk-inducing fibers such as methylcellulose.

Caution

Indeed, producers of some diet aids base the success of their products
on the ability of certain fibers to provide bulk and satiety for the anxious
dieter. If you accept this principle regarding bulk and satiety as a positive approach to managing a low kcalorie diet, you may be relieved to
learn that you do not need to spend extra money on these diet aids.
Selecting fresh fruits and vegetables would represent both an economic
and a nutritious means of adding bulk to your diet.

Fiber in the gastrointestinal tract functions like a sponge, holding water,
binding minerals, and binding acidic materials such as the bile salts used

9   W. D. Holloway, C. Tasman-Jones, and S. P. Lee, Digestion of certain fractions of dietary
fiber in humans, *American Journal of Clinical Nutrition* 31 (1978): 927–930.
10   D. P. Burkitt, Some diseases characteristic of modern Western civilization, *British Medical Journal* 1 (1973): 274–278.

by the body to prepare fat for digestion. The major impact of dietary fiber is on the colon, the last part of the gastrointestinal tract, where colon cancer and diverticular disease can arise, but the addition of fibrous foods to the diet increases the bulk of food all along the intestine.

Some of the ways in which food fibers are thought to prevent disease states are:

● By promoting weight loss (as already mentioned) by enhancing satiety and displacing the kcalories of concentrated fats and sweets—achieved by adding more servings of fruits, vegetables, and whole grains to the diet.

● By attracting water into the digestive tract, thus softening the stools and preventing constipation.

● By preventing increased abdominal pressure and enlargement of veins from prolonged straining on defecation, which may lead to the swollen veins of hemorrhoids. Softer stools allow for decreased straining of rectal muscles.

● By preventing formation of small fecal stones, which could obstruct the appendix, increase abdominal pressure, and allow for bacterial invasion of the appendix, resulting in appendicitis.

● By exercising the muscles of the digestive tract so that they retain their health and tone and resist bulging out into the pouches characteristic of diverticulosis.

● By speeding up the passage of food materials through the digestive tract, thus shortening the "transit time" and helping to prevent exposure of the tissue to cancer-causing agents in food.

● By binding lipids such as cholesterol and carrying them out of the body with the feces so that the blood lipid concentrations are lowered, and possibly the risk of heart and artery disease as a consequence.

● By binding the bile salts and reducing their absorption in the intestinal tract.

● By modulating the body's response to glucose; monosaccharides from complex carbohydrates, in the presence of fiber, produce a more even rise in blood glucose.

However, not all the fibers have similar effects. For example, wheat bran, which is composed mostly of cellulose, has no cholesterol-lowering effect, whereas oat bran and the fiber of apples (pectin) do lower blood cholesterol. On the other hand, wheat bran seems to be one of the most effective stool-softening fibers, especially if a certain particle size is used. Fibers that form gels in water (pectin, guar) prolong the time of transit of materials through the intestine, whereas insoluble fibers (cellulose) tend to decrease the time.

Diverticular disease is very common in Europe and North America but relatively rare among rural Africans. In this disease there is usually high pressure in the intestine and a prolonged transit time. Fiber has recognized medical value in treating diverticular disease because it reduces both pressure and transit time.

Although fiber is considered to be a nonnutritive substance, it does

diverticulosis (dye-ver-tic-you-LOH-sis): outpocketings of weakened areas of the intestinal wall (like blow-outs in a tire). The danger of diverticulosis is that it can give rise to **diverticulitis** (-EYE-tis), in which the pockets become infected or inflamed and may rupture. About one in every six people in Western countries develops diverticulosis in middle or later life.

divertir = to turn

osis = too much

itis = infection or inflammation

Pectin and guar are water-retaining fibers capable of forming gels, delaying gastric emptying time, and slowing the absorption of carbohydrate. They are also called **viscous** (VISS-cuss) fibers.

viscum = thick, sticky gum

influence the metabolism of certain nutrients.[11] Recent reports indicate that diets high in fiber enable the body to handle glucose efficiently, helping to manage diabetes. Persons with mild cases of diabetes, given high fiber diets, have been able to reduce their insulin doses.[12]

The typical Western diet is low in fiber. It permits rapid absorption of carbohydrates with sharper rises in blood glucose and insulin than does a diet high in fiber. A high-fiber diet modulates these rises. In general, the more viscous the fiber, the greater the modulating effect.

The Exchange System teaches the person with diabetes that one food containing available carbohydrate (that is, starch or naturally occurring sugars) may be exchanged for another food on the same list with the same amount of carbohydrate, as long as equivalent portions are used. Fiber studies suggest, however, that the body's insulin response and absorption of monosaccharides from foods may be very much influenced by the type of fiber in the food. The body absorbs glucose more rapidly and produces more insulin in response to potatoes than to rice, for example. The response is also affected by the degree of processing of the food—for example, the insulin response to the sugars from applesauce or apple juice is greater than to the same amount of sugars from whole apples.

In this sense, a half-cup of rice is not necessarily the same as a small potato or a slice of bread, even though they are on the same exchange list. Nor are the following pairs of items the same:

- A slice of white bread versus a slice of whole-grain bread.
- A mashed potato versus a baked potato with the skin.
- A portion of apple juice versus an apple.

The second member of each pair would create less demand for insulin and thus would enhance the diet of the person with diabetes attempting to control the disease without artificial means.

Caution

Before recommending that persons with diabetes increase their intakes of complex carbohydrates, a word of warning is in order. Persons who are currently using artificial agents to control their blood glucose need to check with their physicians before altering their diets. The physician may need to make crucial adjustments, for example, in the amount of insulin used or the type of carbohydrate delivered to regulate the person's blood glucose on a high-fiber diet. Otherwise, too much or too little insulin might be present for appropriate control.

---

11   J. W. Anderson and W. L. Chen, Plant fiber: Carbohydrate and lipid metabolism, *American Journal of Clinical Nutrition* 32 (1979): 346–363.

12   Two kinds of diets are effective: diets high in viscous fiber (pectin or guar), and diets high in polysaccharides and limited in fats and simple sugars. J. W. Anderson and K. Ward, High carbohydrate, high fiber diets for insulin treated men with diabetes mellitus, *American Journal of Clinical Nutrition* 32 (1979): 2312–2321.

The presence of too much insulin in the blood is associated with obesity and heart and artery disease as well as with diabetes. The preventive approach to nutrition would stress a high-fiber diet to guard against diseases in which excessive insulin response is known to be a causative factor. People may not readily accept high-fiber diets, however, because they involve a significant reduction in fat and protein-rich foods.

Some fibers probably help prevent heart and artery disease not only by way of their effect on the insulin response but also by lowering blood cholesterol. Highlight 3 explores these effects.

Population studies have suggested that fiber in the diet also offers protection from cancer of the colon and rectum. The decreased transit time attributed to some fibers shortens the time of exposure of the colon wall to cancer-causing agents that enter the body with food. The fiber-bound compounds (bile, fat, salts) and increased water in the intestine may act as solvents for any potential cancer-causing agents and carry them out of the body.[13]

Too Much Fiber

Most clinical reports are concerned with the influence of the lack of fiber in the diet on health and disease. The questions whether there are any harmful effects to excessive fiber in the diet, and what the ideal range of fiber intakes may be, remain to be answered.

Too much bulk from the diet could impose an overall decrease in the amount of food consumed and cause deficiencies of both nutrients and kcalories. Vegetarian children are especially vulnerable to this chain of events.

The malnourished and elderly, who may have marginal or inadequate intakes of the vitamins and trace minerals, may also be likely to develop nutrient deficiencies on high-fiber diets. Maximum absorption of iron occurs early during digestion. Due to the faster transit of high-fiber foods, there may be a decreased opportunity for maximal absorption of iron and other nutrients.

A compound not classed as a fiber but often found with it in foods is phytic acid. On a high-fiber diet losses of minerals may occur if they become bound to phytic acid. Most of the phytic acid in our diet comes from seeds such as the cereal grains. (The role of phytate in the plant seed may be to store these ions and hold them in plant tissue during germination.)

phytate (FYE-tate) **(phytic acid):** an organic storage compound of plant seeds. Phytic acid is found in the husks of grains, legumes, and seeds and is capable of binding ions such as zinc, iron, calcium, magnesium, and copper in insoluble complexes in the intestine.

Measures of Fiber Amounts

A problem for people trying to sort out the effects of fiber is that the amounts of fiber in food are hard to estimate. Chemists can analyze food for fiber content in the laboratory by digesting it with acids and bases. Whatever remains is called crude fiber. But if you eat the same food, subjecting it

crude fiber (CF): the residue of plant food remaining after extraction with dilute acid followed by dilute alkali in a laboratory procedure; that is, the fiber that remains in food after a harsh chemical digestive procedure.

13   D. P. Burkitt, Colonic-rectal cancer: Fiber and other dietary factors, *American Journal of Clinical Nutrition* 31 (1978): S58–S64.

dietary fiber (DF): the residue of plant food resistant to hydrolysis by human digestive enzymes; that is, the fiber that remains from food after digestion in the body.

➤ *1 g crude fiber ~ 2–3 g dietary fiber.*

TABLE 2–3 **Foods Recommended for a High-Fiber Diet**

Whole-wheat and whole-grain breads and crackers

Cereals with bran as a major ingredient; shredded wheat; oatmeal

Fresh fruits with skin, such as apples, figs, apricots, peaches, pears, plums; bananas; berries

Dried fruits such as apricots, figs, pears, prunes, dates, currants, raisins

Raw vegetables such as cauliflower, carrots, celery, lettuce, spinach, tomatoes, radishes, mushrooms, cabbage; vegetables steamed in small amounts of water

Legumes, nuts, seeds

Bran muffins or cookies; oatmeal cookies

Popcorn

Source: Adapted from B. S. Worthington-Roberts, *Contemporary Developments in Nutrition* (St. Louis: Mosby, 1981), p. 58.

to the action of your own enzymes, the undigested residue will be greater, because the body's enzymes are less harsh than the laboratory treatment. What we really need to know is how much fiber remains in the body after the normal human digestive process: this is dietary fiber. But how can we measure it? One imprecise and unpleasant procedure involves collecting all the stools excreted over a 24-hour period and then drying and weighing them.

Crude fiber contents of food are, for obvious reasons, more often reported than dietary fiber contents. As a rule of thumb, for every gram of crude fiber in a food, there are probably about 2 or 3 grams of dietary fiber.

How much fiber is enough? There is no recommended daily allowance (RDA) for fiber. An average 2 to 3 grams of crude fiber a day is perhaps sufficient for minimum body needs, but in order to receive all the benefits of fiber claimed by high-fiber diet advocates, one would have to eat about three to four times the average intake, as do the populations of people studied in Africa. The question then is whether it is necessary to increase the fiber intake of this nation back to where it was in 1900 (an increase to about 6 grams of crude fiber a day) or to increase it to four or more times that amount (25 to 30 grams crude fiber), as suggested by the African studies, in order to affect health positively. At the present time, the question remains unanswered.

If foods are used as the fiber sources, then 6 grams of crude fiber is probably a safe intake. A study in Europe has shown good health and long life in people consuming twice that much (37 grams, when expressed as dietary fiber).[14] The wholesale addition of purified fiber (for example, bran) to foods is probably ill advised, however, because it can cause dehydration and carry off needed minerals with the lost water. Adding a variety of whole grains, nuts, fruits, and vegetables to your diet adds a mixture of the dietary fiber components and increases the diet's overall nutritive value. Table 2–3 presents a list of foods noted for their fiber content.

The diet can easily supply 10 to 20 grams of dietary fiber daily. One slice of whole-grain bread, two servings of fruit (fresh or dried), and two half-cup servings of vegetables (fresh or cooked) will provide this much fiber. Some people find it useful to learn the approximate fiber content of com-

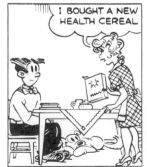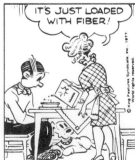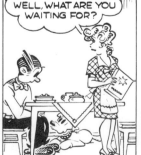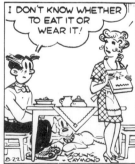

14 D. Kromhout, E. B. Bosschieter, and C. de L. Coulander, Dietary fibre and 10-year mortality from coronary heart disease, cancer, and all causes, *Lancet*, September 4, 1982, pp. 518–522.

mon foods. Table 2–4 offers examples that may help in this endeavor. Using the recommendations of Table 2–4 would provide about 25 grams a day of total dietary fiber. (Appendix K offers fiber contents of additional foods.)

Summing Up

Nutrition status affects our well-being even at the level of the body's cells. The body strives to maintain its blood glucose within a normal range for optimal health and functioning. The hormones insulin, glucagon, and epinephrine function to maintain glucose homeostasis in the body.

At least half our food energy is derived from carbohydrate, principally from starch but also from the simple sugars. Carbohydrates are classified as complex carbohydrates—the polysaccharides—or simple carbohydrates—the monosaccharides and disaccharides. These units are put together by condensation reactions and taken apart by hydrolysis reactions. The most common of the monosaccharides is glucose; the sweetest, fructose. All the monosaccharides share the same chemical formula ($C_6H_{12}O_6$), but their arrangements of atoms are different.

Each of the three disaccharides contains a molecule of glucose paired with either fructose, galactose, or another glucose. Sucrose, or table sugar, can be hydrolyzed to yield glucose and fructose. The source of energy from concentrated sweets such as sodas, cakes, and candy is sucrose. Lactose, or milk sugar, is made up of a molecule each of glucose and galactose. Lactose

TABLE 2–4 **Foods to Provide 25 g Dietary Fiber per Day**

Fruit group: About 2 g fiber per serving; use four or more per day.

Apple, 1 small	Orange, 1 small
Banana, 1 small	Peach, 1 medium
Strawberries, ½ c	Pear, ½ small
Cherries, 10 large	Plums, 2 small

Bread and cereal group: About 2 g fiber per serving; use four or more per day.

Whole-wheat bread, 1 slice	All Bran, 1 tbsp
Rye bread, 1 slice	Corn flakes, ⅔ c
Cracked wheat bread, 1 slice	Oatmeal, dry, 3 tbsp
Shredded wheat, ½ biscuit	Wheat Bran, 1 tsp
Grape-Nuts, 3 tbsp	Puffed Wheat, 1½ c

Vegetable group: About 2 g fiber per serving; use four or more per day. These values are for cooked portions.

Broccoli, ½ stalk	Lettuce, raw, 2 c
Brussels sprouts, 4	Green beans, ½ c
Carrots, ⅓ c	Potato, 2 inch diameter
Celery, 1 c	Tomato, raw, 1 medium
Corn on the cob, 2 inch piece	Baked beans, canned, 2 tbsp

Miscellaneous group: About 1 g fiber per serving

Peanut butter, 2½ tsp	Pickle, 1 large
Peanuts, 10	Strawberry jam, 5 tbsp

Source: Adapted from Recommendation for a high-fiber diet, *Nutrition and the MD*, July 1981, in turn adapted from D.A.T. Southgate, B. Bailey, E. Collinson, and A. Walker, A guide to calculating intakes of dietary fiber, *Journal of Human Nutrition* 30 (1976): 303-313.

is easily digested except by people with lactose intolerance. Milk is recommended as the primary source of nutrition for infants because they are able to digest lactose but not starch from birth. The third disaccharide, maltose, is hydrolyzed during digestion to two molecules of glucose.

The polysaccharides starch, cellulose, and glycogen are composed of chains of glucose units. Starch is the storage form of glucose in the plant. Sources of starch in the diet include seeds, grains, and starchy vegetables. Cellulose is indigestible by humans but is important in the diet as a source of fiber. Glycogen, or animal starch, is more complex than starch and is synthesized in liver and muscle from excess glucose in the bloodstream.

It is recommended that people consume 125 grams or more of carbohydrate a day, preferably from complex carbohydrates. The Exchange System provides a useful guide to estimating the carbohydrate content of a meal. Four of the exchange lists itemize sources of carbohydrate: milk (12 grams per cup), vegetables (5 grams per half cup), fruit (10 grams per portion), and grain (15 grams per slice of bread or equivalent). One must also evaluate the carbohydrate content of concentrated sweet foods. There are 5 grams of carbohydrate per teaspoon of sugar.

The sugar alcohols, mannitol, sorbitol, xylitol, and maltitol, are used as alternatives to sucrose by persons who must restrict their intakes of sugar. Artificial sweeteners, including aspartame, cyclamate, and saccharin, convey a sweet taste to the brain but practically no kcalories to the body.

Plant fibers include the polysaccharides pectin and hemicellulose. There are also noncarbohydrate sources of fiber such as lignin and gums. Researchers are currently studying the beneficial effects of fiber in diet and disease, and fiber has found an important place in diet therapy for diabetes. Intakes of 4 to 7 grams of crude fiber a day (10 to 20 grams of dietary fiber) would seem to be safe and beneficial.

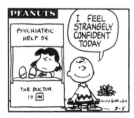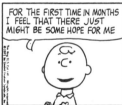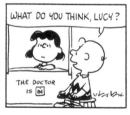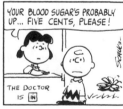

NOTE: References recommended for further reading are in Appendix J; see "Carbohydrates" and "Fiber and Oxalates."

Self-study exercises in Appendix Q show you how to:

● Estimate your carbohydrate consumption and evaluate its quality.
● Learn about the sugar you buy and eat.
● Estimate your fiber consumption.

The *Instructor's Manual* includes three extra transparancy/handout masters: one on blood glucose regulation TH2-2, one to give practice in estimating carbohydrate in meals TH2-6, and one on available and digestible carbohydrate TH2-7. It also includes an entire supplementary lecture, "Hypoglycemia"—diagnosis and treatment.

HIGHLIGHT 2
Sugar Stands Accused

Rabbit said, "Honey or condensed milk with your bread?" [Pooh] was so excited that he said, "Both," and then, so as not to seem greedy, he added, "But don't bother about the bread, please."

A. A. MILNE, *Winnie the Pooh*

Sugar is one of the most controversial items in the diet. People gravitate to it like flies, they eat it by the bowlful, and yet many people seem to feel that it is a positively "bad" substance. It has been accused of causing every human ill from tooth decay to criminal behavior. What, really, is the truth about sugar? This Highlight will examine six of the major charges made against sugar; a later Highlight will delve into its relationship with binge eating.[1]

Arguments against Sugar

Among the arguments that have been leveled against sugar are the following:

1 Concentrated sugar is new in the human diet. The human species evolved without it and does not need it. It isn't a nutrient, it's an additive. As such, it is not natural, and anything not natural is dangerous.

2 If you eat a lot of sugar, you will have to eat a lot less of something else that would have contained essential nutrients. Therefore, sugar causes malnutrition by displacing nutrients in the diet.

3 If you eat a lot of sugar *without* eating less of something else, you will get too many kcalories. Used this way, sugar causes obesity.

4 If you dump a lot of sugar into your bloodstream, your pancreas will overstrain itself trying to produce insulin to handle the load and will wear out. Thus excessive sugar consumption leads to diabetes.

5 Excess sugar is converted to fat and so can cause high levels of fat in the blood (hyperlipidemia). This is a known risk factor for heart and blood-vessel disease (atherosclerosis).

6 Sugar also causes tooth decay.

So go the arguments of those who claim we should eliminate sugar from our diets.

1   This Highlight was adapted, partly, from E. M. N. Hamilton and E. N. Whitney, Controversy 4A: Sugar, in *Nutrition: Concepts and Controversies*, 2nd ed. (St. Paul, Minn.: West, 1981), pp. 101–106.

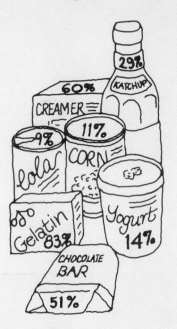

Sugar is concealed in many common products. Source: Adapted from Too much sugar, *Consumers Reports,* March 1978, pp. 137, 139

Evidence

1 Is sugar nonessential in the human diet? Sugar is indeed new in our environment, and we are not biologically adapted to cope with large quantities of it. We do require carbohydrates in our diet, but the body has absolutely no need for sugar itself. Our ancestors only a few hundred years ago lived entirely without it. In the United States, sugar consumption was only about 20 pounds per person per year in 1820, but had reached over 100 pounds per person per year in the 1970s. In Canada it is now between 85 and 100 pounds per person per year.[2] By now, over a third of the kcalories in our diet come from sugars and visible fats, and sugar is today's leading additive.[3] Our consumption of it is thus not voluntary; of the 100-plus pounds that we eat in a year, 70-some pounds are already added to foods during processing.[4] Figures H2–1, H2–2, and H2–3 show the recent increase in sugar consumption and the contributions made by sugar as an additive and by sugar-sweetened beverages.

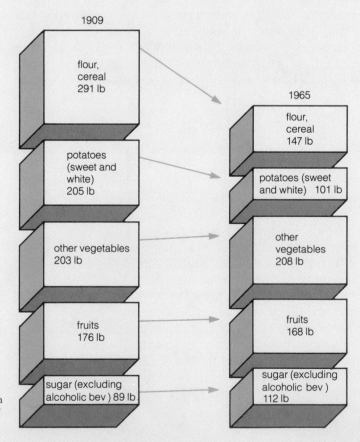

FIGURE H2–1 **Carbohydrate consumption in the United States, 1909 versus 1965.** The figure shows that people are eating less carbohydrate but more sugar. The amounts shown are pounds per person (average) per year.

Source: Adapted from Berta Friend, Nutrients in U.S. food supply, *American Journal of Clinical Nutrition* 201 (1967): 8.

2 *Statistics Canada,* 1980, as cited by E. A. Hamilton, Diabetes, type II (letter to the editor), *Nutrition Today,* March/April 1983, pp. 36–37; E. Newburn, Sugar and dental caries—a review of human studies, *Science* 217 (1982): 418–423.

3 C. W. Lecos, Sugar: How sweet it is—and isn't, *FDA Consumer,* February 1980, pp. 21–23.

4 Institute of Food Technologists' Expert Panel on Food Safety and Nutrition, Sugars and nutritive sweeteners in processed foods, *Food Technology* 33 (May 1979): 101–105.

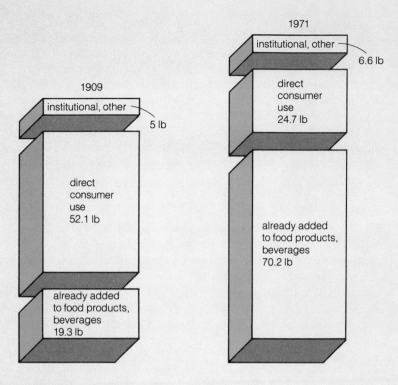

FIGURE H2–2 **Sugar consumption in the United States, 1909 versus 1971.** The figure shows where the sugar of Figure H2–1 is coming from. Most of the increase in people's sugar consumption is from already-added sugar.

Source: Adapted from L. Page and B. Friend, Level of use of sugars in the United States, in *Sugars in Nutrition*, ed. H. L. Sipple and K. W. McNutt (New York: Academic Press, 1974).

FIGURE H2–3 **Soft-drink consumption in Canada and the United States, 1970s.** The figures show average daily intakes of sugar from soft drinks, in grams. One pound is 454 grams, so you can see that teenagers are consuming close to a pound a day, each, of sugar in this form alone.

Source: Figures for Canada adapted from Bureau of Nutritional Sciences, Health Protection Branch, Department of National Health and Welfare, *Food Consumption Patterns Report* (Nutrition Canada, 1970-1972). Figures for the United States from L. Page and B. Friend, Level of use of sugars in the United States, in *Sugars in Nutrition*, ed. H. L. Sipple and K. W. McNutt (New York: Academic Press, 1974), chap. 7.

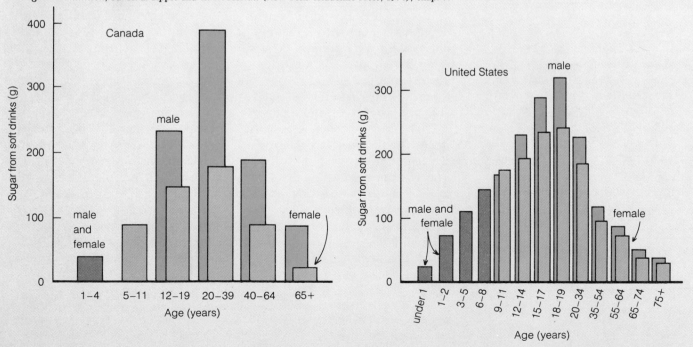

empty-kcalorie food: a popular term used to denote foods that contribute kcalories but are relatively empty of the nutrients protein, vitamins, and minerals. The most notorious empty-kcalorie foods are sugar, fat, and alcohol.

Some of the effects sugar is thought to have on behavior probably come about indirectly, by way of poor nutrition. See note at end of Highlight.

The study of populations, **epidemiology** (ep-uh-deem-ee-OLL-uh-gee), involves collecting and interpreting data on the incidence and distribution of diseases. Epidemiology often can demonstrate a correlation between two variables, but cannot prove a cause.

Sugar is not needed, then, and perhaps we are consuming an excess. Still, carbohydrate has an important role to play in sparing protein. If the only carbohydrate available or acceptable is sugar, then it may perform a much-needed function. It can be beneficial to a child with kidney disease, for example. The feeding of children with kidney disease presents problems. They need protein to grow, but their kidneys can handle only a limited amount of the nitrogen waste from protein. Furthermore, these children often lack appetite. Feeding them sugar permits them to use the protein they receive for growth, rather than for energy, and protein used for growth produces a minimum of waste nitrogen for the kidney to handle. The sugar, then, spares the protein. Starch could be used as well, but sugar is better accepted by these children, who often don't feel like eating much food at all. Like starch, sugar is clean fuel, and taxes the kidneys not at all. Nutritionists therefore offer popsicles and hard candies freely to children with renal disease, knowing it will help their growth.[5] In such a situation, sugar provides a source of valuable needed energy.

2 Does sugar displace nutrients in the diet? Purified, refined white sugar—sucrose—after digestion yields a 50-50 mixture of glucose and fructose. In the body it becomes equivalent to pure glucose. As such, it differs in no way from the glucose that comes from starch. Starch comes in foods with other nutrients, however, while sugar contains no other nutrients—no protein, vitamins, or minerals—and so can be termed an empty-kcalorie food. If you have 200 kcalories to "spend" on something, and you spend them on sugar, you get nothing of value for your outlay. If you spend your 200 kcalories on three slices of whole wheat bread instead, you get 14 percent of the protein, 18 percent of the thiamin, and 12 percent of the niacin recommended for a day, as well as comparable amounts of many other nutrients (Table H2–1). Whether you can afford to eat sugar, then, depends on how many kcalories you have to spend altogether.

It is theoretically possible, with careful food selection, to obtain all the needed nutrients within an allowance of about 1,500 kcalories—but this is not easy for most people. (The Modified Four Food Group Plan requires ingesting about 2,200 kcalories.) A teenage boy needs as many as 4,000 kcalories to get all the energy he needs; if he eats some very nutritious foods, then perhaps the "empty kcalories" of cola beverages are an acceptable addition to his diet. On the other hand, many teenage girls eat only 1,200 kcalories or even less, so they can't afford any but the most nutrient-dense foods. Sugar can clearly cause malnutrition, then—not by any positive action of its own but by displacing nutrients that prevent malnutrition. The appropriate attitude to take is not that sugar is "bad" and that we must avoid it, but that nutritious foods must come first. If the nutritious foods end up crowding sugar out of the diet, that is fine.

3 Does sugar cause obesity? Excess kcalories from any energy nutrient, even protein, are stored in body fat. Evidence from population studies shows that in many countries obesity rises as sugar consumption increases. But sugar cannot be singled out as the sole cause. Where sugar intake

---

5   M. Berger, Dietary management of children with uremia, *Journal of the American Dietetic Association* 70 (1977): 498–505.

TABLE H2–1 **Sugar as Empty kCalories.**
The indicated portion of any of these foods would provide 100 kcalories. Notice what nutrients the eater receives along with those 100 kcalories.

FOOD	SIZE OF 100-kCAL PORTION	PROTEIN	CALCIUM	IRON	VITAMIN A	THIAMIN
Milk, lowfat	¾ c	17	26	—	3	5
Kidney beans	½ c	12	4	13	<1	9
Watermelon	4-by-8-inch wedge	3	3	12	50	9
Bread, whole-wheat	1½ slices	7	4	7	—	9
Sugar, white	2½ tsp	0	0	0	0	0
Molasses, blackstrap	2 tbsp	0	27	35	0	3
Cola beverage	1 c	0	0	0	0	0
Honey, strained or extracted	1½ tbsp	—	<1	1	0	—

The header over PROTEIN...THIAMIN is: PERCENTAGE OF U.S. RDA[a]

[a] Percentages are rounded to nearest whole number. A dash means the percentage has not been determined and is significant. The U.S. RDA are recommended adult intakes (see Highlight 12 and inside back cover).

increases, physical activity usually decreases, while fat and total kcalorie intake rise.[6] Obesity occurs sometimes where sugar intake is low, and in one society it appears that fat people eat less sugar than thin people.[7] Sugar doesn't cause obesity by itself, then, and obesity can occur without it.

4 Does sugar cause diabetes? Here, the evidence is conflicting and interesting. First of all, it should be pointed out that diabetes is not one but several disorders. The predominant type is non-insulin-dependent diabetes (type II diabetes), which may develop only in people who have the genetic tendency for it. Another type of diabetes, insulin-dependent or type I diabetes, is less common. Still another type, caused by chromium deficiency, is described in Chapter 11. Being careful to make the distinction, we can ask whether those who are prone to diabetes (the major type) should eliminate sugar from their diets.

In vast areas of the world, as the diet has changed in the direction of increased sugar consumption, a profound increase—by as much as ten-fold—in the incidence of diabetes has occurred. (This is true for the Japanese, Israelis, Africans, Native Americans, Eskimos, Polynesians, and Micronesians.) Yet in other populations, no relation has been found between sugar intake and diabetes. Wherever starch (or is it the fiber or the chromium that goes with it?) is a major part of the diet, diabetes is rare, and "high rates of diabetes have not been reported in any society where obesity is rare."[8] What does this tangle of associations mean?

correlation: the simultaneous increase or decrease of two variables.

variable: a factor that may vary (increase or decrease). One variable may depend on another; for example, the height of the average child depends partly on his age. One variable may be independent of another; for example, the intelligence of a child is independent of her height.

Diabetes mellitus, the "sugar disease," comes in two main forms. **Type I diabetes,** or **insulin-dependent diabetes mellitus (IDDM),** is the more rare (about 20 percent of cases). Persons with IDDM are usually thin, usually contract the disease suddenly and early in life, and cannot synthesize insulin at all. IDDM used to be called **juvenile-onset diabetes,** but some cases arise in adulthood.

Type II diabetes, or **non-insulin-dependent diabetes mellitus (NIDDM),** is the more common (80 percent of cases). Persons with NIDDM are usually obese and usually contract the disease gradually and later in life. While they can synthesize insulin, their insulin is ineffective. NIDDM used to be called **adult-onset diabetes.**

6   D. F. Hollingsworth, Translating nutrition into diet, *Food Technology* 31 (February 1977): 38–41, 78.

7   K. M. West, Prevention and therapy of diabetes mellitus, in *Nutrition Reviews' Present Knowledge in Nutrition,* 4th ed. (Washington, D.C.: Nutrition Foundation, 1976), pp. 356–364.

8   West, 1976.

This digression is intended to help you learn to evaluate what you read about nutrition in reports of experimental results. The last paragraph said, "High rates of diabetes have not been reported in any society where obesity is rare." Epidemiologists can seldom make this kind of statement—that a *consistent* correlation between two variables has been found. The statement makes a strong case for a causal relationship between obesity and diabetes, but always remember that even a consistent correlation is not proof of a causal relationship. For example, you may notice that the sun always rises shortly after the newspaper girl has made her delivery to your doorstep. This does not mean that she makes the sun rise. Further study would show that the newspaper girl's coming and the sun's rising are independent events; one can happen without the other, although both tend to correlate with a third variable, the time of day. Use caution when you read; note that if A correlates with B, it does not always follow that A causes B. Ask yourself, "Are there other variables with which both A and B may correlate?"

Caution

On the other hand, finding exceptions to a correlation rules out a causal relationship. High intakes of sugar are not *always* found where diabetes is found; diabetes can occur without a high sugar intake. Sugar, then, may *help* to cause, but by itself is not sufficient to cause, diabetes.

When we turn to animal experiments, we find more conflicting evidence. The idea that large amounts of glucose "overstrain" the pancreas appears overly simple in light of the fact that mixed meals stimulate much greater insulin production than sugar alone.[9] Experimenters can induce diabetes in animals by feeding them diets high in fat, protein, *or* sugar and can prevent it by lowering total food intake. From these facts, it is tempting to conclude that excess energy intake—obesity—causes diabetes; however, diets very high in sugar can cause the disease even if the animals do not become obese.[10] One extensive and well-designed study on rats clearly implicated sugar as the cause of diabetes. In this study, one set of animals was fed a starch-based diet, while the other was fed a similar, but sugar-based diet. The rats fed starch did not develop symptoms; those fed sugar did.[11] The fairest conclusion that can be drawn is that obesity is a major factor in the causation of diabetes but that sugar has not been proven innocent as a special factor.

After epidemiological studies have revealed a connection between certain variables (such as sugar and obesity) and a disease (such as diabe-

---

9   West, 1976.

10   West, 1976.

11   A. M. Cohen, High sucrose intake as a factor in the development of diabetes and its vascular complications, in U.S. Senate, Select Committee on Nutrition and Human Needs, *Dietary Sugar and Disease* (Washington, D.C.: Government Printing Office, 1973), pp. 167–198.

tes), researchers often are able to state theories as to the cause of the disease. They then turn to animal studies to test the theories. Experiments using animals with physiological systems similar to the human system under study can often yield much more information than studies of human beings, for many reasons.

For one thing, with humans, there are always many variables present that cannot be separated from one another. When a large population has recently started consuming large quantities of sugar and the incidence of diabetes among its members has also risen dramatically, it is tempting to conclude that the sugar has at least contributed to the disease, but it is impossible to rule out other factors. At the same time that the people have changed their habits with respect to sugar consumption, they are also likely to have bought cars, increased their TV-watching, moved into cities, and welcomed a hundred other changes into their lives. When you read about epidemiological studies, then, you have to remember to ask whether the researcher considered all these confounding variables.

In an animal study, all the subjects share a common heredity, their life span is short compared with that of human beings, and they can be maintained in laboratory conditions, where most variables can be controlled. If both sugar and obesity, for example, are suspected of contributing to diabetes, then sugar alone can be tested in one experiment, and obesity in another. Even then the results are not always clear, as the illustration given here shows, but progress has been made toward defining the relationships among the various possible causal factors. Notice, when reading about animal studies, how the researchers have designed their experiments so that possible causal variables are tested one by one.

Variables that cannot be separated from the one under study are known as **confounding variables**. They greatly complicate the problem of interpreting epidemiological studies.

Caution

One of the earliest symptoms of diabetes is excessive hunger. As the common form of diabetes (type II) develops, the person typically first becomes hungry, then becomes obese, and finally exhibits overt symptoms of diabetes. Thus sugar may contribute, not to diabetes, but to the obesity that brings the disease into the open. Obesity then aggravates the situation by causing resistance to insulin. In fact, in this type of diabetes there is too much, rather than too little, insulin; but the tissues fail to respond to it. Both weight control and avoidance of sugar are therefore recommended for the potential and overt diabetic.

5 Does sugar cause atherosclerosis? The same epidemiological studies that show high sugar intakes correlating with increased obesity also show high sugar intakes correlating with increased blood fat levels and deaths from heart disease. It is found, however, that the deaths are associated more closely with obesity than with sugar intake. Experiments performed using animals as subjects have implicated sugar in heart and artery disease, but they have used diets so high in sugar that they are "unphysiological." A moderate amount of sugar (5 to 10 percent of total kcalories) has not been shown conclusively to affect the disease process, although some evidence suggests that it may raise blood lipid levels in a special subgroup of the population—"carbohydrate-sensitive" individuals. As many as one in five

atherosclerosis: a form of hardening of the arteries. More about atherosclerosis and its causes appears in Highlight 3.

dental caries (CARE-eez): tooth decay, cavities.

A statement of the amount of dental decay a food would produce would be a **cariogenicity** (CARE-ee-oh-jen-ISS-it-ee) **index** for the food.

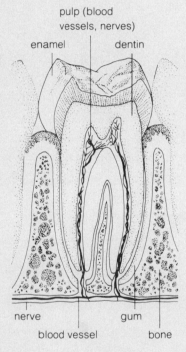

pulp (blood vessels, nerves)

enamel   dentin

nerve   gum

blood vessel   bone

FIGURE H2–4 **A normal tooth**. Bacteria tend to collect in areas where tooth and tooth or tooth and gum are in contact. Given carbohydrate, they multiply, adhere more firmly, and produce acid which eats into the tooth enamel.

adults may fall in this category.[12] Sugar in the amounts usually consumed seems to have no discrete influence on heart disease in most people, however.

6 Does sugar cause tooth decay? Dental caries is a serious public health problem, afflicting nearly everyone in the country, half of them by the time they are two years old. One of the most successful measures taken to reduce the incidence of dental decay is fluoridation of community water (see Chapter 11). But sugar has something to do with dental caries, too.

Dental caries is actually caused by the acid byproduct of bacterial growth in the mouth (see Figures H2–4 and H2–5). Bacteria thrive on food particles, especially if they contain carbohydrate, and so it is logical to implicate sugar as the cause of cavities. However, any carbohydrate, including starch, can support bacterial growth. Equally important is the length of time the food stays in the mouth, and this depends on how soon you brush your teeth after eating and how sticky the food is. Because the damage sugar does is related to both the amount and the stickiness of the sugar, it has been suggested that food labels express their sugar contents in terms of both. Rather than stating simply how much sugar is in a food, the label should state how much dental decay the food causes under defined test conditions. By such a measure, a sticky, sugary food like *raisins* or *granola* would be seen to be more caries-causing than an easily rinsed-off sugary food such as a sweetened beverage.

Sugar can be eaten and then removed from tooth surfaces soon enough to prevent decay, however. A rule of thumb is that bacterial action is maximal within the first 20 minutes after the mouth bacteria have had access to carbohydrate. If immediate brushing is not possible, milk or water drunk with a meal will help wash the carbohydrate off the teeth.

Alternatively, you can remove the bacteria themselves by flossing. It takes 24 hours for a large enough clump of bacteria to accumulate on a tooth to produce caries-causing acid, so once-a-day flossing may effectively prevent formation of caries, regardless of carbohydrate content of the diet. And some people may *never* get cavities because they have inherited resistance to them. In this matter, as in the others, sugar may not be the extreme villain that some have made it out to be. Still, if sugar is guilty of any of the six accusations listed at the start, it is guilty of contributing to tooth decay.[13]

Conclusion

Is sugar "bad" for you? There is no reason to believe that the moderate consumption of sugar (5 to 10 percent of kcalories) is in any way dangerous

12   Nutritionists say reevaluation of sucrose "appears to be warranted," *Food Chemical News*, February 21, 1983, pp. 1–3.

13   Of eight substantial charges against sugar made in 1978 by the Federal Trade Commission (FTC), that agency and several other review organizations concluded in 1980 that only one charge could be upheld: "The *only* demonstrated hazard that sugars pose to the public health . . . remains their contribution to dental decay." The FDA, FTC, and USDA also agreed that sugar is safe at current levels of usage. G. M. Bollenbach, Sugar in health, *Cereal Foods World* 26 (1981): 213–217; Update, *FDA Consumer*, February 1983, pp. 2–5.

to the normal, healthy human being. Clearly, however, it may be associated with other factors that are harmful: obesity, the displacement of needed nutrients and fiber, and dental decay. If on these grounds you conclude that sugar is indeed to be avoided, it is important to recognize that other kcaloric sweeteners, such as honey, are no better.

You should also note that sugar is hidden in many supposedly healthful products. The advertising industry would have us believe that some products provide an excellent replacement for a balanced meal. One such product, advertised as a substitute for breakfast, contains more sugar than any other single ingredient. Labeling laws require that food ingredients be listed on the container in the order of their weight, with the ingredient in the largest amount listed first. In the breakfast substitute just mentioned, the first three ingredients are refined sugar, vegetable shortening, and water. The recommended serving contains 370 kcalories. For only 325 kcalories, you could have a half-cup of orange juice (60), a poached egg on toast (150), a pat of margarine (35), and a cup of skim milk (80). This breakfast of real foods provides complex carbohydrate in contrast to the simple sugar in the substitute. The fat in the foods is less saturated (see Chapter 3) than in the substitute. The protein from eggs and milk is of high quality, and the bread contributes needed fiber. As for the vitamins and minerals, you can be sure that the foods contain many, whereas the substitute probably contains only those listed on the label. In reality, then, although you can't tell from the label, the substitute is far inferior.

The dieter who is limiting kcalories needs especially to choose nutritious foods because he has a smaller kcalorie allowance within which to get his nutrients. Weight Watchers, Inc., recommends refusing foods when the label puts sugar in the first or second place.

Should we switch to the use of artifical sweeteners in place of sugar? The question whether their use incurs any risks is still open, but if it does, those risks have to be weighed against the risks of consuming the sugar you would otherwise use. An interesting calculation using saccharin as an example was presented by B. L. Cohen in *Science*: Assuming (1) that saccharin users consume less sugar than they would otherwise, (2) that people consuming less sugar consume fewer kcalories, and (3) that lower kcalorie consumption promotes longer life, Cohen figured that the risk from using the sweetener is far less than the risk from consuming sugar would be.[14] All three of these assumptions may be false, however,[15] so it may be more prudent to reduce sugar intake without substituting artificial sweeteners.

As for saccharin's competitor, aspartame, it is too early to say whether its use entails any hazard; so far, it seems remarkably free of attendant risk. To be on the safe side, though, authorities are recommending users confine themselves to three to four aspartame doses a day—that is, the equivalent of three to four teaspoons of sugar.[16]

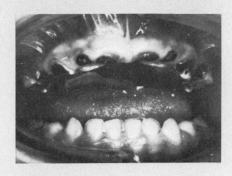

FIGURE H2–5 **An extreme example of tooth decay.** This child was frequently put to bed sucking on a baby bottle filled with apple juice, so that the teeth were bathed in carbohydrate for long periods of time—a perfect medium for bacterial growth. The upper teeth have decayed all the way to the gumline, a phenomenon known as nursing bottle syndrome.

Source: Courtesy of H. Kaplan and V. P. Rabbach.

14   B. L. Cohen, Relative risks of saccharin and calorie ingestion, *Science* 199 (1978): 983.

15   A. R. P. Walter, The relative risks of saccharin and sucrose ingestions (letter to the editor), *American Journal of Clinical Nutrition* 32 (1979): 727–728.

16   G. S. Wong, Position statement (Canadian Diabetes Association): Aspartame and its safe use. Abstract cited in *Journal of the American Dietetic Association 81* (1982): 85.

Recommendations on ways to reduce sugar consumption abound. An American Friends Service Committee publication points out that alternatives to desserts might be "cheese and whole grain crackers and yogurt" and that snacks for children need not be sugar-water drinks. Instead, they can have "fruits, raw vegetables, popcorn, unsalted nuts, home made fruit juice popsicles and other wholesome foods."[17] A government publication makes the following suggestions:

● Substitute fruit juices or plain water for regular soft drinks, punches, fruit drinks, and ades that contain considerable amounts of sugar.
● Go easy on candy, pies, cakes, pastries, and cookies.
● Fruits are often canned in heavy sirup, which is a high-sugar product. Buy fruit canned in its own juice, other fruit juice, or light sirup.
● Many cereals are presweetened. Check the label. Buy *unsweetened* kinds, so you can control the amount of sugar added.
● Experiment with reducing the sugar in your favorite recipes. Some recipes taste just the same even after a 25 percent reduction in sugar content. Others taste different but just as delicious.

The Professional Nutritionist reports that the "sweet spices"—allspice, anise, cardamom, cinnamon, cloves, fennel, and ginger—can replace substantial sugar in recipes. Use half as much sugar and half again as much spice as the recipe calls for.[18]

Many recommend substituting raw or brown sugar or honey for white sugar, because they contain some minerals essential for human health. They contain chromium, for example, although the amount is miniscule. However, it would be absurd to rely on any kind of sugar for its nutrient contributions, because one would have to eat so much to obtain significant amounts. (There is only one significant exception. Blackstrap molasses contains over 3 milligrams of iron per tablespoon. If used frequently, it can make a major contribution of this important and, for women, hard-to-get nutrient. It's not as sweet as the other sweeteners, however, and so doesn't satisfy the "sweet tooth" of people who like sugar.) Rather than go to the extreme of eating large quantities of any sweetener, it makes sense to ensure that the diet is otherwise adequate and then use sugar for its taste appeal in whatever form one prefers. You might then choose honey, correctly, not for its nutrient contributions but for its sweetness.

Should we eliminate sugar from our diets? Moderation in its use is probably the course to adopt. Totally eliminating sugar seems unnecessary, even if it were possible. But those who consume large amounts of sugar should reduce their intake, all who use it should be extra conscientious about brushing and flossing their teeth, and potential diabetics should probably avoid it altogether.

NOTE: Appendix J includes additional references under "Carbohydrates" and "Dental Health."

Sugar is sometimes thought to have harmful effects on behavior, a subject not dealt with here. If it does have harmful effects, they may come about indirectly, by way of poor nutrition. The *Instructor's Manual* includes a supplementary lecture on this subject: "Nutrition and Behavior: Nutrient Deficiencies and Sugar."

17   L. Warschoff, *What Betty Crocker doesn't tell you about sugar!* (Baltimore: American Friends Service Committee, 1976).
18   J. Wylie-Rossett, Spices to the rescue, *Professional Nutritionist*, Spring 1982, pp. 4–6.

CHAPTER 3
The Lipids: Fats and Oils

CONTENTS

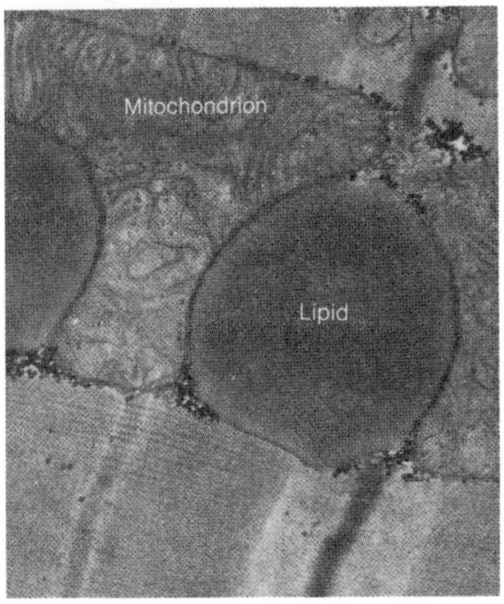

Muscle cells derive their energy from both fat and carbohydrate. Here, two lipid droplets nestle close to a muscle fiber (bottom), while mitochondria surround the droplets and gather energy from them.

The notion that matter is something inert and uninteresting is surely the veriest nonsense. If there is anything more wonderful than matter in the sheer versatility of its behavior, I have yet to hear tell of it.

FRED HOYLE

Most people are conditioned to believe that slim is beautiful. The less fat you carry on your frame, the lovelier (sexier, healthier) you are thought to be. On the other hand, your body fat does things for you that would be hard to do without. If you carry neither too much nor too little body fat, you will enjoy the benefits provided by your body's stores of this very important nutrient.

Although a third of the world's population is underfed, at least a third of the U.S. population is overfed. And indeed, overweight is a major health problem in the developed countries, contributing to the incidence of heart disease, diabetes, and many other ills.

The Importance of Fat

The fats—more properly called the lipids—are actually a family of compounds that include both fats and oils. Both fats and oils occur in your body, and both

85

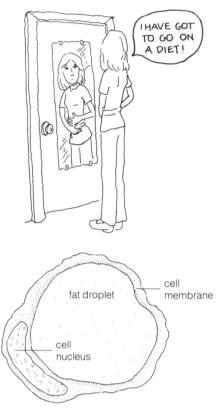

Within the fat cell, lipid is stored in a globule. This globule can enlarge indefinitely, and the fat cell membrane will grow to accommodate its swollen contents.

Fat cells are often called **adipose** (ADD-ih-poce) **cells.**

1 pound body fat = 3,500 kcal (but see Chapter 6).

ketones (KEE-tones): a condensation product of fat metabolism produced when carbohydrate is not available (see Chapter 6).

help to keep it healthy. Natural oils in the skin provide a radiant complexion; in the scalp they help nourish the hair and make it glossy. The layer of fat beneath the skin, being a poor conductor of heat, insulates the body from extremes of temperature. A pad of hard fat beneath each kidney protects it from being jarred and damaged, even during a motorcycle ride on a bumpy road. The soft fat in the breasts of a woman protects her mammary glands from heat and cold and cushions them against shock. The fat that lies embedded in the muscle tissue shares with muscle glycogen the task of providing energy when the muscles are active.

An uninterrupted flow of energy is so vital to life that in a pinch any other function is sacrificed to maintain it. If a growing child is fed too little food, for example, the food she does consume will be used for energy to keep her heart and lungs going, but her growth will come to a standstill. To go totally without an energy supply, even for a few minutes, would be to die. The urgency of the need for energy has ensured, over the course of evolution, that all creatures have built-in reserves to protect themselves from ever being deprived of it. Chapter 2 described one provision against this sort of emergency—the stores of glycogen in the liver that can return glucose to the blood whenever the supply runs short.

However, the liver cells can store only a limited amount of energy as glycogen; once this is depleted, the body must receive new food or start degrading body protein to continue making glucose. Unlike the liver, the body's fat mass has a virtually unlimited storage capacity, and fat supplies two-thirds of the body's ongoing energy need. During a prolonged period of food deprivation, fat stores may make an even greater contribution to energy needs.

A person who fasts (drinking only water to flush out metabolic wastes) will rapidly oxidize body fat. A pound of body fat provides 3,500 kcalories; so a fasting person who expends 2,000 kcalories a day can lose a maximum of 4 pounds of body fat each week. (Actually, the person loses some lean tissue, too, because of the brain's need for glucose, which fat can't supply; so he loses *fat* at a slower rate than this.) In conditions of enforced starvation—say, during a siege or a famine—the fatter person survives longer because of this energy reserve.

If you happen to be acquainted with a polar bear, you may be aware that the same thing is true for him. As he lumbers about on his iceberg, great masses of fat ripple beneath his thick fur coat. When he hibernates, he oxidizes that fat, extracting tens of thousands of kcalories from it to maintain his body temperature and to fuel other metabolic processes while he sleeps. Come spring, he is a hundred or more pounds thinner than when he went to sleep.

Although fat provides energy in a fast, it cannot provide it in the form of glucose, the substance needed for energy by the brain and nerves. After a long period of glucose deprivation, these cells develop the ability to derive about half of their energy from a special form of fat known as ketones, but they still require glucose as well. With the available glycogen long gone, they demand this glucose from the only alternative source—protein. And since no protein is coming in from food, the only supply is in the muscles and other lean tissues of the body. These tissues give up their protein and

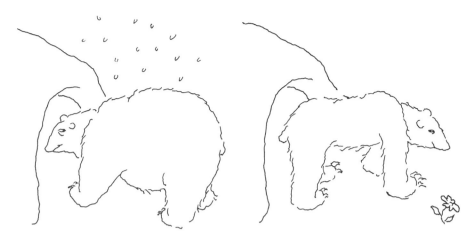

atrophy, bringing on weakness, loss of function, and ultimately—when half the body protein has been used up—death. Death from loss of lean body tissue will occur even in a fat person if he fasts too long.

To sum up the roles of body fat, it helps maintain the health of the skin and hair, protects body organs from temperature extremes and mechanical shock, and provides a continuous fuel supply, helping to keep the body's lean tissue from being depleted. It is oxidized for energy by many body tissues, and when it is being used in the absence of glucose, it forms ketones that can meet about half the energy needs of the brain and nervous system. Protein released from wasting muscle and other lean tissue provides the other half.

Not only is fat important in the body; it is also important in foods. Many of the compounds that give foods their flavor and aroma are found in fats and oils; they are fat-soluble. Four vitamins—A, D, E, and K—are also soluble in fat. Understanding this fact provides insight into many different areas in nutrition, so let us spend a moment here considering fat solubility.

As you know, fats and oils tend to separate from water and watery substances. The oil floats to the top when salad dressing stands. As hot meat drippings cool, the fat separates and hardens on top of the other juices. You can probably think of many other examples of this phenomenon. Whenever a fatty liquid and a watery liquid separate in this manner, the other compounds must go with either the fat or the water. The nutritional significance of this is evident if you think what happens when the fat is removed from a food; many of the fat-soluble compounds are also removed. Significant among these are flavors and vitamins.

In general, foods from which the fat or oil has been removed lack much of their original flavor, aroma, and fat-soluble vitamin content. Chicken meat skinned before cooking, for example, is so tasteless that it is hard to guess what kind of meat it is. If cooked with the skin it soaks up both fat and flavor. Foods cooked with fat are tasty and aromatic; the "good food" smell comes from the fat, too. It is the fat that makes the delicious aromas associated with bacon, ham, hamburger, and other meats, as well as onions being fried, french fries, and stir-fried Chinese vegetables. Milk when skimmed loses much of its buttery flavor; and even more importantly, it loses all its vitamins A and D. To provide skim milk with the desired

atrophy (ATT-ro-fee): to waste away.

a = without

trophy = growth

For more about the dangers of fasting, see Chapter 6.

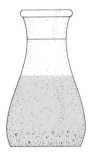

Fat solubility. Oil and water separate; fat-soluble compounds stay dissolved in the oil, water-soluble compounds in the water.

Fortification actually involves adding back more vitamin D than was in the whole milk originally (see Highlight 12).

amounts of these nutrients, vitamins A and D are added to it; hence the "vitamin A and D fortified" label you see on skim milk. (Vitamin D is also added to whole milk, because its natural vitamin D level is low.)

An additional feature is lost when fat is removed: kcalories. A medium pork chop with the fat trimmed to within a half-inch of the lean contains 260 kcalories; with the fat trimmed off completely, it contains 130 kcalories. A baked potato with butter and sour cream (1 tablespoon each) has 260 kcalories; plain, it has 90. So it goes. The single most effective step you can take to reduce the energy (kcalorie) value of a food is to eat it without the fat.

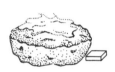

Pork chop with ½-inch fat (260 kcal).

Potato with 1 tbsp butter and 1 tbsp sour cream (260 kcal).

Whole milk, 1 c (170 kcal).

Remember, fat is a more concentrated energy source than the other energy nutrients: 1 g carbohydrate or protein = 4 kcal; but 1 g fat = 9 kcal.

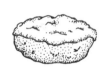

Pork chop with fat trimmed off (130 kcal).

Plain potato (90 kcal).

Skim milk, 1 c (80 kcal).

The Chemist's View of Fats

The lipids in foods are 95% fats and oils (that is, triglycerides) and 5% other lipids (phospholipids and sterols).

"Your blood triglycerides are fine." If a doctor says this, the patient may be reassured. Most of us are aware nowadays that there is a close relationship between the fats in the blood and the health of the heart. A closer look at the fats will lay the foundation for an understanding of this relationship.

When we speak of fats, we are usually speaking of triglycerides. Almost all the lipids in the diet (95 percent) are triglycerides. The other two classes of dietary lipids are the phospholipids (lecithin is one) and the sterols (among them, cholesterol). Because the triglycerides predominate in the diet, the following section focuses on them.

To understand the fats and the beneficial and harmful effects they have on your body, you must understand their molecular structure. It is not so complicated as it may seem at first. If you follow the few steps of reasoning presented here, you can reap an appreciation for the whole subject that you might not otherwise have enjoyed. Those who have grasped the structure of the triglycerides become enthusiasts, ascribing beauty, elegance, and other such praiseworthy attributes to these molecules. See what you think.

The Triglycerides

Triglycerides come in many sizes and several varieties, but they all share a common structure; all have a "backbone" of glycerol to which three fatty acids are attached. All glycerol molecules are alike, but the fatty acids may vary in two ways: length and degree of saturation.

A fatty acid is a chain of carbon atoms with hydrogens attached and with an acid group (COOH) at one end. The fatty acid shown in Figure 3–1 is acetic acid, the compound that gives vinegar its sour taste. This is the simplest of the fatty acids; the "chain" is only two carbon atoms long. A longer fatty acid may have four, six, eight, or more carbon atoms (they mostly come in even numbers). Among those common in dairy products are fatty acids that are six to ten carbons long. Butyric acid, found in butter, is a four-carbon fatty acid. Fatty acids that predominate in meat and fish are 14 or more carbon atoms long.

To illustrate the characteristics of these fatty acids, let us look at the 18-carbon ones (a special one among them deserves attention anyway). Stearic acid is the simplest of the 18-carbon fatty acids (see Figure 3–2). When three stearic acids attach to a glycerol molecule, the resulting structure is a triglyceride (see Figure 3–3).

The triglyceride shown in Figure 3–3 is a saturated fat, because the fatty acids are saturated fatty acids. They are loaded, or saturated, with all the hydrogen (H) atoms they can carry. If some Hs were to be removed, the result would be an unsaturated or even a polyunsaturated fat. The distinction between these kinds of fats is of interest, because people threatened with heart trouble may be told to reduce their intake of saturated fats and to increase their intake of polyunsaturated fats. (Cutting out butter and using soft margarines or vegetable oils instead is one way to do this.)

Vegetable oils are rich in polyunsaturated fats, triglycerides in which the fatty acids are carrying less than their full load of hydrogens. Consider stearic acid once more: if we remove two Hs from the middle of the carbon chain, we are left with a compound like that in Figure 3–4. The two carbon atoms that formerly held the Hs are, in a sense, empty-handed. Each has a bond that is going unused. Such a compound cannot exist in nature. But an extra bond can be formed between the two carbons to satisfy nature's requirement that every carbon must have four bonds connecting it to other atoms. There is then a "double bond" between them (see Figure 3–5).

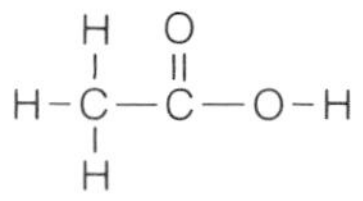

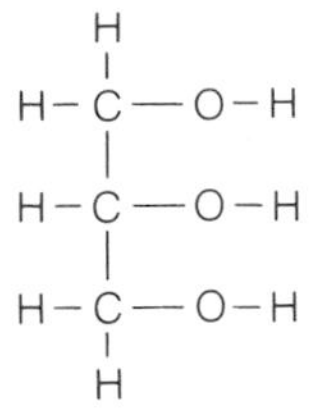

Glycerol

glycerol (GLISS-er-ol): an organic alcohol composed of a 3-carbon chain with an alcohol group attached to each carbon. An alcohol group is a reactive –OH group.

ol = alcohol

acid: a compound that tends to ionize in water solution, releasing H+ ions. The more H+ ions that are free in the water, the stronger the acid (see Appendix B).

acid group: the COOH group of an organic acid, which can also be represented this way:

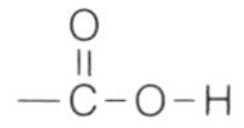

fatty   d: an organic compound mad_ up of a carbon chain with hydrogens attached and an acid group at one end.

triglyceride (try-GLISS-uh-ride): a compound composed of carbon, hydrogen, and oxygen arranged as a molecule of glycerol with three fatty acids attached to it.

tri = three

glyceride = a compound of glycerol

saturated fatty acid: a fatty acid carrying the maximum possible number of hydrogen atoms—for example, stearic acid. A **saturated fat** is composed of triglycerides in which all, or virtually all, of the fatty acids are saturated.

fat: a mixture of triglycerides.

FIGURE 3–1   **Acetic acid (a 2-carbon fatty acid).**

FIGURE 3–2 **Stearic acid (an 18-carbon fatty acid).** TH 3-1

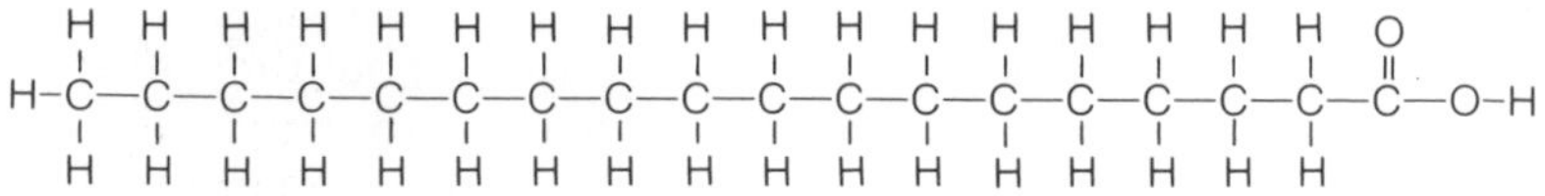

1 The structure with all details.

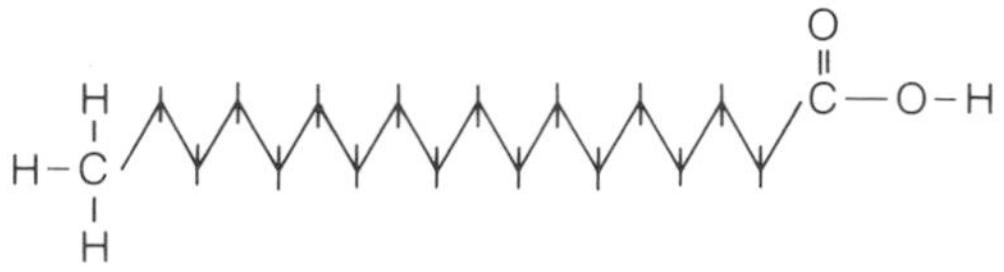

2 A simpler way to depict the same structure. Each "corner" on the zigzag line represents a carbon atom with two attached Hs.

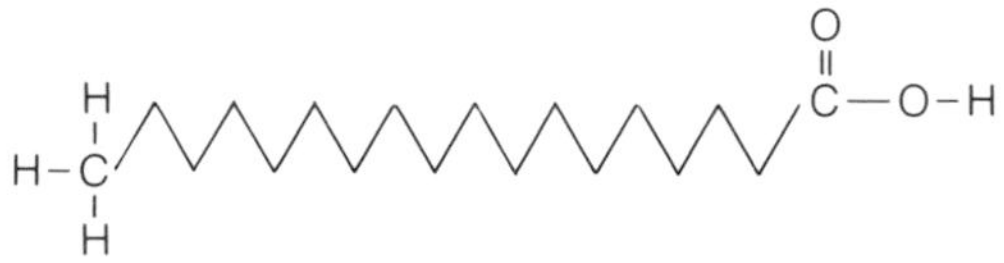

3 Still more simply, the lines representing bonds to the Hs can be left out. If you count the "corners," you will see that this still represents an 18-carbon fatty acid. This is the way fatty acids will be represented in many of the following diagrams.

FIGURE 3–3 **Formation of a fat (triglyceride): Three fatty acids attached to glycerol.** TH3-2

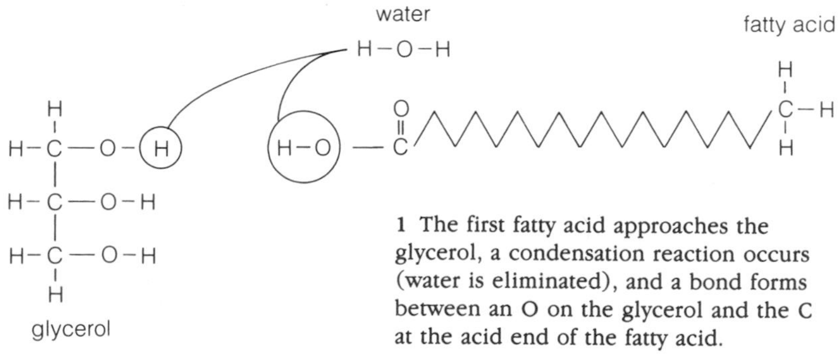

water

fatty acid

glycerol

1 The first fatty acid approaches the glycerol, a condensation reaction occurs (water is eliminated), and a bond forms between an O on the glycerol and the C at the acid end of the fatty acid.

2 Later, two more fatty acids attach themselves to the glycerol by the same means; the resulting structure is a triglyceride.

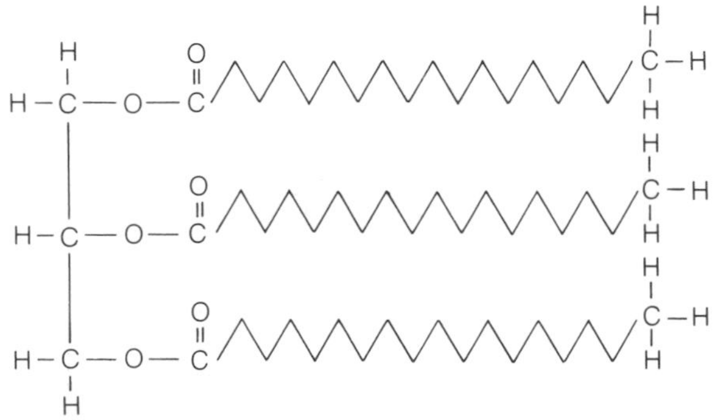

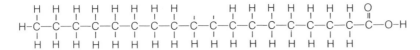

FIGURE 3-4 **A fatty acid lacking two hydrogens—an impossible structure.**

(The same situation exists in the acid group at the end of the chain, where an O is double-bonded to the terminal C. That carbon has its full four bonds, and the oxygen meets its requirement of having two.) The resulting structure is an unsaturated (in this case *mono*unsaturated) fatty acid, oleic acid, which is found abundantly in the triglycerides of olive oil.

The heart patient is advised to eat *poly*unsaturated fats, because they seem to reduce the risk of heart and artery disease. A polyunsaturated fat contains triglycerides in which the fatty acids have two or more points of unsaturation. An example is linoleic acid, which lacks four Hs and has two double bonds, as shown in Figure 3-6. Linoleic acid is found in the triglycerides of most vegetable oils—corn oil, safflower oil, and the like. It is the most common of the polyunsaturated fatty acids in foods and the most important. In fact, it is the special fatty acid we promised you earlier; it has a section of its own later in this chapter.

Having looked at three of the most common fatty acids in foods, you can probably anticipate what the others look like. The fourth member of the family of 18-carbon fatty acids is linolenic acid, which has three double bonds. A similar series of 20-carbon fatty acids exists, as well as a series of 22-carbon fatty acids. These are the long-chain fatty acids. In smaller

monounsaturated fatty acid: a fatty acid that lacks two hydrogen atoms and has one double bond between carbons—for example, oleic acid.

polyunsaturated fatty acid (PUFA): a fatty acid that lacks four or more hydrogen atoms and has two or more double bonds between carbons—for example, linoleic acid (2 double bonds) and linolenic acid (3 double bonds). Thus a **polyunsaturated fat** is composed of triglycerides containing a high percentage of PUFA.

Note: Linoleic acid (18 Cs, 2 double bonds) should not be confused with linolenic acid (18 Cs, 3 double bonds). The shorthand way of describing these two fatty acids is 18:2 and 18:3. For the fatty acid series, names, and structures, see Appendix C.

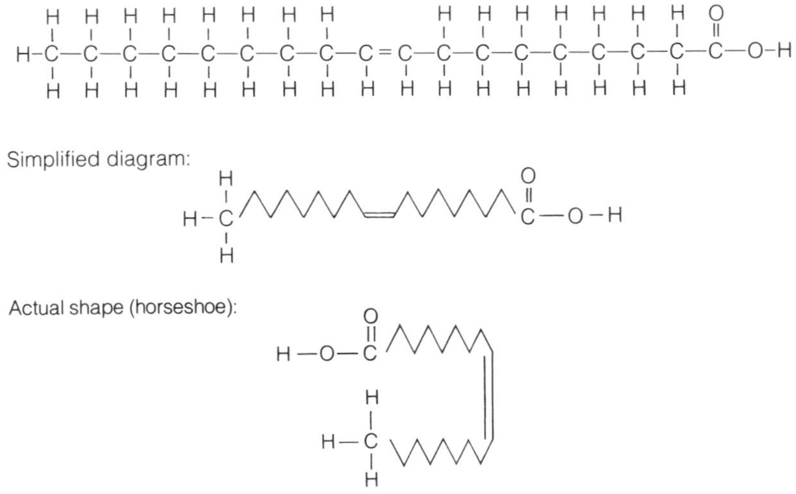

Simplified diagram:

Actual shape (horseshoe):

FIGURE 3-5 **Oleic acid (an 18-carbon fatty acid).** Because it has one point of unsaturation, oleic acid is monounsaturated. For more about the shape of unsaturated fatty acids, see Figure 3-10. TH3-1

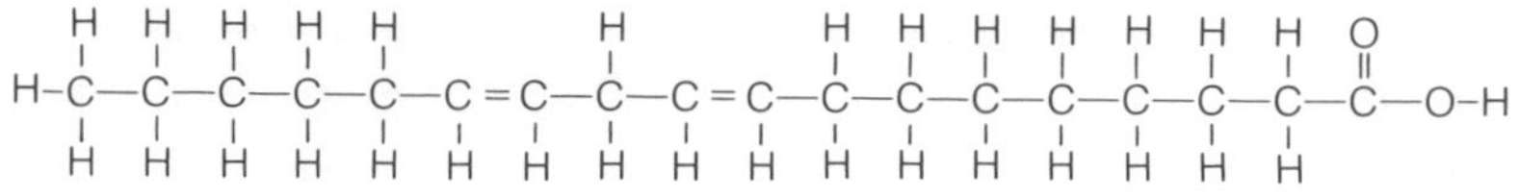

Simplified diagram (the actual shape is bent at the double bonds):

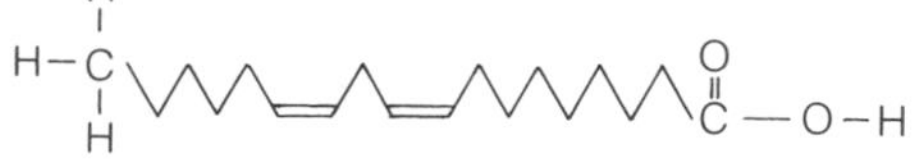

FIGURE 3–6 **Linoleic acid (an 18-carbon fatty acid).** Its two points of unsaturation make it polyunsaturated. Linoleic acid is one of the essential fatty acids. TH3-1

amounts, medium-chain (10 to 14 Cs) and short-chain (6 to 8 Cs) fatty acids are also present in foods.

To sum up what has been said to this point, the fats and oils are mostly (95 percent) triglycerides: glycerol backbones with fatty acids attached. Those that are fully loaded with Hs are the saturated fats; those that have a multitude of double bonds are unsaturated and polyunsaturated fats. To complete the picture, it only remains to say that a fat or oil may contain any combination of fatty acids. A mixed triglyceride, one that contains more than one type of fatty acid, is shown in Figure 3–7.

The Essential Fatty Acids

Linoleic acid is an essential nutrient (see p. 2 for a definition of *essential nutrient*). When linoleic acid is missing from the diet, the skin reddens and becomes irritated, infections and dehydration become more likely, and the liver develops abnormalities. In infants, growth failure also occurs. Adding linoleic acid back to the diet clears up these symptoms. It turns out that what the body cells need is arachidonic acid (20 Cs, four double bonds), and that the body can make this compound if linoleic acid is supplied in the diet. Linolenic acid, thought to be derived from linoleic acid, is needed, too. Linoleic acid has thus come to be known as "the"

The **essential fatty acid** is linoleic acid. The **essential fatty acids** (as some authorities name them) are linoleic, linolenic, and arachidonic acids. See Appendix C for their structures.

Reddening and irritation of the skin are symptoms known as **dermatitis** (derm-uh-TIGHT-us).

derma = skin

itis = infection or inflammation

FIGURE 3–7 **A mixed triglyceride typical of those found in foods.** A "fat" is a mixture of mixed triglycerides. (The shape of the fatty acids is shown straight for ease of viewing.)

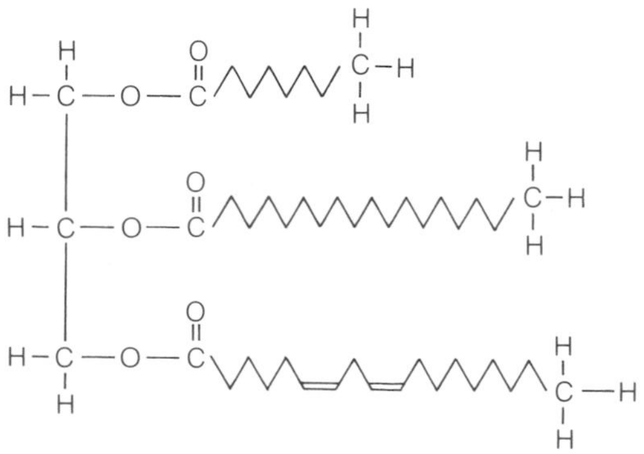

essential fatty acid, on the assumption that the other needed fatty acids can be synthesized from it. Some evidence suggests, however, that at least some linolenic acid must also be supplied by the diet.[1]

The body's cells are equipped with many enzymes that can convert one compound to another. To make body fat or oil—triglycerides—all the enzymes need is a usable food source containing the atoms triglycerides are composed of: carbon, hydrogen, and oxygen. Glucose does perfectly well. In fact, given an excess of blood glucose (and a filled glycogen storage space), this is precisely what some enzymes use. They cleave the glucose to make the 2-carbon compound acetic acid, and then combine many acetic acid molecules, with the appropriate alterations, to make long-chain fatty acids. (This is why most fatty acid carbon chains come in even numbers.) But the cells do not possess an enzyme that can arrange the double-bonding of linoleic acid, so linoleic acid must be supplied in the foods we eat.

Thus, as mentioned, linoleic acid has been called "the essential fatty acid"; but arachidonic acid can alleviate the deficiency symptoms and, to a limited extent, linolenic acid also helps. The three together are known as "the essential fatty acids," sometimes abbreviated EFA. Nearly all diets supply enough EFA to meet the requirement. Deficiencies are usually seen only in infants fed a formula that lacks EFA and in hospital patients who have been fed through a vein for prolonged periods a formula that provides no EFA. Even in an otherwise totally fat-free diet, only one teaspoon (5 grams) of corn oil would be sufficient to supply the needed amount of EFA for an adult.

Compound A ——————▶ Compound B

Compound A is the **precursor** of compound B. Linoleic acid is the precursor of arachidonic acid.

Acetic acid, or acetyl CoA, is formed from glucose (or other compounds; see Chapter 6).

EFA: the essential fatty acids.

The relief of a skin rash by linoleic acid might suggest to the unwary observer that all skin rashes indicate a deficiency of this nutrient. Not so! More than a hundred body compounds besides linoleic acid are needed to ensure the health of the skin, including other oils, vitamins, minerals, and hormones. A deficiency of any of these or an imbalance among them can cause a rash. The lack of some compound might be at fault, but the compound might also be present in excess, or might be improperly handled by the skin cells. Bacterial and viral infections, allergies, physical agents such as radiation, and chemical irritants also cause rashes. There can even be a psychosomatic cause, as when excessive nervous activity in the brain generates a hormone imbalance that affects the skin. For these reasons, when you notice a symptom such as a rash, you can only know that a problem exists; you have no clue as to the cause.

In dealing with nutrition, it is important to remember the distinction being made here—the distinction between a symptom and a disease. A symptom can be alleviated (soothing oils can be applied to irritated skin to make it feel better, for example), but until you have diagnosed the disease, you cannot achieve a cure. The rule for nutritional deficiency

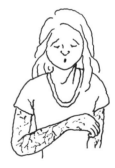

psychosomatic: a term applied to any condition of the body that originates in the mind.

psyche = mind, soul

soma = body

1   P. Budowski, Nutritional effects of ω3-polyunsaturated fatty acids, *Israel Journal of Medical Sciences* 17 (1980): 223–231.

symptoms is that, if a certain nutrient clears up the symptom, then a deficiency of that nutrient *may* have been the cause. (To be certain, you would have to remove the nutrient and see the symptom reappear, then reintroduce the nutrient and see the symptom disappear; and you would have to do the experiment "blind." See Highlight 8B).

The field of nutrition is littered with misunderstandings about the interpretations of symptoms. People may think that if you are going bald, you need pantothenic acid; that if you have wrinkles, you need vitamin C; that if your hair is turning grey, you need zinc; and (yes) that if you have a skin rash, you need linoleic acid. None of these statements is true; in fact, they are all preposterous. When someone tries to persuade you of any such relationships between symptoms and nutrients, beware. Chances are, the person either doesn't see the distinction himself, or is intentionally trying to deceive you. What you need is not a nutrient, but a correct diagnosis.

The same fallacious reasoning sometimes links *foods* with symptoms. Some people think that for prevention of colds, you need to eat oranges; for health of the digestive tract, yogurt; for sexual potency, oysters; for weight loss, grapefruits; for physical strength, beefsteak; for good eyesight, carrots; to keep the doctor away, apples; and (yes) for health of the skin, safflower oil. Actually, of course, these foods are not essential at all, although the *nutrients* in them may be, and the foods may be good sources of those nutrients. In any case, to avoid a deficiency of EFA, all you need is to eat an ordinary mixed diet; it will inevitably include some oils containing polyunsaturated fat.

The distinction between foods and nutrients has been emphasized once before (p. 2). The implication that any specific food has magical, miraculous, or curative powers is false.

For the polyunsaturated fat content of vegetable oils and other foods, see Appendix G.

Caution

The Prostaglandins

Linoleic acid and its relatives also produce prostaglandins—hormonelike compounds—in many body organs, and the prostaglandins have a multitude of diverse effects. Only recently discovered, they do not have names like other hormones (insulin, epinephrine), but are designated by letters and numbers—E_1, E_2, and so forth. One prostaglandin dilates and/or constricts blood vessels. Another alters transmission of nerve impulses. Still another modulates the body tissues' responses to other hormones. Others act on the kidney, affecting its water excretion. Another, in breast milk, helps to protect the infant's digestive tract against injury. About 100 different prostaglandins are known to be produced in the body.

prostaglandins: hormone-like compounds produced in the body from the essential fatty acids; so named because the first one to be discovered was found in association with the prostate gland.

Processed Fat

Ever since researchers first began to realize that saturated fats were linked to heart disease and that polyunsaturated fats might not be, advertisers have been proclaiming their oils and margarines as "high in polyunsaturates." Indeed, margarines made from vegetable oils and plant foods such as peanut butter do contain unsaturated fatty acids, and this is why they spread and melt more easily than foods that contain saturated fats.

Unfortunately, however, although you may gain something in health from polyunsaturated fats, you lose something in keeping quality. The more double bonds there are in a fatty acid, the more easily oxygen can destroy it. The oxidation of a fatty acid is shown in Figure 3–8. An oxygen molecule attacks the double bond and combines with the carbons at that site to yield two aldehydes. Aldehydes smell bad, giving a clue that the product has spoiled. (Other types of spoilage, due to microbial growth, can occur, too.) In general, unsaturated fatty acids are less stable than their saturated counterparts.

Marketers of fat-containing products have three alternative ways of dealing with the problem of spoilage, none perfect. They may keep their products tightly sealed away from oxygen and under refrigeration—an expensive storage system. The consumer then has to do the same, and most people prefer not to buy products that spoil readily. Marketers may also protect their products by adding preservatives such as antioxidants, but these additives, though probably not harmful, are unpopular. Finally, they may increase the products' stability by processing the fat (hardening or hydrogenating it). Figure 3–9 shows Hs being added at a double bond to hydrogenate a fat.

Hydrogenation makes fat more solid, which is often desirable. Margarine made from vegetable oils is solid at room temperature because the oils have been partially hydrogenated, and this makes it easy to work with. Hydrogenation, however, diminishes the margarine's polyunsaturated fat content and possibly, therefore, its health value. Moreover, new evidence suggests that there may be other concerns about hydrogenated oils.

If a vegetable oil is fully hydrogenated—that is, if hydrogen is added at all its double bonds—it becomes indistinguishable from a saturated fat of the same length. If, however, the oil is partially hydrogenated, then a change takes place at some of the double bonds where hydrogen was *not* added: their configuration changes from *cis* to *trans* (see Figure 3–10). One effect of this change is to create a more solid product, but double bonds are still left in the fatty acids; so the manufacturer can still say the product is unsaturated or polyunsaturated. But *trans* fatty acids are not made by the body's cells, and they are rare in foods. It is not clear that our bodies are equipped to deal with large quantities of *trans* fatty acids; the

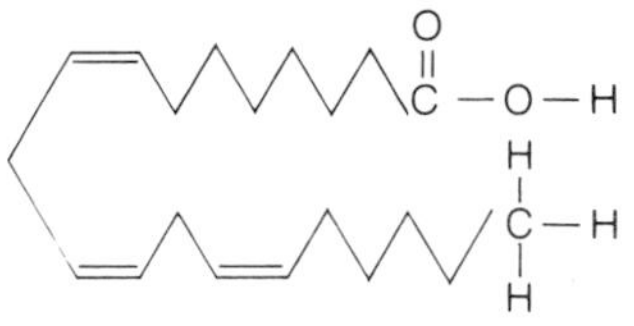

A 20-carbon essential fatty acid related to linolenic acid, from which some of the prostaglandins are made. Notice the similarity of structures.

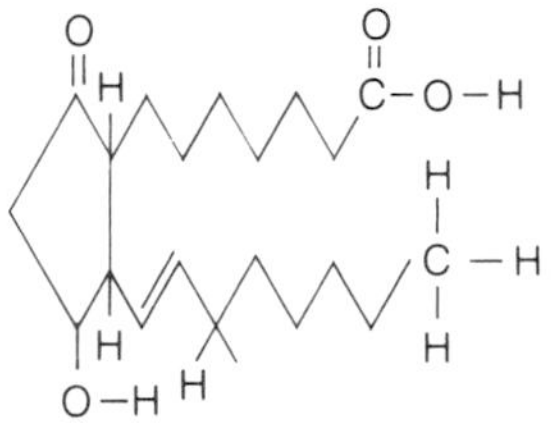

Prostaglandin E₁

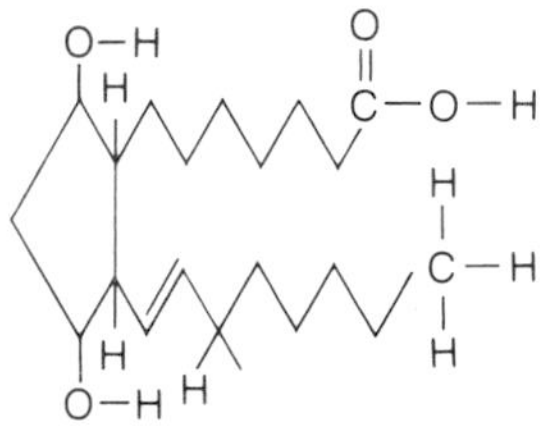

Prostaglandin F₁ₐ

Two of the prostaglandins.

aldehyde (AL-duh-hide): an organic compound containing a CHO group:

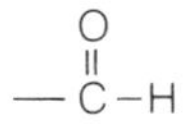

$$\overset{O}{\underset{}{\overset{\|}{-C}}}-H$$

For some questions and answers about additives, see Highlight 10. For some special notes on BHA and BHT, see Highlight 11.

FIGURE 3–8 **Oxidation of a fatty acid.** TH3-3

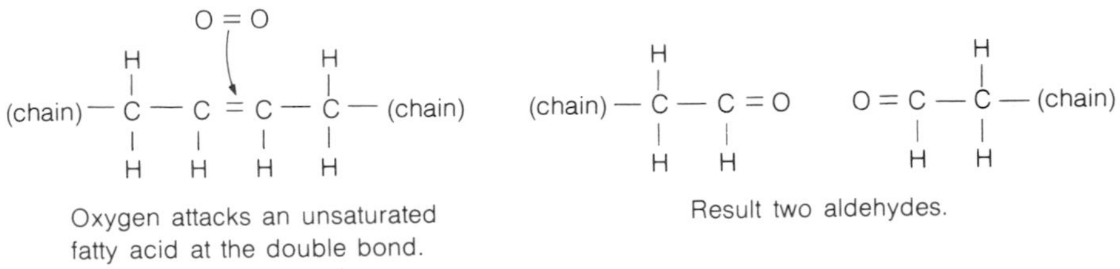

Oxygen attacks an unsaturated fatty acid at the double bond.

Result two aldehydes.

hydrogenation (high-dro-gen-AY-shun): a chemical process by which hydrogens are added to unsaturated or polyunsaturated fats to reduce the number of double bonds, making them more solid and more resistant to oxidation.

cis (sis): same side.

trans: opposite sides.

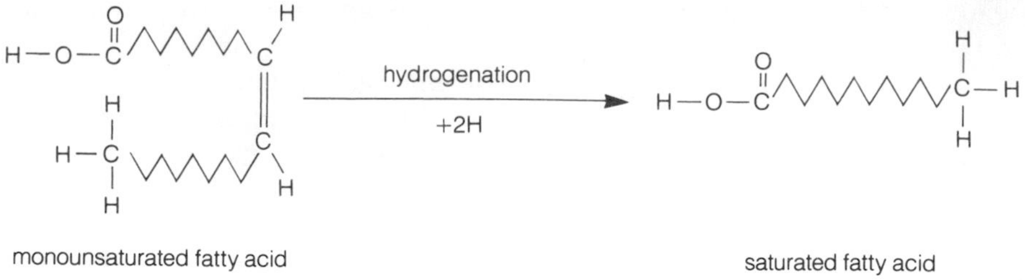

monounsaturated fatty acid

hydrogenation

+2H

saturated fatty acid

FIGURE 3–9 Hydrogenation. Hs are added at the double bond, yielding a saturated fatty acid. TH3-3

FIGURE 3–10 Formation of a *trans*-fatty acid. The starting material was the same as in Figure 3-9, but this fatty acid, instead of adding Hs, went through a *cis-trans* shift.

Almost all unsaturated fatty acids occur in nature in the *cis* form; that is, the hydrogens on the carbons adjacent to the double bond stick out on the same side of the molecule. During processing, the double bonds that do not add hydrogens may shift—something like being broken and reformed. As this happens, the hydrogens become fixed in the *trans* position—across from each other. This changes the molecule from a horseshoe shape to an extended shape that will fit together differently with other molecules in cell membranes.

This kind of change in shape occurs at double, but not at single, bonds. A double bond is like a pair of sticks between two tinker-toy wheels; the wheels can't rotate. If you attach two other structures to the wheels, they will stick out above and below them in a fixed arrangement, maintaining their positions relative to each other. You can create two distinct configurations around a rigid bond. (A single bond is like a single stick between the two wheels. The wheels can rotate around the stick, so that the configurations attached to them become identical.) TH3-3

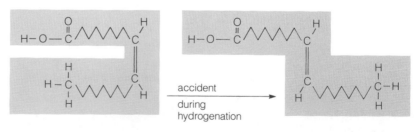

accident
during
hydrogenation

cis-fatty acid

The Hs are on the same side of the double bond, forcing the molecule to assume a horseshoe shape.

trans-fatty acid

The Hs are on opposite sides of the double bond, forcing the molecule into an extended position.

presence of these unusual molecules in our cells and tissues may create problems. As yet, this issue is poorly understood.

Some researchers believe that the presence of *trans*-fatty acids in processed fat may make consumers of that fat prone to develop certain kinds of cancer.[2] However, so many dietary factors are implicated in cancer causation that it is hard to sort them all out or to decide which are significant and which are not. Probably consumers' total fat consumption is more significant than their consumption of *trans*-fatty acids.

While the evidence on processed fats is still being collected, consumers can, if they wish, apply the principle of dilution already referred to in Chapter 1. Rather than margarine, for example, you can mix warm butter with vegetable oil in equal amounts, producing a spread that is cheaper than butter, spreads well, has the same degree of polyunsaturation as margarine but more linoleic acid, and contains no *trans*-fatty acids. As for peanut butter, it is possible to find unhydrogenated varieties on the shelf. The peanut mash and the oil may separate in these products, but you can stir them back together before using them or pour off the oil for a product lower in kcalories.

Ultimately, if fat processors wish to produce margarines free of *trans*-fatty acids, they can use an alternative process that hydrogenates double bonds without producing the *cis*-to-*trans* shift. This process is a little more expensive and technically more difficult than the one presently in use, so it has not yet been employed on a wide scale.

How the Body Handles Fat

The body has a problem in digesting and using fats—how to get at them. Substances that are soluble in fat are called water-fearing, and among these substances are, of course, the fats themselves. Fats are neutral; they carry no net charge. In any compartment of the digestive tract they tend to float to the top, clumping together and separating themselves as far as possible from the watery digestive juices. Water molecules, although they too have no net charge, are polar; that is, they have a positive side and a negative side. Enzymes have positively and negatively charged groups on their surfaces, and so they mix comfortably with the ions in water—they are water-loving. What the body needs to help mix them together is a substance that is friendly with both water-fearing and water-loving substances. The bile acids meet that need.

Manufactured by the liver and stored in the gallbladder until needed, the bile acids are released into the intestine whenever fat arrives there. Not surprisingly, they are made largely from lipids themselves. The system seems to have been designed for maximum efficiency. The more fat you eat, the more is available to manufacture the bile acids needed to prepare the fat for digestion.

Each molecule of bile acid has at one end an ionized group that is

One way to determine the degree of unsaturation of a fat is to perform a chemical test using iodine to obtain the "iodine number." The higher the iodine number, the greater the degree of unsaturation. Common oils, with their iodine numbers, are:

Safflower oil, about 140.

Most other vegetable oils, about 110–120.

Soft margarines, about 90.

Olive oil, about 75.

Hard margarines, about 70.

Butter, about 25–40.

Coconut and palm "oil," about 10–15.

If you mix safflower oil with butter, half and half, you get a spread that is soft like margarine but has no *trans*-fatty acids.

Water-fearing substances are known to chemists as **hydrophobic** or **lipophilic**.

hydro = water

phobia = fear

lipo = lipid

phile = friend

Water-loving substances are **hydrophilic**.

enzyme: a large protein molecule that facilitates the making or breaking of chemical bonds (in this case the breaking, for digestion). Enzymes are fully defined and described in Chapter 4.

bile: the emulsifying compound manufactured by the liver, stored in the gallbladder, and released into the small intestine when fat is present there. Bile contains no enzymes. It appears sometimes in acid form, sometimes in salt form; for our purposes these need not be distinguished.

2   M. G. Enig, R. J. Munn, and M. Keeney, Dietary fat and cancer trends—a critique, *Federation Proceedings* 37 (1978): 2215–2220.

attracted to water and at the other end a fatty acid chain that has an affinity for fat. Just as a skilled hostess who wants you to mix with people at her party will take your hand, draw you away from the company of your old friends, and leave you shaking hands with a new acquaintance, so a molecule of bile acid will attach itself to a lipid molecule in a droplet and draw it into the surrounding solution where it can meet an enzyme. The process is known as emulsification (see Figure 3–11).

Now, after all this preparation, the enzymes can get at the triglycerides. The enzymes digest each triglyceride by removing two of its fatty acids, leaving a monoglyceride, or by removing all three of them, leaving a molecule of glycerol. As with the carbohydrates, the digestive process requires the participation of water, as shown in Figure 3–12. Finally, the monoglycerides, glycerol, and fatty acids form tiny, spherical complexes with the bile acids and pass into the cells of the intestinal wall.

The products of lipid digestion are then released for transport through the body. Some of the larger ones are packaged in protein for this purpose. The protein-wrapped packages, called lipoproteins, are the subject of intensive research as laboratory sleuths seek to detect their structure and their relationships to heart and artery disease. The lipoproteins will appear again later in this chapter and are fully described in Chapter 5.

> **emulsify** (ee-MULL-suh-fye): to disperse and stabilize fat droplets in a watery solution.

> These complexes are the **micelles** (MY-cells). They are so small that they can fit between the tiny, hair-like microvilli of a single intestinal cell (emulsified fat particles are 100 times larger in diameter).

The Phospholipids

The preceding pages have been devoted to one of the three classes of lipids, the triglycerides. The other two classes, the phospholipids and sterols, comprise only 5 percent of the lipids in the diet, but they are nonetheless interesting and important. Among the phospholipids, the best known is lecithin (actually, there are several lecithins).

Like the triglycerides, the lecithins and the other phospholipids have a backbone of glycerol; they are different because they have only two fatty acids attached to them. In place of the third fatty acid is a molecule of choline or a similar compound containing phosphorus (P) and nitrogen (N) atoms. A diagram of a lecithin molecule is shown in the margin (others differ in the nature of the attached fatty acids).

> **phospholipid**: a compound similar to a triglyceride but having choline or another phosphorus-containing acid in place of one of the fatty acids.

> Choline: see also p. 291.

FIGURE 3–11 **Emulsification of fat by bile**. Detergents work the same way (they are also emulsifiers), which is why they are so effective in removing grease spots from clothes. Molecule by molecule, the grease is dissolved out of the spot and suspended in the water, where it can be rinsed away. You can guess where the manufacturers of "detergents with enzymes" got their idea.

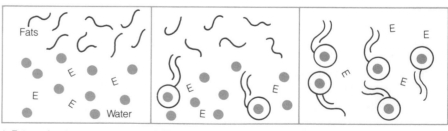

1. Fats and water separate, enzymes (E) are in water.

2. Emulsifier has affinity for fats and for water, so brings them together.

3. Emulsified fat. The enzymes now have access to the fat, which is mixed in the water solution.

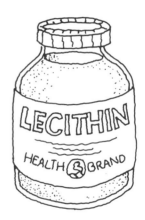

2 fatty acids

from choline

from glycerol

One of the lecithins. Others have other fatty acids on glycerol's first two carbons.

(The plus charge on the N is balanced by a negative ion—usually chloride—that stays nearby.)

"Lecithin" periodically receives noisy attention in the popular press, being credited with great good deeds. You may hear that it is a major constituent of cell membranes (true), that the functioning of all cells depends on the integrity of their membranes (true), and that you must therefore purchase bottles of lecithin and give yourself daily doses (false). You might as well believe that in order to grow healthy hair or to maintain the brain you must eat hair or brains! The enzyme lecithinase in the intestine takes lecithin apart before it passes into the body fluids anyway, so the lecithin you eat does not reach the body tissues intact. The lecithin you need for building cell membranes and for other functions is made from scratch by the liver. In other words, the lecithins are not needed in the diet—that is, they are not essential nutrients. Furthermore, although once thought to be harmless, large doses of lecithin have now been seen to cause GI upsets, sweating, salivation, and loss of appetite.[3] Perhaps these symptoms are beneficial because they serve to warn people to stop self-dosing with lecithin.

Many body compounds carry on remarkable, important functions that are exciting to read about, especially when they first make the headlines. Often hucksters immediately seize on these new discoveries by bottling preparations of these compounds and selling them, on the reasoning that "This does wonderful things for you; you must not allow yourself to become deficient in it." That might be so, but then, no one ever has been deficient in lecithin. The body makes it for itself—and the same can be said for hundreds of other miraculous compounds. Before buying bottles of lecithin or any other wonder substance, ask yourself, "Do I really need this? What is the evidence that my body is likely to be deficient?"

lecithin (LESS-uh-thin): one of the phospholipids; a compound of glycerol attached to two fatty acids and a choline molecule.

Caution

Lecithins and other phospholipids are important constituents of cell membranes. They also act as emulsifying agents, helping to keep other fats in solution in the blood and body fluids. The structure of lecithin reveals

3   J. L. Wood and R. G. Allison, Effects of consumption of choline and lecithin on neurological and cardiovascular systems, *Federation Proceedings* 41 (1982): 3015–3021.

how they can do this; the choline part of the molecule, with its plus and minus charges, is water-soluble, while the fatty acid part is fat-soluble.

FIGURE 3–12   **Digestion (hydrolysis) of a fat (triglyceride).**

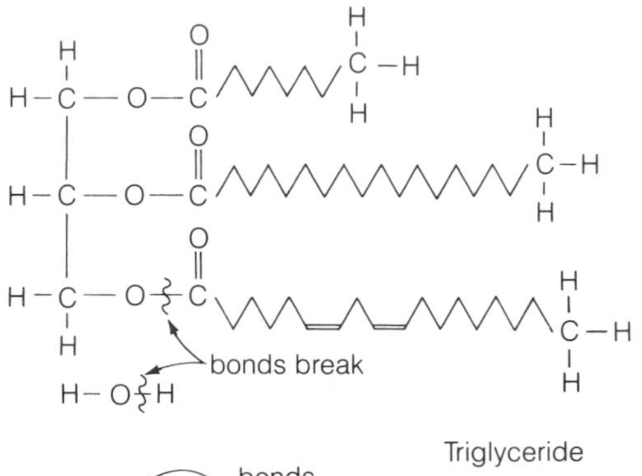

Triglyceride

1 A molecule of water splits, and the parts combine with the parts of the triglyceride, freeing a fatty acid and leaving a diglyceride.

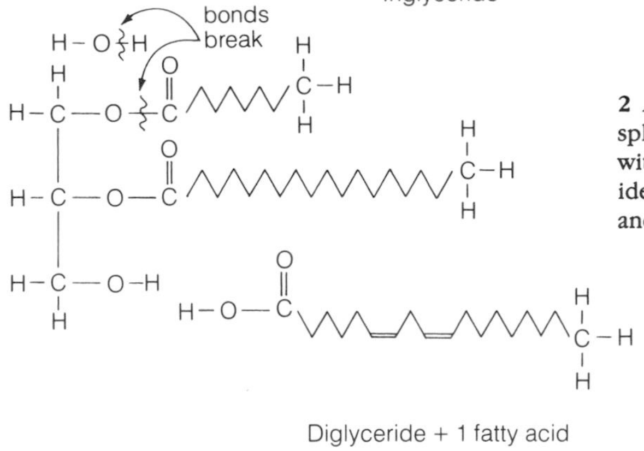

Diglyceride + 1 fatty acid

2 A second molecule of water splits, and the parts combine with the parts of the diglyceride, freeing another fatty acid and leaving a monoglyceride.

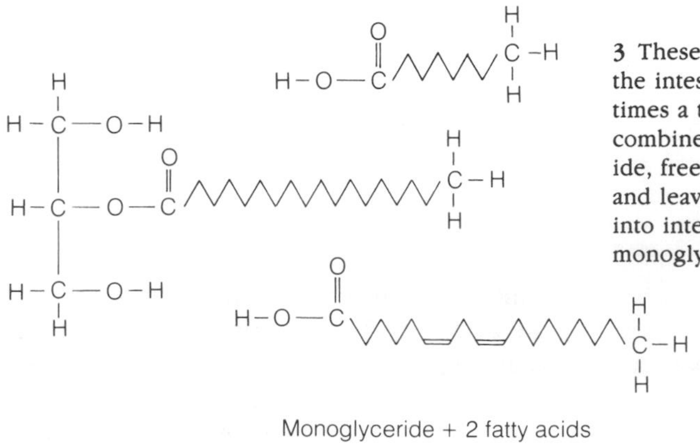

Monoglyceride + 2 fatty acids

3 These products may pass into the intestinal cells, but sometimes a third molecule of water combines with the monoglyceride, freeing a third fatty acid and leaving glycerol. Absorbed into intestinal cells: fatty acids, monoglycerides, and glycerol.

The Sterols: Cholesterol

A student observing the chemical structure of cholesterol for the first time once remarked, "Would you believe pentamethyl hydroxy chicken wire?" He was not far wrong; chemists do remarkable "terminologizing." According to them, cholesterol is a member of the cyclopentanoperhydrophenanthrene family, whose particular designation is 3-hydroxy-5,6-cholestene. Never mind. It is not necessary to memorize a structure as complex as this one. But once having viewed it, you can say, "I have seen the structure of cholesterol."

Cholesterol is not at all an unusual type of molecule. There are dozens of similar ones in the body; all are interesting and important. Among them are the bile acids, the sex hormones (such as testosterone), the adrenal hormones (such as cortisone), and vitamin D.

sterol: a compound composed of C, H, and O atoms arranged in rings like those of cholesterol, with any of a variety of side chains attached.

cholesterol: one of the sterols.

Cholesterol

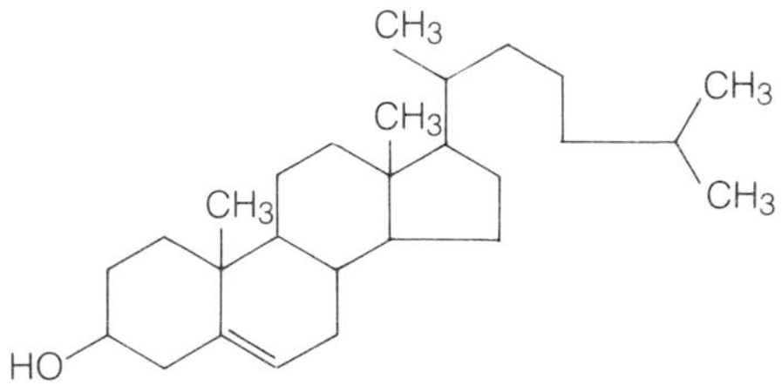

Like the lecithins, cholesterol is needed metabolically but is not an essential nutrient. Your liver is manufacturing it now, as you read, at the rate of perhaps 50,000,000,000,000,000 molecules per second. The raw materials that the liver uses to make cholesterol can all be taken from glucose or saturated fatty acids. (Another way of saying the same thing is that cholesterol can be made from either carbohydrate or fat.)

After manufacture, cholesterol either leaves the liver or is transformed into related compounds like the hormones just mentioned. The cholesterol that leaves the liver has three possible destinations:

All the carbons in cholesterol come from acetyl CoA (see Chapter 6), which in turn can be derived from many other body compounds, glucose and fatty acids among them.

● It may be made into bile and move into the intestine, and some may then be excreted in the feces.
● It may be deposited in body tissues.
● It may wind up accumulating in arteries and causing artery disease.

How Cholesterol Is Excreted

Some of the cholesterol the liver makes becomes part of the bile salts, and these are released into the intestine to emulsify fat. After doing their job, some of them reenter the body with absorbed products of fat digestion. The cholesterol is thus recycled—back to the liver, once again into bile salts, back to the intestine, again into the body, and once more back to the liver.

The recycling of cholesterol and bile is diagramed on p. 180.

Once out in the intestine, however, some of the bile salts can be trapped by certain kinds of dietary fibers, which carry them out of the body with the feces. The excretion of bile salts reduces the total amount of cholesterol remaining in the body.

How Cholesterol Is Deposited in the Body

Lipoproteins are made by both the intestine and the liver. Chapter 5 tells the whole story of lipid transport.

Some cholesterol leaves the liver packaged with other lipids for transport to the body tissues. These packages are the lipoproteins. The blood carries them through all the body's arteries, and any tissue can extract lipids from them; some cells take them up whole. More than nine-tenths of all the body's cholesterol is located in the cells, where it performs vital structural and metabolic functions.[4] To pass into the cells, lipids must first cross the artery walls, and it is in connection with the artery walls that they may be implicated in artery disease.

Artery disease—atherosclerosis—is the subject of Highlight 3.

The Fats In Foods

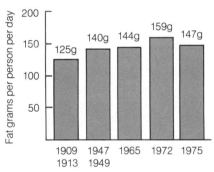

Recently, people have been eating less fat.

It seems more than likely that dietary fat (triglycerides) and possibly cholesterol are among the contributing factors in heart and artery disease. Cholesterol accumulates in arteries, and is manufactured largely from fragments derived from saturated fat. Thus, limiting your consumption of fat will do no harm, and it may do some good. And on the assumption that some of the body's cholesterol may come from the diet, it may make sense to limit your cholesterol intake as well. It is on this reasoning that three of the U.S. *Dietary Goals* and three of Canada's *Dietary Recommendations* were based (pp. 29, 31). When the *Dietary Goals* were translated into the broader *Dietary Guidelines for Americans* (p. 30), the resulting recommendation was simply to avoid excess fat, saturated fat, and cholesterol.

At the turn of the century in this country, people were eating about 125 grams of fat per day, on the average, according to a survey of the period 1909–1913. By 1972, they were eating more, 159 grams of fat each; but by 1975, they had reduced their intake somewhat and were eating 147 grams a day.[5]

This recent downturn in the consumption of total fat has been welcomed by nutritionists. They would like to believe that it has come about at least partly as a result of an intensive campaign to show the public the relationship between dietary fat and the development of cardiovascular disease (Highlight 3). Another benefit is that a lowered fat consumption may mean a reduced risk of certain kinds of cancer, for fat has been implicated in the causation of this disease as well. In the meantime, there is still much concern over the fact that fat consumption today is one-sixth higher than it

---

4   M. S. Brown and J. S. Goldstein, Lowering plasma cholesterol by raising LDL receptors (editorial), *New England Journal of Medicine* 305 (1981): 515–517.

5   C. A. Chandler and R. M. Marston, Fat in the U.S. diet, *Nutrition Program News* (a USDA periodical), May/August 1976.

was in the 1913 survey and that, until recently, heart and blood vessel diseases and cancers had also been increasing.

Food disappearance studies and diet surveys have both produced the same finding. People probably do eat about 40 to 50 percent of their kcalories as fat—more, perhaps, than they should. Those who wish to reduce and alter their dietary fat intakes need to know where the fats are found in foods.

The exchange system presented in Chapter 1 provides a useful means of learning where the fats are (see Table 1–6, p. 16). Three of the six lists in the exchange system—the milk list, the meat list, and the fat list—include foods containing appreciable amounts of fat:

● Items on the milk list contain protein, carbohydrate, and fat.
● Items on the meat list contain protein and fat (legumes contain carbohydrate as well).
● Items on the fat list contain fat only.

Figure 3–13 shows the lists that contain fat, with their portion sizes. Figure 3–14 shows how the exchange system can be used to estimate the amount of fat in a meal or in a day's meals.

The listing of milk's three fat levels emphasizes the importance of being aware of the fat content of milk. Users of the exchange system learn to think of skim milk as milk, and of low-fat and whole milk as milk with added fat.

A person studying the meat list for the first time may be surprised to note how many fat kcalories are in meat. An ounce of lean meat supplies 28

Fat values of milk—0 g for skim, 5 g for low-fat, and 10 g for whole milk (1 c).

Fat values of meat—3 g for lean, 5½ g for medium-fat, and 8 g for fat meat (1 oz); peanut butter has 15½ g in 2 tbsp.

Fat value of fat—5 g per tsp or equivalent.

FIGURE 3–13 **Foods containing fat.**

Milk list

1 c skim milk contains	0 g fat	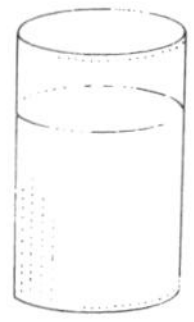
1 c 2% milk contains	5	
1 c whole milk contains	10	

10 g in 1 c whole milk

Meat list

1 oz lean meat contains	3 g fat	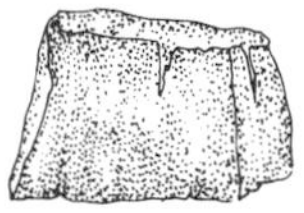
1 oz medium-fat meat contains	5½	
1 oz high-fat meat contains	8	
2 tbsp peanut butter contains	15½	

3 g in 1 oz lean meat

Fat list

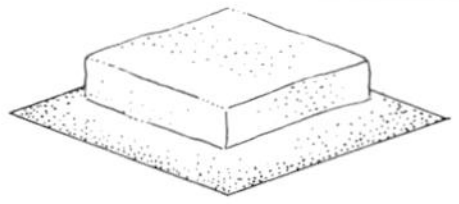

1 tsp butter or margarine (or any other serving of food on the fat list) contributes	5 g fat	

5 g in 1 pat butter or margarine

1 g protein = 4 kcal.
1 g fat = 9 kcal.

1 oz = about 30 g.

Remember that an ounce of meat is not an ounce of protein. An ounce (30 g) of lean meat contains 7 g protein and 3 g fat. The other 20 g are largely water with associated vitamins and minerals.

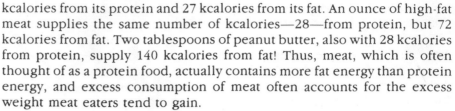

kcalories from its protein and 27 kcalories from its fat. An ounce of high-fat meat supplies the same number of kcalories—28—from protein, but 72 kcalories from fat. Two tablespoons of peanut butter, also with 28 kcalories from protein, supply 140 kcalories from fat! Thus, meat, which is often thought of as a protein food, actually contains more fat energy than protein energy, and excess consumption of meat often accounts for the excess weight meat eaters tend to gain.

Note that the unit by which meat is measured in this system is a single ounce. To use the system you need to be aware of the number of ounces in typical servings. An egg, in this system, is equivalent to 1 ounce of meat. A hamburger is usually 3 or 4 ounces. A dinner steak may be 6 or 8 ounces or even larger.

FIGURE 3–14 **How to estimate fat intake**. The values presented in Figure 3–13 provide a way to estimate the amount of fat eaten at a meal or in a day. Two reminders are needed. First, fat is often hidden in cooked vegetables; as a rule of thumb, vegetables served with butter or margarine can be assumed to contain one fat exchange per half-cup serving. Second, some baked goods also contain appreciable fat; you can find them on the bread list in Appendix L.

Using these values, let us see how much fat was provided by the day's meals described on p. 64. Adding up the meat exchanges for the egg, peanut butter, and steak; taking into account the extra fat in these meats, the whole milk, and the shortcake biscuit; adding the fat used in frying the egg and flavoring the beans and potato; and finally adding a fat exchange for the heavy cream—we reach a total of 109 grams of fat for the day:

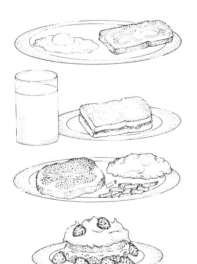

	FAT-CONTAINING EXCHANGES	FAT (g)
Breakfast		
1 egg fried in 1 tsp fat	1 meat + 1½ fat	10½
1 slice toast with 1 tsp margarine	1 fat	5
Lunch		
2 slices bread		
2 tbsp peanut butter	1 meat + 2½ fat	15½
2 tsp jelly		
1 c milk	2 fat	10
Dinner		
6-oz steak	6 meat + 6 fat	48
½ c green beans served with 1 tsp margarine	1 fat	5
1 c mashed potato served with 1 tsp margarine	1 fat	5
Dessert		
2-inch diameter biscuit	1 fat	5
¾ c strawberries		
1 tbsp heavy cream	1 fat	5
6 tsp sugar		
Total		109 g fat (rounded off)

The day's meals thus supplied about 981 kcalories from fat (9 × 109). The day's total from all these foods was about 1,930 kcalories, so the eater consumed about 50 percent of her kcalories from fat.

To focus on the members of the fat list for a moment, everyone knows that butter, margarine, and oil belong there, but it can be a surprise to discover that bacon, olives, and avocados are also on the list. These foods are listed together because the amount of lipid they contain makes them essentially contributors of pure fat. An eighth of an avocado or one slice of bacon contains as much fat as a pat of butter, and like butter, these foods contain negligible protein and carbohydrate. Hence, when you eat them, you are not eating protein-rich foods; you are eating fat-rich foods.

Saturated Fat and Cholesterol in Foods

The fat in milk is mostly saturated fat; the cholesterol content is 25 milligrams per cup of whole milk or 7 milligrams per cup of skim milk. Thus, choosing skim in place of whole milk reduces your intakes of both saturated fat and cholesterol.

The fats in meats and eggs are mostly saturated; those in poultry and fish have a better balance between saturated and polyunsaturated fats. (Tables showing the saturated and unsaturated fats in foods are in Appendix G.) As for cholesterol, the foods that contain the highest amounts are such organ meats as liver and kidneys and such shellfish as lobster, oysters, and shrimp. Lower but still detectable levels of cholesterol are contained in beef, ham, lamb, veal, and pork, followed by poultry and fish. (The cholesterol contents of foods are also shown in Appendix G.) As a general rule, a meat-eater wishing to reduce both saturated fat and cholesterol intake could accomplish these objectives by eating less meat and more poultry and fish (except shellfish). A vegetarian who uses animal products could shift to skim milk and low-fat cheeses, and could limit butter and egg intake. Pure vegetarians eat a diet very low in fat and consume no cholesterol, because plant foods do not contain it.

Eggs contain about 240 milligrams of cholesterol each, all of it in the yolk. For a person trying to adhere strictly to a low-cholesterol diet, the use of eggs has to be curtailed. For most people trying to lower blood cholesterol, however, it is not as effective to limit cholesterol intake as to limit saturated fat intake. Evidence on the blood-cholesterol-raising effect of eggs has been contradictory. Some experiments have seemed to show that subjects could eat several eggs a day for days at a time without their blood cholesterol's changing. Others have seemed to show that blood levels would rise if enough eggs were eaten.[6] In any case, eggs are an inexpensive, high quality protein source, and should probably not be eliminated from most people's diets, only cut back.

The degree of saturation of a fat determines how hard it is at a given temperature. Thus, you can tell one fat is more saturated than another if it is harder, say, at room temperature. Chicken fat, for example, is softer than

A low-cholesterol diet might allow only 300 mg cholesterol a day or less. (The U.S. *Dietary Goals* suggested this limit.)

Saturated fats have a high melting point and are solid at room or body temperature.

Polyunsaturated fats have a low melting point and are liquid at room or body temperature.

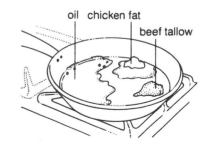
oil   chicken fat   beef tallow

The most polyunsaturated fat melts soonest.

6   The first of these articles says eggs increase serum cholesterol; the second says that, at least in the context of a normal diet, they don't. S. L. Roberts, M. P. McMurry, and W. E. Connor, Does egg feeding (i.e., dietary cholesterol) affect plasma cholesterol levels in humans? The results of a double-blind study, *American Journal of Clinical Nutrition* 34 (1981): 2092–2099; T. R. Dawber, R. J. Nickerson, F. N. Brand, and J. Pool, Eggs, serum cholesterol, and coronary heart disease, *American Journal of Clinical Nutrition* 36 (1982): 617–625.

pork fat, which is softer than beef tallow. Of the three, beef tallow is the most saturated and chicken fat the least saturated. Polyunsaturated fats melt more readily. Generally speaking, vegetable and fish oils are rich in polyunsaturates, whereas the harder fats—animal fats—are more saturated.

If you wish to make choices consistent with the *Goals* or *Guidelines*, you should learn how to read food labels. But beware. Words like *vegetable fat* and *unsaturated fat* can be used to mislead you. Not all vegetable oils are polyunsaturated. Coconut oil, for example, is often used in nondairy creamers, and coconut oil is a saturated fat. Vegetable oils that are hydrogenated may have lost their polyunsaturated character. Another exception to the rule is olive oil, widely used in salad dressings and in Greek and Italian foods. The predominant fatty acid in olive oil is the *mono*unsaturated fatty acid oleic acid. Thus olive oil can claim to be *un*saturated but not to be *poly*unsaturated.

Caution

NONDAIRY CREAMER
contains vegetable fat

Ingredients:
corn syrup solids, hydrogenated vegetable oils (palm kernel, coconut)

Here's the truth. Notice, too, that sugar is listed first!

Each culture has its own favorite food sources of fats and oils. In Canada, rapeseed oil is widely used. The peoples of the Mediterranean (Greeks, Italians, and Spaniards) rely heavily on olive oil, and Orientals use the polyunsaturated oil of soybeans. Jewish cookery traditionally employs chicken fat, whereas U.S. Southerners rely heavily on pork fat—lard and bacon.[7] Elsewhere in the United States, butter and margarine are widely used, and with the recent popularity of fast foods, vegetable oil use has also been increasing.

Artificial Fat: Sucrose Polyester

An artificial fat is beginning to attract public attention, although it is not yet on the market. Invented in the late 1960s, sucrose polyester (SPE) is a synthetic combination of sucrose and fatty acids that looks, feels, and tastes like food fat. Unlike either sucrose or fatty acids alone, however, sucrose polyester is indigestible; the body has no way to take it apart. It can therefore be substituted for fats in meals without adding kcalories or promoting a rise in consumers' blood fat levels.

Tests with animals and human beings so far indicate that SPE is safe. Most human subjects are unable to tell the difference between SPE margarine and regular margarine, or between SPE oil and regular oil. Obese subjects find it as satisfying as regular fat in meals and appear not to increase their

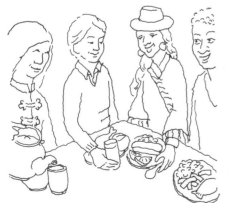

---

7   The saturated fat consumption of blacks is cause for special concern among health authorities, who note a high incidence of heart disease, both atherosclerosis and high blood pressure, among these people. This high rate of heart disease may be diet-related, genetically caused, or both. High blood pressure is related to salt (sodium) intake in some people; thus the *Dietary Goals* and the *Guidelines* recommend limiting salt intake, a matter taken up in Chapter 10.

kcalorie intakes to compensate for the kcalories they lose by not having regular fat.[8]

Undesirable side effects of SPE use have yet to be discovered. It might, for example, carry fat-soluble vitamins out of the body with it, causing deficiencies. Further tests will tell. But given that high blood cholesterol and obesity are two of our major health problems, SPE is being viewed with hope as a possible help in the treatment of both.

Summing Up

Lipids in the body, both fats and oils, function to maintain the health of the skin and hair, to protect body organs from heat, cold, and mechanical shock, and to provide a continuous fuel supply. The oxidation of one pound of body fat supplies 3,500 kcalories to meet energy needs.

In foods, fats and oils act as a solvent for the fat-soluble vitamins and the compounds that give foods their flavor and aroma. About 95 percent of the lipids in the diet are triglycerides; the phospholipids and sterols make up the other 5 percent. Triglycerides are composed of glycerol with three fatty acids attached. The fatty acids may be long-chain, medium-chain, or short-chain fatty acids, and they may be classified as saturated, monounsaturated, or polyunsaturated. Any combination of fatty acids is possible in a fat or oil.

Linoleic acid is both the most common and most important of the polyunsaturated fatty acids in foods. The body is unable to synthesize it; therefore, it is an essential fatty acid. Linolenic acid and arachidonic acid are also classified by some authorities with linoleic acid as essential. Deficiency symptoms of the essential fatty acids include dermatitis, increased incidence of infection and dehydration, and liver abnormalities. The essential fatty acids also serve as precursors for the hormone-like prostaglandins.

Food fats containing unsaturated fatty acids spoil easily. Hydrogenation makes these acids less susceptible to oxidation; but in partial hydrogenation, *trans*-fatty acids, which may have an adverse effect on health, are formed.

During digestion, the triglycerides are emulsified by bile and then hydrolyzed by enzymes to monoglycerides, glycerol, and fatty acids, which then pass into the intestinal cells. After absorption, all three classes of lipids are transported by lipoproteins in the body fluids.

Cholesterol, a sterol, is synthesized in the body by the liver. Most of this cholesterol becomes bile salts, used to emulsify fats. Cholesterol from the liver may be transported to body tissues via the lipoproteins and may also be abnormally deposited in artery walls. A diet high in saturated fat and cholesterol has been implicated as a causative factor in atherosclerosis. Some authorities recommend limiting excess fat, saturated fat, and cholesterol as a preventive measure.

---

8   R. Carol, Sucrose polyester—a synthetic fat substitute? *ACSH News and Views*, March/April 1983, p. 10.

In the exchange system, foods that contain fat are found on the meat list, the milk list, and the fat list. Most of the saturated fat found in the diet comes from meat and animal fats. Cholesterol is contributed by organ meats, shellfish, eggs, meats, and animal fats. No plant product contains cholesterol. Vegetable and fish oils generally contain more polyunsaturated fats than do animal fats.

A new product, sucrose polyester (an artificial fat), is indigestible, and therefore may be substituted in the diet without adding fat or kcalories. Sucrose polyester has not yet been approved for use by the general public.

NOTE: References recommended for further reading are in Appendix J; see "Fats and Oils."

Self-study exercises in Appendix Q show you how to:

● Estimate your fat consumption and evaluate its quality.
● Calculate your intakes of essential fatty acids and cholesterol.
● Discover visually how much fat you consume daily.

The *Instructor's Manual* includes an extra transparency/handout master to give practice in estimating fat in meals. TH 3-4 It also includes a supplementary lecture, "Nutrition and Cancer," which explores some of the relationships between dietary fat and cancer causation.

HIGHLIGHT 3
Nutrition and Atherosclerosis

The single most important approach to alleviating almost any disease is the reduction of stress. . . . Better still is the elimination of constant worry about your heart, plus the restoration of relaxation and pleasure to your mealtimes. Enjoy food rather than fear it.

EDWARD R. PINCKNEY AND
CATHEY PINCKNEY

More than half the people who die in the United States each year die of heart and blood vessel disease. The underlying condition that contributes to most of these deaths is artery disease, which is so widespread it has been called an epidemic. What are its causes? How can it be prevented? Can it be reversed?[1]

Artery disease often begins with a condition called hardening of the arteries, or atherosclerosis. In atherosclerosis, soft mounds of lipid accumulate along the inner walls of the arteries. These plaques gradually enlarge, making the artery walls lose their elasticity and narrowing the passage through them.

Normally, blood surges through the arteries with each beat of the heart, and the arteries expand with each pulse to accommodate the flow. Arteries hardened and narrowed by plaques cannot expand, and so the blood pressure rises. The increased pressure puts a strain on the heart and damages the artery walls further.

As pressure builds up in an artery, the arterial wall may become weakened and balloon out, forming an aneurysm. An aneurysm can burst, and when this happens in a major artery such as the aorta, it leads to massive bleeding and death.

In addition to being elastic, the inner walls of the arteries must be glass-smooth so that the blood can move over the surface with as little friction as possible. Clotting of blood is an intricate series of events triggered when the blood moves past a rough surface, such as the edge of a cut. As long as the inner wall remains smooth, clots will not form in it, but if the plaques encroach on the inside of the vessel, their roughness can cause clotting reactions to begin (see Figures H3–1 and H3–2).

atherosclerosis (ath-er-oh-scler-OH-sis): a type of artery disease characterized by patchy nodular thickenings of the inner walls of the arteries, especially at branch points.

> *athero* = porridge (soft)
>
> *scleros* = hard
>
> *osis* = too much

plaques (PLACKS): mounds of lipid material, mixed with smooth muscle cells and calcium, which are lodged in the artery walls. The same word is also used to describe an entirely different kind of accumulation of material on teeth, which promotes dental caries.

aneurysm (AN-you-rism): the ballooning out of an artery wall at a point where it has been weakened by deterioration.

aorta (ay-OR-tuh): the large, primary artery that conducts blood from the heart to the body's smaller arteries.

1   This Highlight is adapted from E. M. N. Hamilton and E. N. Whitney, Highlight 5A: Atherosclerosis, in *Nutrition: Concepts and Controversies*, 2nd ed. (St. Paul, Minn.: West, 1982), pp. 132–139.

A stationary clot is called a **throm-bus**. When it has grown enough to close off a blood vessel, it is a **thrombosis**. A **coronary thrombosis** is the closing off of a vessel that feeds the heart muscle. A **cerebral throm-bosis** is the closing off of a vessel that feeds the brain.

coronary = crowning (the heart)

thrombo = clot

cerebrum = part of the brain

A thrombus that breaks loose is an **embolus** (EM-boh-luss), and when it causes sudden closure of a blood vessel, it is an **embolism**.

embol = to insert

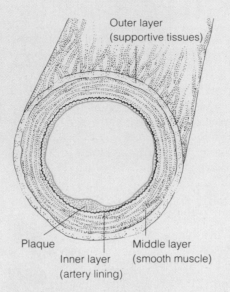
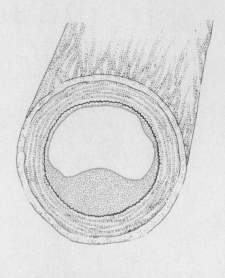
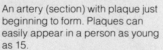

Outer layer (supportive tissues)

Plaque

Inner layer (artery lining)

Middle layer (smooth muscle)

An artery (section) with plaque just beginning to form. Plaques can easily appear in a person as young as 15.

The same artery, years later, half blocked by plaque.

FIGURE H3–1 **Development of atherosclerosis.** For photographs of real arteries with and without plaques, see Figure H3–2.

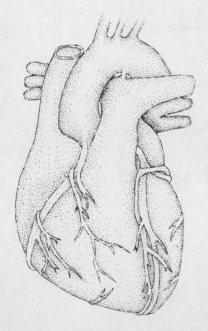

The heart gets its nutrients and oxygen not from inside its chambers but from arteries that lie on its surface. These are the coronary arteries.

The clot thus formed may linger, attached to a plaque, and gradually grow until it shuts off the blood supply to that portion of the tissue supplied by the artery. That tissue may die slowly and be replaced by scar tissue. Or the clot may break loose and travel along the system until it reaches an artery too small to allow its passage. Then the tissues fed by this artery will be robbed of oxygen and nutrients and will die suddenly. When such a clot lodges in an artery of the heart, causing sudden death of part of the heart muscle, we say the person had a heart attack. When the clot lodges in an artery of the brain, killing a portion of brain tissue, we call the event a stroke.

Atherosclerosis begins early. Fatty streaks have been observed in the aortas of infants less than a year old, and plaques are well developed in most individuals by the time they are thirty. No one is free of the condition.[2] The question is not whether you have it but how far advanced it is and what you can do to retard or reverse it.

2   R. L. Holman, H. C. McGill, J. P. Strong, and J. C. Greer, The natural history of atherosclerosis: The early aortic lesions as seen in New Orleans in the middle of the 20th century, *American Journal of Pathology* 34 (1958): 209–234.

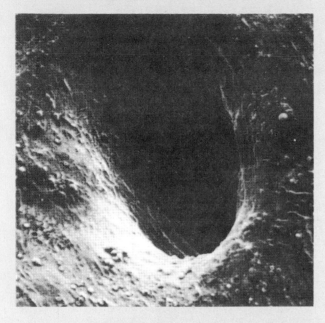

A. A healthy artery provides an open passage for the flow of blood.

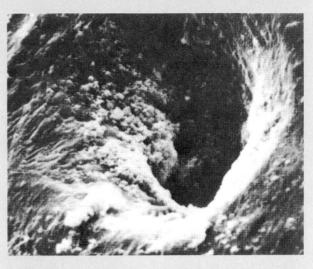

B. Plaques along an artery narrow its diameter and obstruct blood flow. Clots can form, aggravating the problem.

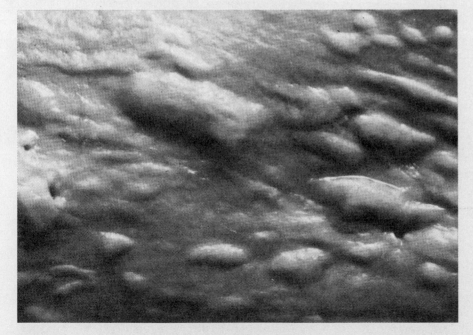

C. Atherosclerotic inner surface of a human artery that has been slit open (magnified 2.5 times). The lumps are the plaques.

FIGURE H3–2 **Plaques in arteries.**

Sources (A and B): Reproduced by permission. Original material provided by Abel L. Robertson, M.D., Ph.D., University of Illinois at Chicago, Dept. of Pathology, College of Medicine, Chicago, IL 60612.

Source (C): From *Scientific American* 236 (1977): 75. Reprinted by permission of Scientific American Inc.

Miniglossary of Heart Disease Terms

angina (an-JYE-nuh; some people say ANN-juh-nuh): pain in the heart region caused by lack of oxygen.

CAD (coronary artery disease): another term for CHD.

CHD (coronary heart disease): atherosclerosis in the arteries feeding the heart muscle.

CVA (cerebrovascular accident): a stroke or aneurysm in the brain.

CVD (cardiovascular disease): a general term for all diseases of the heart and blood vessels. Atherosclerosis is the main form of CVD.

IHD (ischemic heart disease): another term for atherosclerosis and its relatives.

ischemia (iss-SHE-me-uh): the deterioration and death of tissue (for example, of heart muscle), often caused by atherosclerosis.

myocardial infarct (MI) (my-oh-CARD-ee-ul in-FARKT): the sudden shutting off of the blood flow to the heart muscle by a thrombus or embolism; the same as a heart attack.
  myo = muscle
  cardium = heart
  infarct = blocking off

occlusion (ock-CLOO-zhun): shutting off of the blood flow in an artery.

multifactorial: having many causes.

risk factors: factors known to be related to (or correlated with) a disease but not proven to be causal.

Atherosclerosis takes its heaviest toll among men in the most productive period of their lives. Many health agencies have devoted millions of hours to the battle against atherosclerosis, but so far all that can be said for sure about its causes is that it is multifactorial in origin. There are many risk factors—perhaps 30 or so in all. The relationships among these many factors are not at all clear. They are only correlations; we do not know what causes what. Furthermore, we do not know whether reducing any of the risk factors will actually reduce the risk of dying of the disease.

An analogy may help to make clear the point being made here about correlations and causes. Suppose that there is an outbreak of crime in a certain city—arson, for example. Someone is setting fires, and the police are after him. It is observed that a certain person, Mr. A, is always seen in the neighborhoods when the fires start, and he is deemed guilty of the crimes. However, it may be that a very sneaky individual, Ms. B, is the real culprit, and that Mr. A is only following her around. Mr. A is associated with, but is not a causal agent in, the setting of the fires. The evidence against him is only circumstantial (correlational). If the police can show that whenever he is locked up there are no fires and that whenever he is let out the fires start again, the evidence against him will be stronger. Better yet, they will know for sure if they catch him pouring the gasoline and lighting the match. You may recall that this point has been made before; correlation is not cause. Be careful when you interpret data that imply a causal relationship between factors linked only by association.

Caution

Risk Factor Studies

Among the many factors linked to atherosclerosis are: smoking, gender (being male), heredity (including diabetes), high blood pressure, lack of exercise, obesity, stress, high blood cholesterol, many nutrient excesses and deficiencies, personality characteristics, and more. Some of the risk factors are powerful predictors of heart disease. If you have none of them, the statistical likelihood of your developing CVD may be only 1 in 100. If you have three major ones, the chance may rise to over 1 in 20. Table H3–1 shows one way of calculating your risk score.

TABLE H3–1   **Your Risk of Heart Disease**

	H	E	A	R	T
Everyone plays the game of health whether he wants to or not. What is your score? Add up the numbers in each category that most nearly describe you.					
Heredity	1 No known history of heart disease	2 One relative with heart disease over 60 years	3 Two relatives with heart disease over 60 years	4 One relative with heart disease under 60 years	6 Two relatives with heart disease under 60 years
Exercise	1 Intensive exercise, work, and recreation	2 Moderate exercise, work, and recreation	3 Sedentary work and intensive recreational exercise	5 Sedentary work and moderate recreational exercise	6 Sedentary work and light recreational exercise
Age	1 10–20	2 21–30	3 31–40	4 41–50	6 51–65
Lbs.	0 More than 5 lbs below standard weight	1 ±5 lbs standard weight	2 6–20 lbs overweight	4 21–35 lbs overweight	6 36–50 lbs overweight
Tobacco	0 Nonuser	1 Cigar or pipe	2 10 cigarettes or fewer per day	4 20 cigarettes or more per day	6 30 cigarettes or more per day
Habits of eating fat	1 0% No animal or solid fats	2 10% Very little animal or solid fats	3 20% Little animal or solid fats	4 30% Much animal or solid fats	6 40% Very much animal or solid fats

Your risk of heart attack:
 4–9 Very remote   16–20 Average   26–30 Dangerous
10–15 Below average   21–25 Moderate   31–35 Urgent danger—reduce score!
Other conditions—such as stress, high blood pressure, and increased blood cholesterol—detract from heart health and should be evaluated by your physician.

Source: Courtesy of Loma Linda University.

High blood cholesterol is any value over 220 mg/100 ml. Blood cholesterol levels considered normal in the United States range from 140 to 260 mg/100 ml, with younger people having lower values—but while these values are "normal," they may not be desirable.

Blood pressure values between 100/60 and 130/80 are considered normal.

In a **retrospective study**, researchers study a number of people now, and look back at their history to see what may account for the differences among them. In a **prospective study**, researchers take measurements on a number of people now, and then wait for some years to see what differences arise among them.

Three factors have emerged as the major predictors of risk:

- Smoking.
- High blood cholesterol.
- High blood pressure.

From statistics pooled from many studies on these risk factors, the American Heart Association has published the *Coronary Risk Handbook*, a small portion of which is shown in Table H3–2. The table illustrates dramatically that the chances of having a healthy heart and arteries are much greater if you don't smoke and your blood cholesterol and blood pressure are low.[3]

Millions of dollars and decades of effort by hundreds of researchers have yielded many positive findings from risk factor research. Still, as mentioned, the ultimate causes of CVD are unknown. The kind of problem that repeatedly hinders research is illustrated by the story of an investigation conducted in Britain.

The researchers, who wanted to relate physical activity to heart attack risk, chose to study bus drivers and bus conductors. They did find, as expected, that the more active people—the conductors—suffered fewer heart attacks than did the sedentary ones—the drivers. They might have been tempted to conclude that they had found the relationship they were looking for: "Less activity leads to more heart attacks." But they looked further and found that the drivers were also fatter than the conductors. Perhaps the relationship was: "Less activity leads to more obesity leads to more heart attacks." They checked further still, however, and found that the drivers had been fatter than the conductors when they started work years before. The conclusion had to be rephrased: "Fatter people choose less active work." But what, then, caused the heart disease? Conceivably, the drivers might have been headed for CVD as children, even before they became obese. What comes first? Inactivity? No—in this study, it was obesity. What comes before obesity?[4]

The problem illustrated by this study is one that plagues the researcher who is trying to untangle a chain of events and find its beginning. You can see that conclusions drawn from research like this are somewhat shaky. They can always be criticized on the basis that they are retrospective (looking back), so that the researcher cannot tell whether the people who developed the condition might have been self-selected —might have gotten onto the track headed toward heart disease long before the differences (in occupation, for example) were observed. To be free of this criticism, such a study should be "prospective." A matched group of people should be selected for study and then fol-

3 M. F. Oliver, Diet and coronary heart disease, *British Medical Bulletin* 37 (1981): 49–58. Oliver sets the upper limit of normal for blood cholesterol at 220 milligrams per 100 milliliters.

4 J. Gorman, A running argument: Does physical activity help prevent heart attacks? *The Sciences*, January/February 1977, pp. 10–15.

TABLE H3–2 **Risk of Developing CVD within Six Years**.
This portion of the table shows the effect of the three major risk factors alone and in combination for a 45-year-old man.

SMOKER	CHOLESTEROL (mg/100ml[a])	BLOOD PRESSURE (mm mercury[b])	RISK (per 100)
No	185	105	1.5
No	185	195	4.4
No	335	195	16.7
Yes	335	195	23.9

[a]Milligrams of cholesterol per 100 milliliters of blood.
[b]The first of the two numbers recorded (for example, 120 in 120/70). The silver column that rises on a blood-pressure instrument is a column of mercury; the height to which it is pushed is marked off in millimeters.
Source: U.S. Senate, Select Committee on Nutrition and Human Needs, *Diet Related to Killer Diseases II, Part 1, Cardiovascular Disease*, Washington, D.C.: Government Printing Office, 1977.

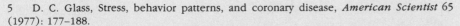

lowed through time to see what differences develop. Understanding this sampling problem in research will help you evaluate the results of other studies like this one.

Caution

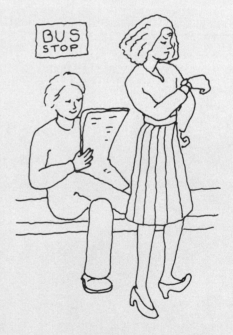

Another complicating factor has already been mentioned in connection with the sugar-and-diabetes relationship discussed in Highlight 2—the problem of interpreting epidemiological studies. It can be demonstrated that in many countries where the diets are low in fat the incidence of heart and artery disease is much lower than it is in the United States and Canada. But to attribute the difference in disease rates to the differing diets would be naive. Many other factors also present in developed countries may play a role: urban life; lack of exercise; indeed, lifestyles that differ in many, many respects.

It can be argued that the risk factors all reflect an underlying prior condition. Psychologists point to personality type, and especially the way the person responds to stress, as a potent predictor of risk.[5] People of the personality type called "Type A" are notorious for being heart-attack prone. A Type A person is competitive, strives for achievement, has a sense of time urgency, is inclined to be hostile, suppresses the feeling of fatigue—in short, is uptight, as compared with the more easygoing Type B person. In one type of research, people are scored A or B first and then followed up. The Type A people are found to have more than twice the rate of heart disease that the Type B people have.[6] This is prospective research, and the A-versus-B difference shows up even when the three major risk factors already mentioned are taken into account.

5   D. C. Glass, Stress, behavior patterns, and coronary disease, *American Scientist* 65 (1977): 177–188.

6   R. H. Rosenman, R. H. Rahe, N. O. Borhanie, and M. Feinleib, Heritability of personality and behavior pattern, *Proceedings of the First International Congress on Twins*, Rome, 1975, as cited by Glass, 1977.

Type A people's heart disease seems to arise in the classic way: by blockage of the arteries. The way they react physically to stress may account for the damage. The stress hormones affect blood pressure and blood lipid levels, so the key to prevention may lie in study of the hormones or of the stress response.

Intervention Studies

While research goes on, people want to know what to do *now* to prevent this devastating disease that kills one out of every two people. To find out what to do, researchers design intervention studies. Studies of this kind involve tinkering with a cluster of factors (like the obesity–inactivity–smoking–high blood pressure–cholesterol cluster) by altering the items one by one and seeing if any of these alterations leads to reduction in deaths from CVD. A successful intervention study is a major step forward in research; it helps to demonstrate that a risk factor not only accompanies but causes a disease.

In some massive intervention studies conducted during the 1970s, thousands of men were persuaded to give up smoking, take medication to reduce their blood pressure (if it was high), and alter their diets to reduce their blood cholesterol levels. These studies were complicated by a curious problem, however: everyone else was doing those same things. Word had gotten around to the whole U.S. population that these measures were beneficial. The intervention studies failed to show significant improvement of the experimental groups over controls, perhaps because there *were* no good controls. A retrospective analysis of the impressive downturn in the rate of deaths from CVD between the late 1960s and the late 1970s suggests that a massive, unintentional intervention study may have been spontaneously conducted by the whole U.S. population.

In any case, something certainly seems to have happened in that ten-year period that saved 200,000 lives.[7] At a major conference held in 1979, the experts who had been following the lifestyle changes and trends among people in the United States reported that as a people:

1 We are smoking less.[8]
2 We are controlling our blood pressure better.[9]
3 Our blood cholesterol levels have fallen slightly.[10]
4 We are exercising more.[11]

7   R. Levy, Introduction, in *Proceedings of the Conference on the Decline in Coronary Heart Disease Mortality*, ed. R. J. Havlik and M. Feinleib, U.S. Department of Health, Education, and Welfare, Public Health Service, National Institutes of Health, NIH publication no. 79-1610, May 1979, p. 1.

8   J. C. Kleinman, J. J. Feldman, and M. A. Monk, Trends in smoking and ischemic heart disease mortality, in Havlik and Feinleib, 1979, pp. 195-211.

9   N. O. Borhanie, Mortality trend in hypertension, United States, 1950–1976, in Havlik and Feinleib, 1979, pp. 218–235.

10   R. Beaglehole and coauthors, Secular changes in blood cholesterol and their contribution to the decline in coronary mortality, in Havlik and Feinleib, 1979, pp. 282–297.

11   R. S. Paffenbarger, Jr., Countercurrents of physical activity and heart attack trends, in Havlik and Feinleib, 1979, pp. 298–311.

In other words, independently of the research studies, people have been taking measures that are paying off in lower mortality.[12]

The evidence from review of this happening suggests that reduction of risk factors is advisable for all members of the population, not just for the most heart-attack prone. If you divide the population into five groups, from the lowest to the highest risk, more than half the preventable heart disease deaths appear to be in the *middle* three groups.

Which of the risk factors is most important? The balance sheet may look like this:

● A fourth of the reduced risk comes from a moderate reduction in blood cholesterol.
● A fourth comes from better control of high blood pressure, primarily by drugs but also by diet.
● Half comes from a decrease in the prevalence of cigarette smoking.[13]

The rest of this Highlight focuses on reducing blood cholesterol (see Chapter 10 for more on blood pressure).

How to Lower Blood Cholesterol

Let us first clarify one point: which cholesterol we are talking about. The public has been very much confused by a failure to distinguish between *dietary* cholesterol and *blood*, or *serum*, cholesterol. We are talking about *blood*, or *serum*, cholesterol.

Two kinds of lipid in foods are emphasized when people talk about CVD:

● Dietary fat (triglycerides, saturated or unsaturated).
● Dietary cholesterol.

Similarly, two kinds of lipid in the blood (serum) are traditionally talked about in connection with CVD:

● Serum triglycerides.
● Serum cholesterol.

We might call the first pair "the fat on the plate" and the second, "the fat in the blood." The question to ask, then, is "What fat on the plate contributes most to the fat in the blood?" The answer is not dietary cholesterol (that in eggs, shellfish, liver, and the like). The important relationship is this: saturated fat (on the plate) raises cholesterol (in the blood). People often fail to understand this point, and the question arises again and again: "Should I eat cholesterol?" When told, "It doesn't matter much," the questioner often jumps to the wrong conclusion, the conclusion that cholesterol doesn't matter. It does matter. High *serum* cholesterol is an indica-

Blood, plasma, and *serum* cholesterol all refer to about the same thing, at least when speaking of cholesterol.

---

12   J. Stamler, reporting for R. Byington and colleagues, Recent trends of major coronary risk factors and CHD mortality in the United States and other industrialized countries, in Havlik and Feinleib, 1979, pp. 340–380.

13   Remember, this refers to the reduced risk from CVD only. If risk of death from all causes is measured, serum cholesterol becomes relatively less important—4 percent—and cigarette smoking considerably more important—65 percent. And exercise is not included because it isn't one of the "big three" in the heart disease picture. Stamler, 1979.

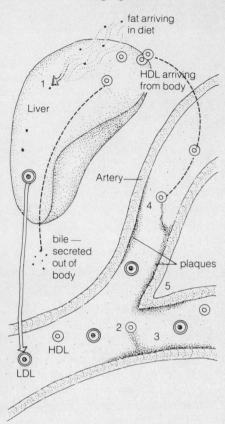

FIGURE H3-3 **Factors influencing plaque formation**. These are a few of the more important factors thought to contribute to atherosclerosis. TH3-5

tor of risk for CVD, and the main food factor associated with it is a high saturated *fat intake*.

Figure H3-3 shows how a plaque is formed and the role blood cholesterol is thought to play in the process. There are two vehicles in the blood that carry this substance, the low-density lipoproteins, or LDL, and the high-density lipoproteins, or HDL (see Chapter 5). It is the LDL that are associated with heart disease risk; and as it turns out, the changes in diet that reduce serum cholesterol concentrations mostly do so by reducing LDL, not HDL.[14]

By far the most influential factor would appear to be:

● Saturated fat—which raises serum cholesterol (LDL).

Next comes:

● Monounsaturated fat and especially polyunsaturated fat—which lower it.

And then comes:

● Cholesterol itself—which raises it slightly, depending on the amount already being eaten and on the body's ability to compensate by making less.

For years, the American Heart Association has been publishing guidelines focusing on these factors:

● Lower your saturated fat intake.
● Partially substitute polyunsaturated for saturated fats. (These two measures will increase your P:S ratio.)
● Reduce your cholesterol intake.

Dietary fiber may also confer benefits. Persons on high-fiber diets have been shown to excrete more bile acids, sterols, and fat than persons on low-fiber diets. One reason for the lowered blood cholesterol levels following a high-fiber regimen is a faster transit time for materials through the GI tract, which allows less time for cholesterol absorption. Also, if the body is losing bile acids bound to fiber components, it must simultaneously synthesize new bile acids from its stores of cholesterol, and some of these will then be excreted, reducing body cholesterol further. Diets high in fiber are typically low in fat and cholesterol anyway—another advantage to emphasizing fiber.

The various dietary fibers have varying effects on blood cholesterol. The soluble fibers pectin and guar gum have greater cholesterol-lowering effects than the insoluble fibers cellulose and lignin. Indeed, rolled oats and oat bran (rich in soluble fiber) have favorable effects on blood choles-

14   Food and Nutrition Board, National Research Council, National Academy of Sciences, *Towards Healthful Diets*, reprinted in *Nutrition Today*, May/June 1980, pp. 7–11.

terol whereas wheat bran (high in cellulose) does not appear effective.[15] Apples, pears, peaches, oranges, and grapes are good sources of pectin.

A dietary approach to prevention and therapy of cardiovascular disease that people often ask about is the Pritikin Diet. Its creator, Nathan Pritikin, has taken the principles espoused by the American Heart Association to an extreme. His diet allows only 10 percent of kcalories from fat, for example, versus the American Heart Association's 30 percent and the 50 percent many people actually consume. Foods high in fats and sugars, as well as caffeine and alcohol, are forbidden. He also recommends vigorous daily activity, pushing the heart rate to 70 or 80 percent of its capacity for half an hour or more twice a day. Some former heart patients swear by his regimen, but authorities are cautious. The diet may be too low in fat, may be deficient in vitamins and minerals, has not yet been adequately tested in long-term studies. It is fairly well agreed, however, that the kinds of dietary changes Pritikin recommends—perhaps not so extreme—are more likely to help than to hurt the person wishing to avoid heart trouble; and certainly the exercise is beneficial. In fact, *the* benefit of the Pritikin program may be conferred by exercise, not diet![16]

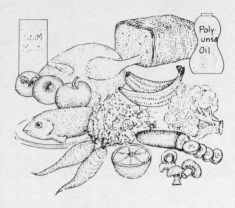

Some foods to enjoy on a prudent diet.

Caution

A less controversial approach to preventive diet is to adopt the "prudent diet" developed by the American Heart Association (see Table H3–3). This diet achieves a total fat intake of 30 percent of kcalories, with 10 percent coming from each type of fat (saturated, monounsaturated, and polyunsaturated), and a cholesterol intake below 300 milligrams per day.

How to Raise HDL

While most of the blood cholesterol is carried in the LDL and correlates *directly* with CVD risk, some is carried in the HDL and correlates *inversely* with risk. In fact, for men over fifty, the most potent single predictor of heart-attack risk may be the HDL level—the higher, the better.[17] While we must exercise the same caution here as formerly (since we don't know for sure if it will have any beneficial effect), we can examine the question how to raise HDL levels.

TABLE H3–3 General Guidelines for a Prudent Diet

1. Limit egg yolks to not more than three a week, including those used in cooking.
2. Limit use of shrimp, organ meats, luncheon meats, bacon, and sausage.
3. Use fish, chicken, turkey, and veal most often. Moderate-sized portions of beef, lamb, pork, and ham can be used less frequently.
4. Use lean meats trimmed of all visible fat and discard fat that cooks out of meat.
5. Avoid frying foods.
6. Use liquid vegetable oils and margarine rich in polyunsaturated fats instead of butter, shortening, or lard.
7. The label on margarine should list *liquid* vegetable oil as the first ingredient and one or more partially hydrogenated vegetable oils as additional ingredients.
8. Use skim milk and skim milk cheeses.

Source: Adapted from American Heart Association, *The Way to a Man's Heart* (Dallas: American Heart Association, 1972).

15   P. A. Judd and A. S. Truswell, The effect of rolled oats on blood lipids and fecal steroid excretion in man, *American Journal of Clinical Nutrition* 34 (1981): 2061–2067; R. W. Kirby and coauthors, Oat-bran intake selectively lowers serum low-density lipoprotein cholesterol concentrations of hypercholesterolemic men, *American Journal of Clinical Nutrition* 34 (1981): 824–829.

16   The Pritikin program—claims vs. facts, *Consumer Reports*, October 1982, pp. 513–518.

17   Dozens of research articles now support this finding. A typical recent one: J. G. Brook and coauthors, High-density lipoprotein subfractions in normolipemic patients with coronary atherosclerosis, *Circulation* 66 (1982): 923–926.

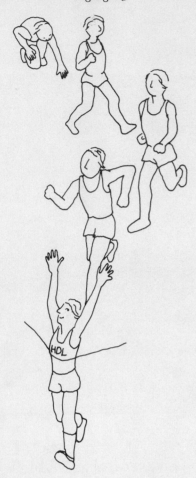

One way (although you can't do much about this) is to be female. Women have higher HDL levels than men. Another, interestingly, seems to be to stop smoking. Nonsmokers have uniformly higher HDL levels than smokers. Still another is to be in the process of losing weight.

If there are dietary factors of any significance, one may be the use of fish rather than meat;[18] another may be the use of certain fibers, which lower LDL levels selectively and leave HDL levels unchanged.[19] A few investigators have reported that the consumption of moderate amounts of alcohol appeared to raise HDL levels; however, it is becoming apparent that there is more than one kind of HDL,[20] and that the kind of HDL affected by alcohol may not be the "good" kind. By far the most powerful influence on HDL levels is not a nutrition-related factor at all, but exercise—prolonged, intense, and frequent.

The discovery that exercise raises HDL levels has given great impetus to the physical fitness movement of the 1970s and 1980s, and especially to the popularity of running as a national pastime. The earliest reports were of raised HDL levels in long-distance runners.[21] At first it was thought that only long-distance, endurance-type running had any significant effect, but subsequent reports have suggested that even moderate exercise may both lower LDL levels[22] and raise HDL levels[23] if consistently pursued. Evidently, then, it is beneficial even for very sedentary people to become only moderately active.[24]

It seems that the factors affecting the health of the heart and arteries are all tangled together. The exact relationships among them have not yet been worked out; but although we don't know which causes what, all evidence points in the same general direction. For good health, and to avoid CVD, stop smoking; reduce blood pressure and weight if necessary; eat a balanced, adequate, and varied diet; reduce fat intake, especially saturated fat; increase activity; and—now that you have it all under control—enjoy life.

18   T. O. Von Lossonczy and coauthors, The effect of a fish diet on lipids in healthy human subjects, *American Journal of Clinical Nutrition* 31 (1978): 1340–1346.

19   J. W. Anderson and W. L. Chen, Plant fiber: Carbohydrate and lipid metabolism, *American Journal of Clinical Nutrition* 32 (1979): 346–363; Dietary fiber, exercise and selected blood lipid constituents, *Nutrition Reviews* 38 (1980): 207–209.

20   J. L. Marx, The HDL: The good cholesterol carriers? (Research news), *Science* 205 (1979): 677–679.

21   P. D. Wood and coauthors, The distribution of plasma lipoproteins in middle-aged male runners, *Metabolism* 25 (1976): 1249–1257.

22   A. Weltman, S. Matter, and B. A. Stamford, Caloric restriction and/or mild exercise: Effects on serum lipids and body composition, *American Journal of Clinical Nutrition* 33 (1980): 1002–1009.

23   D. W. Erkelens and coauthors, High-density lipoprotein-cholesterol in survivors of myocardial infarction, *Journal of the American Medical Association* 242 (1979): 2185–2189; D. Streja and D. Mymin, Moderate exercise and high-density lipoprotein-cholesterol, *Journal of the American Medical Association* 242 (1979): 2190–2192; W. P. Castelli, Exercise and high-density lipoproteins (editorial), *Journal of the American Medical Association* 242 (1979): 2217.

24   Streja and Mymin, 1979.

Although diet and nutrition have been the focus of attention here, it seems important to conclude by taking a broader view of the problem of CVD. Nutrition is obviously not the only factor involved. People die of heart attacks and strokes for many reasons: urbanized living, breakup of the family, alienation, air pollution, and many others. And CVD deaths are falling while others are on the rise: deaths from accidents, homicides, suicides, lung cancer, liver disease. The lifestyle of the whole society is implicated in these deaths—it is an urbanized, competitive, industrial society with built-in stresses that have major impacts on health. While we continue focusing on this book's central concern, nutrition, we must acknowledge that society itself may need to change in fundamental ways before we can arrive at ultimate solutions to some of these problems.

NOTE: Appendix J recommends many readings on diet and cardiovascular disease. See "Atherosclerosis and Diet."

CHAPTER 4
Protein: Amino Acids

CONTENTS

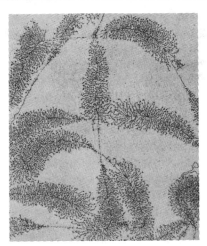

Enzymes work rapidly and systematically. Part of a cell is shown here, in which about 12 genes (segments of DNA) are being copied into RNA. About 50 enzymes are at work in each gene, creating a Christmas-tree-like formation. Each enzyme is moving along the DNA, making an RNA copy. Those that have moved the farthest have made the longest RNA branches.

There is present in plants and in animals a substance which . . . is without doubt the most important of all the known substances in living matter, and, without it, life would be impossible on our planet. This material has been named Protein.

GERARD JOHANNES MULDER (1838)

Everybody knows that protein is important. It is advertised on every cereal box; it is said to "build strong bodies," and to provide "super go power." In fact, as you will see, protein has been so overemphasized that many people eat more than enough, sometimes at the expense of other nutrients that are equally important. An understanding of the quantity and quality of protein needed in the diet will help put it in its proper place as only one—although a very important one—of the nutrients needed in correct proportions to achieve a balanced diet.

This chapter departs from the organization used for the preceding chapters, jumping right into a description of the chemical structure of protein. The reason is that proteins are far more versatile than carbohydrates or fats in the roles they play in the body, and they derive their versatility from their extraordinary structure. Those who have worked on elucidating the chemical structure of protein

123

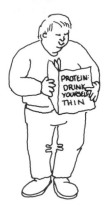

One thing protein does *not* do for you is make you thin! See Chapters 6 and 7.

protein: a compound composed of C, H, O, and N atoms, arranged into amino acids linked in a chain. Some amino acids also contain S (sulfur) atoms.

$$H-N-C-C-O-H$$

amino (a-MEEN-oh) **acid**: a building block of protein; a compound containing an amino group and an acid group attached to a central carbon, which also carries a distinctive side chain.

amino = containing nitrogen

Amino group   Acid group

Glycine

have been rewarded with a profound insight into the elegance of nature's designs.

The Chemist's View of Protein

A protein is a chemical compound that contains the same atoms as carbohydrate and lipid—carbon, hydrogen, and oxygen—but protein also contains nitrogen atoms. These C, H, O, and N atoms are arranged into amino acids, which are linked into chains to form proteins. It is easy to construct a protein once we know what an amino acid looks like, and the unit structure of an amino acid is simpler than that of either carbohydrates (monosaccharides) or lipids (glycerol and fatty acids).

Amino Acid Structure

An amino acid has a backbone of one nitrogen and two carbon atoms linked together. Recall that carbons must form four bonds with other atoms, oxygens two, and hydrogens one. In amino acids, nitrogens must form three bonds with other atoms. The structure all amino acids have in common fulfills these requirements. At one end is an amino group (NH_2); at the other is an acid group (COOH). Both are attached to a central carbon that also carries a hydrogen (H). As you can see, on this drawing one position is left unfilled—the central carbon atom must have another atom or group of atoms attached to it to make a complete structure.

This central carbon atom and the attached structures are what make proteins so varied in comparison to either carbohydrates or lipids. A polysaccharide (starch, for example) is composed of glucose units one after the other. It may be 100 or 200 units long, but every unit in the chain is a glucose molecule just like all the others. In a protein, on the other hand, 22 different amino acids may appear.[1] Each differs from the others in the nature of the side group it carries on the central carbon. The simplest amino acid, glycine, has a hydrogen atom in that position. A slightly more complex amino acid, alanine, has an extra carbon with three attached hydrogen atoms. Other amino acids have still more complex side groups. For example, one amino acid may have an acid group, another may have a basic amino group. Still others may have neutral side groups, including some complicated ring structures. These acidic, basic, and neutral groups confer different characteristics on the amino acids. Thus, although the amino acids all share a common starting structure, their properties differ (see Figure 4–1).

---

1   It is often said that there are 20 amino acids, but if cystine and ornithine are counted, there are 22. Amino acids sometimes occur in related forms (for example proline can add an OH group to become hydroxyproline). Chemists can make still other amino acids, not commonly found in nature. We have elected to present (in Appendix C) the structures of the 22 common amino acids as in Nomenclature policy: Abbreviated designations of amino acids, *Journal of Nutrition* 112 (1982): 15. The structure of hydroxyproline is shown in Chapter 8.

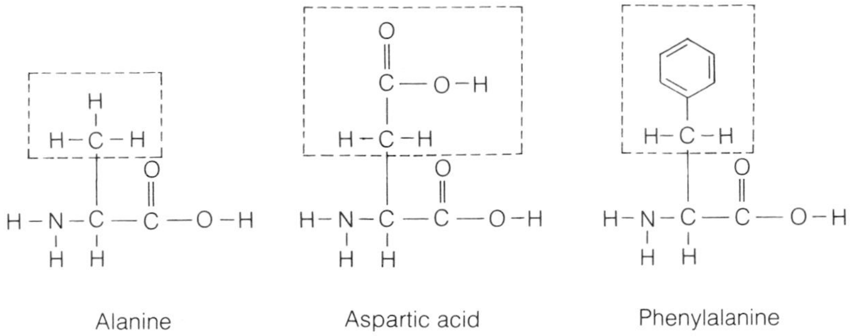

FIGURE 4-1 **Examples of amino acids.**
TH 4-1

Alanine   Aspartic acid   Phenylalanine

Amino Acid Sequence

The 22 common amino acids may be linked together in a great variety of ways to form proteins. They connect by means of a condensation reaction (Figure 4–2). An OH is removed from the acid end of one, and an H is removed from the amino group of another. A bond forms between the two amino acids, and the H and OH join to form a molecule of water. The resulting structure is a dipeptide (see Figure 4–2). By the same reaction, the OH can be removed from the acid end of the second amino acid and an H from the amino group of a third to form a tripeptide. As additional amino acids are added to the chain, a polypeptide is formed. Most proteins are polypeptides, 100 to 300 amino acids long.

It would be misleading, however, to end the description here, because in showing the structures on paper we have drawn a straight, flat chain. Actually, polypeptide chains fold and tangle so that they look not like rods but like crazy jungle gyms. The sequence of amino acids in a protein determines which specific way the chain will fold.

Folding of the Chain

You can best visualize the chain structure by keeping in mind that each side group on the amino acids has special characteristics that attract it to other groups. Some side groups are polar (charged), and are attracted to

dipeptide: two amino acids bonded together. The bond between two amino acids is a **peptide bond**.

di = two

peptide = amino acid

tripeptide: three amino acids bonded together by peptide bonds.

tri = three

polypeptide: many amino acids bonded together by peptide bonds. *Many* refers to ten or more. An intermediate string of between four and ten amino acids is an **oligopeptide**.

poly = many

oligo = few

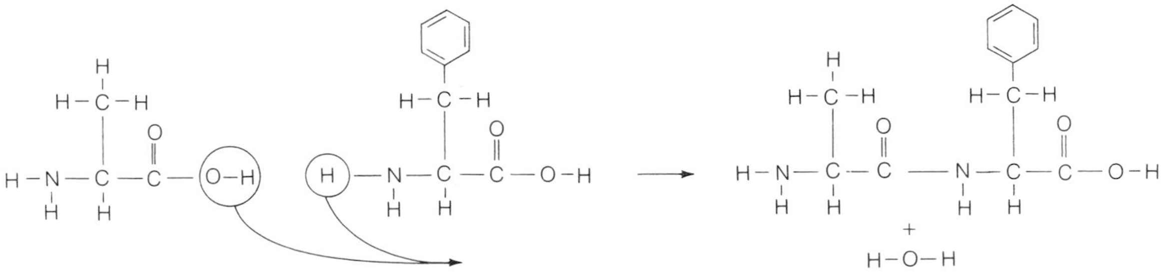

FIGURE 4–2 **Formation of a dipeptide.** A dipeptide forms as two amino acids condense, splitting out a molecule of water. Condensation reactions have already been shown twice before (pp. 55, 90). TH4-1

the charges around water molecules. Other side groups are neutral, and are repelled by water. As amino acids are added to a polypeptide chain and the chain lengthens, the charged groups, being hydrophilic (see p. 97), are attracted to positions on the outer surface of the completed protein. The neutral groups, being hydrophobic (p. 97), tend to tuck themselves inside, away from water. The shape the polypeptide finally assumes is either roughly spherical or fibrous, whichever gives it the maximum stability in water. Finally, two or more of these giant molecules may associate to form a still larger working aggregate. Thus the completed protein is a complex, tangled chain of amino acids, bristling on the surface with positive and negative charges. Sometimes two, three, or four such chains tangle together to make a giant protein molecule. Hemoglobin, shown in Figure 4–3, is one of the big proteins.

When a protein molecule is subjected to heat, acid, or other conditions that disturb its stability, it uncoils or changes its shape, thus losing its function to some extent. That is what happens to an egg when it is cooked; alterations of the egg proteins during cooking largely account for the observable changes in the egg white and yolk.

The change in a protein's shape brought about by heat, acid, or other conditions is known as **denaturation**. Past a certain point, denaturation is irreversible.

The Completed Protein

If you could step onto a carbohydrate molecule like starch and walk along it, the first stepping stone would be a glucose. The next stepping stone would be glucose again, and then glucose, and then glucose, and then

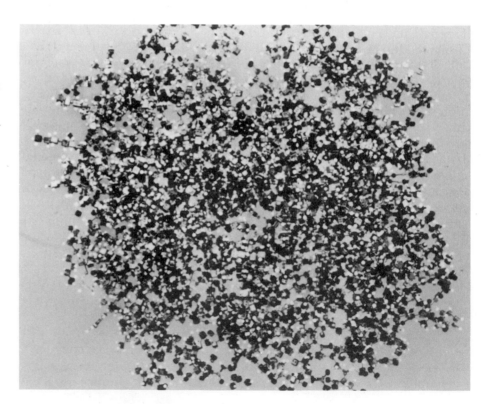

FIGURE 4–3 **The intricate structure of a protein molecule**. This molecule represents one molecule of hemoglobin, magnified 27 million times.

Source: Human hemoglobin model constructed by Dr. Makio Murayama, NIH, Bethesda, Maryland (scaled to ½ inch to angstrom). Atomic coordinates were supplied for the model by Dr. Max F. Perutz, Cambridge, England.

glucose. But if you were to walk along a polypeptide chain, your first stepping stone might be a methionine. Your second might be an alanine. The third might be a glycine, and the fourth a tryptophan, then another alanine, and so on. In other words, the units in a protein are varied in both their nature and the sequence in which they appear.

Another analogy compares the amino acids to letters in an alphabet. If you were to try to make a sentence using only the letter G, you could only speak gibberish: G-G-G-G-G-G-G. But with 20-odd different letters available, you can say, "To be or not to be, that is the question"—or, on a different plane, "The way to a man's heart is through his stomach." The Greek alphabet contains only 24 letters, and all of Homer was written with it.

The variety of sequences in which the 22 amino acids can be linked together is even greater than that possible for letters in a sentence, because proteins do not have to be pronounced as words do. This gives them a tremendous range of possible surface structures, which in turn enables them to perform very distinct, individual, and specialized functions. The human body contains an estimated 10,000 to 50,000 different kinds of proteins. Of these thousands only about 1,000 have been identified,[2] and only about 10 are described in this chapter.

Enzymes: A Function of Protein

When we first mentioned enzymes, we promised that we would look at these magnificent molecules more closely when protein structure had been explained. Let's start by looking at the enzyme maltase.

A typical protein, maltase is a tangled, ball-shaped polypeptide chain, 100 or so amino acids long. The little molecule maltose, on the other hand, is a disaccharide perhaps 100 times smaller. From the point of view of a maltose molecule, then, the enzyme maltase is very large. The small maltose molecule, encountering such an enzyme, would find itself snapping into position on the enzyme's surface, a surface custom-designed to fit maltose's contours. On this surface, maltose would soon encounter a molecule of water, and as its two glucose parts split apart, the water would also be split apart, its H being added to one glucose and its OH to the other. Releasing the free glucose, the enzyme would attract other maltoses into that same position and hydrolyze them the same way.

Enzymes and what they do are so fundamental to all life processes that it seems worthwhile to introduce an analogy to clarify two important characteristics they all share. Enzymes are comparable to the ministers and judges who respectively make and dissolve human matrimonial bonds. When two individuals come to a minister to be married, the couple leaves with a new bond between them. They are joined together—but the minister is only momentarily involved in the process and remains unchanged. One minister can therefore perform thousands of marriage ceremonies. Similarly, a judge, who facilitates the separation of married couples, may decree many divorces before he dies or retires.

2   A. Rosenfeld, The great protein hunt, *Science 81*, January/February 1981, pp. 64–67.

methionine (meth-EYE-oh-neen), **alanine** (AL-uh-neen), **tryptophan** (TRIP-toe-fane): amino acids. A complete list of the amino acids, with their structures, appears in Appendix C.

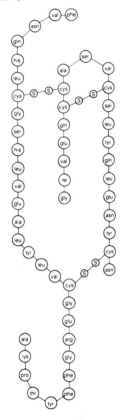

The complete amino acid sequence of insulin, a small protein. S-S represents the cross-links between cysteine molecules, known as disulfide bridges. (For structures and abbreviations of individual amino acids, see Appendix C.)

maltase: the enzyme that hydrolyzes maltose to two glucose units.

maltose: the disaccharide composed of two glucose units (see p. 55).

ase: a word ending denoting an enzyme. The first part of the word usually identifies the compound the enzyme works on. Thus maltase is the enzyme that works on maltose.

An apology for the use of fanciful descriptions appears in the Preface.

Model of enzyme action (maltase).

synthetase (SIN-the-tase): an enzyme that synthesizes compounds.

protease (PRO-tee-ase): an enzyme that hydrolyzes proteins.

lipase (LYE-pase): an enzyme that hydrolyzes lipids.

The definitions of **carbohydrase**, **disaccharidase**, **sucrase**, **lactase**, and **phospholipase** are self-evident.

catalyst (CAT-uh-list): a compound that facilitates chemical reactions without itself being destroyed in the process.

enzyme: a protein catalyst.

The minister represents enzymes that synthesize larger compounds from smaller ones—the synthetases, which build body structures. The judge represents enzymes that hydrolyze larger compounds to smaller ones—the proteases, lipases, carbohydrases, disaccharidases, and others. Maltase is a disaccharidase.

The first point to be learned is that some enzymes put compounds together and others take them apart. Since you yourself are a very put-together kind of organism, superbly organized out of billions of molecules designed to make muscle, bone, skin, eyes, and blood cells, you can imagine how numerous and active in your body are the enzymes that put things together. (Only a naive student thinks of enzymes as being solely digestive enzymes—those that take things apart.)

The second point is that enzymes are not themselves affected in the process of facilitating chemical reactions. They are catalysts. Biologists and chemists define an enzyme as *a protein catalyst.*

What makes you unique and distinct from any other human being is minute differences in your body proteins (enzymes, antibodies, and others). These differences are determined by the amino acid sequences of your proteins, which are written into the genetic code of the DNA you inherited from your parents and ancestors. Each person receives at conception a unique combination of genes (DNA codes for protein sequences). The genes direct the making of all the body's proteins, as shown in Figure 4-4.

Perhaps you have realized by now that the protein story moves in a circle. All enzymes are proteins. All proteins are made of amino acids. Amino acids have to be put together to make proteins. Enzymes put together the amino acids. Only living systems work with such self-renewal. A broken toaster cannot be fixed by another toaster; a car cannot make another car. Only living creatures and the parts they are composed of—the cells—can duplicate themselves.

To follow the circle in nutrition, start with a person eating proteins. The proteins are broken down by proteins (enzymes) into amino acids. The amino acids enter the cells of the body, where proteins (enzymes) put them together in long chains with sequences specified by DNA. The chains fold and become enzymes themselves. These enzymes may then be used to break apart other compounds or to put other compounds together. Day by day, billion reactions by billion reactions, these processes repeat themselves and life goes on.

A Closer Look at Enzyme Action

If you look closely at the details of the reaction sequences governed by enzymes, some additional important facts emerge. The following description is an example of the way enzymes work to alter the structure of a compound. It is this book's only example of the details biochemists actually think about. The object is to give you an insight into the kinds of processes that account for human nutrient needs.

Let's look at part of a biochemical pathway and see how each enzyme

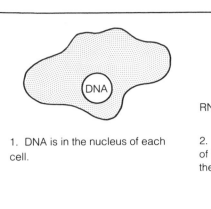

1. DNA is in the nucleus of each cell.

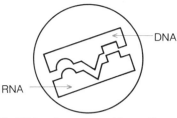

2. DNA makes a copy of the portion of itself that has the instructions for the protein the cell needs.

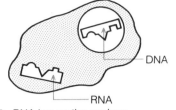

3. RNA leaves the nucleus.

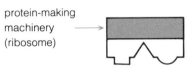

4. RNA attaches itself to the protein-making machinery of the cell.

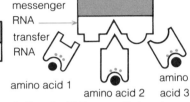

5. Transfer RNAs carry their amino acids to the messenger RNA, where they are snapped into place.

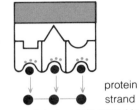

6. The completed protein strand is released.

FIGURE 4-4 **Protein synthesis.** The instructions for making every protein in a person's body are transmitted in the genetic information he or she receives at conception. This body of knowledge is filed away in the nucleus of every cell. The master file is the DNA (deoxyribonucleic acid), which never leaves the nucleus. The DNA is identical in every cell and is specific for each individual. Each specialized cell has access to the total inherited information but calls on only the instructions needed for its own functions.

To inform the cell of the proper sequence of amino acids for a needed protein, a "photocopy" of the appropriate portion of DNA is made. This copy is messenger RNA (ribonucleic acid), which is able to escape through the nuclear membrane. In the cell fluid it seeks out and attaches itself to one of the ribosomes (a protein-making machine, itself composed of RNA and protein). Thus situated, the messenger RNA presents the sequence in which the amino acids should be linked into a protein strand.

Meanwhile, another form of RNA, called transfer RNA, collects amino acids from the cell fluid and brings them to the messenger. For each of the 22 amino acids there is a specific kind of transfer RNA. Thousands of these transfer RNAs, with their loads of amino acids, cluster around the ribosomes, like vegetable-laden trucks around a farmer's market awaiting their turn to unload. When an amino acid is called for by the messenger, the transfer RNA carrying it snaps into position. Then the next and the next and the next loaded transfer RNAs move into place. Thus the amino acids are lined up in the right sequence. Then an enzyme bonds them together.

Finally, the completed protein strand is released, the messenger is degraded, and the transfer RNAs are freed to return for another load. It takes many words to describe the events, but in the cell, 40 to 100 amino acids can be added to a growing protein strand in only a second. TH4-2

Intermediates in glucose metabolism.

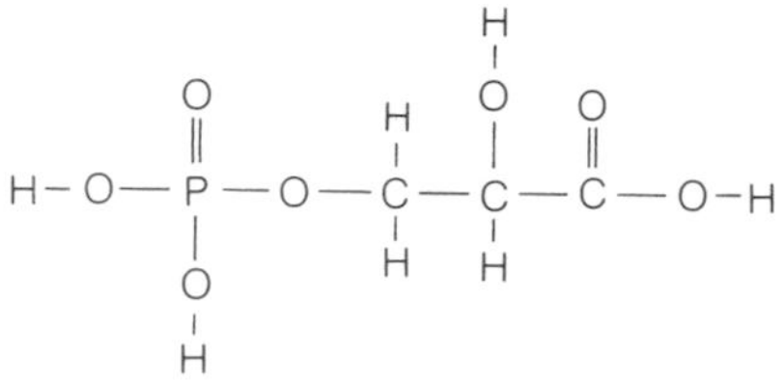

Compound A. (TH4-3)

alters the structure of a compound until one thing has been converted into quite another thing. Beginning with glucose, a six-carbon compound, enzymes have added a phosphate group, have altered the arrangement of the atoms, and then have broken the compound in two so that a three-carbon compound has resulted: compound A.

Compound A floats around until it encounters an enzyme that recognizes it. This enzyme has the specialized function of removing hydrogen atoms from molecules of compound A. The encounter results in the altered compound, compound B.

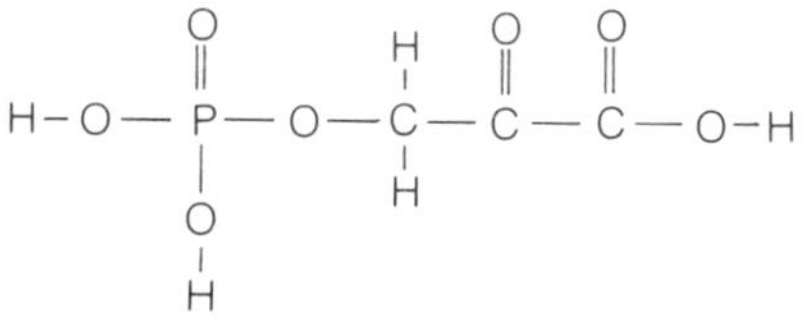

Compound B. (TH4-3)

Compound B is released from the enzyme and encounters another enzyme, whose sole mission in life is to remove oxygens from compound B and to substitute amino groups in their place. What results is compound C. The next enzyme removes the phosphate group from the end carbon and replaces it with a hydrogen, leaving compound D.

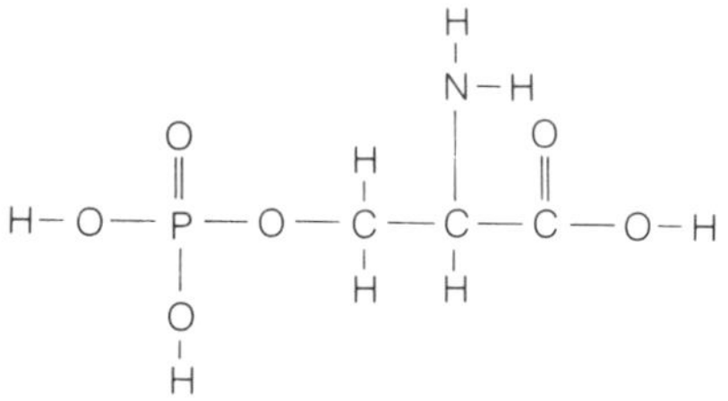

Compound C. (TH4-3)

If you look closely at the picture of compound D, you may recognize its characteristics and not be surprised by the statements that follow. But let us take the process one more step. Another enzyme, whose function is to remove CH_2OH groups from these molecules, forms compound E. Look at this product closely; you have seen it before. It has an amino group at one end, an acid group at the other, and a central carbon carrying two Hs. It is the amino acid glycine (p. 124).[3]

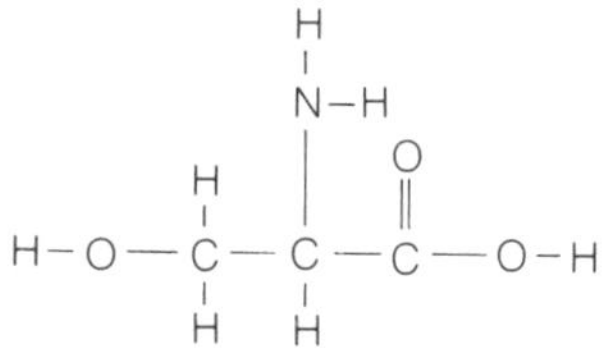

Well, how about that! We started with a molecule of glucose, a derivative of dietary carbohydrate, and by making one minute change after another, we transformed it into an amino acid, a member of the protein family.

The lesson to be learned from this sequence of events is that the body can make, from glucose and nitrogen-containing compounds, many of the amino acids needed to build body proteins. Glycine is one of these. Compound D, which precedes glycine on the pathway, is the amino acid serine (which has a CH_2OH on its central carbon). Serine, too, is an amino acid the body can make.

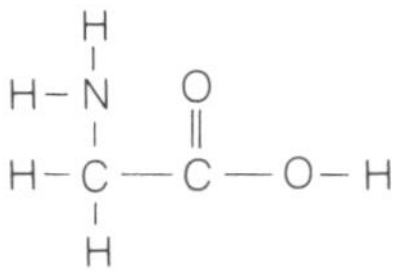

Compound D. (TH4-3)

Protein Quality

It is now clear that the role of protein in food is not to provide body proteins directly but to supply the amino acids from which the body can

Compound E. (TH4-3)

3   The enzyme that produced compound B was a dehydrogenase; the next enzyme, a transaminase; the next, a phosphatase.

make its own proteins. Since the body can make glycine and serine for itself, the proteins in the diet need not contain these two amino acids. But there are some amino acids the body cannot make at all, and some it cannot make fast enough to meet its need. (This is because the body does not possess the genes for the enzymes that could synthesize these amino acids, or because the enzymes it does make work too slowly.) These are the essential amino acids. Eight amino acids are essential for adults; histidine is also essential for infants.[4]

To make body protein, a cell must have all the needed amino acids available simultaneously. The first important characteristic of dietary protein is, therefore, that it should supply at least the eight essential amino acids and enough nitrogen for the synthesis of the others.

A complete protein is a protein that contains all of the essential amino acids in amounts adequate for human use; it may or may not contain all the others. A high-quality protein is not merely complete, but contains the essential amino acids in amounts proportional to the body's need for them, and is digestible, so that these amino acids reach the body's cells in the needed amounts.

Ideally, dietary protein supplies each amino acid in the amount needed for protein synthesis in the body. If one amino acid is supplied in an amount smaller than is needed, the total amount of protein that can be synthesized from the others will be limited. By analogy, suppose that a signmaker plans to make 100 identical signs, each saying LEFT TURN ONLY. He needs 200 Ls, 200 Ns, 200 Ts, and 100 of each of the other letters. If he has only 20 Ls, he can make only 10 signs, even if all the other letters are available in unlimited quantities. The Ls limit the number of signs that can be made. Furthermore, the signmaker has no place to keep leftover letters (the body has no storage place for extra amino acids), so if he doesn't get some more Ls right away, he will have to throw away all his other letters.

When the body uses a protein of poor quality, it wastes many of the amino acids. Enzymes strip off their nitrogen-containing amino groups and fix them into the compound urea, which is excreted in the urine. The carbon skeletons that remain are used to make glucose or fat, or are oxidized for energy; the nitrogen is not stored in the body. The amount of urea excreted is thus a measure of the number of amino acids not retained in body proteins.

The quality of dietary protein, then, depends partly on whether the protein supplies all the essential amino acids and, more importantly, on the extent to which it supplies them in the needed proportions and in a digestible form. An excellent protein by these standards is egg protein, whose nitrogen tends to be retained in the body. Egg protein has been designated the reference protein and has been assigned a biological value of 100 by the Food and Agriculture Organization of the United Nations, which sets world standards.

4   R. E. Olson, Clinical nutrition: An interface between human ecology and internal medicine, *Nutrition Reviews* 36 (1978): 161–178. There is some debate indicating that histidine may, under some conditions, be essential for adults as well: M. R. Jones, J. D. Kopple, and M. E. Swendseid, [14]CO$_2$ expiration after ^{14}C-histidine administration in normal and uremic men ingesting two levels of histidine, *American Journal of Clinical Nutrition* 35 (1982): 15–23.

---

essential amino acid: an amino acid that the body cannot synthesize in amounts sufficient to meet physiological need. See also the definition of *essential nutrient* on page 2. The eight amino acids known to be essential for human adults:

methionine (meh-THIGH-oh-neen)

threonine (THREE-oh-neen)

tryptophan (TRIP-toe-fane)

isoleucine (eye-so-LOO-seen)

leucine (LOO-seen)

lysine (LYE-seen)

valine (VAY-leen)

phenylalanine (fee-nul-AL-uh-neen)

Infants also require **histidine** (HISS-tuh-deen).

Students attempting to learn these by heart often use the device "TV TILL PM" to recall their first letters.

complete protein: a protein containing all the amino acids essential in human nutrition in amounts adequate for human use.

high-quality protein: an easily digestible, complete protein whose amino acids fit the pattern needed by humans.

limiting amino acid: the amino acid found in the shortest supply relative to the amounts needed for protein synthesis in the body.

How urea is made: see Chapter 6.

reference protein: egg protein; used by FAO/WHO as a standard against which to measure the quality of other proteins.

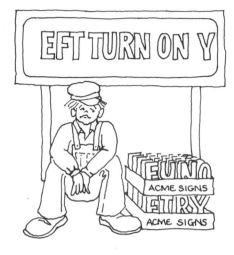

The amino acid composition of a test protein can be compared with the composition of egg protein, and a chemical score can be derived to express the theoretical value of the test protein. A test protein with a chemical score of 70, for example, contains a limiting amino acid, and that amino acid is present in only 70 percent of the amount found in the ideal amino acid pattern. If you fed the test protein to human beings under carefully controlled conditions in which the total protein fed was just enough to meet the requirement, you would expect that 30 percent of its amino acids would not be retained in the body (30 percent of its nitrogen would be excreted in the urine).

In a world where food is scarce and where many people's diets contain marginal or inadequate amounts of protein, it is important to know which foods contain the highest-quality protein. It is possible to determine the amino acid composition of any protein relatively inexpensively, but unfortunately, chemical scoring does not always reflect accurately the way the body will use a protein. The main reason is that proteins differ in digestibility—a characteristic the chemical score does not reflect. If a protein can't be digested to small fragments—amino acids, dipeptides, and tripeptides—then its amino acids will not pass across the intestinal wall into the blood, but will be lost in the feces.

To determine the actual value of a protein as it is used by the body, it is necessary to measure not only urinary but also fecal losses of nitrogen when that protein is actually fed to human beings under test conditions. (Even then, small additional losses from sweat, shed skin, hair, and fingernails will be missed.) This kind of experiment determines the biological value (BV) of proteins, a measure used internationally. The biological values of the proteins in some sample foods are shown below. Generally, a biological value of 70 or above indicates acceptable quality.

chemical score: a rating of the quality of a test protein arrived at by comparing its amino acid pattern with that of a reference protein.

digestibility: a measure of the amount of amino acids absorbed from a given protein intake. To learn why "predigested" protein is less digestible than whole protein, even though it is delivered to the body in small fragments, turn to p. 168.

biological value (BV): the amount of protein nitrogen that is retained from a given amount of dietary protein nitrogen that is digested and absorbed. Appendix D gives more details.

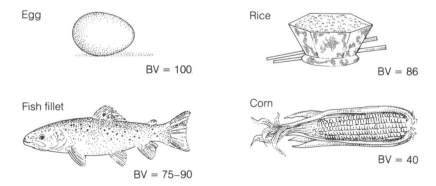

Egg — BV = 100

Rice — BV = 86

Fish fillet — BV = 75–90

Corn — BV = 40

protein efficiency ratio (PER): a measure of protein quality derived by feeding a test protein to growing animals and determining their weight gain. Appendix D gives more details.

As you may well imagine, determining the biological value of a protein is a cumbersome and expensive procedure. A different laboratory test involves feeding a test protein to young animals (usually rats) and measuring their growth rate. This measure, the protein efficiency ratio (PER), is used to qualify statements about daily protein requirements in the United States. You are assumed to eat protein with a PER equal to or better than that of the milk protein casein; if the protein's PER is lower, you need more of the protein.

For those who choose not to tangle with the formulas for BV and PER, a convenient way to distinguish among proteins is to think of animal proteins as being generally of higher quality than plant proteins. However, the educated vegetarian can design a perfectly acceptable diet around plant foods alone.

Diet planning for the vegetarian: see note at end of chapter.

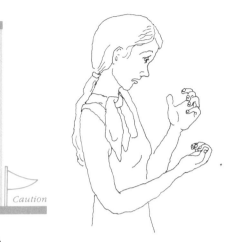

Like all generalizations, the statement that "animal proteins are generally of higher quality" does not quite stand up to close inspection. One animal protein that is not complete is gelatin (it lacks tryptophan). Ironically, this is the protein often recommended for correcting cracked nails and dull or brittle hair. The logic is that, because these tissues are made of protein, a drink of protein will improve their texture. Even if this were the case, however—and a symptom, you remember, is not a deficiency disease—gelatin supplements would help only if protein containing tryptophan had already been supplied. And if that protein were complete, then the gelatin would not be needed!

Caution

Evidently, then, everyone needs some high-quality protein in the diet to support optimal growth and maintenance of body tissues. There is a place for the lesser-quality proteins too, however. Plant proteins, eaten in abundance, serve as an excellent support for the efficient use of high-quality animal proteins. Research has shown that expensive meat protein is far more efficiently used when ample bread, cereal, and vegetable protein accompanies it. An adult needs only 20 percent of total protein as essential amino acids; the rest can be "nonspecific nitrogen."[5]

Carbohydrate and fat allow amino acids to be used to build body proteins. This is known as the **protein-sparing action** of carbohydrate and fat.

There is one circumstance in which dietary protein—no matter how high the quality—will not be used efficiently by the body and will not support growth: when energy from other energy nutrients is lacking. The body assigns top priority to meeting its energy need, and when no kcalories from other sources are available, it will break down protein to meet this need. Stripping off and excreting the nitrogen from the amino acids, it will use their carbon skeletons in much the same way it uses those from glucose or from fat. The major reason why it is necessary to have ample carbohydrate and fat in the diet is to prevent this wasting of protein.

Energy value of protein: 1 g provides 4 kcal.

Other conditions also affect the body's use of protein. In brief, to be used with maximum efficiency, a protein must contain a suitable amino acid pattern, must be digestible, must be consumed with sufficient kcalories from other sources so that it will not be sacrificed for energy; must be accompanied by the needed vitamins and minerals to facilitate its use; and must be received by a body that is healthy and equipped to use it.

Other Roles of Protein

This chapter began by describing the proteins that act as enzymes, in order to show how vitally important they are, and how—among the thousands of

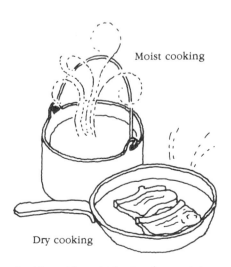

Moist cooking

Dry cooking

Cooking with moist heat makes protein more digestible.

5 M. C. Crim and H. N. Munro, Protein, in *Nutrition Reviews' Present Knowledge in Nutrition*, 4th ed. (Washington, D.C.: Nutrition Foundation, 1976), pp. 43–54.

tasks they perform—they manufacture many of the amino acids they themselves are made of. Before going on to state the amounts of protein people need, we must describe a few of the other tasks proteins perform in the body.

Although the following discussion focuses on protein's role, other nutrients (vitamins and minerals) cooperate in these tasks. The minerals sodium and potassium, for example, help proteins maintain the water balance; vitamin C helps make the protein collagen, which is involved in wound healing. For the present, we suggest that you read with the thought in mind that proteins do all these things. Then you will have the background to appreciate the roles of the helper nutrients, details of which are given in Chapters 8, 9, 10, and 11. Margin references in this section remind you of these helper nutrients.

The space in the blood vessels is the **intravascular space**; the space between the cells is the **intercellular or interstitial space**; the space inside the cells is the **intracellular space**.

intra = inside

inter = between

interstice = space between

Minerals are helper nutrients. The attractiveness of protein and mineral particles to water is osmotic pressure; see Chapter 10.

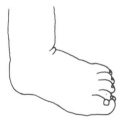

edema (uh-DEEM-uh): accumulation of fluid in the interstitial spaces. Edema in the abdomen is *ascites* (uh-SITE-eez).

diuretic (dye-yoo-RET-ic): a drug that stimulates increased renal water excretion.

renal = kidney

Fluid Balances

Proteins help maintain the water balance. To understand how this extremely important function is managed, you must know that there are three principal compartments for fluids in the body: the space in the blood vessels, the spaces between the cells, and the spaces within the cells. In normal, healthy people, each of these compartments contains the proper amount of fluid. Fluid can flow back and forth across the boundaries between them, but whenever the volume of fluid deviates, it is rapidly brought back to normal. Protein (with certain minerals) helps to maintain water at the proper volume in each compartment.

This process works on a simple principle. Proteins are so large that they cannot pass freely across the walls or membranes that separate the compartments. They are trapped where they are. They are also hydrophilic, or attractive to water molecules, so the water molecules stay with or near them. By regulating the amount of protein (and minerals) in each compartment, the body indirectly regulates the distribution of water.

It has been thought that protein deficiency causes edema, the symptom in which fluid leaks out of the blood vessels into the interstitial space (Figure 4–5 diagrams edema). Recently, however, it has been pointed out that although the two often go together, either can occur without the other.[6] Clearly other nutrients besides protein, as well as hormones that are affected by malnutrition, are involved in the causation of edema.

The uninformed person may believe that the way to prevent the swelling of edema is to drink less water or to increase excretion by taking a diuretic. If edema has become extreme, these measures, as well as salt restriction, may indeed be a necessary part of treatment. Yet you can never cause edema just by drinking too much water. The more you drink, the more the kidneys excrete.

This fact illustrates a principle that pervades physiology. The body

6 M. H. N. Golden, Protein deficiency, energy deficiency, and the oedema of malnutrition, *Lancet* I (1982): 1261–1265.

maintains its own health. Provided that you are healthy to begin with, no drug can render it better able to do so. Drugs are needed only to remedy situations in which body functions have become impaired. Diuretics may be needed only when excess fluid has already accumulated, due to an abnormal physiological state. (The edema of pregnancy is not such a state; see Chapter 13.) Diuretics are not useful as preventive medicine.

Since the taking of a diuretic increases water excretion, it causes a sudden weight loss. A healthy person who fails to distinguish between loss of body fat and loss of water may see this as a desirable effect and start using diuretics for this purpose. But because the only loss induced is water loss, the only achievement gained is dehydration.

In edema from whatever cause, the water that should be held within the bloodstream leaks into the interstitial space and causes swelling. This water is not available to the kidneys to excrete; they can only excrete what is in the bloodstream that travels through them. Hence the remedy is not to drink less water but to obtain an accurate diagnosis of the cause of the edema so that it can be dealt with at its source.

Caution

Another fluid balance proteins help maintain is that between acids and bases. An acid solution is one in which hydrogen ions are floating around. The more hydrogen ions, the more concentrated the acid. Proteins (and minerals), which have negative charges on their surfaces, attract hydrogen ions, and hydrogen ions in turn attract proteins. As long as the concentration of hydrogen ions—that is, the strength of the acid—stays within certain limits, the proteins maintain their integrity. If the acid becomes too

acid-base balance: the balance maintained in the body between too much and too little acid. Blood pH, for example, is regulated normally between 7.38 and 7.42.

pH: the concentration of H^+ ions (see Appendix B). The lower the pH, the stronger the acid. Thus pH 2 is a strong acid; pH 6 a weak acid (pH 7 is neutral). A pH above 7 is alkaline, or basic (a solution in which acid-accepting ions such as OH^- predominate).

ion: see p. 374 and Appendix B.

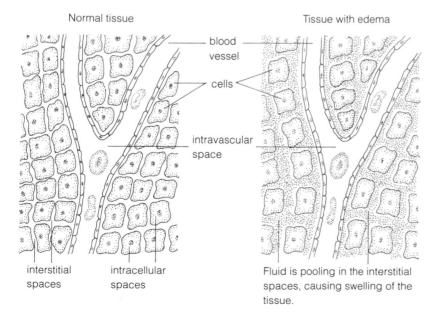

Normal tissue

blood vessel

cells

intravascular space

interstitial spaces

intracellular spaces

Tissue with edema

Fluid is pooling in the interstitial spaces, causing swelling of the tissue.

FIGURE 4–5 **Edema: An accumulation of fluid between the cells.**

Development of immunity.

1 Body is challenged with foreign
invaders.

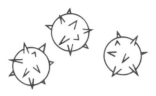

2 Body makes code for manufacturing
antibody.

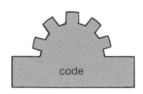

3 Code makes antibody.

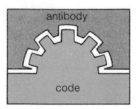

4 Antibody inactivates foreign invader.

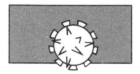

5 Code remains to make antibodies faster
the next time this foreign invader attacks.

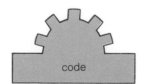

strong, however, the extra positive charges cap some of the negative charges on the proteins, changing their internal attractive forces and, so to speak, pulling them out of shape. When this happens, the proteins can no longer function.

Of all the consequences that stem from exceeding the normal limits of the acid-base balance, the most direct and serious is a disturbance of the shapes of the proteins that carry out so many vital body functions. Acidosis and alkalosis both are lethal if unchecked. The proteins in the plasma, such as albumin, help to prevent these conditions from arising. In a sense, the proteins protect one another by binding or sequestering extra hydrogen ions when there are too many in the surrounding medium and by releasing them when there are too few. This ability to regulate the acidity of the medium is known as the buffering action of proteins.

Antibodies and Hormones

Other major proteins found in the blood—the antibodies—act against disease agents. When a body is invaded by a virus—whether it is one that causes flu, smallpox, measles, or the common cold—the virus enters the cells and multiplies there. One virus may produce a hundred replicas of itself within an hour or so. These burst out and invade a hundred different cells, soon yielding ten thousand virus particles, which invade ten thousand cells. After several hours there may be a million viruses and then a hundred million and so on. If they were left free to do their worst, they would soon overwhelm the body with the disease they cause.

The antibodies, giant protein molecules circulating in the blood, present a defense against viruses, bacteria, and other "foreign agents." Each type of antibody molecule is different and specific, able to combine with and inactivate a specific foreign protein such as that in a virus coat or bacterial cell membrane. The antibodies work so efficiently that in a normal healthy individual the many disease agents that attempt to attack never have a chance to get started. If a million bacterial cells are injected into the skin of a healthy person, fewer than ten are likely to survive for five hours.[7]

Once the body has manufactured antibodies against a particular disease agent (such as the measles virus), the cells never forget how to produce them. The next time that virus invades the body, the antibodies will respond even more quickly. Thus the body acquires immunity against the diseases it is exposed to, by virtue of the molecular memory of the antibody-producing cells.

Hormones are also carried by the blood, and some are made of amino acids. Among them are the thyroid hormone and insulin. The thyroid hormone regulates the body's metabolic rate—the rate of the chemical reactions that yield energy. Insulin regulates the concentration of the blood glucose and its transportation into cells, upon which the functioning of the brain and the nervous system depend. Hormones have many other profound effects, which will become evident as you read further.

7   R. Y. Stanier, M. Doudoroff, and E. A. Adelberg, *The Microbial World*, 3rd ed. (Englewood Cliffs, N.J.: Prentice-Hall, 1970), p. 784.

Transport Proteins

A special group of the body's proteins specializes in moving nutrients and other molecules in and out of cells. These proteins reside in the membranes of every cell of the body, and each is specific for a certain compound or group of related compounds. Most of these proteins are confined to the cell membranes but can rotate or shuttle from one side to the other. Thus they act as "pumps," picking up compounds on one side of the membrane, depositing them on the other, and thereby permitting the cells to "decide" what substances to take up and what to release.

Examples of well-known transport proteins are the glucose, potassium, and sodium pumps. The first two transport glucose and potassium into cells faster than they can leak out; the sodium pump transports sodium out of cells faster than it can leak in. Thanks to these pumps, a higher concentration of glucose and potassium, and a lower concentration of sodium, is maintained inside the cells than in the surrounding medium. Laboratory scientists know they are observing pumps at work whenever they find a cell maintaining a concentration gradient of a substance across its membrane. These gradients are of great importance to cells. For example, the sodium-potassium distribution across the membranes of nerve cells makes it possible for nerve impulses to travel—and so for you to think and act.

The mineral calcium enters the body with the help of a protein, too—the calcium-binding protein in the intestinal tract. In fact, almost every water-soluble nutrient seems to have its own transport system in cell membranes. (By contrast, lipids can cross membranes without the help of pumps. Cells seem to regulate lipids' transport by attaching them to proteins or other molecules so that they *cannot* move across membranes, disconnecting them to move them in or out, and reconnecting them to proteins or other molecules again to keep them in place.)

The cell membranes' protein machinery can be switched on or off in response to the body's needs. Often hormones do the switching, with a marvelous precision. A familiar example is provided by insulin and glucose. When there is too much glucose in the blood, the pancreas steps up its output of the hormone insulin; the insulin stimulates the cells to take up glucose (and is destroyed in the process); the cells pick up the excess glucose; then, when the blood glucose concentration is normal, the pancreas reduces its insulin output. The blood concentration of calcium is regulated in a similar manner by the hormones calcitonin and parathormone. Hundreds of other body proteins maintain the distribution of hundreds of other substances into the various body spaces.

Other transport proteins, not attached to membranes, move about in the body fluids carrying nutrients and other molecules from one organ to another. The lipids are an example. You have already read about the problem these cumbersome molecules pose for the digestive system. They have to be emulsified to be made accessible to the enzymes that hydrolyze them. After absorption, they continue to require special handling; they must be wrapped in protein before they can travel in the blood. The complexes formed for lipid transport are the lipoproteins, giant aggregates much larger than lipids by themselves, but able to travel easily in water because their protein coats are hydrophilic. (Only the smaller lipids—for example, monoglycerides, glycerol, and fatty acids—can travel freely without carri-

acidosis: too much acid in the blood and body fluids.

alkalosis: too much base in the blood and body fluids.

lethal: causing death.

sequester (see-KWESS-ter): to hide away or take out of circulation.

buffer: a compound that can reversibly combine with H⁺ ions to help maintain a constant pH. Figure 10–3 shows how a buffer works.

antibody: a large protein of the blood and body fluids, produced in response to invasion of the body by unfamiliar molecules (mostly proteins); it inactivates the invaders and so protects the body.

The thyroid hormone contains iodine; insulin contains zinc; these minerals are helper nutrients. See Chapter 11.

Hormone: see Chapter 2.

These membrane-associated proteins are variously called **permeases**, **vectorial enzymes**, and **transferases**.

concentration gradient: a difference in concentration of a **solute** (SOLL-yoot)—a dissolved substance—on two sides of a semipermeable membrane.

Calcium concentration is tightly controlled by hormones, as described in Chapter 10.

Lipoproteins are described in full in Chapter 5.

The protein residing in the intestinal wall cells is **ferritin**; the carrier protein, **transferrin**; the storage protein, **ferritin** again; the red-blood-cell protein, **hemoglobin**; and the muscle-cell protein, **myoglobin**.

The protein that relays calcium's messages is **calmodulin**. See Chapter 10.

The chain of events is as follows:

1 A phospholipid **(thromboplastin)** is released from blood platelets (small, cell-fragment-like structures in the blood).
2 Thromboplastin catalyzes the conversion of **prothrombin** (a precursor protein made in the liver that circulates in the blood) to **thrombin**.
3 Thrombin then catalyzes the conversion of **fibrinogen** (another circulating precursor protein) to **fibrin**.

thrombo = clot

fibr = fibers

ogen = gives rise to

Vitamin K (involved in the production of prothrombin) and calcium (needed for the blood to clot) are helper nutrients—see Chapters 9 and 10.

collagen: the protein material of which scars, tendons, ligaments, and the foundations of bones and teeth are made.

kolla = glue

Vitamin C (needed to form collagen) and minerals (to calcify bones and teeth) are helper nutrients. See Chapters 8, 10, and 11.

opsin: the protein of the visual pigments. Vitamin A is a helper nutrient, attached to opsin to form the pigment rhodopsin—see Chapter 9.

ers.) The fat-soluble vitamins are also carried by special proteins, and many carriers for the water-soluble vitamins are also becoming known.

The mineral iron is a nutrient whose handling in the body illustrates especially well how precisely proteins operate. On moving into a cell of the intestinal wall, iron is captured by a protein residing in the cell, which will not let go of it unless the iron is needed in the body. Iron leaving the cell to enter the bloodstream is attached to a carrier protein. The carrier, in turn, can pass iron on to a storage protein in the bone marrow or other tissues, which will hold it until it is called for. Then, when it is needed, iron is incorporated into the structure of still another protein in the red blood cells, where it assists in oxygen transport, or into a muscle protein, which helps muscle cells oxidize their energy fuels. At least one protein is similarly involved in the body's handling of calcium. One of this protein's many roles is to relay to cells a sort of message conveyed from other parts of the body by calcium ions.

Blood Clotting

Blood is unique and wonderful in its ability to remain a liquid tissue even though it carries so many large molecules and cells through the circulatory system. But blood can also turn solid within seconds when the integrity of that system is disturbed. (If it did not clot, a single pinprick could drain your entire body of all its blood, just as a tiny hole in a bucket makes the bucket forever useless for holding water.) When you cut yourself, a rapid chain of events leads to the production of fibrin, a stringy, insoluble mass of protein fibers that plugs the cut and stops the leak. Later, more slowly, a scar forms to replace the clot and permanently heal the cut.

Connective Tissue

Proteins help make scar tissue, bones, and teeth. When the construction of a bone or a tooth begins, bone-building cells first lay down a scaffolding made of the protein collagen. Later, they lay down crystals of calcium, phosphorus, fluoride, and other minerals on this matrix to form the hardened bone. When a bone breaks, the bone-building cells begin mending the break by molding a collagen matrix, then lay down the bony material. Collagen is also the mending material in torn tissue, forming scars to hold the separated parts together. It is the material of ligaments and tendons and is a strengthening glue between the cells of the artery walls that helps enable them to withstand the pressure of surging heartbeats.

Visual Pigments

The light-sensitive pigments in the cells of the retina are molecules of the protein opsin. Opsin responds to light by changing its shape, thus initiating the nerve impulses that convey the sense of sight to the higher centers of the brain.

The list of protein functions here is by no means exhaustive, but it does give some sense of the immense variety and importance of proteins in the body. With this information as background, you are in a position to appreciate the significance of the world's most serious malnutrition problem: protein-kcalorie deficiency.

Protein-kCalorie Malnutrition

Protein and kcalories (energy) are involved in every body function. When children are deprived of food and suffer a kcalorie deficit, they degrade their own body protein for energy and thus indirectly suffer a protein deficiency as well as an energy deficiency. Protein and kcalorie deprivation thus go hand in hand—so often, that public health officials have adopted an abbreviation for the overlapping pair: PCM. Cases are observed at both ends of the spectrum, however. The classic protein deficiency disease is kwashiorkor, and the kcalorie deficiency disease is marasmus.

Kwashiorkor

The word *kwashiorkor* originally meant "the evil spirit which infects the first child when the second child is born." It is easy to see how this superstitious belief arose among the Ghanaians who named the disease. When a mother who has been nursing her first child bears a second child, she weans the first and puts the second on the breast. The first child soon begins to sicken and die, just as if an evil spirit had accompanied the new baby into the world and set out to destroy the older child. What actually happens, of course, is that protein deficiency follows soon after weaning. Breast milk provides a child with sufficient protein, but the child is generally weaned to a starchy, protein-poor gruel. The gruel does not supply enough amino acids even to maintain a child's body, much less enough to enable it to grow.

Kwashiorkor occurs not only in Africa but also in Central America, South America, the Near East, the Far East—and in wealthy, as well as poor, countries on every continent. It is probably a mixture of deficiency symptoms from lack of both protein and zinc and possibly other nutrients as well. Wherever mother's milk is the only reliable and readily available source of protein and zinc for infants, kwashiorkor threatens them at weaning time. It typically sets in at about the age of two, and the child's growth slows down, so that by the time the child is four, he is no taller than he was at two. His hair loses its color, his skin is patchy and scaly, sometimes with ulcers and sores that fail to heal. His limbs and face become swollen with edema; his belly bulges with fatty liver; he sickens easily and is weak, fretful, and apathetic. Figure 4–6 shows a picture of such a child.

The body follows a priority system when there is not enough protein to meet all its needs. It abandons its less vital systems first. When it cannot obtain enough amino acids from dietary sources, the body switches to a "metabolism of wasting"; it begins to digest its own protein tissues. This way, it can supply the amino acids needed to continue maintaining the vital, internal organs and thus keep itself alive. Hair and skin pigments (which are made of amino acids) are dispensable and are no longer manu-

protein-kcalorie malnutrition: a deficiency of protein or kcalories or both, often referred to as **PCM**; also **PEM**, for **protein-energy malnutrition**.

kwashiorkor (kwash-ee-OR-core, kwash-ee-or-CORE): malnutrition caused by protein deficiency in the presence of adequate kcalories.

marasmus (ma-RAZZ-mus): malnutrition caused by simple starvation.

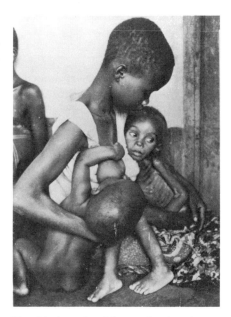

Kwashiorkor: the sickness that invades the first child when the second child is born.

gruel: a thin porridge made by boiling meal of grains or legumes in water.

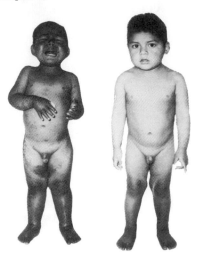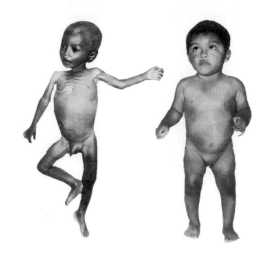

FIGURE 4–6 **Kwashiorkor.** The child at far left has the characteristic "moon face" (edema), swollen belly, and patchy dermatitis (from zinc deficiency) often seen with kwashiorkor. At center left, the same child after nutritional therapy. **Marasmus.** The child at center right is suffering from the extreme emaciation of marasmus. At far right is the same child after nutritional therapy.

Source: Courtesy of Dr. Robert S. Goodhart, M.D.

dysentery (DIS-en-terry): an infection of the gastrointestinal tract caused by an amoeba or bacterium and giving rise to severe diarrhea.

When two variables interact so that each increases the other, they are said to be acting synergistically. Malnutrition and infection are a deadly combination because they work this way.

synergism (SIN-er-jism): the effect of two factors operating together in such a way that their combined actions are greater than the sum of the actions of the two considered separately.

factured. The skin needs less integrity in a life-or-death situation than the heart does, so its maintenance stops and skin sores fail to heal. Many of the antibodies are also degraded so that their amino acids may be used as building blocks for heart and lung and brain tissue. A child with a depleted supply of antibodies cannot resist infection and readily contracts dysentery, a disease of the digestive tract. Dysentery causes diarrhea, leading to rapid loss of any nutrients—including amino acids—that the child may be receiving in food. Thus dysentery worsens the protein deficiency, and the protein deficiency in turn increases the likelihood of a second or third or tenth attack of dysentery.

The water loss in diarrhea increases losses of minerals and of the water-soluble B vitamins and vitamin C. Lack of protein carriers for the fat-soluble vitamins creates a deficiency in vitamins A and D as well. The child's inability to manufacture protein carriers for fat often leaves him with fat accumulated in the liver tissue, from which it would normally be carried away. As the liver clogs with fat, its cells lose their ability to carry out their other normal functions, and gradually they atrophy and die.

A malnourished child who contracts measles cannot fight it off. In our country, where protein deficiency is almost never a problem, the child with measles may expect to recover within five to seven days; the kwashiorkor child often dies within the first two days. Other diseases take a similarly heavy toll.

Marasmus

Textbooks usually describe marasmus and kwashiorkor as the two endpoints on a spectrum—lack of kcalories at one end and lack of protein at the other—with PCM occupying the central region. In practice these distinctions are not so easily made. At all points between marasmus and kwashiorkor, protein deficiency produces symptoms, whether the underlying cause is lack of dietary protein or lack of kcalories to conserve protein. Furthermore, a diet deficient in protein and kcalories is invariably deficient in other nutrients as well.

A marasmic child looks like a wizened little old person—just skin and bones (see Figure 4–6). She is often sick, because her resistance to disease is low. All her muscles are wasted, including the heart muscle, and the heart is weak. Reduced synthesis of key hormones leads to a metabolism so slow that her body temperature is subnormal. Unlike the kwashiorkor child, she has no fat accumulated in her liver, and little or no fat under her skin to insulate against cold. The experience of hospital workers with victims of marasmus is that their primary need is to be wrapped up and kept warm. They also need love, because they have often been severely deprived of maternal attention as well as food.

Unlike the kwashiorkor child, who has been fed milk until weaning, the marasmic child may have been neglected from early infancy. The disease occurs most commonly in children from 6 to 18 months of age in all the overpopulated city slums of the world, and in rural children who have been fed inadequate formulas for too long. Since the brain normally grows to almost its full adult size within the first two years of life, marasmus impairs brain development and so may have a permanent effect on learning ability.

In order to study the effects of PCM on brain growth, one group of researchers analyzed the brain tissue of young children who had died of severe marasmus as well as brain tissue from otherwise healthy accident victims (children of comparable ages). They found that the number of brain cells of the marasmic children was significantly lower than the number in the well-fed children (see Figure 4–7).[8] Since the number of brain cells does not increase significantly after about the first year of life, children with marasmus may never attain their full intellectual potential, even if they are well fed later.[9]

Protein-kcalorie malnutrition particularly affects vulnerable groups in the community, such as pregnant and lactating women, nursing infants, just-weaned children, and children in periods of rapid growth. These groups have a great need for protein because of the new tissues being formed in their bodies. They need ample kcalories to protect that protein from degradation, yet in many cultures they are the very ones who are denied nourishing food.

The extent, severity, and causes of world hunger are reviewed in Highlight 9, together with some approaches to a solution in which individuals can become involved.

8   M. Winick, P. Rosso, and J. Waterlow, Cellular growth of cerebrum, cerebellum, and brain stem in normal and marasmic children, *Experimental Neurology* 26 (1970): 393–400.
9   It is difficult, however, to sort out the effects of nutritional from emotional and intellectual deprivation. J. Cravioto, Nutrition, stimulation, mental development and learning, *Nutrition Today*, September/October 1981, pp. 4–8, 10–15.

FIGURE 4–7 **Malnutrition reduces brain cell number.** The graph shows the total DNA in cerebellums of children who died at ages up to two and a half years. Those that suffered malnutrition in infancy had less DNA (a reflection of brain cell number).

Source: M. Winick, P. Rosso, and J. Waterlow, Cellular growth of cerebrum, cerebellum, and brain stem in normal and marasmic children, *Experimental Neurology* 26 (1970): 393–400.

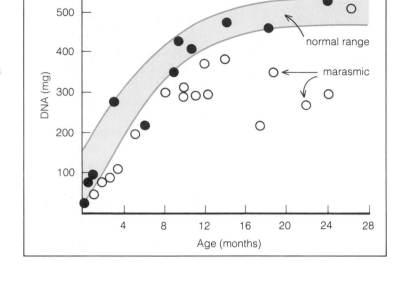

The "beer belly" of the alcoholic is usually rightly attributed to fat, due to an excess intake of kcalories, but it sometimes reflects ascites (edema in the abdomen) or fatty liver.

cirrhosis (seer-OH-sis): irreversible liver damage involving death of liver cells and their replacement by scar tissue.

For more about the effects of alcohol on the liver, see Highlight 8A.

Adult PCM

Kwashiorkor is only one of several diseases associated with protein deficiency. Another that is closer to home for most of us is the nutritional liver disease associated with alcoholism. The alcoholic person, like the kwashiorkor child, consumes abundant kcalories, but up to three-fourths of his kcalories may come from alcohol, a nonprotein substance. Like the kwashiorkor child, the malnourished alcoholic may have a belly swollen with fat; puffy hands, feet, and face; skin sores; and a reduced ability to withstand infection. If the alcoholic's fatty liver goes unremedied for too long, the liver cells ultimately die and are replaced by inert scar tissue. This is the progression to cirrhosis, which is so often caused by alcoholism.

Adult kwashiorkor and marasmus also occur in hospital patients whose diets have been inadequate. A person undergoing surgery or fighting an infection has a greatly increased need of protein and kcalories. At the same time, she may feel too sick to eat or may be fed only liquids or intravenous fluids, which are not nearly nutritious enough even to maintain a healthy body. Hospital malnutrition occurs in up to 50 percent of the patients in some hospitals and increases the risks associated with surgery and infection. Physicians, whose medical school training has until recently almost totally neglected nutrition, are now becoming increasingly aware of its importance in the treatment of the sick. Some hospitals now maintain special staffs to assess the nutrition status of their patients and to provide nutrition support.[10]

10   G. L. Blackburn, B. S. Hopkins, and B. R. Bistrian, The nutrition support service in hospital practice, Ch. 9 in *Nutritional Support of Medical Practice*, 2nd ed., ed. H. A. Schneider, C. E. Anderson, and D. B. Coursin (Hagerstown, Md.: Lippincott, 1983), pp. 111–127.

Recommended Protein Intakes

Proteins are needed for growth and maintenance of all body tissues. Whenever you take a bath, you wash off whole cells from the surface layers of your skin, losing protein. The cells that manufacture hair and fingernails have to synthesize new protein constantly to go into these structures; these processes also result in a net loss of body protein. Protein losses also occur inside your body. When you swallow food, it passes down your intestinal tract. Ultimately, the undigested materials—fiber, water, and waste—leave your body, carrying with them cells that have been shed from the intestinal lining. Both inside and outside you must constantly build new cells to replace those lost from the exposed surfaces. In fact, it is said that a person's skin is replaced totally every seven years.

Given either fat or carbohydrate (composed of C, H, and O) as an energy source, the body can construct many of the materials (also composed of C, H, and O) needed to replace these lost cells. But to replace the protein, it must have protein from food, because food protein is its only available source of the essential amino acids and virtually its only source of nitrogen with which to build the other amino acids.

If the body is growing, it must manufacture more cells than are lost. Children end each day with more blood cells, more muscle cells, more skin cells than they had at the beginning of the day. So protein is needed both for routine maintenance (replacement) and growth (addition) of body tissue.

The quantity of protein you need depends on the amount of lean tissue in your body. Fat tissue requires relatively little protein to maintain itself, but the muscles and blood and other metabolically active tissues must be maintained by a continuous supply of essential amino acids. To determine how much protein people need, laboratory scientists have performed nitrogen balance studies.

Protein is the only one of the three energy-yielding nutrients that contains nitrogen. Nitrogen is easy to measure; so it serves as a convenient indicator of the location and amount of protein in food, in the body, and in excreted waste. Nitrogen balance therefore indirectly reflects the amount of protein retained.

Normally, healthy adults are in nitrogen equilibrium—they have at all times the same amount of total protein in their bodies. When nitrogen-in exceeds nitrogen-out, they are said to be in positive nitrogen balance; when nitrogen-in is less than nitrogen-out, they are in negative balance. These balances reflect a wide variety of physiological states of the body, both in health and in disease.

Growing children and pregnant women are in positive nitrogen balance; they are adding to their bodies every day new blood, bone, and muscle cells that contain protein. (When a woman gives birth, she suddenly loses most of the protein she has helped her baby to accumulate.) When a woman is lactating, she is in nitrogen equilibrium, but it is a sort of enhanced equilibrium: she is both eating more protein, and excreting more protein in her milk, than before she was pregnant. In contrast, people

Positive nitrogen balance.

"I just lost an awful lot of nitrogen!"

Zero nitrogen balance.

nitrogen balance: the amount of nitrogen consumed (N in) as compared with the amount of nitrogen excreted (N out) in a given period of time. The average amino acid weighs about 6.25 times as much as the nitrogen it contains, so the laboratory scientist can estimate the protein in a sample of food, body tissue, or excreta by multiplying the weight of the nitrogen in it by 6.25.

Nitrogen equilibrium (zero nitrogen balance): N in = N out.

Positive nitrogen balance: N in > N out.

Negative nitrogen balance: N in < N out.

who are sick are often in negative nitrogen balance; when they have to rest in bed for a long time, their muscles atrophy and the protein-nitrogen that escapes is excreted in the urine. A circumstance in which positive nitrogen balance might also reflect illness is in kidney disease: accumulation of urea nitrogen in the blood then reflects a failure of excretion. Negative nitrogen balance in such a case would reflect recovery.

Nitrogen balance studies have led to the setting of recommendations for people's protein intakes at various stages of life. Some of these recommendations are described in the following sections.

The Dietary Goal for Protein

The Senate committee that published the *Dietary Goals for the United States* observed that protein intake has been relatively constant in U.S. diets for many decades, representing about 12 percent of the total kcalories consumed. In setting the dietary goals for protein, fat, and carbohydrate, the committee recommended that you continue to consume about 12 percent of your kcalories from protein. They reasoned that your intake need not be higher than it already is, and that a reduction, which might require drastic alterations in your lifestyle, would not pay off in any predictable benefits. The dietary goals for the three energy nutrients, then, were:

To calculate the percentage of kcalories you derive from protein:

1 Use your total kcalories as the denominator (example: 1,900 kcal).
2 Multiply your protein *grams* by 4 kcal/g for the numerator (example: 70 g protein × 4 kcal/g = 280 kcal).
3 Divide to obtain a decimal, multiply by 100, and round off (example: 280/1,900 × 100 = 15% kcal from protein).

- *Protein:* 12 percent of kcalories (more loosely, 10 to 15 percent is fine).
- *Carbohydrate:* 58 percent of kcalories (or more).
- *Fat:* 30 percent of kcalories (or less).

The RDA for Protein

The Committee on RDA of the Food and Nutrition Board of the National Academy of Sciences states that a generous protein allowance for a healthy adult would be 0.8 grams of high-quality protein per kilogram of "ideal" body weight per day. Protein RDA for people of average heights at all ages are presented in the RDA Table (inside front cover). If your height is not average, you can compute your own individualized RDA for protein. Suppose your desirable weight is 50 kilograms, for example; your protein RDA would then be 0.8 times 50, or 40 grams of protein each day.

The committee uses the *average* weight for a given height, not an atypical individual's actual weight, for this calculation because the average weight is proportional to the lean body mass of the average person. Lean body mass determines protein need. If you gain weight, your fat tissue increases in mass; but fat tissue is composed largely of fat—C, H, and O—and, as mentioned, does not require much protein for maintenance.

In setting the RDA, the committee assumes that the protein eaten will be of high quality (a PER equal to or above that of casein), that it will be consumed with adequate kcalories from carbohydrate and fat, and that other nutrients in the diet will be adequate. The committee also assumes you are a healthy individual, with no unusual metabolic need for protein.

To figure your protein RDA:

1 Look up the weight for a person your height (inside back cover). Assume this weight is "ideal" for you (see Chapter 7).
2 Change pounds to kilograms (kg).
3 Multiply kilograms by 0.8 g/kg.

Example (for a 5'8" medium-frame male):

1 "Ideal" weight: about 150 lb.
2 150 lb × 1 kg/2.2 lb = 68 kg (rounded off).
3 68 kg × 0.8 g/kg = 54 g protein (rounded off).

For information on how the RDA was set, see Chapter 1.

The Canadian and FAO/WHO Recommendations
The Canadian recommendation for protein is similar to the RDA (see the Canadian *Dietary Standard* in Appendix O). The protein recommendation of the world agencies FAO/WHO, in contrast, is slightly lower: 0.75 grams per kilogram of ideal body weight.

FAO/WHO have a task somewhat different from that of the U.S. and Canadian agencies, and this accounts for their lower recommendation. They must find acceptable levels of nutrient intakes for a world in which poverty makes generous intakes a luxury. FAO/WHO carefully define their protein recommendation in terms of egg or milk protein and also publish a set of graded recommendations for proteins of lower quality. The difference between the FAO/WHO and the Canadian and U.S. recommendations reflects the different realities in the societies for which they were designed.

The Upper Limit
Is it possible to consume too much protein? Apparently so. Animals fed high-protein diets experience a protein overload effect, seen in the hypertrophy of their livers and kidneys. Infants are placed at risk in many ways if fed excess protein.[11] People who wish to lose weight may be handicapped in their efforts if they consume too much protein.[12] The higher a person's intake of such protein-rich foods as meat and milk, the more likely it is that fruits, vegetables, and grains will be crowded out of the diet, making it inadequate in other nutrients. Diets high in protein necessitate higher intakes of calcium as well, because such diets promote calcium excretion.[13] There are evidently no benefits to be gained by consuming a diet that derives more than 15 percent of its kcalories from protein, and there are possible risks.[14] Even in growing children, only half that amount is all that is needed to support optimal growth, provided the children are healthy and the protein is of high quality.[15]

hypertrophy (high-PURR-tro-fee): growing too large.

hyper = too much

trophy = growth

Protein in Foods

The foods that supply protein in abundance are those on the milk and meat lists of the exchange system. A cup of milk provides 8 grams of protein; an ounce of the average meat, 7 grams, as shown in Table 1–6 (p. 16). A half-cup portion of legumes, used as a meat substitute, is also treated as having 7

11 Infections and undernutrition, *Nutrition Reviews* 40 (1982): 119–128.

12 Dietary protein and body fat distribution, *Nutrition Reviews* 40 (1982): 89–90.

13 Urinary calcium increases with high protein intakes, perhaps because the protein makes the urine more acid than usual. A. A. Licata, Acute effects of increased meat protein on urinary electrolytes and cyclic adenosine monophosphate and serum parathyroid hormone, *American Journal of Clinical Nutrition* 34 (1981): 1779–1784.

14 High protein diets and bone homeostasis, *Nutrition Reviews* 39 (1981): 11–13.

15 *Protein–Energy Requirements* 1981.

FIGURE 4–8 Foods containing protein.

Milk list

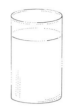

1 c milk contains 8 g protein

Meat list

1 oz meat contains 7 g protein

Vegetable list

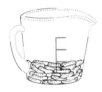

½ c vegetables contains 2 g protein

Bread (starchy vegetables) list

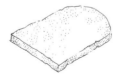

1 slice bread, portion cereal, or starchy vegetable contains 2 g protein

grams of protein in the exchange system. As the table also shows, the foods in the vegetable and bread lists contribute small but significant amounts of protein to the diet.

The exchange system provides an easy way to estimate the amount of protein a person consumes. Figure 4–8 shows the protein contents of foods, and Figure 4–9 demonstrates the calculation of how much protein is in a day's meals.

The protein RDA represents a generous intake; it is set high enough to cover the estimated needs of most people, even those with unusually high requirements. Still, most people in developed countries such as the United States ingest much more protein than the RDA. This is not surprising when you consider that a single ounce of meat or glass of milk conveys 7 or 8 grams of protein and that the RDA for an average-sized person is only about 50 grams a day.

To illustrate this point, suppose *your* recommended protein intake is 50 grams per day. This would divide easily into three meals: 10 grams at breakfast, 20 grams at lunch, and 20 grams at dinner. An egg (7 grams) and a glass of milk (8 grams) at breakfast would exceed the amount allotted for breakfast by half. A chef's salad with only 3 ounces of cut-up meat or cheese (21 grams—no eggs, no vegetables but lettuce, no bread, no milk) would more than cover the amount allotted for lunch. A small piece of chicken (21 grams again) would suffice for dinner. By the time you added a few vegetables (2 grams per half-cup), the recommended second cup of milk (8 grams), and the four bread and/or cereal items suggested by the Four Food Group Plan (8 grams), you would have by far exceeded your protein needs for the day. Finally, if you also consumed two ¾-cup portions of legumes, you would add another 21 grams of protein to your intake. No wonder most people get more than twice as much protein as they need, and most of it of higher quality than necessary.

Chapter 1 introduced the principles of wise diet planning: adequacy, balance, kcalorie control, nutrient density, and variety. To these should now be added another watchword: moderation.

Summing Up

Proteins are composed of carbon, hydrogen, oxygen, and nitrogen atoms arranged as amino acids, which are linked in chains. The sequence of a protein's amino acids determines how it folds, and the final configuration establishes the surface characteristics that enable the protein to act in specific ways.

Many amino acids can be synthesized in the body from other energy nutrients and a nitrogen source. Those that cannot are the essential amino acids. The major role of dietary protein is to supply amino acids for the synthesis of proteins needed in the body, although dietary protein can also serve as an energy source.

FIGURE 4–9 **How to estimate protein intake**. The day's meals shown on pp. 64 and 104 contained approximately 78 grams of protein:

	EXCHANGES	PROTEIN (g)
Breakfast		
1 egg	1 meat	7
1 slice toast	1 bread	2
Lunch		
2 slices bread	2 bread	4
2 tbsp peanut butter	1 meat	7
1 c milk	1 milk	8
Dinner		
6-oz steak	6 meat	42
½ c green beans	1 vegetable	2
1 c mashed potato	2 bread	4
Dessert		
2-inch diameter biscuit	1 bread	2
Total		78 g protein

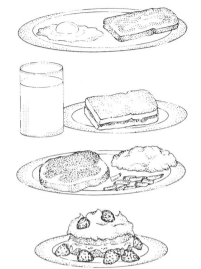

A complete protein supplies all the essential amino acids; a high-quality protein not only supplies them but also provides them in the appropriate proportions. Egg protein is the World Health Organization's reference protein, the standard by which the quality of other proteins is measured. Ways of measuring protein quality include the use of chemical scoring; the protein efficiency ratio, or PER; and the biological value, or BV. Animal protein sources are generally of higher quality than vegetable protein sources, but a vegetarian can design a diet adequate in protein.

In addition to acting as enzymes, proteins perform many other functions in the body. They regulate the distribution of water in the various body compartments (the water balance), and they help to maintain the acid-base balance. Antibodies and some hormones are made of protein. In the cell membrane, protein "pumps" enable the cell to take up specific compounds while excluding others, thus establishing concentration gradients. The absorption of many nutrients from the gastrointestinal tract depends on this function. Protein carriers are necessary to transport nutrients in the circulatory system. The body's oxygen carriers, hemoglobin and myoglobin, are also proteins. Other important body proteins include blood clotting factors, collagen, and the light-sensitive pigments of the retina.

Since all body cells contain protein, routine maintenance and repair of body tissues requires a continual supply of amino acids to synthesize proteins. Growth of new tissue requires additional protein.

Kwashiorkor is the disease in which protein and often zinc are lacking but kcalories are adequate. Kwashiorkor typically occurs in children after weaning, with severest symptoms observed after the age of two, but it also is seen in the alcoholic with nutritional liver disease and in the undernourished hospital patient.

Protein deficiency also can occur when kcalories are inadequate. In this case, amino acids are degraded for energy, causing protein deficiency indirectly. This condition, marasmus, occurs most commonly in children from 6 to 18 months of age. The deficiencies of protein and kcalories, which often go hand in hand, are together called PCM (protein-kcalorie malnutrition); this is the world's most serious malnutrition problem.

The amount of protein needed by humans can be determined by nitrogen balance studies. The RDA for protein for the healthy adult is 0.8 grams of protein per kilogram of "ideal" body weight. The Canadian recommendation is similar; the FAO/WHO recommendation is lower.

In the exchange system, the groups that supply protein in abundance are the milk list and the meat list. Vegetable and bread exchanges also contribute some protein. Most people's average consumption of protein is considerably higher than the RDA. Diets especially high in protein may actually be hazardous.

NOTE: Appendix J recommends additional readings on protein. See "Books" and "Protein."

Self-Study exercises in Appendix Q show you how to:

● Estimate your protein intake, compare it with the recommended intake, and evaluate its quality.
● Notice how your protein intake is distributed throughout the day.
● Calculate the cost of the foods you buy in terms of their protein contributions.

The *Instructor's Manual* includes an extra transparency/handout master (TH4-4) to give practice in estimating protein in meals. It also includes several supplementary lectures. One, "Inborn Errors," reveals the profound effects of disturbed protein metabolism and the life-saving impact of diet therapy based on the understanding of that metabolism. Another supplementary lecture in the *Instructor's Manual* is on "Hormones," another on enzyme adaptation ("Nutrition and Adaptation"), and still another on "Nutrition and Immunity." An appendix presents the nutrient recommendations of FAO/WHO.

HIGHLIGHT 4
Nutrition and the Brain

We . . . have the fascinating prospect that the normal function of the central nervous system may depend on several transmitter substances, some stimulatory and others inhibitory.

KNUT SCHMIDT-NIELSEN

Have you ever wondered if what you eat affects how you think? Do certain foods calm you down? Does any food or nutrient help to put you to sleep? Could a food help to relieve depression or pain? Do people only imagine these things—is it all psychological—or is there a basis of reality beneath the imaginings?

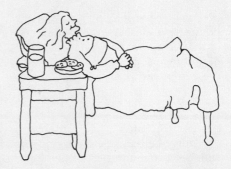

Not long ago, most serious-minded scientists would have pooh-poohed the idea that food could affect mood, behavior, or wakefulness. But recent research not only has shown that it does have such effects but is beginning to show how the effects are brought about at the molecular level. Two of the foremost researchers working in this area are Drs. R. J. Wurtman and J. J. Wurtman, who have been assembling their own and other research into a massive work, *Nutrition and the Brain*, that has been appearing in published form, volume by volume, since 1977.[1] This Highlight focuses on a few of the areas their work has revealed.

How Nutrients Reach the Brain

As the body's master-controller, the brain is more completely protected from harmful influences than any other organ. Three barriers separate the brain from direct exposure to what you eat. First, the GI tract cells themselves are selective; they refuse to absorb materials they don't recognize as nutrients (although they can be fooled sometimes). Second, all the materials absorbed into the blood circulate through the liver, which selectively removes toxins, drugs, and excess quantities of nutrients before allowing the blood to reach other parts of the body (Chapter 5). Thus the blood arriving at the brain has already been twice adjusted and cleansed; but the brain has its own molecular sieve to safeguard it further. Called the blood-brain barrier, this protective device normally lets in only those substances the brain cells particularly need: glucose (or ketones), oxygen, amino acids, nutrients. As for the complex molecules the brain cells themselves are made of, the cells make these molecules for themselves out of the

The blood-brain barrier is composed of the cells lining the blood vessels in the brain, which are so tightly glued to each other that substances can only get through the lining by crossing the cell bodies themselves. Thus the cells can use all their sophisticated equipment and be highly selective in permitting entry.

1   R. J. Wurtman and J. J. Wurtman, eds., *Nutrition and the Brain* (New York: Raven Press, 1977-present).

simple building blocks they accept from the passing blood supply. If there is a *deficiency* of an essential nutrient, the brain's supply falls short, of course. The chapters on vitamins and minerals provide many examples of severe effects of deficiencies on brain function. But if there is an excess, or if substances are circulating in the body that the brain doesn't need, the contents of brain cells do not reflect these fluctuations.

The neurotransmitters, the substances that transmit impulses from one nerve cell to the next, are an exception to the rule that substances in the brain don't reflect blood concentrations. These compounds, or at least some of them, are unusual in being subject to precursor control; that is, the nerve cells respond to a larger or smaller supply of building blocks by making larger or smaller amounts of neurotransmitters. Furthermore, the building blocks (precursors) are able to penetrate the blood-brain barrier; and they are nutrients derived from food. Thus the food you eat can influence your brain chemistry, to the extent that it produces high concentrations of the precursor nutrients in an available form. These facts link nutrition to brain activity in some intriguing ways. Figure H4–1 depicts a neurotransmitter with its precursor, an amino acid available from the diet.

How Neurotransmitters Work

Nerve cells are elongated structures, analogous to the wires or cables in electrical communications equipment. Each nerve cell has a receiving end, where a stimulus may initiate an electrical impulse, and a transmitting end, where the impulse may be passed on to another nerve cell or to a muscle cell (see Figure H4–2). The electrical impulse can in some cases jump unaided from one cell to the next, but in most cases the gap between cells prevents electrical transmission. This gap is the synapse.

neurotransmitter: a substance that is released at the end of one nerve cell when a nerve impulse arrives there, diffuses across the gap to the next nerve cell, and alters the membrane of that cell in such a way that it becomes either less or more likely to fire (or does fire).

precursor: a substance that is converted into another substance.

precursor control: control of a compound's synthesis by the availability of that compound's precursor. (The more precursor there is, the more of the compound is made.)

synapse (SIN-aps): The gap between one nerve cell and the next cell with which it communicates, or between a nerve cell and the muscle cell it stimulates.

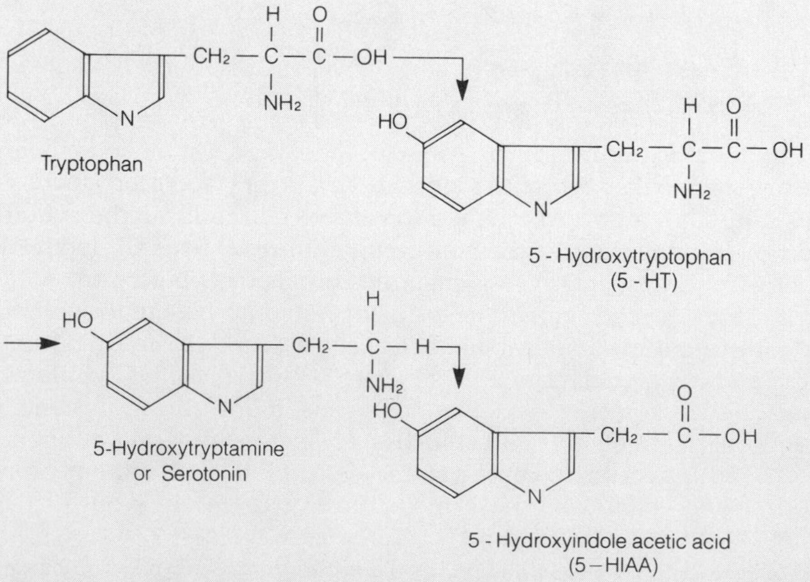

FIGURE H4–1 Tryptophan is converted to the neurotransmitter serotonin in two steps. Serotonin breaks down to the inactive product 5-HIAA when its concentration rises too high, and 5-HIAA leaves the brain to be excreted. The chemical drawings shown here are simplified by omission of the Cs and Hs in the ring structures.

Communication across synapses usually involves neurotransmitters. The first nerve cell (the one sending the impulse) releases a quantity of these molecules, and they diffuse across the synapse to reach the second (receiving) nerve cell. On arrival, they may make the receiving nerve cell either *more* or *less* likely to fire. Thus a neurotransmitter can either *stimulate* or *inhibit* the postsynaptic nerve. If it stimulates it, and the nerve fires, then an electrical impulse starts up and travels along the nerve to the other end, the next synapse. Thus messages are carried along nerves by electrical impulses and from one nerve to the next by chemical compounds, until they result in action (storage or integration of information or contraction of a muscle) or die away.

A nerve cell "decides" to fire based on inputs from all the other cells in contact with it. If the amount of stimulation relative to the amount of inhibition is great enough to initiate an impulse, then the nerve cell will fire. Figure H4–2 shows a nerve cell causing another to fire by dispatching a neurotransmitter to stimulate it.

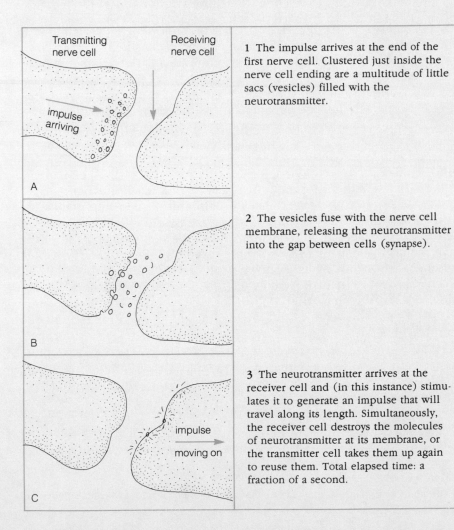

Transmitting nerve cell

Receiving nerve cell

impulse arriving

A

1 The impulse arrives at the end of the first nerve cell. Clustered just inside the nerve cell ending are a multitude of little sacs (vesicles) filled with the neurotransmitter.

B

2 The vesicles fuse with the nerve cell membrane, releasing the neurotransmitter into the gap between cells (synapse).

C

impulse

moving on

3 The neurotransmitter arrives at the receiver cell and (in this instance) stimulates it to generate an impulse that will travel along its length. Simultaneously, the receiver cell destroys the molecules of neurotransmitter at its membrane, or the transmitter cell takes them up again to reuse them. Total elapsed time: a fraction of a second.

FIGURE H4–2 How nerve cells transmit messages.

serotonin: A compound related in structure to (and made from) the amino acid tryptophan; it serves as one of the brain's principal neurotransmitters.

norepinephrine: a compound related in structure to (and made from) the amino acid tyrosine. When secreted by the adrenal gland, it acts as a hormone; when secreted at the ends of nerve cells, it acts as a neurotransmitter.

acetylcholine (ASS-uh-teel COAL-een): a compound related in structure to (and made from) choline (Chapters 3, 8); it serves as one of the brain's principal neurotransmitters.

Nerve cells manufacture and release amounts of neurotransmitters that, at least in some cases, vary in response to diet. Thus dietary factors affect the overall chemical climate of the brain. If a transmitter's action within a cluster of cells is primarily inhibitory, then an increase in the supply of that transmitter will inhibit the cells further. If the same transmitter has an excitatory effect on another group of cells, then an increase will excite them. A change in the supply of a single neurotransmitter could increase some kinds of activity and decrease others, thus altering the balance of activities in the brain. Among the diet-responsive neurotransmitters are serotonin, norepinephrine, and acetylcholine. We'll use serotonin as an example of how they all work.

Serotonin

The neurotransmitter serotonin is made in the brain from the essential amino acid tryptophan (Figure H4–1). The amount of serotonin made normally varies with the amount of tryptophan available. Tryptophan availability, in turn, depends on what is eaten (remember, an essential amino acid can't be made in the body). And a lack of tryptophan flowing into the brain can manifest itself in wakefulness, enhanced sensitivity to pain, and possibly depression.[2] We believe it is serotonin that is being affected by a lack of dietary tryptophan in such cases because sleep, pain sensitivity, and some forms of depression involve nerve cells that use serotonin as their neurotransmitter. In the case of pain, animals that have been made tryptophan-deficient have a lowered threshold for pain; when they are given a single injection of tryptophan they manifest simultaneous restoration of brain serotonin levels and a normalized pain threshold.[3]

Findings like these are of great interest to researchers who seek insight into brain function, because they suggest ways of altering it when necessary. Both sleep and the experience of pain are of great importance in health and in illness. So the question has been asked—and answered—exactly how the diet can be adjusted to alter the amount of tryptophan flowing into the brain. It isn't as simple as you might think at first, but experiments with animals have shown what the key factors are.

If tryptophan is fed or injected by itself, as a single amino acid, its concentration in the blood rises, it flows into the brain, and brain serotonin increases proportionately. If protein containing tryptophan is fed, blood tryptophan also rises, but it does *not* flow into the brain. It turns out that some of the other large amino acids in the protein compete with tryptophan for entry into the brain; they use the same carrier.[4] So protein, even though it contains the amino acid tryptophan, does not effectively enhance brain serotonin synthesis.

2   J. D. Fernstrom, Effects of the diet on brain neurotransmitters, *Metabolism* 26 (1977): 207–223; S. H. Zeisel and J. H. Growdon, Diet and brain neurotransmitters, *Nutrition and the MD*, April 1980.

3   Fernstrom, 1977.

4   The amino acids that share this carrier are tyrosine, phenylalanine, leucine, isoleucine, and valine.

On the other hand, if insulin is injected, or if a diet high in carbohydrate (which raises blood insulin) is fed, blood tryptophan rises and enters the brain. It seems that insulin drives the other amino acids, but not tryptophan, into cells, leaving the tryptophan free to enter the brain without competition. Thus, paradoxically, a meal high in carbohydrate, but not one high in protein, causes a rise in tryptophan in both the blood and the brain and so promotes serotonin synthesis. It's not the total amount of tryptophan, then, but the amount relative to the competing amino acids that affects the brain's serotonin level.[5]

With this knowledge, researchers have some fascinating avenues open to them. Experimentation is active, and its objective is to learn how diet modification can benefit people with sleep disturbances, pain, and depression.

An emphatic caution is in order. *None* of the information presented here is in a form to be used, yet, by the person on the street or even by the very knowledgeable student of nutrition, nursing, or medicine. Much of this information has reached the popular media, and health food stores make available preparations labeled "tryptophan...take two...for sleep" and the like, as if it were possible to use them to treat sleep disorders or other problems just as we self-medicate ourselves for simple cold symptoms. Research into the therapeutic effects of any of the nutrients in such disorders is still very much in the exploratory stage. Anyone who tried to apply what is known, now, in a real-life situation would be opening himself or herself to the double hazard of upsetting the body's balance with unpredictable consequences and of failing to obtain medical attention for what could be a serious—and treatable—condition.

Because this book is intended for an audience of responsible readers, it is expected that the information it contains will not be misused. At this time the only proper uses for the information presented in this Highlight—outside of strictly controlled, clinical investigation—are to shed light on the fascinating interrelationships of nutrients, the brain, and the mind; to enhance your appreciation of the complexity of those interrelationships; and to motivate you to want to learn more.

Caution

Applications

While the research on diet and neurotransmitters progresses, and before its applications and limitations are satisfactorily defined, is there any way we can safely use what we know? Popular magazines have published some suggestions; is it all right to follow them? The Rodale Press's *Executive Fitness Newsletter*, for example, says that if you want to go to sleep easily at

5   Fernstrom, 1977. The reader acquainted with this research may recall that it was at one time thought that *free* tryptophan (tryptophan not bound to albumin) was the key variable and that therefore other substances that bind albumin, such as fatty acids, might affect tryptophan availability to the brain. The paper cited here presents evidence that the binding of tryptophan to albumin is loose and has little or no effect on its availability to the brain.

night, you'd better have a turkey sandwich—turkey for the tryptophan, bread for the carbohydrate to "liberate" it.[6] Is this good advice? The turkey may be superfluous in a body where plenty of tryptophan is already circulating, but the carbohydrate may help to facilitate its entry into the brain. *Health* magazine recommends a cup of warm milk as a nightcap.[7]

There may or may not be a basis in fact for these or other choices, but at least one feature stands out in their favor. They probably will do no harm. Many people feel they can't sleep well on an empty stomach, and babies and animals slumber after eating. The next Highlight will touch on another effect of food on brain chemistry—the production of natural tranquilizers that help to relieve both pain and stress. The increased synthesis of serotonin after a carbohydrate feeding provides a possible explanation for at least part of the soothing effect such a feeding may have. Research presently under way is investigating the possibility that the serotonin-using nerves may even provide feedback control of their own tryptophan supply. When they have enough serotonin neurotransmission going on, they suppress carbohydrate consumption.[8] When they lack serotonin, perhaps they signal a need for carbohydrate.

All these and many other observations hint at answers to the questions raised at the start. Perhaps what you eat does affect how you think and feel. Perhaps carbohydrate plays a special role in modulating these effects. The research reviewed in this Highlight has answered one or two questions but has raised a dozen more. Highlight 7 returns to the subject of carbohydrate once again—specifically, to the fascinating question of sugar addiction.

Research into the roles of nutrients in the brain is relatively new, but has branched out into many lines of investigation. Investigators are studying relationships of several other substances besides tryptophan to neurotransmission: the mineral iron, the compound choline, and the amino acid tyrosine. The more they learn, the more they want to find out, because so much territory remains to be explored. Hopefully, research into these areas will continue to be supported, not only because they are of interest but also because they have great potential for enhancing human life.

NOTE: Appendix J offers additional readings on the subjects discussed in this Highlight. See "Nutrition and the Brain."

6   What to eat if you're going to eat before going to bed, *Executive Fitness Newsletter* 12 (January 10, 1981).

7   News about nightcaps, *Health*, November/December 1981, p. 6.

8   Zeisel and Growdon, April 1980.

CHAPTER 5
Digestion, Absorption, and Transport

CONTENTS

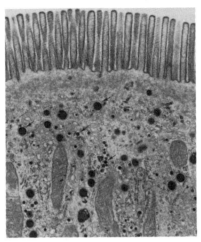

The cells of the GI tract lining display an intricate architecture that supports their function. Part of one cell is shown here with microvilli at top. The round, dark bodies are lipid droplets (chylomicrons) forming within the cell from recently absorbed lipid fragments. These will be coated with protein and released into the body for transport elsewhere. The slim, striped bodies inside the cell are mitochondria, busily producing energy to fuel the cell's work.

Food does not become nutrition until it passes the lips.

RONALD M. DEUTSCH

Lynn, age one, is playing with her mother's necklace of glass beads. As one-year-olds do, she puts it in her mouth and chews on it. The necklace breaks, and Lynn puts the beads into her mouth one by one and swallows them. An hour later her mother finds her with only a few of the hundred beads left on the table. In a panic, her mother calls the doctor. "Doctor," she says, "my daughter has just swallowed a necklace!" "Don't panic," says the doctor. "What was the necklace made of?" "Glass beads," says the mother. "That's all right, then," says the doctor. "You'll get them back. Just watch her diapers for a day or so."

One of the beauties of the digestive tract is that it is selective. Materials that are nutritive for the body are broken down into particles that can be assimilated into the bloodstream. Those that are not are left undigested and pass out the other end of the digestive tract. In a sense, the human body is doughnut–shaped, and

155

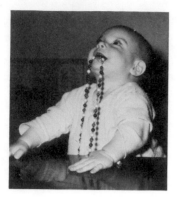

The problems of food contaminants, which may be absorbed defenselessly by the body, are the subject of Highlight 11.

Diaphragm: see p. 158.

the digestive tract is the hole through the doughnut. You can drop beads through the hole indefinitely, and they will never enter the body of the doughnut. Two days after Lynn swallowed them, her mother has recovered and restrung all the beads—and is again wearing the necklace!

The Problems of Digestion

Should you ever accidentally swallow a necklace, you would be protected from any serious consequences by the design of your digestive tract. The system solves many problems for you without your having to make any conscious effort. In fact, the digestive tract is the body's ingenious way of getting the nutrients ready for absorption. Let's consider the problems that are involved:

1 Human beings breathe as well as eat and drink through their mouths. Air taken in through the mouth must go to the lungs; food and liquid must go to the stomach. The throat must be arranged so that food and liquid do not travel to the lungs.

2 Below the lungs lies the diaphragm, a dome of muscle that separates the upper half of the major body cavity from the lower half. Food must be conducted through this wall to reach the abdomen.

3 To pass smoothly through the system, the food must be ground to a paste and must be lubricated with water. Too much water would cause the paste to flow too rapidly; too little would compact it too much, which could cause it to stop moving. The amount of water should be regulated to keep the intestinal contents at the right consistency.

4 When digestive enzymes are working on food, it should be very finely divided and suspended in a watery solution so that every particle will be accessible. Once digestion is complete and all the needed nutrients have been absorbed out of the tract into the body, only a residue remains, which is excreted. It would be both wasteful and messy to excrete large quantities of water with this residue, so some water should be withdrawn, leaving a paste just solid enough to be smooth and easy to pass.

5 The materials within the tract should be kept moving, slowly but steadily, at a pace that permits all reactions to reach completion. The materials should not be allowed to back up, except when a poison or like substance has been swallowed. At such a time the flow should reverse, to get rid of the poison by the shortest possible route (upward). If infection sets in farther down the tract, the flow should be accelerated, to speed its passage out of the body (downward).

6 The enzymes of the digestive tract are designed to digest carbohydrate, fat, and protein. The walls of the tract, being composed of living cells, are made of the same materials. These cells need protection against the action of the powerful juices that they secrete.

7 Once waste matter has reached the end of the tract, it must be excreted, but it would be inconvenient and embarrassing if this function occurred continuously. Provision must be made for periodic, voluntary evacuation when convenient.

The following sections show how the body solves these problems, with elegance and efficiency.

Anatomy of the Digestive Tract

The gastrointestinal (GI) tract is a flexible muscular tube measuring about 26 feet in length from the mouth to the anus. The voyage of the glass beads traces the path followed by food from one end to the other (see Figure 5–1).

When Lynn swallowed the beads, they first slid across her epiglottis, bypassing the entrance to her lungs. This is the body's solution to problem 1: whenever you swallow, the epiglottis closes off your air passages so that you do not choke.

Next the beads slid down the esophagus, which conducted them through the diaphragm (problem 2) to the stomach. There they were retained for a while. The cardiac sphincter at the entrance to the stomach closed behind them so that they could not slip back (problem 5). Then one by one they popped through the pylorus into the small intestine, and the pylorus, too, closed behind them. At the top of the small intestine they bypassed an opening (entrance only, no exit) from a duct (the common bile duct), which was dripping fluids (problem 3) into the small intestine from two organs outside the GI tract—the gallbladder and the pancreas. They traveled on down the small intestine through its three segments—the duodenum, the jejunum, and the ileum—a total of 20 feet of tubing coiled within the abdomen.

Having traveled through these segments of the small intestine, the beads arrived at another sphincter (problem 5 again)—the ileocecal valve, at the beginning of the large intestine (colon) in the lower right-hand side of the abdomen. As the beads entered the colon they passed another opening. Had they slipped into this opening they would have ended up in the appendix, a blind sac about the size of your little finger. They bypassed it, however, and traveled along the large intestine up the right-hand side of the abdomen, across the front to the left-hand side, down to the lower left-hand side, and finally below the other folds of the intestines to the back side of the body, above the rectum.

During passage through the colon, water was withdrawn, leaving semi-solid waste (problem 4). The beads were held back by the strong muscles of the rectum. When it was time to defecate, this muscle relaxed (problem 7), and the last sphincter in the system, the anus, opened to allow their passage.

To sum up, the path followed by the beads is as shown in the margin. This is not a very complex route, considering all that happens on the way.

The Involuntary Muscles and the Glands

You are usually unaware of all the activity that goes on between the time you swallow and the time you defecate. As is the case with so much else

---

GI tract: the gastrointestinal tract or alimentary canal; the principal organs are the stomach and intestines.

gastro = stomach

aliment = food

Epiglottis

Esophagus
Diaphragm
Cardiac sphincter

Pylorus

Common bile duct

Duodenum, jejunum, ileum

Ileocecal valve
Colon

Appendix

Rectum

Anus

See Figure 5–1.

FIGURE 5-1 **The flexible muscular tube called the gastrointestinal tract, with associated structures.** TH5-1

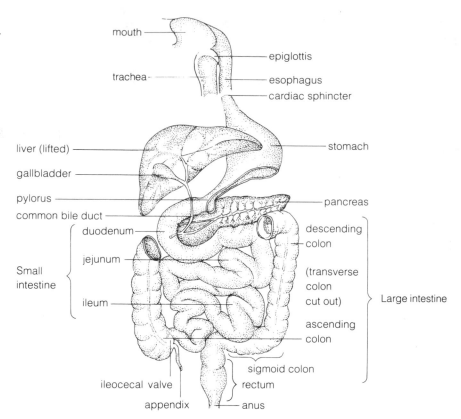

Route followed by nutrients:
MOUTH past epiglottis to ESOPHAGUS through cardiac sphincter to STOMACH through pylorus to SMALL INTESTINE (small intestine, with entrance from gallbladder and pancreas, then jejunum, then ileum) through ileocecal valve to LARGE INTESTINE past appendix to RECTUM ending at ANUS.

gland: a cell or group of cells that secretes materials for special uses in the body. Glands may be **exocrine glands**, secreting their materials "out" (into the digestive tract or onto the surface of the skin) or **endocrine glands**, secreting their materials "in" (into the blood).

exo = outside

endo = inside

krine = to separate

The salivary glands are exocrine glands.

bolus (BOH-lus): the portion of food swallowed at one time.

that goes on in the body, the muscles and glands of the digestive tract meet internal needs without your having to exert any conscious effort to get the work done.

Chewing and swallowing are under conscious control, but even in the mouth there are some automatic processes you have no control over. The salivary glands squirt just enough saliva to moisten each mouthful of food so that it can pass easily down your esophagus (problem 3). After a mouthful of food has been swallowed, it is called a bolus.

At the top of the esophagus, peristalsis begins. The entire GI tract is ringed with muscles that can squeeze it tightly. Within these rings of muscle lie longitudinal muscles. When the rings tighten and the long muscles relax, the tube is constricted. When the rings relax and the long muscles tighten, the tube bulges. These actions follow each other so that

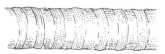

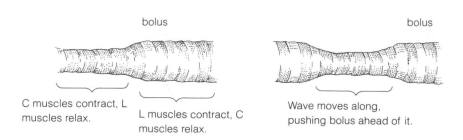

Miniglossary of GI Terms

epiglottis (epp-ee-GLOTT-iss): cartilage in the throat that guards the entrance to the trachea and prevents fluid or food from entering it when a person swallows.

epi = upon (over)
glottis = back of tongue

trachea (TRAKE-ee-uh): windpipe.

esophagus (e-SOFF-uh-gus): food pipe.

cardiac sphincter (CARD-ee-ack SFINK-ter): sphincter muscle at the junction between the esophagus and the stomach.

cardiac = the heart

sphincter: circular muscle surrounding and able to close a body opening.

sphincter = band (binder)

pylorus (pie-LORE-us): sphincter muscle separating the stomach from the small intestine.

pylorus = gatekeeper

Gallbladder and pancreas: see pp. 158, 162–163.

duodenum (doo-oh-DEEN-um, doo-ODD-num): the top portion of the small intestine (about "12 fingers' breadth" long, in ancient terminology).

duodecim = twelve

jejunum (je-JOON-um): the first two-fifths of the small intestine beyond the duodenum.

ileum (ILL-ee-um): the last segment of the small intestine.

ileocecal (ill-ee-oh-SEEK-ul) **valve**: sphincter muscle separating the small and large intestines.

colon (COAL-un): the large intestine. Its segments are the ascending colon, the transverse colon, the descending colon, and the sigmoid colon.

sigmoid = shaped like the letter S (sigma in Greek)

appendix: a narrow blind sac extending from the beginning of the colon; a vestigial organ with no known function.

rectum: the muscular terminal part of the intestine, from the sigmoid colon to the anus.

anus (AY-nus): terminal sphincter muscle of the GI tract.

peristalsis (peri-STALL-sis): successive waves of involuntary muscular contraction passing along the walls of the intestine.

peri = around
stellein = wrap

---

the intestinal contents are continuously pushed along (problem 5). (If you have ever watched a lump of food pass along the body of a snake, you have a good picture of how these muscles work.) The waves of contraction ripple through the GI tract all the time, at the rate of about three a minute, whether or not you have just eaten a meal. Peristalsis, along with the sphincter muscles that surround the tract at key places, prevents anything from backing up.

The intestines not only push but also periodically squeeze their contents at intervals—as if you had put a string around them and pulled it tight. This motion, called segmentation, forces their contents backward a few inches, mixing them and allowing the digestive juices and the absorbing cells of the walls to make better contact with them.

segmentation: a periodic squeezing or partitioning of the intestine by its circular muscles.

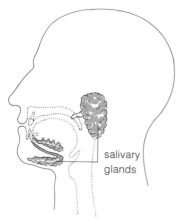

The salivary glands.

gastric glands: exocrine glands in the stomach wall that secrete gastric juice into the stomach.

gastro = stomach

chyme (KIME): the semiliquid mass of partly digested food expelled by the stomach into the duodenum.

chymos = juice

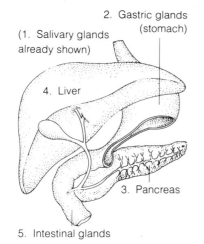

2. Gastric glands (stomach)

(1. Salivary glands already shown)

4. Liver

3. Pancreas

5. Intestinal glands

Organs that secrete digestive juices.

Four major sphincter muscles divide the tract into its principal divisions. The cardiac sphincter prevents reflux of the stomach contents into the esophagus. The pyloric sphincter, which stays closed most of the time, prevents backup of the intestinal contents into the stomach and also holds the bolus in the stomach long enough so that it can be thoroughly mixed with gastric juice and liquefied. At the end of the small intestine, the ileocecal valve performs a similar function. Finally, the tightness of the rectal muscle is a kind of safety device; together with the anus, it prevents elimination until you choose to perform it voluntarily (problem 7).

Besides forcing the bolus along, the muscles of the GI tract help to liquefy it so that the digestive enzymes will have access to all the nutrients in it. The first step in this process takes place in the mouth, where chewing, the addition of saliva, and the action of the tongue reduce the food to a coarse mash suitable for swallowing. A further mixing and kneading action then takes place in the stomach.

Of all parts of the GI tract, the stomach has the thickest walls and strongest muscles; in addition to the circular and longitudinal muscles, it has a third layer of transverse muscles that also alternately contract and relax. While these three sets of muscles are all at work forcing the bolus downward, the pyloric sphincter usually remains tightly closed, preventing the bolus from passing into the duodenum. Meanwhile, the gastric glands release juices that mix with the bolus. As a result, the bolus is churned and forced down, hits the pylorus, and bounces back. When the bolus is thoroughly liquefied, the pylorus opens briefly, about three times a minute, to allow small portions through. From this point on, the intestinal contents are called chyme. They no longer resemble food in the least.

The Process of Digestion

One person eats nothing but vegetables, fruits, and nuts; another, nothing but meat, milk, and potatoes. How is it that they wind up with essentially the same body composition? It all comes down to the fact, of course, that the body renders food—whatever it is to start with—into the basic units that carbohydrate, fat, and protein are composed of. The body absorbs these units and builds its tissues from them. The final problem of the GI tract is to digest the food.

For this purpose five different body organs secrete digestive juices: the salivary glands, the stomach, the small intestine, the liver, and the pan-

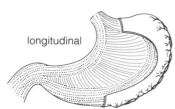

longitudinal

Stomach muscles.

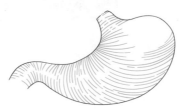

diagonal

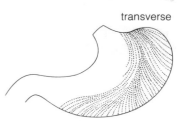

transverse

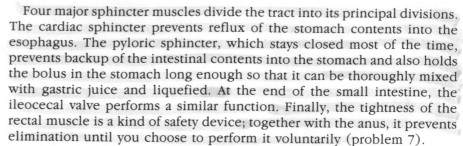

creas. Each of the juices has a turn to mix with the intestinal contents and promote their breakdown to small units that can be absorbed into the body.

Saliva contains not only water and salts, but also amylase, an enzyme that breaks bonds in the straight chains of starch. The digestion of starch thus begins in your mouth. In fact, you can taste the change if you choose. Starch has very little taste, but some maltose is released, conveying a subtly sweet flavor that you may associate with malted milk. If you hold a piece of starchy food like white bread in your mouth without swallowing it, you can taste it getting sweeter as the enzyme acts on it. Saliva also protects the tooth surfaces and linings of the mouth, esophagus, and stomach from attack by molecules that might harm them.[1]

saliva: the secretion of the salivary glands; the principal enzyme is salivary amylase.

amylase (AM-uh-lace): an enzyme that hydrolyzes amylose (a form of starch). An older name for salivary amylase is ptyalin (TY-uh-lin).

hydrolyze (HIGH-dro-lize): to split by hydrolysis (see p. 55).

Digestion in the Mouth

Carbohydrate	Starch $\xrightarrow{\text{amylase}}$ maltose
Fat	No chemical action
Protein	No chemical action
Vitamins	No chemical action
Minerals	No chemical action
Water	Added
Fiber	No chemical action

gastric juice: the secretion of the gastric glands. The principal enzymes are rennin (curdles milk protein, casein, and prepares it for pepsin action), pepsin (acts on proteins), and lipase (acts on emulsified fats).

A pH of 2 is 1,000 times stronger than a pH of 5. See Appendix B.

Gastric juice is composed of water, enzymes, and hydrochloric acid. The acid is so strong (pH 2 or below) that if it chances to reflux into the mouth, it burns the throat. The strong acidity of the stomach prevents bacterial growth and kills most bacteria that enter the body with food. It would kill the cells of the stomach as well, but for their natural defenses. To protect themselves from gastric juice, the cells of the stomach wall secrete mucus, a thick, slimy, white polysaccharide that coats the cells, protecting them from the acid and enzymes that would otherwise digest them (problem 6).

mucus (MYOO-cuss): a mucopolysaccharide (relative of carbohydrate) secreted by cells of the stomach wall. The cellular lining of the stomach with its coat of mucus is known as the mucous membrane. (The noun is *mucus*; the adjective is *mucous*.)

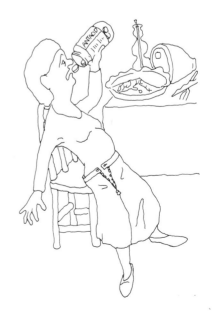

It should be noted here that the strong acidity of the stomach is a desirable condition—television commercials for antacids notwithstanding. A person who overeats or who bolts her food is likely to suffer from indigestion. The muscular reaction of the stomach to unchewed lumps or to being overfilled may be so violent as to cause regurgitation (reverse peristalsis, another solution to problem 5). When this happens, the overeater may taste the stomach acid in her mouth and think she is suffering from "acid indigestion." Responding to TV commercials, she may take antacids to neutralize the stomach acid. The consequence of

1   R. J. Gibbons and I. Dankers, Inhibition of lectin-binding to saliva-treated hydroxyapatite, to buccal epithelial cells, and to erythrocytes by salivary components, *American Journal of Clinical Nutrition* 36 (1982): 276–283.

this action is a demand on the stomach to secrete more acid to counteract the neutralizer and enable the digestive enzymes to do their work. So
the consumer ends up with the same amount of acid in her stomach but
has had to work against the antacid to produce it.

Antacids are not designed to relieve the digestive discomfort of the
hasty eater. Their proper use is to correct an abnormal condition, such as
that of the ulcer patient whose stomach or duodenal lining has been
attacked by acid. Antacid misuse is similar to the misuse of diuretics
already described. To avoid falling into the same trap as our misguided
consumer, remember that what such a person needs to do is to chew
food more thoroughly, eat it more slowly, and possibly eat less at a
sitting.

Caution

pepsin: a gastric protease. It circulates as a precursor, pepsinogen, and
is converted to pepsin by the action
of stomach acid.

Vitamin B_{12} and the intrinsic factor:
see Chapter 8.

intestinal juice: the secretion of the
intestinal glands; contains enzymes
for the digestion of carbohydrate and
protein and a minor enzyme for fat
digestion.

pancreatic (pank-ree-AT-ic) **juice**:
the exocrine secretion of the pancreas, containing enzymes for the
digestion of carbohydrate, fat, and
protein. (The pancreas also has an
endocrine function, the secretion of
insulin and other hormones.) Juice
flows from the pancreas into the
small intestine through the pancreatic duct.

All proteins are responsive to acidity; the stomach enzymes work most
efficiently in a fluid of pH 2 or lower. However, salivary amylase, which is
swallowed with the food, does not work in acid this strong, so the digestion
of starch gradually ceases as the acid penetrates the bolus. In fact, salivary
amylase becomes just another protein to be digested; its amino acids end
up being absorbed and recycled into other body proteins.

The major digestive event in the stomach is the hydrolysis of proteins.
Both the enzyme pepsin and the stomach acid itself act as catalysts for this
reaction. Minor events are the hydrolysis of some fat by a gastric lipase, the
hydrolysis of sucrose (to a very small extent) by the stomach acid, and the
attachment of a protein carrier to vitamin B_{12}.

<table>
<tr><td colspan="2" align="center">**Digestion in the Stomach**</td></tr>
<tr><td>Carbohydrate</td><td>Minor action</td></tr>
<tr><td>Fat</td><td>Minor action</td></tr>
<tr><td>Protein $\xrightarrow{\text{Pepsin, HCl}}$</td><td>Smaller polypeptides</td></tr>
<tr><td>Vitamins</td><td>Minor action</td></tr>
<tr><td>Minerals</td><td>No chemical action</td></tr>
<tr><td>Water</td><td>Added</td></tr>
<tr><td>Fiber</td><td>No chemical action</td></tr>
</table>

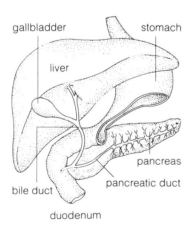

The pancreatic and bile ducts conduct
pancreas and liver secretions into the
duodenum.

By the time food has left the stomach, digestion of all three energy
nutrients has begun. But the action really gets going in the small intestine,
where three more digestive juices are contributed. Glands situated in the
intestinal wall secrete a watery juice containing all three kinds of digestive
enzymes—carbohydrases, lipases, and proteases—and others as well. In
addition, both the pancreas and the liver make contributions by way of
ducts leading into the duodenum. The pancreatic juice also contains
enzymes of all three kinds, plus others.

Food evidently needs to be digested completely. The sharing of the task by several organs underscores the body's determination to get the job done. If the pancreas fails, the intestine can still do its share; if the intestine fails, the pancreas can substitute, at least in part. Such distribution of labor is seen in nature whenever the job to be done is absolutely vital, as it is in this case.

In addition to enzymes, the pancreatic juice contains sodium bicarbonate. The pancreatic juice joins the intestinal contents just after they leave the stomach, and the bicarbonate neutralizes the acidic chyme as it enters the small intestine. From this point on, the contents of the digestive tract are at a neutral or slightly alkaline pH. The enzymes of both the intestine and the pancreas work best at this pH.

Bile, a secretion from the liver, also flows into the duodenum. The liver secretes this material continually, but it is needed only when fat is present in the intestine. The bile is concentrated and stored in the gallbladder, which squirts it into the duodenum on request. Bile is not an enzyme but an emulsifier (see Chapter 3); it brings fats into suspension in water so that enzymes can work on them. Thanks to all these secretions, all the energy nutrients are digested in the small intestine.

When the pancreas fails, however, fat digestion is seriously impaired, since the intestine has no major lipase.

bicarbonate: an alkaline secretion of the pancreas, part of the pancreatic juice. (Bicarbonate also occurs widely in all cell fluids.)

bile: an exocrine secretion of the liver (the liver also performs a multitude of metabolic functions). Bile flows from the liver into the gallbladder, where it is stored until needed. *an emulsifier*

gallbladder: the organ that stores and concentrates bile. When it receives the signal that fat is present in the duodenum, the gallbladder contracts and squirts bile down the bile duct.

Digestion in the Small Intestine

Carbohydrate	All carbohydrates $\xrightarrow{\text{Enzymes}}$ Monosaccharides
Fat	All fats $\xrightarrow{\text{Bile}}$ Emulsified fats
	Emulsified fats $\xrightarrow{\text{Enzymes}}$ Monoglycerides or glycerol and fatty acids
Protein	All proteins $\xrightarrow{\text{Enzymes}}$ Dipeptides, tripeptides, and amino acids
Vitamins	No chemical action
Minerals	No chemical action
Water	Added
Fiber	No chemical action

Most proteins are broken down to dipeptides, tripeptides, and amino acids before they are absorbed. With this in mind, you will be in a position to refute certain untrue claims made about foods—for instance, "Don't eat Food A. It contains an enzyme B that will harm you." Any enzyme you eat becomes but one among thousands of different proteins in your digestive tract. Except for the digestive enzymes whose design prevents them from being digested while they work, enzymes you eat are simply proteins that are broken down to amino acids identical to those from the other proteins you eat. Your body cannot tell the source of a particular amino acid any more than it can tell where its vitamin C

Caution

comes from (Highlight 1B). Don't be fooled by claims that imply that enzymes you eat will not be digested by the body.

The bacterial inhabitants of the GI tract are known as the **intestinal flora.**

flora = plant growth

The intestine, being neutral, permits the growth of bacteria. In fact, a healthy small intestine supports a thriving bacterial population that normally does the body no harm and may actually do some good. Bacteria in the GI tract produce a variety of vitamins; two of them (biotin and vitamin K) may, on occasion, be of significance to the person surrounding the GI tract. (For example, we sometimes rely on some of the vitamin K our bacteria have produced for us.) Provided that the normal intestinal flora are thriving, infectious bacteria have a hard time getting established and launching an attack on the system.

The small intestine—and in fact the entire GI tract—also manufactures and maintains a strong arsenal of defenses against foreign invaders. Several different kinds of defending cells are present there and confer specific immunity against intestinal diseases.[2]

Some minerals and vitamins are slightly altered during digestion. Iron is reduced in the stomach acid to its ferrous state (see Appendix B); Vitamin B_{12} is picked up by a carrier, intrinsic factor (see p. 289).

The story of how food is broken down into nutrients that can be absorbed is now nearly complete. All that remains is to recall what is left in the GI tract. The three energy nutrients—carbohydrate, fat, and protein—are the only ones that must be disassembled to basic building blocks before they are absorbed. The other nutrients—vitamins, minerals, and water—are mostly absorbable as is. The function of undigested residues, such as some fibers, is not to be absorbed but rather to remain in the digestive tract, mainly to provide a semisolid mass that can stimulate the muscles of the tract so that they will remain strong and perform peristalsis efficiently. Fiber also retains water, keeping the stools soft, and carries bile acids, sterols, and fat with it out of the body, as explained in Chapter 2.

Absorption in the Small Intestine

Carbohydrate	Almost completely absorbed (as basic units)
Fat	Almost completely absorbed (as basic units)
Protein	Almost completely absorbed (as basic units)
Vitamins	Almost completely absorbed
Minerals	Mostly absorbed
Water	Remains
Fiber	Remains

The process of absorbing the nutrients into the body presents its own problems, to be discussed in the next section. For the moment, let us assume that the digested nutrients simply disappear from the GI tract as

2   P. L. Ogra, Local defense mechanisms in the gut, in *Inadvertent Modification of the Immune Response, Effects of Foods, Drugs, and Environmental Contaminants,* proceedings of the fourth FDA Science Symposium (Washington, D.C.: Government Printing Office, 1978), pp. 19–21.

soon as they are ready. Virtually all are gone by the time the contents of the GI tract reach the end of the small intestine. Little remains but water, a few dissolved salts and body secretions, undigested materials such as fiber, and an occasional glass bead. These enter the large intestine (colon).

In the colon, intestinal bacteria degrade some of the fiber to simpler compounds (Chapter 2). The colon itself actively retrieves from its contents the materials that the conservative body is designed to recycle—much of the water and the dissolved salts (problem 4).

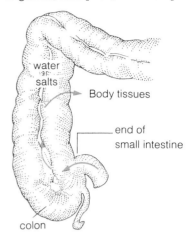

The large intestine reabsorbs water and salts.

Absorption in the Colon

Minerals	Reabsorbed
Water	Some reabsorbed
Fiber	Some digested by bacteria; some remains

The Problem of Absorption

Problem: Given an elaborate production in which 1,000 actors are on stage at once, provide a means by which all can exit simultaneously. This is the problem of absorption. Within three or four hours after you have eaten a dinner of beans and rice (or spinach lasagna, or steak and potatoes) with vegetable, salad, beverage, and dessert, your body must find a way to absorb some two hundred thousand million, million, million amino acid molecules one by one, and an equivalent number of monosaccharide, monoglyceride, glycerol, fatty acid, vitamin, and mineral molecules as well.

For the stage production, the manager might design multiple wings that all the actors could crowd into, a dozen at a time. A mechanical genius might somehow design moving wings that would actively engulf the actors as they approached. The absorptive system is no such fantasy; in 20 feet of small intestine it provides a surface whose extent is comparable to a quarter of a football field in area where the nutrient molecules can make contact and be absorbed. To remove them rapidly and provide room for more to be absorbed, a rush of circulation continuously bathes the underside of these surfaces, washing away the absorbed nutrients and carrying them to the liver and other parts of the body.

The Absorptive System

The small intestine is a tube about 20 feet long and an inch or so across. Its inner surface looks smooth and slippery, but viewed through a microscope, it turns out to be wrinkled into hundreds of folds. Each fold is covered with thousands of nipple-like projections, as numerous as the hairs on velvet

villi (VILL-ee, VILL-eye), singular
villus: fingerlike projections from
the folds of the small intestine.

microvilli (MY-cro-VILL-ee, MY-cro-
VILL-eye), singular **microvillus**: projections from the membranes of the
cells of the villi.

fabric. Each of these small intestinal projections is a villus. A single villus,
magnified still more, turns out to be composed of hundreds of cells, each
covered with microscopic hairs, the microvilli (see Figures 5–2 and 5–3).

The villi are in constant motion. Each villus is lined by a thin sheet of
muscle, so that it can wave, squirm, and wriggle like the tentacles of a sea
anemone. Any nutrient molecule small enough to be absorbed is trapped
in the microvilli and drawn into the cells beneath them. Some partially
digested nutrients are caught in the microvilli, digested further by enzymes
there, and then absorbed into the cells.

Once a molecule has entered a cell in a villus, the next problem is to
transport it to its destination elsewhere in the body. Everyone knows that
the bloodstream performs this function, but you may be surprised to learn

FIGURE 5–2 **Surface features of the small
intestinal wall.** TH5-3

A. Five folds in the wall of the small
intestine. Each is covered with villi.
B. Two villi (detail of A). Each villus is
composed of several hundred cells.
C. Three cells of a single villus (detail of
B). Each cell is coated with microvilli.
Figure 5–3 is a photograph of part of two
cells like these, on neighboring villi.

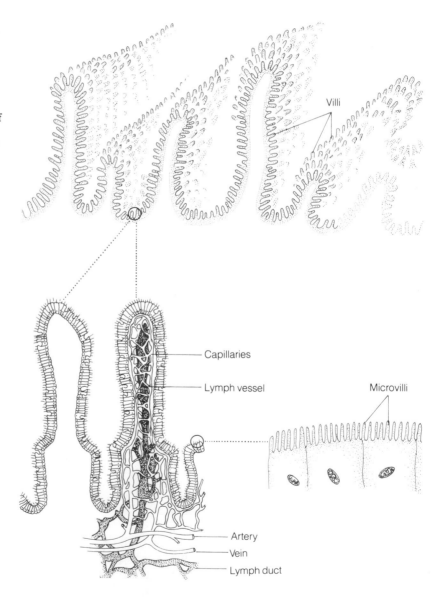

Villi

Capillaries

Lymph vessel

Microvilli

Artery

Vein

Lymph duct

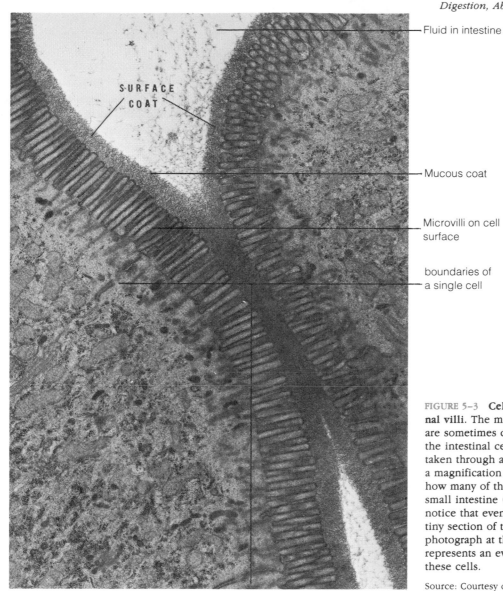

Fluid in intestine

SURFACE COAT

Mucous coat

Microvilli on cell surface

boundaries of a single cell

FIGURE 5–3 **Cells of two adjacent intestinal villi.** The microvilli and mucous coat are sometimes called the brush border of the intestinal cells. This photograph was taken through an electron microscope at a magnification of 51,000 times. Think how many of these cells there are in the small intestine (refer to Figure 5–1 and notice that even part A represents but a tiny section of the intestinal wall). The photograph at the start of this chapter represents an even closer view of one of these cells.

Source: Courtesy of Dr. Susumu Ito.

that there is a second transport system—the lymphatic system. Both of these systems supply vessels to each villus, as shown in Figure 5–2B. When a nutrient molecule has crossed the cell of a villus, it may enter either the lymph or the blood. In either case, the nutrients end up in the blood, at least for a while.

A Closer Look at the Intestinal Cells
The cells of the villi are among the most amazing in the body, for they recognize, select, and regulate the absorption of the nutrients the body

lymph (LIMF): the body's interstitial fluid, between the cells and outside the vascular system. Lymph consists of all the constituents of blood that can escape from the vascular system; it circulates in a loosely organized system of vessels and ducts known as the **lymphatic system.**

needs. (Thanks to these cells, glass beads never enter the body proper to lodge in inconvenient places, but the cells can make far more sophisticated distinctions than this.) A close look at these cells is worthwhile, because it will help to explode a number of common misconceptions about nutrition.

Each cell of a villus is coated with thousands of microvilli, which project from its membrane (Figure 5–2C). In these microvilli and in the membrane lie hundreds of different kinds of enzymes and "pumps," which recognize and act on different nutrients. For example, the enzyme lactase, which breaks apart the disaccharide lactose (milk sugar) lies within the cells' microvilli. The presence of lactase at the cell surface ensures the efficient absorption of this sugar, because as soon as it is broken into its component parts (glucose and galactose), those parts are easily contacted by the nearby pumps, which move them into the interior of the cell. This arrangement makes it easy for a newborn infant to absorb and use milk sugar, even though his gastrointestinal tract may in some ways still be immature.

Enzymes for cleaving dipeptides and tripeptides also lie in the surface structures of the intestinal cells. Whole proteins—long polypeptides—are digested to chains a few amino acids in length out in the fluid of the intestine, but once they have been rendered into dipeptides and tripeptides, these fragments are contacted and trapped by the microvilli, where the last steps of digestion occur. The cells' enzymes then can deliver the final products—amino acids—directly to the pumps, which carry them into the interior of the cells.

There is nothing random about this process. The anatomical arrangement guarantees not only digestion but also delivery of its products into the body. Digestion and absorption are coordinated.

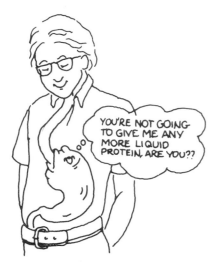

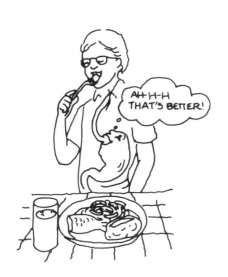

Some people believe that eating predigested protein (amino acid preparations such as the "liquid protein" products sold to dieters) saves the body the work of having to digest protein, so that the digestive system won't "wear out" so easily. Nothing could be further from the truth. As a matter of fact, whole proteins are better absorbed and utilized, even by the body of a very sick, malnourished person, than are hydrolyzed amino acid mixtures.[3] This surprising finding has come to light through actual experiments, not through the exercise of reasoning from what was known before. It has proven wrong the claims of advertisers who try to sell hydrolyzed amino acid preparations to athletes, sick people, dieters, and others. The "best" protein is food protein.

When hydrolyzed proteins (that is, predigested mixtures of amino acids) are consumed, there can be no coordination of digestion and absorption. The amino acids arrive en masse, presenting the intestine

3   The well-meaning attempt to provide predigested amino acids to sick people was based on "a misconception concerning the digestive capacities of the human gastrointestinal tract in emaciation, disease, and after surgery. Actual feeding experiments have proven...that even in extreme starvation proteins can still be digested as long as food can be swallowed." A. A. Albanese and L. A. Orto, The proteins and amino acids, in *Modern Nutrition in Health and Disease*, 5th ed., ed. R. S. Goodhart and M. E. Shils (Philadelphia: Lea and Febiger, 1973), p. 37.

with the problem of trying to absorb them all at once. At first, floating free in the intestinal fluid, they exert an attractive force (remember that charged molecules attract water), so that excess fluid is drawn into the GI tract, causing at least discomfort, and at worst cramping, nausea, and diarrhea. On the other hand, when whole food proteins are delivered to the intestine they are systematically and gradually cleaved to pieces that can be digested and absorbed in sequence. The amino acids that flow into the body also arrive in sequence, perhaps even in the sequence needed to build protein in the cells.[4]

This attractive force is osmotic pressure (see Chapter 10).

In general, it is unwise to try to second-guess the body. It has evolved over millions of years to derive its nutrients efficiently from foods. How could we presume, after five minutes of listening to a salesman or fad diet promoter, that we can improve on this natural capacity?

Caution

An additional refinement of the system for digesting and absorbing protein gives a further reason for not tampering with it. The amino acid transport systems are not specific for individual amino acids but for groups of them. For example, there is one pump for the basic amino acids and another for the neutral ones. Each group of amino acids with similar structures shares a transport system. This means that competition can occur. The amino acids within a group can interfere with each other's absorption.

These groups of amino acids have related chemical structures. See Appendix C.

Normally, no problems arise with this arrangement. Food proteins deliver balanced assortments of amino acids to the GI tract, digestion occurs slowly, fragments are delivered in leisurely fashion to the microvilli, and the final steps of digestion and absorption occur without much mutual interference. If, however, a person takes pure amino acids rather than protein, the competition for carriers is more severe, and some amino acids are lost. If the person still more foolishly presumes to decide that she needs certain specific amino acids and takes an overdose of one, she may precipitate a deficiency of the others that share its carrier.[5] If the lost amino acids are essential ones, the net effect will be to reduce her total supply of usable protein.

Essential amino acids: see p. 131.

This is not to say that some food proteins can't be improved by amino acid supplementation. A plant protein of very poor quality may be better utilized by the body if the limiting amino acids are added to it. In this instance, adding amino acids provides a balance closer to what the body needs. This theory has been scientifically tested and confirmed—for example, in growth experiments on children.

Another common misconception about digestion is that people shouldn't eat certain food combinations (for example, fruit and meat) at the same meal, because the digestive system can't handle more than one

4   E. M. N. Hamilton and E. N. Whitney, Controversy 6: Liquid protein, in *Nutrition: Concepts and Controversies*, 2nd ed. (St. Paul, Minn.: West, 1982), pp. 176–179.

5   A. E. Harper, N. J. Benevenga, and R. M. Wohlhueter, Effects of ingestion of disproportionate amounts of amino acids, *Physiological Reviews* 50 (1970): 428–558.

task at a time. The art of "food combining" is based on this idea, and represents a gross underestimation of the body's capabilities. There is seldom interference, other than the specific molecular competition just mentioned, between the absorption and utilization of one kind of nutrient and that of another. In fact they often seem to enhance each other. For example, sugars taken at the same time as protein (within four hours) seem to promote better retention of the protein. The sugars may slow the digestive process so that it is more complete, or they may provide precursors for some nonessential amino acids so that whole proteins can be produced more readily and retained in the body.

The interaction between the carbohydrate in one food and the protein in another is not unique; there are others that have to do with the vitamins and minerals. For example, the vitamin C in one food enhances the absorption of iron from another. Many other instances of mutually beneficial interactions are presented in later chapters.

Caution

The preceding discussion has illuminated some aspects of the absorption of carbohydrate and protein but has said nothing about lipids. The absorption of lipids differs in that pumps are not involved. Cell membranes dissolve lipids easily because they are made largely of lipid themselves. After the triglycerides have been digested to monoglycerides or to glycerol and fatty acids, for example, they simply diffuse across the cell membrane. The cell retains them by reassembling them.

As you can see, the cells of the intestinal tract wall are beautifully designed to perform their functions. A further refinement of the system is that the cells of successive portions of the tract are specialized for different absorptive functions. The nutrients that are ready for absorption early are absorbed near the top of the tract; those that take longer to be digested are absorbed farther down. Thus the top portion of the duodenum is specialized for the absorption of calcium and several B vitamins, such as thiamin and riboflavin; the jejunum accomplishes most of the absorption of triglycerides; and vitamin B_{12} is absorbed at the end of the ileum. Medical and health professionals who deal with digestion learn the specialized absorptive functions of different parts of the GI tract so that, when one part becomes dysfunctional, the diet can be adjusted accordingly.

The rate at which the nutrients travel through the GI tract is finely adjusted to maximize their availability to the appropriate absorptive segment of the tract when they are ready. The lowly "gut" turns out to be one of the most elegantly designed organ systems in your body.

Release of Absorbed Nutrients

Once inside the intestinal cells, the products of digestion must be released for transport to the rest of the body. The water-soluble nutrients (including the smaller products of lipid digestion) are released directly into the bloodstream. For the larger lipids and the fat-soluble vitamins, however, access directly into the capillaries is impossible because they are insoluble in water. The cells assemble the monoglycerides and long-chain fatty acids into larger molecules, triglycerides. These triglycerides and the other large lipids (cholesterol and the phospholipids) are then wrapped in protein to form chylomicrons. Finally, the cells release the chylomicrons into the lymphatic system. They can then glide through the lymph spaces until they move to a point of entry into the bloodstream near the heart.

Chylomicrons are one kind of lipoprotein. The lipoproteins are described beginning on p. 175.

Transport of Nutrients into Blood

Water-soluble nutrients
  Carbohydrates
    Monosaccharides   Directly into blood
  Lipids
    Glycerol   Directly into blood
    Short-chain fatty acids   Directly into blood
    Medium-chain fatty acids   Directly into blood
  Proteins
    Amino acids   Directly into blood
  Vitamins
    Vitamins B and C   Directly into blood
  Minerals   Directly into blood
Fat-soluble nutrients
  Lipids
    Long-chain fatty acids }
    Monoglycerides   Made into triglycerides* ⌐

    → *Triglycerides }
    Cholesterol   }(in lipoproteins)   To lymph, then blood
    Phospholipids }
  Vitamins
    Vitamins A, D, E, K   To lymph, then blood

Anatomy of the Circulatory Systems

Once a nutrient has entered the bloodstream or the lymphatic system, it may be transported to any part of the body and thus become available to any of the cells, from the tips of the toes to the roots of the hair. The circulatory systems are arranged to deliver nutrients anywhere they are needed. Figure 5–4 shows the various ways in which the nutrients get into cells.

The Vascular System
The vascular or blood circulatory system is a closed system of vessels through which blood flows continuously in a figure-8, with the heart serv-

FIGURE 5–4 **How things get into cells.**

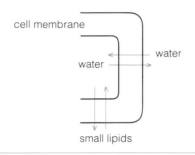

cell membrane

water → water

water

small lipids

Diffusion. Some substances cross membranes freely. Water is an example. The concentration of water tends to equalize on the two sides of a membrane; as long as it is higher outside the cell, it flows in; if it is higher inside the cell, it flows out. The cell cannot regulate the entrance and exit of water directly but can control it indirectly by concentrating some other substance to which water is attracted, such as protein or sodium. Thus the cell can pump in sodium, and water will follow passively. This is the way the cells of the wall of the large intestine act to retrieve water for the body. Since nearly all the sodium is taken into these cells before waste is excreted, nearly all the water is absorbed too. Small lipids also cross cell membranes by diffusion.

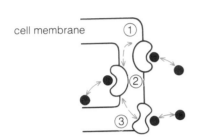

cell membrane

①

②

③

Facilitated diffusion. Other compounds cannot cross the membranes of the intestinal wall cells unless there is a specific carrier or facilitator in the membrane. The carrier may shuttle back and forth from one side of the membrane to the other, carrying its passengers either way, or it may affect the permeability of the membrane in such a way that the compound is admitted. The end result is the same as for diffusion; equal concentrations are reached on both sides. By providing carriers only for the desired compounds, the cell effectively bars all others (except those to which it is freely permeable). Facilitated diffusion is also termed carrier-mediated diffusion or passive transport.

1 Carrier loads particle on outside of cell.
2 Carrier releases particle on inside of cell.
3 Or the reverse.

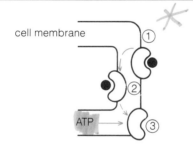

cell membrane

①

②

ATP →

③

Active transport. For compounds that must be absorbed actively, the two types of diffusion systems mentioned above will not suffice. The best a cell can do using only diffusion is to move a compound across its membrane until the concentration inside the cell is equal to that outside. An effective means of concentrating a substance inside or outside the cell is to pump it across the membrane, consuming energy in the process. Glucose, amino acids, and other nutrients are absorbed by intestinal wall cells in this manner.

1 Carrier loads particle on outside of cell.
2 Carrier releases particle on inside of cell.
3 Carrier returns to outside to pick up another, powered by the energy carrier, ATP (see p. 198). (Cells can concentrate substances inside or outside their membranes this way.)

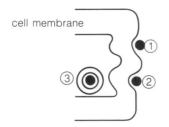

cell membrane

①

③ ②

Pinocytosis. This process involves a large area of the cell membrane, which actively engulfs whole particles and "swallows" them into the cell. Pinocytosis is not of great importance in the GI tract, but this process is one way the white blood cells are able to engulf invading viruses and bacteria in order to dispose of them.

1 Particle touches cell membrane.
2 Membrane wraps around particle.
3 Portion of membrane surrounding particle separates into cell.

ing as a pump at the crossover point. The system is diagramed in Figure 5–5. As the blood circulates through this system it picks up and delivers materials as needed.

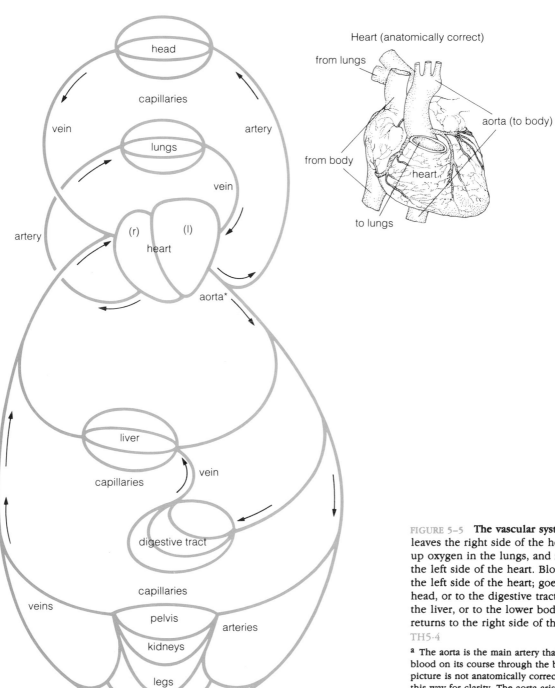

Heart (anatomically correct)

from lungs

from body

aorta (to body)

to lungs

heart

head

capillaries

vein

artery

lungs

vein

artery

(r) (l)

heart

aorta*

liver

capillaries

vein

digestive tract

capillaries

veins

pelvis

kidneys

legs

arteries

FIGURE 5–5 **The vascular system**. Blood leaves the right side of the heart, picks up oxygen in the lungs, and returns to the left side of the heart. Blood leaves the left side of the heart; goes to the head, or to the digestive tract and then the liver, or to the lower body; then returns to the right side of the heart.
TH5-4

a The aorta is the main artery that launches blood on its course through the body. The picture is not anatomically correct but is drawn this way for clarity. The aorta arises behind the left side of the heart and arcs upward, then divides.

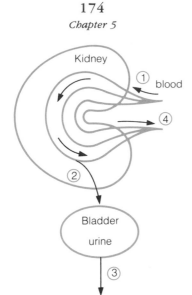

Kidney

① blood

④

②

Bladder

urine

③

1 Blood enters the kidney by way of the arteries.
2 Waste is removed and sent as urine to the bladder.
3 Urine is periodically eliminated.
4 Cleansed blood is returned to the general circulation.

artery: a vessel that carries blood away from the heart.

capillary (CAP-ill-ary): a small vessel that branches from an artery. Capillaries connect arteries to veins. Exchange of oxygen and nutrients and waste materials takes place across capillary walls.

vein: a vessel that carries blood back to the heart.

The blood arriving at the intestines flows through the **mesentery** (MEZ-en-terry), a strong, flexible membrane that surrounds and supports the abdominal organs.

The vein that collects blood from the mesentery and conducts it to capillaries in the liver is the **portal vein**.

portal = gateway

The vein that collects blood from the liver capillaries and returns it to the heart is the **hepatic vein**.

hepat = liver

All the body tissues derive oxygen and nutrients from the blood and deposit carbon dioxide and other wastes into it. The lungs are the place for exchange of carbon dioxide (which leaves the blood to be breathed out) and oxygen (which enters the blood to be delivered to all cells). The digestive system is the place for nutrients to be picked up. The kidneys are the place where wastes other than carbon dioxide are filtered out of the blood to be excreted in the urine.

Blood leaving the right side of the heart circulates by way of arteries into the lung capillaries, where it exchanges materials with the cells, and then back through veins to the left side of the heart. The left side of the heart then pumps the blood out through arteries to all systems of the body. The blood circulates in the capillaries, where it exchanges materials with the cells, and then collects into veins, which return it again to the right side of the heart (see Figure 5–5). In short, blood travels this simple route:

● Heart to arteries to capillaries to veins to heart.

There is something different about the routing of the blood past the digestive system, however. The blood is carried to the digestive system (as to all organs) by way of an artery, which (as in all organs) branches into capillaries to reach every cell. However, blood leaving the digestive system goes by way of a vein, not back to the heart, but to another organ: the liver. This vein *again* branches into capillaries, so that every cell of the liver also has access to the blood it carries. (Blood leaving the liver then returns to the heart by way of a vein.) The route is:

● Heart to arteries to capillaries (in intestines) to vein to capillaries (in liver) to vein to heart.

An anatomist studying this system knows there must be a reason for this special arrangement. The liver is placed in the circulation at this point so that it will have the first chance at the materials absorbed from the GI tract. In fact, the liver has many jobs to do preparing the absorbed nutrients for use by the body. It is the body's major metabolic organ.

You might guess that in addition the liver may stand as gatekeeper to waylay intruders that might otherwise harm the heart or brain. Perhaps this is why, when people ingest poisons that succeed in passing the first barrier (the intestinal cells) and entering the blood, it is the liver that suffers the damage—from hepatitis virus, from drugs such as barbiturates, from alcohol, from poisons, and from contaminants such as mercury. Perhaps, in fact, you have been undervaluing your liver, not knowing what heroic tasks it quietly performs for you. (Highlight 8A offers more information about this noble organ.)

The Lymphatic System

The lymphatic system is an open system that can be pictured simply as being similar to the water-filled spaces in a sponge. If you squeeze one end of a sponge, you can force the water to the other end. Between the cells of the body are spaces similar to those in the sponge, and the fluid circulating in them is the lymph. This fluid is almost identical to that of the blood except that it contains no red blood cells, because they cannot escape through the blood vessel walls. The spaces between the cells are somewhat imprecisely called lymphatic "vessels."

The lymphatic system has no pump; like the water in a sponge, lymph "squishes" from one portion of the body to another as muscles contract and create pressure here and there. Ultimately much of the lymph collects in a large duct behind the heart. This duct terminates in a vein that conducts the lymph into the heart. Thus materials from the GI tract that enter lymphatic vessels in the villi ultimately enter the blood circulatory system and then circulate through arteries, capillaries, and veins like the other nutrients. In short, nutrients that are first absorbed into lymph soon get into the blood.

Once inside the body, the nutrients can travel freely to any destination and can be taken into cells and used as needed. What then becomes of them is the subject of the next chapter. Before leaving the transport system, however, you might be interested in looking more closely at the forms in which lipids travel.

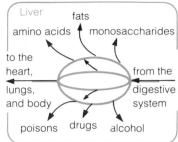

The liver removes many materials from the blood.

The duct that conveys lymph toward the heart is the **thoracic** (thor-ASS-ic) **duct**. The **subclavian vein** connects this duct with the right upper chamber of the heart, providing a passageway by which lymph can be returned to the vascular system.

Transport of Lipids: Lipoproteins

Within the circulatory systems, lipids always travel from place to place wrapped in protein coats—that is, as lipoproteins. Lipoproteins are very much in the news these days. In fact, when the doctor measures a person's blood lipid profile, she is interested not only in the types of fat she finds (triglycerides and cholesterol) but also in the types of protein coats they are wrapped in. Newly absorbed lipids leaving the intestinal cells are mostly packaged in the lipoproteins known as chylomicrons. Lipids that have been processed or made in the liver are released in lipoproteins known as VLDL and LDL. Lipids returning to the liver from other parts of the body are packaged in lipoproteins known as HDL.

In the scientist's laboratory, the lipoproteins are distinguished by their size and density. (The scientist layers the blood on top of a thick fluid in a test tube, and spins the tube in a centrifuge so that the smallest, densest particles (HDL) will settle to the bottom.) But the distinction of greatest interest for the rest of us, because it has implications for the health of the heart and blood vessels, is the distinction between the HDL and the LDL. Raised LDL concentrations are associated with a high risk of heart attack; and raised HDL, with a low risk.

A brief look at each of these types of particles will help you to interpret the news about them as new findings continue to emerge—and to understand the significance of tests the doctor may run to determine your own lipid profile. To help you picture them, an artist has provided an imaginative view of what they look like in Figure 5–6.

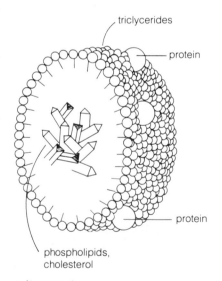

A lipoprotein

Source: Adapted from D. Kritchevsky, An update on lipids, lipoproteins and fat metabolism, in *The Medicine called Nutrition*, Medical Education (Meded) Programs, Ltd. (Englewood Cliffs, N.J.: Best Foods, 1979), p. 61.

Chylomicrons: From the Intestinal Cells
The lipids you eat are in the form of water-insoluble triglycerides, cholesterol, and phospholipids, with the triglycerides predominating (comprising about 95 percent of dietary lipid). As already described, although they

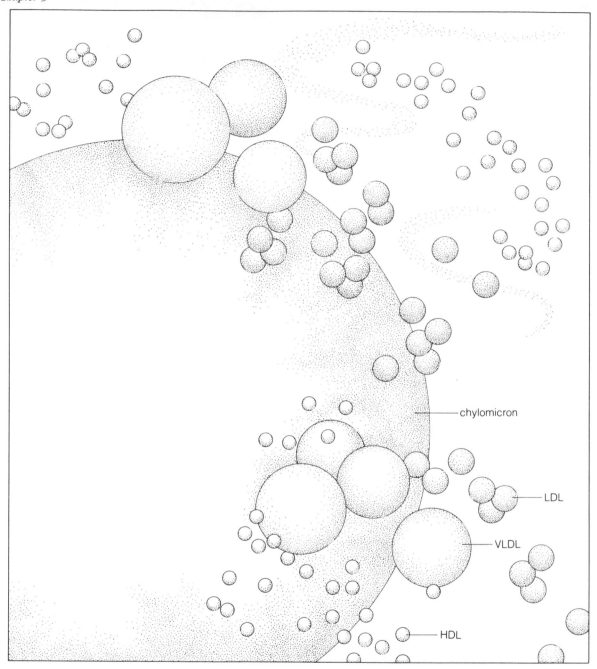

chylomicron

LDL

VLDL

HDL

FIGURE 5–6 **The lipoproteins**. The larger the particle, the higher the lipid content, so the particle floats in water solution. Smaller, protein-dense particles sink.

may be partly disassembled for entry into an intestinal cell, once inside the cell, these lipids are mostly reassembled. The cell then allows them to form a cluster. The hydrophobic tails of the fatty acids position themselves as far away from the water as they can get, some phospholipids and cholesterol arrange themselves nearby, and a thin skin of protein forms around the entire aggregate. In this ingenious configuration, the fat can be released from the intestinal cell and can travel through the lymph to the blood-stream. Figure 5–7 shows the composition of a chylomicron.

The protein of the chylomicron remnants is recognized by protein receptors on the surface of the liver cells, which make it their business to remove the remnants from the circulation, to dismantle them, and to custom-design new lipids for use by other body cells. Chylomicrons are large, fluffy particles that float at the top of a sample of blood in a test tube. This floating layer of fat does not appear if blood is drawn 14 hours after a meal, for after this period of time or less, the body's cells have removed the triglycerides and the liver cells have disposed of the remnants.

VLDL and LDL: From the Liver

The liver cells have the task of metabolizing other fats for the body's use. They pick up fatty acids arriving in the blood and use them to make other fatty acids, cholesterol, and other compounds. (At the same time, if they have quantities of carbohydrates, proteins, or alcohol to deal with, the liver cells may be making lipids from some of these.) Ultimately, some of the lipids they manufacture will need to be used or stored in other parts of the body. To send them there, the liver once again wraps them in proteins, this time as VLDL and LDL (see Figure 5–8).

The VLDL made by the liver carry all three classes of lipids, triglycerides, phospholipids, and cholesterol. The LDL contain few triglycerides but abundant cholesterol (see Figure 5–8). Released from the liver into the blood, these particles circulate throughout the body, making their contents available to all the body cells—muscle, including the heart muscle, adipose tissue, the mammary glands, and others. The body cells can select lipids from these particles to build new membranes, to make hormones or other compounds, or to store for later use. Both VLDL and LDL are much smaller and denser than the chylomicrons, but the VLDL are still large enough to give the blood a milky appearance if there are enough of them.

chylomicron (kye-lo-MY-cron): the lipoprotein formed in the intestinal wall cells following digestion and absorption of fat. Released from these cells, chylomicrons transport ingested fats to all cells of the body, which remove the ones they need, leaving chylomicron remnants to be picked up by the liver cells. The liver cells dismantle the chylomicron remnants and construct other lipoproteins for further transport.

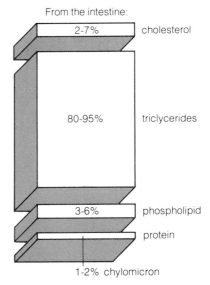

FIGURE 5–7 **A chylomicron.** The density of these particles is very, very low because they contain so little protein and so much triglyceride. You can see how the laboratory report that a person has "high blood triglycerides" might easily reflect a high concentration of chylomicrons in his blood. TH5-6

FIGURE 5–8 **VLDL and LDL.** Compare these particles with the chylomicrons and HDL. Note that "high blood cholesterol" might easily reflect a high LDL concentration. TH5-6

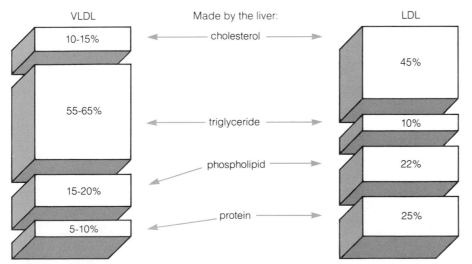

Returned to the liver:

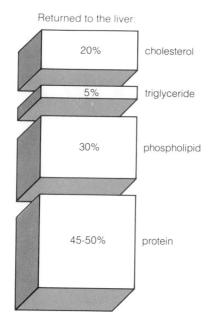

20%	cholesterol
5%	triglyceride
30%	phospholipid
45-50%	protein

FIGURE 5–9 **HDL.** These particles are denser than the others because they contain such a high percentage of protein. TH5-6

VLDL: very-low-density lipoprotein. This type of lipoprotein is made by liver cells (and to some extent by intestinal cells). An alternative name is "pre-beta" (pre-BAY-tuh) lipoprotein.

LDL: low-density lipoprotein. This type of lipoprotein may be made by liver cells or derived from VLDL as cells remove triglycerides from them. An alternative name is "beta" (BAY-tuh) lipoprotein.

HDL: high-density lipoprotein. These lipoproteins seem to transport cholesterol back to the liver from peripheral cells. An alternative name is "alpha" lipoprotein.

HDL: From the Body Cells

When energy is in short supply, the cells may have only their own stored lipids to rely on. At such a time they mobilize lipids; that is, they take them out of storage. They use their triglycerides for energy; and if they need to dispose of cholesterol and phospholipid, they return them to the blood. The packages in which unused cholesterol is found are the HDL (Figure 5–9). It is believed that their function is to return cholesterol to the liver for recycling or disposal.

Atherosclerosis and the Lipoproteins

The lipoproteins have become headline news in recent years, as researchers have discovered that they may be an important clue to the risks of heart and artery disease. In the early years, scientists spoke of "hyperlipidemia" —too much lipid in the blood. Now they refer to "hyperlipoproteinemia," recognizing the carrier in which the lipid appears.

The formation of plaques in the artery walls is described in Highlight 3. The cholesterol deposited in these plaques is available to them from the lipoproteins that carry it in the bloodstream. Those that carry the most cholesterol are the LDL, and the LDL correlate most closely with atherosclerosis. LDL have an affinity for the artery walls, perhaps because of the character of their protein. Generally speaking, *high blood cholesterol* reflects a high LDL concentration. As Highlight 3 made clear, high blood cholesterol is a primary risk factor for atherosclerosis, and prudence dictates that those of us who are susceptible to heart and artery disease should take all possible means of lowering LDL cholesterol.

The HDL also carry cholesterol, but raised HDL concentrations represent lower total body cholesterol, a lower risk of developing atherosclerosis, and a lower risk of heart attack. It is clearly not useful simply to measure the total amount of cholesterol in the blood; it is necessary to know whether the cholesterol is contained in LDL or HDL.

Some people have abnormal lipid profiles (high in chylomicrons, VLDL, or LDL) for genetic reasons, but apparently some may have them due to such poor health habits as overeating, overconsumption of fat, or underactivity. To normalize their blood lipid profiles, such people may need to eat less fat and lose weight. Activities that raise HDL concentrations—such as frequent, intensive, and sustained physical activity—may help to reverse degenerative disease processes such as atherosclerosis.

Excretion of Cholesterol with Fiber

Chapter 2 stated that some types of fiber lower the body's total cholesterol content by carrying bile salts out of the body with the feces. Now that this chapter has described the digestive and circulatory systems, it should be clear exactly how that relationship comes about. Cholesterol is used by the liver to manufacture bile. The bile collects in the gallbladder and stays there until fat arrives in the intestine; then the bile is squirted into the intestine to emulsify the fat.

When emulsified fat is absorbed, some of the bile accompanies it into the intestinal cells. The cells can't use this bile, and they excrete some of it back into the GI tract. They return the rest of the bile to the bloodstream, where it travels by way of the portal vein back to the liver. There it may either be degraded or returned once again to the gallbladder for repeated recycling to the intestine.

The bile that is left in the intestine travels down the GI tract with the waste materials and is excreted from the body with them. Certain kinds of fibers have an affinity for bile, and when the diet is rich in those fibers, more bile is excreted. This effectively reduces the total body cholesterol content and is one reason for interest in dietary fiber as a possible means of retarding the development of atherosclerosis.

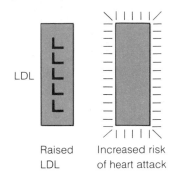

LDL

Raised LDL — Increased risk of heart attack

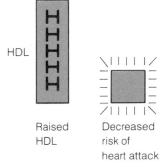

HDL

Raised HDL — Decreased risk of heart attack

People who have learned that "fiber lowers blood cholesterol" have not learned quite enough to take advantage of this knowledge. If you accept oversimplified statements like this one, you may find yourself on a bandwagon like the fiber fad. Faddists have for some years been buying purified fiber to sprinkle onto their foods, in the hope of improving their health. But it happens that the purified fiber they buy most often is wheat bran, the only type to have no cholesterol-lowering effect. (Bran is, however, an excellent stimulator of peristalsis and promotes the maintenance of healthy muscle tone in the GI tract.) Fibers that do lower blood cholesterol include pectin (the fiber of apples and other fruits) and hemicellulose (a fiber found in cereal grains, especially oat bran). Most effective is the fiber of chickpeas and other legumes, providing still another reason why legumes should be emphasized in the diet (see Chapter 1 for more about legumes).

Once again, the lesson seems to be that foods, not purified nutrients or other food components, are most likely to offer the greatest benefits to those who seek good health—and not so much any particular foods as a variety of foods. You may recall that other nutrition knowledge points in the same direction (see pp. 2, 94, 168).

How to control blood cholesterol level:
Control your weight.
Eat less saturated fat.
Exercise intensely and frequently.

Caution

The System at Its Best

We have described the anatomy of the digestive tract on several levels: the sequence of digestive organs, the structures of the villi and of the cells that compose them, and the selective machinery of the cell membranes. The intricate architecture of the GI tract makes it sensitive and responsive to conditions in its environment. Knowing what the optimal conditions are will help you to promote the best functioning of the system.

One indispensable condition is good health of the digestive tract itself. This health is affected by such factors of lifestyle as sleep, exercise, and state of mind. Adequate sleep allows for repair, maintenance of tissue, and removal of wastes that might impair efficient functioning. Exercise pro-

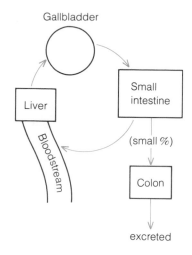

Gallbladder

Small intestine

Liver

Bloodstream

(small %)

Colon

excreted

The circulation of bile from the liver to the gallbladder to the intestine and back to the liver is known as the **enterohepatic circulation** of bile.

enteron = intestine

motes healthy muscle tone. As for mental state, Highlight 5 shows how profoundly it affects digestion and absorption. In a person under stress, digestive secretions are reduced and the blood is routed to the skeletal muscles more than to the digestive tract, so that efficient absorption of nutrients is impaired. To digest and absorb food best, you should be relaxed and tranquil at mealtimes.

Another factor is the kind of meals you eat. Among the characteristics of meals that promote optimal absorption of nutrients are balance, variety, adequacy, and moderation. Balance means having neither too much nor too little of anything. For example, some fat is needed; fat slows down intestinal motility, permitting time for absorption of some of the nutrients that are slow to be absorbed. Too much fat, however, can form an insoluble, soapy scum with calcium and so rob the body of this mineral. A well-planned meal presents you with perhaps 20 to 40 percent of its kcalories as fat.

Another example of balance is already familiar. Fiber stimulates intestinal motility. With too little fiber, the intestines are likely to be sluggish; they may then fail to mix their contents or fail to bring materials into contact with the sites on the intestinal walls where they can be absorbed. Too much fiber, however, can cause the contents of the intestines to move so fast through the tract that they are not in contact with the walls long enough to be absorbed. A well-planned meal delivers a moderate amount of fiber along with a generous assortment of nutrients.

Variety is important for many reasons but partly because some food constituents interfere with the absorption of others. Phytic acid was mentioned in Chapter 2 as a compound that often accompanies fiber in foods, and that interferes with the absorption of minerals. Phytic acid is found in whole-grain cereals and legumes, so the minerals in those foods may be to some extent "unavailable." This does not mean that whole-grain cereals are undesirable; they are rightly praised for their nutrient contributions. It does mean, though, that a person who relies too heavily on cereals and legumes may be deriving less of certain minerals from his diet than he would if he were to vary his choices.

As for adequacy—in a sense this entire book is about dietary adequacy. But here, at the end of this chapter, is a good place to underline the interdependence of the nutrients. It could almost be said that every nutrient depends on every other. Whimsically, we might attempt to sum up this notion in one overlong, oversimplified sentence. (Don't take this seriously; it is not for memorizing. Details we think you should learn are presented more systematically.) The sentence shows the needed nutrients in capital letters and those they interact with in italics.

One Long Sentence

You need PROTEIN to attract *water* into cells, to provide transport systems and diffusion-mediators for *amino acids* and *minerals*, and to provide carriers for *calcium, iron*, the *lipids, fat-soluble vitamins*, and

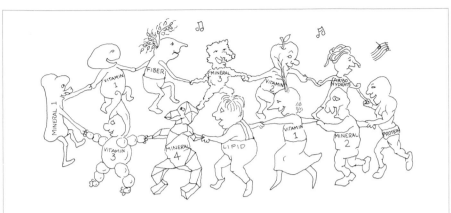

other substances; you need LIPID to stimulate the release of bile to emulsify *lipids* and *fat-soluble vitamins* and to slow down intestinal motility to allow time for absorption of certain *minerals* and *vitamins*; you need CARBOHYDRATE as *glucose* to provide energy for the active transport of many nutrients into cells, and as *cellulose (fiber)* to stimulate the mixing and moving along of *all* the nutrients; you need VITAMIN D for *calcium* absorption; VITAMIN C to facilitate *iron* absorption; and VITAMIN B_6 to help the transport systems for *amino acids*; you need MINERALS such as *chlorine* to make the hydrochloric acid that provides the stomach acidity that facilitates the digestion of *protein* and the absorption of *iron* and *calcium*; *sodium* to provide the sodium bicarbonate secreted by the pancreas to neutralize stomach acid when it reaches the duodenum, to help with the distribution of *water* across cell membranes, and to assist the transport system for *glucose*; and *phosphorus* to assist *vitamin B_6*, which in turn assists the transport systems for *amino acids*; and you need WATER to suspend *all* the nutrients in a finely divided state so that they are accessible to the absorptive machinery.

You need not eat all these nutrients at the same time in every meal, but they all work together and are all present in the cells of a healthy digestive tract. The point of all this must be abundantly clear. To maintain health and promote the functions of the GI tract, you should make adequacy, balance, variety, and moderation features of every day's menus.

Summing Up

Let's follow some food through the digestive tract to the point where all needed nutrients have been absorbed. The food is lubricated by saliva and broken up into particles by chewing. Starch digestion proceeds no farther than maltose in the mouth.

The food is swallowed and carried down the esophagus and through the cardiac sphincter by peristalsis. In the stomach further liquefaction occurs, and the digestion of proteins begins through the action of pepsin and hydrochloric acid. The pylorus releases small portions of the liquefied acidic contents into the duodenum.

In the duodenum the emulsification of fats occurs—thanks to bile, a secretion of the liver that is concentrated and stored in the gallbladder. Pancreatic bicarbonate neutralizes the intestinal contents to allow the enzymes of the intestinal and pancreatic juices to work, and fat, protein, and carbohydrate digestion all proceed further.

As the liquefied mixture passes along the small intestine, the three energy nutrients continue being digested. By the time the mixture reaches the ileocecal valve, these nutrients have been almost completely rendered into simpler compounds—the carbohydrates to monosaccharides; the lipids to monoglycerides, glycerol, and fatty acids; the proteins to dipeptides, tripeptides, and then amino acids—and have been absorbed. The vitamins and minerals have also largely been absorbed by this time. For the most part, only water, fiber, and some dissolved salts remain. In the large intestine, water and salts are reabsorbed, leaving a semisolid waste that is excreted from the rectum when the anus opens.

From carbohydrates, the monosaccharides are absorbed mostly from the small intestinal villi into the capillaries of the mesenteric membrane; the capillaries converge into veins, which in turn converge into the portal vein. The next stop is the liver.

From lipids, the medium-chain and short-chain fatty acids and glycerol follow the same route. The long-chain fatty acids and monoglycerides are reassembled into triglycerides and packaged, together with cholesterol and phospholipids, in protein to form chylomicrons, which leave the intestinal cells by way of the lymphatic system. These lipoproteins later join the general circulation through a vein from the lymphatic system into the heart, and ultimately they deposit their triglycerides into cells and are disposed of by the liver.

From proteins, the amino acids follow the same route as the monosaccharides, traveling through the mesenteric capillaries and veins and finally through the portal vein to the liver. The water-soluble vitamins and the minerals accompany the monosaccharides and amino acids; the fat-soluble vitamins are attached to carriers and follow the path of the larger fats. Some water moves with all these nutrients; the water that remains is retrieved in the large intestine. Undigested fiber remains in the GI tract until it is excreted from the body.

The lipoproteins made in intestinal cells are mostly chylomicrons. The liver makes other lipoproteins—the VLDL and LDL. The VLDL and LDL transport lipids from the liver to the peripheral cells. The LDL may also deposit cholesterol in arterial plaques, contributing to atherosclerosis. Cholesterol returning to the liver for dismantling and disposal is packaged in HDL; a raised HDL level correlates with a reduced risk of atherosclerosis.

The absorption of many nutrients depends on protein; the absorption of many others, on minerals and vitamins. The complex interrelationships among them suggest that for optimal functioning a mixture of nutrients should be taken together at each meal.

NOTE: Appendix J recommends further reading; see "Digestion and Absorption."

The *Instructor's Manual* includes two extra transparency/handout masters. One summarizes the processes of digestion (TH5-2); the other provides details of the kidney nephron (TH 5-5). It also includes a supplementary lecture, "Common Digestive Problems," which offers answers to questions students often have about choking, vomiting, diarrhea, constipation, and ulcers.

HIGHLIGHT 5
Stress and Nutrition

*Stress is not even necessarily bad for you; it is also
the spice of life, for any emotion, any activity
causes stress. But, of course, your system must be
prepared to take it.*

HANS SELYE, M.D.

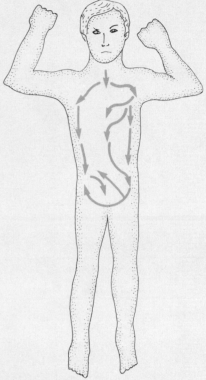

Stress involves hormones that affect all body tissues.

"When I'm under stress, I can't eat a thing," one person says. Another responds, "When I'm under stress, I eat like a horse." And a third notices, "My friend was under severe stress for a while and it took so much out of her. . . . She looks years older."

You may suffer from stress, or you may thrive on it. Whatever your reaction may be, it is virtually certain that your eating behavior is one of the many things affected. And because stress can "take a lot out of you," literally, it is important to know what happens to your body during periods of stress and what you can do before, during, and after, to protect yourself from the most severe effects.

To begin by defining terms, *stress* can be loosely described as anything that you experience as a threat to your stability or equilibrium. Even eating sugar and walking in the cold are stresses, because they demand action to restore the status quo—normal blood glucose level and body temperature. The stresses that are the subject of this Highlight, though, are those that elicit the body's hormonal stress response—major physical and psychological disturbances. Major physical stresses include pain, illness of any kind, surgery, wounds, burns, infections, a very hot or humid climate, toxic compounds, radiation, and pollution. Major psychological stresses are listed in Table H5–1.

The *stress response* is the body's way of responding to such a perceived threat. As you are already aware, it involves hormones that affect all body tissues.

The Stress Response
The stress response readies the body to deal with danger efficiently and effectively. In today's world, it stimulates people to solve problems and achieve great objectives. Yet it can wreak havoc with your health. Stress in the extreme is known to destroy mental and physical health, and to shorten life. To understand why, you have to realize that the stress response is designed to enable the body to cope with *physical* danger, while many of the threats we experience today are psychological. The stress response

stress: any threat to a person's well-being. The threat may be physical or psychological, desired or feared, but the reaction is always the same. See *stress response*.

stress response: the body's response to stress, mediated by both nerves and hormones initially; begins with an *alarm reaction*, proceeds through a stage of *resistance*, and then to recovery or, if prolonged, to *exhaustion*. This three-stage response has also been termed the **general adaptation syndrome**.

TABLE H5-1 **Events People Perceive as Stressful**

People ranked these events, according to how stressful they perceived them to be, on a scale from 1 to 100. Note that some "happy" events are included here. Individual people may score these events higher or lower than the averages shown here.

LIFE EVENT	"STRESS POINTS"
Death of spouse	100
Divorce	73
Marital separation	65
Jail term	63
Death of close family member	63
Personal injury or illness	53
Marriage	50
Being fired at work	47
Marital reconciliation	45
Retirement	45
Change in health of a family member	44
Pregnancy	40
Sex difficulties	39
Gain of new family member	39
Business readjustment	39
Change in financial state	38
Death of close friend	37
Change to different line of work	36
Change in number of arguments with spouse	35
Mortgage over $10,000	31
Foreclosure of mortgage or loan	30
Change in responsibilities at work	29
Son or daughter leaving home	29
Trouble with in-laws	29
Outstanding personal achievement	28
Wife beginning or stopping work	26
School beginning or ending	26
Change in living conditions	25
Revision of personal habits	24
Trouble with boss	23
Change in work hours or conditions	20
Change in residence	20
Change in schools	20
Change in recreation	19
Change in church activities	19
Change in social activities	18
Mortgage or loan less than $10,000	17
Change in sleeping habits	16
Change in number of family get-togethers	15
Change in eating habits	15
Vacation	13
Christmas	12
Minor violations of the law	11

Source: Adapted from T. H. Holmes and R. H. Rahe, The social readjustment rating scale, *Journal of Psychosomatic Research* 11 (1967): 213–218, and updated as published in Lifescore, *Family Health*, January 1979, p. 32.

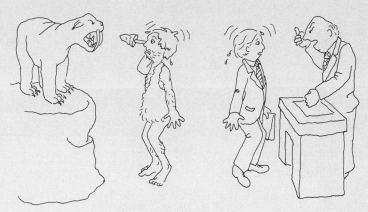

The stress response readies the body for vigorous muscular activity . . . but many of the threats we experience today are psychological.

readies the body for the vigorous muscular activity of fight or flight, not for the uptight, anxious posture of a person holding it all in.

The reaction begins when a threat to your equilibrium is perceived by the brain. The sight of a car hurtling toward you; the terror that an enemy is concealed around a nearby corner; the excitement of planning for a party, a move, or a wedding; the feeling of pain; or any other such disturbance perceived by the brain serves as an *alarm signal*. There follows the chain of events depicted in Figure H5–1, which acts through both nerves and hormones to bring about a state of readiness in every body part. The effects all favor physical action (fight or flight). Notice the tremendous array of target organs in the paragraph that follows.

The pupils of the *eyes* widen so that you can see better; the *muscles* tense up so that you can jump, run, or struggle with maximum strength; breathing quickens to bring more oxygen into the *lungs*, and the *heart* races to rush this oxygen to the muscles so that they can burn the fuel they need for energy. The *liver* pours forth the needed fuel—glucose—from its stored supply, and the *fat cells* release fatty acids and ketones as alternative fuels. Body *protein tissues* break down to supply amino acids to back up the glucose supply and to be ready to heal wounds if necessary. The *blood vessels* of the muscles expand to feed them better while those of the *GI tract* constrict; and GI tract glands shut down (digestion is a low-priority process in time of danger). Less blood flows to the *kidney*, so that fluid is conserved; and less flows to the *skin*, so that blood loss will be minimized at any wound site. More *platelets* form to allow the blood to clot faster if need be. *Hearing* sharpens, and the *brain* produces local opium-like substances, dulling its sensation of pain, which during an emergency might distract you from taking the needed action. And your *hair* may even stand on end—a reminder that there was a time when our ancestors had enough hair to bristle, look bigger, and frighten off their enemies.

This tightly synchronized, adaptive reaction to threat provides superb support for emergency physical action. You probably remember having had to take such action; you may have performed an amazing feat of strength or speed for a few minutes, and only after it was over noticed your heart was hammering, your breathing was fast, your fingers cold, your skin

Figure H5–1 **The stress reaction.**

[1] This hormone is antidiuretic hormone (ADH), which prevents water loss in urine.
[2] This is adrenocorticotropic hormone (ACTH), which stimulates the adrenal glands.
[3] These are the glucocorticoids, hormones from the adrenal glands, affecting the body's management of glucose.
[4] The platelets are small, cell-fragment-like bodies in the blood that help with blood clotting if injury occurs.
[5] This is the hormone aldosterone from the adrenal glands, involved in blood pressure regulation.
[6] This enzyme is renin, from the kidneys, which functions to raise blood pressure by activating angiotensin. (Chapter 10 explains in full.)•
[7] This hormone is angiotensin, which is involved in blood pressure regulation.

Source: Adapted from M. B. Marcinek, Stress in the surgical patient, *American Journal of Nursing* 77, November 1977, 1809–1811, and from M. V. Kaminski, Jr., R. P. Ruggiero, and C. B. Mills, Nutritional assessment, a guide to diagnosis and treatment of the hypermetabolic patient, *Journal of the Florida Medical Association* 66 (1979): 390–395.

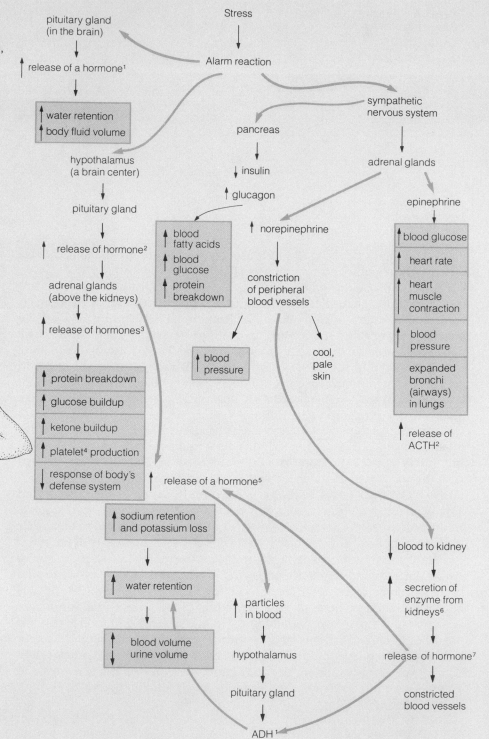

tingling, your mouth dry, and the sensation of pain or exhaustion just beginning to come through as the adrenaline drained away.

Anyone can respond in this magnificent fashion to sudden physical stress for a short time. But if the stress is prolonged, and especially if physical action is not a permitted response to it, then it can drain the body of its reserves and leave it weakened, aged, and susceptible to illness. How can we best prepare to deal with periods of stress? How can we best get through them? And how can we recover most rapidly and completely afterwards?

Body Reserves Drawn on during Stress

All three energy fuels—carbohydrate, fat, and protein—are drawn upon in increased quantities during stress. If the stress requires vigorous physical action, and if there is injury, all three are used. While the body is busy responding and not eating, the fuels must be drawn from internal sources.

The conservation of *water* at such a time is of utmost importance, as you can deduce from a look at Figure H5-1. The body takes several measures to conserve water. One is to retain sodium—but to retain sodium the kidney exchanges, and loses, *potassium*. Thus you need ample stores of potassium to be able to afford this loss.

As for the energy nutrients, *glucose* is taken from stored glycogen in the liver for as long as the supply lasts, but the supply is exhausted within a day. Thereafter, body *protein* provides the only significant continuing glucose supply, and this is drawn primarily from muscle. Amino acids from muscle also have to be used to make scar tissue to heal wounds. Tissues that can do so use *fat* for energy, and in a normally nourished person, fat stores are adequate to meet the need for many days. Chapter 7 displays these processes as they occur during the stress of fasting; for now, what is important to notice is that the body uses not only dispensable supplies (those that are there to be used up, so to speak, like stored fat) but also functional tissue that one doesn't want to lose, like muscle tissue. Two thoughts come to mind. First, in preparation for prolonged periods of stress, one would want to have as much protein in the muscle as possible. Second, one would want to take measures to minimize the wasting of muscle during stress.

Another nutrient lost from the body during stress is *calcium* from the bones. The evidence is not completely clear on this, but it has been observed that people lose widely varying amounts of this important bone mineral, depending partly on their hormonal state.[1] Adult bone loss is a common occurrence anyway, so the same considerations apply here as for protein: one wants to know, first, how to prepare for these losses and second, how to minimize them.

Nutrition prior to Periods of Stress

The body that is healthy, with tissues containing optimal amounts of the needed nutrients, is best prepared for stress. Protein and calcium are

1   W. H. Griffith, Food as a regulator of metabolism, *American Journal of Clinical Nutrition* 17 (1965): 391–398.

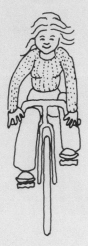

among the nutrients just mentioned; how do you obtain optimal quantities of these nutrients? In both cases the answer is the same: by eating foods that provide ample amounts of these nutrients (easy), and, equally important, by exercising to make them "stick" (takes work). Muscles don't grow and retain protein without activity, even if they are bathed in an amino-acid rich fluid. They don't respond passively to what's in their environment, but actively to the demands that are put upon them. Only when they are called upon to *work* do they grow and accumulate protein. So being healthy, in this sense, means more than just nutrition; it means nutrition and exercise. It means daily or every-other-day workouts, prolonged and demanding enough to bring about the building of muscle. (This can be accomplished pleasantly—with only 20 minutes or so of vigorous exercise every other day at first.) Then when stress hits, even if eating is altogether impossible for a while, the wasting that may inevitably occur will have less severe impact. (And incidentally, in having increased your muscle mass, you will have added significantly to your potassium supplies.)

Bones, like muscles, do not passively accumulate their component nutrients (calcium, in this case). No matter how many glasses of milk you drink a day, the extra calcium will not be deposited in bone but will be excreted as fast as you take it in—unless you *work* your bones. In response to stress (the "good" stress of physical work), bones store calcium and become denser, stronger, and able to carry more weight. Like the muscles, then, when they respond to the weakening effects of the "bad" stress of anxiety, illness, or the like, they can better afford to give up some calcium without becoming dangerously weak.

In short, the best nutritional preparation for stress is a balanced and varied diet as part of a lifestyle in which exercise plays a constant part. Notice that nothing is said here about supplements or gimmicks. Just eat well and work out regularly, and your body will be as well prepared as it can be to withstand the impact of periods of unavoidable stress.

Nutrition during Stress

The appetite is suppressed during severe stress. We've already said why. It's an adaptive reaction to a *physical* threat, the kind of threat that our ancestors experienced during their evolution. Energy at such a time is needed for fight or flight; it would be wasteful and risky to spend it looking for or eating food. The blood supply has been diverted to the muscles to maximize strength and speed; so even if you swallow food you may not be able to digest or absorb it efficiently. (In a severe upset, the stomach and intestines will even reject solid food; vomiting and/or diarrhea are their way of disposing of a burden they can't handle.) All of this means that it is poor advice to someone under severe stress to tell them to eat. They can't; and if they force themselves to eat, they can't assimilate what they've eaten.

On the other hand, fasting is itself a stress on the body, and the longer you go without eating, the harder it can be to get started again. So it can be a no-win situation. It is frightening to see the downward spiral people can get into once they have let stress affect them to the point where they can't eat, and not eating makes it harder for them to handle the stress.

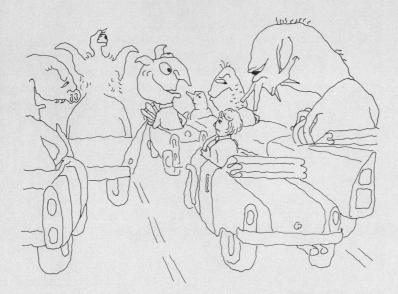

It is therefore desirable not to let stress become so overwhelming that eating becomes impossible. Managing stress so that it does not overwhelm is not only a nutritional but also a psychological task.

If you can eat, do so, of course. Take only a little if that's all you can handle, and eat more often to keep meeting your nutrient and kcalorie needs. Choose a variety of foods. Listen to your body, remember what you know about nutrition, and try to keep in tune with what you need and can handle. Drink fluids, too. Although the body conserves fluids during stress, it will excrete what it does not need, and by taking in water you enable your kidneys to excrete the sodium they might otherwise have to retain.

Whenever someone can't eat, there will inevitably be depletion of nutrients. Aside from the protein, calcium, and potassium already mentioned, the nutrients most susceptible to this depletion are the vitamins and minerals that are not stored in substantial quantities. People are aware that some water-soluble vitamins (B vitamins and vitamin C) fall into this category; they are less likely to know that some two dozen minerals do, too. When the question arises whether one should take vitamin supplements during periods of stress, the answer should probably be: "Yes, if you can't eat—but not just vitamin supplements. Take a vitamin-mineral preparation that supplies a balanced assortment of all the nutrients that might be needed, not in 'megadoses,' but in amounts comparable to the RDA."

The vitamins and minerals occupy four chapters later in the book, but it seems important to say this much about them here. Generally, people consuming less than 1,200 to 1,500 kcalories per day of food need such supplements. The RDA table on the inside front cover shows the amounts to look for, and Appendix P compares national brands.

Stress Eating

All that has been said so far has been directed at the person who loses appetite during stress. What about the one who eats more than usual? It is

stress eating: eating in response to stress; causes unknown as yet.

Substitution of a familiar and comforting behavior such as eating for a frightening behavior such as fighting is a phenomenon biologists call *displacement activity*, and is observed in all kinds of animals.

endogenous opiates: morphine-like compounds produced in the brain in response to a variety of events and activities including stress, eating, and exercise. Also known as **endorphins**.

endo = within (the body)

gen = arising

It has been proposed that peptides with opiate activity be termed **exorphins**. Like endorphins, they have opiate-like effects—but they arise from the diet and probably act within the GI tract, whereas the endorphins arise and work within the brain.

not clear why stress drives some people to eat more, but it certainly does happen.[2] One possible explanation is this sequence of events. Glucose is drawn from stores, the body fails to use it up by way of physical exertion, and instead stores it as fat. The net effect is that glycogen stores have been depleted, but the glucose hasn't been used for energy. Blood glucose will now fall an hour or two sooner than it should, and the person will get hungry and eat sooner.

Another possibility is that the *behavior* of eating helps to relieve stress by occupying the nervous system with a familiar activity that discharges its nerves without doing harm as fighting might do.[3] It may be that eating, or the food eaten, leads to release of substances in the brain that are experienced as soothing. Highlight 4 showed that neurotransmitter levels change when carbohydrate-containing food is eaten. Something else happens, too, that is worth a paragraph of explanation.

It seems that certain stresses lead to the production of substances in the brain that act in the same way as opiates like morphine do. These opiates in the emotion-governing brain centers promote both eating and reduction of activity.[4] Some proteins, on digestion, also apparently release peptides that have hormonal or opiate-like activity.[5] Much remains to be learned about these endogenous and exogenous opiates, but it already seems likely that they may help to explain stress-induced eating. The person who is subject to this behavior and who is threatened with obesity on account of it would be well advised to find an alternative behavior with which to respond to stress—exercise, meditation, listening to music, or the like.

The phenomenon of stress eating shows why exercise is important during stress as well as before. In fact, it may be positively harmful *not* to exercise in response to acute stress. As just described, in the stress response, muscle fuel floods the bloodstream; it needs to be used, or else it will be stored as fat. For psychological reasons, too, it is desirable if you are upset, angry, anxious, or even happy to express those feelings through physical action. Cry, scream, laugh, punch a pillow, pace, run, lift weights, dance, or do whatever else you choose. Actions like these release tensions that otherwise build up and increase stress.

Exercise during stress has at least two other beneficial effects. It builds muscle and bone, as already explained, promoting the retention of needed

2   A. S. Levine and J. E. Morley, Stress-induced eating, in *Food in Contemporary Society*, symposium sponsored by Stokely-Van Camp at the University of Tennessee, Knoxville, May 27–29, 1981, pp. 126–135; J. Slochower and S. P. Kaplan, Anxiety, perceived control, and eating in obese and normal weight persons, *Appetite* 1 (1980): 75–83.

3   Levine and Morley, 1981.

4   This has been demonstrated in experiments using rats and is believed to account for what is seen in humans as well. Levine and Morley, 1981; also J. E. Morley and A. S. Levine, The endorphins and enkephalins as regulators of appetite, in *Food and Contemporary Society*, pp. 136–148; J. E. Morley and A. S. Levine, Stress-induced eating is mediated through endogenous opiates, *Science* 209 (1980): 1259–1261; and A. Mandenoff, F. Fumeron, and M. Apfelbaum, Endogenous opiates and energy balance, *Science* 215 (1982): 1536–1538.

5   J. E. Morley, Food peptides—a new class of hormones? (Commentary), *Journal of the American Medical Association* 247 (1982): 2379–2380.

nutrients. And it may release the same pain-killing chemicals (endorphins) that stress does, helping to heighten mood.[6]

Nutrition in the Recovery Period

When the stressful time is over and the body can recover, the opportunity comes to replenish depleted stores. If you have lost weight you need to gain it back—not just by eating and putting on fat, but by eating and exercising to restore both lean and fat tissue. If you have gained weight, it is time to get back in trim with a combination of diet and exercise. But just as important as nutrition techniques is the learning of mind-control techniques to prevent the next stressful event from being so overwhelming and debilitating.

Stress Management

A clue to the management of stress comes from the fact that it is not the event itself but the individual's reaction to it that determines how much it will strain the body's resources. Remember, stress is defined as anything you *perceive* as a threat to your equilibrium. Divorce is considered extremely stressful by most people (it receives an average score of 73 in Table H5–1), but it may threaten one person much more than another. Happy events like marriage are also stressful. Psychological counselors urge that you learn stress management techniques to ride through the disruptive changes in your life. They suggest that you:

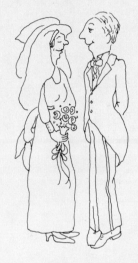

● Change how you perceive the event, so that you will react less violently to it (learn to see it not as a disaster that may destroy you but as a change you can handle).
● Learn to express yourself (ventilate), so that you will not be so uptight. This involves muscular action and deep breathing with vigorous and dramatic demonstration of your feelings (when and where appropriate).
● Take time out. Meet your need for relief from pain, anxiety, or anger by using meditation, relaxation techniques, exercise, or the like.
● Expand your social support system. Much that is exhausting and painful to handle alone is easier to manage when you have understanding from a circle of supportive friends or helpers.

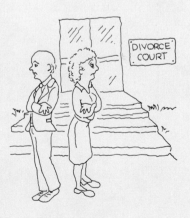

This Highlight necessarily ends by putting nutrition in perspective as part of a much larger picture in which many nonnutritional factors are of great importance. But it has also shown that nutrition *is* important, and has given some practical pointers for everyone to apply.

NOTE: Appendix J suggests additional readings under the heading "Stress and Nutrition."

6   Run-away pain (Breakthrough), *Health*, April 1982, p. 22.

CHAPTER 6
Metabolism: Feasting, Fasting, and Energy Balance

CONTENTS

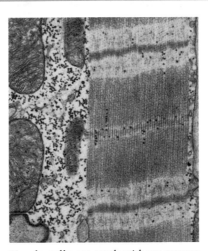

Muscle cells can work without oxygen as long as they have glycogen for fuel. This strand of muscle is peppered with glycogen (dark spots). Nearby are two mitochondria to oxidize both glycogen and fat breakdown products when oxygen is available.

Brain, in its rigid vault, cannot store more than a few minutes' worth of glycogen at the most. . . . Hence, the compliant liver expands and contracts. . . .

G. F. CAHILL, T. T. AOKI, and A. A. ROSSINI

When you eat too much you get fat; when you eat too little you get thin. Everybody knows these simple facts, but nobody knows exactly how to account for them. The mission of this chapter is to shed some light on what we do know and to provide answers to some of the questions people often ask about diets. What makes a person gain weight? Are carbohydrate-rich foods more fattening than other foods? What's the best fuel for an athlete? What's the best way to lose weight? Is fasting dangerous? Are low-carbohydrate diets dangerous? The answers to these and many other questions lie in an understanding of metabolism.

Metabolism could be defined as the way the body handles the energy nutrients; a more precise definition appears in the margin. But before we get into the body cells to see metabolism in progress, a brief review of the energy nutrients themselves may be helpful.

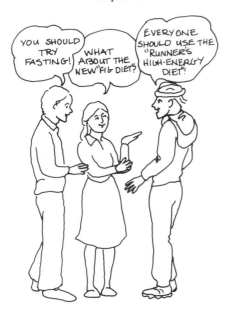

metabolism: the sum total of all the chemical reactions that go on in living cells.

meta = among

bole = change

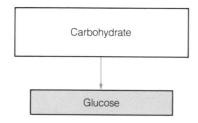

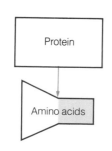

Starting Points

The first four chapters introduced the energy nutrients—carbohydrate, fat, and protein—as they are found in foods and in the human body. Chapter 5 followed the nutrients through digestion to the simpler units they are composed of and showed these units disappearing into the blood. Four of these units will be followed here:

1 *Carbohydrate.* During digestion, all available carbohydrates are broken down to monosaccharides and absorbed into the blood. Fructose and galactose are then mostly taken into liver cells and converted to glucose or to very similar compounds. To follow carbohydrate through metabolism we will simply follow glucose.

2,3 *Lipids.* Most of the dietary lipids are triglycerides. The basic units these are composed of are glycerol and fatty acids. To follow lipids through metabolism we will follow glycerol and fatty acids.

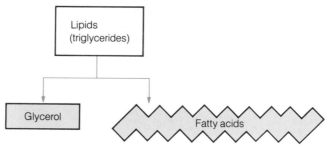

4 *Protein.* Protein is ultimately digested to amino acids; these are the units we will follow through metabolism.

Building Body Compounds

You already know what may happen to some of these basic units when their energy is not needed by the cells. They may be stored "as is," and then

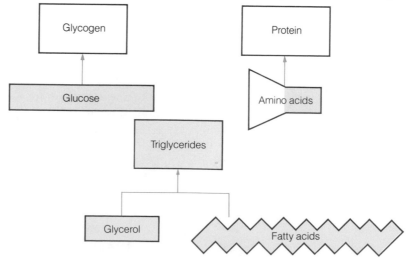

used to build body compounds. Glucose units may be strung together to make glycogen chains. Glycerol and fatty acids may be assembled into triglycerides. Amino acids may be used to make proteins. These building reactions, in which simple compounds are put together to form larger, more complex structures, involve doing work and so require energy. They are called anabolic reactions, and are always represented by "up" arrows in diagrams such as those in this chapter.

anabolism (an-ABB-o-lism): reactions in which small molecules are put together to build larger ones. Anabolic reactions consume energy and often involve reduction (Appendix B).

ana = up

Breaking Down Nutrients for Energy

If the body needs energy, it may break apart any or all of these four units into smaller fragments. The breakdown reactions are called catabolic reactions. They release energy and are represented by "down" arrows in diagrams. Much of the body's catabolic work is done by enzymes in the liver cells, and all the reactions described in this chapter can take place there.

At this point, it must be recalled that although glucose, glycerol, fatty acids, and amino acids are the basic units we get from food, they are composed of still smaller units, the atoms. During metabolism, the body actually separates these atoms from one another. To follow how this takes place, it will help to recall the structures of these compounds, introduced in the first four chapters. There is no need to remember exactly how they are put together; it is enough to remember how many carbons are in their "backbones." Figure 6–1 reviews this information.

The main point to notice in the following discussion is that compounds that have a 3-carbon skeleton can be used to make the vital nutrient glucose. Those that have 2-carbon skeletons cannot.

What happens to these compounds inside of cells can be best understood by starting with glucose. Two new names appear—pyruvate (3 Cs) and acetyl CoA (2 Cs)—and the rest of the story falls into place around them.

catabolism (cuh-TAB-o-lism): reactions in which large molecules are broken down to smaller ones. Catabolic reactions release energy and often involve oxidation (Appendix B).

kata = down

Glucose has 6 Cs.
Glycerol has 3 Cs.
Fatty acids have multiples of 2 Cs.
Amino acids have 2 or 3 or more Cs with Ns attached.
3 Cs can make glucose; 2 Cs cannot.

pyruvate (PIE-roo-vate): pyruvic acid, a 3-carbon compound derived from glucose and certain amino acids in metabolism. The term *pyruvate* means a salt of pyruvic acid. (Throughout this book the ending *ate* is used interchangeably with *ic acid*; for our purposes they mean the same thing.)

The metabolic breakdown of glucose to pyruvate is **glycolysis** (gligh-COLL-uh-sis).

glyco = glucose
lysis = breakdown

FIGURE 6–1 **The products of digestion.** Metabolism centers on these. TH6-1

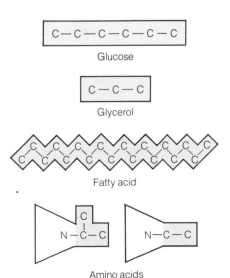

Glucose

Glycerol

Fatty acid

Amino acids

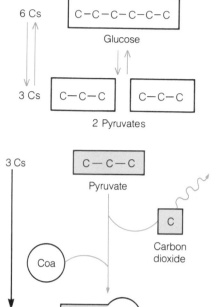

6 Cs

C—C—C—C—C—C

Glucose

3 Cs

C—C—C   C—C—C

2 Pyruvates

3 Cs

C—C—C

Pyruvate

C

Carbon dioxide

Coa

2 Cs

C—C—Coa

Acetyl Coa

CoA (coh-AY): nickname for a compound described further in Chapter 8. As pyruvate loses a carbon and becomes a 2-carbon compound (**acetate**, or **acetic acid**), a molecule of CoA is attached to it, making **acetyl CoA** (ASS-uh-teel, or uh-SEET-ul, co-AY). For our purposes, acetyl CoA is just "a 2-carbon compound"; the CoA will not be discussed further here.

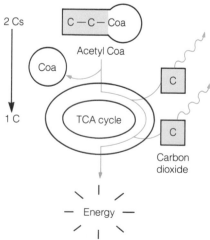

2 Cs

C—C—Coa

Acetyl Coa

Coa

TCA cycle

1 C

C

C

Carbon dioxide

Energy

Glucose

In breaking down, glucose first splits in half, releasing energy. One product is the 3-carbon compound pyruvate, and the other is a 3-carbon compound that is converted to pyruvate, so that two identical halves result from this step.

Should a cell "change its mind" after splitting glucose to pyruvate, it could reverse this step. It could put the two halves back together to make glucose again. For this reason, arrows are shown pointing both up and down between glucose and pyruvate.

If the cell still needs energy, however, it breaks the pyruvate molecules apart further, cleaving a carbon from each. The lone carbon is combined with oxygen to make carbon dioxide, which is released into the blood, circulated to the lungs, and breathed out. The 2-carbon compound that remains is acetate (acetyl CoA).

Should the cell change its mind at this point and want to retrieve the shed carbons and remake glucose, it could not do so. The step from pyruvate to acetyl CoA is metabolically irreversible. It is a one-way step, and it is shown with only a "down" arrow in the diagram.

The carbon removed from pyruvate ends up being combined with oxygen to make carbon dioxide. The person had to breathe oxygen into the lungs, had to attach it to a carrier (hemoglobin) in the red blood cells, and had to bring it to the metabolizing cells to make it available for this purpose. Everyone knows you need to breathe harder when you are using energy faster (exercising), but not everyone "sees" what's happening. Energy nutrients are being broken down to provide that energy, and oxygen is always ultimately involved in the oxidation process.

Finally, acetyl CoA may be split, yielding two more carbon dioxide molecules. The energy released in this step powers most of the cell's activities. The whole sequence is shown in Figure 6–2. (Figures 6–4 and 6–5 then add details to Figure 6–2, while the text explains them. Then they are all put together in Figure 6–7.) In short, the main steps in the metabolism of glucose are: glucose to pyruvate to acetyl CoA to carbon dioxide. Notice (again) that only the first step is reversible.

The process by which acetyl CoA splits and releases its energy is known as the TCA cycle. The details of the cycle are not necessary to the basic understanding of nutrition offered here, but a summary is offered in Figure 6–3.

Most people spend their entire lives without ever making the acquaintance of pyruvate and acetyl CoA, yet chemists and nutritionists can become quite excited talking about them. The behavior of these two compounds explains the most interesting and important aspects of nutrition and makes it possible to answer questions like those asked at the outset. Are carbohydrate-rich foods more fattening than other foods? What's the best energy fuel for an athlete? What's the best way to lose weight? Is fasting dangerous? Are low-carbohydrate diets dangerous?

A person who understands the basics of metabolism can choose what fuel to burn for various purposes. The enlightened athlete knows, for

FIGURE 6–2 **Glucose breakdown**. These are the processes by which energy from glucose is made available to do the cells' work. Many chemical reactions are involved. Ultimately, glucose is completely disassembled to single-carbon fragments, the fragments are combined with oxygen to form carbon dioxide, and most of the freed energy is used to make other compounds such as ATP, glycogen, and fat. ATP is a short-term energy-carrying compound (see Figure 6–3). Glycogen and fat are longer-term energy-storage deposits. TH6-2

[a] In the TCA cycle, acetyl CoA first releases its CoA while the acetate becomes attached to a 4-carbon compound, forming a 6–carbon compound. Then, in a series of reactions, the 6–carbon compound loses one carbon (as carbon dioxide) and then another (as carbon dioxide), reappearing as a 4-carbon compound that can pick up another acetate from acetyl CoA. Details of the TCA cycle and the electron transport chain are shown in Appendix C.

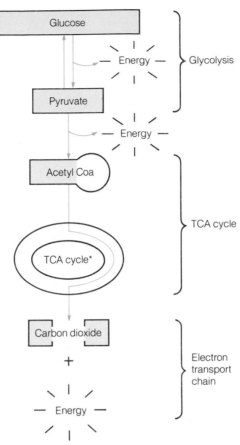

The reactions by which the complete oxidation of acetyl CoA is accomplished are those of the **TCA** (tricarboxylic acid) or **Krebs cycle** (named for the biochemist who elucidated them) and **oxidative phosphorylation**. The net result is that acetyl CoA splits, the carbons combine with oxygen, and the energy originally in the acetyl CoA becomes available for the body's use.

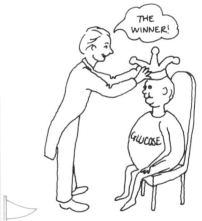

example, that in some athletic events the muscles use fat and glucose, while in others, they require glucose only. The enlightened dieter knows how to encourage the use of fat rather than muscle-protein kcalories during a weight-loss program. It all hinges on which fuels can be converted to glucose and which cannot. The parts of protein and fat that can be converted to pyruvate (3 Cs) *can* provide glucose for the body; those that are converted to acetyl CoA *cannot* provide glucose. And glucose is all important.

Caution

Glycerol and Fatty Acids

Figure 6–4 shows how glycerol and fatty acids enter the pathways of metabolism. The glycerol (3 Cs) is easily converted to pyruvate (also 3 Cs, but with a different arrangement of Hs and OHs on the Cs), and then may go either "up" to form glucose or "down" to form acetyl CoA and finally carbon dioxide. The three fatty acids are taken apart two carbons at a time to make acetyl CoA. Because the arrow from pyruvate to acetyl CoA goes one way (down) only, the fatty acids *cannot* be used to make glucose.

The significance of this is that fat, for the most part, cannot normally provide energy for the organs (brain, nervous system) that require glucose

FIGURE 6–3 **ATP, the energy-carrier compound.**

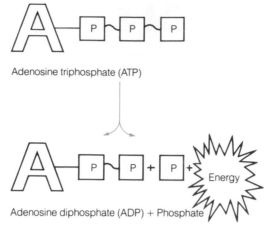

Adenosine triphosphate (ATP)

Adenosine diphosphate (ADP) + Phosphate

Energy

A. The body as a whole stores its excess energy in special storage organs: the liver and muscle (as glycogen) and the fat cells (as fat). However, each cell also has to have a ready supply of "instant energy." This is like storing money in the bank but also keeping pocket money in cash. The cells' cash is adenosine triphosphate (ATP).

When the cell needs energy, each ATP molecule releases one phosphate group. The packet of energy in the broken bond is used, and the phosphate stays in the fluid of the cell along with the adenosine diphosphate (ADP) that is left. Whenever ATP is broken apart like this, its energy is used to do some work for the cell. Part C shows the energy from an ATP being used to add a unit onto a growing cell structure.

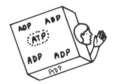

"Help! I need energy! I'm down to my last 2 ATPs"

B. As the cell gradually uses up its energy, the amount of ATP falls, and that of ADP rises. The increased amount of ADP generates a signal that the cell needs energy; so units such as glucose, available in the blood from food, are taken into the cell and broken down to carbon dioxide, water, and energy. The cell deposits the released energy in another high-energy bond, hooking phosphate back onto ADP, reforming ATP. Thus balance is restored.

If no energy units from food are available, glucose and fat drawn from body stores supply the energy to rebuild ATP. In the extreme case of starvation, even body proteins are dismantled in response to the low ATP levels of the cells. Thus "bank" energy is converted to "cash" energy.

An abundance of ATP in the cells also serves as a signal. It tells the liver to route any remaining energy units to storage. Thus "cash" energy can be put back in the "bank."

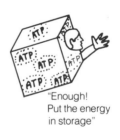

"Enough! Put the energy in storage"

C. Here, ATP energy is doing its work. Note that the energy released from ATP is captured in the growing cell structure (which might be glycogen, fat, protein, a hormone, or any other piece of cellular machinery). A little energy is lost as heat in all such reactions, accounting for the temperature-raising effect of metabolism.

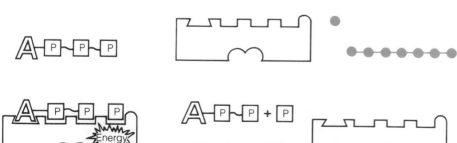

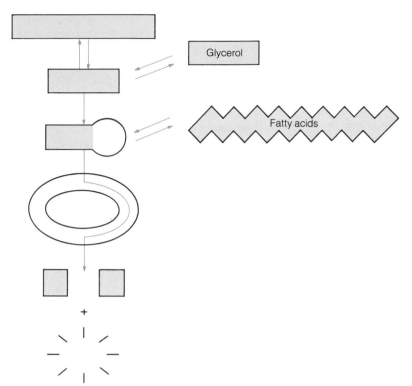

FIGURE 6–4 **How lipids enter the metabolic path**. Glycerol converts to pyruvate; fatty acids to acetyl CoA. TH6-6

as fuel. Remember that almost all dietary lipid is triglyceride, and that the typical triglyceride consists of a molecule of glycerol (3 Cs) and three fatty acids (each about 18 Cs on the average, or about 54 Cs in all). True, the glycerol can yield glucose, but that represents only 3 out of 57 parts of the fat molecule—about 5 percent of its weight. Thus, fat is a very poor, inefficient source of glucose by itself. About 95 percent of it cannot be converted to glucose at all.

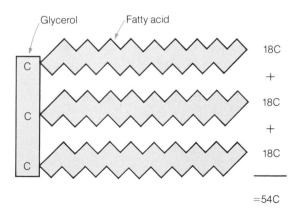

Only 3 of this triglyceride's 57 carbon atoms are in glycerol and can go to glucose.

Amino Acids

Ideally, amino acids will be used to replace needed body proteins, and will not be catabolized at all. But if they are needed for energy, they enter the

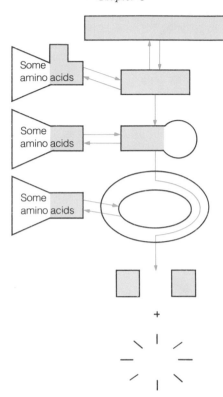

FIGURE 6–5 **How amino acids enter the metabolic path.** About half can convert to pyruvate (and therefore glucose); about half convert to acetyl CoA or go directly into the TCA cycle (and therefore cannot yield glucose). TH6-6

The making of glucose from protein or fat is **gluconeogenesis** (gloo-co-nee-o-GEN-uh-sis). About 5 percent of fat (the glycerol portion of triglycerides) and about 50 percent of protein (the glucogenic amino acids) can be converted to glucose.

gluco = glucose

neo = new

genesis = making

metabolic pathway as shown in Figure 6–5. They are stripped of their nitrogen (see the next section) and then catabolized in a variety of ways.[1] The end result is that about half of the amino acids can be converted to pyruvate; the other half go either to acetyl CoA or directly into the TCA cycle. Those that can be used to make pyruvate can provide glucose for the body. Thus protein, unlike fat, is a fairly good source of glucose when carbohydrate is not available; about 50 percent of it can be used this way.

Amino acids break down when energy needs are not met by carbohydrate and fat, as just described, but they also break down in the same way under another set of conditions: when surplus kcalories and protein are consumed. Surplus protein cannot be stored in the body as such; it has to be converted to other compounds. If you eat more protein than you can use at a given time, the excess amino acids soon lose their nitrogens, and most are converted to acetyl CoA (either directly or indirectly, through pyruvate). This acetyl CoA is not broken down further, because energy is not needed. Instead, it is strung together into chains—fatty acids—and stored in body fat. Thus even the so-called "lean" nutrient, protein, can make you fat if you eat too much of it.

The high-protein dieter objects to the statement above, saying, "Protein makes you thin!" In fact, many weight-loss diets are based on high protein intakes, making the claim that "Protein will give you energy but will not make you fat." "Eat all you want—just stay away from fattening carbohydrates."

The secret of these diets, when they do seem to promote weight loss, is that meals without carbohydrate are in truth so unappetizing that people who ingest them eat much less total food than they normally do. Try eating your breakfast of bacon, eggs, toast, and juice without the toast and juice. Have a ham and cheese sandwich without the bread, and a steak, potatoes, and peas dinner without the potatoes and peas. You'll be surprised how quickly you lose your enthusiasm for the permitted foods. (Some people report, after eating nothing but bacon, eggs, ham, cheese, and steak for a few days, that they start dreaming of toast and juice!)

This method of weight loss may sound fine to the person who wants to lose pounds fast, but the next few sections of this chapter should convince any sane reader otherwise. Meanwhile, it should now be clear that protein, in and of itself, is not nonfattening. People who eat huge portions of meat, even lean meat, and other protein-rich foods may wonder why they have a weight problem. It may be those very foods that are causing the trouble.

There is a message for the athlete in these metabolic facts about protein, too. *Excess* protein is not a muscle-building food, it's a fat-

---

1   Some are rearranged to form pyruvate. Others are 4-carbon compounds that split into two acetyl CoA molecules. One, which contains only two carbons after the nitrogen is removed, is rearranged directly to become acetyl CoA. Still others become compounds that enter the TCA cycle as compounds other than acetyl CoA.

building food. To the extent that protein is used for energy, carbohydrate would do the job just as well. In other words, there is no point to loading up on protein for any reason. Highlight 6 elaborates on nutrition for the athlete.

Caution

What Happens to the Nitrogen?

When amino acids are degraded for energy or to make fat, the first step is removal of their nitrogen-containing amino groups, a reaction called deamination. The product is ammonia, chemically identical to the ammonia in the bottled cleaning solutions used in hospitals and in industry. It is a strong-smelling and extremely potent poison.

A small amount of ammonia is always being produced by liver deamination reactions. Some of this ammonia is captured by liver enzymes and used to synthesize other amino acids, but what cannot be used is quickly combined with a carbon-oxygen fragment to make urea, an inert and less toxic compound.

Urea is released from the liver cells into the blood, where it circulates until it passes through the kidneys. One of the functions of the kidneys is to remove urea from the blood for excretion in the urine (see Figure 6–6). Urea is the body's principal vehicle for excreting unused nitrogen; water is required to keep it in solution and excrete it. This explains why people who consume a high-protein diet must drink more water than usual.

Putting It All Together

After a normal mixed meal, if you do not overeat, the body handles the nutrients as shown in Figure 6–7. The carbohydrate yields glucose; some is stored as glycogen, and some is taken into brain and other cells and broken down through pyruvate and acetyl CoA to provide energy. The protein yields amino acids, and some are used to build body protein. However, if there is a surplus or if not enough carbohydrate and fat are present to meet energy needs, some amino acids are broken down through the same pathways as glucose to provide energy. The fat yields glycerol and fatty acids; some are put together and stored as fat, and others are broken down to acetyl CoA and provide energy.

A few hours after the meal, the stored glycogen and fat begin to be released from storage to provide more glucose, glycerol, and fatty acids to keep the energy flow going. When all the energy supplied from the last meal has been used up and reserves of these compounds are running low, it is time to eat again.

The average person consumes more than a million kcalories a year and expends more than 99 percent of them, maintaining a stable weight for years on end. This remarkable achievement, which many people manage without even thinking about it, could be called the economy of maintenance. The body's energy budget is balanced. Some people, however, eat too little and get thin; others eat too much and get fat. The possible reasons why they do are explored in Chapter 7; the metabolic consequences are discussed here.

deamination: removal of the amino (NH$_2$) group from a compound such as an amino acid.

$$H-\overset{\overset{\displaystyle H}{|}}{N}-H \; + \; -\overset{\overset{\displaystyle O}{||}}{C}- \; + \; H-\overset{\overset{\displaystyle H}{|}}{N}-H$$

Ammonia   Ammonia

$$H-\overset{\overset{\displaystyle H}{|}}{N}-\overset{\overset{\displaystyle O}{||}}{C}-\overset{\overset{\displaystyle H}{|}}{N}-H$$

Urea

When nitrogen is stripped from amino acids, ammonia is produced. The liver detoxifies ammonia by converting it to urea before releasing it into the bloodstream. The diagram greatly oversimplifies the reactions.

urea (you-REE-uh): the principal nitrogen-excretion product of metabolism. Two ammonia fragments are combined with a carbon-oxygen group to form urea.

The Economy of Feasting

Figures 6–8, 6–9, and 6–10 are duplicates of Figure 6–7, and show how metabolism favors fat formation when you eat too much of any energy nutrient. Surplus carbohydrate (glucose) is first stored as glycogen, but there is a limit to the capacity of the glycogen-storing cells. Once glycogen stores are filled, the overflow is routed to fat (note the heavy arrows in Figure 6–8). Fat cells enlarge as they fill with fat, and the body's fat-storing capacity seems to be able to expand indefinitely. Thus excess carbohydrate can contribute to obesity.

In the same way, surplus dietary fat can contribute to the fat stores in the body. It may break down to fragments such as acetyl CoA, but if energy flow is already rapid enough to meet the demand, these fragments will not be broken down further. Instead, they will be routed to the assembly of triglycerides and stored in the fat cells (Figure 6–9, p. 204).

Finally, surplus protein may encounter the same fate (Figure 6–10, p. 205). If not needed to build body protein or to meet present energy

FIGURE 6–6 The liver and kidney each play a role in enabling the body to dispose of excess nitrogen. Can you see why the person with liver disease has high blood ammonia while the person with kidney disease has high blood urea?

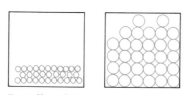

Fat cells enlarge.

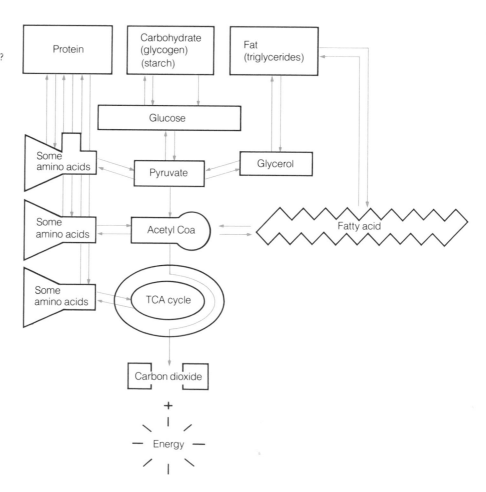

FIGURE 6–7 **The central pathways of metabolism.** TH6-7

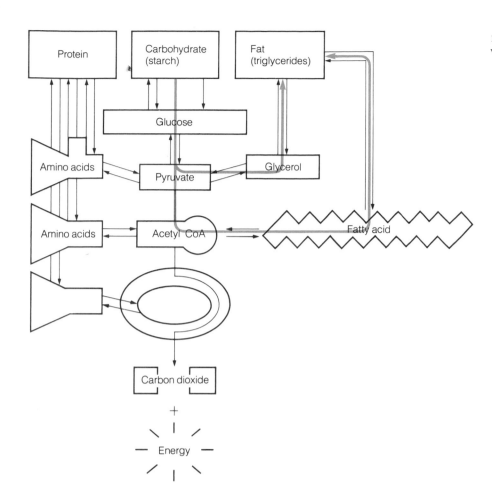

FIGURE 6–8 **Excess carbohydrate is converted to fat.** TH6-8

needs, amino acids will lose their nitrogens and be converted through the intermediates, pyruvate and acetyl CoA, to triglycerides. These, too, swell the fat cells and increase body weight.

The Economy of Fasting

Even when you are asleep and totally relaxed, the cells of many organs are hard at work spending energy. In fact, the work that you are aware of, that you do with your muscles during waking hours, represents only about a third of the total energy you spend in a day. The rest is the metabolic work of the cells, for which they constantly require fuel.

The body's top priority is to meet these energy needs, and its normal way of doing so is by periodic refueling—that is, by eating. When food is withdrawn, the body must find other fuel sources in its own tissues. If people choose not to eat, we say they are fasting; if they have no choice (as in a famine), we say they are starving; but there is no metabolic difference between the two. In either case the body is forced to switch to a wasting

FIGURE 6–9 **Excess dietary fat is converted to body fat.** TH6-9

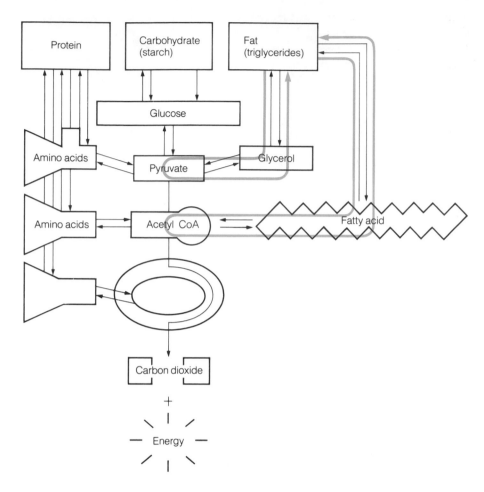

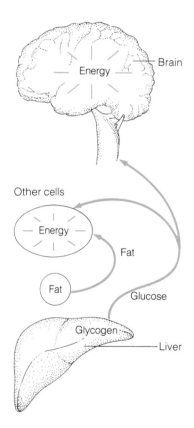

The liver releases glucose and the adipose tissue releases fat to be used as fuel by the body's cells, but the brain can use only the glucose. TH6-14

metabolism, drawing on its reserves of carbohydrate and fat and, within a day or so, on its vital protein tissues as well. Figure 6–11 (p. 207) shows the metabolic pathways operating in the body at the start of a fast.

Fuel must be delivered to every cell. As the fast begins, glucose from the liver's stored glycogen and fatty acids from the body's stored fat are both flowing into cells, breaking down to yield acetyl CoA, and delivering energy to power the cells' work. Several hours later, however, most of the glucose is used up, and the liver glycogen is being exhausted.

At this point, most of the cells are depending on fatty acids to continue providing their fuel. But the brain cells cannot; they still need glucose. (It is their major energy fuel, and even if other energy fuel is available, glucose has to be present to permit their energy-metabolizing machinery to work.) Normally the nervous system (brain and nerves) consumes about two-thirds of the total glucose used each day—about 400 to 600 kcalories' worth.[2]

2   G. F. Cahill, T. T. Aoki, and A. A. Rossini, Metabolism in obesity and anorexia nervosa, in *Nutrition and the Brain*, vol. 3, ed. R. J. Wurtman and J. J. Wurtman (New York: Raven Press, 1979), pp. 1–70.

FIGURE 6–10 **Excess protein is converted to fat.** TH6-10

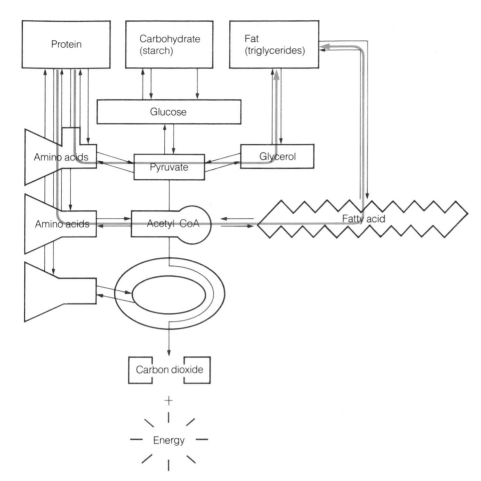

The brain's special requirement for glucose poses a problem for the fasting body. The body can use its stores of fat, which may be quite generous, to furnish most of its cells with energy, but for the brain and nerves it must supply energy in the form of glucose. This is why body protein tissues, such as muscle, always break down to some extent during fasting. Only those amino acids that yield 3-carbon pyruvate can be used to make glucose; and to obtain them, whole proteins must be broken down. The other amino acids, that cannot be used to make glucose, then have to be disposed of. This is an expensive way to gain glucose, but to extract a molecule of glycerol from a triglyceride obligates the body to dispose of some 50 or 60 carbons' worth of fatty acids, which is even more expensive. In the first few days of a fast, body protein provides about 90 percent of the needed glucose, and glycerol about 10 percent. If body protein loss were to continue at this rate, death would ensue within three weeks.

As the fast continues, the body adapts by producing an alternate energy source, ketones, by condensing together acetyl CoA fragments derived from fatty acids. Normally produced and used in only small quantities, ketones can serve as fuel for some brain cells. Ketone production rises until, at the end of several weeks, it is meeting about half or more of the

In fasting, muscle and lean tissue atrophy to supply amino acids for conversion to glucose. This glucose and the ketones produced from fat fuel the brain's activities. TH6-14

nervous system's energy needs. Still, many areas of the brain rely exclusively on glucose, and body protein continues to be sacrificed to produce it.[3]

2 acetyl CoA

A ketone (keto-acid)

Acetone (ASS-uh-tone) is familiar to some as the solvent used in nail-polish remover. "Acetone breath" indicates that a person is in ketosis.

This ketone may lose a molecule of carbon dioxide to become another ketone:

Acetone

During fasting, appetite is suppressed. It has been thought that ketosis caused loss of appetite. The theory was that it would be an advantage to a person in a famine to have no appetite, because the search for food would be a waste of energy. When the person finds food and eats carbohydrate again, the body shifts out of ketosis, the hunger center gets the message that food is again available, and appetite returns. This hypothetical chain of events has served as justification for weight-loss routines, such as fasting and fad diets, that cause ketosis. However, it may be that any kind of food restriction, with or without ketosis, leads a person to adapt by losing appetite. An ordinary low-kcalorie diet can induce the same effect.[4]

Caution

ketone (KEE-tone): a compound formed during the incomplete oxidation of fatty acids. Ketones contain a C=O group between other carbons; when they also contain a COOH (acid) group, they are called keto-acids. Small amounts of ketones are a normal part of the blood chemistry, but when their concentration rises, they spill into the urine. The combination of high blood ketones (ketonemia) and ketones in the urine (ketonuria) is termed **ketosis**.

Figure 6–12 (p. 208) shows the metabolism of late fasting. While the body is shifting to the use of ketones, it simultaneously reduces its energy output and conserves both its fat and lean tissue. As the lean (protein-containing) organ tissue shrinks in mass, it performs less metabolic work, reducing energy needs. As the muscles waste, they do less work, enhancing this effect. Because of the slowed metabolism, the loss of fat falls to a bare minimum—less, in fact, than the fat that would be lost on a low-kcalorie

3   R. A. Hawkins and J. F. Biebuyck, Ketone bodies are selectively used by individual brain regions, *Science* 205 (1979): 325–327.

4   J. C. Rosen, D. A. Hunt, E. A. H. Sims, and C. Bogardus, Comparison of carbohydrate-containing and carbohydrate-restricted hypocaloric diets in the treatment of obesity: Effects on appetite and mood, *American Journal of Clinical Nutrition* 36 (1982): 463–469.

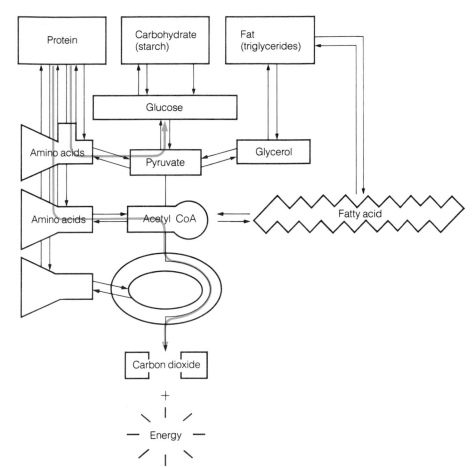

diet.[5] Thus, although weight loss during fasting may be quite dramatic, fat loss may be less than when at least some food is supplied.

The adaptations just described—slowing of energy output and reduction in fat loss—occur in the starving child, the fasting religious person, and the malnourished hospital patient, and help to prolong their lives. The physical symptoms of marasmus include wasting, slowed metabolism, lowered body temperature, and reduced resistance to disease (see Chapter 4).

The body's adaptations to fasting are sufficient to maintain life for a long period. Mental alertness need not be diminished, and even physical energy may remain unimpaired for a surprisingly long time. Still, fasting is not without its hazards, as physician-supervised fasting has revealed. Among the multitude of changes that take place in the body are:

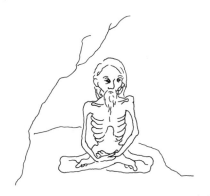

Fasting = Living on (body) fat and (body) protein.

- Sodium and potassium depletion.
- An increase in body uric acid.
- A rise in blood cholesterol.
- A decrease in thyroid hormone.

5   M. F. Ball, J. J. Canary, and L. H. Kyle, Comparative effects of calorie restriction and total starvation on body composition in obesity, *Annals of Internal Medicine* 67 (1967): 60–67.

FIGURE 6–12 **Fasting (late).** Protein breakdown supplies some glucose for the brain. Ketone production helps to support brain function. Darkened arrows show which pathways are speeded up during ketosis. TH6-13

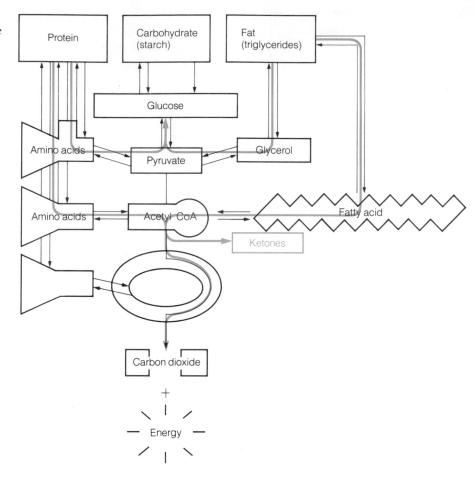

The same alterations are seen in low-carbohydrate dieting (next section). Renewed food intake, especially of carbohydrate, results in dramatic changes in the body's salt and water balance, accounting for most of the wide swings in body weight seen in people on fasts or low-carbohydrate diets.[6]

The Low-Carbohydrate Diet

Low-carbohydrate diet = Living on (dietary and body) fat and protein almost exclusively.

An economy similar to that of fasting prevails if a low-carbohydrate diet is consumed. Advocates of the low-carbohydrate diet would have you believe there is something magical about ketosis, something that promotes faster weight loss than a regular low-kcalorie diet. In fact, the low-carbohydrate diet presents the same problem as a fast. Once the body's available glycogen reserves are spent, the only significant remaining source of energy in the form of glucose is protein. The low-carbohydrate diet provides a little protein from food, but some must still be taken from body tissue. The onset of ketosis is the signal that this wasting process has begun.

6   Cahill, Aoki, and Rossini, 1979.

In a diet that provides fewer than about 900 kcalories (for the average-sized adult), it is pointless to supply any protein at all, because the protein will only be used to provide energy, as carbohydrate would be used. Body protein is lost at the same rate in adults on such a diet whether or not they are given any food protein.[7]

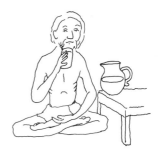

One conclusion to draw from this is that a person who diets at the level of 900 kcalories a day might as well eat carbohydrate without protein, to spare body protein and allow efficient use of body fat. Carbohydrate-containing foods are less expensive than protein-rich foods, and both will serve the same purpose—supplying glucose. This is the choice made by the person on a juice fast, for the only energy nutrient juices contain is carbohydrate. But a wise conclusion is that such a diet is unnecessarily low in kcalories, even dangerously so. The person who wishes to lose body *fat* will select a balanced diet of 1,200 or more kcalories, one containing carbohydrate, fat, *and* protein. At this level, body protein will be spared, ketosis need not occur, vital lean tissues (including both muscle and brain) will not starve, and only the unwanted *fat* will be lost.

People are attracted to the low-carbohydrate diet because of the dramatic weight loss it brings about within the first few days. They would be disillusioned if they realized that much of this weight loss is a loss of glycogen and protein, and with them, quantities of water and important minerals. A dieter who boasts of losing seven pounds in two days on a low-carbohydrate diet must be unaware that at best, a pound or two is fat and five or six pounds are lean tissue, water, and minerals. Once "off" the diet, the dieter's body will avidly devour and retain these needed materials, and the weight will zoom back to within a few pounds of the starting point.

A warning is suggested by these facts. Beware of those who promote quick-weight-loss schemes. Learn to distinguish between loss of *fat* and loss of *weight*.

Juice fasting = Living on (dietary) carbohydrate and (body) fat.

Caution

The Protein-Sparing Fast

A variant on fasting is the technique of ingesting only protein. The hope is that the protein will spare lean tissue and that the person will break down his own body fat at a maximal rate to meet his other energy needs. The protein, together with the body's lean tissues, are used to provide glucose. The idea sounded good when it was first suggested for use with very obese people, but it has met with mixed results. It seems effective only after considerable lean tissue has already been lost, at which time the body may be conserving itself quite efficiently anyway, and the fast has not been

Protein-sparing fast = Living on (dietary) protein, (body) fat, and (body) protein.

7   A. A. Albanese and L. A. Orto, The proteins and amino acids, in *Modern Nutrition in Health and Disease*, 5th ed., ed. R. S. Goodhart and M. E. Shils (Philadelphia: Lea and Febiger, 1973), p. 56.

shown more effective than a mixture of protein and carbohydrate.[8] Furthermore, it doesn't seem to "stick" very well; most people regain the lost weight.[9] Thus the protein-sparing fast has to be judged at best a very moderate success and at worst a failure, for the ultimate criterion of success in any weight-loss program is maintenance of the new low weight.

The idea of a protein-sparing fast originated with some responsible physicians who experimented carefully with it, using whole foods naturally rich in protein, such as fish and lean beef. Unfortunately, the idea was then seized upon and misused with the publication of a popular book, *The Last Chance Diet*, in 1977.[10] Fad dieters, usually without any medical supervision, drank liquid protein potions prepared from low-quality sources, and lost dramatic amounts of weight—including, of course, lean tissue, water, and vital minerals. These "predigested" liquid proteins are of "notably lower quality"[11] than food proteins, and cause dangerous alterations in heart rhythm.[12] Within the year, 11 deaths had been ascribed to the fad, and the FDA had issued a stringent warning about liquid protein preparations.[13] Since then, many more have died on the fast, due to sudden stopping of the heart caused probably by mineral losses.[14]

The term *protein-sparing* has also been used in another connection. Malnourished hospital patients also lose body protein, and this is especially likely, and especially dangerous, if they are simultaneously fighting infection. Physicians make every effort to prevent the loss of vital lean tissue by supplying amino acids as well as glucose in some form—through a vein if the patient can't eat.[15] The effort to provide protein-sparing *therapy* in these circumstances should not be confused with the profiteering of faddists who promote the protein-sparing *fast*.

Caution

8   T. B. Van Itallie and M. U. Yang, Current concepts in nutrition: Diet and weight loss, *New England Journal of Medicine* 297 (1977): 1158–1161.

9   Morbid obesity: Long-term results of therapeutic fasting, *Nutrition Reviews* 36 (1978): 6–7.

10   R. Linn and S. L. Stuart, *The Last Chance Diet* (New York: Bantam Books, 1977).

11   N. L. Marable, M. L. Hinners, N. W. Hardison, and N. L. Kehrberg, Protein quality of supplements and meal replacements, *Journal of the American Dietetic Association* 77 (1980): 270–276.

12   R. A. Lantigua and coauthors, Cardiac arrhythmias associated with a liquid protein diet for the treatment of obesity, *New England Journal of Medicine* 303 (1980): 735–738.

13   "These liquid protein diets are made from hydrolyzed (predigested) collagen or gelatin obtained from animal hides, tendons, and bones.... None is nutritionally complete.... Liquid protein diets are neither registered nor approved by FDA. FDA is responsible for the labeling of such products, but generally the labeling does not give directions for weight-loss regimens. Such claims are made in books, by word of mouth, or in the media, which are beyond FDA's control. FDA can take action, such as seeking recall or seizing the product, only if the product has become adulterated." Predigested protein drinks and "modified fasting" diets, *Journal of the American Dietetic Association* 71 (1977): 609.

14   T. B. Van Itallie, Liquid protein mayhem, *Journal of the American Medical Association* 240 (1978): 144–146.

15   Giving amino acids *instead of* glucose is based on the rationale that amino acids will stimulate insulin secretion less, thus permitting body fat to come out of storage and help spare body protein. However, amino acids stimulate insulin secretion, and results of this therapy do not uniformly support the rationale. R. L. Landau, H. Rochman, P. Blix-Gruber, and A. H. Rubenstein, The protein-sparing action of protein feeding: Absence of relationship to insulin secretion, *American Journal of Clinical Nutrition* 34 (1981): 1300–1304.

Moderate Weight Loss

The body's cells and the enzymes within them make it their task to convert the energy nutrients you eat into those you need. They are extraordinarily versatile. They relieve you of having to compute exactly how much carbohydrate, fat, and protein to eat at each meal. As you have seen, they can convert either carbohydrate (glucose) or protein to fat. To some extent, they can convert protein to glucose. To a very limited extent, they can even convert fat (the glycerol portion) to glucose. But a grossly unbalanced diet or one that is severely limited in kcalories imposes hardships on the body. If kcalorie intake is too low or if carbohydrate and protein kcalories are undersupplied, the body is forced to degrade its own lean tissue to meet its glucose need.

Someone who wants to lose body fat must reconcile himself to the hard fact that there is a limit to the rate at which this tissue will break down. The maximum rate, except for a very large, very active person, is one to two pounds a week. To achieve weight loss that actually reflects body-fat loss, the most effective means is to adopt a balanced, low-kcalorie diet supplying all three energy nutrients in reasonable amounts while increasing energy expenditure by getting more exercise. In effect, this means adjusting the energy budget so that intake is 500 to 1,000 kcalories per day less than output. A person who wants to gain weight needs to make the opposite adjustment.

It might seem that the effort to lose or gain weight would involve tedious counting of kcalories, but this is not the case. The next two sections show how kcalorie input and kcalorie output can be estimated and balanced to achieve weight loss, gain, or maintenance.

Estimating kCalorie Intake from Food

To find out how many kcalories are in a food, a laboratory scientist can burn the food in a bomb calorimeter. This device can reveal kcalorie values in two ways. Either it directly measures the heat given off (and kcalories are units of energy defined in terms of heat, as explained on p. 4) or it measures the amount of oxygen consumed in the burning, an indirect measure of the kcalories produced.

The number of kcalories in a food as determined by direct calorimetry, however, is higher than the number of kcalories that same food would give to the human body. This apparent discrepancy is explained by the fact that the body does not metabolize all the food all the way to carbon dioxide and water as the calorimeter does. When the calorimeter-derived values are corrected for this discrepancy, they state accurately the number of kcalories a food provides to the body, thus permitting researchers to make useful tables presenting the energy values of foods.

Another way to arrive at food energy values is to compute them from the amounts of protein, fat, and carbohydrate (and alcohol, if present) found in them. The Table of Food Composition (Appendix H) presents kcalorie values for about 800 foods, some of which were derived by bomb calorimetry, and many by calculation from their energy-nutrient contents.

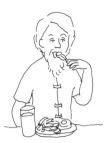

Low-kcalorie diet = Living on food and body fat.

1 lb = 3,500 kcal. A pound of body fat (adipose tissue) is actually composed of a mixture of fat, protein, and water and yields 3,500 kcal on oxidation. A pound of pure fat (454 g) would yield 4,086 kcal at 9 kcal/g.

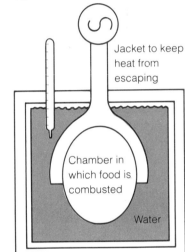

Bomb calorimeter

calorimetry (cal-o-RIM-uh-tree): the measurement of energy as heat.

calor = heat

metron = measure

1 g carbohydrate = 4 kcal.
1 g fat = 9 kcal.
1 g protein = 4 kcal.
1 g alcohol = 7 kcal.

When an organic substance such as food is burned, the energy in the chemical bonds that held its carbons and hydrogens together is released in the form of heat. The amount of heat released can be measured; this direct measure of the amount of energy that was stored in the food's chemical bonds is termed **direct calorimetry**.

As the chemical bonds in food are broken, the carbons (C) and hydrogens (H) combine with oxygen (O) to form carbon dioxide (CO_2) and water (H_2O). Measuring the amount of oxygen consumed in the process gives an indirect measure of the amount of energy released, termed **indirect calorimetry**.

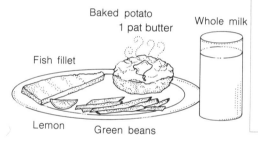

FIGURE 6–13 In case you'd like to try guessing how many kcalories are in the meal depicted here, the answer is provided in Figure 6–14.

But looking up every food in kcalorie charts is boring and inconvenient, and only the most motivated will persist at it for long. For the rest of us who may want to keep track of kcalories, some acquaintance with an exchange system, such as the one described at the end of Chapter 1, provides a simpler method. The foods depicted in Figure 6–13, for example, could be found one by one in Appendix H, but it is quicker to translate them into exchanges and add up the kcalorie values to get a rough idea of the number. With some practice, you can look at any plate of food and "see" the number of kcalories on it. Only seven values need be learned as a start towards gaining this new skill.

Food kCalorie Values

1 c skim milk (for whole milk, add 2 fat)	80 kcal
½ c vegetable[a]	25 kcal
1 portion[a] fruit	40 kcal
1 portion bread or starchy vegetable	70 kcal
1 oz lean meat (for medium-fat meat add ½ fat) (for high-fat meat add 1 fat)	55 kcal
1 fat (1 tsp fat or oil)	45 kcal
1 tsp sugar	20 kcal

[a] For the distinction between vegetables and starchy vegetables, the sizes of fruit portions, and other details, see the exchange lists in Appendix L. An introduction to the exchange system was given in Chapter 1.

Before leaving the subject of the energy in food it is only fair to mention another way of thinking about energy in relation to food. We normally ask, "How many kcalories are *in* that food?" Dr. Jean Mayer, formerly professor of nutrition at Harvard School of Public Health, has pointed out that the average consumer in the United States uses three times as much energy to bring food to the table as the average citizen of developing countries uses for *all* purposes. It's a complicated thought, because more than just electric or gas heat in your kitchen goes into the production of a food. Foods that cost little energy in your kitchen may cost incredible amounts of energy in the field or in processing.[16]

Along the same lines, the nutrition educator Dr. Isobel Contento suggests that we should be teaching people to understand the "energy costs, ecological consequences, and moral implications of their food choices; to analyze the impact of the food system on society as a whole; and to act self-reliantly in providing nourishing meals for themselves

16 J. Mayer, Saving energy in the food system, *Professional Nutritionist*, Winter 1981, pp. 1–4.

and others."[17] In view of the contrast between a third world in which starvation is rampant, and the domestic scene in which the aluminum container for a 1-kcalorie diet soda costs 400 kcalories to produce, perhaps our awareness does indeed need to be raised.

Caution

Estimating kCalorie Output by the Body

Counting the kcalories in your food tells you your energy income, but to balance your budget you also need to know your expenditure. How can you count the kcalories you expend in a day? One way is to assume you are a "typical citizen" of the United States or Canada, and to use the numbers their governments use as standards for population studies.

Government Recommendations

The U.S. Committee on RDA and the Canadian Ministry of Health and Welfare have published recommended energy intakes for various age-sex groups in their populations. These are useful for population studies, but the range of energy needs for any one group is so broad that it is impossible even to guess an individual's needs from them without knowing something about the person's lifestyle. The U.S. recommendation for a woman, for example, assumes she is 20 years old, 5 feet 4 inches tall, weighs about 120 pounds, and typically engages in light activity. A woman who fits all these descriptors is said to need between 1,700 and 2,500 kcalories a day to maintain her weight. The man used as a reference figure is 20 years old, 5 feet 10 inches tall, weighs 154 pounds, engages in light activity, and needs 2,500 to 3,300 kcalories a day. Taller people need proportionately more, and shorter people proportionately fewer, kcalories to balance their energy budgets. Older people generally need fewer kcalories, with the number diminishing about 5 percent per decade beyond 30. Light activity, for both women and men, means sleeping or lying down for eight hours a day, sitting for seven hours, standing for five, walking for two, and spending two hours a day in light physical activity.

Although very few people fit these descriptions exactly, most fall close to the mean. The total span of needs is broad. For adults it is believed that an 800-kcalorie range covers most individuals, but some have energy needs outside this range. Clearly, it is impossible to pinpoint any person's energy need within such a wide range without knowing more.

Diet Record Method

To obtain an individualized estimate of your energy needs, the best means would be to monitor your food intake and body weight over a period of

For the U.S. and Canadian energy allowances, see Appendix O.

FIGURE 6–14 We figure about 530 kcalories for the meal:

1 c milk (80) plus 2 fat (90)	170 kcal
½ c beans	25
1 small potato (1 starchy vegetable)	70
1 pat butter (1 fat)	45
4 oz fish (4 lean meat, assuming no fat is added), at 55 kcal/oz	220
Lemon wedge	0
	530 kcal

Appendix H values yield a total of about 500 kcalories, lower because these foods are low-kcalorie choices within the exchange groups. Any answer within about 50 to 100 kcalories of this is a good estimate.

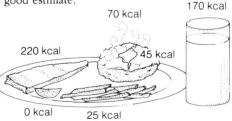

170 kcal

70 kcal

220 kcal   45 kcal

0 kcal   25 kcal

17   I. Contento, Thinking about nutrition education: What to teach, how to teach it, and what to measure, *Teachers College Record* 81, Summer 1980, pp. 421–447.

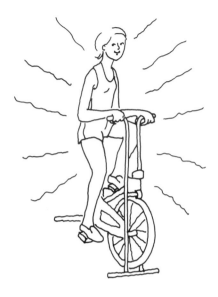

time in which your activities are typical of your lifestyle. If you keep a strictly accurate record of all the food and beverages you consume for a week or two, and if your weight does not change during that time, you can assume that your energy budget is balanced. Records have to be kept for at least a week, however, because intakes fluctuate from day to day. (On about half the days you eat less, on the other half more, kcalories than the average.) If during a week you gain a pound of fat, you can deduce that you expended 3,500 kcalories less than you consumed, or an average of 500 kcalories per day for the seven days.

Laboratory Methods

Energy expenditures can also be accurately measured using laboratory equipment designed for the purpose. Two principles underlie the design of such machines. First, because heat is always a byproduct of energy expenditure, a device that measures escaping heat gives a direct measure of the kcalories being spent. Early efforts to make this kind of measurement involved putting a person inside an insulated, tightly sealed room with water circulating in pipes in the ceiling. The rise in the water's temperature indicated the number of kcalories being generated by the person's body. Inside the room, the person could be at rest or engaged in an activity such as studying or bicycle riding.

This clumsy and expensive method was replaced by a portable and much less expensive machine using the principle that the amount of oxygen consumed or carbon dioxide expelled is in direct proportion to the heat released. If twice as much heat is generated in one instance as another, then twice as much oxygen will also be used. This advance made it possible to measure the kcalories expended during a wider range of physical activities. Laboratory studies of energy output by humans have been so extensive that tables are now available giving averages for people engaged in different activities. Individuals differ, however, and kcalorie expenditures derived from these tables do not always apply to individuals.

Estimating from Basal Metabolism, Activities, and SDE

Human energy is spent in two major ways—on the basal metabolic processes and on voluntary activities. (A third component, the so-called SDE, is minor but is often added in and will be explained below.) A way of estimating the total energy you spend is to estimate each of these components individually, then add them together.

The first component, basal metabolic energy, is by far the largest item in most people's energy budgets. It consists of the energy spent to keep the heart beating, the lungs inhaling and exhaling air, the cells conducting their metabolic activities, the nerves generating their continuous streams of electrical impulses—in short, to keep all the processes going on that support life. The energy needs for basal metabolic activity must be met before any kcalories can be used for physical activity or for the digestion of food.

The basal metabolic rate (BMR) is the rate at which kcalories are spent for these maintenance activities, usually expressed as kcalories per hour. The BMR varies from one person to the next, and may vary for one individ-

basal metabolism: the total energy output of a body at rest after a 12-hour fast. Also called **basal metabolic rate** or **BMR**.

ual with a change in circumstance, physical condition, or age. The BMR is lowest when you are lying down in a room with a comfortable temperature and not digesting any food, and these are the conditions under which it is measured. (During deep sleep, metabolic energy is slightly lower, but periodic muscular activity raises average energy expenditure. The differences associated with sleep can be discounted in all but the most precise laboratory measurements.)

The BMR is surprisingly large, normally amounting to at least two-thirds of the energy spent in a day. (A woman who uses 2,100 kcalories a days uses 1,400 of them just for BMR; a man who uses 3,000 kcalories a day uses 2,000 for BMR.) People often do not realize that so much of their energy is going to support the basic work of their bodies' cells, because they are unaware of all the work these cells do to maintain life.

The BMR is highest in the young, and decreases by about 2 percent per decade after growth has stopped (a decrease in voluntary activity as well brings the total reduction in energy expenditure to 5 percent per decade). It is also higher in people with larger surface areas; of two people who weigh the same, the taller, thinner person will have the faster BMR, reflecting a greater skin surface through which heat is lost by radiation.

The metabolic rate is lower in general in older people and in females, but it is untrue to say that "age always decreases BMR" or that "males always have a faster metabolic rate." The key to the difference is the amount of lean body tissue, or fat-free mass, because lean tissue is more active metabolically than fat tissue, even during rest. A young woman, an older woman, and an older man can have as rapid a metabolic rate as a young man if they have the same amount of lean tissue.[18]

Fever also increases the energy needs of cells, raising the basal metabolic rate by 7 percent for each degree (F). By the same token, fasting and constant malnutrition lower the BMR, due to the shutdown of functions the body can't afford to support. Prolonged starvation also reduces the total amount of metabolically active lean tissue in the body.

The hormones epinephrine and thyroxin also affect the basal metabolic rate. During stress, the body reacts by marshaling all its forces to meet emergencies; the cells' responses to epinephrine increase their energy needs and thus raise the BMR. As for thyroxin, it is the chief hormone that governs the basal metabolic rate. The less thyroxin secreted, the lower the energy used to support the cells' basal activities. Some people move about their tasks in a slow, deliberate fashion, due in part to the lower activity of their thyroid glands. Others race through the day, breaking dishes and becoming irritable, due to thyroid oversecretion. The difference in basal metabolic rates is reflected in the difference in personalities.

To sum up, basal metabolic rate is higher in people with greater lean body mass, in people with a large surface area, in people with fever or

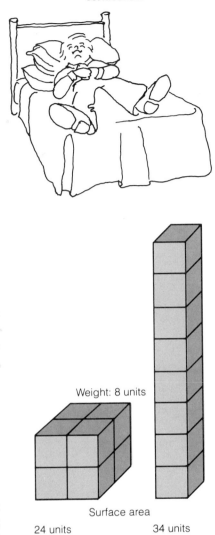

Weight: 8 units

Surface area

24 units   34 units

Both weigh the same, but the tall, thin structure will lose more heat to its surroundings.

thyroxin (thigh-ROX-in): a hormone secreted by the thyroid gland; regulates the basal metabolic rate.

18   "Energy expenditure for 24 hours varied directly with fat-free mass; neither age nor sex affected the relationship." P. Webb, Energy expenditure and fat free mass in men and women, *American Journal of Clinical Nutrition* 34 (1981): 1816–1826. The same conclusion is reached by J. J. Cunningham, A reanalysis of the factors influencing basal metabolic rate in normal adults, *American Journal of Clinical Nutrition* 33 (1980): 2372–2374.

under stress, and in people with high thyroid gland activity. It is lowered by loss of lean tissue due to inactivity, fasting, or malnutrition. The following box shows how basal metabolic energy can be estimated from a person's weight and sex; for a more accurate method, see the Self Study for this chapter (Appendix Q).

Shortcut for Estimating Energy Output: 1. Basal Metabolism

Use the factor 1.0 kcalorie per kilogram of body weight per hour for men, or 0.9 for women. Example (for a 150-pound man):

1 Change pounds to kilograms:

$$150 \text{ lb} \times \frac{1.0 \text{ kg}}{2.2 \text{ lb}} = 68 \text{ kg.}$$

2 Multiply weight in kilograms by the BMR factor:

$$68 \text{ kg} \times 1.0 \frac{\text{kcal}}{\text{kg}} \text{ per hour} = 68 \frac{\text{kcal}}{\text{hr}}.$$

3 Multiply the kcalories used in one hour by the hours in a day:

$$68 \frac{\text{kcal}}{\text{hr}} \times 24 \frac{\text{hr}}{\text{day}} = 1{,}632 \frac{\text{kcal}}{\text{day}}.$$

Energy for BMR equals 1,632 kcalories per day.

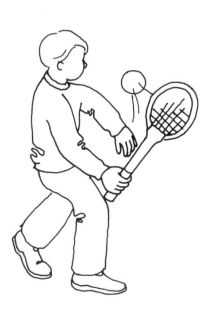

The second of the three components of energy output is physical activity voluntarily undertaken and achieved by use of the skeletal muscles. The amount of energy needed for an activity like playing tennis or studying for an exam depends on the involvement of the muscles, on the amount of weight being moved, and on the length of time the activity is engaged in.

As disheartening as it may be to discover, intense mental activity requires only slightly more energy than normal nervous system activity, even though it may make you very tired. Contraction of muscles, on the other hand, uses up a great many kcalories. In addition to the muscles involved in moving the body, the heart must beat faster to send nutrients and oxygen to the muscles, and the lungs must move faster to get rid of the carbon dioxide and bring in additional oxygen.

The amount of energy needed for a physical activity depends on two factors: body weight and time. The heavier person obviously needs more kcalories when performing the same task in the same time as a lighter person, because it takes extra effort to move the additional body weight. Also, the longer the activity continues, the more kcalories will be used.

You can estimate the energy needed for activities by using the rules of thumb offered in the following box. A more precise calculation of energy expenditure is suggested in the Self Study for this chapter (see Appendix Q).

Shortcut for Estimating Energy Output: 2. Voluntary Muscular Activity

The figures below are crude approximations based on the amount of muscular work a person typically performs in a day. To select the one appropriate for you, remember to think in terms of the amount of *muscular* work performed; don't confuse being *busy* with being *active*.

● For sedentary (mostly sitting) activity (a typist), add 50 percent of the BMR.

● For light activity (a teacher), add 60 percent.

● For moderate activity (a nurse), add 70 percent.

● For heavy work (a roofer), add 100 percent or more.

If the man we used for an example earlier was a typist, we would estimate the energy he needs for physical activities by multiplying his BMR kcalories per day by 50 percent:

$$1,632 \ \frac{kcal}{day} \ \times \ .50 \ = \ 816 \ \frac{kcal}{day}.$$

Energy for activities equals 816 kcalories per day.

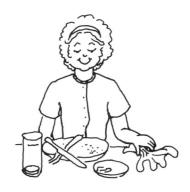

The third component of energy expenditure has to do with processing food. When food is taken into the body, many cells that have been dormant begin to be active. The muscles that move the food through the intestinal tract speed up their rhythmic contractions; the cells that manufacture and secrete digestive juices begin their tasks. All these cells and others need extra energy as they come alive to participate in the digestion, absorption, and metabolism of food. This stimulation of cellular activity is the specific dynamic effect (SDE) of food, and is generally thought to represent about 6 to 10 percent of the total food energy taken in. Contrary to what the advocates of some fad diets would like you to believe, SDE is not significantly higher after a high-protein meal than after a normal, mixed meal.

The SDE for a day is usually calculated by taking 10 percent of the total kcalories used for BMR and physical activity that day. The assumption is that kcalories used for BMR plus activity are about equal to kcalories ingested in food, so the calculation is equivalent to taking 10 percent of food kcalories consumed. (The assumption is also made that the person ate enough that day to maintain weight.) However, if you know the actual food kcalories consumed, you can approximate SDE by taking 10 percent of those kcalories. The box shows a sample calculation.

SDE, or specific dynamic effect, is the energy for metabolizing food; it is sometimes called SDA (specific dynamic activity).

Shortcut for Estimating Energy Output:
3. SDE

If the man in our example ate an average of 2,500 kcalories in a day, his SDE kcalories would amount to:

$$2,500 \ \frac{\text{kcal}}{\text{day}} \times 0.10 = 250 \ \frac{\text{kcal}}{\text{day}}.$$

If we didn't know how many kcalories he ate we could assume they were about enough to support the sum of his BMR energy and his activity energy and calculate as follows:

$$1,632 \ \frac{\text{kcal}}{\text{day}} + 816 \ \frac{\text{kcal}}{\text{day}} = 2,448 \ \frac{\text{kcal}}{\text{day}}.$$

$$2,448 \ \frac{\text{kcal}}{\text{day}} \times 0.10 = 245 \ \frac{\text{kcal}}{\text{day}}.$$

Energy for SDE equals about 250 kcalories per day.

The total energy a person spends in a day is derived by adding the three components together:

Shortcut for Estimating Energy Output:
Total

The man in our example spends, in a day:

$$1,632 \ \frac{\text{kcal}}{\text{day}} + 816 \ \frac{\text{kcal}}{\text{day}} + 250 \ \frac{\text{kcal}}{\text{day}} = 2,708 \ \frac{\text{kcal}}{\text{day}}.$$

Because the exact figure is based on several estimates, it's probably best to express his needs as falling within a 50-kcalorie range:

Total energy equals about 2,685 to 2,735 kcalories per day.

Energy Balance: Weight Loss and Gain

In the average person, a deficit of 500 kcalories a day brings about loss of body fat at the rate of a pound a week; of 1,000 kcalories, two pounds a week. Extraordinarily active people, by virtue of their high energy expenditures, or extremely obese persons, by virtue of the metabolic demands made by the sheer bulk of their body cells and the energy cost of moving their bodies, can lose weight faster. For those who are only moderately obese, the maximum possible rate of fat loss is one to two pounds a week, which for most people means an intake of about 1,000 to 1,500 kcalories a day. Below 1,200, the dieter will be losing lean tissue, and at such a restricted kcalorie level, the diet planner is hard put to achieve adequacy for all the vitamins and minerals. (The person of below-average height will need to adjust these numbers in proportion to his or her height.)

These principles are simple, but putting them into practice is more difficult than you might imagine. Obesity and underweight are complex problems with social and psychological ramifications, as well as the metabolic ones just described. Chapter 7 first deals with the factors that contribute to the problems of overweight and underweight and then provides some practical pointers for the person who wants to lose or gain weight.

Summing Up

Figure 6–7 summarizes the central pathways of metabolism. The principal compounds derived from carbohydrate, fat, and protein in the diet are glucose, glycerol, fatty acids, and amino acids. Glucose may be anabolized to glycogen or catabolized to pyruvate, which in turn yields acetyl CoA. Glycerol and fatty acids may be anabolized to triglycerides or catabolized (glycerol to pyruvate, fatty acids to acetyl CoA). Amino acids may be anabolized to protein or catabolized (after deamination) to pyruvate, acetyl CoA, or TCA cycle intermediates.

Pyruvate is reconvertible to glucose, but the reaction yielding acetyl CoA from pyruvate is irreversible. Hence fatty acids cannot serve as a source of glucose in the body. All three energy nutrients are convertible to acetyl CoA, however, and hence can be used to manufacture body fat.

If a person fasts or if carbohydrate is undersupplied, lean body tissue is catabolized to meet the brain's need for glucose. Within a day or so ketosis sets in. Fatty acids are metabolized to ketones, which can meet some of the brain's energy need. The nitrogen removed from protein is combined with carbon and oxygen to form urea and excreted. Below about 900 kcalories a day, a diet imposes lean tissue loss and ketosis, and the protein kcalories in such a diet are equivalent in the body to carbohydrate kcalories in their protein-sparing effect. Weight loss may be dramatic, but fat loss may be slower than on a moderate, balanced low-kcalorie diet. To design such a moderate diet requires adjusting energy balance so that the intake is reduced, the output is increased, or both.

Energy intake can be computed by adding up the kcalorie values of the foods consumed or can be estimated by using exchange system values. The energy available from food was originally determined by measuring the heat lost when the food was completely burned, with adjustments to account for the incomplete breakdown of food in the body.

Energy output for various age-sex groups are provided by recommendations such as the RDA, but lifestyle has to be taken into account when estimating an individual's energy needs. Machines designed to measure energy expenditure work by measuring heat lost from the body or oxygen used. Data collected in this way have yielded tables from which you can estimate your energy needs quite accurately.

The body's total energy output falls into three categories: energy to support the basal metabolism, energy for muscular activity, and energy to digest, absorb, and metabolize food (SDE, the specific dynamic effect of food). Basal metabolic activities are estimated to require about 1.0 kcalorie per kilogram of body weight per hour for men, and 0.9 for women. Muscular activity requires an additional 50 to 100 percent, and SDE adds about another 10 percent to the total energy expenditure.

The basal metabolic rate is influenced primarily by amount of lean body mass and by body shape. It is also affected by fever, fasting, and hormonal secretions (especially epinephrine and thyroxin).

An energy deficit of 3,500 kcalories is necessary for the loss of a pound of body fat. Loss of body fat in excess of two pounds a week can rarely be sustained. A diet supplying fewer than 1,200 kcalories per day can be made adequate in vitamins and minerals only with great difficulty.

NOTE: References recommended for further reading are in Appendix J; see "Metabolism."

Self-study exercises in Appendix Q show you how to:

● Estimate your energy output, using tables to compute energy spent on BMR and activities.
● Estimate your energy input, using Exchange System kcalorie values for foods.

Appendix C shows details of the metabolic pathways—glycolysis, the TCA cycle, and the electron transport chain, and the *Instructor's Manual* includes transparency/handout masters for these three pathways so that they can be viewed and discussed in class (TH6-3, 6-4, and 6-5).

The *Instructor's Manual* has two additional figures (TH6-11 and 6-12) to show where the body obtains glucose and how it uses ketones during the course of a fast.

HIGHLIGHT 6
Nutrition for the Athlete

The body wants to be fit. Given the chance, it will respond with the strength and vigor that comes from proper exercise, nutrition, and rest.

ELLINGTON DARDEN, Ph.D.

Anyone with a keen interest in athletics is bound to be interested in nutrition as well. Athletes know nutrition affects their performance. Trainers often have had no nutrition education, however, and they pass on much misinformation. Much of what athletes learn from them dates from centuries back and is a mixture of tradition, superstition, and fact. Athletes can easily obtain the nutrients they need from food, because their high kcalorie outputs enable them to eat more food than nonathletes. But they can still make poor food choices, and they need sound nutrition information. This section summarizes the minimum knowledge that a trainer, athlete, or nutrition teacher who deals with athletes should have.

Protein Needs of Athletes

Athletes often believe that their diets should be extremely high in protein. The bodies of athletes contain more muscle than the bodies of nonathletes, and muscles contain more protein than other tissues. Athletes do, in fact, use a little more protein in their activities than nonathletes, but only a little more—perhaps 10 percent. The margin of safety built into the protein recommendation for all people is high enough to cover the athlete's need, so the recommended protein intake is not higher for the athlete than for anyone else.

To protect muscle protein (to avoid losing more than they can easily replace), athletes need to be sure to eat enough protein-sparing kcalories to meet their energy needs, which are higher than most people's. What they need, then, is extra kcalories, not extra protein.

To *build* muscle requires positive nitrogen balance (this was explained in Chapter 4), but even that doesn't mean eating more protein. Most young people's diets already contain about twice as much protein as they can possibly use, and they are actually wasting about half the protein they eat, in the sense that they are using it not to build body protein but rather for energy—a purpose any other energy nutrient could serve just as well, and less expensively.

There is no way to force extra protein into the muscles to make them grow just by eating more protein. Cells don't respond to what's given to

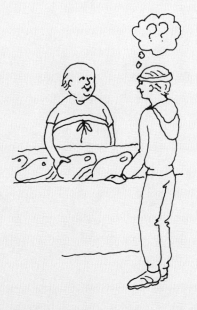

221

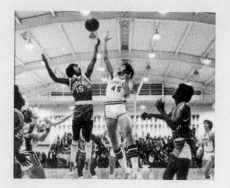

Muscles grow in response to work, not to protein feeding alone.

them by helplessly accepting it—they respond to the hormones that regulate them and to the demands put upon them, and they select the nutrients they need from what is offered. So the way to make muscle cells grow is to put a demand on them—that is, to make them work. They will respond by taking up nutrients, amino acids included, so that they can grow. In summary, don't *push* protein at them, but exercise them in order to demand that they *pull* protein in for themselves. Then make sure that protein is available by eating a diet adequate in protein. There's no advantage to eating excess protein.

kCalorie Needs of Athletes

Depending on the sport, an athlete in active training and competition may have extraordinarily high energy needs. Football players, for example, seem to average close to 6,000 kcalories a day during the football season, with some days' intakes topping 10,000 kcalories.[1] With the increased kcalorie intake goes increased need for the B vitamins (especially thiamin) used to generate energy in metabolism. The increased intake, therefore, shouldn't be just any high-kcalorie food but should be food rich in B vitamins as well—breads, cereals, fruits, vegetables, and other protective foods. It is a rare individual who can eat over 5,000 kcalories of nutrient-dense food in only three meals a day; five to six meals make the task easier.[2]

Gaining and Losing Weight

Another issue athletes need to understand has to do with gaining and losing weight. An athlete who wants to gain weight in a hurry and doesn't care whether it is muscle or fat can add kcalories of any kind to the diet to achieve the desired gain. Because fat in foods is more kcalorie-dense than protein or carbohydrate, the athlete can most easily gain weight by eating a high-fat diet. This technique is said to be one of the most widespread nutrition-related abuses in sports; and it increases the risk of heart disease, to which athletes are not immune. The healthy way to gain weight is to build oneself up by patient and consistent training and at the same time to eat enough kcalories (of nutritious foods) to support the weight gain.

To gain a pound of muscle mass, the athlete has to eat about 3,000 kcalories more than he expends. An athlete who adds a big snack of protective foods (for example, a quarterpound hamburger on a bun, french fries, and a soft drink) between meals can eat 700 to 800 extra kcalories a day this way, thus achieving a healthful weight gain of 1 to 1½ pounds per week.

The athlete must remember to cut *down* on kcalories between and after training periods. Muscles respond to reduced demand by losing mass. It would be magical thinking to believe that the mass simply disappears. In fact, the cells slowly atrophy, and the materials they are made of (mostly carbohydrate, fat, and protein) become available as potential fuel for other

1   S. Short and W. R. Short, Four-year study of university athletes' dietary intake, *Journal of the American Dietetic Association* 82 (1983): 632–645.

2   Energy intake and exercise, *Nutrition and the MD*, August 1981.

body cells. Of course, this fuel will be stored as fat unless it is expended in activity. It should be no surprise, then, that a heavily muscled individual of 20 who stops working out but keeps on eating like a football player in training can become an oversized, flabby, and obese person at 30. There's actually some truth in the notion that his "muscle turned to fat," even though it's a slight oversimplification; muscle has been lost and fat has been gained.

The athlete who wants to lose weight, like the one who wants to gain, can choose a wise or unwise course. To achieve ideal body composition—the optimum ratio of muscle strength to body mass—people must reduce only body fat, and they can't do this for more than a very few weeks at a rate faster than about two pounds a week. Hurry-up techniques, such as sauna bathing, exercising in a plastic suit (to sweat it off), using diuretics or cathartics, or inducing vomiting, achieve faster weight loss only by causing dehydration, and dehydration seriously impairs performance. The hazards of fasts and fad diets are described in Chapter 6, but a reminder should be repeated here. What is achieved by quick-weight-loss dieting is loss of lean tissue, glycogen, bone minerals, fluids—all materials vital to healthy body functioning. Abnormal heart rhythms have been seen in healthy adults after only ten days of fasting.[3]

> Ideal body composition for the athlete: the optimum ratio of muscle strength to body mass.

Even if it is achieved by healthy methods, extreme weight loss can be hazardous to the athlete, as to any person. Occasionally one hears that an "elite runner"—in superb physical condition and at the peak of his career—has died suddenly at the end of an intensive exercise session. These deaths were a mystery until recently, but now a reason for them seems to be emerging. In each case, the person had been severely restricting kcalories and had reached a new, all-time-low weight, while at the same time breaking his own previous records for distance or time. Exactly what causes the deaths is still not known, but severe kcalorie restriction and weight loss combined with hard training seem to be contributing factors.[4]

Women athletes sometimes experience menstrual irregularity or even complete stoppage of the menstrual cycle. Athletic amenorrhea resembles the amenorrhea seen in women with anorexia nervosa or in the world's undernourished women and has been thought to be due to loss of body fat. The theory is that a certain minimum amount of body fat is necessary to support the making and using of the female hormones, which are fat-like compounds themselves. However, low body fat may not be the only cause; a change in the brain's regulation of sex hormone output may be responsible for athletic amenorrhea. In any case, the possible relationship of amenorrhea to body weight serves as a reminder that all athletes should keep in mind the definition of ideal weight already mentioned: the optimum ratio of muscle strength to body mass. *Optimum* means neither too much *nor too little* body mass.

> **athletes' amenorrhea** (ay-men-or-REE-uh): the failure in women athletes to menstruate.
>
> *a* = without
>
> *menor* = menstrual cycle

3   Nutrition and athletic performance, *Dairy Council Digest* 46 (1976). Sometimes, however, an athlete obviously has heart disease, either hereditary or acquired. Diet can't always be blamed for sudden deaths in athletes.

4   T. J. Bassler, Body build and mortality (letter to the editor), *Journal of the American Medical Association* 244 (1980): 1437.

Energy for Muscle Work

Still another question has to do with the foods an athlete should eat to derive energy for training or competition. The fuel of muscle work is not protein but carbohydrate and fat. Muscles normally use a mixture of the two; but during intensive exercise they require glucose, and during rest they store it as glycogen within their cells so that it will be available when needed. (Two-thirds of the body's glycogen is in the muscles, and only one-third is in the liver to serve the rest of the body's needs for blood glucose.) When a muscle uses glycogen, it first derives many glucose units from it, then breaks them down. The breakdown of glucose is a multistep process that releases energy at several of its steps. (You may be aware that the energy from glucose isn't used directly but goes to make ATP. It also can go to CP, creatine phosphate, a special energy carrier of muscle. The subsequent breakdown of these compounds provides the energy for the muscle to contract.) After glucose has released its energy, only water and carbon-dioxide gas are left—tiny waste products that are excreted by way of urine and exhaled breath.

When you exert yourself extremely vigorously without relaxing for a moment, you experience muscle fatigue or even exhaustion and can't work your muscles at all. This effect results from the buildup of lactic acid—and knowing where it comes from can help athletes to improve their endurance.

The first few steps of glucose breakdown take place without oxygen, until pyruvate (pyruvic acid) has been produced (see Figure H6–1).

The next few steps require oxygen and end with the complete breakdown of pyruvic acid to carbon dioxide and water (Figure H6–2). To break down glucose completely, then, and release the waste products, the muscle cells need abundant oxygen.

If the circulation can't bring them oxygen fast enough, the cells break glucose down as far as they can, to pyruvic acid, and then convert the pyruvic acid to the temporary waste product lactic acid (Figure H6–3). That is all they can do without oxygen. This acid accumulates and changes the acid balance in the muscle.

The body's disposal of lactic acid is of great interest to the athlete who knows that its accumulation in her muscles will cause fatigue. A strategy for dealing with lactic acid is to relax the muscles at every opportunity, so that the circulating blood can carry it away and bring oxygen to support aerobic metabolism.

Breathing is important to performance. The more oxygen you can bring to the muscle, the longer it can work aerobically, getting all the available energy from its stored glucose. This is why athletes, to get in the best possible shape, have to condition their cardiovascular and respiratory systems—that is, do aerobic exercise that requires speeded-up breathing and a rapid heartbeat, and not just weight-lifting or exercises that increase muscle strength only.

At the end of an event, the athlete continues to breathe fast, and the heart continues pounding for some time, because oxygen is still being circulated to the tissues to help break down the accumulated lactic acid (Figure H6–4). The carbon dioxide that results stimulates the brain to make the

anaerobic (AN-air-OH-bic): requiring no oxygen.

an = without

aer = oxygen

pyruvic (pie-ROO-vic) **acid** or **pyruvate**: a breakdown product of glucose that can be produced anaerobically. To dispose of pyruvic acid without using oxygen, the cells convert it to lactic acid; see below.

aerobic: requiring oxygen.

lactic acid or **lactate**: a temporary product of anaerobic glucose oxidation. Lactate is completely oxidized or reconverted to glucose as soon as oxygen becomes available.

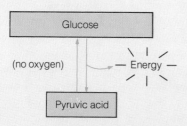

FIGURE H6–1 The first steps in glucose breakdown require no oxygen, release energy, and produce pyruvic acid (pyruvate). These steps are known as anaerobic glycolysis. TH6-15

heart and lungs stay speeded up until the waste products have been disposed of.

This description has shown what provides fuel for intense muscular activity: glycogen, that is, carbohydrate. The message for the athlete is that meals high in protein not only don't help build muscle but also don't help fuel its activity. Many experiments have shown that extra protein in the diet confers no advantage on the athlete in terms of strength, endurance, or speed.

Fat is also used for fuel by muscles but can be broken down only as long as oxygen is available. Fat deposits therefore supply energy for moderate, but not for strenuous, muscular work. Long, slow, moderately intense activities such as long walks can be very effective as an adjunct to a weight-loss effort, because fat is continuously oxidized for the duration of these activities.

A great advantage to muscle conditioning is that it increases the muscles' ability to burn fat as fuel; they build up more fat-metabolizing machinery in response to demand. So people whose muscles are in good shape find it easier to keep off excess fat. Conditioned muscles will burn fat longer during activity, or at a higher-intensity exercise level, than poorly conditioned muscles. In competition, too, conditioned muscles will go much longer before starting to use glycogen. The point at which the body starts using glycogen is the beginning of the end, because glycogen stores are limited, whereas fat stores are (in effect) unlimited.

Athletes in training for an endurance activity such as long-distance running, cycling, or swimming may experience increasing fatigue as the days of training go on. One reason for this is that it takes 48 hours or more to restore muscle carbohydrate to its pre-exercise level after it has been completely exhausted. To replace the used-up carbohydrate, the athlete must eat a diet high in carbohydrate. Two pointers for the athlete in training, then, are to take a periodic day's rest, if possible, during training, and to rest for a day or so before the event and eat a carbohydrate-rich diet.

Athletes who compete in long-distance endurance events naturally want to have as much stored energy in their muscles as they can. Glycogen loading is a technique of tricking the muscles into storing more glycogen than they normally have the capacity for. When the technique was first introduced, athletes were taught to reduce their carbohydrate intake for several days by eating meals high in protein and fat and simultaneously to exercise heavily to deplete the muscle glycogen stores. The second step

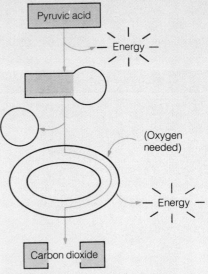

FIGURE H6–2 The breakdown of pyruvic acid to carbon dioxide and energy via the TCA cycle requires oxygen. This is known as aerobic metabolism. TH6-15

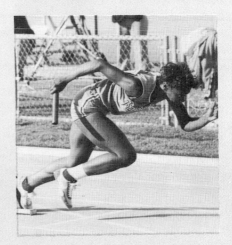

glycogen loading: a technique of inducing muscles to store more glycogen than they normally do, by manipulating the diet's carbohydrate levels.

FIGURE H6–3 Pyruvic acid is shunted temporarily to lactic acid if oxygen isn't available to help oxidize it further. TH6-15

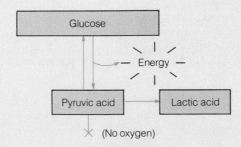

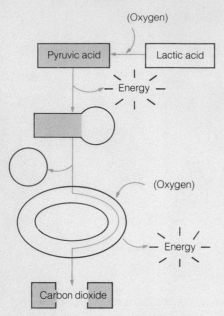

FIGURE H6-4 **When oxygen is available again, lactic acid is reconverted to pyruvic acid and then completely oxidized. TH6-15**

was to reduce exercise intensity and switch abruptly to a diet high in carbohydrate. Muscle glycogen stores rebounded to about two to four times the normal level and thus provided fuel that would last longer in an endurance event.

Until the mid-1970s, the hazards of this practice were unknown. Now, unfortunately, it is clear that there are hazards. Many athletes feel that the side effects of tampering with their diets—muscle and cardiac pain and weight gain—cancel the benefits conferred by loaded glycogen. It is also strongly suggested that this not be done more than about three times a year, due to the effects on heart function. Some athletes feel they can get away with it without ill effects, but most exercise physiologists recommend a different routine. Don't restrict carbohydrate and then rebound, they say; just eat a diet generally high in carbohydrate, and especially high before competition. This method also keeps muscle glycogen high.

Marathon racers can tell when they've run out of glycogen (they "hit the wall" and suddenly slow down); those who have "loaded" can keep going longer and so have the edge in the competition. In a hot climate, glycogen loading may confer an additional advantage, because glycogen holds a lot of water. As it breaks down, it releases this water, helping to meet the athlete's fluid needs.[5]

To maximize endurance, the athlete pays attention not only to fuel reserves in the muscle (that is, glycogen) but also to the muscle's ability to use that fuel. That means maximizing all of the following:

● Aerobic capacity (by heart and lung conditioning).
● Hemoglobin levels (by optimal iron and protein nutrition).
● Metabolic regulators (by optimal vitamin and mineral nutrition).
● Muscular fat-using ability (by muscular conditioning).[6]

The Pre-Game Meal

Athletes also want to know what food is best before an event. There seems to be no special food that should be eaten before an athletic contest. A meal of steak may boost morale, but a meal too high in fat can stay on the stomach long enough to hinder performance. There's no need to avoid milk; the idea that it causes "cotton mouth" is pure superstition. Olympic training tables are laden with carbohydrate foods such as fruit, and this is the best choice, for the reasons described in the previous section.

A competitor who gets very excited before an event may be unable to digest any food very well. For this reason, many athletes tolerate liquid meals best. But there is no magic ingredient in a liquid meal, in spite of what advertisements may claim. Any meal should be finished a good two or even three or four hours before the event, because digestion requires routing the blood supply to the GI tract. By the time the contest begins, the circulating blood should be freed from the task of picking up nutrients

5   G. R. Hagerman, Nutrition in part-time athletes, *Nutrition and the MD*, August 1981.

6   We are indebted to Dr. Sam Smith of the University of New Hampshire for suggesting this summary.

from the GI tract, and should be available instead to carry oxygen and fuel to the muscles.

The notion is widespread that it is smart to eat a candy bar or a few teaspoons of honey right before the event, for "quick energy." It may feel good to do this, but it probably confers a disadvantage physically, at least for aerobic exercise, if it has any effect at all. The body's response is to secrete insulin, which retards fat use at a time when fat use should be maximal. Other foods athletes may choose to eat before events may have special, personal meanings associated with them, but none has any special power to promote speed, coordination, or endurance.

"*None* has any special power? Not even bee pollen? Surely this book must be out of date. Bee pollen has been shown in careful experiments to improve athletic performance."

This book, like any book, can contain erroneous information. When it does, it will be apologetically corrected. But so far, bee pollen is looking like any other health fad. Although one Finnish runner claimed it gave him the edge in the 1972 Olympics, in which he won a gold medal, others have gained no benefits from using it, and a six-month controlled study of swimmers (not yet published) showed no difference in performance between bee-pollen takers and control subjects. Bee pollen does cause allergies in susceptible people, varies widely in composition from area to area and from one harvest to the next, is composed of at least 50 percent sugar, and sells for up to $24 per pound.[7]

What will "the latest" energy booster be, *next* year?

ergogenic: a term referring to foods that are supposed to have unusual energy-producing power. Actually, no foods are ergogenic.

ergo = energy

genic = gives rise to

Caution

The Athlete's Liquid Needs

Muscles heat up during heavy exertion. With inadequate circulation, the exercising muscle cramps. An adequate fluid intake is most important to prevent heat disorders from disabling the athlete. Fluid is needed to maintain the plasma volume so that blood can penetrate the muscles and carry the heat away, and also to permit sweating. The evaporation of sweat is the body's primary means of releasing heat during exercise in a hot climate.

Dehydration can disable the athlete more seriously than any other nutritional factor. Maintaining fluid balance is crucial to successful performance, because the first symptom of dehydration is fatigue. A rapid water loss equal to 5 percent of the body weight can reduce muscular work capacity by 20 to 30 percent.[8] According to the Food and Nutrition Board, a person should begin replacing salt as well as water after having drunk more than four quarts of water to replace that lost in heavy sweating; but according to recent research, the replacement need not be immediate and shouldn't be

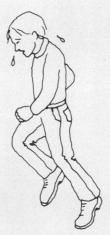

7   K. Cobb, Bee pollen—old diet fads never die, *American Health*, May/June 1983.

8   J. Bergstrom and E. Hultman, Nutrition for maximal sports performance, *Journal of the American Medical Association* 221 (1972): 999.

by way of salt tablets.[9] A person can sweat away as much as nine pounds of fluid and still perform well, provided he or she drinks enough water, even without salt. A rule of thumb is to drink close to a pound of fluid (14 to 16 ounces) for each pound of body weight lost during an activity.[10] When the event is over, eating regular food can make up the salt loss. At that point, replacement of magnesium and potassium may be more important than replacement of sodium.

You may be wondering how this statement can be made when the makers of Gatorade and other "sweat replacers" claim that their mixtures of water with glucose, sodium, chloride, potassium, magnesium, and calcium enter the system "faster than water" and help football players win games. Actually, although such mixtures do resemble sweat in composition (except for the glucose) and do satisfy thirst, they are probably absorbed less rapidly, not more rapidly, than water, because the glucose in them delays absorption.[11] Moreover, the body of a trained athlete stores extra amounts of the minerals in question and can replenish them perfectly well with ordinary food and fluids after the competition is over.[12] Furthermore, a person who sweats heavily (say, two liters) during competition *cannot* replace the lost fluid even by drinking that much, because the stomach can't absorb more than one liter in an hour. The best fluid for a marathon event is *diluted* juice (for example, one part orange juice plus four parts water) or plain, cool water in small quantities. However, there is probably no great harm in the moderate use of sweat replacers. The sugar in them provides a boost; they taste good; and most importantly, they bolster morale.

Some athletes, like the rest of us, enjoy meeting some of their fluid needs with beverages containing caffeine (especially coffee and cola beverages) or alcohol (notably beer). Both practices are safe *in moderation*, but both can be abused. The alcohol in beer actually promotes water loss from the body (see Highlight 8A). So does the caffeine in coffee.[13]

Athletes' Anemia

Some athletes have anemia. It is not known whether this is always the result of iron deficiency, or whether in some cases it may be an adaptation to the athlete's way of life. It is possible that the athlete only appears to be anemic but in fact has a greater than normal number of red blood cells and an even greater plasma volume as a result of conditioning, so that the red blood cells are, in effect, diluted. This effect is enhanced when, during repeated days of heavy training, plasma volume may increase by almost a third

9   S. Wintsch, Beading the heat, *Science 81,* February 1981, pp. 80–82.

10   Hagerman, 1981.

11   Wintsch, 1981. Also, some people think the sugar would elicit the secretion of insulin, which opposes release of both glycogen and fat for use as fuel. However, once an athlete is warmed up and working out, dilute glucose solutions at intervals apparently do not increase insulin secretion. Hagerman, 1981.

12   Wintsch, 1981.

13   Coffee makes longer easier, *Runners World,* July 1978, p. 52.

because the kidney conserves sodium and water at these times.[14] Thus there may be two kinds of anemia in athletes—one, the adaptation just described, and the other, an occasional anemia caused by iron deficiency. Women athletes who are menstruating normally would be especially likely to have iron-deficiency anemia because of their monthly iron loss, and it may be a good idea for them to take iron supplements.

The case of athletes' anemia brings up a point that everyone should keep in mind. Not all apparent abnormalities are "bad." The body is a magnificent system that shows a remarkable ability to adapt to different life-styles and situations. Athletes' anemia may be a case in point; it may be an adaptation to the athlete's way of life, an advantage rather than a disadvantage. We don't know yet, and we can't know what to do about it, if anything, until the research is done.

There are many differences between the bodies of athletes and nonathletes. Often the finger is pointed at nutrition: "You wouldn't be that way if you would eat right." But the athlete being told this should keep in mind that the body may be wiser than the accuser and that the reason the body is different may be because of the different tasks it is called upon to perform.

This note is intended as a general note of caution. When new findings turn up in relation to nutrition and athletics, give them a chance to be responsibly investigated before jumping to conclusions and especially before going to any extremes in terms of food choices. In this field as in all fields of science, you can't find truth by a reasoning process, no matter how good the logic may be. Experimental testing must come first. Meanwhile, before the data are in and analyzed, be moderate in your eating habits. Don't underestimate the body's resources. It may know better than you do.

 Caution

The recommendations made here are simple, common-sense suggestions. To sum up, a normal, varied diet is best for the athlete, as for anyone else. Athletes eat more food to get the extra kcalories they need, and if they choose their foods with reasonable good judgment, they can easily get the protein, vitamins, and minerals they need as well. An adequate fluid intake is indispensable to successful performance.

NOTE: Appendix J contains additional references on nutrition for the athlete; see "Athlete."

14   D. L. Costill, A scientific approach to distance running, *Track and Field News* (Los Altos, Calif.: 1979), p. 22.

CHAPTER 7
Overweight and Underweight

CONTENTS

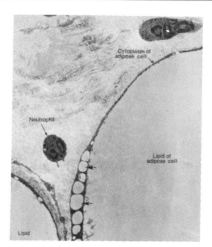

Fat cells can expand immensely as their fat stores increase. Here are two neighboring fat cells. The cell material (cytoplasm) is pushed to the very edge of the cell; the center is a giant fat reservoir. New fat being synthesized first forms small droplets near the edge of the cell (arrows); then the droplets merge into the central reservoir.

No matter how much you huff and puff, you can't just shake it off, rock it off, roll it off, knock it off or bake it off . . . . The only way is to eat less and exercise more.

AMERICAN MEDICAL ASSOCIATION

Obesity is a major malnutrition problem. It is one of the most important and least understood areas in the science of nutrition. Everyone knows roughly what it is. If you are too fat, you are overweight; if much too fat, you are obese. But why and how obesity occurs and what can be done about it are matters for much speculation, debate, and frustration. For the obese person who has earnestly tried every known means of losing weight only to fail, frustration can turn to despair.

Less well recognized is the problem of underweight, which can be equally mysterious. A "skinny" person finds it as hard to gain a pound as a fat person does to lose one.

This chapter emphasizes the problems of overweight and obesity, partly because they have been more intensively studied and partly because they are a more widespread health problem in the developed countries. This does not imply that the underweight person faces a less difficult problem. The concluding section shows that what we know about the one extreme sometimes applies equally well to the other. Two subjects are not covered fully in this chapter but are reserved for Chapter 14: anorexia nervosa and bulimia.

Overweight and underweight both result from unbalanced energy budgets. The overweight person has consumed more food energy (kcalories) than he has expended and has banked the surplus in his fat cells. The underweight person has not consumed enough and so has depleted his fat stores. Energy itself doesn't weigh anything and can't be seen, but when it exists in the form of chemical bonds in nutrients or body fat, the material that it holds together is both heavy and visible.

The amount of fat you might deposit or withdraw from "savings" on any given day depends on your energy balance for that day—the amount you consume (energy-in) versus the amount you expend (energy-out). As Chapter 6 shows, you can reduce your fat deposits by withdrawing more energy from them than you put in. A pound of body fat stores 3,500 kcalories. To lose a pound of body fat you must experience a deficit; you must take in 3,500 kcalories less than you expend. To lose that pound in a week, you need to achieve an average deficit of 500 kcalories a day.

Ideal Weight and Body Fatness

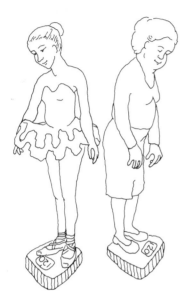

ideal weight: a misnomer; not the desirable but the average weight given in insurance tables for persons of a given sex and height in the United States—not necessarily ideal for a given individual.

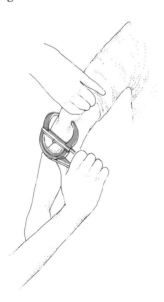

How fat is too fat? And how thin is too thin? It isn't always possible to tell from the bathroom scales, because body weight says nothing about body composition. The relative amounts of lean and fat tissue vary widely from one person to the next. A dancer or an athlete, whose muscles are well developed and whose bones have become dense from constant stress, may weigh much more than a sedentary person with a similar figure. What is needed is a measure of body fatness—not of body weight. Ideally, by a very rough approximation, fat makes up about 18 percent of a man's body weight and about 22 percent of a woman's, with the remainder contributed by water (55 to 60 percent), muscle and other lean tissue (10 to 20 percent), and bone minerals (6 to 8 percent). But there is no easy way to look inside a person and see the bones and muscles.

Several laboratory techniques for estimating body fatness have been developed. One way is to determine the body's density (weight compared with volume). Lean tissue is denser than fat tissue, so the more dense a person's body is, the more lean tissue it must contain. Weight is easy to measure with a scale, but volume measurement involves submerging the whole body in water and measuring the amount of water displaced; this requires a large tank and takes up too much space to be practical for use in, say, a doctor's office. Another way is to inject a water-soluble substance that is easy to detect and measure, and allow it to penetrate into the lean tissues (it will not mix into the fat tissues). A blood sample taken soon after will show the extent to which the substance has been diluted, providing an estimate of the amount of lean tissue.

A direct measure of the amount of body fat can be obtained by lifting a fold of skin from the back of the arm, from the back, or from other body surfaces and measuring its thickness with a caliper that applies a fixed amount of pressure. The fat under the skin in these regions is roughly proportional to total body fat. A fold over an inch thick indicates overfat-ness; under a half-inch reflects underweight. This technique—the fatfold test—is a practical diagnostic tool in the hands of trained people and is in increasingly wide use.

A still simpler test is the mirror test. Undress and stand before a mirror. If you look too fat, you may be too fat. (A notoriously poor judge of this, however, is the teenage girl, who often thinks any amount of fat, no matter how small, is a serious blemish. It may be that she needs to change her self-image—not to go on a diet.)

The scales are not necessarily an accurate indicator of body fatness, then, but you most probably use them anyway. After weighing yourself, you turn to the tables published by the insurance companies (see inside back cover). You then discover that for a person your height and sex, three weight ranges are suggested: one for a small frame, one for medium, and one for large. Don't forget your shoes: you are assumed to be wearing one-inch heels. (Thus a person who stands 5 feet 10 inches tall in bare feet would look up the range for a person 5 feet 11 inches.) Finally, if you weigh yourself nude, you must adjust for clothing (the tables assume five pounds for clothes).

All these steps involve a lot of guesswork. How do you decide on your frame size, for example? As of 1983, the first standards had been provided, but their validity is not yet established. Table 7–1 presents a means of estimating your frame size.

fatfold test: a clinical test of body fatness in which the thickness of a fold of skin on the back of the arm (triceps), below the shoulder blade (subscapular), or in other places is measured with an instrument called a caliper. The older, less preferred, term for this is **skinfold test**.

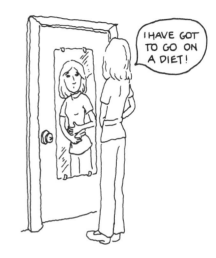

I HAVE GOT TO GO ON A DIET!

frame size: the size of a person's bones and musculature. A person with a large frame should weigh more than one with a small frame.

TABLE 7–1 **How to Determine Your Body Frame by Elbow Breadth**
To make a simple approximation of your frame size:
Extend your arm and bend the forearm upwards at a 90-degree angle. Keep the fingers straight and turn the inside of your wrist away from the body. Place the thumb and index finger of your other hand on the two prominent bones on *either side* of your elbow. Measure the space between your fingers against a ruler or a tape measure.[a] Compare the measurements with the following standards.

These standards represent the elbow measurements for medium-framed men and women of various heights. Measurements smaller than those listed indicate you have a small frame and larger measurements indicate a large frame.

	MEN
Height in 1-in Heels	*Elbow Breadth*
5 ft 2 in to 5 ft 3 in	2½ to 2⅞ in
5 ft 4 in to 5 ft 7 in	2⅝ to 2⅞ in
5 ft 8 in to 5 ft 11 in	2¾ to 3 in
6 ft 0 in to 6 ft 3 in	2¾ to 3⅛ in
6 ft 4 in and over	2⅞ to 3¼ in
	WOMEN
Height in 1-in Heels	*Elbow Breadth*
4 ft 10 in to 4 ft 11 in	2¼ to 2½ in
5 ft 0 in to 5 ft 3 in	2¼ to 2½ in
5 ft 4 in to 5 ft 7 in	2⅜ to 2⅝ in
5 ft 8 in to 5 ft 11 in	2⅜ to 2⅝ in
6 ft 0 in and over	2½ to 2¾ in

[a] For the most accurate measurement, have your physician measure your elbow breadth with a caliper.
SOURCE: Metropolitan Life Insurance Company. An alternative means of measuring frame size appears in Appendix E.

After finding the applicable weight, you have to apply the most important judgment factor of all. Ask yourself whether the weight range you have singled out is really ideal for *you*. At what weight are you most healthy? Does your family tend to be most healthy at the heavier, or lighter, end of the weight ranges? A recent reinterpretation of the insurance company statistics suggests that many people are healthiest at weights slightly *above* those thought to be ideal in the past.

Ideal weight probably changes with age. Many people typically become less active as they grow older. Their muscles get smaller, and their bones decrease in density. Thus a person who at 25 was lean and muscular might weigh the same at 65 and yet have become considerably fatter. Such a person should either gradually lose weight as time goes on or, preferably, maintain a program of vigorous physical activity to preserve muscle mass and bone strength. Not much is known about ideal weights at older ages, but clearly, people do tend to gain about 20 to 30 pounds during adulthood. Perhaps for a person who maintains muscle mass, this weight gain may be consistent with good health if it does not precipitate high blood pressure.

With all their limitations, the weight tables are often used to draw arbitrary lines between too much and too little body weight. A person who is more than 10 percent above the weight on the table is considered overweight; if 20 percent or more, obese. (Some authorities say obesity is 15 percent above the table weight, some say 25 percent.) Similarly, a person who is more than 10 percent below the table weight is considered underweight.

The Problem of Obesity

However you define it, obesity does occur to an alarming extent and is increasing in the developed countries. For example, in the United States some 10 to 25 percent of all teenagers and some 25 to 50 percent of all adults are obese.

Some people become fat in childhood, and others later on. Few of either type lose the excess weight. There is no specific age that divides juvenile-onset obesity from adult-onset obesity, but as the terms imply, there is a distinction between the two types. A child who is obese will develop sturdy muscles and bones as she grows, to support her excess weight. Thus as an adult she will have more lean body mass and more body fat than the average person and will likely always be stocky, even after losing her excess fat. People who become obese as children are also less likely to be able to reduce successfully than people who become obese as adults.

Research on fat cells suggests a possible reason why early-onset obesity is especially resistant to treatment. Simply stated, early overfeeding is thought by some researchers to stimulate fat cells so that they increase abnormally in *number*. The number of fat cells is thought to become fixed by adulthood; if it is, then a gain in weight thereafter can take place only through an increase in the *size* of the fat cells. A person with an abnormally

---

overweight: body weight more than 10 percent above average (insurance company table) weight.

obesity: excessive body fatness; often loosely defined as a condition of being overweight by 15 or 20 percent or more.

underweight: body weight more than 10 percent below normal or average weight.

juvenile-onset obesity: obesity arising in childhood; also called **developmental obesity**.

adult-onset obesity: obesity arising after adolescence; sometimes called **reactive obesity** if it appears to arise in response to a specific traumatic life event.

large number of fat cells is thought likely to be abnormally hungry and to overeat for that reason. On the other hand, a person who gains weight in adulthood supposedly has a normal number of fat cells and needs only to reduce the size of the cells.

This theory has been heavily criticized on several grounds. Fat cells are hard to count, and researchers disagree as to whether new cells are being formed at certain periods or small, empty fat cells are being recruited as new storage cells.[1] Even the critics agree, however, that there are certain periods in life when body fat increases more rapidly than lean tissue: early infancy (up to about two years), again during preadolescence (and throughout adolescence in girls), and possibly again during the third trimester of pregnancy. These are critical periods, in the sense that some developmental events that take place at these times are irreversible. Prevention of obesity would be most important during these times. There is also agreement that fat is hard to lose no matter when it is gained.

Hazards of Obesity

Insurance companies report that fat people die younger from a host of causes including heart attacks, strokes, and complications of diabetes. In fact, gaining weight often appears to precipitate diabetes. Fat people more often suffer high levels of blood fat, hypertension, coronary heart disease, postsurgical complications, gynecological irregularities, and the toxemia of pregnancy. The burden of extra fat strains the skeletal system, causing arthritis—especially in the knees, hips, and lower spine. The muscles that support the belly may give way, resulting in abdominal hernias. When the leg muscles are abnormally fatty, they fail to contract efficiently to help blood return from the leg veins to the heart; blood collects in the leg veins, which swell, harden, and become varicose. Extra fat in and around the chest interferes with breathing, sometimes causing severe respiratory problems. Gout is more common and even the accident rate is greater for the severely obese.

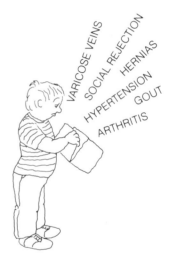

Beyond all these hazards is the risk incurred by millions of obese people throughout much of their lives—the risk of ill-advised, misguided dieting. Some fad diets are more hazardous to health than obesity itself. One survey of 29,000 claims, treatments, and theories for losing weight found fewer than 6 percent of them effective—and 13 percent dangerous![2]

Once a person becomes obese, the situation tends to perpetuate itself. When fat cells enlarge, they become sluggish in responding to insulin, the hormone that promotes the making and storage of fat. The excess glucose remains in the bloodstream longer than normal and stimulates the insulin-producing cells of the pancreas to multiply and secrete more insulin. When the fat cells finally respond, they store more fat than normal in response to

1   R. T. Jung, M. I. Gurr, M. P. Robinson, and W. P. T. James, Does adipocyte hypercellularity in obesity exist? *British Medical Journal* 2 (1978): 319–321; J. Kirtland and M. I. Gurr, Adipose tissue cellularity—a review: 2. The relationship between cellularity and obesity, *International Journal of Obesity* 3 (1979): 15–55.

2   M. Simonton, An overview—advances in research and treatment of obesity, *Food and Nutrition News*, March–April 1982.

A linear (straight-line) relationship:

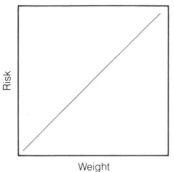

The actual relationship of risk to weight:

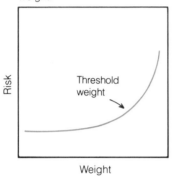

FIGURE 7–1 **Threshold weight**. The relationship of risk to weight is not linear (A), but curvilinear (B). At the threshold weight, risk rises abruptly.

SOURCE: Adapted from C. C. Seltzer, Some reevaluations of the *Build and Blood Pressure Study*, 1959, as related to ponderal index, somatotype and mortality, *New England Journal of Medicine* 274 (1966): 254–259.

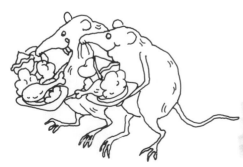

the raised insulin level. As if this were not enough, the enlarged fat cells are also less sensitive to other hormones that promote fat breakdown. Weight loss restores insulin levels to normal, but it first has to be achieved against these odds.

Not only physical but also social and economic disadvantages plague the fat person, who is less often sought after for marriage, pays higher insurance premiums, meets discrimination when applying for a job, can't find attractive clothes so easily, and is limited in choice of sports. Fat girls have only a third the chance of being accepted into college that lean girls have. The fat child often suffers ridicule from his classmates and the unbearable humiliation of having the captain choose him last for the team.

The many disadvantages justify our calling obesity a severe physical handicap. However, it is unlike other handicaps in two important ways. First, mortality risk is not linearly related to excess weight. Instead, there is a threshold at which risk dramatically increases. Being only a few pounds above this threshold weight may cause blood pressure, blood glucose, and blood lipids to zoom upwards. The concept of a danger zone of weight is illustrated in Figure 7–1. Second, obesity is reversible, and if it is corrected in time, some of its risks are, too. Mortality rates (from insurance data) are no higher for the formerly obese than for the never obese.

Ideally a person would never have to struggle with the problem of obesity, because he would never have become obese to begin with. Preventive efforts are needed, especially in vulnerable groups: infants, preadolescents, adolescents, and women before they are pregnant. (This is in no way meant to imply that a woman who is pregnant should attempt to lose weight. Weight loss during pregnancy requires skilled medical supervision if it is done at all.) Where prevention has failed, treatment is urgently needed. But how to treat? Before turning to the matters of diet, drugs, exercise, and other means of attacking the problem, it is necessary to try to figure out what causes obesity.

Causes of Obesity

kCalories are not stored in fat until the body's energy needs have been met. Excess body fat can accumulate only when kcalories are eaten beyond those needed for the day's metabolic, muscular, and digestive activities. To put it bluntly, obesity results from overeating.

In fact, however, this statement neither explains the cause of obesity nor suggests a cure. Why do people overeat? Is it a hunger problem? An appetite problem? A satiety problem? Is it genetic? Metabolic? Environmental? Is it a matter of habits learned in early childhood? Is it psychological? Might all these factors play a role? To tell the truth, we do not know the cause.

In general, two schools of thought address this problem. One attributes it to inside-the-body causes, the other to environmental factors. One currently popular inside-the-body theory is the so-called set-point theory. Noting that many people who lose weight on reducing diets subsequently return to their original weight, some researchers have suggested that the

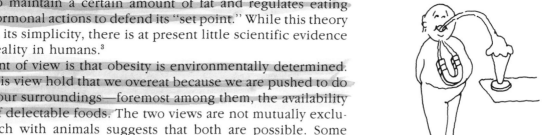

body "wants" to maintain a certain amount of fat and regulates eating behaviors and hormonal actions to defend its "set point." While this theory is compelling in its simplicity, there is at present little scientific evidence supporting its reality in humans.[3]

The other point of view is that obesity is environmentally determined. Proponents of this view hold that we overeat because we are pushed to do so by factors in our surroundings—foremost among them, the availability of a multitude of delectable foods. The two views are not mutually exclusive, and research with animals suggests that both are possible. Some obesity may arise from one, some from the other, cause. The two possibilities were humorously illustrated years ago by two obesity researchers (see Figure 7–2); there is no reason why they should not both be operating, even in the same person.

The inside-the-body idea is supported by the fact that animal strains do exist that are genetically fat, and they tend to be fat in any environment—that is, no matter what kind or variety of food is offered. The environmental obesity model is supported by experiments with "cafeteria rats." Ordinary rats, fed regular rat chow, are of normal weight (for rats), but if those very same rats are offered free access to a wide variety of tempting, rich, highly palatable foods, they greatly overeat and become obese.[4]

It seems likely that both environmental and hereditary factors influence obesity in humans. The average adult in our society gains about 30 pounds between the ages of 20 and 50, but people in non-Western societies do not. This suggests that all people may have inherited the capacity or tendency to gain weight, but that our surroundings have allowed it to be realized, while conditions in other countries prevent it.

One way to test whether human obesity is inherited is to study identical twins raised in different families, one family fat and the other thin. If genes determine fatness, then both twins will become equally fat or thin. But if the environment is responsible, the twins will resemble their respective families. Another approach is to study adopted children, to see whether they resemble their natural or adoptive parents. Studies of both kinds suggest that the tendency to obesity is inherited, but that the environment is influential in the sense that it can prevent or permit the development of obesity when the potential is there.

Inheritance of the tendency to obesity is probably very complex and governed by many different genes. To complicate the situation further, these genes probably occur with different frequencies in different populations.

A related question is, "Do fat babies become fat adults?" Ten years ago, most nutrition experts might have answered "Yes (probably)." Today, however, the results of several longitudinal studies are available that suggest the answer "Not necessarily; some do, some don't." Clearly, not all fat babies are fated to become fat adults; many grow up elegantly thin. Nor is a thin baby immune to becoming fat later on.

A. The "pull" theory of obesity proposes that a subtle disorder inside the person increases food intake either by affecting signals transmitted to a "satiety center" or by altering the sensitivity of the satiety center to such signals.

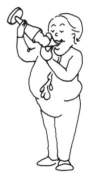

B. The "push" theory proposes that the obese person "force-feeds" himself, overeating for nonphysiological reasons.

FIGURE 7–2 **"Pull" versus "push" theories of obesity.**

SOURCE: Adapted from T. B. Van Itallie and R. G. Campbell, Multidisciplinary approach to the problem of obesity, *Journal of the American Dietetic Association* 61 (1972): 385–390.

A longitudinal study is one in which the subjects are studied over time—for example, in 1960 and again in 1970 and in 1980.

3   The evidence for the set-point theory and its implications for ideal weight are the subject of a separate publication. See note at end of chapter.

4   T. B. Van Itallie, Obesity, the American disease, *Food Technology*, December 1979, pp. 43–47.

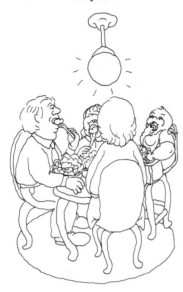

hunger: the physiological need to eat; a negative, unpleasant sensation.

appetite: the desire to eat, which normally accompanies hunger; by itself a pleasant sensation.

satiety (sat-EYE-uh-tee): the feeling of fullness or satisfaction at the end of a meal, which prompts a person to stop eating.

glucostatic theory of hunger regulation: the theory that blood levels of glucose determine when people eat.

gluco = glucose

stasis = staying the same

lipostatic theory: the theory that the body's total fat stores are fixed and that when they are depleted, eating behavior is turned on.

lipo = fat

purinergic theory: the theory that circulating purines regulate eating behavior.

erg = driving force

Still, if obesity is not programmed in by inheritance or by early, critical developmental events, it nonetheless seems to persist from childhood in many instances. Many researchers have the impression that early food habits exert a powerful influence on lifelong tendencies to overeat. Food-centered families encourage such behaviors as overeating at mealtimes, rapid eating, excessive snacking, and eating to meet needs other than hunger. Children readily imitate overeating parents, and their behavior at the table tends to persist outside the home. Obese children have been observed to take more bites of food per interval of time and to chew them less thoroughly than their nonobese schoolmates.

People who eat small but frequent meals may tend to store less fat than those who eat large meals at irregular intervals. Thus families that allow their children to skip meals may be promoting obesity.

Hunger and Appetite Regulation

Whatever sets the stage for excess fat accumulation, the fat is gained because we put food into our mouths. A vast amount of research has been devoted to finding out what stimulates and governs eating behavior. Why do we start to eat? Why do we eat as much as we do? Why do we stop?

An important distinction was made early between hunger, appetite, and satiety. Hunger is said to be physiological—an inborn instinct—whereas appetite is psychological—a learned response to food. The two are not the same. We have all experienced appetite without hunger: "I'm not hungry, but I'd love to have a piece." The too-thin person may often experience the reverse, hunger without appetite: "I know I'm hungry, but I don't feel like eating." Hunger is a negative experience (and we may eat in order to avoid it); appetite is positive. As for satiety, which signals that it is time to stop eating, it vies with hunger and appetite for the distinction of being recognized as the primary regulator of eating behavior. One view holds that eating behavior is turned "on" all the time, except when the satiety signal turns it off. But the exact nature of the satiety signal is not known.

The stomach participates in signaling satiety. Nerves responsive to stretching of the stomach wall fire when the stomach is full, transmitting a message to the brain. Even animals without stomachs get hungry, though, so it is clear that an empty stomach is not the only cue to hunger.

Whether hunger, appetite, or satiety regulates eating behavior (and there are other possibilities discussed below), two questions arise. First, what molecular or other messengers make us feel these sensations? Second, where in the body are they received? Many theories have been put forth to answer the first question. The glucostatic theory of hunger regulation proposes that the blood glucose level determines whether we are hungry or sated; the lipostatic theory states that the size of our fat stores dictates how much we eat; and the purinergic theory proposes that the circulating levels of purines, molecules found in DNA and RNA, govern hunger.[5] Careful measurement of blood levels of glucose show that it does not account for the starting and stopping of eating, however, and glucose

5   A. S. Levine and J. E. Morley, Purinergic regulation of food intake, *Science* 217 (1982): 77–79.

researchers are now pursuing the possibility that exhaustion of liver glycogen may somehow convey the signal "Eat." If fat stores regulate hunger in some way, the messenger they send to the brain to do so has yet to be identified. As for the purinergic theory, its proponents confess that they proposed it "somewhat tongue in cheek"; it is new, and the other three are old, familiar, and frustratingly unsatisfactory to account for what is observed.

The theories just described (at least the first two) have been discussed and researched for several decades. Newer ideas as to what molecules might be the regulators of eating behavior include the endogenous opiates (more about them under "Stressors and Arousal," below) and a variety of hormones. It has long been known that the GI tract produces several hormones that serve to notify the pancreas, the gallbladder, and the intestine that food is present and must be dealt with. A flurry of findings during the early 1980s brought forth many reports that these same hormones, now numbering some 20 or 30, are also produced in the brain after meals. Perhaps, in the brain, they signal satiety.

That brings us to the second question: where in the brain are these messages received (whatever they are)? One brain area stands out as a regulator for food behavior—the hypothalamus—but it is not the only one involved. At one time, it was thought that the front-central hypothalamus was the "satiety center," and that the sides were the "hunger centers." Now, however, that idea has been exposed as an oversimplification. The hypothalamus integrates many kinds of signals received from the rest of the body, including information about the blood's temperature, sodium content, and glucose content. It is certainly important in regulating eating, because damage to the hypothalamus produces derangements in eating behavior and body weight—in some cases causing severe weight loss, in others vast overeating. In the person with a normal hypothalamus, however, eating behavior seems to be a response not to a single signal arriving at some one location in the hypothalamus but to a whole host of signals. Somehow these many inputs become integrated into a "final common path"—the act of eating.

The Behavior of Eating

The word *behavior* has been used many times in this discussion as if it were a simple thing that everybody understands, but the study of behavior offers unique insight into the problem of overeating by viewing it as a conditioned response to a variety of stimuli.

To begin with, certain behavior patterns, whether innate or learned, occur appropriately in response to certain stimuli. For example, dogs salivate in response to the smell of food—but, as everyone knows, they can "learn" (be conditioned) to respond the same way to the sound of a bell. As another example, an appropriate self-care behavior of animals is grooming, which can involve quite a complex pattern of motions—licking, scratching, nibbling the fur—but grooming behavior can suddenly appear unexpectedly at an inappropriate time. In the midst of a hostile confrontation, for example, one contestant will suddenly stop posturing and begin to groom himself intensively as if the wrong switch had been accidentally

Related to body weight regulation, there is also a **thermogenic theory**—but this deals with how energy is spent, not how hunger is regulated. The thermogenic theory suggests that the amount of heat generated in response to food determines how much fat is stored.

thermo = heat

genic = arising from

Among the hormones produced in the brain as well as the GI tract after meals are cholecystokinin (COAL-ee-sis-to-KINE-in), the messenger that communicates the arrival of fat to the gallbladder and pancreas, and calcitonin, a hormone that responds to blood calcium level (see Chapter 10).

hypothalamus (high-po-THALL-uh-mus): a brain center that integrates signals about the blood's temperature, glucose content, and other conditions.

Biologists give the name **displacement activity** to the substitution of one behavior for another under stress.

pushed. It is possible that people also displace one behavior with another when they are threatened. Rather than grooming, the behavior selected may be eating—and if this response occurs often enough, the consequence is obesity.

Displacement may explain some cases of obesity, but even if it doesn't, the view given here is useful. It presents a picture of eating as a sort of package of behavior that can be triggered by any of many different stimuli. Some researchers focus on "external cues" as the triggers; others on "stressors," with connection to the production of endogenous opiates.

External Cues

Some obese people are unconscious eaters. Rather than responding only to internal, visceral hunger cues, they seem to respond helplessly to such external factors as the time of day ("It's time to eat") or the availability, sight, and taste of food.[6] This is the basis of the external cue theory.

external cue theory: the theory that some people eat in response to such external factors as the presence of food or the time of day rather than to such internal factors as hunger.

Of interest in this connection is the report of an experiment in which lean and fat people were housed in a metabolic ward and were offered their meals in monotonous liquid form from a feeding machine. The lean people ate enough to maintain their weight, but the fat people drastically reduced their food intake and lost weight. When kcalories were added to the formula, the lean people adjusted their intake to continue maintaining weight as if they had an internal kcalorie counter. The obese people were unaware of the change, continued drinking the same amount of formula as before, and stopped losing weight.[7] External cues were the only signals the obese people had to go by, and they responded the same way to the same environmental situation, regardless of how many kcalories they were getting.

For the person who responds to external cues, today's environment provides abundant stimuli to promote eating behavior. Restaurants, TV commercials, the display of food in our markets, vending machines in every office building and gas station—all prompt us to eat and drink high-kcalorie foods. There are no "vegetable houses" on our main streets, only steak houses. Kitchen appliances such as the hamburger cooker and the doughnut maker make high-kcalorie foods easy to prepare and thus quickly available.

Stressors and Arousal

Anything that excites or disturbs the equilibrium of an organism can be termed a stressor. The terms *stressor* and *stress response* have specific meanings, as explained in Highlight 5, but they are being used differently by some researchers today to apply to many of the subjects being discussed here. "Stressors" include pain, anxiety, arousal, excitement, even the presence of food.

6   J. F. Schumaker and M. K. Wagner, External-cue responsivity as a function of age at onset of obesity, *Journal of the American Dietetic Association* 70 (1977): 275–279.

7   T. B. Van Itallie and R. G. Campbell, Multidisciplinary approach to the problem of obesity, *Journal of the American Dietetic Association* 61 (1972): 385–390.

The brain seems to respond to many of these stimuli by producing endogenous opiates. They soothe pain and lessen arousal, and they have two effects on energy balance. They enhance appetite for palatable foods, and they reduce activity.[8] Combine these effects with a tendency to be supersensitive to particular stressors anyway, and you are all the more likely to gain weight in response to stress.

The psychiatrist Dr. Hilde Bruch, who has devoted as much attention to the human hunger drive as Freud did to the sex drive, sees other links between eating behavior and human experience. She states that hunger and appetite are understandably mixed up together because both are intimately connected to deep emotional needs. Two factors that she finds most important in this connection are the fear of starvation and "the universal experience in the early life of every individual that food intake requires the cooperation of another person." Feeding behavior is a response not only to hunger or appetite but also to complex human sensations such as "yearning, craving, addiction, or compulsion."[9]

Others agree that food is widely used for nonnutritive purposes, especially in a culture like ours where food is abundant. An emotionally insecure person might eat as a substitute for seeking love or friendship. Eating is less threatening than calling a friend and risking rejection. Often, especially in adolescent girls, eating is used to relieve boredom or to ward off depression. Some obese people respond to anxiety, or in fact to any kind of arousal, by eating. Significantly, however, if they are able to give a name to their aroused condition, thereby gaining a feeling that they have some control over it, they are not as likely to overeat.[10]

Stress may act in another way to promote obesity. The hormones secreted in response to physical stress favor the rapid metabolism of energy stores (glycogen and fat) to fragments such as glucose and fatty acids that can be used to fuel the muscular activity of fight or flight. Under emotional stress the same hormones are secreted and blood concentrations of these same fuels rise. If a person fails to use the fuel in violent physical exertion, the body has no alternative but to turn many of these fragments to fat. If glucose has been used this way, and transferred into fat, then the lowered glucose level or exhausted glycogen will signal hunger, and the person will eat again soon after.[11]

Stress eating may appear in different patterns; some people eat excessively at night, while others characteristically go on an eating binge during an emotional crisis. The overly thin often react oppositely. Stress causes them to reject food and thus become thinner. It is not yet known why these behaviors occur, but clearly investigations of the chemical, hormonal, and neural mechanisms involved in the body's responses to different stimuli hold much promise for a future understanding of eating behavior.

The term **arousal** has been used several times. The general meaning is self-evident, but in the sense in which it is used here, it refers to heightened activity of certain brain centers associated with excitement and anxiety.

8   A. Mandenoff, F. Fumeron, and M. Apfelbaum, Endogenous opiates and energy balance, *Science* 215 (1982): 1536–1538.

9   H. Bruch, Role of the emotions in hunger and appetite, *Annals of the New York Academy of Sciences* 63, part 1 (1955): 68–75.

10   J. Slochower and S. P. Kaplan, Anxiety, perceived control, and eating in obese and normal weight persons, *Appetite* 1 (1980): 75–83.

11   W. H. Griffith, Food as a regulator of metabolism, *American Journal of Clinical Nutrition* 17 (1965): 391–398.

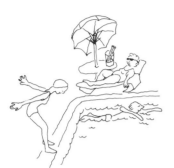

Inactivity

The many possible causes of obesity mentioned so far all relate to the input side of the energy equation. What about output? A person may be obese because he eats too much, but another possibility is that he spends too little energy. It is probable that the most important single contributor to the obesity problem in our country is underactivity. The control of hunger/appetite actually works quite well in active people and only fails when activity falls below a certain minimum level.[12] Obese people under close observation are often seen to eat less than lean people, but they are sometimes so extraordinarily inactive that they still manage to have a kcalorie surplus. One authority has noted that normal people actually swim 35 minutes during "an hour of swimming," whereas obese people swim only 7 minutes during that hour. Most of their time is spent sitting, standing, or lying in the sun.[13]

Individuality

No two people are alike either physically or psychologically, and the causes of obesity may be as varied as the people who are obese. Many causes may contribute to the problem in a single person. Given this complexity, it is obvious that there is no panacea. The top priority should be prevention, but where prevention has failed the treatment of obesity must involve a simultaneous attack on many fronts.

Treatments of Obesity: Poor Choices

The only means of reducing body fat is to shift the energy budget so that energy-in is less than energy-out. This is most effectively done by eating less and exercising more.

This cruel fact is one many of us would like to circumvent. Isn't there an easier way? No, the hard truth is that the only way to lose body fat is to eat fewer kcalories than you spend. Magical alternatives that have been offered time and again over the centuries—ways to "shrink the stomach," to eat "negative kcalories," to "eat all you want and lose weight"—prove to be born of wishful thinking. They are effective only when they directly affect the kcalorie balance. The success of these plans is not in their achievements but in their popularity. They sell easily to susceptible people who want something for nothing, who become enthusiastic practitioners (but only briefly), and who pass on the word to the next person. This type of reaction reflects a human characteristic that for all

12   J. Yudkin, Prevention of obesity, *Royal Society of Health Journal* 81 (1961): 221–224.

13   J. Mayer, as quoted by M. Kernan, Inactivity places burden of obesity on America's youth, *St. Petersburg Times*, August 12, 1973.

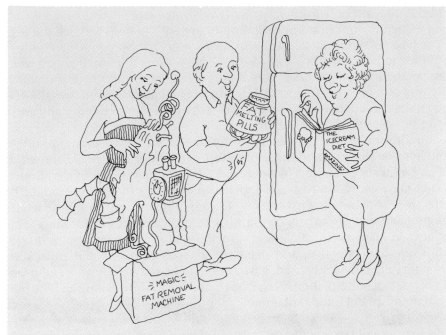

our scientific rationality we have failed to outgrow. We love magic. Many writers of fad diet books and sellers of fraudulent diet pills and formulas use this characteristic to their advantage. Watch out for such frauds. A sign of their presence is the appeal they make to magical thinking and the promise of something for nothing.

Caution

A later section of this chapter addresses appropriate strategies for losing weight, but because rumors of other means fly about, they will first be dispensed with briefly.

Water Pills

For the obese person, the idea that excess weight is due to water accumulation may be an attractive one. Indeed, temporary water retention, seen in many women around the time of the menstrual period, may make a difference of several pounds on the scale. Oral contraceptives may have the same effect. (They may also promote actual fat gain in some women. A woman who has this problem should consult her physician about switching brands.) In cases of severe swelling of the belly, as much as 20 pounds of excess body water may accumulate.

If water retention is a problem, it can be diagnosed by a physician, who will prescribe a diuretic (water pill) and possibly a mild degree of salt restriction. But the obese—that is, overfat—subject has a *smaller* percentage of body water than the person of normal weight. If she takes a self-prescribed diuretic, she has done nothing to solve her fat problem, although she may lose a few pounds on the scale for half a day and suffer from dehydration.

diuretic (dye-you-RET-ic): a drug that promotes water excretion.

dia = through

ure = urine

Diet Pills, Starch Blockers, and Glucomannan

Some doctors prescribe amphetamines ("speed") to help with weight loss. (The best known are dexedrine and benzedrine.) These reduce appetite— but only temporarily. Typically the appetite returns to normal after a week or two, the lost weight (and often more) is regained, and the user then has the problem of trying to get off the drug without gaining more weight. It is generally agreed that these drugs cause a dangerous dependency and are of little or no usefulness in treating obesity.[14]

A multitude of other drugs are presently under investigation: hormones and hormone-like compounds, inhibitors of nutrient absorption, inhibitors of fat synthesis, promoters of fat breakdown, other modifiers of metabolism —in short, every kind of agent that researchers can imagine might be effective in any way against obesity. Tests in humans of any of these would be premature at present, and results in animals are not encouraging. Side effects, in many cases, are severe.[15] In short, at present, no known drug is both safe and effective, and many are hazardous. Even diet pills, long thought safe and widely used, have been shown not to be safe for all users. Two cases of serious illness have been ascribed to the taking of diet pills containing phenylpropanolamine.[16] The only effective appetite-reducing agent to which tolerance does not develop in time is cigarette smoking— and that, of course, entails hazards of its own too numerous to mention.

Among popular drugs recently on the market, starch blockers not long ago attracted a lot of attention. They sounded like a dieter's dream come true—eat your favorite carbohydrate foods and derive no kcalories from them. Unfortunately, although the principle seems sound enough, it doesn't work out in practice. It has been known since 1943 that uncooked wheat and kidney beans contained inhibitors of the starch-digesting enzyme amylase. The inhibitor from kidney beans has been purified and fed to rats, with the result that they excreted some starch and gained less weight than controls. However, tests on humans have shown no inhibition of starch digestion whatsoever.[17]

Neverthless, 100 different starch blocker preparations were on the market as of the end of 1982, and at the peak of their success people were swallowing over a million pills a day. Some people were even stockpiling the pills, expecting that the FDA soon would ban them![18] As expected, FDA has prohibited their being marketed; they have been found to cause nausea, vomiting, diarrhea and stomach pains, and not to block starch digestion.[19]

14   A. C. Sullivan, C. Nauss-Karol, and L. Cheng, Pharmacological treatment, in *Obesity*, ed. M. R. C. Greenwood (New York: Churchill Livingston, 1983), pp. 123–158.

15   Sullivan, Nauss-Karol, and Cheng, 1983.

16   R. D. Swenson, T. A. Golper, and W. M. Bennett, Acute renal failure and rhabdomyolysis after ingestion of phenylpropanolamine-containing diet pills, *Journal of the American Medical Association* 248 (1982): 1216.

17   G. W. Bo-Linn, C. A. Santa Ana, S. G. Morawski, and J. S. Fordtran, Starch blockers—their effect on calorie absorption from a high-starch meal, *New England Journal of Medicine* 307 (1982): 1413–1416.

18   Bo-Linn, Santa Ana, Morawski, and Fordtran, 1982.

19   Starch blockers questioned, *FDA Consumer*, September 1982, p. 2.

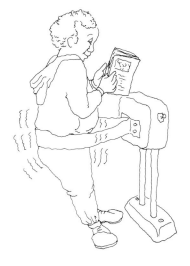

People who don't want to use starch blockers are trying glucomannan, a preparation derived from a vegetable (konjac tuber) used in Japanese cuisine. The Japanese are said to have used konjac for weight control for 1,500 years—but in a controlled experiment reported in 1982, glucomannon was ineffective.[20]

Some day a pill may be developed that is effective against overeating and obesity. None of those described here is a likely candidate. One that may be promising is the opiate antagonist naloxone, which blocks stress-induced eating in animals, and possibly also in humans.[21] Extensive testing will be required to determine whether naloxone can be safely used for this purpose.

Perhaps the most promising anti-obesity agent presently being tested is the artificial fat (sucrose polyester) described in Chapter 3. It remains to be seen, however, whether long-term use will facilitate permanent weight loss or whether, like artificial sweeteners, sucrose polyester will become a mere addition to the diet.

Health Spas

One of the biggest money-making schemes that profits from people's desires to lose weight the easy way is the health spa. The spa can be used to advantage. People who really exercise there reap the expected benefits. But health spas can be extremely costly, and most of their gimmicks offer no real health advantage other than the psychological boost the consumer herself supplies. Hot baths do not speed up the basal metabolic rate so that pounds can be lost in hours. Steam and sauna baths do not melt the fat off the body, although they may dehydrate a person so that his weight on the scales changes dramatically. Machines intended to jiggle parts of the body while the person leans passively on them provide pleasant stimulation but no exercise and so no expenditure of kcalories.

Some people believe there are two kinds of body fat: regular fat and "cellulite." Cellulite is supposed to be a hard and lumpy fat that yields to being "burned up" only if it is first broken up by methods like the massage or the machine typical of the health spa. The notion that there is such a thing as cellulite received wide publicity with the publication of a book by a certain Madame R of Paris, which sold widely during the 1970s. The *Journal of the American Medical Association* has published the statement that cellulite is a hoax.[22]

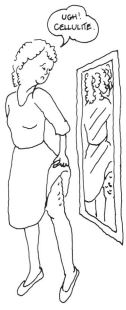

cellulite (SELL-you-leet): supposedly a lumpy form of fat; actually, a fraud. The skin sometimes appears lumpy in fatty areas of the body because strands of connective tissue attach the skin to underlying structures. These points of attachment may pull tight where the fat is thick, making lumps appear between them. The fat itself is not different from fat anywhere else in the body. So, if you lose the fat there, you lose the lumpy appearance.

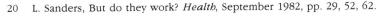

20   L. Sanders, But do they work? *Health*, September 1982, pp. 29, 52, 62.

21   A. S. Levine and J. E. Morley, The shortening pathways to appetite control, *Nutrition Today*, January/February 1983, pp. 6–14.

22   D. C. Fletcher, What is cellulite? (letter to the editor), *Journal of the American Medical Association* 235 (1976): 2773. FDA concurs, in its leaflet: L. Fenner, Cellulite: Hard to budge pudge, HHS publication no. FDA 80–1078 (Washington, D.C.: Government Printing Office), reprinted from *FDA Consumer*, May 1980.

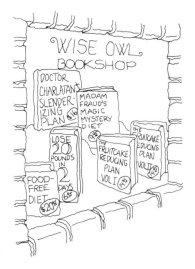

Books like the one by Madame R are often written to make money, and they vary widely in reliability. Madame R probably earns a sizable income from the proceeds of her spa, and her book has enticed many people to spend their money there. She is under no legal obligation to publish only confirmed research findings, and she has not done so. She has published misinformation. Yet she can't be sued unless a customer of hers can prove that her book has caused him bodily harm.

The First Amendment, which guarantees freedom of the press, makes it possible for people like Madame R to express whatever view they like, whether sound, unsound, or dangerous. This freedom is a cornerstone of the U.S. Constitution, and to deny it would be to move hazardously near to totalitarianism. But it puts the burden on consumers to read books skeptically and critically and to use their own judgment in evaluating them. Quacks may hesitate to sell products that are outright frauds, because they can readily be punished for misrepresentation, but they do not hesitate to sell books. Don't let them fool you.

The public is not generally aware that books on nutrition are so unreliable that most professional organizations have had to form committees to combat the misinformation they publish. An example is the Committee on Nutritional Misinformation of the Food and Nutrition Board, National Academy of Sciences/National Research Council. If there is a reward for working on these committees, it is not a dollar reward. On the contrary, it costs time and energy for people to serve on them and money for the organizations to publish their statements.

What about textbooks? Perhaps we, the authors, stand too close to the subject to speak without bias about them, but it is our impression that they sell better if other professors find them factual and reliable. We also stand close enough to know that science professors who write textbooks welcome, even seek, criticism from others in the field. One of the sources of our motivation is plain curiosity, which drives us to keep reading and studying in the hope of getting satisfactory answers to our own and our students' questions.

By far the most reliable of all publications on nutrition are the scientific journals. But even among them there are differences. Those that we rely on most heavily are what we call reputable journals. They are the publications of such organizations as the American Medical Association and the American Dietetic Association, which require confirmed credentials and training for membership. Articles are published in them only after a rigorous review by peers of the authors, people who know how to do research and who are familiar with the area under study. The general reader may find journal articles unspeakably dull, but the motivated reader finds them a gold mine of information. Once the purposes and methods are understood, a journal article can be more exciting than a detective story.

▷ *Caution*

Hormones

Because hormones are powerful body chemicals and many affect fat metabolism, it has long been hoped that a hormone might be found that would promote weight loss. Several have been tried. With testing, all have proven ineffective and often hazardous as well. Thyroid hormone, in particular, causes loss of lean body mass and heart problems except when medically prescribed for the correction of a thyroid deficiency—and thyroid deficiency is very seldom the cause of obesity.

Among the hormones advertised as promoting weight loss is HCG (human chorionic gonadotropin), a hormone extracted from the urine of pregnant women. HCG has legitimate uses; for example, it can stimulate ovulation in a woman who has had difficulty becoming pregnant. But it has no effect on weight loss and does not reduce hunger.[23] A rash of "clinics" run by "doctors" that sprang up on the West Coast during the 1970s advertised tremendous success using HCG in the treatment of obesity. These outfits seem to have had one element in common. They prescribed an extremely rigid low-kcalorie diet, which accounted for their apparent effectiveness. The American Medical Association and the California Medical Association have concluded that the claims made for HCG are groundless and that the side effects are unknown and probably dangerous.[24]

human chorionic gonadotropin (core-ee-ON-ic go-nad-o-TROPE-in), or **HCG**: a hormone extracted from the urine of pregnant women; believed (incorrectly) to promote fat breakdown.

Surgery

Sheer desperation prompts some obese people to request surgery. One operation, bypass surgery, involves removing or disconnecting a portion of the small intestine to reduce absorption. Another involves stapling the stomach to make it smaller.

After a bypass operation, the person can continue overeating but will absorb considerably fewer kcalories. Side effects from this procedure are many and highly undesirable, including liver failure, massive and frequent diarrhea, urinary stones, intestinal infection, and malnutrition. Reports of mortality range from 2 to 10 percent. Still, in the United States, surgery has been reported to be effective more than half the time for treating the massively obese where all other methods have failed. It should probably be attempted only in otherwise healthy and cooperative people under 30 who weigh more than 300 pounds and who have tried everything else.

Gastric stapling is in increasing use in preference to bypass surgery, because it forces the person to eat less rather than causing malabsorption. Still, although the theory is pleasingly simple, stapling involves hazards in practice; stomach tissue is damaged, scars are formed, staples pull loose. The person contemplating surgery should think long and hard before submitting to it.

Fad Diets

Last but not least among poor choices in obesity treatment are the fad diets. The next section shows how to design a healthful weight-loss diet, and Table 7–2 rates presently popular diets according to sound nutrition principles.

23 U.S. Department of Health and Human Services, Food and Drug Administration, *FDA Consumer Memo*, HHS publication no. FDA 77–3035 (Washington, D.C.: Government Printing Office, 1977.)

24 HHS, 1977.

TABLE 7–2 **Weight-Loss Diets Compared**

With a balanced perspective on foods and a sense of what's important in diet planning and what's not, you can evaluate the many different diets people consume. Here's a summary of the questions you might ask. Start with 100 points and subtract if any of these criteria are not met:

1. Does the diet provide a reasonable number of kcalories (enough to maintain weight; not too many; and if a reduction diet, not fewer than 1,200 kcalories for the average-sized person)? If not, give it a **minus 10**.
2. Does it provide enough, but not too much, protein (at least the recommended intake or RDA but not more than twice that much)? If not, **minus 10**.
3. Does it provide enough fat for satiety but not so much fat as to go against current recommendations (say, between 20 and 35 percent of the kcalories from fat)? If not, **minus 10**.
4. Does it provide enough carbohydrate to spare protein and prevent ketosis (100 grams of carbohydrate for the average-sized person)? Is it mostly complex carbohydrate (not more than 20 percent of the kcalories as concentrated sugar)? If no to either, **minus 5**, if no to both, **minus 10**.

DIET NAME AND DESCRIPTION	QUESTION 1: kCALORIES	QUESTION 2: PROTEIN
Dr. Atkin's Diet Revolution. A low-carbohydrate/high-protein diet that allows unlimited protein and fat, but severely limits carbohydrate. See p. 208 for hazards of a very low carbohydrate intake. In addition to these hazards, the diet is high in total fat, saturated fat, and cholesterol. The omission of breads and cereals and the large reduction of fruits, vegetables, and milk characterize the diet. Similar to this diet are *Dr. Atkins' Superenergy Weight Reduction Diet* and others.	Yes	No, excessive protein **MINUS 10**
Banana-Milk Diet (also called the *Johns Hopkins Diet).* Six bananas and three glasses of milk plus vitamin and mineral supplements are eaten daily.	No, provides less than 1,000 kcal **MINUS 10**	No, low protein **MINUS 10**
Beverly Hills Diet. For the first ten days, no food other than specific fruits are allowed. Timing and combining foods are claimed to cause weight loss, with no scientific basis for the claims. Sometimes causes diarrhea and excess gas in the digestive tract because of laxative nature of fruit. Physicians warn that shock, low blood pressure, and perhaps death may result.	No, low kcalories **MINUS 10**	No, low protein **MINUS 10**
Complete Scarsdale Medical Diet plus *Dr. Tarnower's Lifetime Keep-Slim Program.* Touted as a no-hunger, no-pills way to lose 20 pounds in two weeks. The plan is a two-weeks-on, two-weeks-off low-carbohydrate, ample protein diet of about 1,100 kcalories/day.	Yes	No, provides approximately 216% of the protein needs **MINUS 10**
Cambridge Diet. A powdered formula sold directly to the public through "counselors" (nonmedical people who have used the diet) for use three times daily. One day's worth of the formula provides 33 g protein, 40 g carbohydrate, and 3 g fat. Any diet of such low kcaloric value carries serious health hazards (p. 209) in addition to the low-carbohydrate diet effects. The powder is fortified with vitamins and minerals.	No **MINUS 10**	No, low protein **MINUS 10**
Fasting (ZIP Diet). Water is allowed. See pp. 203–208 for a complete discussion of effects.	No **MINUS 10**	No **MINUS 10**
High Roughage Reducing Diet (Dr. David Rubin). The diet requires the addition of two teaspoons of bran to be taken with water at each mealtime. The foods provided by the menus are low-fat, low-kcalorie items, with few milk products. Closely related is *Dr. Siegal's Natural Fiber Permanent Weight-Loss Diet,* but he requires nine "heaping" tablespoons of bran daily. The diarrhea that may result from high bran levels can cause serious medical problems if it continues for several days.	Yes	Yes

5. Does it offer a balanced assortment of vitamins and minerals from whole food sources in all four food groups (see Chapter 1)? If a food group is omitted (for example, meats), is a suitable substitute provided? (There's a discussion of suitable substitutes in Chapter 12). The four food groups are: milk/milk products; meat/fish/poultry/eggs/legumes; fruits/vegetables; grains. For *each* food group omitted and not adequately substituted for, **minus 10 points**.

6. Does it offer variety, in the sense that different foods can be selected each day? If you'd class it as "monotonous," give it a **minus 10**.

7. Does it consist of ordinary foods that are available locally (for example, in the main grocery stores) at the prices people normally pay? Or does the dieter have to buy special, expensive, or unusual foods to adhere to the diet? If you'd class it as "bizarre" or "requiring unusual foods," **minus 10**.

The Self-Study for this chapter (Appendix Q) shows you how to analyze diets not shown here so that you can score them according to this system.

QUESTION 3: FAT	QUESTION 4: CARBOHYDRATE	QUESTION 5: FOOD GROUPS	QUESTION 6: VARIETY	QUESTION 7: ORDINARY FOODS	TOTAL SCORE
No, excessive fat **MINUS 10**	No, inadequate carbohydrate **MINUS 10**	No, three food groups omitted **MINUS 30**	No, monotonous **MINUS 10**	Yes	30 POINTS
No, low fat **MINUS 10**	Yes	No, two food groups omitted **MINUS 20**	No, monotonous **MINUS 10**	Yes	40 POINTS
No, low fat **MINUS 10**	No, no starch **MINUS 10**	No, three food groups omitted **MINUS 30**	No, monotonous; omits most food groups other than fruits **MINUS 10**	No, requires tropical fruits in large quantities and later suggests lobster and steak **MINUS 10**	10 POINTS
No, meat has a high fat percentage **MINUS 10**	No, carbohydrate level is 30% of need **MINUS 5**	No, milk group is omitted **MINUS 10**	Yes	Yes	65 POINTS
No, low fat **MINUS 10**	No, low carbohydrate **MINUS 10**	No food allowed on a regular basis **MINUS 40**	No variety **MINUS 10**	No ordinary food; expensive formula required **MINUS 10**	0 POINTS
No **MINUS 10**	No **MINUS 10**	No **MINUS 40**	No **MINUS 10**	No **MINUS 10**	0 POINTS
Yes	Yes	½ the milk allowance **MINUS 5**	Yes	Requires bran **MINUS 5**	90 POINTS

DIET NAME AND DESCRIPTION	QUESTION 1: kCALORIES	QUESTION 2: PROTEIN
I Love New York Diet (Myerson and Adler).[a] A diet based on a New York City Health Department plan. A strict diet built around the Four Food Group Plan. Alternates periods of 700 kcal/day and 1,500 kcal/day.	Although the average intake is 1,100 kcal/day, periods of severe restriction are included. **MINUS 5**	Yes
Kempner's Rice Diet. The diet was originally developed to treat hypertension and involves eating rice and fruit. Blood pressure can be reduced by the diet, which may be dangerous for normal individuals. Vitamin and mineral supplements are recommended.	Yes	No, low protein **MINUS 10**
Magic Mayo Diet (Grapefruit Diet). Very low carbohydrate, high-fat, high-meat, very-low-kcalorie diet with no milk, doubtless a diet less than magic. One half grapefruit is required before each meal and false claims are made about this food's ability to "burn" kcalories in other foods. The diet is in no way associated with the Mayo Clinic.	No **MINUS 10**	No, too high **MINUS 10**
Nathan Pritikin's Maximum Weight Loss Diet. Originally aimed at curing ills, this diet severely restricts fats, limits proteins to below the recommended levels, and limits dairy products severely. Several levels of kcalories are available from 700 to 1,200 per day.	Choosing any plan except 1,200 kcal will not provide the recommended level. **MINUS 5**	No, too low **MINUS 10**
New Canadian High Energy Diet. Written by a professional dietitian, the diet uses the exchange system to insure adequate nutrient intake, while emphasizing complex carbohydrate foods. High energy comes from nutritional adequacy and from the carbohydrate.	Yes	Yes
Simeons' HCG (Human Chorionic Gonadotrophin) Diet. A. T. W. Simeons claimed that HCG, a hormone obtained from pregnant women's urine, would promote weight loss. Injections accompany a 500 kcal/day diet. For a discussion of hazards associated with very low-kcalorie diets, see p. 209.	No **MINUS 10**	No **MINUS 10**
Dr. Stillman's Quick Inches Off Diet. A high-carbohydrate, low-protein diet that is claimed by the author to allow dieters to reduce fat in desired body areas. No meats or milk products are allowed.	?	No, too low **MINUS 10**
UCLA Diet (California Slim). Developed at the UCLA Center for Health Enhancement, Education, and Research, the diet is basically a low-fat, controlled-portion diet of 1,200 kcal/day that allows unlimited salads and emphasizes fresh vegetables and fruits.	Yes	Yes
Weight Watchers. Emphasis on behavior change and support groups accompany a balanced diet based on the four food groups and exchange system. Processed, prepared dishes such as frozen entrees and other products can be used instead of home prepared foods.	Yes	Yes

Other (name): _____

[a] P. H. Harper, R.D., The I love New York diet (book review), *Journal of Nutrition Education* 14 (1982): 127.

QUESTION 3: FAT	QUESTION 4: CARBOHYDRATE	QUESTION 5: FOOD GROUPS	QUESTION 6: VARIETY	QUESTION 7: ORDINARY FOODS	TOTAL SCORE
Yes	Yes	Yes	Yes	Yes	95 POINTS
No, low fat **MINUS 10**	Yes	No meat or milk allowed **MINUS 20**	No, monotonous **MINUS 10**	Yes	50 POINTS
Yes, but so low in kcalories that total fat is low **MINUS 10**	No, too low **MINUS 10**	No milk or grains allowed **MINUS 20**	No, monotonous **MINUS 10**	Yes	30 POINTS
No, too low **MINUS 10**	Yes	No, meat and milk groups are restricted **MINUS 5** **MINUS 5**	Yes	No, dieters are urged to use "Pritikin breads" and other products **MINUS 10**	55 POINTS
Yes	Yes	Yes	Yes	Yes	100 POINTS
No, too low **MINUS 10**	No **MINUS 10**	No, milk omitted and meat only every other day; no grains **MINUS 25**	Yes, if dieter uses all the latitude allowed	No, the foods may be ordinary, but the shots are hazardous, unnecessary, and very expensive **MINUS 10**	25 POINTS
No **MINUS 10**	Yes	No, meat and milk omitted **MINUS 20**	No, monotonous **MINUS 10**	Yes	50 POINTS
Yes	Yes	Yes	Yes	Yes	100 POINTS
Yes	Yes	Yes	Yes	Yes. Although Weight Watchers produces a line of prepared foods, they are not aggressively marketed and the program is designed to be followed without them.	100 POINTS

The Successful Treatment of Obesity

"The greatest dietary challenge is caloric discipline. Several methods can help but none can substitute for the respect for one's own body and the responsibility for one's health."[25] It seems that the only realistic and sensible way for the obese person to achieve and maintain ideal weight is to cut kcalories, to increase activity, and to maintain this changed lifestyle to the end of his life. This is a tall order. Fewer than a third of those who lose weight manage to keep it off in the long run. To succeed means modifying all the attitudes and behaviors that have contributed to the problem in the first place, sometimes against internal and external pressures that can't be changed. Still, it can be and has been done successfully, as many former "fatties" can attest. A three-pronged approach usually accounts for their success: diet, exercise, and behavior modification.

The way a person loses weight is a highly individual matter. Two weight-loss plans may both be successful and yet have little or nothing in common. To heighten the sense of individuality, the following sections are written in terms of advice to "you." This is not intended to put you under pressure to take it personally but to give you the illusion of listening in on a conversation in which an obese person (with, say, 50 pounds to lose) is being competently counseled by someone familiar with the techniques known to be effective. Notes in the margin highlight the principles involved.

Diet

No particular diet is magical, and no particular food must either be included or avoided. You are the one who will have to live with the diet, so you had better be involved in its planning. Don't think of it as a diet you are going "on"—because then you may be tempted to go "off." The diet can be called successful only if the pounds do not return. Think of it as an eating plan that you will adopt for life. It must consist of foods that you like, that are available to you, and that are within your means.

Dr. Bruce Bistrian, who has worked extensively with weight loss, reports that to be successful, people have to learn not one, but two sets of behaviors: first weight loss, then maintenance of the lost weight. They are separate problems, and of the two, maintenance is the more difficult to manage.[26] If you adopt an "eating plan" rather than "a diet," you can be practicing maintenance behaviors all the time you are losing weight. You will be ready to succeed for the rest of your life, once you arrive at your goal weight.

Choose a kcalorie level you can live with. If you maintain your weight on 2,000 kcalories a day, then you can certainly lose a pound a week on a 1,200-kcalorie diet. A deficit of 500 kcalories a day for seven days is a 3,500-kcalorie deficit—enough to lose a pound of body fat. But make a slightly larger deficit, if the expected weight-loss rate means a lot to you. There is

Diet Counseling Principles

Keep in mind that you will want to maintain your lost weight. Practice the needed behaviors as you go.

Be involved in planning the program.

Adopt a realistic plan.

25   G. B. Gori, The cancer and other connections...if any, *Nutrition Today*, January/February 1981, pp. 14–22.

26   B. R. Bistrian, The medical treatment of obesity (editorial), *Archives of Internal Medicine* 141 (1981): 429–430.

Planning a Weight Loss Diet

When you are maintaining weight on, say, 2,400 kcalories a day, the following balance is suggested:

- 15 percent of kcalories from protein.
- 30 percent or less from fat.
- 55 percent or more from carbohydrate.

These kcalorie amounts translate into grams as follows:

- Protein, 360 kcalories or 90 grams.
- Fat, 720 kcalories or about 80 grams.
- Carbohydrate, 1,320 kcalories or 330 grams.

Now suppose you want to reduce weight. You could cut your kcalorie amount in half, to 1,200 kcalories per day. To avoid getting too hungry, for "satiety value," you must have ample protein and fat. But for health reasons, fat should not supply more than about a third of your kcalories. You must therefore cut the fat grams in half. For maximum satiety, then, leave the protein amount as is. (Protein intake, of course, should never be cut much below the RDA or recommended intake. Nor should it be too high.[27])

So far, you have:

- Protein, 90 grams or 360 kcalories.
- Fat, 40 grams or 360 kcalories.

This gives a total of 720 kcalories and therefore leaves only 480 to be supplied by carbohydrate. This means:

- Carbohydrate, 120 grams or 480 kcalories.

Thus you have cut your carbohydrate down to about a third of what it was formerly. This balance is typical of successful, nutritious weight-loss plans.[28] The protein may be raised and the carbohydrate lowered a little more, so that each of the three energy nutrients delivers about a third of the kcalories. Alternatively, the protein and fat may be slightly lowered and the carbohydrate raised, to deliver 25 percent of the kcalories from protein, 25 from fat, and 50 percent from carbohydrate. A plan based on the latter alternative is shown in Table 7–3. This pattern is one of many that offers a suitable balance.

The design of a weight-reduction diet—with nearly all the protein, about half the fat, and only about a third the carbohydrate of a regular diet—may be responsible for many people's belief that cutting carbohydrate is necessary for weight loss. In a sound weight-loss diet, however, carbohydrate kcalories are not cut below about a third of the total kcalories. To eliminate carbohydrate altogether would be to invite a host of health hazards. Nor should you fast, except under a doctor's supervision.

For the hazards of the low-carbohydrate diet, see Chapter 6.

27   Excess protein can actually cause weight gain, so keep the amount moderate. Dietary protein and body fat distribution, *Nutrition Reviews* 40 (1982): 89–90.

28   A. J. Vergroesen, Physiological effects of dietary linoleic acid, *Nutrition Reviews* 35 (January 1977): 1–5.

TABLE 7–3 **A Sample Balanced Weight-Loss Diet**[a] TH7-1

EXCHANGE ITEM	NUMBER OF EXCHANGES	CARBOHYDRATE (g)	PROTEIN (g)	FAT (g)
Milk (skim)	2	24	16	0
Vegetables	3	15	6	0
Fruit	4	40	0	0
Bread	4	60	8	0
Meat (lean)	7	0	49	21
Fat	3	0	0	15
Total		139 g	79 g	36 g

[a] In this 1,200-kcalorie diet, carbohydrate supplies 556 kcalories, protein 316 kcalories, and fat 324 kcalories. When the dieter returns to a maintenance plan by adding (mostly) carbohydrate foods, the ratio will resemble the recommended 15 percent protein, 30 percent fat, 55 percent carbohydrate.

not much point in hurrying, because you will never go "off" this eating plan (you will only modify it)—and nutritional adequacy can't be achieved on fewer than 1,200 kcalories—1,000 at the very least.

This recommendation is made for the reference woman, 5 feet 4 inches tall, goal weight about 120 pounds. A smaller woman (5 feet tall) with a goal weight of 100 pounds could perhaps go proportionately lower (100 is 5/6 of 120, so she could take 5/6 of the kcalories—900 to 1,000). A larger man (5 feet 10 inches, goal weight 160 pounds) should perhaps not go as low (160/120 of 1,200, or 1,600 kcalories, might be a better kcalorie level for him). No nutrient intake recommendations have been made for non-standard-sized people; the appropriate assumption might be that smaller people need smaller amounts of nutrients and so can get by on fewer kcalories.

Make the diet adequate.

Put diet adequacy high on your list of priorities. This is a way of putting yourself first. "I like me, and I'm going to take good care of me" is the attitude to adopt. This means including low-kcalorie foods that are rich in valuable nutrients—tasty vegetables and fruits; whole-grain breads and cereals; a limited amount of lean protein-rich foods like poultry, fish, and eggs; nutritious meat substitutes like dried beans and peas; and low-fat dairy products such as cottage cheese and skim milk. Within these categories, learn what foods you like and use them often. If you plan resolutely to include a certain number of servings of food from each of these categories each day, you may be so busy making sure you get what you need that you will have little time or appetite left for high-kcalorie or empty-kcalorie foods.

Emphasize high nutrient density.

Individualize. Use foods you like.

Stress do's, not don'ts.

Select carbohydrate foods high in bulk.

The carbohydrate-containing foods you eat should be largely unrefined, complex-carbohydrate foods of low energy density. People who eat these foods in abundance have been observed to spontaneously eat for longer times and to eat 33 percent fewer kcalories than when eating foods of high energy density.[29]

29   K. H. Duncan, J. A. Bacon, and R. L. Weinsier, The effects of high and low energy density diets on satiety, energy intake, and eating time of obese and nonobese subjects, *American Journal of Clinical Nutrition* 37 (1983): 763–767.

At least a fourth of the kcalories in your diet should come from fat, to make your meals more satisfying. At least a third of the fat should be polyunsaturated—soft margarine, salad dressing, mayonnaise, or the like. Read the label to be sure of the kind of fat. And measure your fat with extra caution. A slip of the butterknife adds even more kcalories than a slip of the sugar spoon. And speaking of empty kcalories, omit sugar, pure fat and oil, and alcohol altogether—if you are willing. Let your carbohydrate come from starchy foods and your fat from protein-rich foods. Table 7-3 shows how you can plan a diet using the exchange system.

If at all possible, give up alcohol until you have reached your goal, then add a conservative amount to your daily maintenance plan. If you insist on including alcohol in your diet plan, limit it strictly to no more than 150 kcalories a day (see Table 7–4). Add this amount to the allocated kcalories and reconcile yourself to a slower rate of weight loss. On no account should the empty kcalories of alcohol be allowed to displace the nutritious kcalories of the foods in the plan.

Eat regularly, and if at all possible, eat before you are very hungry. When you do decide to eat, eat the entire meal you have planned for yourself, so that you won't get hungry again too soon. Then don't eat again until the next meal. Save "free" or favorite foods or beverages for the end of the day, in case you are hungry once more.

Eat regular meals, no skipping—at least three a day.

You may have blamed yourself for eating compulsively in the past. That very character trait can work to your advantage. Compulsive people finish what they have started. So diet compulsively. Keep a record of what you have eaten each day for at least a week or two until your habits are beginning to be automatic.

Take a positive view of yourself.

It may seem at first as if you have to spend all your waking hours thinking about and planning your meals. Such a massive effort is always required when a new skill is being learned. (You spent hours practicing writing the alphabet when you were in the first grade.) But after about three weeks, it will be much easier. Your new eating pattern will become a habit. Many sound and helpful books and booklets are available to help you get started, some of which are listed in Appendix J.

Visualize a changed future self.

TABLE 7–4 **Alcoholic Beverages and Mixers—kCalorie Values**

BEVERAGE	AMOUNT (oz)	ENERGY (kcal)
Beer	12	150
Gin, rum, vodka, whiskey (86 proof)	1½	105
Dessert wine	3½	140
Table wine	3½	85
Tonic, ginger ale, other sweetened carbonated waters	8	80
Cola, root beer	8	100
Fruit-flavored soda, Tom Collins mix	8	115
Club soda, diet drinks	8	1

100 proof means 50% alcohol; 86 proof means 43%.
One oz is 28 g, 1½ oz is 42 g.
One g alcohol = 7 kcal.

Take well-spaced weighings to avoid discouragement.

Weigh yourself only once every week or two and always on the same scale, so that you can see clearly the progress you are making. Although 3,500 kcalories roughly equals a pound of body fat, there is no simple relationship between kcalorie balance and weight loss over short intervals. Gains or losses of a pound or more in a matter of days reverse themselves quickly; the smoothed-out average is what is real. Don't expect to lose continuously as fast as you did at first. A sizable water loss is common in the first week, but it will not happen again.

Anticipate a plateau (realistic expectations from the start).

If you see a weight gain and you know you have strictly followed your diet, this probably represents a shift in water weight. Many dieters experience a temporary plateau after about three weeks—not because they are slipping but because they have gained water weight temporarily while they are still losing body fat. The fat you are hoping to lose must be combined with oxygen (oxidized) to make carbon dioxide and water if it is to leave the body. The oxygen you breathe in combines with the carbons of the fat to make carbon dioxide and with the hydrogens to make water. The carbon dioxide will be breathed out quickly, but the water stays in the body for a longer time. The water takes a while to leave the cell, then enters the spaces between the cells, then works its way into the lymph system, and finally enters the bloodstream. Only after the water arrives in the blood will the kidneys "see" it and send it to the bladder for excretion. While water is making its way into the blood, you have a weight gain, because the water weighs more than the fat that was oxidized.[30] If you faithfully follow your diet plan, one day the plateau will break. You can tell from your frequent urination.

Control external cues.

You may find it helpful to control your environment, to avoid situations that prompt you to eat. Begin at the grocery store. Shop when you aren't hungry, and buy only the foods you plan to use on your diet. Purge from your pantry all forbidden items. If you must keep them on hand for other members of your family, surrender them into someone else's possession and ask that they be kept out of your sight as much as possible. Have low-kcalorie foods ready to eat; prepare ahead. To help with your motivation, post reminders on the refrigerator door.

Discourage magical thinking.

It is easier to exclude a food than to exercise away its kcalories. To remind yourself of the reality that kcalories eaten must be spent in physical activity, post Table 7–5 conspicuously in a place where you might otherwise be tempted to eat.

After losing 20 to 30 pounds, expect to reach a stable plateau. Take this as a good sign. It means you have lost so much weight that you now require fewer kcalories to maintain your weight. Take a deep breath (you knew this was coming and you are courageous) and institute a change. Increase your activity, cut your kcalories further, or both.

Use positive reinforcement. Never blame, never punish.

If you slip, don't punish yourself. Positive reinforcement is very effective at changing behavior, but punishment seldom works. If you ate an extra 1,000 kcalories yesterday, don't try to eat 1,000 fewer kcalories today. Just go back to your plan. On the other hand, you can plan ahead and budget for special occasions (two or three times a year). If you want to celebrate your

---

30   Water weight accumulates during fat oxidation because one fatty acid weighing 284 units leaves behind water weighing 324 units, 14 percent more.

TABLE 7-5 **Activity Equivalents of Food kCalorie Values**

FOOD	kCALORIES	ACTIVITY EQUIVALENT TO WORK OFF THE kCALORIES (minutes)		
		Walk[a]	*Jog*[b]	*Wait*[c]
Apple, large	101	19	5	78
Beer, 1 glass	114	22	6	88
Cookie, chocolate chip	51	10	3	39
Ice cream, 1/6 qt.	193	37	10	148
Steak, T-bone	235	45	12	181

SOURCE: Adapted from M. V. Krause and M. A. Hunscher, *Food, Nutrition and Diet Therapy*, 5th ed. (Philadelphia: Saunders, 1972), p. 431.
[a] Energy cost of walking at 3.5 mph, for a 70-kg person, is 5.2 kcal/min.
[b] Energy cost of running is 19.4 kcal/min.
[c] Energy cost of reclining is 1.3 kcal/min.

birthday with cake and ice cream, cut the necessary kcalories from your bread and milk allowance for several days *beforehand*. Again, if you do this compulsively, your weight loss will be as smooth as if you had stayed with the daily plan.

You may have to get tough with yourself if you stop losing weight or start gaining unexpectedly. You may be slipping on portion sizes. Many a dieter has let herself, in time, measure out her meat exchanges too carelessly—and added an extra 500 kcalories to the day's intake. Equally common is the "just this once" substitution of high-fat meat like steak for a fish fillet that was in the plan. You can get away with this only if you scrupulously omit the right amount of fat from other foods the same day. Ask yourself honestly (no one is listening in), "What am I doing wrong?" Very, very seldom does an unpredicted weight plateau of any duration have no explanation in the dieter's own choices.

Identify your problem and correct it. Watch portion sizes.

Learn kcalorie values and fat contents of foods.

Finally, if you stop losing weight or begin to gain, be aware that you may be choosing to do so. Your weight is under your control, and you are entirely free to gain if you wish. You may find you are choosing to take a break, to go into a holding pattern, and to get adjusted before going on. Rather than letting yourself suffer from guilt feelings and feelings of failure, hold your head high and take the attitude, "This is me, and this is the way I am choosing to be right now."

Stress personal responsibility.

Honor the individual.

Exercise

Weight loss is possible without exercise. Obese people often—and understandably—do not enjoy moving their bodies very much. They feel heavy, clumsy, even ridiculous. The choice of whether to exercise regularly, informally, or not at all is a strictly individual matter. But even if you choose not to alter your habits at first, let your mind be open to the possibility that you will want to take up sports, dancing, daily walking, or another activity later on. As the pounds come off, moving your body becomes a pleasure, as does letting others see you move. And the health advantages of regular exercise are well documented. It can truly make you look, feel, and be healthier.

Pave the way for later changes.

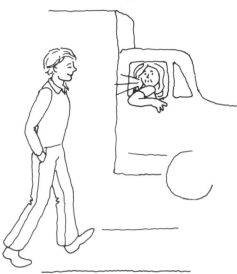

Ultimately, exercise will help with weight loss, too—not so much by virtue of the kcalories spent on the exercise itself as by the changes it brings about in the body. The "lean body" of a chronically inactive person, even a large person, is weak, underdeveloped, and metabolically inactive, whereas a fit lean body is strong, muscular, and metabolically active. Becoming fit means developing a healthier lean body, permitting you to eat more kcalories without gaining weight. As your muscles, heart, and lungs gain in strength, they draw more nourishment from your food, and because you can eat more kcalories, you can give them more nutrients. Now, if you restrict kcalories for a period, your metabolism will not decline but will remain rapid in support of your lean tissues. The person who takes up a regular exercise routine and sticks to it faithfully may start as someone who finds it hard to lose weight, but can become someone for whom it is easier. The fit body, instead of converting kcalories to fat, burns them as fuel.

You must keep in mind that if exercise is to help with weight loss, it must be active exercise—voluntary moving of muscles. Being moved passively, as by a machine at a health spa or by a massage, does not increase kcalorie expenditure. The more muscles you move, the more kcalories you spend. And incidentally, no exercise enables you to "spot reduce." Fat is mobilized by a hormonal mechanism that calls it forth from fat cells all over the body, not from any one particular place. You can change your body shape only to the extent that you can improve your posture and muscle structure.

When you reach your weight plateau and decide to take up regular exercise, let your choice of activity be one that you enjoy—or that you feel you can most likely learn to enjoy in time. What fits best with your self-image? Rapid walking? Bicycling? Running errands for friends? Many people find that after two or three weeks of effort, exercise becomes as habitual as binge eating was before. You can get addicted to it.

Behavior Modification

Everybody is different, but people who overeat are often seen to behave in certain ways at the table, hence the need for behavior modification. Most of us are only faintly aware of our eating behavior and can find it interesting, even funny, to observe ourselves. Notice your own table style and compare it to someone else's. How often do you put down your fork (if at all)? How often do you interrupt your eating to converse with a friend? How fast do you chew your food? Do you always clean your plate? Several good books and other resources (check Appendix J) can help you not only to observe yourself closely but also to set about systematically and effectively retraining yourself to eat like a thin person.

For many people, learning to eat slowly is one of the most important behavior changes to adopt. The satiety signal indicating that you are full is sent after a 20-minute lag. You may eat a great deal more than you need before the signal reaches your brain. Conversely, underweight people need to learn to eat more food within the first 20 minutes of a meal.

Confirming these statements, one research study reported that the eating of soup at either lunch or dinner reduces people's rate of eating. People who eat fewer than 20 kcalories per minute tend to lose more weight. The single suggestion that they include soup in their meals helped the subjects to lose a pound a week.[31]

You may find it helpful to join a group such as TOPS (Take Off Pounds Sensibly), Weight Watchers, or Overeaters Anonymous. A modest expenditure for your own health and well-being is well worth while (but avoid expensive, quick-weight-loss, "magical" ripoffs, of course). Many dieters find it helpful to form their own self-help groups structured around some of the resources already mentioned. Sometimes it also helps to enlist a family member's participation and cooperation.

In case you are a person who eats in response to external cues rather than internally felt hunger, you may need to keep a record for a while of all the circumstances surrounding your eating—the time, the place, the person you are with, the emotions you have at the time, the physical sensations, and other things. An example of such a record is shown in Figure 7–3. Looking back, you can see what stimulates you to eat and learn to control these stimuli. If you find that you are indeed eating for the "wrong" reasons—for example, boredom—this discovery will pave the way for adopting behaviors better suited to your needs than compulsive eating. You can begin to make rules for yourself, like "Never eat when you're bored."

> Keep records to increase your personal investment in success.

If you are especially sensitive to pressure from your family or friends or hosts (can't say no), it will help to have some assertiveness training. Learning not to clean your plate might be one of your first objectives.

From all the behavior changes available to you, you can choose the ones to begin with. Don't try to master them all at once. No one who attempts too many changes at one time is successful. Set your own priorities. Pick one trouble area that you think you can handle, start with that, practice your strategy until it is habitual and automatic. Then you can select another trouble area to work on.

> Use small-step modification.

> FIGURE 7–3 **Food diary**. The record reveals problem areas, the first step towards solving problems.

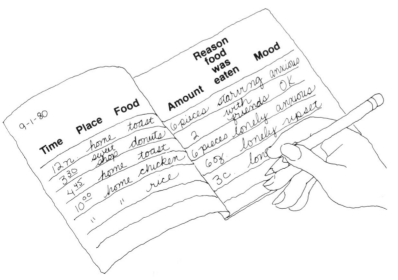

31   H. A. Jordan, L. S. Levitz, K. L. Utgoff, and H. L. Lee, Role of food characteristics in behavioral change and weight loss, *Journal of the American Dietetic Association* 79 (1981): 24–29.

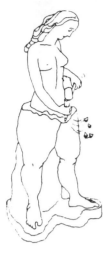

Enjoy your new, emerging self. Inside of every fat person a thin person is struggling to be freed. Get in touch with—reach out your hand to—your thin self, and help that self to feel welcome in the light of day.

Weight Maintenance

As mentioned earlier, it is harder to maintain weight loss than to lose weight. People who lose weight often regain all that they have lost—and more. Paradoxically, those who lose the most (more than 40 pounds) have the greatest tendency to zoom up to levels higher above their starting points than people who have lost less weight.[32] On arriving at the goal weight after months of self-discipline and new habit formation, the victorious weight loser must at all costs avoid "celebrating" by resuming old eating habits. They are gone forever—remember? Membership in an ongoing weight-control organization such as Overeaters Anonymous (OA) or Weight Watchers, and continued participation in regular sports or other physical activity can provide indispensable support for the formerly fat person who wants to remain trim.

The Problem of Underweight

Much of what has been said about obesity applies to underweight as well. No serious hazards accompany mild degrees of underweight. In fact, the only causes of death seen more often in thin people than in normal-weight people are wasting diseases such as tuberculosis and cancer. (Suicide is more common among underweight people, but the underweight is not thought to be a cause. The severe depression probably came first and caused anorexia, or lack of appetite.)

anorexia (an-o-REX-ee-uh): lack of appetite.

an = not

orexis = appetite

The causes of underweight may be as diverse as those of overeating. Hunger, appetite, and satiety irregularities may exist; there may be contributory psychological factors in some cases and metabolic ones in others. Clearly there is a genetic component. Habits learned early in childhood, especially food aversions, may perpetuate themselves. The demand for kcalories to support physical activity and growth often contributes to underweight; an extremely active boy during his adolescent growth spurt may need more than 4,000 kcalories a day to maintain his weight. Such a boy may be too busy to eat. The underweight person states with justification that it is as hard for him to gain a pound as for an obese person to lose one. So much energy may be spent adapting to a higher food intake that as many as 750 to 800 extra kcalories a day may be needed to gain a pound a week.[33]

32   A. J. Stunkard and S. B. Penick, Behavior modification in the treatment of obesity, *Archives of General Psychiatry* 36 (1979): 801–806.

33   Questions doctors ask, *Nutrition and the MD*, June 1978.

Strategies recommended for weight gain center mostly on increasing food intake, using foods that provide as many kcalories in as small a volume as possible so as not to get uncomfortably full. Recommended are nutritious, high-kcalorie milkshakes; liberal servings of meat, bread, and starchy vegetables; and desserts. Whereas the weight loser is urged to select the lowest-kcalorie items from each category, the gainer is encouraged to pick the highest-kcalorie items. Moreover, while the weight loser is taught to eat slowly and fill up on bulky foods at the beginning of a meal, the person who wants to gain weight must do the opposite: eat faster, and eat the higher-kcalorie items first.

An effective strategy for gaining weight is to snack systematically between meals. A 400-kcalorie milkshake at midmorning and a 700-kcalorie sandwich plus shake between lunch and dinner can help to promote a weight-gain rate of 1½ to 2 pounds a week. No known pill, shot, hormone, or surgical procedure will increase weight safely, and a reduction in activity is not recommended unless the condition is so severe as to threaten overall health.

As with weight loss, the person attempting a weight gain must anticipate a plateau. At that time a further increase in food intake will be necessary to continue to gain.

Anorexia Nervosa

An extreme underweight condition is sometimes seen, usually in young women who claim to be exercising self-denial in order to control their weight. They actually go to such an extreme that they become severely undernourished, finally achieving a body weight of 70 pounds or even less. The distinguishing feature of the anorexic, as opposed to other very thin people, is that she intentionally starves herself. Often there is a whole cluster of accompanying "typical" characteristics of the family and the girl's attitudes.

Anorexia nervosa is an extremely serious disorder. It has a higher mortality rate than any other psychiatric disease. From 5 to 20 percent of anorectic persons die. The disorder demands diagnosis and treatment by an experienced doctor or clinic. Even if temporarily reversed by force-feeding, it can reappear. Victims who do not die may suffer permanent brain damage.

A related condition, bulimia, is a disorder in which a person alternately starves herself and binges. Often bulimia escalates into a cycle in which the person eats enormous quantities of food, then vomits, then repeats the process—the so-called binge-purge syndrome. This, too, can lead to serious medical, psychiatric, and social problems.

Anorexia nervosa and bulimia are well known among young people, especially young women. Many older people, however, are former anorexics or bulimics who may retain abnormal eating behaviors and fearful attitudes toward food throughout their adult lives. Chapter 14 presents more details on both conditions and expands on the view that our society promotes these disorders by placing a high value on thinness in the midst of abundant food.

anorexia nervosa (nerv-OH-sah): a severe, self-imposed limitation of food intake sometimes seen in adolescents; a dangerous condition requiring skilled professional treatment.

A person with no appetite is **anorectic** (adjective). A person with anorexia nervosa is an **anorexic** (noun).

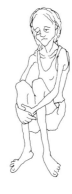

Anorexia nervosa and bulimia: see Chapter 14.

Summing Up

People of the same sex, age, and height may differ in weight due to differing densities of their bones and muscles. The weight compatible with good health depends on the individual. Obesity is sometimes defined as body weight more than 20 percent above desirable weight. More precisely, obesity is excessive body fatness, which can be accurately diagnosed using the fatfold test.

Obesity sometimes arises in early life (juvenile onset) and sometimes later (adult onset); the former is harder to correct and both need to be prevented. Obesity entails a host of health hazards, in addition to social and economic disadvantages. By contrast, underweight (weight more than 10 percent below desirable weight) is associated with an increased risk from wasting diseases. Mortality risk in obesity is not linear and is reversible.

In general there are two schools of thought regarding the cause of obesity. According to one theory, people are locked into a certain weight range by inside-the-body factors such as inherited enzyme or hormonal differences. The other viewpoint suggests that obesity is environmentally determined. It is likely that both hereditary and environmental factors influence obesity in humans. An important contributor to obesity in this country is the extreme physical inactivity that characterizes a sedentary lifestyle.

Since causes of obesity vary widely, treatment must be individualized and multifaceted. Ineffective and dangerous treatments include the use of diuretics, amphetamines, hormones, and—except as a last resort—surgery. The most important step in successful treatment is the adoption of a balanced and nourishing low-kcalorie diet, and fat loss is greatly enhanced by regular exercise and behavior modification. Major criteria for success are a permanent change in eating habits and maintenance of the goal weight over the long term.

Diet can also help the underweight person. Behavior modification and other strategies that facilitate weight loss can be adapted to promote weight gain. But the special case of anorexia nervosa requires skilled professional attention. In all weight-control problems—obesity, underweight, and anorexia—real success is achieved only when new, adaptive eating and coping behaviors have permanently replaced the old ones.

NOTE: Appendix J recommends many interesting readings on obesity and weight control. See "Weight Control."

The Self-Study for this chapter (Appendix Q) shows you how to:

● Plan a diet for weight maintenance, gain, or loss, using the Exchange System.

The *Instructor's Manual* includes two extra transparency-handout masters (TH 7-2; TH7-3) to illustrate diet planning using the exchange system, and a supplementary lecture on the set point theory of body weight regulation.

HIGHLIGHT 7

Sugar Addiction

If Lenny and my parents wouldn't give me any attention, I would turn to someone who could love me back. Food loved me back.

RICHARD SIMMONS

Deep inside there had always been a small child begging for my attention. . . . All I gave her was food. Now I give her love.

EDA LeSHAN

Scene: Your place. *Time of day:* afternoon or evening. You are doing nothing in particular, when suddenly you feel like eating something sweet. You resist, but the feeling gnaws at you. With guilt fluttering in your conscience you head for the cookie jar, telling yourself, "Just one. Maybe two. Not more than three. Or four." But you already have calculated about how many cookies are in the jar. . . . A few minutes later, the jar is empty.

Not all people see themselves in this description, but many more do than you might think—probably the majority of people in our society. We all have a complex and intense relationship with our food that no one completely understands. Many factors are involved, from the body's purely chemical interaction with food to the emotional involvement of the self with food and the consciousness of its social meaning. One factor is the tiny entity, the sugar molecule itself, which provides the sweet taste we all find so attractive.

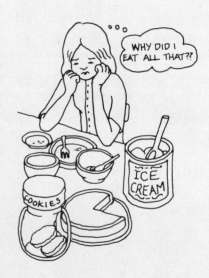

The Sweet Taste

We all love sweets, from the very first time we taste them. The taste for sweetness is innate, as the photos of Figure H7–1 testify—and the reward of eating sweet foods is immediate pleasure. As a result we quickly learn what to eat to obtain the same pleasure again. If you happen to be hungry when you eat sweets, you experience a second reward shortly after the first—the satisfaction of your hunger.

The attractiveness of sugar is therefore very great. In fact, it possesses some of the same characteristics addictive drugs do: opiates, too, are supernormal, immediate, positive reinforcers. If you start eating a sugary food

The reward of sweetness makes sugar an **immediate**, **positive reinforcer**. The pleasure is intense, so sugar is known as a **supernormal** immediate reinforcer. The later satisfaction of hunger is sugar's **postingestive effect**, another reinforcer.

263

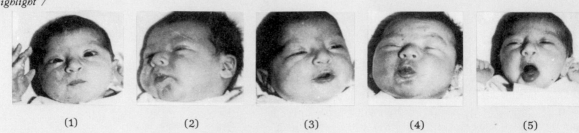

(1)   (2)   (3)   (4)   (5)

FIGURE H7–1 **The innate preference for sugar**. This newborn baby is resting (1), and tasting distilled water (2), sugar (3), something sour (4), and something bitter (5).

SOURCE: Taste-induced facial expressions of neonate infants from the studies of J. E. Steiner in *Taste and Development*, ed. J. M. Weiffenbach, HHS publication no. NIH 77-1068 (Bethesda, Md.: USDHHS, 1977), pp. 173–189, with permission of the author.

when you are very hungry, you are likely to overeat it until your appetite is sated and you are then too full for a nutritious meal. For your health's sake, then, it is important not to eat sugar's empty kcalories when your body's need is for nutritious food, but to save sugary foods for after the meal when hunger has been satisfied, food has provided much of the desired pleasure, and a moderate dose of sugar's sweetness can just serve to top it off. All established, long-lived human societies have developed customary modes of eating that assign a limited place to sugary foods and do not allow them to push aside nutritious foods. In our culture, we refuse to let ourselves or our children eat sugary foods close to mealtimes; we save them for "dessert." But our customary ways of eating family meals are breaking down, and many individuals develop their own eating patterns without models to follow. The results are often unsatisfactory, and sometimes sugary foods assume a far-too-large place in the diet. Some people turn to sugar so often, and with such damaging results, that they feel it is a truly addictive substance.

The Case for Sugar as an Addictive Drug

A member of the board of Overeaters Anonymous, who calls herself a "recovered sucroholic," says she is convinced that refined sugar can be as addictive as alcohol:

> Many of us use sugar like a drug. It is our lover, friend, comforter, and when stress comes into our lives we reach for it automatically. Giving it up is terribly difficult; many people go through withdrawal and get the shakes. For some of us, complete abstinence is the only way out. We cannot be social sugar eaters just the way other people cannot be social drinkers.[1]

Another person who calls himself an "addict" is William Dufty, the author of the bestseller *Sugar Blues*.[2] Dufty describes how he kicked the sugar habit:

> I threw out everything that had sugar in it, cereals and canned fruit, soups and bread.... In about forty-eight hours, I was in total agony, overcome with nausea, with a crashing migraine.... I had it very rough for about twenty-four hours, but the morning after was a revelation. I went to sleep with exhaustion, sweating and tremors. I woke up feeling reborn.[3]

1   J. Pekkanen and M. Falco, Sweet and sour, *Atlantic Monthly*, July 1975, as quoted in The Great American Nutrition Hassle, ed. L. Hofmann (Palo Alto, Calif.: Mayfield, 1978), pp. 252–259.

2   W. Dufty, *Sugar Blues* (New York: Warner Books, 1975).

3   Dufty, 1975, pp. 22–23.

According to *Sugar Blues*, if you allow yourself to get "hooked" on sugar, your addiction can lead to physical and mental ruin. The front cover describes sugar as "the killer in your diet," while the back cover states, "Like opium, morphine and heroin, sugar is an addictive, destructive drug."

Is sugar an addictive drug? Can it lead to total destruction? Can it kill? Some intricate reasoning from experiments with animals sheds some needed light on the question. Figure H7–2 provides the details, in case you are interested. The outcome was that animals can appear addicted to sugar under certain artificial circumstances; but when allowed access to normal food, they will not eat too much sugar. On a poor diet (low-protein), however, their reliance on sugar becomes excessive. *Addiction*, then, is too strong a term to use for their relationship to sugar, but they certainly could be said to indulge in sugar *abuse*.

Furthermore, as has been mentioned in several previous chapters, sugar can displace from the diet foods that contain needed nutrients—to the point where deficiencies of these nutrients arise. Nutrient deficiencies spell malnutrition. While the sugar doesn't cause the malnutrition directly in these cases, it certainly contributes indirectly. The result can be physically and psychologically harmful.

Besides being attractive as a physical reinforcer, sugar offers psychological rewards as well. The next section suggests that the child who wants to rebel against authority can use sugar-eating as one means of doing so.

addiction: a compulsive physiological need for a habit-forming drug such as alcohol or heroin. To express the conviction that some people are addicted to carbohydrate, particularly sugar, the terms **carboholic** and **sucroholic** are in popular use.

Sugar Eating and Puritanism

The sociologist Margaret Mead first observed that the people of our culture take a puritanical attitude towards food. She wrote these three paragraphs in 1943, but what she describes is still true today:

> People feel that they ought to eat correctly, or, less abstractly ("it's wrong to eat too much sweet stuff"), that, in fact, foods that are good for you are not good to eat, and foods that are good to eat are not good for you. So ingrained is this attitude that it may come as a surprise to learn that in many cultures there is no such contrast, that the foods which are thought to make people strong and well are also exclusively the foods which they like to eat, which they boast of eating, and without which they would be most unhappy. . . .

> In the average home, the right food and the wrong food are both placed on the table; the child is rewarded for eating the "right" food and so taught that the right food is undesirable—for parents do not reward children for doing pleasant things. At the same time children are punished by having the "wrong" food taken away from them; here again the lesson is taught to the child that the delicious is an indulgence—for which one is punished or with which one can be rewarded. A dichotomy is set up in the child's mind between those foods which are approved and regarded by adults as undelicious and those foods which are disapproved but recognized as delightful. A permanent conflict situation is established which will pursue that child through his life—each nutritionally desirable choice is made with a sigh or rejected with a sense of guilt; each choice made in terms of sheer pleasure is either accepted with guilt or rejected with a sense of puritanical self-righteousness. Every meal becomes an experience in which an individual must decide between doing right or enjoying himself. Furthermore, as doing right is closely associated with parental supervision, a secondary association is made linking autonomy, adulthood

FIGURE H7-2 **Effects of sugar on animals: Addiction or abuse?**

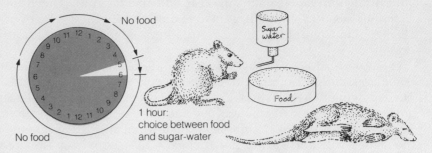

A. One experiment seemed to imply that rats could become addicted to sugar and could kill themselves eating it, even when good food was available to them. This kind of experiment has been widely misinterpreted to signify that if sugar is available to human beings, they will destroy themselves with it, as if it were a drug. What has been overlooked is the feeding schedule on which the rats were maintained. They were allowed access to food for only an hour a day and starved the other 23 hours. During the hour, they were given a choice between nutritious food and pure sugar (in water). They chose the pure sugar every time, and starved themselves to death. Subsequent experiments showed that it wasn't just the sweet taste but also the postingestive effects of the sugar that reinforced the rats' choice. In other words, when they were starving, the rats consistently made the choice that most promptly gave them the feeling that their hunger was being relieved. Sugar is quickly absorbed and detected by the nervous system, so it wins the race.

SOURCE: From L. W. Hamilton, Starvation induced by sucrose ingestion in the rat, *Journal of Comparative and Physiological Psychology* 77 (1971): 59–69.

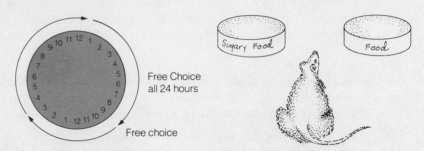

B. Maintaining animals on such a schedule and allowing them to eat only when they are starving is different from allowing them free access at all times to a diet presenting a choice between sugary and more nutritious foods. With free access and free choice between sugar and other foods, rats eat enough nutritious food to stay healthy and grow, although they also eat considerable sugar. Thus, sugar alone doesn't kill rats. Rather, it is sugar administered on a weird schedule to starving rats that has this effect.

SOURCE: From S. Muto, Dietary sweet: Exposure and preference among Japanese children and in laboratory rats, in *Taste and Development, the Genesis of Sweet Preference*, ed. J. M. Weiffenbach (Washington, D.C.: Government Printing Office, 1977), pp. 249–265.

and masculinity with eating what one likes instead of what mother approved of.

This situation is an eternally self-defeating one, for as long as materials for making the wrong food choice are as accessible as those for making the right, many individuals will make the wrong choice, fairly often...we will never have a population which eats, unquestioningly, food based on the best nutritional science which we have. For each generation it has to be done all over again. The mother who has, with a great moral effort, learned to drink milk herself, does not merely place a pitcherful of milk on the table and let her children follow her example as she pours it out—although this is the simple method—but she, because of the conflict within her own personality, will

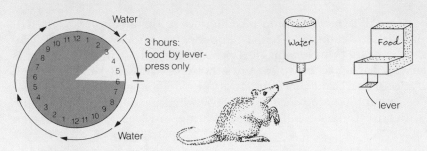

C. An unnatural schedule can even induce a rat to overuse a harmless substance like water. An underfed rat, given access to food only 3 hours a day and made to press a lever for it, will drink about half his body weight in water during that 3-hour period, even though he has plenty of water for the other 21 hours as well. The experimenter who discovered this behavior in rats named it "water abuse." On returning to a normal schedule, the rats drank water normally again.

   Alcohol abuse can be made to appear in rats by a similar manipulation of feeding time (rats normally refuse to become even interested in alcohol, much less abusers of it). After consuming large amounts of alcohol under these artificial conditions for many days, the rats are "hooked" (addicted). They react differently to alcohol now. Even when returned to a normal schedule, they continue to drink alcohol as long as they have access to it.

   A rat that is hooked on alcohol by the weird-schedule technique and then given the choice between alcohol and a sugar solution (still on the weird schedule), will gradually shift his preference to the sugar solution. This experiment has been widely misinterpreted to mean that "sugar is even more addicting than alcohol," but sugar addiction is not what is seen here. It is sugar-preference-on-a-weird-schedule. In the words of the experimenter, "It takes unusual environmental arrangements for [water and sugar] to be abused and to become hazards to health, while ethanol and other agents with addiction liability produce their effects much more directly.... Further, addictive agents are viewed as instituting biochemical changes in the central nervous system which, functioning in a vicious circle, maintain a craving for the particular agent." Sugar preference in animals to the point of extreme self-harm does not persist when they are back on a normal schedule. Sweet abuse, then, is not addiction.

SOURCE: From J. L. Falk, Sweet abuse and the addiction model, in *Taste and Development*, 1977, pp. 374–386, quote from p. 383.

---

argue, threaten, cajole, bribe and punish her children to make them "drink their milk."[4]

   The puritanically raised child who decides to break the rules is likely to think in these terms: "This is for you, mother (the spinach), and this is for me (ice cream)." Part of the pleasure comes from the feeling of getting away with eating a forbidden food.

   Combine this reward with the others already mentioned and you have an impressive combination. First there is the pleasure of rebelling itself; then, the immediate, intense pleasure of the sweet taste; then, especially if the person is hungry (perhaps dieting), the intense postingestive satisfaction.

   No wonder sugar is seen as so all-powerful by those who hate and fear it. Precisely because they hate and fear it, it is especially powerful. Perhaps those who fear it less are less under its spell. How can we help ourselves and our children not to fear sugar but to put it in its proper place in the diet?

   If sugar is a poison, then what to do is to avoid it like—well, like poison. This notion may contribute to the beliefs that are so destructive to the binger, or person with bulimia. The bulimic thinks, "If I touch this forbid-

bulimia, bulimarexia: binge eating (see Chapter 14).

4   M. Mead, Dietary patterns and food habits, *Journal of the American Dietetic Association* 19 (1943): 1–5.

den food, it will overwhelm me. Like alcohol to the alcoholic, sugar will cause me to lose control." Then he touches it—and loses control. The substance appears to have a magical power. Not only that, the bulimic is also starving, having accepted society's thinness standard. The hunger felt in starvation is real and powerful. It is no coincidence that many binge episodes in bulimics are preceded by strict dieting and that many unsuccessful dieters (bingers) believe that dieting involves severely limiting food intake.[5]

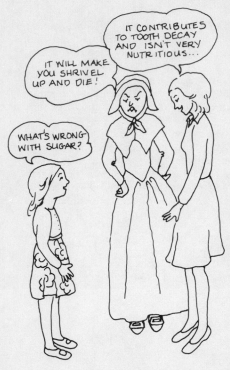

FIGURE H7–3 **The puritanical versus the truthful view of sugar.**

How Can We Cope with Sugar?

If we gave sugar less status in our foodways, perhaps it would have less power. We should demote it from a powerful, evil substance to a harmless but unneeded substance, one for which there is only a little room in a kcalorie-restricted diet. If binge eaters could see it this way, they might then bend their efforts towards figuring out where and how to use their restricted sugar allowance most effectively to enhance their eating pleasure. They could learn to think positively—not "I must never eat those foods," but rather "I must eat *these* (nutritious) foods and I may add a little sweetness where it pleases me the most." A cookie eaten at the end of a nourishing meal has considerably less power to precipitate a binge than a cookie eaten after 24 hours without food.

Both the binge eater and the child, in fact, need to learn the same things to facilitate their developing healthful eating habits. In the conversation of Figure H7–3, the person giving truthful answers (TA) is being much more helpful than the person giving puritanical answers (PA).

One teacher of children put it this way: "Be sure they eat the foods they need first. Children live for the present. *You* protect their future." But this strategy by itself does nothing to prepare children for the time when they themselves will make the choices. It needs two words added: "Be sure they *learn to* eat the foods they need first." Our task as nutrition educators is not to teach children (ourselves included) *not* to eat foods. Our task is to teach them *how* to choose foods wisely.

NOTE: Appendix J recommends an additional reading on binge-eating, and provides the address of Overeaters Anonymous, an organization especially for compulsive overeaters. See "Weight Control."

Two optional lectures in the *Instructor's Manual* are devoted to Nutrition and Behavior. The second one focuses on the effects of nutrient deficiencies caused by sugar's (or other empty kcalories') displacement of nutrients.

5   G. R. Leon, L. Roth, and M. I. Hewitt, Eating patterns, satiety and self-control behavior in obese persons during weight reduction, *Journal of Obesity and Bariatric Medicine* 6 (1977): 172–181.

CHAPTER 8

The Water-Soluble Vitamins: B Vitamins and Vitamin C

CONTENTS

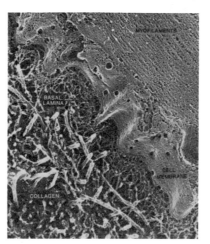

Collagen—made with the help of vitamin C—is the body's major connective material. Here, strands of collagen lie tangled near a muscle fiber membrane disrupted by freezing and chemical etching.

Tests were initiated by the results of my studies on a chicken disease similar to beriberi. I was able to establish that that disease is caused by feeding certain grains, especially rice. Only polished rice (raw or boiled) proved to be harmful; unpolished rice was tolerated quite well by the chickens. . . . From these experiments I drew the conclusion that the cuticles probably contain a substance or substances which neutralize the harmful influence of the starchy nutriment. . . .

C. EIJKMAN, 1897

A television commercial broadcast widely some years ago shows a middle-aged businessman shuffling weakly out of his bedroom with his bathrobe slung loosely around his sagging paunch. He sinks into his chair at the breakfast table and wearily lifts the morning paper to screen his face from the daylight and from his bright-eyed, energetic wife. As she places his coffee cup before him, she observes sympathetically, "Sweetie, you look so tired. Did you forget to take your vitamin pill today?" (Fadeout, with the voice of the announcer saying, "Are you tired in the morning? Do you hate to face the day? What you need is Brand A Vitamins.") Repeat: The same man, transformed, trim and bouncy, waltzes into the breakfast nook, pirouettes gaily around the table, kisses his wife affectionately, takes two hasty sips of coffee, and strides humming out the door. She turns cheerfully to the camera and smiles, "Brand A Vitamins have done wonders for my Harry."

True? No. Poor Harry. If he tries to live on only coffee and vitamins, he will remain a wreck. Like all the organic nutrients found in foods, the B vitamins are

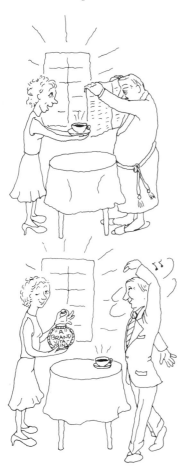

composed of carbon, hydrogen, oxygen, and other atoms linked together by chemical bonds. Of course, these bonds contain energy, but that energy cannot be used to fuel activities or to do the body's work. The energy Harry needs comes from carbohydrate, fat, and protein; the vitamins will only help him burn the fuel if he has the fuel to burn.

It is true, however, that without B vitamins you would certainly feel tired. You would lack energy. Why is this? Some of the B vitamins serve as helpers to the enzymes that release energy from the three energy nutrients—carbohydrate, fat, and protein. The B vitamins stand alongside the metabolic pathways and help to keep the disassembly lines moving. In an industrial plant they would be called expediters. Some of them help manufacture the red blood cells, which carry oxygen to the body's tissues; the oxygen must be present for oxidation and energy release to occur.

So long as B vitamins are present, their presence is not felt. Only when they are missing does their absence manifest itself as a lack of energy. A child who learned this defined vitamins on a test as "what if you don't eat you get sick." The definition is one of the most insightful we've seen.

Water-Soluble Vitamins

The B vitamins and vitamin C are entitled to individual attention, but the whole array of them is presented here first to show you the "forest" in which they are the trees. They come together in foods, they work together in the body, and there is much to be learned from viewing them as a group.

First of all, together with vitamin C, the B vitamins form a natural group of nutrients known as the water-soluble vitamins. They are present in the watery compartment of foods, and they distribute into the water-filled compartments of the body. They can easily be excreted in the urine if their blood concentration rises too high—in contrast to the fat-soluble vitamins, which tend to be hidden away in storage places. As a consequence, the water-soluble vitamins are less likely to reach toxic levels (a plus), but are also more easily depleted (a minus), than the fat-soluble vitamins.

The B vitamin riboflavin is a yellow compound so bright that it is easy to see in a water solution. Since excesses of the B vitamins are excreted, bright yellow urine may signify the presence of this vitamin. If you are in the habit of taking a multivitamin supplement "to avoid deficiencies" and your diet is otherwise adequate in riboflavin, you may notice this effect.

Some vitamin supplements are inexpensive, but others are absurdly costly. Most people don't need them. As you read on, you may discover that it is easy to make your diet adequate by eating nutritious foods alone. If you do consume an adequate diet, the following statement may apply to you. Overdosing with B vitamins will do nothing for you but increase the dollar value of your urine.

Caution

In summary, the water-soluble vitamins are:

- Carried in the bloodstream.
- Excreted in urine.
- Needed in frequent small doses.
- Unlikely to be toxic.

The B Vitamins: Coenzymes

Each of the B vitamins is part of an enzyme helper known as a coenzyme. A coenzyme is a small nonprotein molecule that associates closely with an enzyme. Some coenzymes form part of the enzyme structure, in which case they are known as prosthetic groups; others are associated more loosely with the enzyme. Some participate in the reaction being performed and are chemically altered in the process, but they are always regenerated sooner or later. Others are unaltered but form part of the active site of the enzyme. Thus although there are differences in details, one thing is true of all. Without the coenzymes, the enzymes cannot function.

The consequences of a failure of metabolic enzymes can be catastrophic, as you will realize if you restudy the central pathway of metabolism by which glucose is broken down (Figure 8–1). The nicknames for some of the coenzymes that keep the processes going (NAD^+, TPP, FAD, and CoA) are listed beside the reactions they facilitate; the vitamin names are given in Table 8–1.

Look at the first step. Some of the enzymes involved in the breakdown of glucose to pyruvate require the coenzyme NAD^+. Part of this molecule is a

coenzyme (co-EN-zime): small molecule that works with an enzyme to promote the enzyme's activity. Many coenzymes have B vitamins as part of their structure.

co = with

prosthetic (pros-THET-ic) **group**: a coenzyme that is physically part of (attached to) its enzyme.

prosth = in addition to

active site: that part of the enzyme surface on which the reaction takes place.

To review the structures and functions of enzymes, see Chapter 4.

TABLE 8–1 **B–Vitamin Terminology**
Many of the vitamins have both names and numbers, a mixture of terminologies that confuses newcomers to the study of nutrition. As of 1979, a single set of names for the vitamins had been agreed on and was published, and those names are used in this book.[a] Still, to read the many worthwhile writings published prior to 1979, you have to be aware of the alternative names:

CORRECT NAME	OTHER NAMES COMMONLY USED[b]
Thiamin	Vitamin B_1
Riboflavin	Vitamin B_2
Niacin	Nicotinic acid, nicotinamide, niacinamide
Vitamin B_6	Pyridoxine, pyridoxal, pyridoxamine
Folacin	Folate, folic acid
Vitamin B_{12}	Cobalamin
Pantothenic acid	(None)
Biotin	(None)

[a] The vitamin names used here are those agreed on and published by the Committee on Nomenclature of the American Institute of Nutrition, in Nomenclature policy: Generic descriptors and trivial names for vitamins and related compounds, *Journal of Nutrition* 112 (1982): 7–14.
[b] Also see Appendix C.

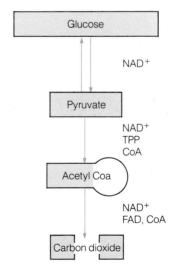

FIGURE 8–1 **The central pathway of metabolism with the coenzymes that facilitate its reactions.**

niacin (NIGH-uh-sin): a B vitamin. Niacin can be eaten preformed or can be made in the body from tryptophan, one of the amino acids (see p. 283).

A compound that can be converted to a nutrient in the body is known as a **precursor** of that nutrient. Thus tryptophan is a precursor of niacin.

thiamin (THIGH-uh-min): a B vitamin.

pantothenic (PAN-to-THEN-ic) **acid**: a B vitamin.

riboflavin (RIBE-o-flay-vin): a B vitamin.

The four B vitamins named above are parts of coenzymes in the glucose-to-energy pathway. Some of these coenzymes have other functions too (see Appendix C for names and structures).

structure the body cannot make. Hence it must be obtained from the diet; it is an essential nutrient (Chapter 1). This essential part is the B vitamin niacin. The way niacin works is shown in Figure 8–2.

In other words, to take glucose apart the cells must have certain enzymes. For the enzymes to work, they must have the coenzyme NAD^+. To make NAD^+, the cells must be supplied with niacin (or a closely related compound they can alter to make niacin). The rest of the coenzyme they can make without outside help.

The next step in glucose catabolism is the breakdown of pyruvate to acetyl CoA. The enzymes involved in this step require NAD^+ plus another coenzyme, TPP. The cells can manufacture the TPP they need from thiamin, but thiamin is a compound they cannot synthesize; so it must be supplied in the diet. Thiamin is the vitamin part.

Another coenzyme needed for this step is coenzyme A, or CoA for short. As you have probably guessed, the cells can make CoA except for an essential part of it that must be obtained in the diet. This essential part—the vitamin part—is pantothenic acid.

The next step in glucose catabolism is breakdown of acetyl CoA to carbon dioxide. The enzymes involved in this process require two of the three coenzymes mentioned above—NAD^+ and coenzyme A—and, in addition, another—FAD. Again, FAD is synthesized in the body, but part of its structure, the vitamin riboflavin, must be obtained in the diet.

Now suppose the body's cells lack one of these B vitamins—niacin, for example. Without niacin, the cells cannot make NAD^+. Without NAD^+, the

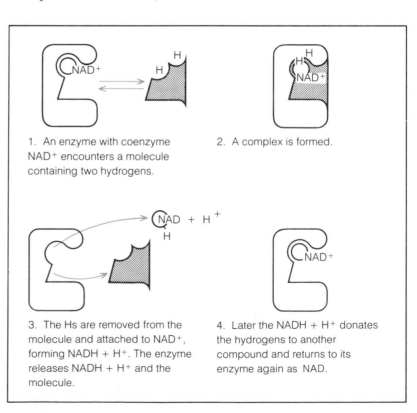

1. An enzyme with coenzyme NAD^+ encounters a molecule containing two hydrogens.

2. A complex is formed.

3. The Hs are removed from the molecule and attached to NAD^+, forming $NADH + H^+$. The enzyme releases $NADH + H^+$ and the molecule.

4. Later the $NADH + H^+$ donates the hydrogens to another compound and returns to its enzyme again as NAD.

FIGURE 8–2 **Coenzyme action.** Each coenzyme is specialized for certain kinds of chemical reactions. NAD^+ (containing niacin), for example, can accept hydrogen atoms removed from other compounds and can lose them to compounds that ultimately pass them to oxygen. In many steps during the catabolism of glucose, hydrogens are removed and NAD^+ participates this way. A model of the way NAD^+ works with an enzyme to remove hydrogens is shown here. TH8-1

enzymes involved in every step of the glucose-to-energy pathway will fail to function. Since it is from these steps that energy is made available for all the body's activities, everything will begin to grind to a halt. This is no exaggeration. The symptoms of niacin deficiency are the devastating "four Ds": dermatitis, which reflects a failure of the skin to maintain itself; dementia (insanity), a failure of the nervous system; diarrhea, a failure of digestion and absorption; and death. These are only the most obvious, observable symptoms. Every organ in the body, being dependent on the energy pathways, is profoundly affected by niacin deficiency. As you can see, niacin is a little like the horseshoe nail for want of which a war was lost.

For want of a nail, a horseshoe was lost.
For want of a horseshoe, a horse was lost.
For want of a horse, a soldier was lost.
For want of a soldier, a battle was lost.
For want of a battle, the war was lost,
And all for the want of a horseshoe nail!

MOTHER GOOSE

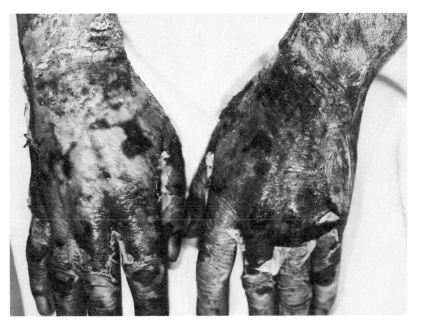

The dermatitis of pellagra. The skin darkens and flakes away as if it were sunburned. In kwashiorkor there is also a "flaky paint" dermatitis but the two are easily distinguishable. The dermatitis of pellagra is bilateral and symmetrical, and occurs only on those parts of the body exposed to the sun.

Source: Courtesy of Dr. Samuel Dreizen, D.D.S., M.D.

The complete breakdown of amino acids and fat, as well as that of glucose, depends on the coenzymes just described. You may remember that a major product of the breakdown of amino acids and fat is acetyl CoA and that this product is processed in exactly the same way as the acetyl CoA from glucose. Thus the release of energy from all foods depends on the same vitamins.

Not only the breakdown (catabolism) but also the building (anabolism) of compounds in the body requires coenzymes. For example, one step in the manufacture of a nonessential amino acid is the step in which the nitrogen-containing amino group is attached to a carbon skeleton—a process called transamination. Enzymes performing this function require a coenzyme made from the essential nutrient vitamin B_6.

Two other B vitamins—folacin and vitamin B_{12}—are together involved in building the units that form part of DNA. Folacin aids directly in the synthesis of one of the purines, and vitamin B_{12} indirectly in the synthesis of the folacin coenzymes. Whenever a cell divides, it must make a whole new copy of its DNA; thus these two coenzymes are necessary for making all new cells. They also serve other functions. (Folacin, for example, is a

transamination: the transfer of an amino group from one compound to another, as when nonessential amino acids are manufactured in the body.

vitamin B_6: a family of compounds—pyridoxine, pyridoxal, pyridoxamine—that act as part of the coenzymes in amino acid metabolism. The step that begins the breakdown of stored glycogen to glucose also depends on these coenzymes; and a crucial step in the making of the iron-containing portion of hemoglobin for red blood cells does, too.

folacin (FOLL-uh-sin): a B vitamin that acts as part of the coenzyme in the manufacture of new DNA and new cells; it transfers single-carbon groups.

vitamin B$_{12}$: a vitamin whose coenzyme helps make the active forms of folacin.

biotin (BY-o-tin): a B vitamin; a coenzyme involved in shifting single-carbon (CO_2) groups, necessary for fat synthesis and other metabolic reactions. The TCA cycle intermediate produced with the help of biotin is oxaloacetate (see Appendix C).

coenzyme in the reaction shown on p. 130, in which one amino acid is converted to another by removing a CH_2OH group.)

Finally, biotin, another B vitamin, serves as a helper in many reactions in which single-carbon groups are shifted from one structure to another. Many reactions involve this activity, including those of fatty acid synthesis and the reaction that converts pyruvate into a compound used in the TCA cycle.

In summary, these eight B vitamins play many specific roles in helping the enzymes to perform thousands of different molecular conversions in the body. They are active in carbohydrate, fat, and protein metabolism and in the making of DNA and thus new cells. They are found in every cell and must be present continuously for the cells to function as they should. It must now be abundantly clear why poor Harry needs the B vitamins to make him feel well, even though without food they do nothing for him. No matter what he eats, he needs B vitamins to help him process it.

B Vitamins and Prescription Drugs

Like the coenzymes, drugs are small but potent molecules, and they often work in the body by altering the actions of its proteins. However, although the body is equipped by eons of evolutionary time to accommodate the vitamins and to use them appropriately, it has had no such long experience with drugs. Most of the prescription drugs are new compounds, synthesized in the laboratory, which affect body functions in ways that may be useful to fight disease. But many drugs have side effects. While they work in one area to counteract the disease process or to correct an abnormality, they may also work in other areas to interfere with normal body processes. Sometimes they interfere with the action of the B vitamins.

For example, a potent drug that inhibits the growth of the tuberculosis bacterium, nicknamed INH, has saved countless lives because of its efficacy against tuberculosis. But INH is also a vitamin B$_6$ antagonist; it binds and inactivates the vitamin, inducing a deficiency. Whenever INH is used to treat tuberculosis, supplements of vitamin B$_6$ must be given to protect the patient from deficiency.

Another example is aspirin, the most frequently prescribed pain reliever. It is very effective against pain, but it also interferes with the binding of folacin to carrier proteins and increases folacin excretion.[1] (It has an impact on vitamin C and iron nutrition, too.) This doesn't imply that aspirin should never be used but rather that people using drugs and physicians prescribing them should be aware that they may affect nutrition.

It is important for someone new to the study of nutrition to be reminded at this point that this is a book about healthy people. The nutrient needs of people who are ill or who are using large amounts of drugs—includ-

1   D. R. Roe, *Drug-Induced Nutritional Deficiencies* (Westport, Conn.: Avi, 1976), pp. 150–151.

ing nonprescription drugs like alcohol—are not discussed here. Nor are the special needs of people with inborn genetic defects that may greatly increase their individual needs for certain nutrients. The statements about recommended intakes and about foods that provide the recommended amounts apply to most people, normally, but there are exceptions that are outside our province. References in Appendix J point the way toward learning more about nutrition in disease, and Highlight 8A is devoted to the special effects of alcohol.

Caution

B-Vitamin Deficiency

Removing a number of "horseshoe nails" can have such disastrous and far-reaching effects that it is difficult to imagine or predict the results. Oddly enough, although we know a great deal about their individual molecular functions, we are unable to say precisely why a deficiency of one B vitamin produces the disease beriberi whereas the deficiency of another produces pellagra. We do know, however, that with the deficiency of any B vitamin, many body systems become deranged, and similar symptoms may appear.

A deficiency of any one B vitamin seldom shows up in isolation. After all, people do not eat nutrients singly; they eat foods, which contain mixtures of nutrients. If a major class of foods is missing from the diet, the nutrients contributed by that class of foods will all be lacking to varying extents. In only two cases, dietary deficiencies associated with single B vitamins have been observed on a large scale in human populations, and diseases have been named for them. One of these diseases, beriberi, was first observed in the Far East when the custom of polishing rice became widespread. Rice contributed 80 percent of the kcalories consumed by the people of those areas, and rice hulls were their principal source of thiamin. When the hulls were removed, beriberi spread like wildfire. It was believed to be an epidemic, and medical researchers wasted much time and energy seeking a microbial cause before they realized that the problem was not what was present in the food but what was absent from it.

The other disease, pellagra, became widespread in the U.S. South in the early part of this century, in people who subsisted on a low-protein diet whose staple grain was corn. This diet was unusual in that it supplied neither enough niacin nor enough of its amino acid precursor tryptophan to make up the deficiency.

Even in these cases, the deficiencies were not pure. When foods were provided containing the one vitamin known to be needed, the other vitamins that may have been in short supply came as part of the package.

beriberi: the thiamin-deficiency disease; pointed the way to discovery of the first vitamin, thiamin.

pellagra (pell-AY-gra): the niacin-deficiency disease.

pellis = skin

agra = seizure

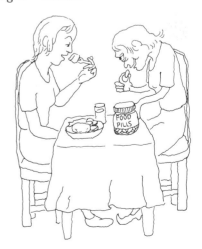

Significantly, these deficiency diseases were eliminated by supplying foods—not pills. Although both diseases were attributed to single B vitamins, both were likely to have been B-complex deficiencies in which

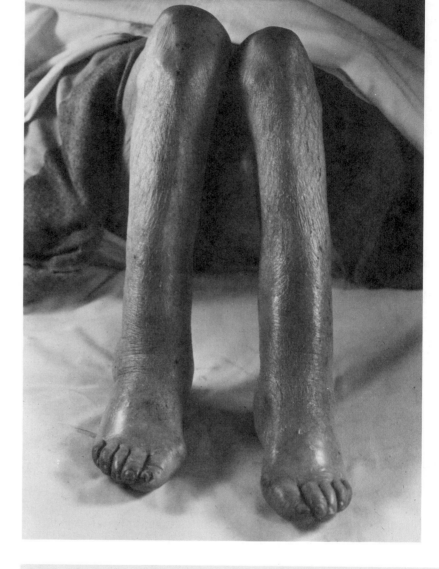

The edema of beriberi. Thiamin deficiency also sometimes produces a "dry" beriberi, without edema, for reasons not well understood. Another marked symptom is inability to walk, manifested by collapse of the lower limbs when the person tries to stand.

Source: Courtesy of Dr. Samuel Dreizen, D.D.S., M.D.

one vitamin stood out above the rest. Giving one B vitamin to people with a B-complex deficiency may make latent deficiencies of other B vitamins become overt.

Pushers of vitamin pills make much of the fact that vitamins are vital and indispensable to life. But life went on long before there were vitamin pills, and human beings thrived on exactly the same kinds of foods as are available now. If your diet lacks a vitamin, the natural solution is to adjust it so that food supplies that vitamin.

Pushers of so-called natural vitamins would have you believe that their pills are the best of all because they are purified from real foods rather than synthesized in a laboratory. But if you think back on the course of human evolution, you may conclude that it really is not natural to take any kind of pills at all. In reality, the finest, most complete vitamin "supplements" available are meat, fish, poultry, eggs, legumes, nuts, milk and milk products, vegetables, fruits, and grain products. Any time you hear the suggestion made that you should meet your vitamin needs by taking pills, look out. Someone may be trying to sell you something you don't need.

Caution

Once vitamin research was well under way and other B vitamins had been discovered, the clarification of their function was often greatly helped by laboratory experiments in which animals or human volunteers were fed diets devoid of one vitamin. The effect of the deficiency of that vitamin could then be studied to determine what functions it normally performed. Other deficiency diseases were discovered in this way and have since been observed to occur outside the laboratory.

Table 8–2 sums up a few of the better-established facts about B vitamin deficiencies. A look at the table will make another generalization possible. Different body systems depend to different extents on these vitamins. Processes in nerves and in their responding tissues, the muscles, depend heavily on glucose metabolism and hence on thiamin; thus paralysis sets in when this nutrient is lacking. The replacement of red blood cells and GI tract cells occurs at a rapid pace and involves much making of DNA; the making of new cells depends on a folacin coenzyme and the making of this coenzyme depends on vitamin B_{12}, so two of the first symptoms of a deficiency of either of these nutrients are a type of anemia and GI deterioration. But again, each nutrient is important in all systems, and these lists of symptoms are far from complete.

The skin and the tongue appear to be especially sensitive to vitamin B deficiencies, but you should note that the listing of these items in Table 8–2 gives them undue emphasis. Remember that in a medical examination these are two body parts that are visible. If the skin is degenerating, other tissues beneath it may be, too. Similarly, the mouth and tongue are the visible part of the digestive system; if they are abnormal, there may well be an abnormality throughout the GI tract. What is really happening in a vitamin deficiency happens inside the cells of the body; what the doctor sees and reports are its outward manifestations.

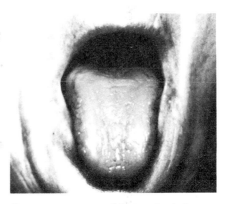

Tongue symptoms of B-vitamin deficiency. The tongue is smooth due to atrophy of the tissues (glossitis). This person has a folacin deficiency.

Source: Courtesy of Dr. Samuel Dreizen, D.D.S., M.D.

It is more and more apparent that you cannot observe a symptom and automatically jump to a conclusion regarding its cause. The warning was given earlier (in Chapter 3) that skin rashes are a symptom, not a disease. As you have seen, deficiencies of linoleic acid, riboflavin, niacin, and vitamin B_6 can all cause rashes. A deficiency of vitamin A can, too. Because skin is on the outside, where you and your doctor can easily look at it, it is a useful indicator of things-going-wrong-in-cells. But by itself a skin symptom tells you nothing about its possible cause.

The same is true of anemia. We often think of anemia as being caused

TABLE 8–2 **B Vitamins—Deficiency Symptoms**

VITAMIN	DISEASE	DEFICIENCY SYNDROME		Technical Terms for Symptoms
		Area Affected	*Main Effects*	
Thiamin B₁	Beriberi	Nervous system	Mental confusion	
			Peripheral paralysis	
		Muscles	Weakness	
			Wasting	
			Painful calf muscles	
		Cardiovascular system	Edema	
			Enlarged heart	
			Death from cardiac failure	
Riboflavin B₂	Ariboflavinosis	Facial skin	Dermatitis around nose and lips	**cheilosis** (kee-LOH-sis)
			Cracking of corners of mouth	
		Eyes	Hypersensitivity to light	**photophobia**
			Reddening of cornea	
Niacin	Pellagra	Skin	Bilateral symmetrical dermatitis, especially on body parts exposed to sun	
		Tongue	Loss of surface features, swelling, edema	**glossitis** (gloss-EYE-tis)
		GI tract	Diarrhea	
		Nervous system	Irritability	
			Mental confusion, progressing to psychosis or delirium	
Vitamin B₆	(No name)	Skin	Dermatitis	
			Cracking of corners of mouth	**cheilosis**
			Irritation of sweat glands	
		Tongue	Smoothness (atrophy of surface structures)	**glossitis**
		Nervous system	Abnormal brain wave pattern	
			Convulsions	
Folacin	(No name)	Tongue	Smoothness, swelling, cracks	**glossitis**
		GI tract	Diarrhea	
		Blood	Anemia (characterized by large cells)	**macrocytic anemia**
Vitamin B₁₂	Pernicious anemia	Blood	Anemia (characterized by large cells)	**macrocytic anemia**
		Nervous system	Degeneration of peripheral nerves	
Pantothenic acid	(No name)	GI tract	Vomiting, GI distress	
		Nervous system	Insomnia, fatigue	
Biotin	(No name)	Skin	Scaly dermatitis, drying, loss of hair	
		Nervous system	Depression, lassitude, muscle pains	
		GI tract	Anorexia, nausea	
		Cardiovascular system	Abnormal heart action	

by an iron deficiency, and often it is. But anemia can also be caused by a folacin or vitamin B_{12} deficiency, by digestive tract failure to absorb any of these nutrients, or by such nonnutritional causes as infections, parasites, cancer, or loss of blood. So be careful. You can often recognize a false claim by the implication that a specific nutrient will always cure a given symptom.

A person who feels chronically tired may be tempted to diagnose herself as having anemia. Knowing only enough to associate iron deficiency with this condition, she may decide to take an iron supplement. But the iron supplement will relieve her tiredness only if the symptom is caused by iron-deficiency anemia. If she has a folacin deficiency (and folacin deficiency is probably the most widespread vitamin deficiency in the world), taking iron will only prolong the period in which she receives no relief. If she is better informed, she may decide to take a vitamin supplement with iron, covering the possibility of a vitamin deficiency. But now she is forgetting that there may be a nonnutritional cause of her symptom. If the cause of her tiredness is actually hidden blood loss due to cancer, the postponement of a diagnosis may be equivalent to suicide.

Caution

Major, epidemic-like deficiency diseases such as pellagra and beriberi are no longer seen in the United States and Canada, but lesser deficiencies of nutrients, including the B vitamins, sometimes are observed. They occur in people whose food choices are poor because of poverty, ignorance, illness, or poor health habits like alcohol abuse. They are especially likely if the staple grain food is refined, as were most bread and cereal products chosen by U.S. consumers during the 1930s and before. One way to protect these people is to add nutrients to their staple food, a process known as fortification or enrichment. The enrichment of refined breads and cereals, required by law in most Eastern states since the late 1940s and in many Western states since the early 1970s, has increased many people's iron and B-vitamin intakes.[2]

fortification: the addition of nutrients to a food, often in amounts much larger than might be found naturally in that food.

enrichment: now considered synonymous with fortification; previously, the addition of four specific nutrients—iron, thiamin, riboflavin, and niacin—to refined breads and cereals in amounts approximately equivalent to those originally present in the whole grain.

The B Vitamins in Foods

The preceding sections have shown both the great importance of the B vitamins in promoting normal, healthy functioning of all body systems and the severe consequences of deficiency. Now you may want to know how to be sure you are getting enough of these vital nutrients. This section offers some practical pointers regarding food intake.

2   A more detailed discussion of the differences between enriched and whole-grain bread is available. See note at end of chapter.

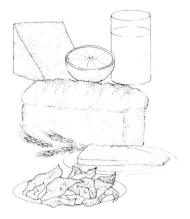

Thiamin: Most nutritious foods contribute about 10 percent of daily need per serving.

Thiamin

The recommended daily thiamin intake for adults is about 1.5 milligrams for men and about 1.0 for women (plus an extra half-milligram during pregnancy). Infants require about half a milligram and children about three-fourths.

Because thiamin is used for energy production, more is needed when energy expenditure is high. (In fact, the thiamin requirement can be stated in terms of milligrams per 1,000 kcalories.) Provided that you are consuming enough kcalories to meet your energy needs—and obtaining those kcalories from thiamin-containing foods—your thiamin intake will adjust automatically to your need. However, people who derive a large proportion of their kcalories from empty-kcalorie items like sugar or alcohol may suffer thiamin deficiency. A person who is fasting or who has adopted a very low-kcalorie diet needs the same amount of thiamin as he did when he was eating more; needs change very little during fasting because they are proportional to energy expenditure, not to energy intake.[3]

Table 8–3 shows the thiamin amounts in different types of foods. If you study the table while thinking about your own food habits, you will probably conclude that many of the foods you like and eat daily contribute some thiamin, but none by itself can meet your total need for a day. A useful guideline is to eliminate empty-kcalorie foods from your diet and to include ten or more different servings of nutritious foods each day, assuming that on the average each serving will contribute about 10 percent of your need. Foods chosen from the bread and cereal group should be either whole-grain or enriched. Thiamin is not stored in the body to any great extent, so daily intake is best.

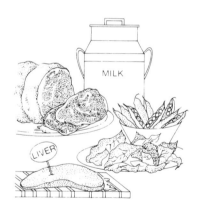

Riboflavin: Milk contributes about 50 percent, meat about 25 percent, whole-grain or enriched breads and cereals additional amounts. The person who does not drink milk should substitute large amounts of dark greens.

Riboflavin

The recommended daily riboflavin intake for adults is about 1.4 to 1.8 milligrams for men and about 1.1 to 1.3 for women (plus about 0.3 milligrams during pregnancy), depending on how much energy they expend daily. (Like thiamin, riboflavin needs can be stated in terms of milligrams per 1,000 kcalories.) Young children's needs begin at about 1 milligram a day and rise rapidly during their growing years. Teenagers, because they are very active, need more riboflavin than adults.

Unlike thiamin, riboflavin is not evenly distributed among the food groups. Table 8–4 shows the riboflavin amounts in different types of foods, and reveals that the major contributors are milk and meat. The need for riboflavin provides a major reason for including milk in some form in every day's meals; no other food that is commonly eaten can make such a substantial contribution. People who don't use milk products can substitute generous servings of dark-green leafy vegetables, because a cup of greens—collards, for example—provides about the same amount of riboflavin as a cup of milk. Among the meats, liver and heart are the richest sources, but all lean meats, as well as eggs, provide some riboflavin. Most people derive

3   M. Brin and J. C. Bauernfeind, Vitamin needs of the elderly, *Postgraduate Medicine* 63, no. 3 (1978): 155–163.

TABLE 8–3 **Thiamin—Average Amounts in Groups of Foods** TH8-2

	THIAMIN (mg)
Milk and Milk Products	
1 c milk[a]	0.10
1 c kefir	0.45
1 c soy milk	0.55
1 oz cheese[b]	-0-
Meat and Legumes	
3 oz meat, fish, or poultry[c]	0.05
3 oz liver[d]	0.20
3 oz ham or pork[e]	0.60
1 egg	0.05
¾ c dried legumes, cooked[f]	0.20
Fruits and Vegetables	
1 portion fruit	0.05
½ c vegetables[g]	0.05
Grains	
1 slice bread, enriched or whole grain[h]	0.10
1 portion cereal[i]	0.10
½ c rice or pasta, enriched or whole grain	0.10
Other	
⅛ avocado	0.05
1 tbsp fat or oil	-0-
2 slices bacon	0.10
1 tbsp sugar or sweets	-0-
1 c soup[j]	0.05
1 tbsp brewer's yeast	1.25

According to the values in the table, a person following the modified four food group plan would obtain:

2 c milk	0.20 mg
2 (3-oz) portions meat	0.10
2 (¾ c) portions legumes	0.40
4 portions fruits and vegetables	0.20
4 portions enriched or whole grains	0.40
Total (compare the U.S. RDA of 1.5 mg)	1.30 mg

For a guarantee of adequacy, any additional foods selected should also be foundation foods such as soups, ice cream (made from milk), cookies or other desserts made from wholesome ingredients like oatmeal or fruit, and the like. To boost thiamin intakes, eat liver and pork products occasionally and add brewer's yeast to milkshakes, baked goods, meatloaf, and other dishes.

This table was made by consulting Appendix H, averaging the thiamin amounts in standard portions of the commonly used foods in each category, and rounding off each average to the nearest 0.05 mg. (Thus, 0 doesn't mean no thiamin, but rather, less than 0.03 mg thiamin.) Values agree approximately with the USDA table, Nutrients furnished by servings of foods, *Essentials of an Adequate Diet*, Bulletin no. 160, 1956. Use of these numbers will provide a rough approximation of the amount of thiamin on a plate or in a day's meals. However, the person who wants maximum accuracy will refer to Appendix H.

[a] 1 c milk or any milk product such as yogurt, ice milk, custard, soft-serve ice cream, milkshake. Malted milk powder raises thiamin content. Cream has half as much thiamin per cup; nondairy creamers have none.

[b] 1 oz any hard cheese, shredded cheese, or cottage cheese (1 c cottage cheese has only 0.05 mg).

[c] Values range from about 0.03 to 0.11 mg. Canned and fried products are much lower in thiamin.

[d] Liver or other organ meat such as heart.

[e] Whole ham or pork, not sausages or lunch meats, which are similar in thiamin content to beef.

[f] Canned beans have less thiamin—about 0.10 mg per ¾ c serving.

[g] Fresh blackeyed peas, green peas, and lima beans have about 0.25 mg thiamin per ½ c serving.

[h] 1 slice bread, enriched or whole-grain; or 1 portion pastry made with enriched or whole-grain flour.

[i] Cereals with added vitamins have higher thiamin contents. Read the label.

[j] 1 c bean soup with pork offers 0.15 mg; 1 c split pea soup offers 0.25 mg.

TABLE 8–4 **Riboflavin—Average Amounts in Groups of Foods** TH8-3

	RIBOFLAVIN (mg)
Milk and Milk Products	
1 c milk[a]	0.40
1 c soy milk	1.20
1 oz cheese[b]	0.10
Meat and Legumes	
3 oz meat, fish, or poultry[c]	0.15
3 oz liver[d]	3.55
1 egg	0.15
¾ c legumes, cooked	0.10
Fruits and Vegetables	
1 portion fruit	0.05
1 c dark green or other riboflavin-rich vegetables[e]	0.25
½ c other vegetables	0.05
Grains	
1 slice bread, enriched or whole grain[f]	0.05
1 portion cereal[g]	0.05
½ c rice or pasta, enriched or whole grain	0.05
Other	
1 tbsp fat or oil	-0-
1 tbsp sugar or sweets	-0-
1 c cream soup	0.25
1 c broth-base soup	0.05
1 tbsp brewer's yeast	0.35

According to the values in the table, a person following the modified four food group plan would obtain:

2 c milk	0.80 mg
2 (3-oz) portions meat	0.30
2 (¾ c) portions legumes	0.20
4 portions fruits and vegetables (assuming no dark green vegetables)	0.20
4 portions enriched or whole grains	0.20
Total (compare the U.S. RDA of 1.7 mg)	1.70 mg

For a guarantee of adequacy, any additional foods selected should also be foundation foods such as soups, ice cream (made from milk), and dark green vegetables. To boost riboflavin intakes, eat liver occasionally and add brewer's yeast to milkshakes, baked goods, meatloaf, and other dishes.

This table was made in the same way as Table 8-3, rounding off averaged riboflavin values to the nearest 0.05 mg.

[a] 1 c any milk or any milk product such as yogurt, kefir, ice milk, cream, custard, soft-serve ice cream, milkshake, milk pudding. 1 c ice cream has about 0.35 mg.

[b] 1 c creamed cottage cheese is equivalent to 1 c milk in riboflavin content.

[c] Fried products are lower in riboflavin content.

[d] Other organ meats are rich in riboflavin too; 3 oz beef heart has about 1.00 mg.

[e] We are using 1 c, not ½ c, as a serving size for dark green vegetables to encourage people to eat larger quantities of these vegetables, especially when substituting them for milk. "Dark green vegetables," here, means: asparagus, beet greens, broccoli, collard greens, dandelion greens, kale, mustard greens, spinach, turnip greens. Other vegetables that offer about 0.25 mg riboflavin per cup are fresh cooked blackeyed peas, brussels sprouts, mushrooms, okra, soy bean sprouts, summer squash, and winter squash.

[f] 1 slice bread, enriched or whole-grain; or 1 serving cake or other pastry made with enriched or whole-grain flour. 1 serving pie offers about 0.10 mg (0.05 for the pastry; 0.05 for the fruit).

[g] Cereals with added vitamins have higher riboflavin contents. Read the label.

about half their riboflavin from milk and milk products, about a fourth from meats, and most of the rest from leafy green vegetables and whole-grain or enriched bread and cereal products.

Riboflavin is light-sensitive; it can be destroyed by the ultraviolet rays of the sun or of fluorescent lamps. For this reason milk is seldom sold (and should not be stored) in transparent glass containers. Cardboard or plastic containers protect the riboflavin in the milk from ultraviolet rays.

Niacin

Recommended niacin intakes are stated in "equivalents," a term that requires explanation. Niacin is unique among the B vitamins because it can be obtained from another nutrient source—protein. The amino acid tryptophan can be converted to niacin in the body: 60 milligrams of tryptophan yields 1 milligram of niacin. Thus a food containing 1 milligram of niacin and 60 milligrams of tryptophan contains the equivalent of 2 milligrams of niacin, or 2 milligram equivalents.

Recommended daily intakes for men are about 15 to 20 milligram equivalents and for women about 12 to 15 (plus 2 to 5 milligram equivalents during pregnancy and lactation). Infants', children's, and teenagers' needs are proportional not to their size but to their energy output.

Tables of food composition list only the preformed niacin in foods, although people actually derive the vitamin from both niacin itself and dietary tryptophan. However, tryptophan is also used to build needed body proteins, so not all of it is used to make niacin. Thus calculating the amount of niacin available from the diet is a complicated matter. A means of obtaining a rough approximation is shown in the margin, but the simplest assumption is that if the diet is adequate in complete protein, it will supply enough niacin equivalents to meet the daily need.

Milk, eggs, meat, poultry, and fish contribute about half the niacin equivalents consumed by most people, and about a fourth come from enriched breads and cereals. Vegetarians are well advised to emphasize nuts and legumes in their diets, as these are good sources of niacin and protein. A look at the nutrient contents of foods (in Appendix H) will reveal other good sources.

Most people in Canada and the United States presently consume a lot of animal protein, so niacin deficiency is a problem only where protein deficiency occurs. The widespread pellagra that was seen during the early part of this century in the U.S. South arose from two causes. First, the predominantly cornmeal–salt pork–molasses diet of the people of that area was lacking in both niacin and protein. Second, what little protein they consumed was corn protein, which is unusually low in tryptophan. The meat product that they ate was salt pork, which is not really a meat but a fat. Symptoms of niacin deficiency are no longer observed very often, except in people like alcohol abusers and undernourished hospital patients, whose protein intakes are unacceptably low.

At the time that pellagra was widespread in the South, half the cases in insane asylums were caused by niacin deficiency. Unfortunately, not all insanity is caused by a lack of niacin; if it were, it would be wonderfully easy to cure. Insanity induced by niacin deficiency has symptoms very like

niacin equivalents: the amount of niacin present in food, including the niacin that can theoretically be made from its precursor tryptophan present in the food.

To obtain a rough approximation of your niacin intake:

1 Calculate total protein consumed (g).
2 Subtract your recommended protein intake to obtain "leftover" protein usable to make niacin (g).
3 Divide by 100 to obtain the amount of tryptophan in this protein (g).
4 Multiply by 1,000 to express this amount of tryptophan in milligrams (mg).
5 Divide by 60 to get niacin equivalents (mg).
6 Finally, add the amount of niacin obtained preformed in the diet (mg).

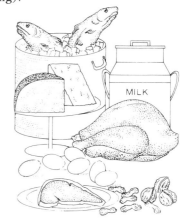

Niacin is adequate if protein is adequate.

schizophrenia (skitz-oh-FREN-ee-uh): a kind of mental illness.

schizo = split

phren = mind

orthomolecular psychiatry: a branch of psychiatry that attempts to treat mental illness by correcting nutrient imbalances and deficiencies.

ortho = right

megavitamin therapy: the administration of huge doses (ten times the normal intake or more) of vitamins in the attempt to cure disease.

mega = huge

those of schizophrenia, but it clears up miraculously when niacin or tryptophan is given. The hope that large doses of niacin would cure schizophrenia has led to some important research and a whole new area of study—orthomolecular psychiatry—but the results have been disappointing. There is no evidence that large doses of niacin have any effect whatever on mental disease other than the dementia of pellagra.

Large doses of niacin have been observed to lower blood cholesterol levels in some cases, and for a while interest ran high in exploring the possible value of niacin therapy in the prevention of atherosclerosis. Both niacin and niacinamide (an alternative form of the vitamin) have been extensively tested for their cholesterol-lowering effects, but the test results have been disappointing. Niacin causes irritation of the intestines and possibly liver damage, and niacinamide is ineffective altogether. This line of research has given way to other, more promising approaches.

One problem with large therapeutic doses of niacin (but not niacinamide) is that they produce flushed skin and a painful, stinging sensation that may be alarming, although megadoses seem to cause no permanent harm if taken only a few times. Some people who believe in the therapeutic power of niacin even enjoy this "niacin flush."

Vitamin B_6 need: 0.02 mg/g protein.

Vitamin B_6

Because the vitamin B_6 coenzymes play many roles in amino acid metabolism, dietary needs are roughly proportional to protein intakes. Adults need about 2 milligrams a day; this is enough to handle 100 grams of protein. Pregnant and lactating women need about half a milligram more. Infants probably receive enough vitamin B_6 either from breast milk or cow's milk formula. There is some possibility that older people have a greater need for vitamin B_6 than young adults.

Pregnant women often show low blood concentrations of vitamin B_6 even though the foods they eat are rich sources of the vitamin. It is thought that this is due to the high demand for vitamin B_6 by the fetus, whose blood normally has about five times more than the mother's. Vitamin B_6 is often prescribed for relief of the nausea and vomiting of pregnancy as well as for depression felt by women taking oral contraceptives.

Measurement of the amounts of vitamin B_6 in foods is under way currently. Complete data are not yet available, so vitamin B_6 has not been included in the table of food composition in Appendix H. Averaged amounts of vitamin B_6, derived from the available data, are shown in Table 8-5, which reveals that the richest food sources are muscle meats, liver, vegetables, and whole-grain cereals.

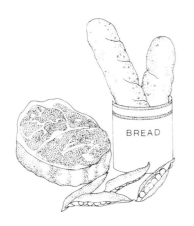

Vitamin B_6 is found in meats, vegetables, and whole-grain cereals.

Note: Recommended folacin intakes are stated in micrograms (μg). A microgram is a thousandth of a milligram or a millionth of a gram. The RDA for folacin, 400 μg, can also be stated as 0.4 mg.

Folacin

Folacin occurs in foods in both bound and free forms; the free form is better absorbed. Canada's recommendation for daily intake, stated in terms of "free folate (folacin)," is 200 micrograms a day for adults, with 50 micrograms added for pregnancy. The U.S. recommendation for adults is stated in terms of all forms of folacin and is 400 micrograms a day. The need

TABLE 8–5 Vitamin B₆—Average Amounts in Groups of Foods (Tentative Values)

	VITAMIN B$_6$ (mg)
Milk and Milk Products	
1 c milk[a]	0.10
1 oz cheese[b]	-0-
1 c cottage cheese	0.15
Meat and Legumes	
3 oz meat, fish, or poultry[c]	0.20
1 egg	0.05
¾ c legumes, cooked[d]	0.60
Fruits and Vegetables	
1 portion fruit[e]	0.05
1 banana	0.50
½ c vegetables[f]	0.15
Grains	
1 slice enriched white bread[g]	-0-
1 slice whole-grain bread[g]	0.05
1 portion cereal or pasta, refined or enriched[g,h]	-0-
1 portion whole-grain cereal or pasta[g]	0.05
½ c rice	0.15
Other	
⅛ avocado	0.15
1 tbsp wheat germ	0.05
1 tbsp fat or oil	-0-
1 tbsp sugar or sweets	-0-
1 c soup[i]	0.05
1 tbsp brewer's yeast	0.20

According to the values in the table, a person following the modified four food group plan would obtain:

2 c milk	0.20 mg
2 (3-oz) portions meat	0.40
2 (¾ c) portions legumes	1.20
4 portions fruits and vegetables	0.40
4 portions grains (whole grains only)	0.20
Total (compare the U.S. RDA of 2.0 mg)	2.40 mg

Without the legumes and whole grains, the total would be 1.00 mg. For a guarantee of adequacy, any additional foods selected should also be foundation foods such as soups, vegetables, and whole-grain breads and cereals. A banana now and then would boost vitamin B₆ intake.

This table was made by consulting Appendix G, Nutrient value of foods and beverages, in H. A. Guthrie, *Introductory Nutrition*, 5th ed. (St. Louis: Mosby, 1983), pp. 608–641; and *Vitamin B₆, A Brief Summary* (Washington, D.C.: United Fresh Fruit and Vegetable Association, 1976). Average values were obtained for groups of foods and rounded off to the nearest 0.05 mg. Values are tentative.

[a] 1 c milk or any milk product including cream, milk drinks, milk shakes, ice cream, ice milk, milk custard, pudding, yogurt.

[b] Average values for 10 varieties of cheese come to less than 0.03 mg.

[c] Values for fish range from 0.12 to 0.34 mg; canned tuna and canned salmon are the highest. Values for meats including meat sausages range from 0.13 to 0.46 mg; lightmeat turkey and lean ground beef are the highest.

[d] Based on one value only: canned red kidney beans.

[e] Values range from 0 to about 0.15 mg except for bananas.

[f] Values range from about 0.05 to 0.30 mg; greens are the highest.

[g] Vitamin B₆ is not added back to refined grains in the enrichment process (only iron, thiamin, riboflavin, and niacin are). Thus the distinction has to be made between enriched and whole-grain bread.

[h] Fortified cereals may have added vitamin B₆. Read the label. See also wheat germ (under "Other").

[i] Values range from about 0.05 to 0.15 mg; tomato and minestrone soups are the highest.

for folacin rises dramatically during pregnancy, more than the need for any other nutrient; the RDA table doubles the folacin recommendation to 800 micrograms a day during pregnancy. This increased need reflects the role folacin plays in cell multiplication. The blood volume in a pregnant woman increases by 50 percent, for example, and the folacin coenzymes are used to manufacture the new blood cells.

Tables of the folacin contents of foods, published before 1973, relied on data derived from experiments that are now known to have yielded incorrect, low values. The measurement of folacin depended on a method in which up to half of the folacin was destroyed. The method now in use involves adding vitamin C to protect the folacin, and new, more accurate data are now available. Still, many uncertainties beset the researcher attempting to estimate folacin intakes from foods. Folacin appears in several forms in foods, and the efficiency of absorption and of conversion of different forms to active folacin in the body varies widely.

The folacin content of foods, derived only from the new method of analysis, has been incorporated into this book's table of food composition for the first time in this edition (see Appendix H). The best food sources of the vitamin are organ meats such as liver; green, leafy vegetables (the name of the vitamin is related to the word *foliage*); beets; and members of the cabbage family such as cauliflower, broccoli, and brussels sprouts. Among the fruits, oranges, orange juice, and cantaloupe are the best sources; among the starchy vegetables, corn, lima beans, parsnips, green peas, pumpkin, and sweet potato are good sources. Whole-wheat bread, wheat germ, and milk also supply folacin.

The presence of folacin in dark-green leafy vegetables is one reason for the Four Food Group Plan recommendation that these vegetables be included in the diet at least every other day. Some forms of folacin are readily destroyed by cooking; hence the advisability of including *raw* vegetables like salad greens and fruits like citrus fruits in daily menus. Table 8–6 shows the amounts of folacin in different types of foods.

Folacin deficiency affects all rapidly dividing cells because of the need for folacin to make new DNA. The most rapidly dividing cells in the body are those in the GI tract, where the intestinal villi are completely regenerated every three days, and in the body's blood-making sites, where new blood cells are being born by the millions every minute. In a folacin deficiency, the villi atrophy, and GI enzymes and secretions are suppressed, so that the absorption of all other nutrients is soon impaired. Also, the blood cells, both red and white, fail to form normally, so that transport of nutrients and oxygen is impaired as well. The white cells are the chief components of the body's immune system, so folacin deficiency depresses immunity, making infectious disease more likely.

Folacin deficiency also affects the brain, nervous system, and behavior by a mechanism as yet unknown;[4] the effect is seen before the deficiency has

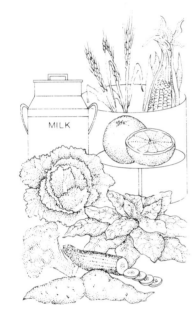

Folacin is the "foliage" vitamin.

4   J. H. Pincus, E. H. Reynolds, and G. H. Glaser, Subacute combined system degeneration with folate deficiency, *Journal of the American Medical Association* 221 (1972): 496–497. Possibly, because folacin is required for many steps in amino acid metabolism, its lack causes altered amino acid levels in the blood, and therefore altered neurotransmitter levels in the brain. Neurological disease in folic acid deficiency, *Nutrition Reviews* 39 (1981): 337–338.

TABLE 8-6   Folacin—Average Amounts in Groups of Foods TH8-4

	FOLACIN (μg)			FOLACIN (μg)
Milk and Milk Products			*Other*	
1 c milk[a]	20		⅛ avocado or 2 tbsp peanut butter	20
1 c soy milk	60		1 tbsp fat or oil	-0-
1 oz cheese[b]	10		1 c soup	10
1 c cottage cheese[c]	30		1 tbsp wheat germ	20
			1 tbsp sugar or sweets	-0-
Meat and Legumes			¼ c soybean flour	60
3 oz meat, fish, or poultry	10		1 serving nuts (1 fat exchange)	10
3 oz liver	120		¼ c sunflower seeds	110
1 egg	20		¼ c sesame seeds	30
¾ c legumes, cooked[d]	80		1 tbsp brewer's yeast	310
			1 c tea	10
Fruits and Vegetables				
1 portion melon[e]	70			
½ c fresh or frozen orange juice	60			
1 portion other fruit[f]	10			
1 c folacin-rich vegetables[g]	120			
½ c other vegetables	20			

According to the values in the table, a person following the modified four food group plan who selected one folacin-rich fruit and one folacin-rich vegetable a day would obtain:

2 c milk	40 μg
2 portions (3 oz) meat, fish, poultry	20
2 (¾ c) portions legumes	160
4 portions fruits and vegetables	200
4 portions enriched or whole grains	40
Total (compare the U.S. RDA of 400 μg)	460 μg

Grains

1 slice bread or ½ c rice[h]	10
1 portion cereal[i]	10
1 piece pie	10

Without the folacin-rich fruits and vegetables and the legumes, the total would be 200 μg. This table was made by consulting Appendix H, averaging the folacin amounts in standard portions of the commonly used foods in each category, and rounding off each average to the nearest 10 μg. (Thus, 0 doesn't mean no folacin, but rather, less than 5 μg.) The values in this table will provide an approximation of the folacin on a plate or in a day's meals. However, refer to Appendix H for maximum accuracy.

[a] 1 c milk or any milk product such as custard, pudding, yogurt, kefir, buttermilk, malted milk, milkshake. Ice cream, ice milk, commercial egg-nog, and cream are lower—average 5 μg. Goat's milk has only 2 μg per cup.

[b] Values range from 2 to 34 μg; riper cheeses such as blue, camembert, liederkrantz, and limburger are the highest; process cheeses and cheese spreads are the lowest.

[c] Ricotta cheese is lower: 10 μg per cup.

[d] Values range from about 40 to about 170; broad beans and limas are the highest. ¾ c split peas has only 10 μg.

[e] ¼ cantaloupe or 1/10 honeydew.

[f] Fresh fruits have more folacin than canned or otherwise processed fruits.

[g] Asparagus, blackeyed peas (cooked from fresh or frozen), fresh beets, greens (except kale), broccoli, brussels sprouts, corn, lettuce (raw endive or looseleaf), green peas or lima beans (cooked from frozen), winter squash, mixed vegetables (cooked from frozen). We have listed a 1-cup serving to remind the user of this table that generous servings of folacin-rich vegetables will help meet the folacin requirement. Values range from about 70 to 240 μg; blackeyed peas, green peas, greens, beets, and asparagus are the highest.

[h] ½ c pasta has much less folacin. ¼ c barley has 10 μg.

[i] Fortified cereals often have 100 μg folacin added per serving. Read the label.

progressed to the point of causing severe changes in the blood. Among the signs are fatigue, mild depression, abnormal intellectual functioning, and abnormal nerve function (reflexes), including disorientation, confusion, poor memory, and inability to perform simple calculations.

Folacin deficiency may result not only from an inadequate intake, but also from impaired absorption or unusual metabolic need for the vitamin. Deficiencies from all three causes are common.

An inadequate intake is seen in babies fed goat's milk, which is notoriously low in folacin. But a too-low intake is also theoretically possible in anyone whose diet does not include generous amounts of folacin-rich foods. Overconsumers of alcohol or other empty-kcalorie items are especially vulnerable. The RDA for folacin is probably not met by the average American diet, but possibly, one can have a folacin intake below the RDA, or even below two-thirds of the RDA, without developing deficiency symptoms.

As for folacin absorption, it varies so widely and depends on so many factors that the vitamin's availability from specific foods is difficult or impossible to predict. For example, absorption from breast milk is good, and perhaps from raw milk as well; but when milk is pasteurized, the folacin-binding proteins are altered, affecting absorption to an extent not yet clear.

Metabolism of folacin can be greatly altered by many conditions. Many drugs affect it and cause deficiencies. Many inherited disorders (all of them rare, fortunately) cause derangements in folacin metabolism severe enough to bring about tragic mental and physical abnormalities. Alcohol abuse increases the need for folacin as well as reducing the intake, and some of the neurological abnormalities seen in alcoholism are ascribed to folacin deficiency. A deficiency can also be precipitated by any condition that requires cell multiplication to speed up: multiple pregnancies (twins, triplets), cancer, skin-destroying diseases such as chicken pox and measles, burns, blood loss, GI tract damage, and more.

Among the poor and in other parts of the world, folacin deficiency due to inadequate intake is probably the most common of all vitamin deficiencies. Folacin deficiency anemia is especially common among pregnant women. Some authorities recommend that in pregnancy, a folacin supplement, as well as an iron supplement, should be given as a preventive measure.

The risks of overdosing with folacin are greater than those for the other B vitamins discussed so far. They arise from the close relationship between folacin and vitamin B_{12}.

Vitamin B_{12}

Note: Recommended vitamin B_{12} intakes are stated in micrograms; 3 μg is .003 mg, 3 millionths of a gram.

According to both the U.S. and Canadian recommendations, adults need about 3 micrograms of vitamin B_{12} a day (plus 1 microgram during pregnancy). This is the tiniest amount imaginable—three-millionths of a gram, and a gram would not even fill a quarter-teaspoon. The ink in the period at the end of this sentence probably weighs about 3 micrograms. But what seems like such a tiny amount to the human eye contains billions of molecules of vitamin B_{12}, enough to provide coenzymes for all the enzymes that need its help.

Vitamin B$_{12}$ is unique among the nutrients in being found almost exclusively in animal flesh and animal products. Anyone who eats meat is guaranteed an adequate intake, and lacto-ovo-vegetarians (who use milk, cheese, and eggs) are also protected from deficiency. But vegans must use vitamin B$_{12}$-fortified soy milk or other such products or take vitamin B$_{12}$ supplements.[5]

A second special characteristic of vitamin B$_{12}$ is that it requires an "intrinsic factor"—a compound made inside the body—for absorption from the intestinal tract into the bloodstream. The design for this factor is carried in the genes. The intrinsic factor is now known to be synthesized in the stomach, where it attaches to the vitamin; the complex then passes to the small intestine and is gradually absorbed.

Certain people have in their genetic makeup a gene for the intrinsic factor that becomes defective, usually in midlife. Without the intrinsic factor, they can't absorb the vitamin even though they are taking enough in their diets, and so they develop deficiency symptoms. In such a case, or when the stomach has been injured and cannot produce enough of the intrinsic factor, vitamin B$_{12}$ must be supplied to the body by injection to bypass the block in the intestinal tract.

One of the most obvious vitamin B$_{12}$-deficiency symptoms is the anemia of folacin deficiency, characterized by large, immature red blood cells. (Vitamin B$_{12}$, remember, is needed to enable folacin to help manufacture red blood cells.) Either vitamin B$_{12}$ or folacin will clear up this condition. However, vitamin B$_{12}$ also functions in maintaining the sheath that surrounds and protects nerve fibers and in promoting their normal growth, as well as in producing mature red blood cells. Thus a deficiency of vitamin B$_{12}$ causes not only anemia but also a creeping paralysis of the nerves and muscles, which begins at the extremities and works inward and up the spine. This symptom is not detectable from a blood test, and the paralysis cannot be remedied by administering folacin. Early detection and correction are necessary to prevent permanent nerve damage and paralysis. The name *pernicious* anemia comes from the hidden, sneaky, and frightening way in which vitamin B$_{12}$ deficiency damages nerves without revealing itself in a blood symptom. Because of the danger of folacin's masking a lack of vitamin B$_{12}$, the amount of folacin in over-the-counter vitamin preparations is limited by law to 400 micrograms, an amount too low to have this effect.[6]

Vitamin B$_{12}$ is adequate if animal foods are included in the diet. Among vegetable products only a few (those that include microorganisms) contain vitamin B$_{12}$, most notably yeast and some fermented soy products.

A vegan is a strict vegetarian, one who excludes not only meat, poultry, and fish but also animal products such as milk, cheese, and eggs.

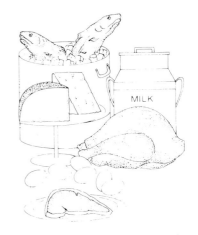

Vitamin B$_{12}$ is found only in animal flesh and animal products.

intrinsic: inside the system. The intrinsic factor necessary to prevent pernicious anemia is now known to be a mucopolysaccharide, made in the stomach, that aids in the absorption of vitamin B$_{12}$.

The way folacin masks pernicious anemia underlines a point already made several times. It takes a skilled diagnostician to make a correct diagnosis, and the risk you take when you diagnose yourself on the basis of a single observed symptom is clearly serious.[7]

5   Guidelines for vegetarian diet planning are available. See note at end of chapter.

6   Committee on Safety, Toxicity, and Misuse of Vitamins and Trace Minerals, National Nutrition Consortium, *Vitamin-Mineral Safety, Toxicity, and Misuse* (Chicago: American Dietetic Association, 1978).

7   Both folacin and vitamin B$_{12}$-deficiency anemias are now known to occur on occasion without red cell enlargement but only with enlargement of certain bone marrow cells. J. L. Spivak, Masked megaloblastic anemia, *Archives of Internal Medicine* 142 (1982): 2111–2114.

> A second point should also be underlined here. Since vitamin B_{12} deficiency in the body may be caused either by a lack of the vitamin in the diet or by a genetically caused inability to absorb the vitamin, a change in diet alone may not correct it. You might wish to think about this in relation to the cautions offered on pp. 93, 274–275 and 277–279.

Caution

Strict vegetarians are at special risk for undetected vitamin B_{12} deficiency for two reasons—first, because they receive none in their diets; and second, because they consume large amounts of folacin from the vegetables they eat. The amount of vitamin B_{12} that can be stored in the body is 1,000 times the amount used each day; so it may take years for a deficiency to develop in a new vegetarian. When it does, it may be masked by the high folacin intake. Sometimes the damage is first seen in the breast-fed infant of a vegan mother.[8]

The history of the discovery of vitamin B_{12} makes an intriguing story. In the 1920s, researchers discovered that pernicious anemia could be controlled but not cured by eating large amounts of calf liver. (Researchers concluded that liver contained a factor—the "extrinsic factor"—needed to prevent the disease, and later they identified the factor as vitamin B_{12}.) The concentration of vitamin B_{12} in liver was so great that people who ate liver absorbed some of the vitamin even without the help of the intrinsic factor. At one time people who suffered from pernicious anemia had no choice but to eat about a pound of liver a day, but now they can be cured by the injection of a few micrograms of the purified vitamin every three weeks.

extrinsic: outside the system. The extrinsic factor first detected in raw liver and found necessary to prevent pernicious anemia is now known to be vitamin B_{12}.

Pantothenic Acid and Biotin

The six best-known B vitamins have already been discussed. Two other B vitamins—pantothenic acid and biotin—are needed for the synthesis of coenzymes that are active in a multitude of body systems. These are just as important as the vitamins discussed so far, but both pantothenic acid and biotin are widespread in foods, and there seems to be no danger that people who consume a variety of foods will suffer deficiencies. Claims that they are needed in pill form to prevent or cure disease conditions are at best unfounded and at worst intentionally misleading.

Pantothenic acid and biotin: deficiencies unlikely in humans.

In a very few instances under unusual circumstances, biotin deficiencies have been seen in human adults. Invariably they have been associated with artificial feeding—that is, feeding mixtures of purified nutrients, lacking biotin, into a vein in hospital patients who could not eat. Even under such circumstances, a patient would normally not experience deficiency because the bacteria in the GI tract can synthesize enough biotin to meet the host's needs. However, in the hospital, antibiotics are often given, and these kill the intestinal bacteria.

The protein **avidin** in egg whites binds biotin.

avid = greedy.

Researchers can induce a biotin deficiency in animals or human subjects by feeding them raw egg whites, which contain a protein that binds biotin.

8   Vitamin B_{12} deficiency in the breast-fed infant of a strict vegetarian, *Nutrition Reviews* 37 (1979): 142–144.

However, it takes more than two dozen raw egg whites to produce the effect; and cooking denatures the protein. Occasional drinkers of eggnog have nothing to fear from raw egg whites.

Biotin is important metabolically, and some genetic disorders greatly increase the need for it. Individuals born with an inherited metabolic disorder involving biotin can develop deficiency symptoms and will benefit from therapeutic doses.

Non–B Vitamins

A trio of compounds sometimes called B vitamins are inositol, choline, and lipoic acid. These are not essential nutrients for humans, although deficiencies can be induced in laboratory animals in order to study their functions. Like the B vitamins described above, they serve as coenzymes in metabolism. Even if they were essential for humans, supplements would be unnecessary, because they are abundant in foods.

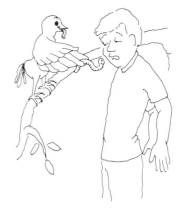

Health-food purveyors make much of inositol, choline, and lipoic acid, insisting that we must supplement our diets with them. Some vitamin companies include them in their formulations in hopes that you will read the label and conclude that their vitamin pill is more "complete" than someone else's. These incorrect notions arise from an unjustified application of findings from animal studies to human beings. Animals are very useful for nutrition research, but their nutrient needs are not the same as ours. Before concluding what an animal research finding means to us, we have to perform the needed tests directly on human beings. To weigh the reliability of nutrition information derived from animal studies, ask yourself if the finding has been proved applicable to human beings.

For a rational way to compare different vitamin-mineral supplements, turn to Appendix P.

 Caution

When used as drugs, choline and its relative lecithin have some important beneficial effects on several disease conditions that affect memory and muscular coordination.[9] These particular diseases are responsive, not because they are caused by deficiencies of choline or lecithin, but because large doses of these nutrients act in a different way altogether from normal doses.

The beneficial effects of choline and lecithin on these diseases have led to many false claims—"Lecithin improves memory" and the like—with a consequent rush to buy and consume bottles of it. As a result, medical practitioners have been able to witness and report on the effects of overdoses of these compounds. They can cause not only short-term discomforts such as GI distress, sweating, salivation, and anorexia, but also long-term

Lecithin, remember, contains choline as part of its structure. See Chapter 3.

When a normal dose of a nutrient clears up a deficiency condition, it is having a **physiological effect**. When a megadose (100 times larger) overwhelms some system and acts like a drug, the nutrient is having a **pharmacological effect**.

9   The two diseases most intensively investigated have been Alzheimer's disease and tardive dyskinesia. Some five others may be ameliorated by choline, lecithin, or phosphatidyl choline. J. L. Wood and R. G. Allison, Effects of consumption of choline and lecithin on neurological and cardiovascular systems, *Federation Proceedings* 41 (1982): 3015–3021.

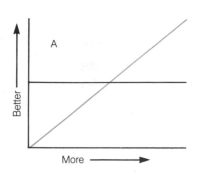

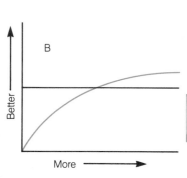

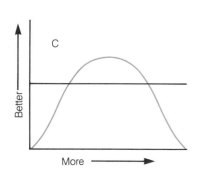

health hazards from disturbance of the nervous and cardiovascular systems.[10]

If you read or hear a report of a substance having a beneficial or harmful effect, it is an oversimplification to conclude that the substance is "good" or "bad." You must ask what dose was used. Two corollaries to this statement might be the following:

- A substance that is poisonous at a high concentration may be an essential nutrient at a lower concentration.
- A nutrient needed at a low concentration may be toxic at a high concentration.

The drawings in the margin show three possible relationships between dose levels and effects. In drawing A, as you progress in the direction of more, the effect gets better and better, with no end in sight. (Real life is seldom if ever like this.) In drawing B, as you progress in the direction of more, the effect reaches a maximum and then a plateau, becoming no better with higher doses. In drawing C, as you progress in the direction of more, the effect reaches an optimum at some intermediate dose and then declines, showing that too much is as bad as too little. Drawing C represents the situation with nutrients—and nonnutrients such as choline and lecithin.

Caution

In addition to choline, inositol, and lipoic acid, other substances have been mistaken for essential nutrients for humans because they are needed for growth by bacteria or other forms of life. These substances include:

- PABA (para-aminobenzoic acid).
- Bioflavonoids (vitamin P or hesperidin).
- Ubiquinone.

Other names you may hear are "Vitamin B_5" (another name for pantothenic acid), "Vitamin B_{15}" (a hoax[11]), "Vitamin B_{17}" (laetrile, a fake "cancer cure" and not a vitamin by any stretch of the imagination), "Vitamin B_T" (carnitine, an important piece of cell machinery but not a vitamin), and more. There is another water-soluble vitamin, however, of great interest and importance—vitamin C.

Vitamin C

Two hundred years ago, any man who joined the crew of a seagoing ship knew he had only half a chance of returning alive—not because he might be slain by pirates or die in a storm but because he might contract the dread

---

10 Wood and Allison, 1982.

11 The quackery surrounding "vitamin B_{15}" is fully exposed in a supplementary reading. See note at end of chapter.

disease scurvy. As many as two-thirds of a ship's men might die of scurvy on a long voyage. Only ships that sailed on short voyages, especially around the Mediterranean Sea, were safe from this disease. It was not known at the time that the special hazard of long ocean voyages was that the ship's cook used up his provisions of fresh fruits and vegetables early and relied for the duration of the voyage on cereals and live animals brought along as provisions.

The first nutrition experiment conducted on human beings was devised in 1747 to find a cure for scurvy. Dr. James Lind, a British physician, divided 12 sailors with scurvy into six pairs. Each pair received a different supplemental ration: vinegar, sulfuric acid, sea water, orange, lemon, or none. The ones receiving the citrus fruits were cured within a short time. Sadly, it was 50 years before the British Navy made use of Lind's experiment by requiring all vessels to carry sufficient limes for every sailor to have lime juice daily. British sailors are still nicknamed "limeys" as a result of this tradition.

The antiscurvy "something" in limes and other foods was dubbed the antiscorbutic factor. Nearly 200 years later, the factor was isolated from lemon juice and found to be a six-carbon compound similar to glucose. It was named ascorbic acid. Shortly thereafter it was synthesized, and today hundreds of millions of vitamin C pills are produced in pharmaceutical laboratories each year and sold for a few dollars a bottle.

Human needs for vitamin C are the subject of much disagreement among experts. The publication of Linus Pauling's controversial book *Vitamin C and the Common Cold* thrust this vitamin into the limelight in 1970 and persuaded thousands of readers that they should be taking doses much higher than the 45 or 60 milligrams a day cited as adequate in published recommended intakes. Highly respected nutritionists and other scientists have taken positions at both extremes on this issue. The controversy over the common cold has largely died down in the popular press (see Highlight 8B), but the question of how much is enough is still being hotly debated.

There is also a controversy over the risks of taking large doses of vitamin C. Some argue for megadoses on the grounds that the risks of excess are negligible but the risks of deficiency are great. Others argue against megadoses because the risk of deficiency is negligible but the risks of toxicity are great! Both positions are based on reasoning from small amounts of evidence and large numbers of words.

We face a difficult task in trying to sort out what is known about vitamin C, what is likely to be shown true, and what claims are clearly unfounded. This chapter deals with the vitamin's known roles and debunks the obvious myths, leaving matters that are in the realm of uncertainty to Highlight 8B.

Metabolic Roles of Vitamin C

Vitamin C is a mysterious vitamin. Like all the vitamins, it is a small organic compound needed by human beings in minute amounts daily. Being organic, it is convertible to several different forms, two of which are active (see Figure 8–3). Like the B vitamins, it is water-soluble, and so it is excreted rapidly when excesses are taken. But unlike the B vitamins

scurvy: the vitamin C deficiency disease.

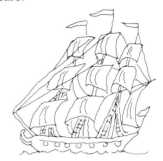

antiscorbutic factor: the original name for vitamin C.

anti = against

scorbutic = causing scurvy

ascorbic acid: one of the two active forms of vitamin C (see Figure 8–3). Many people consistently (and incorrectly) refer to all vitamin C by this name.

a = without

scorbic = having scurvy

Doses of 10 to 30 or more times the recommended intake of a nutrient are termed **megadoses**. In the case of vitamin C, any amount over 1 g (1,000 mg) is considered a megadose.

FIGURE 8-3 **Active forms of vitamin C.** The reduced form can lose two hydrogens with their electrons, becoming oxidized. The electrons may then reduce some other compound. TH8-1

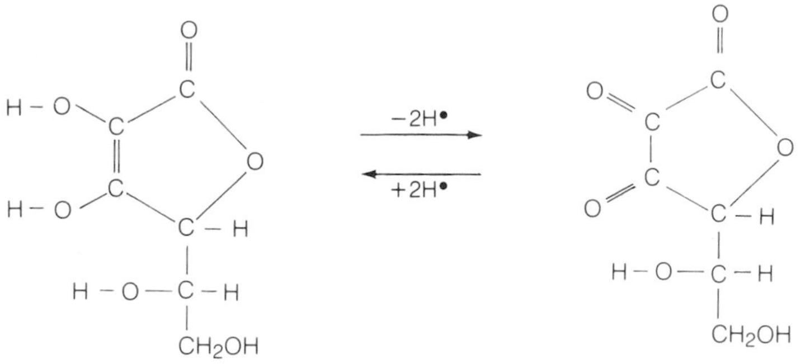

Ascorbic acid
(reduced form)

Dehydroascorbic acid
(oxidized form)

collagen: the characteristic protein of connective tissue.

kolla = glue

gennan = to produce

Collagen is unique among body proteins, because it contains large amounts of the amino acid hydroxyproline, the hydroxy derivative of proline.

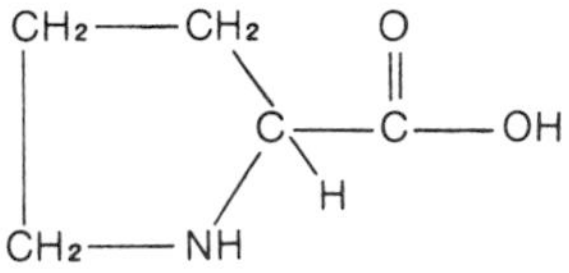

Proline

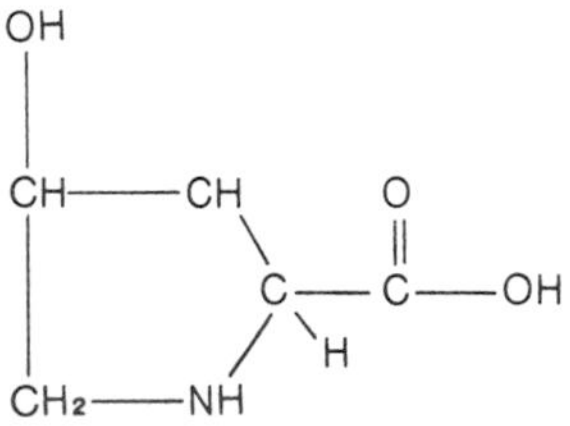

Hydroxyproline

Ion: see Appendix B. Iron is an atom that can exist in two ionic states, ferric (Fe^{+++}, lacking 3 electrons) or ferrous (Fe^{++}, lacking 2).

(which for the most part have clearly defined roles as coenzymes), vitamin C acts in ways that are imperfectly understood. It plays many different important roles in the body, and the secret may be that its mode of action is different in each case. In some settings it may act as a coenzyme or cofactor, assisting a specific enzyme in the performance of its job. In others, it may act in a more general way—for example, as an antioxidant. Often the conclusion reached by investigators studying vitamin C is that it has to "be present" for certain reactions to occur but that the mechanism of its action will require further research.

Collagen Formation

The best-understood metabolic role of vitamin C is its function in helping to form the protein collagen. Brief mention was made of this protein in Chapter 4; it is the single most important protein of connective tissue. It serves as the matrix on which bone is formed. It forms scars; when you have been wounded, collagen glues the separated tissue faces together. The cement that holds cells together is largely made of collagen; this function is especially important in the artery walls, which must expand and contract with each beat of the heart, and in the walls of the capillaries, which are thin and fragile and must withstand a pulse of blood every second or so without giving way.

Collagen, like all proteins, is formed by the stringing together of a chain of amino acids. An amino acid used in abundance to make collagen is proline. After proline is added to the chain, an enzyme adds an OH group to it, making hydroxyproline. This step, which completes the manufacture of collagen, requires oxygen and a special form of iron—the ferrous ion. This iron has a tendency to convert to another form (ferric ion), which the enzyme can't use. Vitamin C stands by to catch ferric ions and reconvert them to the ferrous form so that the enzyme can keep on working.[12] Figure 8-4 shows how this process is believed to occur.

12 The role of ascorbic acid in the hydroxylation of peptide-bound proline, *Nutrition Reviews* 37 (1979): 26-28.

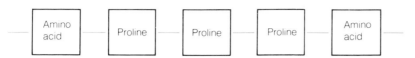

1. Amino acids are strung together in a chain that includes many prolines.

FIGURE 8–4 **How vitamin C helps form collagen.**

2. An enzyme, with the help of iron (Fe^{++}), adds OH groups to the prolines. Vitamin C stabilizes the iron in the ferrous form.

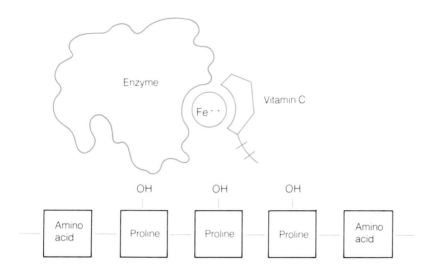

3. The completed collagen molecule contains many hydroxyproline units.

Antioxidant Action

Chemists call the two forms of iron just described oxidized and reduced iron. The oxidized (ferric) form has lost three electrons (see Appendix B); the reduced (ferrous) form has lost two. Any substance that can donate electrons to another is a reducing agent; when it donates its electrons it reduces another compound and simultaneously becomes oxidized itself. Vitamin C is such a compound.

The technicalities of oxidation-reduction reactions are not within our province, and the object of mentioning them is only to make one point clear. Many substances found in foods and important in the body can be altered or even destroyed by oxidation. (An example in Chapter 3 was oils that turn rancid when exposed to air.) Vitamin C—because it can be oxidized itself—can protect other substances from this destruction. Vitamin C is like a bodyguard for oxidizable substances; it stands ready to sacrifice its own life to save theirs. Unemotionally, the chemists call such a bodyguard an antioxidant.

Because of its antioxidant property, vitamin C is sometimes added to food products, not only to improve their nutritional value but also to protect important constituents from oxidation. In the intestines, it protects ferrous iron in this way. In the cells and body fluids, it probably helps to

For a picture of the way oxygen destroys the double bonds in an unsaturated fatty acid, see p. 95.

antioxidant: a compound that protects others from oxidation by being oxidized itself.

Chemists describe this action of vitamin C as maintaining the "oxidation-reduction equilibrium" or "redox state" and as participating in "electron transport."

chelating (KEE-late-ing) **agent**: a molecule that can assume a form suitable for trapping positive ions.

chele = claw

Chelation. The negative "arms" of the chelating agent are attracted to the positive charges of the ferrous ion.

The typical U.S. diet supplies only 5–6 mg iron in every 1,000 kcal. Children need 10 mg per day, and women need 18 mg (see Chapter 11).

protect other molecules—including the fat-soluble compounds vitamin A, vitamin E, and the polyunsaturated fatty acids—by maintaining their watery neighborhood in the appropriately reduced state. Vitamin E and the polyunsaturated fatty acids are important constituents of cell membranes, and these membranes house much of the cells' machinery. This machinery must be meticulously maintained so that the cells can live and work and so that they will discriminate successfully among the things that should cross their membranes and those that should be excluded. Vitamin C—perhaps by way of its ability to alternate between the oxidized and the reduced state—helps maintain these vital functions.

The Absorption of Iron

Vitamin C eaten at the same time as iron helps to promote the absorption of the iron. It is not yet known how the vitamin performs this service, but one intriguing possibility is entitled to an explanation.

You can't pick up a screw with a screwdriver—unless the screwdriver is magnetic. Even then, the screw may fall off at the slightest jolt. You can pick up a screw with a pair of pliers, but then you have to hold it tightly or it will fall out of their grip. But if you have a magnetic pair of pliers, you can hold the screw so securely that the only problem may be that you can't let it go. A chelating agent is the molecular equivalent of a magnetized pair of pliers, and vitamin C is an outstanding example of such a molecule. These molecules are especially good at holding onto positive ions such as ferrous iron (Fe^{++}). Vitamin C can grab and hold such an ion because it has two negative arms (see the diagram in the margin). Thus vitamin C can not only reduce iron but can also surround it. The resulting complex is more easily absorbed by the intestinal cells than iron alone.

It is now well known that eating foods containing vitamin C at the same meal with foods containing iron can double or triple the absorption of iron from those foods. This strategy is highly recommended for women and for children, whose kcalorie intakes are not large enough to guarantee that they will get enough iron from the foods they typically eat.

Some people try to protect the body from overwork by serving it different foods separately so that it can concentrate on handling those foods one at a time. Some evidence against this notion has already been presented (Chapter 5). The cooperation between vitamin C and iron, which seldom appear together in any one food, provides another argument against this simplistic notion. You can recognize many false claims by the implication that foods should be ingested singly to ease the body's work. On the contrary, multicolored, mixed dishes are probably those to which the body, as well as the eye and the palate, responds most gratefully.

Caution

Amino Acid Metabolism

Vitamin C is involved in the metabolism of several amino acids. In at least some instances it probably functions as it does during collagen formation, by keeping iron in a reduced state to aid an enzyme in adding OH groups to other compounds. Some of these amino acids may end up being converted to hormones of great importance in body functioning, among them norepinephrine and thyroxin.

The adrenal glands contain a higher concentration of vitamin C than any other organ in the body, and during stress they release large quantities of the vitamin together with the stress hormones epinephrine and norepinephrine. What the vitamin has to do with the stress reaction is unclear, but it is known that stress increases vitamin C needs.

Vitamin C is also needed for the synthesis of thyroxin, which regulates the rate of metabolism. The metabolic rate speeds up under extreme stress and also when you need to produce more heat—for example, in fever or cold weather. Thus infections and exposure to cold increase your needs for vitamin C. Perhaps its involvement in the fever response to infection explains the vitamin's possible effects on cold prevention and symptom reduction. (Highlight 8B explores these effects as well as the relationship between vitamin C and cancer.)

In scurvy, protein metabolism may be altered, resulting in negative nitrogen balance. No one knows why this occurs, but the involvement of vitamin C with amino acids provides a notable example of the way nutrients of different classes cooperate with one another to maintain health.

Vitamin C Deficiency

In both the United States and Canada, vitamin C deficiency is still seen, despite the past century's explosion of nutrition knowledge. In the United States, the Ten-State Survey showed evidence of unacceptable serum levels of vitamin C in about 15 percent of all age groups studied, with symptoms of outright scurvy showing up in 4 percent. The more recent National Food Consumption Survey showed intakes below two-thirds of the RDA for 20 to 30 percent of all persons surveyed (see Chapter 12). Especially in infants, teenagers, and people over 60 years of age, intakes of vitamin C were much lower than the RDA (less than 50 percent). In Canada, many Eskimos and Indians and some members of the general population have deficiency symptoms. Evidently we all need to be alerted to the symptoms that can result and to make efforts to obtain enough of this vitamin.

With an adequate intake, the body maintains a fixed pool of vitamin C and rapidly excretes any excess in the urine. With an inadequate intake, the pool becomes depleted at the rate of about 3 percent a day. Obvious deficiency symptoms don't begin to appear until the pool has been reduced to about a fifth of its optimal size, and this may take two months or more to occur. Thus the first sign of a developing vitamin C deficiency is a

latent: the period in disease when the conditions are present but before the symptoms have begun to appear.

latens = lying hidden

overt: out in the open, full-blown.

ouvrire = to open

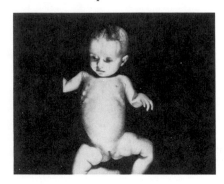

Infant scurvy. This is the characteristic "scorbutic pose," with legs bent and thighs rotated open. The infant's joints are painful and she will cry if made to move.

Source: From C. Conn, *The Specialities in General Practice*, 2nd ed. (Philadelphia: Saunders, 1957).

Early skin symptoms of scurvy. There is a tiny hemorrhage around each hair follicle. These pinpoint hemorrhages are called **petechiae** (pet-EEK-ee-eye).

Source: Courtesy of Dr. Samuel Dreizen, D.D.S., M.D.

lowered serum or plasma vitamin C concentration.[13] A low intake as revealed by the diet history is the cue that prompts the diagnostician to request a clinical test to measure the body's vitamin C levels.

As the pool size continues to fall, latent scurvy appears. Two of the earliest signs have to do with the role of the vitamin in maintaining capillary integrity. The gums around teeth bleed easily, and capillaries under the skin break spontaneously producing pinpoint hemorrhages. If the vitamin levels continue to fall, the symptoms of overt scurvy appear. Failure to promote normal collagen synthesis causes further hemorrhaging. Muscles, including the heart muscle, may degenerate. The skin becomes rough, brown, scaly, and dry. Wounds fail to heal because scar tissue will not form. Bone rebuilding is not maintained; the ends of the long bones become softened, malformed, and painful, and fractures appear. The teeth may become loose in the jawbone and fillings may loosen and fall out. Anemia is frequently seen, and infections are common. There are also characteristic psychological signs, including hysteria and depression. Sudden death is likely, perhaps because of massive bleeding into the joints and body cavities.

Once diagnosed, scurvy is readily reversed by vitamin C. It can be cured within about five days. Moderate doses in the neighborhood of 100 milligrams per day are all that are needed.

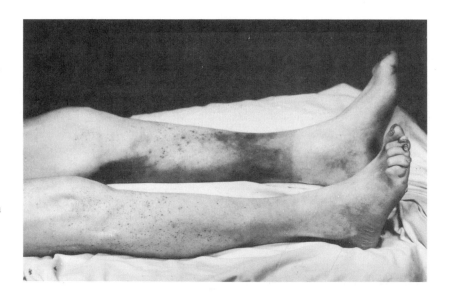

13   Vitamin C shifts unpredictably between the plasma and the white blood cells known as leukocytes; thus a plasma or serum determination may not accurately reflect the body's pool. The appropriate clinical test may be a measurement of leukocyte vitamin C. A combination of both tests may be more reliable than either one alone. Chapters 1 and 12 discuss general principles of clinical testing.

Recommended Intakes of Vitamin C

How much vitamin C is enough? Allowances recommended by different nations vary from as low as 30 milligrams per day in Britain and Canada to 60 milligrams per day in the United States and 75 in Germany. The requirement—the amount needed to prevent the appearance of the overt deficiency symptoms of scurvy—is well known to be only 10 milligrams, but 10 milligrams a day apparently do not saturate all the body tissues, because larger intakes have been observed to increase the body's total vitamin C pool. At about 60 milligrams per day the pool size in the average person stops responding to further increases in intake, and at 100 milligrams per day, 95 percent of the population probably reach tissue saturation. After the tissues are saturated, all added vitamin C is excreted.[14]

It may seem strange that of the United States and Canada, two similar industrialized nations, one should recommend twice the vitamin C intake of the other. In view of the wide range of possible intakes, however, the Canadian and U.S. recommendations are not so far apart. Both are generously above the minimum requirement, and both are well below the level at which toxicity symptoms might appear. The range of possible intakes, illustrated in the margin, shows that the Canadian and U.S. allowances are in the same ballpark. In contrast, the recommendation by Dr. Pauling and others that people should take 2 to 4 grams a day (or even 10 grams) is clearly 'way up in the clouds.

It is important to remember that recommended allowances for vitamin C, like those for all the nutrients, are amounts intended to maintain health in healthy people, not to restore health in sick people. Unusual circumstances may increase nutrient needs. In the case of vitamin C, a variety of stresses deplete the body pool and may make intakes higher than 50 milligrams or so desirable. Among the stresses known to increase vitamin C needs are infections; burns; extremely high or low temperatures; toxic levels of heavy metals such as lead, mercury, and cadmium; and the chronic use of certain medications, including aspirin, barbiturates, and oral contraceptives.[15] After a major operation (such as removal of a breast) or extensive burns, when a tremendous amount of scar tissue must form during healing, the amount needed may be as high as 1,000 milligrams (1 gram) a day or even more.

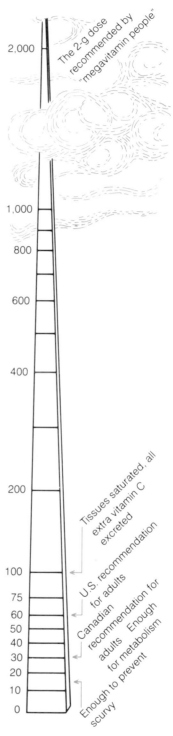

Recommendations for vitamin C intake (mg).

14   A. Kallner, D. Hartmann, and D. Hornig, Steady-state turnover and body pool of ascorbic acid in man, *American Journal of Clinical Nutrition* 32 (1979): 530–539.

15   F. Clark, Drugs and vitamin deficiency, *Journal of Human Nutrition* 30 (1976): 333–337; Committee on Safety, Toxicity, and Misuse of Vitamins and Trace Minerals, National Nutrition Consortium, *Vitamin-Mineral Safety, Toxicity, and Misuse* (Chicago: American Dietetic Association, 1978). Cigarette smoking may increase the need for vitamin C. One experiment suggests that an intake of at least 140 milligrams per day is required for one-pack-a-day smokers to reach steady-state body pools comparable to those of nonsmokers: A. B. Kallner, D. Hartmann, and D. H. Hornig, On the requirements of ascorbic acid in man: Steady-state turnover and body pool in smokers, *American Journal of Clinical Nutrition* 34 (1981): 1347–1355.

Vitamin C Toxicity

Remember the distinction between the *requirement* and the recommended *allowance or standard* (see pp. 19, 21).

When vitamin C is inactivated and degraded, a product along the way is oxalate, which can form stones in the kidneys. People can also have oxalate crystals in their kidneys that are not due to vitamin C overdoses.

The anticlotting agents with which vitamin C interferes are such anticoagulants as warfarin and dicoumarol.

gout (gowt): a metabolic disease in which crystals of uric acid precipitate in the joints.

The easy availability of vitamin C in pill form and the publication of Dr. Pauling's book recommending intakes of over 2 grams a day have led thousands of people to take vitamin C megadoses. Not surprisingly, instances have surfaced of vitamin C's causing harm.

Some of the suspected toxic effects of megadoses have not been confirmed. Among these are formation of stones in the kidneys, upset of the body's acid-base balance, destruction of vitamin B_{12} resulting in a deficiency, and interference with the action of vitamin E. Research and reasoning have demonstrated that these effects are theoretically possible, but no cases of their actual occurrence in human beings have yet been seen with intakes as high as 3 grams a day.

Other toxic effects, however, have been seen often enough to warrant concern. Nausea, abdominal cramps, and diarrhea are often reported. Several instances of interference with medical regimens are known. The large amounts of vitamin C excreted in the urine obscure the results of tests used to detect diabetes, giving a false positive result in some instances and a false negative result in others. People taking medications to prevent their blood from clotting may unwittingly abolish the effect of these medicines if they also take massive doses of vitamin C. Vitamin C megadoses can also enhance iron absorption too much, resulting in iron overload (see Chapter 11).

People of certain genetic backgrounds are more likely to be harmed by vitamin C megadoses than others. Some black Americans, Sephardic Jews, Orientals, and certain other ethnic groups have an inherited enzyme deficiency that makes them susceptible to any strong reducing agent. Megadoses of vitamin C can make their red blood cells burst, causing hemolytic anemia. Those with sickle-cell anemia may also be more vulnerable to megadoses of vitamin C. In sickle-cell anemia, the hemoglobin protein is abnormal; it responds to a reducing agent by assuming a shape that distorts the red blood cells, making them clump and clog capillaries. Those who have a tendency toward gout and those who have a genetic abnormality that alters the way they break down vitamin C to its excretion products are more prone to forming stones if they take megadoses of C.

The proponents of vitamin C megadoses argue that these conditions are very rare and that the "normal" person need not worry about them. Opponents angrily retort that they are *not* rare and that nobody is "normal." The enzyme abnormality mentioned above occurs in about 13 percent of black Americans and in a higher percentage of Sephardic Jews and Orientals.[16] If you have few acquaintances among these ethnic

16 The risks of vitamin C overdosing for special genetic types are spelled out by V. Herbert, Facts and fictions about megavitamin therapy, *Journal of the Florida Medical Association* 66 (April 1979): 475–481.

groups, then this condition may seem rare to you, but if you know more than ten such people, or if you are a member of any of these groups yourself, the risks of taking massive doses of vitamin C may apply directly to you or to one of your friends.

No two people have the same genetic heritage. Nobody has a complete set of "normal" genes and enzymes. No two people's nutrient needs—or nutritional risks—are exactly alike. There are doubtless some whose needs for vitamin C are higher than the average, and there are also some for whom the risks are more severe. Perhaps the greatest risk in speculating about megadosing with vitamin C or any other nutrient is the risk of generalizing. What is safe for your friend many not be safe for you.

A statement that applies to nearly all people does not apply to all people.

Caution

The body of a person who has taken large doses of vitamin C for a long time adjusts by limiting absorption and destroying and excreting more of the vitamin than usual.[17] If the person then suddenly reduces her intake to normal, the accelerated disposal system can't put on its brakes fast enough to avoid destroying too much of the vitamin. Some case histories have shown that adults who discontinue megadosing develop scurvy on intakes that would protect a normal adult. An innocent victim of this kind of error is the newborn baby of a megadoser. In his mother's womb he has adjusted to high levels of vitamin C; once born into an environment providing much smaller amounts, he develops scurvy, a withdrawal reaction.

vitamin C dependency: a temporary condition manifested in the withdrawal symptoms experienced by the person who stops overdosing; the body has adjusted to a high intake and so "needs" a high intake until it can readjust.

withdrawal reaction: a reaction to withdrawal (usually of a drug) that reveals that the user has become dependent, as when an infant born of a mother who took massive doses of vitamin C develops scurvy on an intake that would be adequate for the average infant.

The experience of a person who stops megadosing and then manifests vitamin C deficiency symptoms on a normal intake may lead him to the wrong conclusion. "I took 3 grams a day," he may say, "and then when I stopped my gums started to bleed and I knew I was vitamin C–deficient. Don't you see, that proves I need very high doses? The recommended 30 to 60 milligrams are not nearly enough for me."

In reality, this person has deceived himself. To see whether the recommended, moderate intake of vitamin C is sufficient, he will have to taper off, reducing his large intakes gradually and allowing his body to adjust back to the normal condition. The emergence of withdrawal symptoms from drug doses of vitamin C does not prove a need, any more than the emergence of withdrawal symptoms in a person giving up heroin or alcohol proves that he needs heroin or alcohol. The addict's body appears to need the drug only because it has adapted in order to cope with the drug, not because the drug is an essential nutrient. The consequences of drug abuse cannot be used to justify continued drug use. In these cases, though, medical help may be needed to assist in withdrawal.

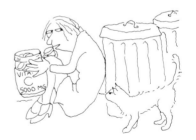

Caution

A **pharmacological dose** is higher than the intake needed to prevent deficiency symptoms and may have unexpected effects, as it may be working by a mechanism different from the one by which the preventive or **physiological dose** works. See the discussion on p. 291.

After reviewing the published research on large doses of vitamin C, the National Nutrition Consortium reported in 1978 that there are probably very few instances in which taking more than 100 to 300 milligrams a day is beneficial. Adults may not be exposing themselves to very severe risks if they choose to dose themselves with 1 to 2 grams a day, but above 2 grams, "genuine caution should be exercised," and amounts above 8 grams per day may be "distinctly harmful. It is irresponsible and inexcusable to proclaim that ascorbic acid is safe in any amounts that may be ingested."[18]

In conclusion, the range of safe vitamin C intakes seems to be broad, as is typical for water-soluble vitamins. Between the absolute minimum of 10 milligrams a day and the reasonable maximum of 1,000 milligrams, nearly everyone should be able to find a suitable intake. People who venture outside these limits do so at their own risk.

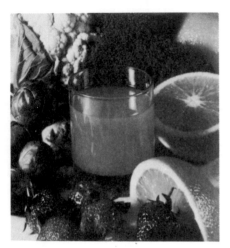

Foods rich in vitamin C.

Vitamin C in Fruits and Vegetables

The inclusion of intelligently selected fruits and vegetables in the daily diet guarantees a generous intake of vitamin C. Even those who wish to ingest amounts well above the recommended 30 to 60 milligrams can easily meet their goals this way. If you drink a double portion of orange juice at breakfast, choose a salad for lunch, and include a stalk of broccoli and a potato on your dinner plate, you will exceed 300 milligrams even before counting the contributions made by incidental other sources. Clearly, then, you would have no need for vitamin C pills unless you wanted to join the ranks of the megadosers.

Table 8–7 shows the amounts of vitamin C in various common foods and reveals that the citrus fruits are rightly famous for being rich in vitamin C. But certain vegetables and some other fruits are in the same league: broccoli, brussels sprouts, cantaloupe, and strawberries. A single serving of any of these provides more than 30 milligrams of the vitamin.

staple: a food kept on hand at all times and used daily or almost daily in meal preparation.

The humble potato is an important source of vitamin C in Western countries, not because a potato by itself meets the daily needs but because potatoes are such a popular staple and are eaten so frequently that overall they make substantial contributions. They provide about 20 percent of all the vitamin C in the U.S. diet. Some young men report french fries as their only regular source of vitamin C, and yet because they eat so many, they receive the recommended amount.

Hexose: see p. 55.

One factor influencing the amount of vitamin C found in a fruit or vegetable is the amount of sun it is exposed to. The reason for this is clear if you realize that the vitamin, being a hexose, is a member of the carbohydrate family and that carbohydrates are produced by photosynthesis. No vitamin C is found in seeds, only in growing plants. Thus grains (breads and cereals) contain negligible amounts of the vitamin. Milk is also a notoriously poor source, and this is why food sources of vitamin C are added early to an infant's diet.

18   Committee on Safety, Toxicity, and Misuse of Vitamins and Trace Minerals, 1978, p. 17.

TABLE 8–7 **Vitamin C—Average Amounts in Groups of Foods** TH8-5

	VITAMIN C (mg)
Milk and Milk Products	
1 c milk or 1 oz cheese	-0-
Meat and Legumes	
3 oz meat, fish, or poultry	-0-
3 oz liver	25
1 egg	-0-
¾ c legumes, cooked	-0-
Fruits and Vegetables	
1 portion citrus or other vitamin C-rich fruit[a]	50
1 portion or piece other fruit	15
1 portion vitamin C-rich vegetable[b]	55
1 portion other vegetable (including lettuce, tomatoes, potatoes)	15
Grains	
1 slice bread or ½ c rice or pasta	-0-
1 portion cereal[c]	-0-
Other	
1 tbsp fat or oil	-0-
1 tbsp sugar or sweets	-0-
1 c soup	5
1 tbsp brewer's yeast	-0-

A person who follows the four food group plan recommendation of consuming one vitamin C-rich vegetable or fruit a day is guaranteed an adequate intake of vitamin C. (The U.S. RDA is 60 mg.)

This table was made by consulting Appendix H, averaging the vitamin C amounts in standard portions of the commonly used foods in each category, and rounding off each average to the nearest 5 mg. (Thus, 0 doesn't mean no vitamin C but rather, less than 3 mg.) Values agree approximately with the USDA table, Nutrients furnished by servings of foods, *Essentials of an Adequate Diet*, Bulletin no. 160, 1956.
[a] ½ c orange or grapefruit juice or cranberry juice cocktail; 1 orange or ½ grapefruit; ¼ cantaloupe; ¾ c papaya; ⅔ c strawberries.
[b] ½ c broccoli, brussels sprouts, cauliflower, collards, kale; or 1 pod raw sweet pepper.
[c] Fortified cereals contain added vitamin C. Read the label.

No animal foods other than the organ meats contain vitamin C. For this reason, if for no other, fruits and vegetables must be included in any diet to make it adequate.

Summing Up

The B vitamins serve as coenzymes assisting many enzymes in the body. Thiamin, riboflavin, niacin, and pantothenic acid are especially important in the glucose-to-energy pathway; they are active in the coenzymes TPP, FAD, NAD^+, and CoA respectively. Vitamin B_6 facilitates amino acid transformations and thus protein metabolism; folacin is involved in pathways leading to the synthesis of new cells, and vitamin B_{12} in the making of folacin coenzymes; and biotin is involved in lipid synthesis. Coenzymes have many other roles.

B-vitamin deficiencies seldom occur in isolation; all have multiple symptoms affecting each body organ and tissue in proportion to the roles they play there. A lack of thiamin causes beriberi; a lack of niacin (unless compensated for by its amino acid precursor tryptophan) causes pellagra; a lack of vitamin B_{12} causes pernicious anemia. Human deficiencies of the other B vitamins, although not given names, have been observed for riboflavin, vitamin B_6, and folacin.

Thiamin is widely distributed in foods, but no food contributes a very great amount of it; a balanced and varied diet of nutritious food will best assure an adequate intake. Riboflavin is concentrated in milk and meats. Niacin is found wherever protein is found and can also be made from the amino acid tryptophan. These three vitamins (and iron) also are added to all enriched breads and cereals. Vitamin B_6 is most abundant in meats, vitamin B_{12} is found only in animal products, and folacin is supplied best by green, leafy vegetables. Any diet plan that includes moderate amounts of all these foods assures probable adequacy for these nutrients.

Vitamin C acts as an antioxidant, helping to maintain iron in its reduced (ferrous ion) form and thus cooperating with enzymes that require this form of iron as a cofactor. The vitamin also helps regulate the overall oxidation-reduction state of the body cells and fluids. In cooperation with iron it promotes the formation of the protein collagen, which is needed for scar tissue, intercellular cement, connective tissues (especially those of capillaries and other blood vessels), and the matrix of bones and teeth. It is involved in the metabolism of several amino acids, including the precursors of the hormones norepinephrine and thyroxin.

Deficiency of vitamin C causes scurvy, but scurvy is prevented by the daily intake of only 10 milligrams of vitamin C and can be cured by a few days of 100-milligram doses.

Recommended daily intakes of vitamin C range from 30 milligrams (Canada) to 60 milligrams (United States) or slightly higher (Germany). Toxic effects of megadoses (3 to 10 grams) have been reported. The sudden discontinuance of megadoses may unveil an induced dependency, and scurvy may occur when intake is reduced to normal.

The best food sources of vitamin C are the citrus fruits, strawberries and cantaloupe, broccoli and other members of the cabbage family, and greens. Important "fair" sources include tomatoes, green peas, and (because they are eaten frequently by many people) potatoes.

NOTE: Appendix J offers additional readings. See "Nutrition and Disease," "Nutrition and Drugs," and "Vitamins," as well as the general references.

Optional lectures in the *Instructor's Manual* offer details on the differences between enriched and whole-grain bread ("Foods in the Home"), vitamin B_{12} in vegetarian diets ("Vegetarian Diet Planning"), and the scandalous story of vitamin B_{15} ("Ripoffs").

The Self-Study for this chapter (in Appendix Q) shows you how to:

● Estimate and evaluate your dietary intakes of thiamin, riboflavin, niacin, folacin, and vitamin C.
● Plan a diet adequate in riboflavin for someone who doesn't drink milk.
● Identify non-fruit sources of vitamin C.
● Detect false claims about vitamins.

HIGHLIGHT 8A
Alcohol and Nutrition

> *Narcotics diminish the oxidation of sugar by the brain. . . . Thought and behavior alter. If the conditions be prolonged, unconsciousness ensues, and if prolonged further the brain-cells are permanently damaged.*

SIR CHARLES SHERRINGTON

If liver cells could talk, they would describe the alcohol of intoxicating beverages as demanding, egocentric, and disruptive of the liver's normally efficient way of running its business. For example, liver cells prefer fatty acids as their fuel, but when alcohol is present, they are forced to use it and let the fatty acids accumulate in huge stockpiles.

Alcohol affects every organ of the body, but the most dramatic evidence of its disruptive behavior appears in the liver. This is the only organ whose cells can oxidize alcohol for fuel to any great extent. All other cells are affected by the presence of alcohol but can do practically nothing about getting rid of it. Liver cells make nearly all of the body's alcohol-processing machinery—namely, the enzyme alcohol dehydrogenase and the MEOS, described below. Alcohol dehydrogenase can convert alcohol to acetaldehyde, which can in turn be converted to acetyl CoA, the compound that all energy nutrients become on their way to being used as fuel. But we are getting ahead of our story. Let's start at the beginning, when alcohol first enters the body in a beverage, and follow it until it leaves or is made into useful acetyl CoA.

Alcohol Enters the Body

To the chemist, *alcohol* refers to a class of compounds containing reactive hydroxyl (OH) groups. The glycerol to which fatty acids are attached in triglycerides is an example of an alcohol to a chemist. But to the average person, *alcohol* refers to the intoxicating ingredient in beer, wine, and hard liquor (distilled spirits). The chemist's name for this particular alcohol is *ethanol*. Glycerol has three carbons with three hydroxyl groups attached; ethanol has only two carbons and one hydroxyl group. For the remainder of this Highlight we will be discussing "alcohol," but you will know that we are really talking about a particular alcohol—ethanol.

From the moment alcohol enters the body in a beverage, it is treated as if it has special privileges. Foods sit around in the stomach for a while, but not alcohol. The tiny alcohol molecules need no digestion; they can diffuse as soon as they arrive, right through the walls of the stomach, and they

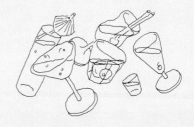

alcohol dehydrogenase: a liver enzyme that converts ethanol to **acetaldehyde** (ass-et-AL-duh-hide). The MEOS also oxidizes alcohol; see below.

Glycerol is an alcohol.

Ethanol is the alcohol in beer, wine, and distilled spirits.

305

euphoria (you-FORE-ee-uh): a feeling of great well-being, that people often seek through the use of drugs such as alcohol.

eu = good

phoria = bearing

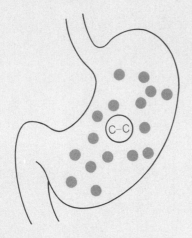

The alcohol (C-C) in a stomach filled with food has a low probability of touching the walls and diffusing through.

V.I.P. (Very Important Person): a person with special privileges.

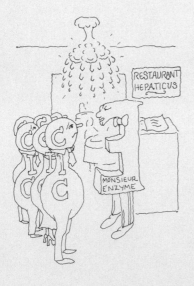

If more molecules of alcohol arrive at the liver cells than the enzymes can handle, the extra molecules must wait.

reach the brain within a minute. You can feel euphoric right away when you drink, especially if your stomach is empty. When your stomach is full of food, the molecules of alcohol have less chance of touching the walls and diffusing through, so you don't feel the effects of alcohol so quickly. If you don't want to become intoxicated at parties, then, eat the snacks provided by the host. Carbohydrate snacks are best suited for slowing alcohol absorption. High-fat snacks help too, because they slow peristalsis.[1] But when the stomach contents are emptied into the duodenum, it doesn't matter that plenty of food is mixed with the alcohol. The alcohol is absorbed rapidly anyway, "as if it were a V.I.P."[2]

Alcohol Arrives in the Liver

The capillaries that surround the digestive tract merge into the veins that carry the alcohol-laden blood to the liver. Here the veins branch and rebranch into capillaries that touch every liver cell. As already mentioned, liver cells are the only cells in the body that can make enough alcohol dehydrogenase to oxidize alcohol at an appreciable rate.

There is a limit to the amount of alcohol anyone can process in a given time. This limit is set by the number of molecules of the enzyme alcohol dehydrogenase that reside in the liver. If more molecules of alcohol arrive at the liver cells than the enzymes can handle, the extra alcohol must wait. It enters the general circulation and moves on past the liver. From the liver it is carried to all parts of the body, circulating again and again through the liver until enzymes are available to convert it to acetaldehyde.

The rate at which alcohol dehydrogenase can work limits the rate of the body's handling of alcohol. The type of enzyme produced varies with individuals, depending on the genes they have inherited. Some racial groups—for example, Orientals—have genetic information that causes them to produce atypical forms of alcohol dehydrogenase and its partner enzyme acetaldehyde dehydrogenase. The difference explains why some persons are made too uncomfortable by alcohol to become addicted.[3]

The amount of alcohol dehydrogenase is also affected by whether you eat or not. Fasting for as little as a day causes degradation of the enzyme (protein) within the cells, and can reduce the rate of alcohol metabolism by half. Drinking on an empty stomach thus not only lets the drinker feel the effects more promptly but also brings about higher blood alcohol levels for longer periods of time and increases the effect of alcohol in anesthetizing the brain.

1   A. B. Eisenstein, Nutritional and metabolic effects of alcohol, *Journal of the American Dietetic Association* 81 (1982): 247–251.

2   F. Iber, In alcoholism, the liver sets the pace, *Nutrition Today*, January/February 1971, pp. 2–9.

3   Alcohol dehydrogenase, although atypical, works as fast as normal in Orientals, but their acetaldehyde dehydrogenase works more *slowly* so that they suffer from a kind of acetaldehyde poisoning. D. P. Agarwal, S. Harada, and H. W. Goedde, Racial differences in biological sensitivity to ethanol—the role of alcohol dehydrogenase and acetaldehyde dehydrogenase enzymes, *Alcoholism: Clinical and Experimental Research* 5 (1981): 12–16.

Alcohol dehydrogenase converts alcohol to acetaldehyde. Simultaneously it converts a molecule of NAD^+ to $NADH + H^+$. (You may recall that the N in NAD^+ is a form of niacin, one of the B vitamins.) The related enzyme acetaldehyde dehydrogenase converts another NAD^+ to $NADH + H^+$ while it converts acetaldehyde to acetyl CoA, the compound that enters the TCA cycle to generate energy.[4] Thus whenever alcohol is being metabolized in the body, NAD^+ is consumed, and NADH accumulates. Chemists describe the consequence by saying that the body's "redox state" is altered, because NAD^+ can reduce, and NADH can oxidize, many other body compounds. During alcohol metabolism, NAD^+ becomes unavailable for the multitude of reactions for which it is required.

Figure 8A–1 is a drawing of the pathway from glucose to energy, showing the many places along the way that require NAD^+. The drawing of pathways like this one seems to be a favorite pastime of chemists and a most

The conversion of ethanol to acetyl CoA. TH8-6

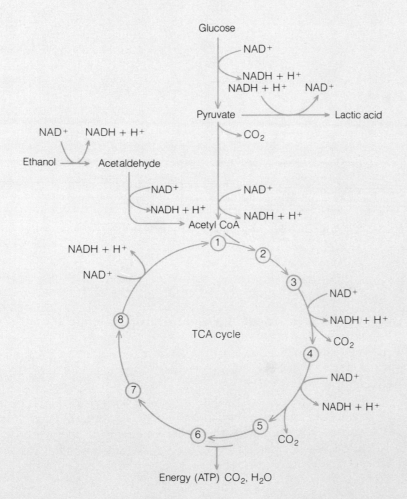

FIGURE H8A–1 **A simplified version of the glucose-to-energy pathway, showing the entry of ethanol into the pathway.** The coenzyme NAD^+ that is the active form of niacin is the only one included. TH8-7

4   All cells possess acetaldehyde dehydrogenase, so this step can take place elsewhere besides the liver.

unfavorite activity for beginning nutrition students. If you are such a student, take a moment with us to look carefully at this map. It should be pleasing to see how an acquaintanceship with the basics of metabolism enables you to gain insight into processes like the body's handling of alcohol.

Maps can be simple or complex, according to need. Sometimes when you ask for directions, the names of the streets don't matter, but certainly you need to be told of possible obstacles. Figure 8A–1 names only the "streets" that are crucial to your understanding, and shows where there may be obstacles that will cause traffic to back up or necessitate an alternate route.

The map shows that for glucose to get completely metabolized the TCA cycle must be operating, and NAD^+ must be present. If they are not (and when alcohol is present they may not be), the road will be blocked and traffic will back up—or an alternate route will be taken. There are physical consequences to such changes in the normal flow of traffic from glucose to available energy. Think about some of these as you follow the diagram.

Acetyl CoAs are blocked from getting into the TCA cycle by the high level of NADH. Instead of being used for energy, they become building blocks for fatty acids.

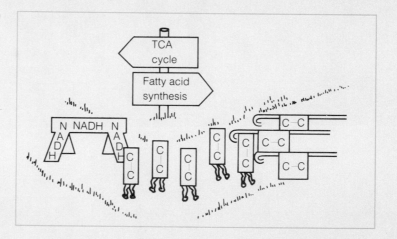

In each step where NAD^+ is converted to $NADH + H^+$, hydrogen ions accumulate. (As a result, the acid-base balance shifts toward acid; this is dangerous.) The accumulation of NADH depresses the TCA cycle, so that pyruvate and acetyl CoA build up. The excess acetyl CoA then takes the route to the synthesis of fatty acids. (Fat clogs the liver so it cannot function.[5])

The body's altered redox state interferes with the process by which the liver generates glucose from protein. The unavailability of glucose from this source, together with the overabundance of acetyl CoA molecules blocked from getting into the TCA cycle, set the stage for a shift into ketosis. The making of ketones consumes acetyl CoA, but some ketones are acids, so they push the acid-base balance further toward acid.

5   C. S. Lieber, Liver adaptation and injury in alcoholism, *New England Journal of Medicine* 288 (1973): 356–361.

The surplus of NADH also favors the conversion of pyruvate to lactic acid, which serves as a temporary storage place for hydrogens from NADH. The conversion of pyruvate to lactic acid relieves the accumulation of NADH + H⁺, but a lactic acid buildup has serious consequences of its own. It adds still further to the body's acid burden and interferes with the excretion of uric acid, causing goutlike symptoms.

The presence of alcohol alters amino acid metabolism in the liver cells. Synthesis of some proteins important in the immune system slows down, weakening the body's defenses against infection. Synthesis of lipoproteins speeds up, increasing blood triglyceride levels.

Protein deficiency develops, both from the depression of protein synthesis in the cells and from poor diet. Normally the cells would at least use the amino acids that a person happened to eat, but the drinker's liver deaminates the amino acids and channels their carbon backbones into fat or ketones. Eating well does not protect the drinker from protein depletion. One has to stop drinking alcohol for complete protection.

The synthesis of fatty acids also accelerates as a result of the liver's exposure to alcohol. Fat accumulation can be seen in the liver after a single night of heavy drinking. Fatty liver, the first stage of liver deterioration seen in heavy drinkers, interferes with the distribution of nutrients and oxygen to the liver cells. If the condition lasts long enough, the liver cells will die and the area will be invaded by fibrous scar tissue—the second stage of liver deterioration, called fibrosis. Fibrosis is reversible with good nutrition and abstinence from alcohol, but the next (last) stage—cirrhosis—is not.

Alcohol affects every tissue's metabolism of nutrients in other ways as well. Stomach cells oversecrete acid and histamine, becoming vulnerable to inflammation and ulcer formation. Intestinal cells fail to absorb thiamin, folacin, and vitamin B_{12}. Liver cells lose efficiency in activating vitamin D, and alter their production and excretion of bile. Rod cells in the retina, which normally process vitamin A alcohol to its aldehyde form needed in vision, find themselves processing ethanol to acetaldehyde instead. The kidney excretes increased quantities of magnesium, calcium, potassium, and zinc.

Acetaldehyde interferes with metabolism, too. It dislodges the vitamin B_6 coenzyme pyridoxine from its protective binding protein, so that it is destroyed, causing a vitamin B_6 deficiency and, thereby, lowered production of red blood cells.

The liver's V.I.P. treatment of alcohol is reflected in its handling of drugs, as well as nutrients. In addition to the enzyme alcohol dehydrogenase, the liver possesses an enzyme system that metabolizes *both* alcohol and drugs—any compounds that have certain chemical features in common. Called the MEOS, this system handles only about one fifth of the total alcohol a person consumes, but the MEOS enlarges if repeatedly exposed to alcohol. This may not make the drinker able to handle much more alcohol at a time than before, because the total alcohol-metabolizing ability of the MEOS is small, but the effect on the ability to metabolize drugs is considerable.

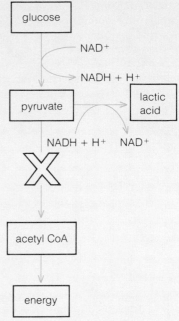

Pyruvate is converted to lactic acid if the pathway to acetyl CoA is blocked. TH8-6

gout (GOWT): accumulation of uric acid crystals in the joints.

fatty liver: an early stage of liver deterioration seen in several diseases, including kwashiorkor and alcoholic liver disease. Fatty liver is characterized by accumulation of fat in the liver cells.

fibrosis: an intermediate stage of liver deterioration seen in several diseases, including viral hepatitis and alcoholic liver disease. In fibrosis the liver cells lose their function and assume the characteristics of connective tissue cells (fibers).

cirrhosis (seer-OH-sis): advanced liver disease, in which liver cells have died, hardened, and turned orange; usually associated with alcoholism.

cirrhos = an orange

MEOS (microsomal ethanol oxidizing system): a system of enzymes in the liver that oxidizes not only alcohol but also several classes of drugs. (The microsomes are tiny particles of membranes with associated enzymes that can be collected from broken-up cells.)

micro = tiny

soma = body

When the MEOS enlarges, it makes the body able to metabolize drugs much faster than before. This can make it confusing and tricky to work out the correct doses of medications. The doctor may prescribe sedatives every four hours, for example, assuming the patient does not drink, and expecting the MEOS to dispose of the drug at a certain predicted rate. Well and good; but if the patient does drink and uses the drug at the same time, the drug will be much more potent. The MEOS is busy disposing of alcohol, the drug can't be handled till later; and the dose may build up to where it greatly oversedates, even kills, the patient.

The opposite effect is seen if the prescription is written for a drinker whose liver is adapted to metabolizing large quantities of alcohol. When this patient takes the drug (and does *not* drink simultaneously), the drug's effects wear off unexpectedly fast, leaving the patient undersedated. Imagine the doctor's alarm if the patient wakes up on the table during an operation! (A skilled anesthesiologist always asks the patient about his drinking pattern before putting him to sleep.)

Ethanol Arrives in the Brain

narcotic (nar-KOT-ic): any drug that dulls the senses, induces sleep, and becomes addictive with prolonged use.

Alcohol is a narcotic. It was used for centuries as an anesthetic because of its ability to deaden pain. But it wasn't a very good anesthetic, because one could never be sure how much a person would need and how much would be a lethal dose. As new, more predictable anesthetics were discovered, they quickly replaced alcohol. However, alcohol continues to be used today as a kind of anesthetic on social occasions, to help people relax or to relieve anxiety. People think that alcohol is a stimulant, because it seems to make them lively and uninhibited at first. Actually, though, the way it does this is by sedating *inhibitory* nerves, which are more numerous than excitatory nerves. Ultimately, it acts as a depressant, because it affects all the nerve cells.

When alcohol flows to the brain it reaches the frontal lobe first, the reasoning part. As the alcohol molecules diffuse into the cells of this lobe, they interfere with reasoning and judgment. If additional molecules continue to enter the bloodstream from the digestive tract before the liver has had time to oxidize the first ones, then the speech and vision centers of the brain become narcotized, and the area that governs reasoning becomes more incapacitated. Later the cells of the brain responsible for large-muscle control are affected; at this point, people "under the influence" stagger or weave when they try to walk. Finally, the conscious brain is completely subdued and the person "passes out." Now, luckily, he can drink no more; if he could, he might die, because the anesthetic effect could reach the deepest brain centers that control breathing and heartbeat. Table 8A–1 shows the blood alcohol levels that correspond with progressively greater intoxication.

In one way, you might consider it lucky that the brain centers are organized as they are, and respond to alcohol in the order just described. One passes out before one can drink a lethal dose. It is possible, though, to drink fast enough that the effects of alcohol continue to accelerate after one has gone to sleep. The occasional death that takes place during a

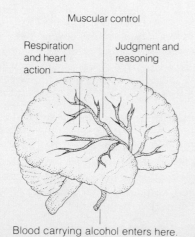

Muscular control

Respiration and heart action

Judgment and reasoning

Blood carrying alcohol enters here.

TABLE H8A–1 **Alcohol Doses and Brain Responses**

NUMBER OF DRINKS	BLOOD ALCOHOL	EFFECT ON BRAIN
2 drinks	0.05%	Judgment impaired
4 drinks	0.10%	Control impaired
6 drinks	0.15%	Muscle coordination and reflexes impaired
8 drinks	0.20%	Vision impaired
12 drinks	0.30%	Drunk, out of control
14 drinks or more	0.50–0.60%	Amnesia, finally death

drinking contest is attributed to this effect. The drinker drinks fast enough, before he passes out, to receive a lethal dose.

Liver cells are not the only cells that die with excessive exposure to alcohol; brain cells are particularly sensitive. When liver cells have died, others may later multiply to replace them, but there is no regeneration of brain cells. This is one reason for the permanent brain damage observed in some heavy drinkers.

Alcohol depresses production of antidiuretic hormone (ADH) by the pituitary gland in the brain. All people who drink have observed the increase in urination that accompanies drinking, but they may not realize that they can easily get into a vicious cycle as a result. Loss of body water leads to thirst. Thirst leads to more drinking—but drinking of what? The only fluid that will relieve dehydration is water, but the thirsty person welcomes any cold fluid, even concentrated alcohol, because it relieves the dry mouth associated with thirst. If a person tries to use concentrated alcoholic beverages to quench thirst, it only becomes worse. The smart drinker, then, either drinks beer (which contains plenty of water), or drinks wine or hard liquor with mixers or chasers.

antidiuretic hormone (ADH): a hormone produced by the pituitary gland in response to dehydration (or a high sodium concentration in the blood); stimulates the kidneys to reabsorb more water and so excrete less. This ADH should not be confused with the enzyme alcohol dehydrogenase, which is sometimes also abbreviated ADH.

The water loss caused by depression of antidiuretic hormone involves loss of more than just water and some alcohol. With water loss there is a loss of such important minerals as magnesium, potassium, calcium, and zinc (see Chapters 10 and 11). These minerals are vital to the maintenance of fluid balance and to many chemical reactions in the cells, including muscle contraction. Repletion therapy has to be instituted early in the recovering alcoholic to bring magnesium and potassium levels back to normal as quickly as possible.

With these changes in mind, it is time to take a look at alcohol consumption from the social view and at the malnutrition that results from excessive drinking.

Drinking and Drunkenness

If you want to drink socially, you should drink slowly, with food, and should sip, not gulp, your drinks. If the alcohol molecules dribble slowly enough into the liver cells, the enzymes will be able to handle the load.

Spacing of drinks is important too. It takes about an hour and a half to metabolize one drink, depending on your body size, on previous drinking experience, on how recently you have eaten, and on how you are feeling at the time.

If a friend has drunk too much and you want to help her sober up, there is no reason to wear yourself out walking her around the block. The muscles have to work harder; but since they can't metabolize alcohol, they can't help clear it from the blood. Time is the only thing that will do the job; each person has a particular level of the enzyme alcohol dehydrogenase, and it clears the blood at a steady rate. This is not true for most nutrients. If you bring in more of a nutrient, generally the body can promptly step up the rate at which it metabolizes that nutrient. But not with alcohol.

Nor will it help your friend to give her a cup of coffee. Caffeine is a stimulant, but it won't speed up the metabolism of alcohol. The police say ruefully, "If you give a drunk a cup of coffee you won't make him sober, but you may make him a wide-awake drunk."

So far we have mentioned only one way that the blood is cleared of alcohol—metabolism by the liver. However, about 10 percent of the alcohol is excreted through the breath and in the urine. This fact is the basis for the breathalyzer test for drunkenness administered by the police. The amount of alcohol in the breath is in proportion to that still in the bloodstream. In most states legal drunkenness is set at 0.15 percent, although many states are lowering the criterion to 0.10 percent—especially as statistics accumulate that show a relationship between alcohol use and industrial and traffic accidents.

The lack of glucose for the brain's function and the length of time needed to clear the blood of alcohol account for some diverse consequences of drinking. Responsible aircraft pilots know that they must allow 24 hours for their bodies to clear alcohol completely, and refuse to fly any sooner. Major airlines enforce this rule. Women who may become pregnant are warned to abstain from the use of alcohol because it severely threatens the development of the fetus's central nervous system. One of the effects of an acute dose in experimental animals is to collapse the umbilical cord temporarily, depriving the developing fetus of oxygen.[6] This can occur even before the woman is aware that she is pregnant.

You may have heard the story of the country woman who kept saying "Amen!" as the preacher ranted about one sin after another; but when he got to her favorite sin, she whispered to her husband that the preacher had "quit preachin' and gone to meddlin'." We've tried to stick to scientific facts, so the only "meddlin'" that we will do is to urge you to look again at the accompanying drawing of the brain and note that judgment is affected first when someone drinks. A person's judgment may tell him that he should limit himself to two drinks at a party, but the first drink may take his judgment away, so that he has many more. The failure to stop drinking as planned, on repeated occasions, is a danger sign that indicates that the person should not drink at all.

The fetal brain grows at the rate of 100,000 new brain cells a minute.

6   A. B. Mukherjee and G. D. Hodgen, Maternal ethanol exposure induces transient impairment of umbilical circulation and fetal hypoxia in monkeys, *Science* 218 (1982): 700–702.

Drinking and Malnutrition

It has been estimated that more than 9 million people in the United States abuse alcohol to the point that their personal relationships, their jobs, or their health are impaired. One of the health hazards is malnutrition. Alcohol depresses appetite by the euphoria it produces as well as by its attack on the mucosa of the stomach, so that heavy drinkers usually eat poorly if at all. With a large portion of their energy fuel coming from the empty kcalories of alcohol, they find it difficult to obtain the essential nutrients. Thus some of their malnutrition is due to lack of food—but even if they eat well, the direct effects of alcohol will take their toll. Alcohol hinders the absorption, alters the metabolism, and increases the excretion of many nutrients, so that malnutrition can occur even in the well-fed drinker.

Ethanol interferes with a multitude of chemical and hormonal reactions in the body, many more than have been enumerated here. The point of this Highlight, however, was not to summarize every effect of alcohol; the longer and more technical references in Appendix J do that. The point was to offer a reward to the reader for learning the basics of metabolism (Chapter 6) and the roles of the vitamins (Chapter 8). The understandings gained permit a profound appreciation of processes like those described here.

NOTE: Appendix J offers recommendations for further reading; see "Alcohol." The *Instructor's Manual* provides an extra transparency/handout master (TH8-8) on alcoholism—a quiz to help people recognize the danger signs.

HIGHLIGHT 8B

Vitamin C:
Rumors Versus Research

I have seen a paper with some writing on it strung round the neck heal such illness of the whole body and in a single night. I have seen a fever banished by pronouncing a few ceremonial words. But such remedies do not cure for long. We have to be on the watch. Illness can be fictitious, so also can cure. Human nature is perverse.

PLATO

When Dr. Linus Pauling published his book *Vitamin C and the Common Cold* in 1970, he started a storm of controversy that raged for a decade.[1] Newspaper headlines screamed VITAMIN C CURES COLDS; others yelled back VITAMIN C NO EFFECT. One "famous scientist" said this, another that. Meanwhile, behind the scenes, teams of researchers in laboratories and hospitals across the world went to work designing and executing experiments to determine whether in fact vitamin C has any therapeutic or preventive effect against the viruses that cause the myriad disorders collectively called the cold.

Since then some hundreds of articles have been published in the research journals, numbering several thousands of pages. Hundreds of people have been tested in a variety of experimental designs and some conclusions have been reached. Meanwhile, Dr. Pauling has gone on to make additional claims for vitamin C; he urges that any patient diagnosed with cancer should immediately start taking 10 grams a day.[2] More research studies have followed, and the cancer question is generating as much controversy as the common cold.

The purpose of this Highlight is twofold. First, it is intended to make you aware of the difficulties inherent in attempting to discover whether a nutrient (or any therapeutic approach) remediates symptoms or cures a disease. The second purpose—because vitamin C may actually be involved in some way with cures of colds and cancer—is to show you the kinds of research questions that will have to be answered before we can know what it does.

1   L. C. Pauling, *Vitamin C and the Common Cold* (San Francisco: W. H. Freeman, 1970).
2   L. Pauling, Vitamin C therapy of advanced cancer (letter to the editor), *New England Journal of Medicine* 302 (1980): 694; N. Horwitz, Now Japanese report 6-fold survival jump in terminal cancer with ascorbate megadoses, *Medical Tribune* (July 22, 1981).

314

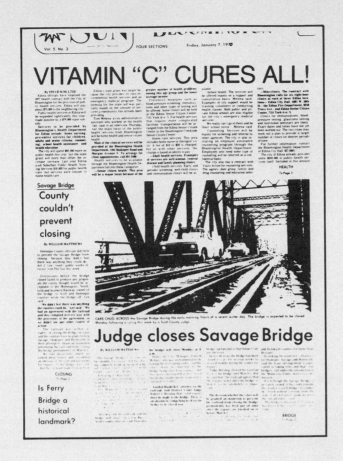

In most studies on the efficacy of vitamin C, two groups of people are selected. Only one group is given vitamin C; both are followed to determine whether the vitamin C group does better in terms of colds or cancer than the control group. A number of pitfalls are inherent in an experiment of this kind; they must be avoided if the results are to be believed.

Controls

First, the two groups must be similar in all respects except for vitamin C dosages. Most important, both must have the same track record with respect to colds, to rule out the possibility that an observed difference might have occurred anyway. (If group A would have caught twice as many colds as group B anyway, then the fact that group B happened to receive the vitamin proves nothing.) Also, in experiments involving a nutrient it is imperative that the diets of both groups be similar, especially with respect to that nutrient. (If those in group B were receiving less vitamin C from their diet, this fact might cancel the effects of the supplement.) Similarity of the experimental and control groups is one of the characteristics of a well-controlled experiment and is accomplished by randomization, a process of choosing the members from the same starting population by throws of the dice or some such method involving chance.

control group: a group of individuals similar in all possible respects to the group being experimented on, except for the experimental treatment. Ideally the control group receives a sham treatment while the experimental group receives a real one.

randomization: a process of choosing the members of the experimental and control groups in a random fashion.

Sample Size

To ensure that chance variation between the two groups does not influence the results, the groups must be large. (If one member of a group of five people catches a bad cold by chance, he will pull the whole group's average toward bad colds; but if one member of a group of 500 catches a bad cold, it will not unduly affect the group average.) In reviewing the results of experiments of this kind, always ask whether the number of people tested was large enough to rule out chance variation. Statistical methods are useful for determining the significance of differences between groups of various sizes.

Placebos

placebo (pla-SEE-bo): an inert, harmless medication given to provide comfort and hope.

placere = to please

placebo effect: the healing effect that faith in medicine, even inert medicine, often has.

If a person takes vitamin C for a cold and believes it will cure him, his chances of recovery are greatly improved. The administration of any pill that the taker believes is medicine hastens recovery in about half of all cases.[3] This phenomenon, the effect of faith on healing, is known as the placebo effect. In experiments designed to find out whether vitamin C actually affects prevention of or recovery from colds or cancer, this mind-body effect must be rigorously controlled.

A blind experiment is one in which the subjects do not know whether they are members of the experimental or the control group.

To control for this effect, the experimenters must give pills to all participants, some containing vitamin C and others, of similar appearance and taste, containing an inactive ingredient (placebos). All subjects must believe they are receiving the vitamin so that the effects of faith will work equally in both groups. If it is not possible to convince all subjects that they are receiving vitamin C, then the extent of unbelief must be the same in both groups. An experiment conducted under these conditions is called blind.

Double Blind

A double-blind experiment is one in which neither the subjects nor those conducting the experiment know which subjects are members of the experimental group and which are serving as control subjects, until after the experiment is over.

The experimenters, too, must not know which subjects are receiving the placebo and which are receiving the vitamin C. Being fallible human beings and having an emotional investment in a successful outcome, they tend to hear what they want to hear and so to interpret and record results with a bias in the expected direction. This is not dishonest but is an unconscious shifting of the experimenters' perceptions of reality to agree with their expectations. To prevent it, the pills given to the subjects must be coded by a third party, who does not reveal to the experimenters which subjects received which medication until all results have been recorded quantitatively.

In discussing these subtleties of experimental design, our intent is not to make a research scientist out of you but to show you what a far cry real scientific validity is from the experience of your neighbor, Mary (sample

3   This finding is widely agreed on; it is discussed, among other places, in the debate on vitamin C in *Nutrition Today* (March/April 1978). See "Vitamins" in Appendix J.

size, one; no control group), who says she takes vitamin C when she feels a cold coming on and "it works every time." (She knows what she is taking, she has faith in its efficacy, and she tends not to notice when it doesn't work.) Before concluding that an experiment has shown that a nutrient cures a disease or alleviates a symptom, you have to ask yourself these questions:

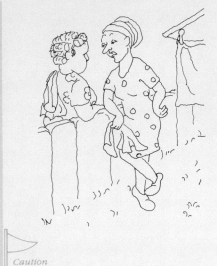

● Was there a control group similar in all important ways to the experimental group?
● Was the sample size large enough to rule out chance variation?
● Was a placebo effectively administered (blind)?
● Was the experiment double blind?

These are a few but not all of the important variables involved in researching a "cure." With them in mind, let us review the literature to see how successfully Dr. Pauling's vitamin C theory has stood the test of experimentation.

Caution

Reviewing the Evidence

Dr. Thomas C. Chalmers, a physician, reviewed the data from 14 clinical trials of vitamin C in the treatment and prevention of the common cold.[4] Of the trials, 5 were poorly controlled, in Chalmers's judgment; and 9 were reasonably well controlled in that the subjects given vitamin C and those given placebos were randomly chosen. In addition, 8 of these 9 studies were double blind. When the data from these 8 studies were pooled, there was a difference of 1/10 of a cold per year and an average difference in duration of 1/10 of a day per cold in favor of those subjects taking vitamin C. In two studies, the effects of vitamin C seemed to be more striking in girls than in boys.

In one study, a questionnaire given at the conclusion revealed that a number of the subjects had correctly guessed the contents of their capsules. A reanalysis of the results showed that those who received the placebo *who thought they were receiving vitamin C* had fewer colds than the group receiving vitamin C *who thought they were receiving the placebos!*

Other reviewers who have assembled and looked at all the evidence, as Dr. Chalmers did, have reached the same conclusions. At the start of the 1980s, reports of additional experiments were still coming out, and most were consistent with previous findings. The balanced picture emerging from the reviews seems to indicate that the effects of the vitamin, if any, are small.

The writer of popular science articles rarely reports on such reviews of literature because they are cold, objective, and give many viewpoints,

4   T. C. Chalmers, Effects of ascorbic acid on the common cold, *American Journal of Medicine* 58 (1975): 532–536.

rarely stressing one. They are not, therefore, sensational enough to sell in the marketplace. Who wants to read a scholarly, conservative, textbooklike report in a newspaper? What usually appears in the newspaper or on TV is the report of one experiment that obtained a significant result. "Professor So-and-So of the Such-and-Such Lab at the Etcetera University," the commentator may say, "has found that vitamin C does make a difference after all, at least for little girls. In a double-blind, cotwin study, in which one of each pair of twins received vitamin C and the other a placebo, the youngest girls, but not the boys, receiving vitamin C had significantly shorter and less severe illnesses than their twins. . . ."

If you chose to look up the source of the report, you would probably find that the study had been conducted as described and that the little girls had indeed had fewer colds than the little boys.[5] But the researchers themselves did not jump to the conclusion that vitamin C makes a difference. In an admirable effort to put their finding in perspective, they pointed out: "One should be aware that, as the number of tests increases, the possibility of obtaining a 'significant' result by chance alone is also increased." In other words, the experiment would have to be repeated and the same result seen several times more before it could be accepted as real. The general public may be made uneasy by scientists who admit that their results are inconclusive, but the scientific community prefers total honesty to dogmatic statements.

The scientist who reports a "significant" finding from a single experiment is not being dishonest. The term *significant* means that statistical analysis suggests that her findings probably didn't arise from a chance event but from the experimental treatment she was testing. The human significance, or meaning, of her findings is apparent only after her piece of research is added into the total picture. Sources you should turn to for a broad and balanced picture of the available information are the journals, the indexes, and the reviews of literature (see Figure 8B–1). If you are relying on a single source for your information, ask yourself, "Is this one viewpoint? Or is it a balanced picture?"

Repeating an experiment and getting the same results is called **replication**. The skeptical scientist, on hearing of a new, exciting finding will ask, "Has it been replicated yet?" If it hasn't, he will withhold judgment regarding its validity. (For a definition of *validity*, see p. 20.)

Caution

The statistical effect of vitamin C on colds in the kinds of populations studied has been small. Meanwhile, what has the research on cancer shown so far?

Vitamin C and Cancer

In 1976, Dr. Pauling and his associate Dr. Cameron reported that they had administered vitamin C to 100 cancer patients in the Vale of Leven, Scotland, and had prolonged their survival rate. As compared with 1,000 similar patients who had been in the same hospital in earlier years and who had lived only 50 days, these patients lived 210 days.[6] In response, a group of

5   J. Z. Miller and coauthors, Therapeutic effect of vitamin C: A co-twin control study, *Journal of the American Medical Association* 237 (1977): 248–251.

6   E. Cameron and L. Pauling, Supplemental ascorbate in the supportive treatment of cancer: Prolongation of survival times in terminal human cancer, *Proceedings of the National Academy of Science USA* 73 (1976): 3685–3689.

FIGURE 8B–1 Sources of reliable nutrition information.

Nutrition Reviews

Volume 37 May 1979 Number 5

Reviews To find a critique of all the important work on a subject, you can turn to a journal of reviews like the one shown here. One major review appears in *Nutrition Reviews* every month. It is followed by a bibliography that provides references to all of the original work reviewed.

Subject Context	▼ Keyword	Ref. No.
HABILITY/ INFLUENCE OF	VITAMIN B-6 UPON REPRODUCTION AND	50647
VITAMIN B-1 VITAMIN B-2	B-6 VITAMIN A VITAMIN C VITA	18486
AGNESIUM COPPER ZINC	B-6 VITAMIN B-12 AND FOLIC-A	69163
ASTIC-DRUG VITAMIN B-1	B-6 VITAMIN B-12 DIAGNOSIS L	23040
E CHANGES VITAMIN B-1	B-6 VITAMIN B-12 METABOLIC-D	49852
M VITAMIN A VITAMIN B-1	B-6 VITAMIN B-12 VITAMIN C P	7317
ITAMIN K FOLACIN NIACIN	B-6 VITAMIN B-12 VITAMIN C P	24026
VITAMIN B-1 VITAMIN B-2	B-6 VITAMIN B-12 VITAMIN C/	24030
VITAMIN B-1 VITAMIN B-2	B-6 VITAMIN C VITAMIN P EPIN	43638
E METABOLIC-DRUG ANTI	B-6 4 AMINO BUTYRATE 2 OXO	62889
ROL BILE ACID VITAMIN C	B-6/ EFFECT OF THE ALIMENTAR	42968
LORIDE IN RAT JEJUNUM	B-6/ IN-VIVO ABSORPTION AND	7806
BROMINE THEOPHYLLINE	BIOGENIC AMINE PSYCHOTROPIC	75520
UCTIVITY IN COWS GRASS	BUTTER FAT/ EFFECT OF A MICR	51809
SYNERGISTIC EFFECT OF	C AND ASPIRIN ON GASTRIC LES	12698
ENTATION OF DIETS WITH	C AND ASPIRIN TO IMPROVE THE	57020
T FOOD/ NITRATE NITRITE	C AND IN-VITRO MET HEMO GLO	25613
TH ON PECTIN ESTERASE	C AND PROTEIN CONTENTS OF T	63379
ATURAL COMPOUNDS OF	C AND THE POSSIBILITY OF ITS	71403
NTENTS OF DRY MATTER	C AND VITAMIN B-1 THERMOLABI	8724
M/ INHIBITING EFFECT OF	C AND VITAMIN B-12 ON THE MI	62091
PONSE TO A MIXTURE OF	C AND VITAMIN E AND CHOLINE	69403
LOVECH BULGARIA WITH	C AND VITAMIN P BY THE METH	57246
IN B-2 VITAMIN D-3 AND	C BY DENSITOMETRY OF THIN LA	24199
RATE CALCIUM THIAMINE	C CALORIC VALUE/ NUTRIENT C	53439
FLAVINE PYRIDOXINE AND	C CHILD VITAMIN K VITAMIN D	43033
RMONE DRUG VITAMIN A	C COENZYME Q-10 ZYMOSAN P	4081
TION ON VITAMIN A AND	C CONTENT OF WHEY SOY DRIN	30295
NEY HYDROXY PROLINE/	C DEFICIENCY IN GUINEA-PIGS	62414
YPER CHOLESTEROLEMIA	C DEFICIENCY/ FUNCTION OF VI	68530
SED CONDITIONS HUMAN	C DEFICIENT GUINEA-PIGS INFL	32645
ISEASE CZECHOSLOVAKIA	C DRY MATTER SPECIFIC GRAVIT	22052

Index You can look up a large number of experiments on a single topic in an index of abstracts. The part of a page shown here, from *Biological Abstracts*, lists all recently published titles containing the term *vitamin C* and gives each one a reference number. The number refers to a short summary of the reported work, which also tells exactly where it was published. The indexes will lead you to reports of experiments in many different journals. New volumes of *Biological Abstracts* come out semimonthly. *Nutrition Abstracts and Reviews*, a monthly publication, would also contain titles including the word *vitamin C.*

researchers at the Mayo Clinic in Rochester, Minnesota, conducted a study to test the validity of this finding. The Mayo Clinic researchers criticized the earlier study on several grounds. It was not legitimate to use former patients as controls; most importantly, they said the control subjects should have been chosen randomly from the *same* population as those given vitamin C, to make sure they were similar. They therefore conducted a randomized, controlled, double-blind trial, giving vitamin C to 60 patients and a placebo that tasted and looked similar to 63 patients. Patients in both groups worsened at the same rate and died at the same times. The authors concluded, "We cannot recommend the use of high-dose vitamin C in patients with advanced cancer who have previously received irradiation or chemotherapy."[7]

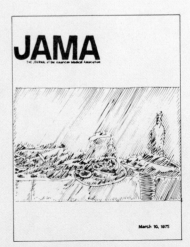

Journals Reports of single experiments are presented in journals like the *Journal of the American Medical Association.*

7   E. T. Creagan and coauthors, Failure of high-dose vitamin C (ascorbic acid) therapy to benefit patients with advanced cancer, *New England Journal of Medicine* 301 (1979): 687–690.

polyp (POLL-ip): in this case, a mushroom-like growth that can progress to cancer.

Dr. Pauling angrily jumped on the authors for their conclusion, pointing out that they had not fairly tested his hypothesis. His patients had relatively strong immune systems because they had not had the debilitating cancer treatments (radiation, chemotherapy) that the Mayo patients had had. The question whether large doses of vitamin C prolong survival time in cancer patients whose immune systems are not already severely damaged remains to be tested in a randomized, controlled, double-blind trial.[8]

Since the Mayo study a few other reports have trickled in, relating to the vitamin's effect on cancer. According to the *Medical Tribune* (a newspaper, not a journal), a Japanese researcher administered various doses of vitamin C to 99 terminal cancer patients who were "untreatable by any conventional forms of cancer therapy." Those receiving 5 to 30 grams a day lived an average of 6.1 times longer than those receiving 4 grams a day or less.[9] No mention was made of whether the study was double blind, so its validity is impossible to assess. It is mentioned here in hopes that the reader will be reminded to view it, and all other such studies, with skepticism unless the full details are given and stand up to close inspection. The question remains open whether vitamin C helps with cancer at all, but one result is clear from the Mayo study. It did not help with advanced cancer patients who had received radiation or chemotherapy.

As this is written, a further attempt to define the effect of vitamin C, if any, on cancer is being made by researchers using a randomized, controlled, double-blind design. Because cancer takes so long (20 years) to develop, the researchers are studying a cancer precursor instead: polyps in the colon. Within a few years, enough data should be in to indicate whether the vitamin C approach to cancer treatment is a hopeful one.[10]

The big questions—Does vitamin C prevent or cure colds? Does it cure cancer or prolong the survival of cancer victims?—remain to be answered. Researchers are hard at work in many labs and clinics pursuing greater understanding of what the vitamin does and doesn't do. This Highlight cannot give a final answer on such a subject, but it has fulfilled its two promises: to make you aware of the difficulties inherent in this kind of research, and to show you the kinds of research questions that will have to be answered before we know what vitamin C does.

While you await reports of the next controlled, double-blind studies on carefully defined and randomized groups of patients, you may wonder what doses of vitamin C to take, yourself, in the light of what is already known. The decision is entirely up to you, but in case you should choose to aim for an intake of several hundred milligrams a day (say, ten times the RDA), this reminder is in order. You can easily obtain this amount of vitamin C by including many vitamin C–rich vegetables and fruits in your daily diet. There is no need to take any kind of pills.

NOTE: Appendix J offers recommendations for further reading; see "Vitamins." The *Instructor's Manual* includes a supplementary article on nutrition and cancer.

8   Pauling, 1980.

9   Horwitz, 1981.

10   W. R. Bruce, G. M. Eyssen, A. Ciampi, P. W. Dion, and N. Boyd, Strategies for dietary intervention studies in colon cancer, *Cancer* 47 (1981): 1121–1125.

CHAPTER 9
The Fat-Soluble Vitamins: A, D, E, and K

CONTENTS

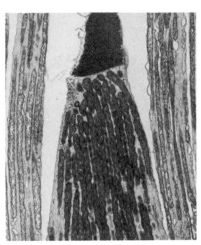

The eye's light-sensitive pigments lie in layers in the rods and cones. This is a cone cell between two rod cells. At the tip of the cone (top) is a stack of discs packed with pigment containing vitamin A (retinal). Beneath the tip lies a bundle of spaghetti-like mitochondria prepared to produce the energy needed to send a nerve impulse when light hits the cone.

I remember well the time when the thought of the eye made me cold all over.

CHARLES DARWIN

Has it ever occurred to you how remarkable it is that you can see things? As an infant you were enchanted with the power this gave you. You closed your eyes and the world disappeared. You opened them and made everything come back again. Later you forgot the wonder of this, but the fact remains that your ability to see brings everything into being for you, more so than any of your other senses. Light reaching your eyes puts you in touch with things outside your body, from your friend sitting near you to stars in other galaxies.

Has it ever occurred to you how extraordinary it is that a child grows? From a mere nothing, a speck so tiny that it is invisible to the naked eye, each person develops into a full-size human being with arms and legs, teeth and fingernails, a beating heart and tingling nerves. Years go into the making of an adult human being, with each day bringing changes so gradual they seem undetectable. Only if you are absent during a part of this process do you notice it on your return and remark to a child, "My, how you've grown!"

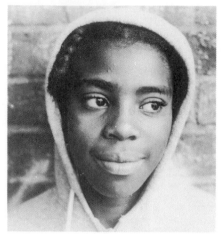

...how remarkable it is that you can see things.

retina (RET-in-uh): the layer of light-sensitive cells lining the back of the inside of the eye; consists of rods and cones.

pigment: a molecule capable of absorbing certain wavelengths of light, so that it reflects only those that we perceive as a certain color.

rhodopsin (ro-DOP-sin): the light-sensitive pigment of the rods in the retina.

iodopsin (eye-o-DOP-sin): the light-sensitive pigment of the cones in the retina. Both rhodopsin and iodopsin contain retinal; the proteins are different.

retinal (RET-in-al): the aldehyde form of vitamin A, active in the eye. For the structure of this and other forms, see Appendix C.

cones: the cells of the retina that respond to bright light and are responsible for color vision.

rods: the cells of the retina that respond to dim light and convey black-and-white vision.

And when did you last think about your breathing? In, out, in, out, day and night, year after year, you take in the oxygen you need and release it, disposing of the used-up carbons whose energy moves you and keeps you alive. The nutrients discussed in this chapter—vitamins A, D, E, and K—are vital for these and other processes that you may often take for granted.

The Roles of Vitamin A

Vitamin A has the distinction of being the first fat-soluble vitamin to be recognized. It may also be one of the most versatile, because of its role in several important body processes.

Vision

At the place where light hits the retina of the eye, profoundly informative communication occurs between the environment and the person. The eye receives the light and transforms it into signals that travel to the interior of the brain. There a mental picture forms of what the light conveys (Figure 9-1). For this to happen, the eye must perform a remarkable transformation of light energy into nerve impulses. The transformers are the molecules of pigment (rhodopsin, iodopsin, and others) in the cells of the retina. A portion of each pigment molecule is retinal, a compound the body can synthesize only if vitamin A or its relatives are supplied by the diet.

A mechanical genius could not have designed such a system better. Light itself cannot be conducted through the solid material of the brain, so it is changed into signals transmitted by nerves. But light comes in different colors (wavelengths), which convey needed information. To keep the colors sorted out, the eye uses different light-sensitive cells (cones) to receive them. Blue light is absorbed by one set of cells, green by another, and yellow-red by a third. By day, combinations of these give the full range of color vision. By night, the light entering the eye is of low intensity, and the set of cells (rods) that can receive this light are of one kind only; so by night a person can normally discern only the presence of light but not its color.

The pigment molecules inside the cells absorb the light. Each pigment molecule is composed of a protein called opsin bonded to a molecule of retinal. When a particle of light (a photon) enters the eye, it is absorbed into the retinal molecule, which responds by changing shape (it actually changes color too, becoming bleached). In its altered form retinal cannot remain bonded to opsin and so is released. This disturbs the shape of the opsin molecule.

This shape change disturbs the cell membrane, permitting charged ions to enter and leave the cell. The cell hyperpolarizes (that is, the electrical charge across its membrane changes), and an electrical impulse travels along the cell's length. At the other end of the cell, the impulse is transmitted to a nerve cell, which conveys it deeper into the brain. Thus the message is sent.

Meanwhile, back in the retina and once again in the dark, the changed molecule of retinal is converted back to its original form and rejoined to opsin to regenerate the pigment rhodopsin. Many molecules of retinal are involved in this process. There are about 6 to 7 million cone cells and 100 million rod cells in the retina, and each contains about 30 million molecules of visual pigment. Repeated small losses incurred by visual activity necessitate the constant replenishment of retinal from the blood, which brings a new supply from the body stores. Ultimately, vitamin A and its relatives in food are the sources of all the retinal in the pigments of the eye.

Bright light seen suddenly, when the eyes are dark-adapted, destroys much more retinal than light seen by day, for three reasons. First, the pupil is wide-open at night, to allow as much light as possible to enter the eye. Second, a shadowing pigment that protects the rods by day withdraws at night, leaving them exposed. Third, there are many more rods than cones. Hence if a bright light suddenly shines at night through the wide-open pupil onto the unprotected rods, much of the pigment in them is bleached and momentarily inactivated. More retinal than usual is freed, and more is lost. A moment passes before the pigments regenerate and sight returns. You no doubt remember being "blinded" on occasion by a flashlight shining directly into your eyes. People who must do a lot of night driving, facing headlights from oncoming cars, thus need an increased amount of vitamin A.

The eye is not designed for night driving or, in general, for accommodating itself to bright light at night. The mechanisms of vision evolved over millions of years, before humankind had harnessed electricity and lit up the night with headlights, beacons, and streetlights. In nature, animals in the wilderness have no need to adapt to sudden flashes of bright light at night, because they occur so seldom.

Vitamin A is undeniably an important nutrient, if for no other reason than that it plays a vital role in vision. But only one-thousandth of the vitamin A in the body is in the retina. The vitamin does other things as well.

opsin (OP-sin): the protein portion of the visual pigment molecule.

photon (FOE-ton): a particle of light energy. Depending on its wavelength, a photon conveys different colors of light.

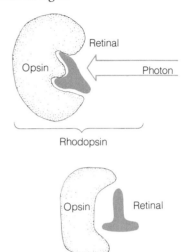

Light (photon) hits pigment. Retinal changes shape and is released from opsin. Opsin changes shape.

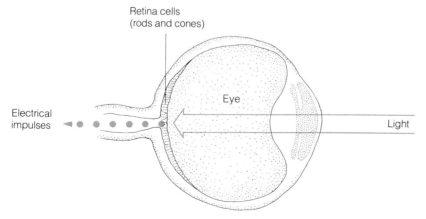

FIGURE 9-1 As light enters the eye, pigments within the cells of the retina absorb the light and generate nerve impulses that travel into the brain.

mucosa (myoo-COH-suh): the membranes, composed of cells, that line the surfaces of body tissues.

urethra (you-REE-thruh): the tube through which urine from the bladder passes out of the body.

The cells on the surface are known as **epithelial** (ep-i-THEE-lee-ul) **cells**.

mucus (adjective **mucous**): a substance secreted by the epithelial cells of the mucosa; mucopolysaccharide (see also p. 161).

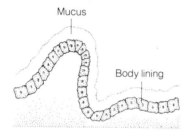

Mucus

Body lining

Healthy body lining.

keratin (KERR-uh-tin): a water-insoluble protein; the normal protein of hair and nails. Keratin may be produced under abnormal conditions by cells that normally produce mucus.

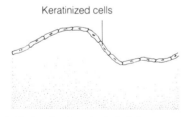

Keratinized cells

Body lining in vitamin A deficiency.

The cells are osteoclasts (see p. 330).

These sacs of degradative enzymes are **lysosomes** (LYE-so-zomes).

lyso = to break

soma = body

Maintenance of Linings

Fortunately for you, your mucosa are all intact. You may not properly appreciate what these membranes do for you, but consider how important it is that each of these surfaces should be smooth: the linings of the mouth, stomach, and intestines; the linings of the lungs and the passages leading to them; the linings of the urinary bladder and urethra; the linings of the uterus and vagina; the linings of the eyelids and sinus passageways. The cells of all these surfaces—epithelial cells—secrete a smooth and slippery substance (mucus) that coats and protects them from invasive microorganisms and other harmful particles. The mucous lining of the stomach also shields its cells from digestion by the gastric juices. In the upper part of the lungs, these cells possess little whiplike hairs (cilia), which continuously sweep the coating of mucus up and out, so that any foreign particles that chance to get in are carried away by the flow. (When you clear your throat and swallow, you are excreting this waste by way of your digestive tract.) In the vagina, similar cells sweep the mucus down and out. During an infection in any of these locations, these surface cells secrete more mucus and become more active, so that a noticeable discharge occurs; when you cough it up, blow your nose, or wash it away, you help to rid your body of the infective agent.

Vitamin A plays a role in maintaining the integrity of the mucous membranes. When vitamin A is not present, the cells cannot produce the carbohydrate normally found in mucus (they produce a protein called keratin instead). Within the body, the mucous membranes line an area larger than a quarter of a football field; so this function of vitamin A accounts for most of the body's vitamin A need. As you might predict, greater losses of vitamin A occur during infection than under normal conditions.

Vitamin A is also essential for healthy skin, another one or two square meters of body surface. Thus all surfaces, both inside and out, are maintained with the help of vitamin A. It has still another role to play during growth.

Bone Growth

"Growth is when everything gets bigger all together" is a child's definition. Certainly that is how it looks from the outside. Actually, however, the organs and body parts all grow at different rates with different timings. The brain, for instance, reaches 90 percent of its adult size by the time a child is two, but the testes are still baby-size when a male enters his teens. Furthermore, body parts do not just "get bigger"; bones are a case in point.

To enlarge the interior of a brick fireplace, the first thing you have to do is remove some of the old bricks. Similarly, to make a bone larger requires remodeling, as Figure 9–2 shows. To convert a small bone into a large bone, the bone-remodeling cells must "undo" some parts of the small bone as they go.

Vitamin A is required for the undoing. Some of the cells involved in bone formation are packed with sacs of degradative enzymes that can take apart the structures of bone. With the help of vitamin A in a sensitively regulated process, these cells release their enzymes, which eat away at selected sites in the bone, removing the parts that are not needed as the bone grows longer. (A similar process occurs when a tadpole loses its tail and becomes a frog. As you know, the tail doesn't simply fall off; rather it is resorbed, "growing" shorter and shorter until it disappears. As a fetus you also had a tail and lost it, a process that depended on vitamin A.)

Vitamin A's roles in promoting good night vision, the health of mucous membranes and skin, and the growth of bone are well known. Others include parts it plays in:

- Reproduction.
- Maintaining the stability of cell membranes.
- Helping the adrenal glands to synthesize a hormone (corticosterone).
- Helping to ensure a normal output of the hormone thyroxin from the thyroid gland.
- Helping to maintain nerve cell sheaths.
- Assisting in immune reactions.
- Helping to manufacture red blood cells.
- Many others.

Vitamin A research still in progress is yielding many new details of how this nutrient functions in the body. Three different forms of vitamin A are active in the body: retinol (an alcohol), retinal (an aldehyde), and retinoic acid (see Figure 9–4). Each has its own special binding proteins in the cells in which it works. There is also a special zinc-containing binding protein to pick up vitamin A from the liver, where it is stored, and to carry it in the blood. Cells that will receive and use vitamin A also have special receptors for it, as if it were fragile, and had to be passed carefully from hand to hand without being dropped.

Each form of vitamin A triggers specific reactions in cells that are set up to respond to it. Retinol and retinoic acid, for example, act like hormones; they travel into cells, cross the nuclear membrane, and interact with DNA, causing certain genes to express their coded instructions and make specific proteins.[1]

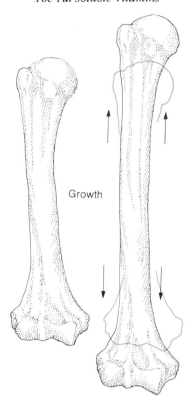

Growth

FIGURE 9–2 As bone lengthens, vitamin A helps remove old bone. TH9–5

Vitamin A Deficiency

Either zinc deficiency or vitamin A deficiency can cause the symptoms of vitamin A deficiency, because zinc is part of the protein that mobilizes vitamin A from the liver (see Chapter 11). Zinc is also part of the enzyme that converts retinol to retinal in the eye. If zinc status is adequate, vitamin A deficiency depends on the adequacy of vitamin A stores.

Up to a year's supply of vitamin A may be stored in the body, 90 percent of it in the liver. If you stop eating good food sources of the vitamin, deficiency symptoms will not begin to appear until after your stores are depleted. Then, however, the consequences are profound and severe.

1   Interaction of retinol and retinoic acid with the nucleus, *Nutrition Reviews* 38 (1980): 23–25.

Table 9–1 itemizes some of them. Some have to do with the role of vitamin A in vision, some with its functions in epithelial tissue, and some with its part in growth; others are as yet unexplained.

Impaired Night Vision

If the blood bathing the cells of the retina does not supply sufficient retinal to rapidly regenerate visual pigments bleached by light, then a flash of bright light at night will be followed by a prolonged spell of night blindness. This is one of the first detectable signs of vitamin A deficiency. Because night blindness is easy to test, it aids in diagnosis of the condition. (Of course it is only a symptom, and may indicate some condition other than vitamin A deficiency.) Figure 9–3 shows how night blindness can be tested.

night blindness: slow recovery of vision after flashes of bright light at night; an early symptom of vitamin A deficiency.

enamel: the hard mineral coating of the outside of the tooth, composed of calcium compounds embedded in a fine network of keratin fibers.

dentin: the softer material underlying the enamel of the tooth, composed of calcium compounds embedded in a network of collagen fibers.

For a picture of tooth structure, see p. 82.

TABLE 9–1   **Vitamin A Deficiency**

AREA AFFECTED	MAIN EFFECT	TECHNICAL NAME FOR SYMPTOMS
Eye		
Retina	Night blindness	
Membranes	Failure to secrete mucopolysaccharide causes changes in epithelial tissue and hyperkeratinization	
General[a]	Drying (mildest form)	**Xerosis**
	Irreversible drying and degeneration of the cornea, causing blindness (most severe)	**Keratomalacia**
Skin	Hair follicles plug with keratin, forming white lumps	**Hyperkeratosis**
GI tract	Changes in lining; diarrhea	
Respiratory tract	Changes in lining; infections	
Urogenital tract	Changes in lining favor calcium deposition, resulting in kidney stones, bladder disorders	
	Infections of bladder and kidney	
	Infections of vagina	
Bones	Bone growth ceases; shapes of bones change	
Teeth	Enamel-forming cells malfunction; teeth develop cracks and tend to decay; dentin-forming cells atrophy	
Nervous system	Brain and spinal cord grow too fast for stunted skull and spine; injury to brain and nerves causes paralysis	
Immune system	Depression of immune reactions	
Blood	Anemia, often masked by dehydration	

[a] The eye's symptoms of vitamin A deficiency are collectively known as *xerophthalmia*.

FIGURE 9–3 **Night blindness.**

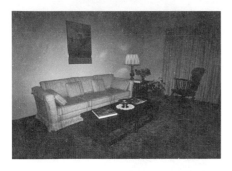

In dim light, you can make out the details in this room. You are using your rods for vision.

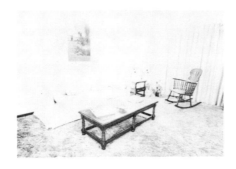

A flash of bright light momentarily blinds you as the pigment in the rods is bleached.

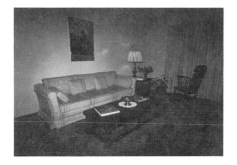

You quickly recover, and can see the details again in a few seconds.

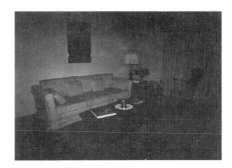

With inadequate vitamin A, you do not recover but remain blind for many seconds.

The epithelial cells fill with keratin in a process known as **keratinization**. The progression of this condition to the extreme is **hyperkeratosis**.

hyper = too much

Roughened Surfaces

Instead of staying smooth and well rounded and producing normal mucus, the epithelial cells flatten and harden with vitamin A deficiency, losing their protective mucous coating and filling with keratin instead. In the eye this process leads to drying and hardening of the cornea, which may progress to permanent blindness. In the mouth, drying and hardening of the salivary glands makes them susceptible to infection; failure of mucous secretion in the mouth may lead to loss of appetite. Mucous secretion in the stomach and intestines is reduced, hindering normal digestion and absorption of nutrients, causing diarrhea, and so indirectly worsening the deficiency. Infections of the respiratory tract, the urinary tract, and the vagina are also made more likely by vitamin A deficiency. On the outer body surface, the cells also harden and flatten, making the skin dry, rough, scaly, and hard. Around each hair follicle an accumulation of hard material makes a lump.

In the eye, the symptoms of vitamin A deficiency are collectively known as **xerophthalmia** (zer-off-THAL-mee-uh).

xero = dry

ophthalm = eye

An early sign is **xerosis** (drying of the cornea); the latest and most severe stage is **keratomalacia** (total blindness).

malacia = softening, weakening

cornea (KOR-nee-uh): the transparent membrane covering the outside of the front of the eye.

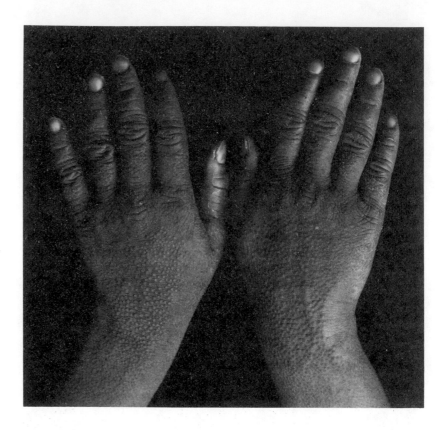

The accumulation of this hard material, keratin, around each hair follicle is **follicular hyperkeratosis**.

follicle (FOLL-i-cul): a group of cells in the skin from which a hair grows.

Follicular hyperkeratosis.

Photo courtesy of Dr. Samuel Dreizen, D.D.S., M.D.

Abnormal Growth

Because growth and development of the brain and eyes are most rapid in the unborn and in the very young, the effects of vitamin A deficiency are most severe at and around the time of birth. For example, in a child of one or two, stunted growth of the skull may cause crowding of the brain (which is growing rapidly at that age), mimicking the signs of a brain tumor. Tooth growth may also be abnormal. Crooked teeth in a child may reflect a vitamin A deficiency suffered by its mother while its jawbones were forming during her pregnancy. Damage to the eyes is also most pronounced in the young, with blindness the result in thousands of cases of vitamin A deficiency throughout the world. Among nutrition problems afflicting the young of the world, vitamin A deficiency is second in extent only to protein-kcalorie malnutrition.

Naivete on the part of the well-intentioned can cause more harm than good, a result often observed when attempts are made to remedy the problem of malnutrition in the underdeveloped countries. An awareness of the way nutrients function in the body and of their interdependence must precede efforts to correct malnutrition problems, as the case of vitamin A illustrates.

Vitamin A depends on proteins, notably the retinol-binding protein, and on the mineral zinc for its functions and transport in the body. In protein-kcalorie malnutrition, when vitamin A stores are also low, there is a balance of a kind. But when protein is given without supplemental vitamin A, protein carriers that are synthesized in response deplete the liver of the last available stores of vitamin A, thus precipitating a deficiency. Administration of protein has been observed to cause an epidemic of blindness, as when skim milk was offered by UNICEF to children in Brazil. Vitamin A capsules were supplied with the milk, but the parents often ate the capsules or sold them, giving only the milk to the children.[2]

The mineral zinc is also needed, both to free vitamin A from liver storage for transport, and to help an enzyme in the retina to convert retinol to retinal.[3] An apparent vitamin A deficiency may reflect an underlying zinc deficiency that must first be corrected. These examples illustrate the point that whenever nutrition help is given, knowledge must accompany that help.

retinol-binding protein (RBP): the protein that carries retinol in the blood. Measurement of RBP is a sensitive indicator of vitamin A status.

Caution

In the United States as well, the problem of vitamin A deficiency is all too common. The Ten-State Survey (described in Chapter 12) revealed that a third of the children under six who were examined had less than the recommended vitamin A intakes. Spanish-Americans and blacks exhibited the most pronounced evidence of deficiency. In the more recent Nationwide Food Consumption Survey, similarly, about a third of the population surveyed had intakes below two-thirds of the RDA. Some subgroups of the Canadian population are also deficient, notably Canadian and Eskimo women, especially during their pregnancies.

A major source of vitamin A is vegetables, and a probable reason for widespread deficits of vitamin A in children is their refusal to eat vegetables. A section of Chapter 14 emphasizes the importance of encouraging children to like vegetables and suggests practical ways to ease their acceptance.

Vitamin A Toxicity

Vitamin A toxicity occurs when all the binding proteins for vitamin A are swamped and free vitamin A attacks the cells. Such effects are not likely if you depend on foods for your nutrients, but if you take pills or supplements containing the vitamin, toxicity is a real possibility. Overdoses have serious effects on the same body systems that exhibit symptoms in vitamin A

2   O. A. Roels, Vitamin A physiology, *Journal of the American Medical Association* 214 (1970): 1097–1102.

3   Mobilization of hepatic vitamin A by zinc supplementation in zinc deficiency associated with protein-energy malnutrition, *Nutrition Reviews* 38 (1980): 275–277.

deficiency (see Table 9–2). Children are most likely to be affected, because they need less, they are smaller and more sensitive to overdoses, and it is easy to give them too much in pill form or in other concentrates. The availability of breakfast cereals, instant meals, fortified milk, and chewable candy-like vitamins, each containing 100 percent of the recommended daily intake of vitamin A, makes it possible for a well-meaning parent to provide several times the daily allowance of the vitamin to a child in a few hours. Serious toxicity is seen in small infants when they are given more than ten times the recommended amount every day for weeks at a time. A child herself may also overdose. Liking vitamin pills and thinking of them as candy, she may eat several.

There is a wide range of vitamin A intakes in which neither deficiency nor toxicity symptoms appear. Recommended intakes in both the United States and Canada are set at about double the minimum necessary to prevent deficiency. Doubtless, many people need not consume amounts this high. The exact upper limit of safety can't be determined exactly, because people's tolerances to overdoses vary. Probably the amount of added vitamin A that anyone can tolerate depends on the length of time he takes it and on how much of the vitamin has already accumulated in his body stores before he begins to overdose. Alcohol use makes vitamin A toxicity more likely.

osteoclasts: the cells that destroy bone during its growth. Those that build bone are **osteoblasts**.

osteo = bone

clast = break

blast = build

jaundice (JAWN-diss): yellowing of the skin; a symptom of liver disease, in which bile and related pigments spill into the bloodstream.

TABLE 9–2 **Vitamin A Toxicity**

DISEASE	AREA AFFECTED	MAIN EFFECTS
Hypervitaminosis A	Bones	Increased activity of osteoclasts causes decalcification, joint pain, fragility, stunted growth, thickening of long bones; pressure increases inside skull, mimicking brain tumor.
	Blood	Red blood cells lose hemoglobin and potassium; menstruation ceases; clotting time slows; bleeding is easily induced
	Immune system	Stimulation of immune reactions
	Nervous system	Loss of appetite, irritability, fatigue, restlessness, headache, nausea, vomiting, muscle weakness, interference with thyroxin
	GI tract	Nausea, vomiting, abdominal pain, diarrhea, weight loss
	Skin	Dryness, itching, peeling, rashes, dry scaling lips, loss of hair, brittle nails
	Liver	Jaundice, enlargement, massive accumulation of fat and vitamin A[a]
	Spleen	Enlargement
Hypercarotenemia	Skin	Yellow color

[a] If liver impairment is severe, the "classic" signs seen in skin and hair may be masked. Masked hypervitaminosis A and liver injury, *Nutrition Reviews* 40(1982): 303–305.

In one case, toxic effects were reported in a person who took daily doses 10 times the recommended intake for only one month;[4] but in others it may take 40 times the recommended intake for several months to elicit symptoms of toxicity.[5] The National Nutrition Consortium advises that adults should avoid intakes of more than 5 to 10 times the recommended amounts to ensure safety.[6] In general, it makes sense to get your vitamin A from natural, mostly plant, sources.

Adolescents should be warned that massive doses of vitamin A taken internally will have no beneficial effect on acne but may cause the miseries itemized in Table 9–2. The belief that vitamin A cures acne arises from the knowledge that it is needed for the health of the skin. As with all nutrients, however, the vitamin promotes health when enough is supplied; more than enough has no further beneficial effects.

However, a relative of vitamin A, vitamin A acid, does sometimes help relieve the symptoms of acne when applied directly to the skin surface. The acid helps loosen the plugs that may accumulate in pores, allowing the skin to cleanse itself naturally. Such a treatment should of course be undertaken only on a doctor's recommendation.[7]

Some of vitamin A's relatives may have a preventive role with respect to cancer. Retinol itself is not one of these, but this doesn't stop gullible people from taking massive doses of vitamin A in the hope of preventing cancer. It is expected that more cases of vitamin A toxicity will be reported in the years to come, but hopefully no reader of this book will be among them.[8]

Caution

It is possible to suffer toxicity symptoms only when excess amounts of the preformed vitamin from animal foods or supplements are taken. The precursor, beta-carotene, which is available from plant foods, is not converted to vitamin A rapidly enough in the body to cause toxicity but is instead stored in fat depots as carotene. Being yellow in color, it may accumulate under the skin to such an extent that the overdoser actually turns yellow.

preformed vitamin A: vitamin A in its active form.

precursor: a compound that can be converted into active vitamin A (see also p. 93).

beta-carotene: a vitamin A precursor found in plants.

4   S. J. Yaffe and L. J. Filer, Jr., American Academy of Pediatrics, Joint Committee Statement on Drugs and on Nutrition, The use and abuse of vitamin A, *Pediatrics* 48 (1971): 655–656.

5   D. R. Davis, Using vitamin A safely, *Osteopathic Medicine* 3 (October 1978): 31–43.

6   Committee on Safety, Toxicity, and Misuse of Vitamins and Trace Minerals, National Nutrition Consortium, *Vitamin-Mineral Safety, Toxicity, and Misuse* (Chicago: American Dietetic Association, 1978).

7   For further information on nutrition and acne, read E. M. N. Hamilton and E. N. Whitney, Controversy 14A: Acne, in *Nutrition: Concepts and Controversies*, 2nd ed. (St. Paul, Minn.: West, 1979), pp. 481–484.

8   Masked hypervitaminosis A and liver injury, *Nutrition Reviews* 40 (1982): 303–305. The relationship of vitamin A to cancer is fully explored elsewhere; see note at end of chapter.

Vitamin A in Foods

Vitamin A terminology is in a period of transition. Vitamin A occurs in a number of different forms, and these convert to the active forms in the body with different efficiencies. In animal foods, vitamin A occurs as retinol-like compounds which convert to retinol and its relatives in the body with high efficiency. In plant foods, no biologically active, preformed vitamin A occurs, but plant pigments known as carotenoids can be converted to vitamin A in the body with a lower efficiency. The most active of the carotenoids is beta-carotene. When beta-carotene is split, it yields two molecules which are converted to retinol. Figure 9–4 diagrams the common forms of the vitamin A family.

The active form of vitamin A used for reference is retinol, and the recommended amounts of vitamin A are stated in terms of retinol equivalents (RE). As of 1980, both U.S. and Canadian authorities were using this terminology and were recommending 1,000 RE per day for adult men and 800 RE for women.

retinol: one of the active forms of vitamin A, similar to retinal. Retinol is an alcohol; retinal is an aldehyde (see pp. 305, 95, and Appendix C).

RE (retinol equivalent): a measure of vitamin A activity; the amount of retinol that a vitamin A compound will yield after conversion in the body.

FIGURE 9–4 **Vitamin A and beta-carotene.**
TH9-1

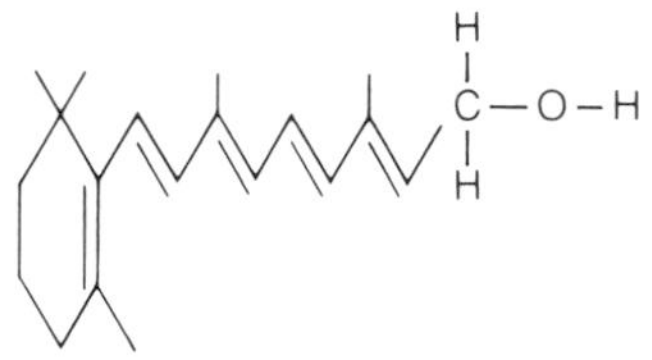

Retinol, the alcohol form

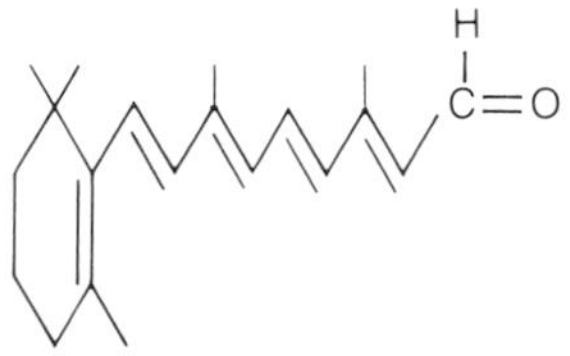

Retinal, the aldehyde form

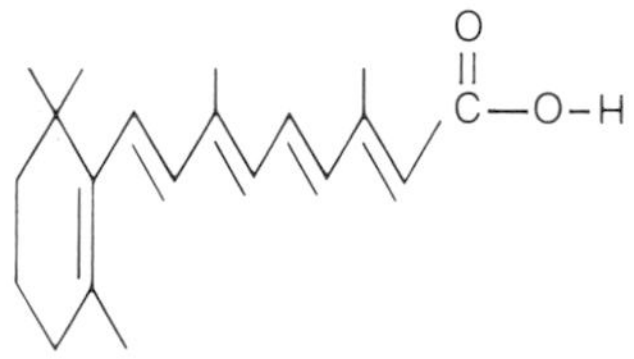

Retinoic acid, the acid form

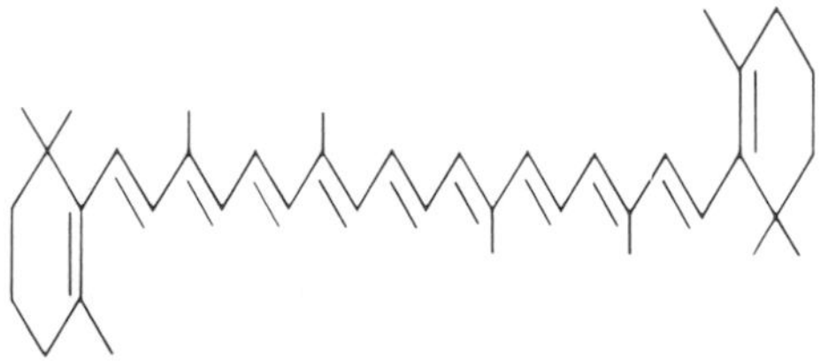

Beta-carotene

The amounts of vitamin A found in *foods*, however, are often still reported using an older system of measurement, international units (IU), which are based on some assumptions now known to be not completely correct. In the future, tables of food composition will report the vitamin A activity of foods in RE. Until they do, you will have to do some computing if you wish to use a table of food values expressed in IU to estimate your vitamin A intake. You will have to remember both terms, RE and IU, and the fact that 1 RE is roughly equivalent to 3.33 IU of vitamin A from animal tissues or 10 IU from plant tissues.[9] This book's Table of Food Composition (Appendix H) presents vitamin A in RE.

Table 9–3 shows the vitamin A contents of various kinds of foods, expressed in RE. The vitamin A value of plant foods is not as great as it appeared to be when they were expressed in IU, but still, the plant foods stand out as major contributors of vitamin A activity to the diet.

The major vitamin A contributors among foods are almost all brightly colored—green, yellow, orange, and red. Any plant food with significant vitamin A activity must have some color, since the vitamin and its plant precursor carotene are colored compounds themselves (vitamin A is a pale yellow; carotene is a rich, deep yellow, almost orange). The dark-green, leafy vegetables contain abundant amounts of the green pigment chlorophyll, which masks the carotene in them. A skilled hostess or restaurateur knows that an attractive meal includes foods of different colors that complement one another, but may not be aware that such a meal probably ensures a good supply of vitamin A as well.

On the other hand, food with a yellow or orange color does not invariably contain vitamin A or carotene. Many of the compounds that give foods their colors, such as the yellow and red xanthophylls, are unrelated to vitamin A and have no nutritional value.

On the third hand (this chapter has three hands), if a plant food is white or colorless, you can be sure it contains little or no vitamin A. Notice that many of the low-vitamin A foods in Table 9–3 are in this category.

About half of the vitamin A activity in foods consumed in the United States comes from fruits and vegetables, and half of this comes from the dark leafy greens (not iceberg lettuce or green beans) and the rich yellow or deep orange vegetables, such as squash, carrots, and sweet potatoes (not corn). The other half comes from milk, cheese, butter, and other dairy products; eggs; and meats. Since vitamin A is fat-soluble, it is lost when milk is skimmed. Skim milk is often fortified with 2,000 IU (or about 40 percent of the intake recommended for men) of vitamin A per quart to compensate.[10] The butter substitute, margarine, is usually fortified with 15,000 IU (4,500 RE) per pound. Milks and margarines may also be fortified with vitamin D; read the label to find out.

IU (international unit): a measure of vitamin activity, determined by such biological methods as feeding a given compound to vitamin-deprived animals and measuring the number of units of growth produced. This system was used to measure vitamin A before chemical analysis of the vitamin A compounds and their precursors was possible.

1 RE = 3.33 IU from animal foods or 10 IU from plant foods. (On the average, 1 RE = about 5 IU.)

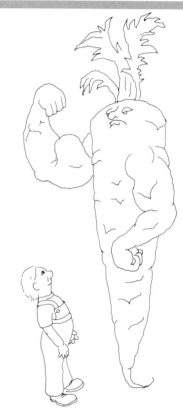

The vitamin A contents of plant foods may look greater than they are.

---

9   J. G. Bieri and M. C. McKenna, Expressing dietary values for fat-soluble vitamins: Changes in concepts and terminology, *American Journal of Clinical Nutrition* 34 (1981): 289–295; Food and Nutrition Board, Committee on Recommended Allowances, *Recommended Dietary Allowances*, 9th ed. (Washington, D.C.: National Academy of Sciences, 1980), pp. 56–57.

10   In Canada, 1,500 IU (about 450 RE) per liter.

TABLE 9–3 **Vitamin A—Average Amounts in Groups of Foods** TH9-2

	VITAMIN A (RE)
Milk and Milk Products	
1 c *unfortified* whole milk or creamed cottage cheese[a]	100
1 c *unfortified* skim milk	-0-
1 c buttermilk or skim milk yogurt or cottage cheese	25
1 c *fortified* whole or skim milk or milk product[b]	150
1 oz cheese[c]	75
Meat and Legumes	
3 oz fish[d] or chicken	25
3 oz most other meat, fish, or poultry	-0-
3 oz liver	15,000
1 egg	100
¾ c legumes, cooked	-0-
Fruits and Vegetables	
1 portion or piece vitamin A-rich fruit[e]	400
1 portion pink, orange, or yellow fruit[f]	125
1 portion pink grapefruit[g]	50
1 portion or piece other fruit[h]	10
1 c or piece dark green or deep orange vegetable[i]	1,000
½ c green vegetable or tomato[j]	50
½ c other vegetable	25
Grains	
1 slice bread or ½ c rice or pasta[k]	-0-
1 portion cereal[l]	-0-
Other	
1 tbsp butter or fortified margarine	125
1 tbsp other fat or oil	-0-
1 tbsp sugar or 1 candy or sweet	-0-
2 tbsp tomato catsup	50
1 c soup with carrots or tomatoes	200
1 c other soup including cream soup	50
1 tbsp brewer's yeast	-0-

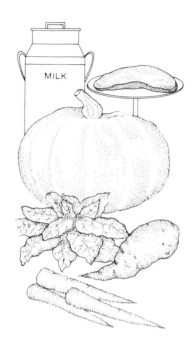

Foods rich in Vitamin A.

According to the values in the table, a person following the four food group plan recommendation to consume one vitamin A-rich vegetable every day would easily meet the U.S. RDA of 1,000 RE. A person who did not would be well advised to use only vitamin A-fortified milk and milk products and to select vitamin A-rich fruits often. A meal of liver every week or two would boost vitamin A intakes.

This table was made by consulting Appendix H, averaging the vitamin A contents in standard portions of the commonly used foods in each category, and rounding off each average to the nearest 25 RE. Values agree approximately with the USDA Handbook, Nutrients furnished by servings of foods, *Essentials of an Adequate Diet*, Bulletin no. 160, 1956. Use of these numbers will provide a rough approximation of the amount of vitamin A on a plate or in a day's meals. However, the person who wants maximum accuracy will refer to Appendix H.

[a] 1 c milk (but not cream); whole milk yogurt, goat's milk, commercial milkshake; ice milk; milk drinks, custards, and puddings made with unfortified milk.

[b] 1 c vitamin A-fortified milk; kefir; ice cream; milk drinks, custard, and puddings made with fortified milk.

[c] 1 c ricotta cheese has about 325 RE.

[d] 3 oz sardines contain 60 RE; 1 c oysters has 225 RE.

[e] 4 medium fresh or ¼ c dried apricots; or ¼ cantaloupe.

[f] ½ c papaya, 1 yellow peach, or a 4 x 4 in wedge of watermelon.

[g] ½ pink grapefruit or ½ c pink grapefruit juice.

[h] Values range from 0 to 35 RE; oranges, tangerines, and prunes are the highest.

[i] 1 c dark greens; 1-2 carrots; 1 c pumpkin or winter squash; ½ c sweet potato; or 1 c mixed vegetables.

[j] Values range from 10 to 110 RE; tomatoes and darker lettuces are the highest.

[k] Cakes and pies may be made with vitamin A-rich ingredients. 1 piece of pumpkin or sweet potato pie contains ½ the U.S. RDA.

[l] Breakfast cereals may be fortified with half or more of the vitamin A RDA per serving. Read the label.

The safest and easiest way to meet your vitamin A needs, then, is to consume generous servings of a variety of dark-green and deep-orange vegetables and fruits. A one-cup serving of carrots, sweet potatoes, or dark greens such as spinach would provide such liberal amounts of carotenoids that, even allowing for inefficient absorption and conversion, intake would be sufficient. Alternatively, a diet including more or larger servings of medium sources would ensure an ample intake. No doubt you can find food sources of the vitamin that appeal to you and can easily calculate the minimum amounts you should eat to meet your needs.

The fruit and vegetable family is, of course, one of the four food groups. Its importance for meeting vitamin A needs is reflected in the recommendation that adults have at least four servings a day, including "at least one dark-green or deep-orange" item every other day.

Fast foods are notable for their *lack* of vitamin A. Anyone who dines frequently on hamburgers, french fries, shakes, and the like is advised to emphasize vegetables heavily—and not just salads—at other meals.

One animal food notable for its vitamin A content is liver. A moment's reflection should reveal the reason for this. Vitamin A not needed for immediate use is stored in the liver.[11] Some nutritionists recommend that people include a serving of liver in their diets every week or two, partly for this reason.

People sometimes wonder if vitamin A toxicity can result from using liver too frequently. This problem has never been observed except in the arctic, where explorers who have eaten large quantities of polar bear liver have become ill with symptoms suggesting vitamin A toxicity. Liver is an extremely nutritious food, and its periodic use is highly recommended.

chlorophyll: the green pigment of plants, which absorbs photons and transfers their energy to other molecules, initiating photosynthesis.

photosynthesis: the synthesis of carbohydrates by plants from carbon dioxide and water, using the sun's energy.

Recall that folacin, too, is found most abundantly in dark-green vegetables.

The Roles of Vitamin D

Vitamin A helps to remodel bones; vitamin D helps to mineralize them. It is a member of a large and cooperative bone-making and maintenance team made up of nutrients and other compounds, including vitamin C; the hormones parathormone and calcitonin; the protein collagen, which underlies and supports bone; and the minerals calcium, phosphorus, magnesium, fluoride, and others, which compose the inorganic part of bone.

Blood calcium is very active metabolically. It has been estimated that about a fourth of the calcium in the blood is exchanged with bone calcium every minute. The special function of vitamin D is to help make calcium and phosphorus available in the blood that bathes the bones, to be deposited as the bones harden (mineralize).

Vitamin D raises blood concentrations of these minerals in three ways: by stimulating their absorption from the GI tract; by helping to withdraw calcium from bones into the blood; and by stimulating calcium retention by the kidneys. The star of the show is calcium itself; vitamin D is a director.

Parathormone and calcitonin: see p. 385.
Collagen: see pp. 294–295.

mineralization (calcification): the process in which calcium, phosphorus, and other minerals crystallize on the collagen matrix of a growing bone, hardening the bone.

---

11   Liver is not the only organ that stores vitamin A. The kidneys, adrenals, and other organs do too, but liver is the only one commonly eaten.

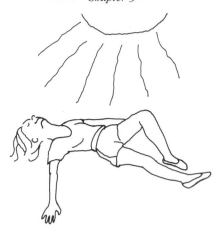

The precursor of vitamin D made in the liver is 7-dehydrocholesterol, which is made from cholesterol. This is one of the body's many "good" uses for cholesterol.

The technical name for the final product, active vitamin D, is 1,25-dihydroxycholecalciferol—dihydroxy vitamin D for short.

A description of how calcium moves from food into the blood and into and out of bone is reserved for Chapter 10, where a closer view of the whole system is provided. The object here is to make you aware of the importance of vitamin D, the risks of deficiency and toxicity, and the ways in which the vitamin can be obtained.

Vitamin D is different from all the other nutrients in that the body can synthesize it with the help of sunlight. Therefore, in a sense, vitamin D is not an essential nutrient. Given enough sun, you need consume no vitamin D at all in the foods you eat. Rather, it is like a hormone—a compound manufactured by one organ of the body that has effects on another. And like certain hormones, it can actually enter a cell, cross the nuclear membrane, attach to specific receptors on the DNA or its protein wrapping, and promote the synthesis of specific proteins.

The liver manufactures a vitamin D precursor, which is released into the blood and circulates to the skin. When ultraviolet rays from the sun hit this compound, it is converted to previtamin D_3, which works its way back into the interior of the body. Slowly, then, over the next 36 hours, the previtamin is converted with the help of the body's heat to vitamin D_3. Two more steps occur before the vitamin becomes fully active. First, the liver adds an OH group, and then the kidney adds another OH group at specific locations to produce the active vitamin.[12] (This is why diseases affecting either the liver or the kidney exhibit symptoms of bone deterioration.) Active vitamin D then promotes the making of several proteins that help with calcium transport into the intestinal cell, and assists them in their action.[13] It also has specific attachment sites in the brain, parathyroid glands, bone, and kidney, where it is thought to regulate the production of proteins that manage calcium homeostasis.[14] In the pancreas, it affects insulin secretion.[15]

There are two ways to meet your vitamin D needs. You can synthesize it yourself with the help of sunlight, or you can eat foods containing the preformed vitamin—chiefly animal foods.[16]

12 The whole story is told by one of the principal investigators in this area, whose meticulous work has revealed many more details than are presented here. See DeLuca, 1979, in Appendix J, "Vitamins."

13 A vitamin D–dependent, membrane-derived intestinal calcium-binding protein, *Nutrition Reviews* 39 (1981): 175–177.

14 Presence of 1,25-dihydroxyvitamin D_8 receptor in rat pituitary, *Nutrition Reviews* 39 (1981): 140–142.

15 A. W. Norman, B. J. Frankel, A. M. Heldt, and G. M. Grodsky, Vitamin D deficiency inhibits pancreatic secretion of insulin, *Science* 209 (1980): 823–825; Vitamin D and insulin, *Nutrition Reviews* 40 (1982): 221–222.

16 A plant version of vitamin D (ergosterol) may also yield an active compound, vitamin D_2 (ergocalciferol), on irradiation, but less is known about the body's further use of this compound. Thus animal sources of vitamin D are considered the only reliable ones.

Vitamin D Deficiency and Toxicity

Both inadequate and excessive vitamin D intakes take their toll in the United States and Canada, despite the fact that the vitamin has been known for decades to be essential for growth and toxic in excess. The Ten-State Survey conducted in the late 1960s revealed that nearly 4 percent of the children under six who were examined showed evidence of vitamin D deficiency, with several cases of overt rickets. (The more recent Nationwide Food Consumption Survey did not assess vitamin D.) The National Nutrition Survey in Canada revealed low intakes of vitamin D in women and children but no overt cases of rickets—although they may exist in persons not tested. Worldwide, rickets still afflicts large numbers of children.

The symptoms of an inadequate intake of vitamin D are those of calcium deficiency, shown in Table 9–4. The bones fail to calcify normally and may be so weak that they become bent when they have to support the body's weight. A child with rickets who is old enough to walk characteristically develops bowed legs, often the most obvious sign of the disease.

Adult rickets, or osteomalacia, occurs most often in women who have low calcium intakes and little exposure to sun, and who go through

rickets: the vitamin D-deficiency disease in children. A rare type of rickets, not caused by vitamin D deficiency, is known as **vitamin D refractory rickets**.

osteomalacia (os-tee-o-mal-AY-shuh): the vitamin D deficiency disease in adults.

osteo = bone

mal = bad (soft)

Osteomalacia may also occur in calcium deficiency; see Chapter 10.

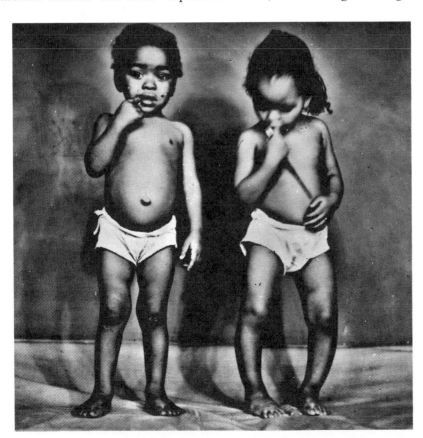

Rickets

Source: Courtesy of Parke-Davis & Company.

Bowing of the ribs causes the symptom known as **pigeon breast**. The beads that form on the ribs resemble rosary beads; thus this symptom is known as **rachitic** (ra-KIT-ik) **rosary** (the rosary of rickets).

Fontanel: the open space in the top of a baby's skull before the skull bones have grown together.

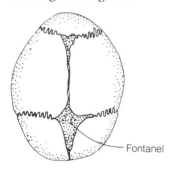

Fontanel

thorax: the part of the body between the neck and the abdomen.

alkaline phosphatase: an enzyme in blood.

Vitamin D activity was previously expressed in international units (IU) but as of 1980 is expressed in micrograms of cholecalciferol. To convert, use the factor:

100 IU = 2.5 µg

400 IU = 10 µg

TABLE 9–4 **Vitamin D Deficiency**

DISEASE	AREA AFFECTED	MAIN EFFECTS
Rickets	Bones	Faulty calcification, resulting in misshapen bones (bowing of legs) and retarded growth
		Enlargement of ends of long bones (knees, wrists)
		Deformities of ribs (bowed, with beads or knobs)
		Delayed closing of fontanel, resulting in rapid enlargement of head
	Blood	Decreased calcium and/or phosphorus
	Teeth	Slow eruption; teeth not well-formed; tendency to decay
	Muscles	Lax muscles resulting in protrusion of abdomen
	Excretory system	Increased calcium in stools, decreased calcium in urine
	Glandular system	Abnormally high secretion of parathyroid hormone
Osteomalacia	Bones	Softening effect: deformities of limbs, spine, thorax, and pelvis; demineralization; pain in pelvis, lower back, and legs; bone fractures
	Blood	Decreased calcium and/or phosphorus, increased alkaline phosphatase
	Muscles	Involuntary twitching, muscle spasms

repeated pregnancies and periods of lactation. The bones of the legs may soften to such an extent that a girl who grows up tall and straight becomes bent, bowlegged, and stooped by the end of her second or third pregnancy.

Vitamin D deficiency depresses calcium absorption and results in low blood calcium levels and abnormal mineralization of bone. An excess of the vitamin does the opposite, as shown in Table 9–5. It increases calcium absorption, causing abnormally high concentrations of the mineral in the blood, and promotes return of bone calcium into the blood as well. The excess calcium in the blood tends to precipitate in the soft tissue, forming stones. This is especially likely to happen in the kidneys, which concentrate calcium in the effort to excrete it. Calcification or hardening of the blood vessels may also occur and is especially dangerous in the major arteries of the heart and lungs, where it can cause death.

The range of safe intakes of vitamin D is narrower than that of vitamin A. Half the recommended intake is too little, but over a few times the recommended intake may be too much. Intakes of 100 micrograms per day cause high blood calcium levels in infants, and some infants are sensitive to lower doses than this. Intakes of 250 micrograms per day for four months or 5,000 micrograms per day for two weeks cause toxicity in children and, if further prolonged, in adults. The amounts of vitamin D found in foods available in the United States and Canada are well within these limits, but pills containing the vitamin in concentrated form should definitely be kept out of the reach of children.

TABLE 9–5 **Vitamin D Toxicity**

DISEASE	AREA AFFECTED	MAIN EFFECTS
Hypervitaminosis D	Bones	Increased calcium withdrawal
	Blood	Increased calcium and phosphorus concentration
	Nervous system	Loss of appetite, headache, excessive thirst, irritability
	Excretory system	Increased excretion of calcium in urine; kidney stones; irreversible renal damage
	Tissues	Calcification of soft tissues (blood vessels, kidneys, lungs), death

Vitamin D from Sun and Foods

In rapidly growing children, an intake of close to 10 micrograms (400 IU) of vitamin D a day is recommended; mature adults need half as much. Only a few animal foods supply significant amounts of the vitamin, notably eggs, liver, and some fish, and even these vary greatly, depending on the animal's exposure to sun and on its consumption of the vitamin in its foods. Neither cow's milk nor human breast milk supplies enough vitamin D to reliably meet human needs; hence cow's milk is fortified, and infants must be given either fortified formula or supplements. The fortification of milk with 400 IU per quart (360 IU per liter in Canada) is the best guarantee that children will meet their vitamin D needs and underscores the importance of milk in children's diets.

Significant amounts of vitamin D can be made with the help of sunlight. It is generally agreed that most adults, especially in the sunnier regions, need not make special efforts to obtain vitamin D in food. If children are taken out in the sun for a while each day at noon, they will receive a protective dose of vitamin D. However, people who are not outdoors much or who live in northern or predominantly cloudy or smoggy areas are advised to make sure their milk is fortified with vitamin D, to drink at least 2 cups a day, and to make frequent use of eggs and periodic use of liver in menu planning.

Darker-skinned people make less vitamin D on limited exposure to the sun. By 3 hours of exposure, however, vitamin D synthesis in strongly pigmented skin arrives at the same plateau as that at 30 minutes in fair skin. The difference may account for the fact that darker-skinned people in northern, smoggy cities are more prone to rickets. The experiments revealing these findings also suggest that overexposure to sun cannot cause vitamin D toxicity, because synthesis of vitamin D is limited to a fixed maximum on each exposure.[17]

The RDA for vitamin D for adults over 22 is 5 μg cholecalciferol (200 IU).

Canadian *Dietary Standard:* 2.5 μg cholecalciferol.

Exposure to sun should be reasonable. Excessive exposure may cause skin cancer.

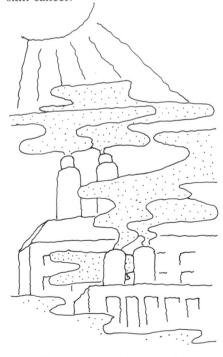

Smog filters out ultraviolet rays of the sun.

17   M. F. Holick, J. A. MacLaughlin, and S. H. Doppelt, Regulation of cutaneous previtamin D_8 photosynthesis in man: Skin pigment is not an essential regulator, *Science* 211 (1981): 590–593.

The Roles of Vitamin E

Antioxidant: see pp. 295–296.

oxidant: compound (such as oxygen itself) that oxidizes other compounds.

Vitamin E is an antioxidant like vitamin C, but fat-soluble. If there is plenty of vitamin E in the membranes of cells exposed to an oxidant, chances are this vitamin will take the brunt of the oxidative attack, protecting the lipids and other vulnerable components of the membranes. Vitamin E is especially effective in preventing the oxidation of the polyunsaturated fatty acids (PUFA), but it protects all other lipids (for example, vitamin A) as well.

One of the most important places in the body in which vitamin E exerts its antioxidant effect is in the lungs, where the exposure of cells to oxygen is maximal. At least two kinds of cells benefit from the vitamin's protection: the red blood cells that pass through the lungs, and the cells of the lung tissue itself. The vitamin acts to:

radicals: unstable molecular intermediates that arise during oxidation reactions. They are highly reactive and readily oxidize other molecules with which they come in contact; see Appendix B.

- Detoxify oxidizing radicals that arise during normal metabolism.
- Stabilize cell membranes.
- Regulate oxidation reactions.
- Protect vitamin A and polyunsaturated fatty acids from oxidation.

peroxidation: production of unstable molecules containing more than the usual amount of oxygen. Hydrogen peroxide, H_2O_2, for example, may be produced from water, H_2O. Appendix B explains the chemistry of free radical formation.

scavenger: a clean-up agent; for example, a garbage collector or an animal that feeds on refuse and waste.

Some similar roles are played by an enzyme containing the trace element selenium. See Chapter 11.

Lungs are sometimes also exposed to air pollutants that are strong oxidizing agents, such as nitrogen dioxide or ozone. Ozone causes peroxidation of the cell membrane lipids. A product of this peroxidation can be measured in expired air, and some people produce more of the product when exercising in air contaminated with ozone.[18] Vitamin E supplements restore the normal level, suggesting that vitamin E acts as a scavenger of free radicals.

Follow-up studies using animals have investigated the possibility that peroxidation can occur not only in lungs, but also in liver and adrenal tissue. In these locations, too, vitamin E seems to exert a protective effect.[19]

The role of vitamin E in protecting red blood cell membranes has led researchers to ask whether it might protect white blood cells as well, and perhaps participate in the body's immune defenses. Indeed, deficiency of vitamin E suppresses the immune system and supplementation stimulates it in several species of animals.[20] The effect may be direct, by way of the vitamin's action in the membranes of the white blood cells when they interact with antigens, or may be indirect by way of PUFA and prostaglandins.[21]

18   One group of experimenters found that some human subjects exercising in an ozone-contaminated environment breathed out more pentane (an index of peroxidation). Taking vitamin E supplements for two weeks (about 1,000 IU per day) restored pentane production to normal. C. J. Dillard and coauthors, Effects of exercise, vitamin E, and ozone on pulmonary function and lipid peroxidation, *Journal of Applied Physiology* 45 (1978): 927–932.

19   F. Umeda and coauthors, Inhibitory effect of vitamin E on lipoperoxide formation in rat adrenal gland, *Tohoku Journal of Experimental Medicine* 137 (1982): 369–377.

20   C. F. Nockels, Protective effects of supplemental vitamin E against infection, *Federation Proceedings* 38 (1979): 2134–2138; B. E. Sheffy and R. D. Schultz, Influence of vitamin E and selenium on immune response mechanisms, *Federation Proceedings* 38 (1979): 2139–2143.

21   Vitamin E does affect prostaglandin synthesis. Effect of vitamin E on prostanoid biosynthesis, *Nutrition Reviews* 39 (1981): 317–320.

Vitamin E Deficiency

Studies related to vitamin E's effects have seldom revealed any carryover of animal findings to humans. In fact, of 12 possible diseases associated with vitamin E deficiency in animals, only one has been demonstrated in human beings. When the blood concentration of vitamin E falls below a certain critical level, the red blood cells tend to break open and spill their contents, probably due to oxidation of the polyunsaturated fatty acids (PUFA) in their membranes.

Except to correct erythrocyte hemolysis, no need for vitamin E supplements has been demonstrated in normal human beings under normal environmental conditions. However, abnormal environmental conditions such as air pollution may increase human vitamin E needs. Also, a great many diseases can affect people's vitamin E needs. Among individuals who benefit from vitamin E supplementation are:

● Premature infants, because the transfer of vitamin E across the placenta becomes maximal only right before full-term delivery.[22]
● Infants, children, or adults who can't absorb fats and oils because of liver, pancreas, or gallbladder disease; GI surgery; or inherited diseases.[23]
● Individuals with certain blood disorders.[24]

Two other conditions seen in humans appear to be remediable by large doses of vitamin E. One, a harmless breast disease, is characterized by painful lumps in the breasts, which can be relieved with vitamin E therapy. The other, a leg problem, causes pain on walking and cramps in the calves at night, and also responds to vitamin E therapy.

Many extravagant claims have been made for vitamin E. It has been such a popular "miracle vitamin" that it vies with the snake-oil medicines of past times. But while research has revealed possible roles for vitamin E, it also has shown clearly some things that vitamin E does *not* do. During the 1960s and 1970s, vitamin E was said to improve athletic endurance and skill, to increase potency and enhance sexual performance, to prolong the life of the heart, and to reverse the damage caused by atherosclerosis and even heart attacks. An immense amount of experimentation has discredited

The breaking open of red blood cells is **erythrocyte** (eh-REETH-ro-cite) **hemolysis** (he-MOLL-uh-sis): the vitamin E deficiency disease in human beings.

erythrocyte: red blood cell.

erythro = red

cyte = cell

hemolysis: bursting of red blood cells.

hemo = blood

lysis = breaking

Both diseases have unwieldy names. One is **fibrocystic breast disease**, the other is **intermittent claudication**.

fibr = fibrous lumps

cystic = in sacs

intermittent = at intervals

claudicare = to limp

Caution: other very serious conditions can cause lumps in the breasts and cramps in the legs. Don't self-diagnose; see a doctor.

22   It seems that oxygen damage to the retina in these infants may be reduced or prevented by vitamin E given in time. Vitamin E in clinical nutrition, *Nutrition and the MD*, October 1982.

23   These conditions include cirrhosis, cystic fibrosis, biliary obstruction, abetalipoproteinemia, and gastrectomy. In biliary atresia, a problem with bile secretion in children, vitamin E given by injection prevents a long list of neurological problems that otherwise develop, suggesting that normal nerve development depends on vitamin E. M. A. Guggenheim, Vitamin E deficiency diseases, *Vitamin Nutrition Information Service*, RCD 3813A/III, Hofmann–La Roche, Inc., Nutley, NJ 07110. In adults with severe malabsorption of fat, neurological dysfunction is improved by vitamin E. D. P. R. Muller, J. K. Lloyd, and O. H. Wolff, Vitamin E and neurological function, *Lancet*, January 29, 1983, pp. 225–228.

24   These include sickle-cell anemia, beta thalassemia, and G6PD (a red-blood-cell enzyme) deficiency.

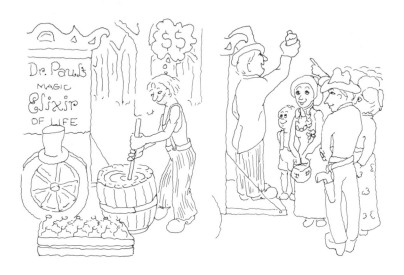

these and many similar claims.[25] To give one example: Doses of 1,600 IU a day given to 48 heart patients for six months had no effect on chest pain (angina), exercise capacity, heart function, or other factors related to heart disease.[26] Vitamin E also does not help with:

- Lowering high blood lipids, including cholesterol.[27]
- "Hot flashes."[28]
- Bladder cancer.[29]
- Preventing heart attacks.
- Restoring or improving sexual potency.
- Improving athletic ability.

Nor does it have any effect on other processes of aging, such as graying of the hair, wrinkling of the skin, and reduced activity of body organs.

Another thing vitamin E does *not* do is prevent or cure muscular dystrophy in humans. Hereditary muscular dystrophy is a disease afflicting children, who usually die at an early age when their respiratory muscles deteriorate. Nutritional muscular dystrophy, however, is the muscular weakness produced in many animals by a deficiency of vitamin E. This

muscular dystrophy (DIS-tro-fee): a hereditary disease in which the muscles gradually weaken; its most debilitating effects arise in the lungs.

nutritional muscular dystrophy: a vitamin E deficiency disease of animals, characterized by gradual paralysis of the muscles.

25   Expert Panel on Food Safety and Nutrition, Committee on Public Information, Institute of Food Technologists, Vitamin E, *Contemporary Nutrition* 2 (November 1977); A. L. Tappel, Vitamin E, *Nutrition Today*, July/August 1973, pp. 4–12; H. H. Draper and coauthors, A further study of the specificity of the vitamin E requirement for reproduction, *Journal of Nutrition* 84 (1964): 395–400.

26   R. E. Gillilan, B. Mondell, and J. R. Warbasse, Quantitative evaluation of vitamin E in the treatment of angina pectoris, *American Heart Journal* 93 (April 1977): 444–449; Vitamin E: A scientific status summary by the Institute of Food Technologists' Expert Panel on Food Safety and Nutrition and the Committee on Public Information, *Food Technology* 31 (1977): 77–80.

27   E. T. G. Leonhardt, Effects of vitamin E on serum cholesterol and triglycerides in hyperlipidemic patients treated with diet and clofibrate, *American Journal of Clinical Nutrition* 31 (1978): 100–105.

28   Questions readers ask, *Nutrition and the MD*, May 1980.

29   Questions, 1980.

deficiency leads to atrophy of the muscles; it can be cured by reintroducing vitamin E into the diet. At no time has there been any evidence in reliable literature that links this condition to hereditary muscular dystrophy.

Two steps are necessary in both animal and human research to show that lack of a nutrient is causing a certain symptom. First, a diet lacking that nutrient and only that nutrient must be fed. The administration of this diet must result consistently in the appearance of the deficiency symptom. Then, when the nutrient is returned to the diet, the deficiency symptom must disappear. Furthermore, nutrient research using animals requires several preparatory steps.

● An animal must be found that does not synthesize the nutrient. For example, research on vitamin C deficiency cannot be carried out on rats, because rats synthesize vitamin C. Guinea pigs have to be used instead.

● A laboratory feed must be prepared that contains all essential nutrients except the one under study. This entails the time-consuming task of mixing the nutrients in the correct proportions—usually synthetic nutrients, since natural foods would very likely contain traces of the nutrient being excluded. Moreover, chemical analysis must show that the mixture is indeed free from the nutrient and that it is not lacking in another essential nutrient. (Alternatively an antinutrient can be used to bind, inactivate, or compete with the nutrient in question, but then the researcher must distinguish between the effects of the nutrient's lack and those of the antinutrient's presence.)

● The animals must have a common heredity and be maintained on similar diets for the same length of time prior to the start of the experiment.

● Other variables may need to be controlled for specific nutrients. For example, if it has been shown in other work that a nutrient's absorption is under seasonal hormone control, that fact will need to be considered in the design of the experiment.

When the deficiency symptom has been produced in the laboratory animal and alleviated with the addition of the missing nutrient, researchers can say that in that species they have found the lack of a particular nutrient to cause a particular symptom. When other laboratories have replicated these results, they are accepted—for that species. Until laboratory research has shown this relationship to be true for another species of animal, researchers can only theorize that the relationship may be true in both.

It is much trickier to apply knowledge gained from research with laboratory animals to humans than to transfer knowledge gained from one species to another in the laboratory. The experimental animal is caged, thus assuring that feed, fluid, temperature, and most of the factors in his environment will be controlled. It is also possible to allow the experiment to continue until the animals die, after which an autopsy can

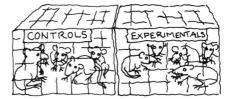

show the effects of the nutrient deficiency on the internal organs.

In research with humans, the intake of food and fluid cannot be controlled except in short-term experiments. In addition, there is no way of knowing that all subjects are in a similar nutritional state prior to the beginning of the experiment. This fact necessitates the use of large numbers of human subjects so that the results can be averaged. Finding a large enough population hinders the launching of such an experiment and adds to the cost. Experimentation on human beings must also depend on subjects who are free to break the restrictions of the diet or to drop out of the experiment at any time, even if they are being paid to be subjects.

In the case of vitamin E research on human beings, there have been several unique obstacles in addition to these:

● Vitamin E is widely distributed in foods. It is, therefore, difficult to compose a diet totally devoid of it.

● Vitamin E is one of the fat-soluble vitamins and as such is stored in abundance in the tissues of the body, particularly in adipose tissue. Therefore, it takes a long period of deficiency for the body to be depleted.

Another type of study that can be carried out with humans involves pooling results from many case studies involving possible vitamin E deficiency to see if there is a common thread. It is by these means that vitamin E has been shown to be ineffective in the treatment of such diseases as muscular dystrophy, reproductive failure, and heart disease.

In summary, when a symptom has been shown to be caused by a nutrient deficiency in several species of laboratory animals, this fact can be used as a pointer toward the existence of the same relationship in humans. However, until a deficiency symptom can be produced in human subjects by a diet deficient in the nutrient and then cured by the restoration of that nutrient, it cannot be claimed that the symptom is caused by the lack of that nutrient.

Caution

Vitamin E Toxicity

All kinds of people take vitamin E supplements for all kinds of reasons. As a result, many signs of toxicity are now known or suspected, including disturbances of the action of many hormones, interference with vitamin K, alteration of the mechanism of blood clotting, alteration of blood lipid levels, impairment of white blood cell activity, GI distress, and many, many more.[30] Doses of 100 IU, or certainly of 300 IU, should be considered megadoses and should only be taken on a physician's advice, with caution, or not at all.[31]

30   H. J. Roberts, Perspective on vitamin E as therapy (commentary), *Journal of the American Medical Association* 246 (1981): 129–131.

31   Roberts, 1981.

Vitamin E Intakes and Food Sources

Vitamin E is a kind of alcohol, namely a tocopherol. Several tocopherols occur in foods; the most active is alpha-tocopherol. Alpha-tocopherol occurs in two mirror-image forms, D and L (remember D and L sugars in Chapter 2), of which the D form is more active. Different forms of vitamin E differ in their activity; to reconcile them the recommended intake is, as of 1980, expressed in terms of "the amount of vitamin E activity equivalent to that of 10 milligrams of D-alpha-tocopherol." Many people were surprised when, in 1980, the RDA for vitamin E appeared to have dropped from the 15 units recommended in 1974 to 10 units. Actually, the units changed, and 15 of the old units give the same activity as 10 of the new ones. The amount of vitamin E recommended is the same.[32]

A person's need for vitamin E is higher if the amount of PUFA he consumes is higher. Fortunately, vitamin E and the polyunsaturates tend to occur together in the same foods.

Vitamin E is widespread in foods. About 60 percent of the vitamin E in the diet comes directly or indirectly from vegetable oils in the form of margarine, salad dressings, and shortenings; another 10 percent comes from fruits and vegetables; smaller percentages come from grains and other products. Soybean oil and wheat germ oil have especially high concentrations of vitamin E; cottonseed, corn, and safflower oils rank second, with a tablespoon of any of these supplying more than 10 milligrams (more than the RDA) of the vitamin. Other oils contain less (for example, peanut oil supplies about half as much per tablespoon). Animal fats such as butter and milk fat have negligible amounts of vitamin E.

Vitamin E is readily destroyed by heat processing and oxidation, so fresh or lightly processed foods are preferable as sources of this vitamin. The processed and convenience foods often used by the elderly and nursing homes may contribute to a vitamin E deficiency if their use continues over several years.[33]

tocopherol (tuh-KOFF-er-all): a kind of alcohol (see Appendix C). Alpha-tocopherol is one of several forms of tocopherol, and D-alpha-tocopherol is the "right-handed" version.

The RDA for vitamin E for adults: 10 mg for men, 8 mg for women.

Canadian *Dietary Standard:* 8–9 mg for men, 6 mg for women.

Vitamin E units: 1 mg = 1 IU D-alpha-tocopherol.

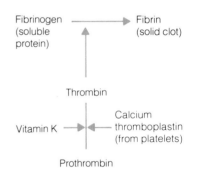

The clotting process. TH9-3

Vitamin K

Vitamin K seems to act primarily in the blood clotting system. There, its presence can make the difference between life and death. At least 13 different proteins and the mineral calcium are involved in making a blood clot, and vitamin K is essential for the synthesis of at least 4 of these proteins, among them prothrombin, the precursor of the protein thrombin.[34]

K stands for the Danish word *koagulation* (coagulation or clotting).

Prothrombin and thrombin: see p. 138.

32 Bieri and McKenna, 1981.

33 H. H. Koehler, H. C. Lee, and M. Jacobson, Tocopherols in canned entrees and vended sandwiches, *Journal of the American Dietetic Association* 70 (1977): 616–620.

34 It has recently been learned that vitamin K also participates with vitamin D in synthesizing a bone protein that helps to regulate blood calcium levels. The active form of vitamin D stimulates the synthesis of a vitamin K–dependent bone protein, *Nutrition Reviews* 39 (1981): 282–283.

hemorrhagic (hem-o-RAJ-ik) **disease**: the vitamin K deficiency disease.

hemophilia: a hereditary disease having no relation to vitamin K but caused by a genetic defect that renders the blood unable to clot because of lack of ability to synthesize certain clotting factors.

hemolysis: see p. 341.

jaundice: yellowing of the skin, due to spillover of bile pigments from the liver into the general circulation.

The bacterial inhabitants of the digestive tract are known as the **intestinal flora**.

flora = plant inhabitants

Provisional RDA for vitamin K (1980): 70–140 µg.

sterile: free of microorganisms, such as bacteria.

The synthetic substitute usually given for vitamin K is **menadione** (men-uh-DYE-own); see Appendix C.

When any of these factors is lacking, blood cannot clot and hemorrhagic disease results; if an artery or vein is cut or broken under these circumstances, bleeding goes unchecked. (As usual, this is not to say that the cause of hemorrhaging is always vitamin K deficiency. Another cause is hemophilia, which is not curable by vitamin K.) Deficiency of vitamin K may occur under abnormal circumstances when absorption of fat is impaired (that is, when bile production is faulty, or in diarrhea). The vitamin is sometimes administered before operations to reduce bleeding in surgery but is only of value at this time if a vitamin K deficiency exists. Toxicity is not common but can result when water-soluble substitutes for vitamin K are given, especially to infants or to pregnant women. Toxicity symptoms include red cell hemolysis, jaundice, and brain damage.[35]

Vitamin K can be made within your GI tract—but not by you. In your intestinal tract there are billions of bacteria, which normally live in perfect harmony with you, doing their thing while you do yours. One of their "things" is synthesizing vitamin K that you can absorb. You are not dependent on bacterial synthesis for your vitamin K, however, since many foods also contain ample amounts of the vitamin, notably green leafy vegetables, members of the cabbage family, and milk.

The body resists vitamin K deficiency, and it is seldom seen except when an unusual combination of circumstances conspire to bring it about. When it does occur, however, it can be fatal. The scenario goes like this: a patient is in the hospital; he has been given antibiotics to prevent or overcome infection; and he is being fed a formula diet that does not include vitamin K. The antibiotics have killed his intestinal bacteria, and his vitamin K stores are depleted. Now he goes into surgery, and when he bleeds, his blood fails to clot normally; so he bleeds to death. The combination of antibiotics, unsupplemented formula diet, and surgery raises a warning flag and requires that clotting time be checked before surgery is performed.[36]

Brand new babies are commonly susceptible to a vitamin K deficiency, for two reasons. First, a baby is born with a sterile digestive tract; he has his first contact with intestinal bacteria as he passes down his mother's birth canal, and it takes the bacteria a day or so to establish themselves in the baby's intestines. Second, a baby may not be fed at the very outset (and breast milk is a poorer source of vitamin K than cow's milk). A dose of vitamin K (usually in a water-soluble form similar but not identical to the natural vitamin) may therefore be given at birth to prevent hemorrhagic disease of the newborn; it must be administered carefully to avoid toxic overdosing. People taking sulfa drugs, which destroy intestinal bacteria, may also become deficient in vitamin K.

---

35 A toxic dose of a vitamin K compound causes the liver to release a bile pigment into the blood (hyperbilirubinemia), and leads to jaundice of certain areas of the brain (kernicterus). Vitamin K, in *Vitamin-Mineral Safety*, 1978, pp. 11–12.

36 Intestinal microflora, injury and vitamin K deficiency, *Nutrition Reviews* 38 (1980): 341–343.

Summing Up

Vitamin A as a part of visual pigments is essential for vision, especially in dim light. Vitamin A is involved in maintaining the integrity of mucous membranes throughout the internal linings of the body and thus in promoting resistance to infection. It helps maintain the skin and is essential for the remodeling of bones during growth or mending; it also plays a part in cell membranes, in hormone synthesis, in reproduction, and in other functions.

Deficiency of vitamin A causes night blindness due to the failure to regenerate rhodopsin; a failure of mucous secretion, which can lead by way of keratinization of the cornea to blindness; disorders of the respiratory, urogenital, reproductive, and nervous systems; and abnormalities of bones and teeth. Toxicity symptoms are caused by large excesses (ten times the recommended intake or more) taken over a prolonged period and result only from the preformed vitamin (from supplements or animal products such as liver)—not from the precursor carotene and its relatives, the yellow pigments found in plants.

The recommended intake for vitamin A (800 RE for women, 1,000 RE for men) is easily met by periodically consuming the vitamin's richest food sources, such as liver or dark-green leafy vegetables, or by consuming other concentrated sources daily, such as carrots, cantaloupe, yellow squash, or broccoli. All plant food sources of the carotenoids have some color.

Vitamin D promotes intestinal absorption of calcium, mobilization of calcium from bone stores, and retention of calcium by the kidneys, and is therefore essential for the calcification of bones and teeth. Given reasonable exposure to sun, humans can synthesize this vitamin in the skin from a precursor manufactured by the liver. Deficiency of vitamin D causes the calcium deficiency diseases (rickets in children and osteomalacia in adults); excesses cause abnormally high blood calcium levels, due to excessive GI absorption and withdrawal from bone, and result in deposition of calcium crystals in soft tissues, such as the kidneys and major blood vessels. The recommended adult intake of 200 IU (5 micrograms cholecalciferol) per day is best met by drinking fortified milk; food sources of vitamin D are unreliable. However, exposure to sunlight probably ensures vitamin D adequacy for the average adult.

The best-substantiated role of vitamin E in humans is as an antioxidant that protects vitamin A and the polyunsaturated fatty acids (PUFA) from destruction by oxygen. Although many vitamin E deficiency symptoms have been observed in animals, only one has been confirmed in humans: erythrocyte hemolysis. Vitamin E also protects the lungs against oxidizing air pollutants.

The recommended intake of vitamin E is 6 to 10 milligrams per day for adults. The human requirement for vitamin E is known to vary with PUFA intake; since the vitamin occurs with PUFA in foods, it is normally supplied in the needed amounts. Deficiencies are seldom observed, but there is some concern that the overuse of processed foods may make deficiencies more likely. Toxicity symptoms are seen with intakes above 300 milligrams per day.

Vitamin K, the coagulation vitamin, promotes normal blood clotting; deficiency causes hemorrhagic disease. The vitamin is synthesized by intestinal bacteria and is available from foods such as green vegetables and milk. Deficiency is normally seen only in newborns, whose intestinal flora have not become established, in people taking antibiotics or sulfa drugs, or in people whose fat absorption is impaired.

NOTE: Appendix J suggests additional readings on vitamins A and D: See "Vitamins." The Self-Study for this chapter (Appendix Q) shows you how to:

● Evaluate your intakes of vitamins A, D, E, and K.
● Detect nutrition misinformation with respect to the fat-soluble vitamins.

An optional lecture in the *Instructor's Manual* delves into the connections between vitamin A and other nutrients and cancer.

HIGHLIGHT 9
World Hunger

The light of curiosity absent from children's eyes. Twelve-year-olds with the physical stature of eight-year-olds. Youngsters who lack the energy to brush aside flies collecting about the sores on their faces. Agonizingly slow reflexes of adults crossing traffic. Thirty-year-old mothers who look sixty. All are common images in developing countries; all reflect inadequate nutrition; all have societal consequences.

ALAN BERG

Hunger wastes the most precious of all the world's resources—the human being. Despite numerous development programs, malnutrition is not disappearing; the tragic number of malnourished people continues to grow. Nutrition planners are rightly concerned with increased food production, better storage facilities, access to markets, more stable supplies, better nutritional quality of foodstuffs, and ultimately food consumption itself. In addition, these fundamental questions have to be asked. What is restricting the poor's access to food? How can these restrictions be removed? Adequate nutrition can be achieved only when the economic, political, and social structures which hinder food consumption become the targets of change.

The term **hunger** as used here means a continuous lack of the nutrients necessary to achieve and maintain optimum health, well being, and protection from disease.

Prevalence of Malnutrition

The United Nations Food and Agriculture Organization (FAO) estimates that there are at least a half-billion malnourished people in the world today. These people lack the nutrients to support healthy, active lives. The marks of undernutrition include blind eyes, swollen bellies, skin irritations, general listlessness, and stunted physical growth. Table H9–1 lists the nations described by the United Nations as most seriously affected.

Of all population groups, children are most seriously affected by malnutrition.[1] The United Nations World Health Organization (WHO) reports that there are 10 million severely malnourished children under the age of five; these children are below 60 percent of the standard body weight for their age. Another 240 million preschoolers are also estimated to be suffering from malnutrition. Additional millions of children die yearly from the

"Leila is a girl of seven in the urban slums of Dacca, Bangladesh. During the last two years her eyes have been growing dim. Today she is stone blind not by accident or birth defect but because of a lack of vitamin A in her daily diet. For this malady there is no cure. Now sightless, Leila is looked upon by her parents as a sign of the curse of Allah. She is kept in the back room and no longer plays with other children. In her isolation from her past playmates and from the lost sights of the world around her, she cries."

1   The stories of the children Leila and Ishmael, told in the margin, are from D. Burgess, The future of hungry children abroad, *Journal of Current Social Issues*, Summer 1975, p. 36.

349

TABLE H9–1 **Countries Most Seriously Affected by Hunger**

Afghanistan	Guatemala	Nepal
Bangladesh	Guinea	Niger
Benin	Guinea-Bissau	Pakistan
Burma	Guyana	Rwanda
Burundi	Haiti	Samoa
Cameroon	Honduras	Senegal
Cape Verde	India	Sierra Leone
Central African Empire	Ivory Coast	Somalia
Chad	Kenya	Sudan
Democratic Yemen	Laos	Sri Lanka
Egypt	Lesotho	Tanzania
El Salvador	Madagascar	Uganda
Ethiopia	Mali	Upper Volta
Gambia	Mauritania	Yemen Arab Republic
Ghana	Mozambique	

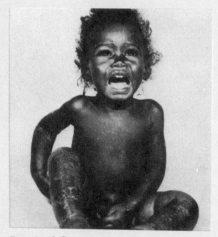

Protein deficiency.

Marasmus and kwashiorkor: see Chapter 4.

indirect effects of marginal malnutrition—parasites and infectious diseases with accompanying diarrhea, which interact with poor nutrition in a vicious cycle. For example, measles, a relatively mild disease in industrialized countries, has a high fatality rate in Africa. Among poorly nourished children, the mortality rate for measles may be several hundred times the rate among well-nourished children.[2] Chronic diarrhea, whooping cough, tuberculosis, malaria, and parasites also aggravate sickness and mortality in malnourished children.

The most widespread form of malnutrition among children in the developing world today is protein-kcalorie malnutrition, or PCM. Children who are thin for their height may be suffering from acute PCM or recent severe food restriction, whereas children who are short for their age have experienced long-term chronic PCM. Stunted growth due to PCM, rather than symptoms of vitamin and mineral deficiency diseases, may be the most common sign of malnutrition in developing countries.[3] Breastfeeding permits infants in many developing countries to achieve weight and height gains equal to children in developed countries until about six months of age, but then the majority of these children, too, fall behind in weight and height. Failure of children to grow is a warning that one of the extreme forms of PCM, marasmus or kwashiorkor, may soon follow.

Mother-Child Malnutrition

Pregnant or lactating women, together with their small children, have a greater need for nutrients for their size than other groups because of the higher demand for nutrients during periods of rapid growth (see Chapter 13). When family food is limited, these women and their children are the first to show the signs of undernutrition.

2   D. Morley, *Pediatric Priorities in the Developing World* (London: Butterworth, 1973), p. 207.

3   S. N. Gershoff, Science—neglected ingredient of nutrition policy, *Journal of the American Dietetic Association* 70 (1977): 471.

Maternal weight gain during pregnancy is necessary for normal fetal growth and development. Women in developed countries gain an average of 12.5 kilograms (about 27 pounds). Studies among poor women show a weight gain often limited to 5 to 7 kilograms (11 to 15 pounds).[4] Women with lower weight gains in pregnancy more often have low-birthweight babies. Infection, congenital defects, and death are often seen in low-birthweight infants.

In India, several studies show that a significant number of pregnant women are underweight and experience a deficit of 500 to 600 kcalories a day.[5] Women in developing countries are responsible, even during their pregnancies, for most of the physical labor required to procure food for their families. The poor nutrition of these women is also the result of the distribution of food in the family. A mother will feed her husband, children, and other family members first, eating only whatever is left. Cultural and social beliefs also limit food intake.[6]

Other instances of malnutrition can be traced to inappropriate "modernization," such as replacing breast milk with formula feeding in environments and economic circumstances that make it impossible to formula feed safely. Breast milk, the recommended food for infants, is sterile and contains antibodies that enhance an infant's resistance to disease. Formula in bottles, however, in the absence of sterilization and refrigeration, is an ideal breeding ground for bacteria. More than 1,300 million people in developing countries do not have access to safe drinking water.[7] Mixing contaminated water with milk powder and feeding this to infants often causes infections leading to diarrhea, dehydration, and decreased absorption of nutrients from the foods the children are given. Malnourished children cannot fight these infections effectively, and many die.

The infant mortality rate ranges from about 50 (Sri Lanka) to over 200 (Afghanistan) in the poorest of the developing countries as compared with an average of 13 to 20 in the developed countries. The death rate for children from one to four years old is no more favorable; it ranges from 20 to 30 times higher in developing countries than in developed countries.[8] This age span includes the weaning period, one of the most dangerous periods for all children. Infection, delayed at first by breastfeeding, appears inevitable after weaning. Causes include ingesting infected water, gruel, or other materials.

In developing countries, the diet's basis is formed by bulky grains such as wheat, rice, millet, sorghum, and corn and by starchy root crops such as cassava, sweet potatoes, plantain, and bananas. These may be supple-

A low-birthweight baby is one that weighs less than 2,500 grams (5.5 pounds) at birth.

"Ishmael, age four, was taken by his parents during the terrible drought last year from their two acres of parched farmland to a refugee camp in Wollo Province of Ethiopia in order to get food, medicine, and shelter. Because his mother had a sparse diet when she was carrying Ishmael in her womb, and because he was not fed enough nutritious food for his first four years, Ishmael acts deranged at times, apathetic at others. He grunts instead of talking. His parents will never know that his mother's deficient diet four years ago and his subsequent lack of enough food in his early years have damaged his brain permanently. If Ishmael lives through the current famine, he will never learn to read or write. He will be destined to become the village idiot."

infant mortality rate: the number of deaths during the first year of life per thousand live births.

In the Indian Punjab, Dr. Carl Dyer, director of the Johns Hopkins Narangwal Program, aimed at reducing malnutrition in local villages, found that a malnutrition rate of 10 to 15 percent persisted even after a major effort to provide supplementary foods. The majority of those affected were very young females, least able to demand their share and least recognized by other family members as deserving a fair share. In other areas of India, a child may be forbidden to eat curds and fruit because they are "cold," and bananas because they "cause convulsions."

---

4   M. Cameron and Y. Hofvander, *Manual on Feeding Infants and Young Children*, 2nd ed., Protein Advisory Board of the United Nations, 1976, p. 1.

5   S. Ghosh, *The Feeding and Care of Infants and Young Children*, 2nd ed. (New Delhi: Voluntary Health Association of India, 1976), pp. 3–4.

6   Dr. Carl Dyer's findings related to social and cultural beliefs about food in India, described in the margin, are from A. Berg, *The Nutrition Factor* (Washington, D.C.: Brookings Institute, 1973), p. 46.

7   I. Rozov, The decade: Not just pumps and pipes, *World Health*, April–May 1983, p. 29.

8   World Bank, *World Development Report 1981*, Table 21.

Legumes are also sometimes called **pulses**.

mented with legumes (peas or beans) and, rarely, with animal proteins. An infant has a small stomach and can't eat enough of these staples (grains or root crops) to meet its daily energy and protein requirements. A great need exists to develop more adequate and inexpensive weaning foods in the developing countries. The most promising weaning foods are usually concentrated mixtures of grain and locally available peas or beans.[9] Mothers are advised to continue breastfeeding while they introduce weaning foods.

Limited Success in Local Efforts

Infants and children need not be raised in middle-class homes to be protected from PCM. Slight modifications of the children's own diets can be immensely beneficial. Encouraging examples are provided by recent experiences in Sierra Leone, Nepal, and Southeast Asia.

In Sierra Leone, "Bennimix" was developed from subsistence crops and introduced as a supplement to infants' diets. Rice, sesame (benniseed), and ground nuts were hand-pounded to make a flour meal and then cooked. The local children found it tasty—and, whereas they had been malnourished before, they thrived when Bennimix was added to their diets. The village women formed a cooperative to reduce the household drudgery of preparation, and they rotated the work on a weekly or monthly basis.[10] The government also established a manufacturing plant to produce and market the mixture at subsidized prices. The success of the venture appeared to lie in involving the local people in the process of identifying the problem and devising its solution. It was not considered enough only to accomplish the goals of an agency; the needs of the people were remembered.

A similar success was achieved in Nepal by maximizing use of local resources and facilities to prepare a supplementary food. Ingredients for the food were soybeans, corn, and wheat, mixed in a 2:1:1 proportion, and yielding a concentrated "super-flour" of high biological value suitable for infants and children. A Nutrition Rehabilitation Center tested this super-flour by giving the undernourished children and their mothers two cereal-based meals a day, and giving the children three additional small meals of super-flour porridge daily. Within ten days the undernourished children had gained weight, lost their edema, and recovered their appetites and social alertness. The mothers, who saw with their own eyes the remarkable recoveries of their children, were motivated to learn how to make the tasty supplementary food and incorporate it into their local foodstuffs and customs.[11]

Another success story is the research surrounding the winged bean plant, cultivated in Southeast Asia for years, but only recently studied by the

9   P. Pellet, The role of food mixtures in combating childhood malnutrition, in *Nutrition in the Community*, ed. D. McLaren (New York: Wiley, 1978), pp. 185–202.

10   J. M. Steckle, Improving food utilization in developing countries, *Canadian Home Economics Journal* 27 (1977): 34–39.

11   *National Conference on Primary Health Care* (Kathmandu: Ministry of Health, Health Services Coordination Committee, WHO, UNICEF, 1977), pp. 9, 25, as cited by M. E. Frantz, Nutrition problems and programs in Nepal, *Hunger Notes* 2 (1980): 5–8.

National Academy of Sciences. The plant is easily cultivated, even in sandy soil and tropical climates, needs no fertilizer, and is completely edible. The winged bean is similar to the soybean, but is much easier to grow. Complemented with corn, it can be made into a weaning food with the protein quality of milk and a high vitamin A content.[12]

These three examples offer hope that the world food situation can be improved by simple means, but they do not fully address the issue of poverty. One-shot intervention programs—offering nutrition education, food distribution, food fortification, and the like—are not enough. It is difficult to describe the misery a mother feels when she has received education about nutrition but is unable to purchase the foods her family needs. She now knows *why* her child is sick and dying but is helpless in *applying* her new knowledge.

Major Problems Still to Solve

The discussion thus far illustrates a major fact that many people are unaware of. World hunger is *not* the result of a world food shortage. The rest of this Highlight will show you the realities underlying world hunger and will invite you to become personally involved in bringing about the end of hunger in our lifetime. An understanding of what causes hunger in the world is basic to deciding what must be done.

The world food problem is many things. It is an economic problem, because supply and demand for food are not balanced. It is a technological and environmental problem. It is a demographic problem as well as a moral scandal in which there is unequal access to resources, extremes of dietary patterns, and an unjust economic system. The status of the world food situation is poignant even when presented statistically (see Table H9–2). Some of the causes of the problem are shown in Table H9–3. Two generalizations and an important question are suggested by these tables:

1 The underlying causes of global hunger and poverty are complex and interrelated.
2 Hunger is a product of poverty resulting from the ways in which governments and businesses manage national and international economies.
3 The question "Why are people hungry?" has been answered: "Because they are poor." The question that remains to be answered is "Why are people poor?"

A diagram of the poverty-hunger web is presented in Figure H9–1.

Solutions and Alternatives

Experts assure us that we possess the knowledge, technology, and resources to end hunger. As individuals, therefore, we can take action to respond to this human suffering. Hunger and poverty in a world that has

---

12   The Hunger Project, *A Shift in the Wind* 13 (1982): 3. A new report, *The Winged Bean: A High Protein Crop for the Tropics*, is available from: Commission on International Relations, National Research Council, 2101 Constitution Avenue, Washington, DC 24018.

TABLE H9–2 **The Realities of Hunger**

The United Nations reports that there are 520 million malnourished people in the world.

Fifteen to twenty million people die each year of hunger-related causes, including diseases brought on by lowered resistance due to malnutrition. Of every four of these, three are children.

Over 40 percent of all deaths in poor countries occur among children under five years old.

UNICEF states that 17 million children died last year from preventable diseases—one every two seconds, 40,000 a day. (A vaccination immunizing one child against a major disease costs 7 cents.) At least 50 million children are permanently blinded each year simply through lack of vitamin A.

More than 500 million people in poor countries suffer from chronic anemia due to inadequate diet.

Every day, the world produces 2 pounds of grain for every man, woman, and child on earth. This is enough to provide everyone with 3,000 kcalories a day, well above the average need of 2,300 kcalories.

A person born in the rich world will consume 30 times as much food as a person born in the poor world.

The poor countries have nearly 75 percent of the world's population, but consume only about 15 percent of the world's available energy.

Almost half the world's people earn less than $200 a year—many use 80 to 90 percent of that income to obtain food.

Of nearly 5 billion people on earth, more than 1 billion drink contaminated water. Water-related disease claims 25 million lives a year. Of these, 15 million are under five years of age.

There are 800 million illiterates. In many countries, half of the population over 15 is illiterate. Two-thirds of these are women.

The money required to provide adequate food, water, education, health, and housing for everyone in the world has been estimated at $17 trillion a year. It is a huge sum of money —about as much as the world spends on military expenditures every two weeks.

Sources: *World Hunger: Facts*, Oxfam America, 115 Broadway, Boston, MA 02116; Office on Global Education, Church World Service, 2115 North Charles Street, Baltimore, MD 21218.

the means to alleviate them are intolerable and unacceptable—even for one more day. The rest of this Highlight will discuss some of the changes necessary, on the international, national, and personal levels, to end world hunger. The issues to be addressed in more detail are:

● *Birth rates:* The importance of realizing that overpopulation is caused, not by food abundance, but by hunger.
● *Land reform:* The need for aggressive redistribution of resources.
● *Multinational corporations:* The need for a change in their role in the developing countries.
● *Lifestyle:* How *we* can avoid contributing to world hunger.
● *Agenda for action:* How *you* can become part of the solution to the world food problem.

Overpopulation and Hunger

The current world population is approximately 5 billion, and for the year 2000 the projected United Nations figure is 6 billion. These facts justify

TABLE H9–3 **Causes of the World Food Problem**

WORLDWIDE PROBLEMS	PROBLEMS OF DEVELOPING WORLD
1. Natural catastrophes—drought, heavy rains and flooding, crop failures	1. Underdevelopment
2. Environmental degradation—soil erosion and inadequate water resources	2. Excessive population growth
3. Food supply-and-demand imbalances	3. Lack of economic incentives—farmers using inappropriate methods and laboring on land they may lose or can never hope to own
4. Inadequate food reserves	4. Parents lacking knowledge of basic nutrition for their children
5. Warfare and civil disturbances	5. Insufficient government attention to the rural sector
6. Migration—refugees	
7. Culturally based food prejudices	
8. Declining ecological conditions in agricultural regions	

PROBLEMS OF INDUSTRIALIZED WORLD	PROBLEMS LINKING INDUSTRIAL AND DEVELOPING WORLDS
1. Excessive use of natural resources	1. Unequal access to resources
2. Pollution	2. Inadequate transfer of research and technology
3. Inefficient, animal-protein diets	3. Lack of development planning
4. Inadequate research in science and technology	4. Insufficient food aid
5. Excessive government bureaucracy	5. Excessive food aid
6. Loss of farmland to competing uses	6. Politics of food aid and nutrition education
	7. Inappropriate technological research
	8. Inappropriate role of multinational corporations
	9. Insufficient emphasis on agricultural development for self-sufficiency

Source: Adapted from C. G. Knight and R. P. Wilcox, *Triumph or Triage? The World Food Problem in Geographical Perspective*, Resource paper no. 75–3 (Washington, D.C.: Association of American Geographers, 1976), p. 4.

concern over the world's capacity to produce adequate food in the future. It does not necessarily follow, however, that "too many people" is the cause of the world food problem. Actually, poverty seems to be at the root of the problem, and both hunger and overpopulation are caused by poverty. Three factors affect population growth: birth rates, death rates, and standards of living. Low-income countries have high birth and death rates and a low standard of living. When a people's standard of living rises, giving them better access to health care, family planning, and education, the death rate falls first, but then the birth rate also falls. As the standard of living continues to improve, the family earns sufficient income to risk having smaller numbers of children. A family depends on its children to cultivate the land, to secure food and water, and to make the adults secure in their old age. If a family is confronted with ongoing poverty, parents will choose to have many children to ensure that some will survive to adulthood. Therefore, the improvement of poor people's economic status is a most effective means of contraception.

Evidence supports the idea that we first have to reduce the infant mortality rate if we want to reduce the birth rate.[18] Families will only choose to

13   The human tide ebbs a little, *New York Times*, 29 July 1983.

FIGURE H9-1 **Behind hunger stands poverty.**

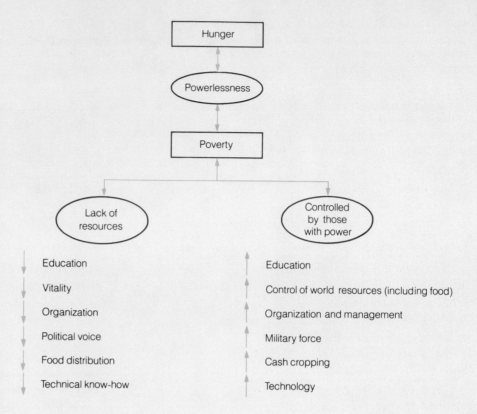

"Fernando is a child of 5 in Bolivia. His father, a hardworking copper miner, and his mother care for him and his six brothers and sisters. Fernando has rickets, is anemic, is small in stature and weak in body. Because of the lack of clean water in his village, he and other members of his family suffer from continual diarrhea. If Fernando is lucky enough to become an adult, he will remain small in stature and weak in body. If Fernando dies soon, his parents will feel impelled to bring another child into the world in the hope that a new child will live to adulthood and be able to care for the parents in old age."

have fewer children if they feel sure their children will *live*. Table H9–4 shows the relationships between infant mortality rate and population growth rate. These statistics reveal that hunger and poverty in a nation reflect not only the level of national development but also the people's sense of security.[14]

In many countries where economic growth has occurred and resources have been distributed relatively equally among all groups, the rates of population growth have decreased. Examples include China, Costa Rica,

TABLE H9-4 **Infant Mortality Rate and Birth Rate in Hungry and Nonhungry Countries**
TH9-4

	HUNGRY COUNTRIES	NONHUNGRY COUNTRIES
Average infant mortality rate	113	35
Total infant deaths per year	10.6 million	1.4 million
Size of population	2.3 billion	2.3 billion
Average rate of increase	2.4%	1.0%
Total births per year	86.4 million	38.6 million

Source: Adapted from *The Ending Hunger Briefing Workbook*, 1982, available from The Hunger Project, 2015 Steiner Street, San Francisco, CA 94115, pp. 26, 30.

14 The story of Fernando, told in the margin, is from Burgess, 1975.

South Korea, Sri Lanka, Taiwan, and West Malaysia. In countries where economic growth has occurred but the resources have been unevenly distributed, population growth has remained high. Examples are Brazil, Mexico, the Philippines, and Thailand, where a large family continues to be a major economic asset for the poor.[15]

Distribution of Resources/Land Reform

Land reform—giving people a more meaningful stake in food production, development, and the benefits of society—can combine with population control to increase everyone's assets. To introduce this section, a few facts must be presented:[16]

● Much of the world's agriculture is very primitive. More than 50 percent of all food consumed in the world is still hand-produced.
● In many countries, up to 90 percent of the population lives on rural land.
● Of the more than 150 nations of the world, fewer than 24 are democracies. Most governments dictate the day-to-day lives of their people.
● Securing enough food on a day-to-day basis is a problem for as many as a billion human beings.
● The land in many parts of the world does not support the growing of food, even by the wealthy. Furthermore, the poor are often crowded onto mountainous slopes that are even less arable.

arable: capable of being plowed.

arare = to plow

The problem of unequal distribution of resources exists not only between rich and poor nations but also between rich and poor people within nations. The FAO estimates that world food production averages about 3,000 kcalories per person per day, but that food is distributed unequally. Huge amounts of grains are fed to livestock to produce protein foods the poor cannot afford to purchase. Also, by some estimates, at least 20 percent of the total food produced is lost to pests and spoilage.[17]

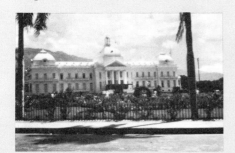
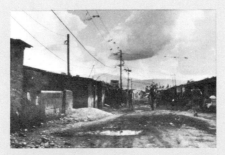
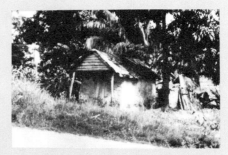

The stark contrasts between rich and poor within a single developing country are depicted here in the homes of the people. The ruler maintains a palace while the majority of the population live in city tenements or rural huts.

15   J. Kocher, Not too many but too little, in *The Feeding Web: Issues in Nutritional Ecology*, by J. D. Gussow (Palo Alto, Calif.: Bull Publishing, 1978), pp. 81–83.

16   R. R. Spitzer, *No Need for Hunger* (Danville, Ill.: Interstate Printers and Publishers, 1981), pp. 20–23.

17   *Nutrition Week* 13 (Washington, D.C.: CNI, 1983), pp. 4–5.

If you give a man a fish, he will eat for a day. If you teach him to fish, he will eat for a lifetime.

Again, the problem is poverty; the symptom is inability to purchase basic food for sustenance. But the wealthy nations cannot simply give to the poor; it weakens them further not to fend for themselves. The question of policy makers and nutrition planners is: How do we increase the productivity and self-reliance of the rural poor in a nonpaternalistic fashion? Much is involved, but four things are basic and are required simultaneously. The poor must have greater opportunities for access to land, capital, technology, and knowledge.[18] International food aid is also required during the development period.

Governments have learned from recent history the importance of developing local agricultural technology. A major effort made in the 1960s—the Green Revolution—failed because it was not in harmony with local realities. It was an effort to bring the genetic-engineered, petroleum-demanding agricultural technology of the industrial world to the developing countries, but the high-yielding strains of wheat and rice that were selected required irrigation, chemical fertilizers, and pesticides—all costly, and beyond the economic means of too many of the farmers in the developing world.

Instead of transplanting industrial technology into the developing countries, there is a need to develop small, efficient farms and local structures for marketing, credit, transportation, food storage, and agricultural education. International research centers need to examine the conditions of tropical countries and orient their research towards labor-intensive rather than energy-intensive agricultural methods.

Environmental concerns must be taken more seriously as well. As important as the amount of land available for crop production is the condition of the soil. Soil erosion is now accelerating on every continent, at a rate that threatens the world's ability to continue feeding itself. Erosion of soil has always occurred; it is a natural process—but in the past it has been compensated for by processes that build the soil up. Farmers should alternate soil-building crops with soil-devouring crops, a practice known as crop rotation. An acre of soil planted one year in corn, the next in wheat, and the next in clover loses 2.7 tons of topsoil each year, but if it is planted only in corn it will lose 19.7 tons a year.[19] When a farmer must choose whether to make three times as much money planting corn year after year or rotate crops and go bankrupt, naturally he chooses the profits. Ruin may not follow immediately, but it will follow.[20]

Multinational Corporations: Coordinators of World Hunger?
Businesspeople, economists, and some development specialists often extol the benefits to Third World countries deemed to result from the investments of multinational corporations, especially in fostering eco-

Third World: the underdeveloped nations of the world that are aligned with neither the communist nor the noncommunist blocs.

18   M. R. Langham, L. Polopolus, and M. L. Upchurch, *World Food Issues* (Gainesville, Fla.: University of Florida Press, 1982), pp. 18–20.

19   National Agricultural Lands Study, *Soil Degradation: Effects on Agricultural Productivity, Interim Report No. 4* (Washington, D.C.: USDA, November 1980), as cited by L. R. Brown, World population growth, soil erosion, and food security, *Science* 214 (1981): 995–1002.

20   Brown, 1981.

nomic growth. Other observers, however, are convinced that the multinationals have done more harm than good. Because the negative effects have included malnutrition, the topic of this Highlight, they are emphasized here. (Other views are presented in Appendix J and elsewhere.[21])

The opponents of multinational corporations suggest that hunger is the result of political and economic systems that exploit the poor. A multinational corporation's primary concern is profit.

> Agribusiness is now buying or renting more and more arable land. Decisions on what to plant and where to distribute the harvest are made with the balance sheet in mind. Thus it is profitable in poor countries to use land for exportable luxuries even while the people are suffering severe malnutrition because it does not grow enough grain.[22]

Multinational corporations are international organizations with direct investments and/or operative facilities in more than one country. The U.S. oil companies are an example.

The classical example of the subtle exploitation of the poor, related to nutrition, is the competition for farmland between cash crops and food crops. The tragic scenario unfolds this way: Large landowners and multinational corporations control the best farmlands, and they use them mainly to grow crops that can be exported at considerable profit. Native persons work for below-subsistence wages and are forced onto marginal lands to do their own farming. The poor work hard, but they are cultivating crops for other people, rather than for themselves. The money they earn is not enough even to buy the products they help produce. The poor never acquire their share of the profits realized from the marketing of their products. The results: imported foods—bananas, beef, cocoa, coconut, coffee, pineapple, sugar, tea, winter tomatoes, and others—fill *our* grocery stores, while the poor who grow these foods have even less food and resources than before. Additional cropland is diverted for nonfood cash crops—tobacco, rubber, cotton, and other agricultural products.

The rural poor in many countries subsidize the diets of the more affluent.

Export-oriented agriculture thus uses the labor, land, capital, and technology that is needed to help local families produce their own food. For example, the effort required to produce bananas for export could be reallocated to provide food for the local people. It has been suggested that one solution to the world food problem is not that the developed countries should *give* more food aid, but that they should *take* less food away from the poor countries.[23] Truly, imported foods raised on land from which thousands of small farmers have been displaced symbolizes the exploitation of the poor as vividly as does a bottle of contaminated formula in the mouth of a dying infant.

Countless examples can be cited to illustrate how natural resources are diverted from producing food for domestic consumption to producing luxury crops for those who can afford them. A few such examples are included here:[24]

21 For the other side of the argument—offering multinationals as part of the solution rather than the problem—see M. L. Kastens, Harvest of hunger: How government meddling threatens the world's food supply, *Futurist* 15, no. 5 (1981): 5–10.

22 R. J. Barnet, Multinationals: A dissenting view, *Saturday Review* 3 (1976): 11, 58.

23 G. Kent, Food trade: The poor feed the rich, *Food and Nutrition Bulletin* 4 (1982): 25–33.

24 F. M. Lappe and J. Collins, *Food First: Beyond the Myth of Scarcity* (Boston: Houghton Mifflin, 1978), p. 15.

● Africa is a net *exporter* of barley, beans, peanuts, fresh vegetables, and cattle (not to mention luxury crop exports such as coffee and cocoa), yet it has a higher incidence of PCM among young children than any other continent. . . .

● Mexico now supplies the United States with over half its supply of several winter and early spring vegetables, while infant deaths associated with poor nutrition are common. . . .

● Half of Central America's agricultural land produces food for export, while in several of its countries the poorest 50 percent of the population eat only half the protein they need. (The richest 5 percent, on the other hand, consume two to three times more than they need.)

Besides diverting acreage away from the traditional staples of the diet, multinationals may also contribute to hunger by way of their marketing techniques. Their advertisements lead many consumers with limited incomes to associate products like cola beverages, cigarettes, infant formula, and snack foods with good health and prosperity. These promotions are tragically inappropriate for these people. A poor family's nutrition status suffers when its tight budget is pinched further by purchase of such goods.

The United Nations has commissioned several studies in the hopes of establishing an international code of conduct for the multinational corporations.[25] These powerful organizations can have an immense impact on national economies, for good or for ill. They can, if they choose, increase the credit and capital available to the developing world; and these resources, if properly used, can help to eliminate hunger. The multinationals also possess the scientific knowledge and organizational skills needed to help develop improved food and agricultural systems. However, experience reveals that wise control of these corporations is mandatory to ensure that human needs do not become subordinate to political and financial gains.

Lifestyle: Influencing World Hunger

How we choose to live our individual lives is ultimately a personal matter; however, our choices have an impact on the way the rest of the world's people live and die. Our nation, with 6 percent of the world's population, consumes about 40 percent of the world's food and energy resources. The food problem depends partly on the demands we place on the world's finite natural resources. In a sense, we therefore contribute to the world food problem. People in affluent nations have the freedom and means to choose their lifestyles; people in poor nations do not. We can find ways to reduce our consumption of the world's nonrenewable resources; we can use only what is absolutely required. The admonition, so familiar in childhood, to "clean your plate," as if that would alleviate the suffering of some starving stranger, could well be replaced with the mandate simply to "consume less food." Choosing a diet at the level of necessity, rather than excess, would decrease the resource demands made by our industrial agri-

25 *Identifying a Food Policy Agenda for the 1980s: A Working Paper*, Interreligious Taskforce on U.S. Food Policy, January 1980, p. 30.

culture. Humanitarian and economic benefits could be achieved, as well.

One major way to reduce the demands we make on world resources is to depend less on animal-based protein and to use more plant-based proteins. Even one meal a week per person would make a difference. Meat does not necessarily have to be eliminated totally from the diet, because ruminants —cattle, sheep, and goats—can use forage crops and crop residues produced on land not suitable to other crops.[26] In so doing, these animals convert plants indigestible by humans into high-quality animal protein. Today, however, much rich cropland is used to grow animal feed instead of foods for humans. The animals are then fed these grain and protein feeds in feedlots, where they are fattened much faster than if they had grazed on pastureland. Figure H9–2 shows the different rates at which animals convert feed to edible animal protein. As shown, chickens require about 3 pounds of grain to produce one pound of meat, whereas cattle require 16 pounds of grain to do the same. An argument, therefore, is that by simply cutting back on our beef consumption and substituting less land-costly plant protein sources, we could make large amounts of land available for human food production. We would also realize other ecological benefits, including decreased water and fertilizer requirements. Irrigation for beef alone requires 4 to 45 times more water than for other field crops.[27] To understand some of the inefficiency in the consumption of protein and kcalories from animal rather than plant sources, one needs to examine the dynamics of the food chain, as shown in Figure H9–3.

A second way in which the developed world can foster betterment of the quality of life in the developing countries is to shift to a less energy-dependent lifestyle. This type of private commitment stems from the reali-

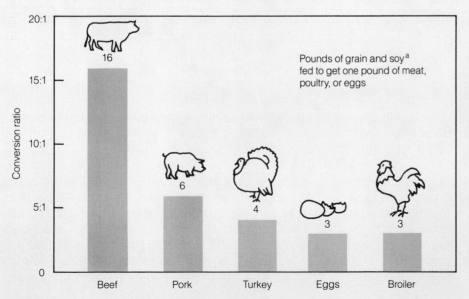

FIGURE H9–2 **A protein factory in reverse.** TH9-5

[a]Soy constitutes only 12% of steer feed and 20–25% of poultry feed.
Source: F. M. Lappé, *Diet for a Small Planet* (New York: Ballantine Books, 1975), p. 11. Institute for Food and Development Policy, 1885 Mission Street, San Francisco, CA 94103.

26   The argument in favor of maintaining animal agriculture is discussed in Spitzer, 1981, pp. 183–202.

27   C. G. Knight and R. P. Wilcox, *Triumph or Triage? The World Food Problem in Geographical Perspective*, Resource paper no. 75–3 (Washington, D.C.: Association of American Geographers, 1976), p. 53.

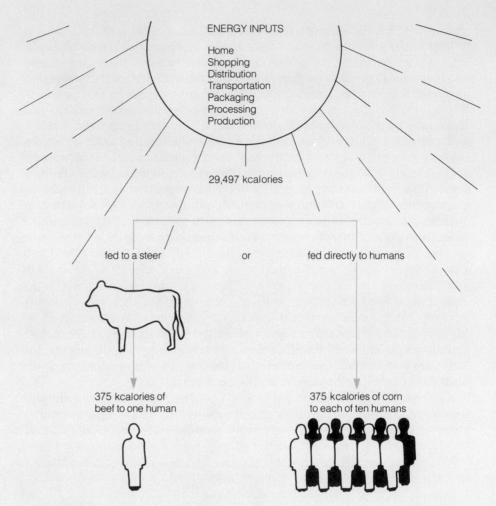

ENERGY INPUTS

Home
Shopping
Distribution
Transportation
Packaging
Processing
Production

29,497 kcalories

fed to a steer   or   fed directly to humans

375 kcalories of
beef to one human

375 kcalories of corn
to each of ten humans

FIGURE H9-3 **The food chain**. It takes
3,011 kcalories to bring to a consumer a
1-pound can of sweet corn that has a
food value of 375 kcalories. It takes
29,497 kcalories to supply 140 grams of
beef, also worth 375 kcalories. TH9-6

Source: Adapted from D. Pimentel and
M. Pimentel, *Food, Energy and Society* (New
York: Wiley, 1979).

zation that hunger can be eliminated. Table H9–5 lists several suggestions
for reducing our energy consumption, and the last section of this Highlight
offers more ways to become further involved in ending world hunger.

This Highlight has suggested that the availability of food is dependent
on many interrelated factors: population, lifestyle, available arable land,
water, fertilizer, energy supply, and others. The present food and energy
resources will not meet the needs of the future. A world planning objective
might therefore be to balance food supply, energy expenditures, and population growth. Two steps we might take toward achieving this objective
might be to use more plant foods in the diet and, as already mentioned, to
reduce our energy use. These measures, by themselves, would do nothing
to solve the world hunger problem, but they would help create the potential for a solution.

The primary reason to alter our food and energy consumption patterns is
not to redistribute our food to underdeveloped countries, but to reduce the
demand we make on their resources. This would make those resources
available to them for their own self development.

TABLE H9–5 **Lifestyle: Reducing Energy Consumption**

1. Choose to eat lower on the food chain. Learn the basis of plant protein complementarity.

2. If you eat beef, look for sources of forage-fed or grass-fed, rather than grain-fed, cattle.

3. Grow your own fruits and vegetables whenever possible. This reduces energy needed in commercial transport of these products. Use organic fertilizer and biological pesticides to further reduce energy consumption.

4. Choose an adequate, not an excessive, diet. Avoid having to throw food away after meals.

5. Reduce use of heavily processed foods—frozen specialty and convenience foods.

6. Avoid nonreturnable beverage containers. Recycle glass, aluminum, paper, and other goods.

7. Whenever possible, purchase staple goods in bulk containers. Join or start a food cooperative.

Source: Adapted from D. Katz and M. T. Goodwin, *Food: Where Nutrition, Politics, and Culture Meet* (Washington, D.C.: Center for Science in the Public Interest, 1976), p. 155.

It follows, of course, that careful planning is required so that the poor themselves realize the potential benefits being suggested here. Guidelines must be developed, to divert to needy markets the resources this country would make available, and these guidelines must be reflected in the policies of our government. In the words of an author who has devoted intensive study to world hunger:

> We somehow have failed to recognize that doing good for the sake of doing good is self-interest. To most people, ethical concerns are of value. Compassion and human decency may not lend themselves neatly to cost-benefit analysis, but the desire for sound moral values is a legitimate rationale for government action. Somehow, affluent societies must learn to accept this kind of self-interest as a basis for public policy.[28]

Agenda for Action

To summarize what is known about the world food situation, let us examine the conclusions of the Presidential Commission on World Hunger. The members of the commission believe that the 1980s must be a decade of concern for human life. They are convinced that worldwide efforts to overcome hunger and malnutrition and to foster self-reliant development must be intensive. Their major conclusions are listed in Table H9–6.

Reducing personal consumption, eliminating food waste, and more equitably distributing existing food sources are immediate short-range solutions to end hunger. Long-range solutions are necessary as well, and you may use the resource list in Appendix J to find the books and organizations that will provide you not only with food for thought but also with the will to chart your course of action.

Now is an opportune time to exercise our global citizenship on behalf of the poor. One of the most important steps individuals can take is to urge government and corporate policy makers to make hunger a priority item,

28   A. Berg, The trouble with triage, *New York Times Magazine*, June 15, 1975, pp. 26–35.

TABLE H9–6 **Presidential Commission on World Hunger: Conclusions**

- The major world hunger problem today is the prevalence of chronic undernutrition—which calls for a political as well as a technical solution.
- The world hunger problem is getting worse rather than better.
- A major crisis of global food supply—of even more serious dimensions than the present energy crisis—appears likely within the next 20 years, unless steps are taken now to facilitate a significant increase in food production in the developing nations.
- Rising global demand for food must be met within resource limits—of land, water, energy, and agricultural inputs.
- There is no ideal food, no perfect diet, no universally acceptable agricultural system waiting to be transplanted from one geographic, climatic, or cultural setting to another. Assistance programs must focus on self-reliance and respond to the needs of each country. Needs and requirements cannot be generalized.
- In addition to action by the industrialized nations, decisive steps to build more effective national food systems must be taken by the developing countries.
- The outcome of the war on hunger, by the year 2000 and beyond, will be determined not by forces beyond human control, but by decisions and actions well within the capability of nations and people working individually and together.

Source: Presidential Commission on World Hunger, *Overcoming World Hunger: The Challenge Ahead* (Washington, D.C.: Government Printing Office, 1980), pp. 180–185.

just as the issues of energy, inflation, and nuclear arms are. Three of the most powerful social movements of this century began with moral outrage against dehumanized situations—sex discrimination, slavery, and the war in Vietnam. Vigorous voices are needed to influence the policies of our governments and corporations, since their present policies of food trade, aid, and investment appear to be keeping the Third World *underdeveloped*. To remain silent is to render support to the status quo. To urge change is to make it known that the way to achieve food adequacy for everyone in a sensible time span is with a detailed, monitored, aggressive policy of redistribution, both at the international and national levels.

At this printing our government had recently formed a National Task Force on Hunger. It is up to those committed to ending hunger to make their intentions known to this task force. Further suggestions for your personal contribution to the solution are listed here:

- Read more about national and international food issues. Discuss these issues with a group of friends or coworkers. Be able to articulate them to others.
- Help raise money for volunteer agencies working abroad. Their projects directly affect some portion of the poor at the grassroots level, and are more likely to get food and funds into the hands of the poor than are those of top-heavy bureaucracies.
- Examine the sources of foods and products you buy. You may decide to join in boycotting products imported from developing countries as cash crops or products of companies that market goods inappropriately in the Third World. What we choose to eat affects not only our lives but also the lives of those who produce it.

● Attend or organize an event to raise your community's awareness of world food issues. World Food Day occurs annually on October 16, commemorating the founding of FAO, the United Nations agency responsible for improving global access to food. Oxfam America sponsors the Fast for a World Harvest each year in November.

● Support local groups such as food banks and soup kitchens. Donate time, funding, or food.

● Write letters, as often as possible. Ask your government legislators what they are doing to end world hunger. Share your knowledge with them. Write to local newspapers—provide them with information on hunger issues to be shared with their readers. Oxfam America and Bread for the World have guidelines to help you write effectively to these people.

How may we move closer to the ideal of an adequate diet every day for all men, women, and children? Many avenues are open. People can make a difference in the world food problem. We have the technology and resources available to feed everyone on earth. All that is needed is the will to do so.

NOTE: Recommended resources and references for further reading are given in Appendix J. See "World Hunger." Information and addresses are also provided for you to contact organizations actively involved in the world food problem.

The *Instructor's Manual* has two supplementary transparency/handout masters related to world hunger. One describes what it is like to live on one hundred dollars a year and the other gives tips on effective letter writing. TH9-7, TH9-8

"Hunger exists not because we can't end it, but simply because we haven't."—World Runners

CHAPTER 10

Water and the Major Minerals

CONTENTS

The mineral phosphorus abounds in DNA. The tremendous, orderly tangle shown here is part of a chromosome consisting of long loops of DNA attached to a core of protein (dark area at bottom).

It was assuredly not chance that led Thales to found philosophy and science with the assertion that water is the origin of all things.

LAWRENCE J. HENDERSON

Water and dissolved minerals provide the medium in which nearly all of the body's reactions take place, participate in many of these reactions, and supply the means for transporting vital materials to cells and waste products away from them. Every cell in the body is bathed in a fluid of the exact composition that is best for it. Each of these fluids is constantly undergoing loss and replacement of its constituent parts as cells withdraw nutrients and oxygen from them and excrete carbon dioxide and other waste materials into them. Yet the composition of the body fluids in each compartment remains remarkably constant at all times. Every important constituent of body fluids is similarly regulated. The interstitial fluid, for example, always has a high concentration of sodium and chloride ions and lower concentrations of about eight other major ions. The intracellular fluid always has high potassium and phosphate concentrations and lower concentrations of other ions. These special fluids regulate the functioning of cells; the cells in turn regulate the composition and amount of the fluids. The entire system of cells and fluids remains in a delicate but firmly maintained state of dynamic equilibrium.

367

The maintenance of this balance is so important that it is credited with our ability and that of other animals to live on land. It is thought that we had single-celled ancestors that depended on the sea water they lived in to provide nutrients and oxygen and to carry away their waste. We have managed over the course of our 2-billion-year evolutionary history to internalize the ocean—to continue bathing our cells in a warm nutritive fluid that keeps them alive. The amounts of salts in our body fluids, and their temperature, are believed to be the same as in the ocean—not as it is now, but as it was at the time when our ancestors emerged onto land. The ocean has since become more salty, but we still carry the ancient ocean within us.

This chapter first introduces you to water itself; then to the minerals that contribute to salt balance; and then to the body's other major minerals.

Water in the Body

Water in the body is a river coursing through the arteries, capillaries, and veins, carrying a heavy traffic of nutrients and waste products. Water molecules also nestle inside the body's giant proteins, glycogen, and other macromolecules, helping to form their structure. It constitutes about 55 to 60 percent of an adult's body weight.

Water also serves many other functions:

- It participates actively in many chemical reactions.
- It serves as the solvent for minerals, vitamins, amino acids, glucose, and a multitude of other small molecules.
- It acts as a lubricant around joints.
- It serves as a shock absorber inside the eyes, spinal cord, and amniotic sac in pregnancy.
- It aids in the body's temperature maintenance.

Salt does not refer only to sodium chloride but also to ionic compounds, as defined in Appendix B:

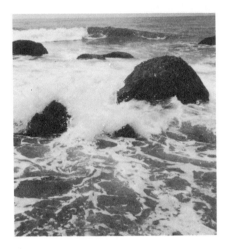

The Constancy of Total Body Water

The total amount of water in the body remains constant, thanks to the delicate balancing mechanisms that regulate intake and excretion.

Thirst governs water intake; when you need water, you drink. The evidence from experiments with thirst points to the possibility that several mechanisms operate in its regulation. One is in the mouth itself. When the blood is too salty (having lost water but not salts), water is withdrawn from the salivary glands into the blood. The mouth becomes dry as a result, and you drink to wet your mouth. Another thirst mechanism is in a brain center, where cells sample and monitor the salt concentration in the blood. When they find it too high, they initiate impulses that travel to brain centers that in turn stimulate drinking behavior. The stomach may also play a role. Thirsty animals drink until nerves in their stomachs, known as stretch receptors, are stimulated enough to turn off the drinking. More must be learned about these mechanisms, but it is clear from what we know already that thirst is finely adjusted to provide a water intake that exactly meets the need.

Water follows salt, moving in the direction of higher osmotic pressure (see pp. 375–377).

The brain center described here is the **hypothalamus** (hy-po-THAL-a-mus).

The mechanism of water excretion involves the brain and the kidneys. The cells of the hypothalamus, which monitor salt concentration in the blood, stimulate the pituitary gland to release a hormone, ADH, whenever the body's salt concentration is too high. ADH stimulates the kidneys to hold back (actually, reabsorb) water, so that it recirculates rather than being excreted. Thus the more water you need, the less you excrete. There are also cells in the kidney itself that are responsive to the salt concentration in the blood passing through them. When they sense a too-high salt concentration, they too release a substance. By a roundabout route, this substance also causes the kidneys to retain more water (see Figure 10–6, later in this chapter). Again, the effect is that when more water is needed, less is excreted.

These renal excretion mechanisms cannot work by themselves to maintain water balance unless you drink enough water. This is because the body must excrete a minimum amount of water each day—the amount necessary to carry away the waste products generated by a day's metabolic activities. Above this amount (a minimum of about 500 milliliters a day), the amounts of water you excrete can be adjusted to balance your intake. The urine merely becomes more dilute. Hence drinking plenty of water is never a bad idea.

In addition to the obvious dietary source, water itself, nearly all foods contain water (see p. 3). In addition, water is generated from the energy nutrients in foods (recall that the Cs and Hs in these nutrients combine with oxygen during metabolism to yield CO_2 and H_2O). Daily water intake from these three sources totals on the average about 2½ liters (about 2½ quarts). Similarly, in addition to the water excreted via the kidneys, some water is lost from the lungs as vapor, some in feces, and some from the skin. The losses of all of these also total about 2½ liters a day on the average. Table 10–1 shows how intake and excretion naturally balance out.

ADH (antidiuretic hormone): a hormone released by the pituitary gland in response to high osmotic pressure of the blood. The kidney responds by reabsorbing water.

This substance is the enzyme **renin** (REEN-in). See Figure 10–6 for its action leading to the release of **aldosterone**.

A liter is roughly the same size as a quart. A U.S. quart is a little smaller and a Canadian (imperial) quart a little bigger than a liter.

The Water Supply

When you draw water from the tap into a glass and drink it, it is not only water that you are drinking. Chlorine may have been added to it, to kill microorganisms that might otherwise convey disease. Fluoride may have been added to it, if your community has adopted fluoridation. In addition, it contains naturally occurring minerals, toxic heavy metals, live microorganisms, and a miscellany of organic compounds. Most people in the more developed countries take their water supply for granted and assume that it is pure and safe. At the same time, they may be very much concerned over the presence of incidental additives in food. Actually, water may contain "incidental additives" of greater significance to human health than those in foods.

The quality of water varies, depending on its source. To learn about the water in your area, you may want to consult your local health department. The variables affecting water quality fall into four groups: minerals, heavy metals, microorganisms, and organic compounds. In addition, there are important questions to ask about water quantity.

TABLE 10–1 **Water Balance**

WATER INTAKE	ML
Liquids	550–1,500
Foods	700–1,000
Metabolic water	200– 300
	1,450–2,800

WATER OUTPUT	ML
Kidneys	500–1,400
Lungs	350
Feces	150
Skin	450– 900
	1,450–2,800

hard water: water containing high concentrations of calcium and magnesium.

soft water: water containing a high sodium concentration.

cation: see p. 374.

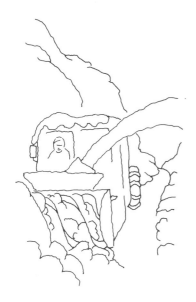

Minerals in the Water Supply

All the 20-odd major and trace minerals discussed in this chapter and the next are present in various ground waters in different concentrations. Often they make significant contributions as nutrients to the health of the people who drink the water. A case in point is fluoride, which in some areas occurs naturally at the concentration that precisely meets the human need for fluoride. Few communities have yet analyzed their water supplies completely enough to state which mineral needs they may be helping to meet, but most at least have information about the major minerals.

The distinction between hard and soft water, which has some important health implications, is based on three of these minerals. Hard water usually comes from shallow ground, and it contains high concentrations of the cations calcium and magnesium. Soft water usually comes from deep in the earth, and its principal cation is sodium. Well water is hard or soft, depending on the area. Most people distinguish between these two types of water in terms of their practical experience. Soft water dissolves soap better and leaves less of a ring on the tub; hard water leaves a residue of rocklike crystals in the teakettle after a while, and turns clothes gray in the wash. Hence consumers often consider soft water to be the more desirable and may even purchase water-softening equipment, which removes magnesium and calcium and replaces them with sodium. However, as far as we know today, hard water seems to support health better.

Soft water can add appreciable sodium to people's diets, and it appears to contribute to a higher incidence of high blood pressure and heart disease in areas where it is used. The National Academy of Sciences has suggested a standard for public water allowing no more than 100 milligrams of sodium per liter. This limit would ensure that the water supply would add not more than 10 percent to the average person's total sodium intake. The American Heart Association has recommended a more conservative standard of 20 milligrams per liter, to protect heart and kidney patients whose sodium intakes must be restricted. At present, about half the U.S. population drinks water containing more than 20 milligrams per liter. Where snowy roads are salted, the salt running off into the water supply may raise its sodium content considerably higher than this.

Soft water also dissolves certain metals, such as cadmium and lead, from pipes. Cadmium is not an essential nutrient. In fact, it can harm the body, affecting at least some enzymes by displacing zinc from its normal sites of action. Cadmium has been found in high concentrations in the kidneys and urine of patients with high blood pressure and is suspected of having some causal connection with the condition. A normal intake of zinc may protect against cadmium-induced high blood pressure. Lead is another toxic metal, and the body seems to absorb it more readily from soft than from hard water—possibly because the calcium in hard water protects against its absorption.[1]

---

1   Soft water and heart disease, *Nutrition and the MD*, November 1975.

The examples just given show that the choice to install a water softener in your home may be unwise, especially if your family is heart-disease prone. (One family we know solves the problem by connecting the water softener only to the hot-water line, then using hot water for washing and bathing, and only cold water for cooking and drinking.) These examples also show that the minerals in water interact in unpredictable ways. Someday we may be able to fortify our water with the ideal amounts of minerals for human consumption. But before that time arrives, we have much to learn about what is in the water already and what is ideal for humans.

Caution

Toxic Metals in the Water Supply

In the wilderness, water cycles rapidly through living systems, undergoing a natural purifying process in every cycle. Animal waste excreted onto the earth is filtered out by the soil before the water arrives underground. Pollutants entering rivers quickly disappear back into the earth as the rivers flow along, leaving the water pure. But neither the earth nor its rivers can purify completely the heavily polluted water expelled as city sewage or industrial waste. Water leaving a factory may contain concentrations of toxic metals so high that some are still present when it is recycled to become drinking water. And if the water is cycled through the same factory again, it will contain still higher concentrations the next time around.

Human technology bears the burden of purifying water contaminated by human technology. The Public Health Service sets drinking water standards (upper limits for the amounts of toxic metals permitted in water), and public law distributes the responsibility for adhering to these standards among the industries and the water-processing plants.

The metals of greatest concern are mercury, cadmium, and lead. These metals may be absorbed into the body, where they change cell membrane structure, alter enzyme or coenzyme functions, or even change the structure of the genetic material, DNA, causing cancer or birth defects. If they happen to alter the DNA in the germ cells (eggs or sperm), the changes (mutations) will become hereditary. When combined into complexes with organic compounds, these metals may be absorbed especially rapidly and may damage body tissue even more.[2]

Mercury is one of the rarer elements in the earth's crust, but has been mined extensively for industrial use; and so it is present in our environment in unnaturally high concentrations. Much of it ends up in the water supply as mercury compounds. By far the most toxic of these is methyl mercury, which is efficiently (90 percent) absorbed in the GI tract and accumulates in red blood cells, the brain, and the nerves. In a pregnant woman, methyl mercury becomes concentrated in the growing fetus. Thus

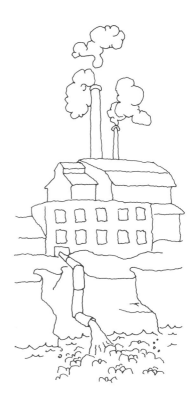

2   M. M. Varma, S. G. Serdahely, and H. M. Katz, Physiological effects of trace elements and chemicals in water, *Journal of Environmental Health* 39 (1976): 90–100.

it can cause mental and physical defects in the newborn even though the mother has shown no symptoms.

Nerve damage occurs with mercury intakes as low as 300 micrograms per day, so the Food and Drug Administration (FDA) has set a limit of one-tenth that amount on the mercury levels in foods and drugs.[3] (Monitoring mercury concentrations in water is a task of the public health agencies, such as the Environmental Protection Agency.) Two serious outbreaks of mercury poisoning have occurred in Japan, where people have eaten fish that grew near industrial plants that discharged mercury wastes into the water (see Highlight 11). Rising levels of environmental mercury have been observed in other industrial countries, including the United States.

Cadmium has its most toxic effects in the kidney, causing chronic renal disease; in the lungs, causing emphysema; and in the bones, causing osteoporosis and osteomalacia. It has been in commercial use since 1910 and has caused severe outbreaks of disease in Japan. Cadmium in contaminated water can be absorbed into vegetables and grains and so can find its way into human consumers of these foods.[4]

Lead, another highly toxic material, enters the water supply mostly by being captured in rain falling from atmospheres polluted with automobile exhaust. It is a metabolic poison that interferes with the action of several enzymes. Symptoms of mild lead poisoning include lowered hemoglobin, intestinal cramps, fatigue, and kidney abnormalities. These may be reversible if exposure stops. More severe exposure causes irreversible nerve damage, paralysis, mental retardation in children, abortions, and death.[5]

These are only three examples of metal pollutants, but they are enough to illustrate how the purity of the water supply can be threatened by industrial use. Both government and consumer environmental protection groups have to be vigilant in detecting, reporting, and preventing dangerous levels of contamination, because our water is a vital resource.

Microorganisms in the Water Supply

Many harmless, even beneficial, bacteria dwell in the human digestive tract and are excreted into sewage. If these were the only inhabitants of sewage, there would be no concern about their presence in drinking water. But disease organisms are also excreted into sewage, and others are introduced into it by flies and other carriers. Before a sewage treatment plant releases its effluent into the water supply, it must reduce the bacterial count enough so that the further dilution that follows will make recycled water safe for human use.

An efficient secondary sewage plant may remove 99 percent of the bacteria in the water, which sounds pretty good for a start. But there are typically 10 million bacteria in a milliliter (⅕ teaspoon) of sewage. After 99 percent

The first step in sewage treatment allows the solids to settle out. This is **primary treatment**.

secondary treatment: removes the suspended matter, including bacteria and some viruses.

tertiary treatment: removes dissolved compounds, both organic and inorganic.

3   The acceptable mercury content of water is 0.5 micrograms per liter. U.S. Public Health Service standard, in Varma, Serdahely, and Katz, 1976.

4   Varma, Serdahely, and Katz, 1976.

5   Varma, Serdahely, and Katz, 1976.

removal there will still be 100,000 bacteria left in each milliliter. Chlorination then kills another 99 percent, leaving 1,000 bacteria per milliliter. Most of these are harmless, and the few that are harmful can be diluted below the danger point if the water leaving the plant enters a large river.[6] Alternatively, the facility may give the water tertiary treatment, sprinkling it over a large land area so that it will be filtered before reentering the general water supply.

High standards for sewage treatment in the developed countries ensure that most people have potable water, but for the rest of the world, microbial contamination remains the primary cause of human diseases and epidemics. Two of the most basic public health needs of the world's people are safe drinking water and an acceptable standard of waste disposal.[7]

potable (POTE-uh-bul): suitable for drinking.

potare = to drink.

Organic Compounds in the Water Supply

The fourth class of substances that may occur in water are the organic compounds from sewage, insecticides, petroleum-based and other industries, and other sources. Research on these substances is less than 20 years old, and few of them have been identified, but many are known to be toxic. Some cause birth defects, some are carcinogenic, some cause permanent alterations of the inherited genetic material.[8] Many contain chlorine, and some may be formed during the chlorination of water. No information is available on the risks now presented by water containing these compounds; standards are only now being established, and new filtering systems may be called for if public water exceeds these standards. The study of organics in the water supply is an increasingly important research area.

In some regions, consumers have become sufficiently alarmed about their local water supplies to turn to buying bottled water for their personal consumption. The choice is an individual matter, and we take no position regarding its appropriateness. However, in buying water, as in buying any other product, the consumer needs to be alert to fraudulent claims. Mineral waters from "famous spas" offer no known health advantages and may be undesirably high in sodium. On the other hand, bottled water sold in the United States must be tested by the producers once a year for safety and must meet standards set by the FDA for its contents of many chemical substances.

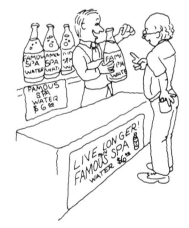

Water Quantity

The matter of water quantity still must be discussed. Is there enough to meet our needs? Water is an abundant natural resource, and until recently its availability has been unquestioned. But the use of water in the industrial countries is putting a strain on the supply. Used by agriculture for irrigating and by industry for transporting, dissolving, washing, rinsing, cooling,

6   K. Kawata, Water and other environmental interventions: The minimum investment concept, *American Journal of Clinical Nutrition* 31 (1978): 2114–2123.

7   Kawata, 1978.

8   Varma, Serdahely, and Katz, 1976.

flushing away waste, and many other purposes, water in huge quantities is diverted from its original, ordinary uses. Processed and fast foods cost much more, in water, than do whole foods from the farm. In the future the water supply may limit human progress. It has been estimated, for example, that if the U.S. population increases by another 20 percent or so, the water supply will be unable to continue meeting all the demands placed on it. We will therefore have to compromise our living standards in order to meet the top-priority need for safe, pure water for human use.

This book is about individual nutrition and has dealt little with the economic and ecological problems of worldwide supply and demand. This discussion of water brings those problems into the foreground. To continue surviving and to maintain a desirable quality of life in an increasingly crowded and complicated world may mean making some hard choices in the near future.

The Body's Salts

Table 1–2 in Chapter 1 listed the major minerals; Figure 10–1 shows the amounts found in the body. As you can see, the most prevalent are calcium and phosphorus, the chief minerals of bone (discussed later). Four of the major minerals—potassium, sodium, chlorine, and (again) phosphorus—strongly influence the water balance. These form salts that are abundant in the body fluids.

To understand how cells regulate the amount of water they contain, it is necessary to take a closer look at the minerals as ions, the form in which cells use them for water regulation. Cell membranes are freely permeable to water molecules, which are neutral, and which flow in and out of cells all the time. Yet the cells never lose all their water nor do they overfill. Along the evolutionary path they have contrived a method of keeping their water constant; they do this beautifully by employing the salts to assist them. They make use of the principle that water follows salt.

Chemists use the term *salt* to include many inorganic substances, not just ordinary table salt. The chemist refers to table salt as sodium chloride, $NaCl$. In this salt, sodium and chlorine atoms are bound together by strong electrostatic forces in a rigid crystalline structure. Outwardly, the crystals exhibit no electrical charge. However, when dissolved in water, the rigid structure relaxes. Some of the sodium moves about freely as positively charged ions, and some of the chloride also dissociates and moves about as negatively charged ions. The salt thus reveals itself as a compound composed of charged particles. The positive ions are cations; the negative, anions.

A salt that partly dissociates in water, as sodium chloride does, is known as an electrolyte. Since the fluids of the body are composed of water and partly dissociated salts, they are electrolyte solutions.

Electrolyte solutions are always electrostatically balanced. There is no such thing as a test tube filled with sodium ions. Sodium ions are always positively charged, and they cannot exist apart from negatively charged

salt: a compound composed of charged particles (ions). Exceptions: a compound in which the cations are H^+ is an acid; a compound in which the anions are OH^- is a base.

cation (CAT-eye-un): a positively charged ion.

anion (AN-eye-un): a negatively charged ion.

For a closer look at ions, see Appendix B.

Na = sodium.
Cl = chlorine.

chloride: the ionic form of chlorine.

dissociation: physical separation of the ions in an ionic compound. A salt that partly dissociates in water is an **electrolyte**.

electrolyte solution: a solution that can conduct electricity.

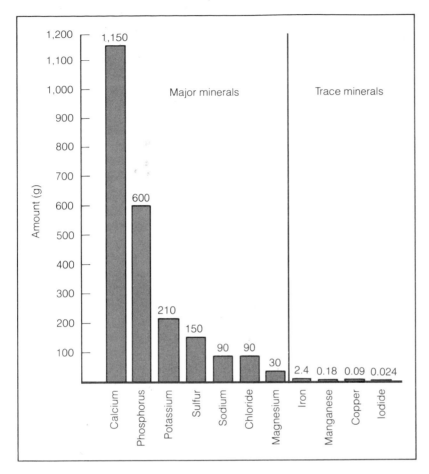

FIGURE 10-1 **The amounts of minerals in a 60-kilogram human body.** A line separates the major minerals from the trace minerals. The major minerals are those present in amounts larger than 5 grams (a teaspoon). A pound is about 454 grams; thus only calcium and phosphorus appear in amounts larger than a pound. There are more than a dozen trace minerals, although only four are shown here.

ions. Therefore, in any fluid with dissolved electrolytes there will always be the same number of positive and negative ions.[9] If an anion enters a cell, a cation must accompany it or another anion must leave so that electroneutrality will be maintained.

Water Balance

We stated above that water follows salt. More precisely, there is a force that moves water into a place where a solute, such as sodium chloride, is concentrated. This force can operate only if the divider separating the two fluid solutions is permeable to water but not permeable (or less freely This force is known as the **osmotic pressure** of a solution. Water flows *toward* the higher osmotic pressure. The substances dissolved in the water that create this pressure are the **solutes** (SOLL-yutes).

9   For instance, in serum, the numbers of cations and anions both equal 155 milliequivalents per liter (mEq/l). Of the cations, sodium ions make up about 140 mEq/l; and potassium, calcium, and magnesium ions make up the remainder. Of the anions, chloride ions number 104 mEq/l, bicarbonate ions number 27, and the rest are provided by phosphate ions, sulfate ions, organic acids, and protein. A milliequivalent is the number of ions equal to the number of H^+ ions in a milligram of hydrogen. This is a useful measure, because when we are considering ions we are usually interested in the number of positive or negative charges present in a solution rather than in their weight.

Other terms used to describe electrolyte solutions: **isotonic** (having the same osmotic pressure as a reference solution), **hypertonic** (having a higher osmotic pressure than a reference solution), and **hypotonic** (having a lower osmotic pressure than a reference solution). The salty water on the outside of the lettuce cells is hypertonic to the water inside the cells, so it attracts water out of the cells. Saline (salt) solutions used in the hospital are made isotonic to human blood.

The cell membrane is **semipermeable**—that is, more permeable to some substances (such as water) than to others (such as sodium and potassium). This is the condition necessary for osmotic pressure to operate.

permeable) to the solute. Figure 10–2 shows this force in operation. In the top part, equal amounts of solute on both sides of the divider cause the amounts of water to be equal also. In the bottom part, the presence of more solute on Side B has drawn water across the divider so that the *concentration* of solute on both sides becomes equal (see Figure 10–2). The total *amount* of water is now greater on Side B.

You have seen this force at work if you have ever salted a lettuce salad an hour before eating it. When you came back to the salad, the lettuce was wilted and there was water in the salad bowl. The high concentration of salt (and therefore low concentration of water) on the outside of the lettuce cells caused water to move out of the cells. They collapsed (the lettuce wilted), and the water puddled in the salad dish. Sugar would have caused the same reaction. There is one way you could have prevented this (here's a cooking lesson for the novice). You could have coated the lettuce lightly with oil before salting it or put salad dressing on it. The oil would have acted as a barrier against the salt, keeping it from attracting water out of the lettuce.

The divider between the water inside and outside a cell is the cell membrane. The cell cannot pump water directly across its membrane, but it does have proteins in its membrane that can attach to sodium ions and move them from one side of the membrane to the other. When these sodium pumps are active, they pump out sodium faster than it can diffuse into the cell. Water follows the sodium. When potassium pumps are active,

FIGURE 10–2 **Osmotic pressure.** Water flows in the direction of the added solute.

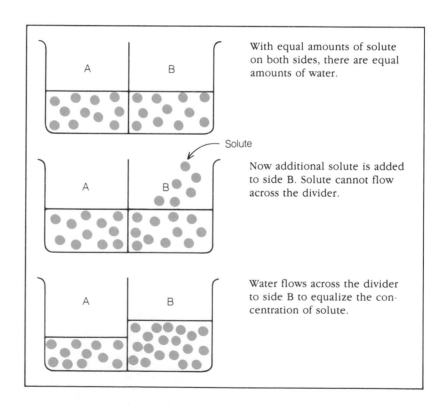

With equal amounts of solute on both sides, there are equal amounts of water.

Solute

Now additional solute is added to side B. Solute cannot flow across the divider.

Water flows across the divider to side B to equalize the concentration of solute.

they pump in potassium, and water follows this ion. By maintaining a certain amount of sodium outside and potassium inside, the cell can exactly regulate the amount of water it contains.

For more about the cell-membrane pumps, see Chapter 4.

Acid-Base Balance

The body uses its ions not only to help maintain water balance but also to help regulate the acidity (pH) of its fluids. Some of the electrolyte mixtures in the body fluids, as well as the proteins, protect the body against changes in acidity by acting as buffers—substances that act to neutralize newly introduced acids or bases. The action of a buffer is shown in Figure 10-3.

Surprisingly, although one person may eat more or less of certain minerals than another person, the body's total content of electrolytes remains very nearly constant. The job of regulating the body's salt population is largely delegated to the kidneys, under the supervision of several monitoring systems, notably the adrenal and pituitary glands. The net effect of all the homeostatic balancing systems is to help ensure that output balances intake. A person who eats a lot of table salt, for example, excretes more sodium and chloride in his urine than one who eats only a little. Thus, except for a transient rise immediately after ingestion, the *body's* total

buffer: a substance or mixture capable in solution of neutralizing both acids and bases and thereby capable of maintaining the original acidity of the solution.

A buffer is a large molecule, usually protein, that can accommodate excess plus or minus charges (ions).

FIGURE 10–3 **Action of a buffer.**

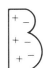 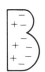

A buffer can be neutral (an equal number of plus and minus charges).

A buffer can be acidic (an excess of plus charges).

A buffer can be alkaline, or basic (an excess of minus charges).

In a solution, a buffer helps maintain the acid-base balance by soaking up excess plus or minus charges or by giving them up to the solution.

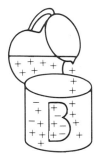

If the solution receives excess plus charges, tending to make it acidic,

If the solution loses plus charges, tending to make it alkaline (basic),

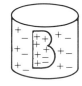

the buffer will pick these up. The solution keeps its acid-base balance.

the buffer will give up its plus charges. The solution keeps its acid-base balance.

Kidney stones are deposits of mineral and other salts that have crystallized within the kidney. Technically, they are termed **renal calculi** (REE-nul CAL-kyoo-lie).

renal = of the kidney

calculus = a small stone.

acid ash diet: a diet of acid-forming foods (foods that, if burned to ash, would be found to contain acid-forming minerals). Such a diet contributes to acidity of the urine, because the kidney collects the excess acid-forming minerals into the urine for excretion.

alkaline ash diet: a diet of base-forming foods.

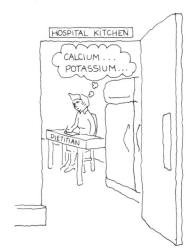

electrolytes remain constant, and it is the composition of the *urine* that is affected by what you eat.

Some foods are classed as acid-formers, others as base-formers, depending on the amount of acid they donate to the urine after their metabolism. It has been thought (but it is not clear) that their acid-forming or base-forming nature derives partly from the balance of mineral salts they contain. The distinction becomes important when kidney stones form, because excesses of many metabolites flow through the kidneys on their way to being excreted (some are excluded from absorption and leave the body with the feces). Some stones tend to form in acid, others in basic solutions, so when a person has a tendency to form kidney stones, she is advised to eat the foods least likely to aggravate that tendency. She is instructed, then, to eat either an acid-ash or an alkaline-ash diet. Figure 10–4 shows the acid-forming and base-forming foods.

Diseases of the kidney more serious than stones impair the body's ability to regulate its fluid and electrolyte balances. To keep a renal patient alive, in addition to many medical procedures, the physician may order adjustment of the patient's electrolyte input from food. The burden then falls on the dietitian to calculate a diet that precisely specifies sodium, potassium, calcium, water, and many other constituents. (A dietitian in this sophisticated medical specialty requires several years of schooling.)

FIGURE 10–4 **Acid-forming and base-forming foods.**

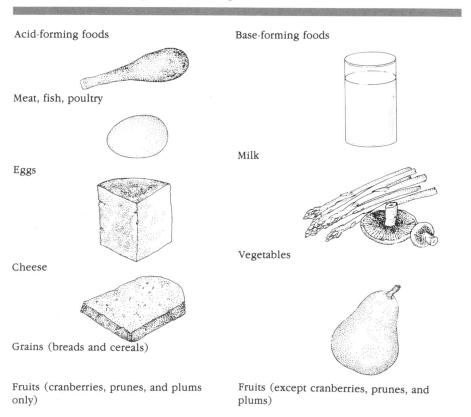

Acid-forming foods

Meat, fish, poultry

Eggs

Cheese

Grains (breads and cereals)

Fruits (cranberries, prunes, and plums only)

Base-forming foods

Milk

Vegetables

Fruits (except cranberries, prunes, and plums)

It is not known whether any regulating system other than the kidneys governs the body's salt contents. We have thirst, to govern our intake of water, but do we have a salt hunger to govern our intake of sodium? Salt hunger is well known in plant-eating animals like cattle, which will travel long distances to a salt lick when they have been depleted of sodium. The tongue, in both animals and humans, is equipped with taste receptors that respond only to the salty taste. Animals know instinctively when to seek this stimulus, but humans may seek it when they have no need. Future research may determine whether a true salt hunger operates in humans.

There are four kinds of taste receptors on the tongue: those sensitive to salt, sweet, sour, and bitter flavors.

Water and Salt Imbalances

The activity of the kidneys in regulating the body's contents of sodium and water is remarkable. Sodium is absorbed easily from the intestinal tract, then travels in the blood, where it ultimately passes through the kidneys. The kidneys filter all the sodium out, then with great precision return to the bloodstream the exact amount needed. Normally, the amount excreted equals the amount ingested that day. About 30 to 45 percent of the body's sodium is thought to be stored on the surface of the bone crystals, where it is easy to recover if the blood level drops.

When the blood level of sodium rises, as it does after a person eats heavily salted foods, the thirst receptors in the brain are stimulated. The fluid intake increases to make the sodium-to-water ratio constant. Then the extra water is excreted by the kidneys along with the extra sodium.

Thus you are well protected from imbalances of water and electrolytes. However, you may be thrown into situations for which your kidneys, thirst instinct, and cell membranes cannot compensate. This is the case when large amounts of fluid and electrolytes are suddenly lost. Vomiting, diarrhea, heavy sweating, burns, wounds, and the like may incur such great fluid losses that a medical emergency results.

Technically, these kinds of imbalances are known as **fluid-and-electrolyte imbalances**.

The details of electrolyte balance are among the most important ones that medical students must learn. Mastery of these details is appropriately left to them and to their medical associates. For the general reader and the student of nutrition, it is necessary only to appreciate the importance of this balance and the principles by which it is maintained and to be aware of the situations that threaten it. When any of these gets out of control, the appropriate action is to call the doctor. Water and salts, which we take for granted and usually ignore, are more vital to life than any of the other nutrients considered in this book.

Sodium, Other Minerals, and High Blood Pressure

The body has to maintain a certain blood pressure to sustain the lives of its cells. The pressure of the blood against the walls of the arteries ensures that fluids carrying nutrients and oxygen move out of the arteries into the tissues to deliver their cargo. By the time blood reaches the veins, much of

Atherosclerosis is the subject of Highlight 3.

hypertension: high blood pressure. People sometimes confuse hypertension with stress, but hypertension is an internal and stress an external condition. Stress may cause hypertension in sensitive people, however.

Secondary hypertension is high blood pressure caused by kidney disease (10 percent of cases). Primary, or essential, hypertension is of unknown origin (90 percent of cases) and can cause kidney disease.

"High" blood pressure is defined differently for different purposes. Here, if the higher of the two numbers is over 140 or if the lower is over 90, it is considered to be too high.

its fluid has exited, and the concentration of cells and solutes in the remaining blood is at a maximum. Fluids from the tissues, attracted by the concentrated plasma, then seep back into the veins, now carrying carbon dioxide and other waste materials. Thus the cells' needs for supply and removal of materials are met. The blood pressure also helps ensure good filtration of wastes into the urine as blood passes through the kidneys.

When the blood pressure falls, the lives of all the body's cells are threatened. The kidneys detect the lowered pressure and immediately set in motion a mechanism to raise the blood pressure again. Figure 10–5 shows how this mechanism works.

Normally, this response of the kidneys is highly adaptive. In dehydration, for example, a "water deficiency" exists. By constricting the blood vessels and conserving water and sodium, the kidney-initiated mechanism ensures that blood pressure is maintained until more water can be drunk.

Sometimes, however, the kidneys are fooled. They experience a "water deficiency" when there is none. Then they raise the blood pressure with harmful effects—a maladaptive response. Most often, the cause is atherosclerosis (hardening of the arteries), which deprives the kidneys of water just as if there were a water deficiency. In response to poor circulation of blood fluid, the kidneys raise the blood pressure and the heart has to pump extra hard to push the extra fluid around against resistant arteries. Added weight (obesity) raises the pressure further, and the extra adipose tissue means miles of extra capillaries through which the blood must be pumped. The combination of high blood pressure, obesity, and hardened arteries is deadly.

In 10 percent of cases, hypertension is caused by recognized kidney disease, and is called secondary hypertension, but in 90 percent, the cause is unknown. The vast majority of cases are called *essential* hypertension, meaning that the disease process must be primary.

FIGURE 10-5 Blood pressure regulation. Renin from the kidney splits the plasma protein angiotensinogen to form angiotensin I; in the presence of another enzyme, angiotensin I is activated to angiotensin II, which acts as a vasoconstrictor and also stimulates aldosterone secretion. The net effect is to raise blood pressure. TH10-1

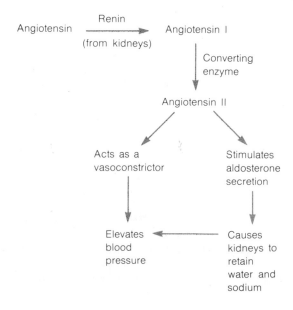

The mineral sodium has been implicated so strongly in the causation of high blood pressure that many people have been led to believe it alone is to blame. Findings such as these incriminate sodium (but withhold judgment for a moment):

1 Populations with high intakes of sodium have more high blood pressure (for example, the Japanese).

2 Populations that eat little or no salt have normal blood pressure (even some vegetarian groups in our society).

3 Severely restricting sodium reduces high blood pressure; adding sodium back to the diet restores high blood pressure.[10]

4 A nationwide program to control blood pressure, including sodium reduction, has seemed to lower blood pressure in many individuals.[11]

5 People in areas with soft water have higher (average) blood pressure than people in areas with hard water.

6 Genetically sodium-sensitive strains of animals are known; their blood pressure is greatly affected by dietary sodium, some humans (perhaps 20 percent) are genetically sensitive also.[12]

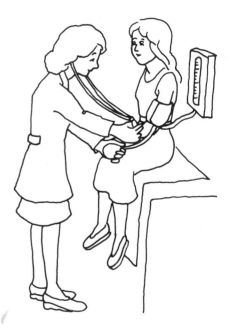

Blood pressure regulation is not simple, however. Other factors are involved. Items 1 and 2, above, show correlations, not evidence of cause. With respect to Item 3, people with *normal* blood pressure usually do not show an increase when fed large amounts of salt. With respect to Item 4, drugs were used to lower blood pressure, and the independent effect of sodium restriction, if any, is unknown. As for Item 5, who is to say that it is the sodium in soft water that accounts for the difference? Perhaps it is some other mineral; or perhaps the minerals in *hard* water protect against high blood pressure.

The only findings that seem to hold up strongly are that some people are sensitive to sodium and tend to have high blood pressure, and that they can lower it by reducing their salt intakes. Since not all those people know who they are (and you can't tell by "feel" when you have high blood pressure) some authorities contend that the whole population should be encouraged to reduce its salt intakes. The government's *Dietary Goals*, the *Dietary Guidelines for Americans*, and the Canadian government's guidelines all recommend reducing sodium intakes based on this assumption.

We'll come back to sodium shortly, but first, what are the other diet-related factors that affect blood pressure? Obesity is one, as already mentioned (see Chapter 7, especially). Several other minerals are also involved —notably, potassium, calcium, magnesium, and cadmium.

When sodium is retained in the body, potassium is traded for it. Even subjects with normal blood pressure, if fed very large quantities of sodium, ultimately show a rise in blood pressure—but at the same time, their

10   Institute of Food Technologists' Expert Panel on Food Safety and Nutrition, Dietary salt, *Food Technology*, January 1980, pp. 85–91.

11   Joint National Committee on Detection, Evaluation, and Treatment of High Blood Pressure, *1980 Report*, NIH publication no. 81–1088 (Washington, D.C.: Government Printing Office, 1980).

12   Institute, 1980; A. M. Altschul and J. K. Grommet, Sodium intake and sodium sensitivity, *Nutrition Reviews* 38 (1980): 393–402.

potassium excretion is increasing. Fed potassium simultaneously with the sodium, they do not have a rise in blood pressure.[13]

Population studies show sodium being traded for potassium in a different sense. People who eat many foods high in sodium (processed foods, for example), necessarily eat fewer potassium-containing foods (such as fruits and whole vegetables) at the same time.

Calcium and magnesium are implicated because of the hard water versus soft water observation already mentioned above. It has also been reported that calcium in the blood is low in people with high blood pressure.[14] The contaminant cadmium is leached from pipes into water, especially soft water, and may contribute to high blood pressure.[15] Other factors mentioned have been chloride, alcohol, and protein.[16]

Still, the use of highly salted foods probably contributes to hypertension for those who have a genetic tendency to develop it anyway. How many people this represents is a much-debated question, but one in five seems to be a conservative estimate. Black Americans are significantly more at risk than other groups. It is possible that, by the age of 65, as many as three out of four people have high blood pressure.[17] This being the case, perhaps we should all curtail our sodium intakes, as the authorities mentioned earlier suggest.

There is certainly no sodium shortage in the diet. Foods almost always include more salt than is needed. Intakes vary widely, especially because of cultural differences in diets. Orientals, who liberally use soy sauce and monosodium glutamate (MSG or Accent) for flavoring, consume about 30 to 40 grams of salt per day; most people in the United States average about 6 to 18 grams per day. Vegetarians, depending on their food preferences, can consume much less.

The *Dietary Guidelines* recommend that we limit our sodium intake to not more than 5 grams of added salt a day (that is, salt added by manufacturers and consumers above and beyond that already in the food as grown). In practice, this would mean avoiding highly salted foods and removing the salt shaker from the table. Table 10-2 shows a sampling of the sodium contents of commonly eaten foods, and the notes in the margin provide general suggestions for avoiding sodium in foods for the person who wishes to do so.

Persons who wish to avoid salt need to know that what they pour from the salt shaker may be only a third of the total salt they consume. One-fourth to one-half comes from processed food, to which salt is added as a preservative and flavoring agent. This makes eating something of a guessing game,

5 g salt is about 2 g sodium.

1 g salt = ⅙ tsp.

Estimated safe and adequate daily dietary intake of sodium (Committee on RDA): 1.1–3.3 g (1,100–3,300 mg).

13   G. Kolata, Value of low-sodium diets questioned (Research News), *Science* 216 (1982): 38–39.

14   D. A. McCarron, Low serum concentrations of ionized calcium in patients with hypertension, *New England Journal of Medicine* 307 (1982): 226–228.

15   S. J. Kopp and coauthors, Cardiovascular actions of cadmium at environmental exposure levels, *Science* 217 (1982): 837–839; R. Masironi and A. G. Shaper, Epidemiological studies of health effects of water from different sources, *Annual Reviews of Nutrition* 1 (1981): 375–400.

16   L. Newman, More "salt" talks: Diet and hypertension (medical news), *Journal of the American Medical Association* 248 (1982): 2949–2951.

17   M. Jacobson and B. F. Liebman, Dietary sodium and the risk of hypertension (correspondence), *New England Journal of Medicine* 303 (1980): 817–818.

TABLE 10–2 **Sodium—Average Amounts in Groups of Foods** TH10-2

	Sodium (mg)
Milk and Milk Products	
1 c milk[a]	100
1 c buttermilk	250
½ c instant pudding	450
½ c homecooked pudding	200
1 oz natural cheese[b]	250
1 oz process cheese	400
1 c cottage cheese	700
Meat and Legumes	
1 egg	50
3 oz meat, fish, or poultry (cooked without added salt)[c]	50
3 oz cured ham	800
3 oz commercial sausage or lunchmeat	1,100
3 oz canned tuna, salmon, or sardines	500
¾ c dry cooked legumes[d]	-0-
¾ c canned beans	550
¾ c canned peas	450
¾ c fresh peas	-0-
Fruits and Vegetables	
1 portion fresh or canned fruit	-0-
½ c fresh vegetable, cooked without salt	-0-
½ c canned vegetable, drained[e]	300
1 c fresh greens, cooked	100
½ c sauerkraut	550
1 large pickle	1,450
½ c raw celery or carrots cooked without salt	50
Grains	
1 slice bread[f]	150
1 slice low-sodium bread	-0-
1 portion quick bread (70 kcal)	400
1 piece chocolate cake	350
1 c hot cereal or rice, cooked without salt	-0-
1 c spaghetti, macaroni, or noodles, cooked without salt	-0-
1 oz cornflakes or other processed cereal	250
1 oz puffed wheat or rice, plain	-0-
Other	
1 c drinking water[g]	0-75
1 small portion salty snack[h]	200
2 strips broiled bacon	250
1 portion nuts without added salt	-0-
1 tsp unsalted butter or margarine	-0-
1 tsp regular butter or margarine	50
1 frozen chicken TV dinner	1,150
1 pot pie	800
1 toaster pastry	300
1 fried chicken dinner (fast food)	2,250
1 large fast food hamburger[i]	1,500
2 tbsp peanut butter	50
1 tsp salt	1,950
1 tbsp soy sauce	1,000

Values are averaged to the nearest 50 mg. Many more foods are high in sodium; this table represents a sampling sufficient to demonstrate the rule: the more processed a food, the higher its sodium content.
[a] 1 c milk or any milk product including whole or skim milk, half and half, yogurt, goat's milk, malted milk, milk shake, custard, ice cream (hard and soft serve), chocolate milk, and hot chocolate.
[b] 1 oz mozzarella or gruyere has less than average, about 100 mg.

To avoid too much sodium:

Learn to enjoy the unsalted flavors of foods.

Cook with only small amounts of added salt.

Add little or no salt to food at the table.

Cut down on:

Foods prepared in brine, such as pickles, olives, and sauerkraut.

Salty or smoked meats, such as bologna, corned or chipped beef, frankfurters, ham, luncheon meats, salt pork, sausage, smoked tongue.

Salty or smoked fish, such as anchovies, caviar, salted and dried cod, herring, sardines, smoked salmon.

Snack items such as potato chips, pretzels, salted popcorn, and salted nuts and crackers.

Bouillon cubes; seasoned salts (including sea salt); soy, Worcestershire, and barbecue sauces.

Cheeses, especially processed types.

Canned and instant soups.

Prepared horseradish, catsup, and mustard.

Read labels. You may be surprised to learn that some processed foods that contain no table salt and don't taste salty have lots of sodium. Look for the word *soda* or *sodium* or the symbol *Na* on labels. Examples are *sodium* bicarbonate (baking *soda*), mono*sodium* glutamate, most baking powders, di*sodium* phosphate, *sodium* alginate, *sodium* benzoate, *sodium* hydroxide, *sodium* propionate, *sodium* sulfite, and *sodium* saccharin.—USDA

c Values range from 26 to 94 mg sodium. The higher values are for calf's liver and dark meat of turkey or chicken. Shrimp meat contains 118 mg per 3 oz; hardshell clams contain 172 mg per 3 oz. meat.

d Salt added during the canning process varies with the brand. The values range from 250 mg for soybeans to 869 for canned white beans with pork and tomato sauce.

e The amounts of salt added to canned vegetables varies. Low- sodium varieties contain about the same amount of sodium as the fresh cooked products.

f Yeast–leavened, as almost all breads are. Values for bread range from 100 for Boston brown bread to 182 for pumpernickel. Read the label.

g Softened water. The harder the water is initially, the more sodium it takes to soften it. If the original water hardness was 1.0 grains per gallon, it will contain about 8 mg/qt after softening, or about 2 mg/c. If it was 40 grains per gallon, it will contain 300 mg/qt or about 75mg/c.

h All products that have a salty taste are high in sodium: 10 chips, 2 regular twist pretzels, and 1 c commercial popcorn have 200 mg each.

i Big Mac from McDonalds.

Sources: Adapted from Institute of Food Technologists' Expert Panel on Food Safety and Nutrition, Dietary salt, *Food Technology*, January 1980, pp. 85–91; Water Quality Association, *Sources of Sodium in the Diet*, Technical Paper 2/78, available from 477 East Butterfield Road, Lombard, IL 60148; A. C. Marsh, R. N. Klippstein, and S. O. Kaplan, *The Sodium Content of Your Food* (Washington, D.C.: USDA, 1980); C. F. Church and H. N. Church, *Bowes and Church's Food Values of Portions Commonly Used*, 12th ed. (Philadelphia: Lippincott, 1975); Salt and high blood pressure, a reprint from *Consumer Reports*, March 1979, available from CU Reprints, Consumers Union, Orangeburg, NY 10962.

because labels do not necessarily declare the sodium contents of foods. The serious sodium-avoider must stay away from fast-food places and Oriental restaurants and stop using many canned, frozen, and instant foods at home.[18] (On the positive side, unprocessed, whole foods are lower in sodium—and higher in potassium—than most people realize.)

Processed foods don't always taste salty. Most people are surprised to learn that a serving of cornflakes contains more sodium than a serving of cocktail peanuts—and that a serving of chocolate pudding contains still more.[19] A perusal of the sodium contents of foods in Appendix I and other references is well worth while for anyone wishing to curtail sodium and increase potassium intakes.

Avoiding sodium is hard to do, not only because sodium is often hidden, but also because foods are far less tasty without salt. With practice, however, people can learn to enjoy the flavors of many unsalted foods and, where spices are needed, to make liberal use of sodium-free spices like those listed in Table 10–3. If you persist long enough (say, two months) in eating a low-salt diet, your taste threshold for salt will actually change so that your preferred level is lower.[20]

In summary, the person who wishes to use diet to prevent high blood pressure should probably not only reduce sodium intake but emphasize positive actions as well:

● Eat plenty of fresh fruits and vegetables, because they are rich in potassium.
● Be sure to eat a balanced diet, including good food sources of calcium and magnesium.
● Maintain ideal weight.
● Be moderate in the use of alcohol.

TABLE 10–3 **Sodium-Free Spices and Flavorings**

Allspice	Onion powder
Almond extract	Paprika
Bay leaves	Parsley
Caraway seeds	Pepper
Cinnamon	Peppermint
Curry powder	extract
Garlic	Pimiento
Garlic powder	Rosemary
Ginger	Sage
Lemon extract	Sesame seeds
Mace	Thyme
Maple extract	Turmeric
Marjoram	Vanilla extract
Mustard powder	Vinegar
Nutmeg	Walnut extract

18   L. Fenner, Salt shakes up some of us, *FDA Consumer*, March 1980, reprint.

19   Salt and high blood pressure, *Consumer Reports*, March 1979, reprint.

20   M. Bertino, G. K. Beauchamp, and K. Engelman, Long-term reduction in dietary sodium alters the taste of salt, *American Journal of Clinical Nutrition* 36 (1982): 1134–1144.

Calcium

Unlike sodium, calcium is not so abundant in the diet, and deficiencies are widespread in human societies. The price you pay for neglecting to obtain enough calcium throughout early and middle life is extensive degeneration of the skeleton in old age—adult bone loss, which leads to crippling deformities, irreparable fractures, and even death. Nearly all people suffer some bone loss as they grow older, and it causes serious fractures in about one of every three people over 65. It is therefore urgent to understand the necessity of obtaining adequate calcium in food from the early years on throughout adulthood.

The urgency of obtaining enough calcium has to be learned through education, because the body sends no signals saying it is deficient. Most nutrient deficiencies make themselves known by way of symptoms that can be felt or seen, such as pain, skin lesions, tiredness, and the like. But a developing calcium deficiency is utterly silent; it becomes apparent only when a hip or pelvic bone suddenly shatters into fragments that cannot be reassembled. No evidence of a developing calcium deficiency can be found in a blood sample, because blood calcium remains normal no matter what the bone content may be. Nor does depletion of bone calcium show up on an x-ray until it is so far advanced as to be virtually irreversible.

Figure 10–6 shows a hip bone sliced lengthwise so that you can see the lacy network of calcium-containing crystals inside the bone. These are the deposits in the body's calcium bank, which are drawn on whenever the supply from the day's diet runs short. Invested in savings during the milk-drinking years of childhood, these calcium deposits provide a nearly inexhaustible fund of calcium; 99 percent of the body's calcium is stored in the bones.

The other 1 percent of the body's calcium is in the blood and body fluids, where its concentration is tightly controlled by a system of hormones and vitamin D. Whenever the blood calcium concentration rises too high, these agents promote its deposit into bone. Whenever the blood concentration falls too low, the regulatory system acts in three locations to correct it:

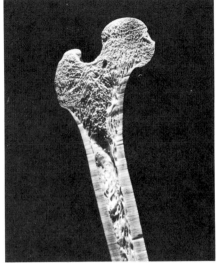

FIGURE 10–6 **Cross section of bone**. The lacy structural elements are **trabeculae** (tra-BECK-you-lee), which can be drawn on to replenish blood calcium.

The regulators are hormones from the thyroid and parathyroid glands, as well as vitamin D. One, **parathormone**, raises blood calcium. Others, **calcitonin** and **thyro-calcitonin**, lower it by inhibiting release of calcium from bone. The hormone-like **vitamin D** raises blood calcium by acting at the three sites listed.

- Intestine: increase calcium absorption.
- Bone: increase calcium release.
- Kidney: reduce calcium excretion.

Thus blood calcium returns to normal.

To say that food calcium never affects blood calcium is not to say that blood calcium never changes. In fact, sometimes blood calcium does rise above normal, causing a condition known as calcium rigor. When this happens, the muscle fibers contract and cannot relax. Similarly, calcium levels may fall below normal in the blood, causing calcium tetany—also characterized by uncontrolled contraction of muscle tissue, due to a change in the stimulation of nerve cells. These conditions do not reflect a dietary lack or excess of calcium; they are caused by a lack of vitamin D or by glandular malfunctions that result in abnormal amounts of the hormones that regulate blood calcium concentration.

calcium rigor: hardness or stiffness of the muscles caused by high blood calcium.

calcium tetany: intermittent spasms of the extremities due to nervous and muscular excitability caused by low blood calcium.

Collagen: see pp. 138, 294.

cofactor: a mineral element that, like a coenzyme, works with an enzyme to facilitate a chemical reaction.

Coenzyme: see pp. 271–274.

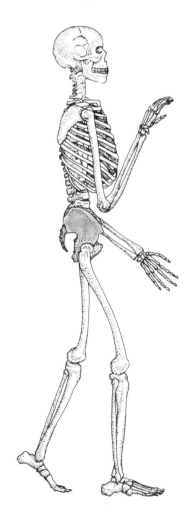

On the other hand, a chronic *dietary* deficiency of calcium or a chronic deficiency due to poor absorption over the course of years can diminish the savings account in the bones. Because this is an important concept, we repeat: it is the bones, not the blood, that are depleted by calcium deficiency.

Roles of Calcium

The calcium that circulates in the body fluids plays many roles. Some calcium is found in close association with cell membranes, where it appears to be essential for their integrity. It helps to regulate the transport of other ions into and out of cells. It is essential for muscle action and so helps maintain the heartbeat. Calcium must be present between nerve and nerve, and between nerve and muscle, for the transmission of nerve impulses; and when it enters cells, it delivers important messages to intracellular receptors (see Figure 10–7).

Calcium must also be present if blood clotting is to occur, because it is one of the 14 factors directly involved in this process. (The other 13 are proteins; vitamin K is needed, too, for the synthesis of some of these proteins.) Calcium also acts as a cofactor for several enzymes.

As for the calcium in bone, it plays two important roles. One, as already mentioned, is to serve as a bank to prevent alteration of the all-important blood calcium concentration. And the bones, of course, hold the body upright and serve as attachment points for muscles, making motion possible.

FIGURE 10–7 **How calcium delivers messages.** Calcium is over 1,000 times more concentrated outside of cells than inside, and normally, it can't get in. When it does, however (for example when an electrical impulse arrives along a nerve, altering the membrane), it finds molecules of the protein **calmodulin** (cal-MOD-YOU-lin) waiting inside. Calcium binds to calmodulin, changing its shape. Now, calmodulin activates other proteins, which take action. Thus calcium has "delivered" the message transmitted along the nerve, and the appropriate action is taken (calcium, meanwhile, is rapidly expelled from the cell by membrane pumps).

Calcium is abundant; so is calmodulin. The reaction is one of the fastest in the body. Even hormones cannot work so fast. TH10-3

Source: W. Y. Cheung, Calmodulin, *Scientific American* 246 (1982): 62–70.

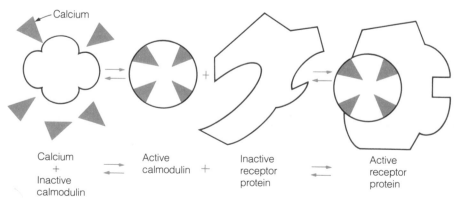

Calcium

Calcium + Inactive calmodulin → Active calmodulin + Inactive receptor protein → Active receptor protein

Calcium Deficiency

The disease rickets has been mentioned in connection with vitamin D deficiency. Often in rickets the amount of calcium in the diet is adequate, but it passes through the intestinal tract without being absorbed into the body, leaving the bones undersupplied. Vitamin D deficiency, by depressing the production of the calcium-binding protein, is the most common cause of rickets. (The symptoms were listed in Table 9–4.) In children, the failure to deposit sufficient calcium in bone causes growth retardation, bowed legs, and other skeletal abnormalities. In adults, the disease may set in after a normal childhood during which calcium intake and absorption were adequate, and after the skeleton has become fully calcified. Prolonged inadequate calcium uptake during adulthood, often due to vitamin D deficiency, may cause the gradual and insidious removal of calcium from the bones. The result is altered composition or reduced density of the bones in old age, which makes them fragile.

Many older people are severely afflicted with osteoporosis. The causes seem to be multiple, but inadequate storage of calcium during the growing years is a factor always in the background. This fact underscores the importance of prevention: drink plenty of milk while you are young to have strong bones in later life, and continue drinking milk throughout adulthood, to avoid losing calcium.

A net calcium loss occurs in many adults, especially women after menopause or hysterectomy, suggesting that hormonal changes are responsible. Many minerals and vitamins are required to form and stabilize the structure of bones, including magnesium, fluoride, vitamin A, and others. Any of these may be essential for preventing osteoporosis. One obvious line of defense, however, is to maintain a lifelong adequate intake of calcium.

Food Sources of Calcium

The recommended intake of calcium, arrived at by way of balance studies, is 700 to 800 milligrams (0.7 to 0.8 grams) per day for adults in both the United States and Canada. Adults can stay in balance on intakes lower than this if they adapt over a long period of time to lower intakes, and the World Health Organization recommends only 400 to 500 milligrams per day for adults. However, high protein intakes increase calcium excretion, and in the United States and Canada, where diets are rich in protein, 700 to 800 milligrams for adults and 1,200 for pregnant and lactating women seems to be a protective recommendation. Authorities are considering raising this recommendation to 1,000, or even 1,200, milligrams a day for women over 50.

Calcium is found almost exclusively in a single class of foods—milk and milk products—as shown in Table 10–4. For this reason, if for no other, members of this group must be included in the diet daily or *wise* substitutions must be made. Because a cup of milk contains almost 300 milligrams of calcium, an intake of 2 cups of milk provides a good start towards meeting the amount recommended for an adult for a day. A pregnant or lactating woman should have 3 to 4 cups; and an older woman, 3 cups. The other dairy food that contains comparable amounts of calcium is cheese.

rickets: the calcium deficiency (or vitamin D deficiency) disease in children.

Altered composition of the bones is reflected in **osteomalacia,** the condition in which the bones become soft (see pp. 337–338). Osteomalacia is sometimes called **adult rickets.**

Reduced density of the bones results in **osteoporosis** (oss-tee-oh-pore-OH-sis)—literally, porous bones.

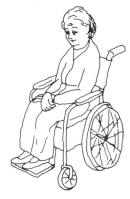

Chapter 15 shows that exercise, too, is important in the prevention of osteoporosis.

The RDA for calcium: 800 mg.

Canadian *Dietary Standard:* 800 mg for men, 700 mg for women.

TABLE 10–4 **Calcium—Average Amounts in Groups of Foods** TH10-4

	Calcium (mg)
Milk and Milk Products	
1 c milk[a]	300
1 c cottage cheese or ½ c ricotta	200
1 c other milk products[b]	200
1 c soy milk[c]	25
1 oz cheese[d]	200
Meat and Legumes	
3 oz canned salmon or sardines (with bones)	275
3 oz fish or shellfish[e]	50
3 oz meat or poultry	-0-
2 eggs	50
¾ c legumes, cooked, or ¼ c soy flour	50
4 oz soybean curd (tofu)	150
Fruits and Vegetables	
1 portion or piece fruit[f]	0-25
1 c calcium-rich vegetables[g]	200
½ c other vegetables	25
Grains[h]	
1 slice bread or ½ c rice or pasta	0-25
1 portion bread or cereal product made with calcium-rich cornmeal[i]	100
1 piece cake or pie or 1 muffin	50
Other	
1 portion nuts[j]	0-25
1 tbsp fat or oil	-0-
1 tbsp sugar or 1 candy[k]	-0-
1 oz milk chocolate candy	50
1 tbsp blackstrap molasses	150
1 c cream soup	175
1 tbsp brewer's yeast	-0-
1 tbsp wheat germ	-0-

According to the values in the table, a person following the modified four food group plan would obtain:

2 c milk	600 mg
2 (3-oz) portions meat, fish, poultry (including periodic use of salmon and sardines)	50
2 (¾ c) portions legumes	100
1 c calcium-rich vegetables[g]	200
3 servings other fruits or vegetables	75
4 portions enriched or whole grains	75
Total (compare the U.S. RDA of 1,000 mg)	1,100 mg

A person who doesn't use canned salmon or sardines frequently, and who doesn't consume calcium-rich vegetables daily can obtain adequate calcium by adding a third cup of milk to the day's intakes.

This table was made by consulting Appendix H, averaging the calcium amounts in standard portions of the commonly used foods in each category, and rounding off each average to the nearest 25 mg. (Thus, 0 doesn't mean no calcium, but rather, less than 13 mg.) Values agree approximately with the USDA table, Nutrients furnished by servings of foods, *Essentials of an Adequate Diet*, Bulletin no. 160, 1956. Refer to Appendix H for further details.

[a] 1 c milk or any milk drink or custard or pudding made with milk; 1 c soft serve ice milk; or 1 c yogurt. 1 c yogurt made from skim milk with added milk solids has 450 mg.

[b] 1 c ice cream or ice milk; 1 c cream or sour cream; ½ c ricotta; 1 c cottage cheese.

[c] Unfortified. Soy-based infant formula is calcium fortified.

[d] Not including cream cheese, which has only 20 mg calcium per ounce.

[e] Values range from 10 mg for tuna to 100 mg for canned shrimp.

f 40 kcalories (1 exchange) of any fruit except oranges contains less than 25 mg calcium; 40 kcalories of orange has a little more.

g 1 c dark leafy greens, broccoli, bokchoy (white mustard cabbage). All of these, except broccoli, also contain large amounts of a calcium binder—oxalic acid—which renders the calcium it binds unabsorbable. The extent of the binding is, at present, being determined; it seems probable that none of the calcium in most dark greens is absorbable, but that the oxalate in greens does not interfere with absorption of calcium from other foods eaten at the same meal. L. H. Allen, Calcium bioavailability and absorption: A review, *American Journal of Clinical Nutrition* 35 (1982): 783–808.

h Grain products with milk in the mix or recipe have more calcium, of course. The fiber and phytates in whole grains reduce calcium absorption to an extent that may be significant (Allen, 1982).

i Stone-ground or self-rising cornmeal is calcium-rich.

j 1 portion (1 fat exchange, or 45 kcalories) of any of the 8 varieties of nuts listed in Appendix H contains about 5 to 20 mg calcium.

k Candies containing milk (caramels, milk chocolate) can contain as much as about 50 mg calcium per ounce. Chocolate-flavored beverage powders made with milk can contain up to about 150 mg calcium per ounce.

One slice of cheese (1 ounce) contains about two-thirds as much calcium as a cup of milk. (Cottage cheese, however, is a poor source.) For people who don't drink enough milk, dark-green leafy vegetables have been thought to be an important calcium source, but the calcium binder—oxalate—renders the calcium in most greens except broccoli unabsorbable. (Greens are still a valuable source of riboflavin, folacin, vitamin A, iron, and other nutrients, however.)

The absurdity of attempting to meet calcium needs in any way other than by consuming two or more servings a day of these foods can be demonstrated by listing the amounts of some other foods you would have to consume instead: 6 heads of iceberg lettuce, 10 cups of cooked green beans, 12 oranges or eggs, or 20 cups of strawberries!

The amount of calcium recommended for the daily diet is so great that it won't fit in a single pill that can be swallowed. To make it absorbable, the manufacturers combine the calcium into a large organic salt such as calcium gluconate or calcium lactate, making an extremely bulky pill. To get 600 milligrams of calcium in this salt you would have to take six pills that might each be the diameter of a quarter and the thickness of four quarters. You therefore never find significant amounts of calcium in vitamin-mineral supplements of the type that are to be taken once a day. Many vitamin-mineral supplements do contain some calcium, however.

There are two ways to read a label. One is to read what it contains, and the other is to read how much. A list of the ingredients in a pill that contains calcium might mislead unaware consumers into believing that their calcium needs would be met by the pill. However, often the label lists the calcium content of each pill as 20 milligrams. Only when you compare this amount with the recommended intake (800 milligrams) do you realize that you would have to take 40 of these pills a day to meet your calcium needs. This discussion should remind you that you should always use a yardstick when reading nutrient amounts on labels.

It is important to remember, too, that pills do not supply the relative amounts of nutrients that are in the best balance for your overall health. A typical calcium supplement, for example, is labeled with the instructions to take six a day. Yet six of these pills a day supply less than 50

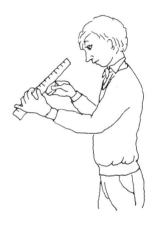

Appendix P compares the formulations of many commonly used vitamin-mineral supplements.

percent of the recommended intake of calcium and 500 percent of the vitamin D—and vitamin D is toxic in excess. (Vitamin D is added to the pill to enhance the absorption of calcium.)

In contrast, 2 cups of skim milk fortified with vitamins A and D would supply the following percentages of the nutrients an adult man needs: calcium, 60 percent; vitamin D, 50 percent; protein, 40 percent; vitamin A, 50 percent; thiamin, 12 percent; and riboflavin, 50 percent; plus 24 grams of carbohydrate in the form of lactose. Calcium absorption is enhanced by several of these other nutrients. Once again, a point made previously (p. 40) is relevant: there are fringe benefits to eating a nutrient in a natural food as opposed to a purified nutrient preparation.

Caution

The Four Food Group Plan recommends daily milk servings:

Children under 9	2–3 cups
Children 9-12	3+ cups
Teenagers	4+ cups
Adults	2 cups
Pregnant women	3+ cups
Lactating women	4+ cups
Older women	3 cups

milk allergy: the most common food allergy; caused by the protein in raw milk. Milk allergy is sometimes overcome by cooking the milk to denature the protein, sometimes "cured" by abstinence from and gradual reintroduction to milk. See also the discussion of lactose intolerance, p. 59.

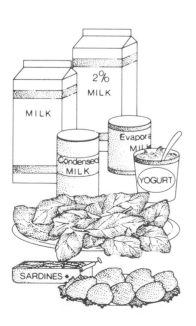

For most people, then, the obvious way to meet calcium needs is to include milk and milk products in the diet daily. This is especially important for pregnant and lactating women, older women, and children in the growing years (their calcium balance must be positive to permit good skeletal growth). Adults concerned with feeding children who dislike milk may find it helpful to learn how to conceal milk in foods. Ice cream, ice milk, and yogurt are acceptable substitutes for regular milk, and puddings, custards, and baked goods can be prepared in such a way that they also contain appreciable amounts of milk. Powdered skim milk, which is an excellent and inexpensive source of protein, calcium, and other nutrients, can be added to many foods (such as cookies and meatloaf) in preparation. For children with a milk allergy, a calcium-rich substitute such as fortified soy milk must be found. Butter and cream contain negligible calcium, because calcium is not soluble in fat. Figure 10–8 presents a decision tree for persons seeking a milk substitute.

The word *daily* should be stressed with respect to food sources of calcium. Because of its limited ability to absorb calcium, the body cannot handle massive doses periodically but instead needs frequent opportunities to take in small amounts.

Many factors affect calcium absorption. The stomach's acidity favors it by helping to keep calcium soluble. Vitamin D aids in calcium absorption by helping to make the necessary calcium-binding protein. (It is no accident that milk is chosen as the vehicle for fortification with vitamin D.) The lactose in milk also seems to facilitate calcium absorption by a mechanism as yet unknown.[21] Calcium levels are lower in breast milk than in cow's milk, but babies absorb calcium better from breast milk, possibly because of its higher lactose content.

Some foods contain binders that combine chemically with calcium (and other minerals such as iron and zinc) to prevent their absorption, carrying them out of the body with other wastes. For example, phytic acid renders the calcium, iron, and zinc in certain foods unavailable; oxalic acid binds calcium and iron; and uronic acid binds calcium. Phytic acid is found in

21   L. H. Allen, Calcium bioavailability and absorption: A review, *American Journal of Clinical Nutrition* 35 (1982): 783–808.

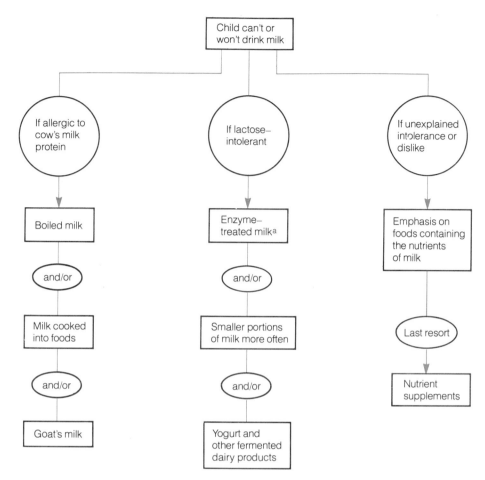

FIGURE 10–8 **Choosing a milk substitute.**
TH10-5

Source: Adapted from E. N. Whitney and C. B. Cataldo, Choosing Formulas and Milk Substitutes, in *Understanding Normal and Clinical Nutrition* (St. Paul, Minn.: West, 1983), pp. 559–568.

[a] You can buy milk already treated or add the enzyme (LactAid) yourself. Enzyme treatment may not reduce lactose content sufficiently to relieve symptoms, and you may have to try the other alternatives.

whole grains; oxalic acid in beets, rhubarb, and dark green leafy vegetables; and uronic acid in the fiber of grains, fruits, and vegetables.[22] Fiber in general seems to hinder calcium absorption, so the higher the diet is in fiber, the higher it should be in calcium. This fact in no way affects the overall value of high-fiber foods. Whole grains, legumes, greens, other vegetables, and fruits are nutritious for so many reasons that no one should hesitate to include them in menu planning.

The body is able to regulate its absorption of calcium by altering its production of the calcium-binding protein. More of this protein is made if more calcium is needed. Thus you will absorb more when you need more. This system is most obviously reflected in the increased absorption by a pregnant woman, who absorbs 50 percent of the calcium from the milk she drinks instead of only 30 percent, as she formerly did. Thus her body's calcium intake almost doubles, even if her food intake does not change at all. Similarly, growing children absorb 50 to 60 percent of ingested calcium; when their growth slows or stops (and their bones no longer demand a net increase in calcium content each day), their absorption falls to the adult level of about 30 percent.

binders: chemical compounds occurring in foods that can combine with nutrients (especially minerals) to form complexes the body cannot absorb. **Phytic** (FIGHT-ic) and **oxalic** (ox-AL-ic) **acids** are examples of such binders. See Chapter 2 for more about phytic acid.

22   Oxalate content of common foods, *Nutrition and the MD*, September 1979.

An important relationship exists between calcium and phosphorus. Each is better absorbed if they are ingested together. Authorities differ on the ratio that might best favor health, but it seems probable that most would agree on a 1:1 ratio; perhaps any ratio from 3:1 to 1:3 is all right.

Protein also affects calcium status, as already mentioned, but not by affecting absorption. The higher the diet is in protein, the greater the amount of calcium excreted.[23] This is why people in the United States and Canada are told to ingest more calcium than people in countries whose protein intakes are lower.

A generalization that has been gaining strength throughout this book is supported by the information given here about calcium. A balanced diet that supplies a variety of foods is the best guarantee of adequacy for all essential nutrients. All food groups should be included, and none should be overused. Calcium is found lacking wherever milk is underemphasized in the diet—whether through ignorance, simple dislike, lactose intolerance, or allergy. By contrast, iron is found lacking whenever milk is overemphasized, as Chapter 11 shows.

Caution

Phosphorus

Phosphorus is the mineral in second largest quantity in the body. About 85 percent of it is found combined with calcium in the crystals of the bones and teeth. There it occurs as calcium phosphate, one of the compounds in the crystals that give strength and rigidity to these structures.[24]

The concentration of phosphorus in blood plasma is less than half that of calcium: 3.5 milligrams per 100 milliliters of plasma. But as part of one of the body's major acids (phosphoric acid), it is found in all body cells. It is a part of DNA and RNA, the genetic code material present in every cell. Thus phosphorus is necessary for all growth, because DNA and RNA provide the instructions for new cells to be formed.

Phosphorus also plays many key roles in energy transfers occurring during cellular metabolism. Many enzymes and the B vitamins become active only when a phosphate group is attached. (The B vitamins, you will recall, play major roles in energy metabolism.) ATP itself, the energy carrier of the cells, contains three phosphate groups and uses these groups to do its work.

Some lipids contain phosphorus as part of their structure. These phospholipids help to transport other lipids in the blood; they also reside

23   Allen, 1982.

24   The suffix *ate* in *calcium phosphate* indicates that the phosphorus has undergone a chemical reaction with oxygen and is bonded to it.

in cell membranes, where they affect transport of nutrients into and out of the cells. The phosphate ion also helps in one of the blood's most important buffering systems.

Animal protein is the best source of phosphorus, because phosphorus is so abundant in the energetic cells of animals. The recommended intakes for phosphorus are the same as those for calcium: 700 to 800 milligrams per day for adults. Deficiencies are unknown.

The RDA for phosphorus: 800 mg.

Canadian *Dietary Standard:* 800 mg for men, 700 mg for women.

Chlorine

The element chlorine occurs as a poisonous gas, but when it combines with sodium in salt, it is not poisonous but is part of a life-giving compound. It occurs in salt as the negative chloride ion.

The chloride ion is the major negative ion of the fluids outside the cells, where it is found mostly in association with sodium. Chloride can move freely across membranes and so is also found inside the cells in association with potassium. Its role in balancing the pH of the blood has already been described.

In the stomach, the chloride ion is part of hydrochloric acid, which maintains the strong acidity of the stomach. The cells that line the stomach continuously expend energy to push chloride into the stomach fluid. One of the most serious consequences of vomiting is the loss of acid from the stomach, which upsets the acid-base balance.

A chlorine compound is added to public water to reduce its bacterial count before it flows through pipes into people's homes. The compound turns to the deadly poisonous gas chlorine, kills dangerous microorganisms that might otherwise spread disease, and then evaporates, leaving the water safe for human consumption. The addition of chlorine to public water is one of the most important public health measures ever introduced in the developed countries and has eliminated such water-borne diseases as typhoid fever, which once ravaged vast areas, killing thousands of people.

Estimated safe and adequate daily dietary intake of chloride (Committee on RDA): 1,700–5,100 mg.

Potassium

Potassium is critical to maintaining the heartbeat. The sudden deaths that occur in severe diarrhea and in children with kwashiorkor may often be due to heart failure caused by potassium loss. As the principal positively charged ion inside body cells, it plays a major role in maintaining water balance and cell integrity. When water loss from the body involves sodium loss, the ultimate damage comes when potassium is pulled out of the cells and excreted. Dehydration is especially scary, because potassium deficiency affects the brain cells early, making the victim unable to perceive that she needs water.

During nerve transmission and muscle contraction, potassium and

Estimated safe and adequate daily dietary intake of potassium (Committee on RDA): 1,875–5,625 mg (1.9–5.6 g).

Potassium-rich foods include bananas and many other whole, fresh fruits; orange juice and many other fruit juices; and potatoes, tomatoes, and many other vegetables. For details, see Appendix I.

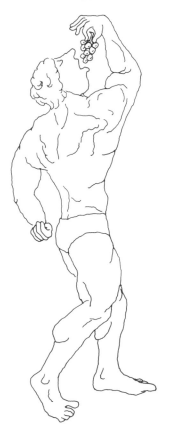

Amino acids containing sulfur are methionine and cysteine. Cysteine in one part of a protein chain can bind to cysteine in another part of the chain by way of a sulfur-sulfur bridge (see p. 127). Two cysteine molecules linked this way are called cystine (see Appendix C).

sodium briefly exchange places across the cell membrane. Nerve and muscle cells, then, are especially rich in potassium, but all cells must contain some. Potassium is also known to play a catalytic role in carbohydrate and protein metabolism, but the exact nature of this role is not known.

A deficiency of potassium from getting too little in the diet is unlikely, but high-sodium diets low in fresh fruits and vegetables make it a possibility. Abnormal conditions such as diabetic acidosis or loss of large volumes of water can cause potassium deficiency. One of the earliest symptoms is muscle weakness.

Gradual potassium depletion can occur when a person sweats profusely day after day and fails to replenish his potassium stores. A study of this effect shows that up to about 3 grams of potassium can be lost in a day. The average diet in this country supplies about 1.5 to 2.5 grams. The authors of one study recommend that a person who sweats heavily and often should eat five to eight servings of potassium-rich foods each day.[25]

> It has been pointed out several times previously that there are advantages to eating foods instead of taking supplements. Salt tablets contain sodium and chloride, but foods contain a multitude of minerals. The body evolved in dependence on foods, not supplements. Also, men who think fruit is only for dainty ladies might take note that because of the potassium it contains, fruit may do more for their muscles than meat.

Caution

Potassium supplements are not advisable except when prescribed, because too much potassium is as dangerous as too little. Even salt substitutes containing potassium should be avoided, especially by heart patients, except as recommended by a physician.

Sulfur

Sulfur is present in all proteins and plays its most important role in determining the contour of protein molecules. Sulfur helps the strands of protein to assume a particular shape and hold it—and so to do their specific jobs, such as enzyme work. Some of the amino acids contain sulfur in their side chains; once built into a protein strand, one of these amino acids can link to each other by way of sulfur-sulfur bridges. The bridges stabilize the protein structure. Skin, hair, and nails contain some of the body's more rigid proteins, and these have a high sulfur content.

There is no recommended intake for sulfur, and no deficiencies are known. Only if a person lacks protein to the point of severe deficiency will he lack the sulfur-containing amino acids.

25   H. W. Lane and J. J. Cerda, Potassium requirements and exercise, *Journal of the American Dietetic Association* 73 (1978): 64–65.

Magnesium

Magnesium barely qualifies as a major mineral. Only about 1¾ ounces of magnesium are present in the body of a 130-pound person, most of it in the bones. Bone magnesium seems to be a reservoir to ensure that some will be on hand for vital reactions regardless of recent dietary intake.

Magnesium also acts in all the cells of the soft tissues, where it forms part of the protein-making machinery and where it is necessary for the release of energy. Its major role seems to be as a catalyst in the reaction that adds the last high-energy phosphate bond to ATP. Magnesium also helps relax muscles after contraction and promotes resistance to tooth decay by holding calcium in tooth enamel.

A dietary deficiency of magnesium does not seem likely, but deficiency may occur as a result of vomiting, diarrhea, alcohol abuse, or protein malnutrition; in postsurgical patients who have been fed incomplete fluids into a vein for too long; or in people using diuretics. A severe deficiency causes tetany, an extreme and prolonged contraction of the muscles very much like the reaction of the muscles when calcium levels fall. Magnesium deficit is also thought to cause the hallucinations experienced by alcoholics during withdrawal.

Recommended intakes of magnesium are 300 to 350 milligrams a day for adult males, 250 to 300 for females. Good food sources include nuts, legumes, cereal grains, dark-green vegetables, seafoods, chocolate, and cocoa. The kidney acts to conserve magnesium; the magnesium not absorbed is excreted in the feces.

The RDA for magnesium: 350 mg for men, 300 mg for women.

Canadian *Dietary Standard:* 300 mg for men, 250 mg for women.

Summing Up

Water in the body participates in many chemical reactions, and serves as a solvent, transportation medium, and lubricant. It makes up 55 to 60 percent of the body's weight.

Public water may contain significant quantities of minerals, depending on the source and locale. Hard water is rich in calcium and magnesium; soft water is rich in sodium.

Industrial waste may add toxic heavy metals like mercury, cadmium, and lead to the water supply, creating a health hazard. A second threat from water is microbial contamination, which can be controlled by sewage treatment that includes chlorination. A third concern is that highly toxic organic compounds may enter the water supply from agricultural and industrial use; little is known about these. A need may arise in the future to limit technological uses of water in order to continue providing a sufficient and safe supply to sustain human life.

The principal electrolytes in body fluids are sodium, chloride, phosphorus, and potassium; each is maintained at a constant concentration by means of renal excretion. The electrolytes are involved in moving body water from place to place, thus maintaining the water balance. They also help determine the pH of body fluids, maintaining the acid-base balance. Fluid and electrolyte imbalances are medical emergencies.

The body maintains a certain blood pressure to sustain the lives of its cells. When blood pressure falls, as in dehydration, the kidneys raise it by conserving water and sodium. However, the kidneys also respond to poor circulation of blood fluid, as in atherosclerosis, by raising blood pressure. Ten percent of hypertension cases are attributed to kidney disease; all others result from unknown causes, but several diet-related factors affect blood pressure.

Sodium is abundant in the diet, as part of salt. Deficiencies are rare except in dehydration. Genetically sensitive people may develop high blood pressure in response to too-high sodium intakes.

About 99 percent of the body's calcium is a structural component of the bones and teeth. The 1 percent of calcium found in body fluids helps maintain cell membrane integrity, intercellular cohesion, transport of substances into and out of cells, and transmission of nerve impulses. It is also essential for blood clotting and acts as a cofactor in some enzyme systems. Calcium concentration in the blood is held constant.

Calcium deficiency may be caused directly by inadequate calcium intakes over a prolonged period or indirectly by vitamin D deficiency. The diseases that result are rickets, osteomalacia, and osteoporosis.

A substantial portion of the recommended calcium intake is easily supplied by 2 cups of milk or equivalent dairy products such as cheese; fortified soy milk is an alternative in the case of milk allergy or lactose intolerance. The only other rich food source of calcium is dark-green leafy vegetables, but their calcium may be unabsorbable, being bound to oxalate.

Phosphorus, another major mineral, is so abundant in foods that deficiencies are unlikely. It participates with calcium in forming the crystals of bone and therefore is found in large quantities in the body. Chlorine, which occurs in salt as the negative chloride ion, also contributes to the formation of the stomach's hydrochloric acid. Potassium is primarily involved in the working of nerve and muscle cells. A deficiency caused by protein deprivation or dehydration can stop the heart; excess potassium is also dangerous. Sulfur, like phosphorus, is a major mineral constituent of body tissues. It is abundant in the diet, and deficiencies are unknown. Magnesium plays a role in the synthesis of body proteins and so is important to all body functions. It is found lacking in human beings in conditions that aggravate dietary protein deficiency, such as kwashiorkor and alcoholism. A deficiency of magnesium causes tetany.

NOTE: References recommended in Appendix J provide further information on water and the water supply, and on high blood pressure. See "Water," and "Sodium and High Blood Pressure."

The Self-Study for this chapter in Appendix Q shows you how to:

● Estimate and evaluate your calcium and sodium intakes.
● Find alternative calcium sources for someone who doesn't drink milk.

The *Instructor's Manual* includes a supplementary lecture with a diagram illustrating fluid and electrolyte imbalances.

HIGHLIGHT 10
Food Additives

Food is a fantastically complex mixture of chemicals, probably numbering in the hundreds of thousands.

F. M. STRONG

If you are curious to know what substances are in the foods you eat and what they do, you can't help wondering about additives. Reading labels is all very well (see Highlight 12), but it takes you only so far. The most a label tells you about additives is what they do to the foods they are in—but what do they do to *you*? This question may especially concern you if you have heard some of the stories that implicate additives in the causation of cancer, birth defects, and other frightening conditions.

For example, cyclamate, a widely used artificial sweetener, was banned from use in the United States in 1969 because of some tests suggesting that it could cause cancer. Since then, five other substances have been banned for similar reasons: red dye no. 2, violet no. 1, carbon black, diethylpyrocarbonate, and salts of cobalt (used in beer). Two others, saccharin and nitrite, have also been banned, but the bans have been suspended—a situation some consumers find confusing and troubling. Some 20 other

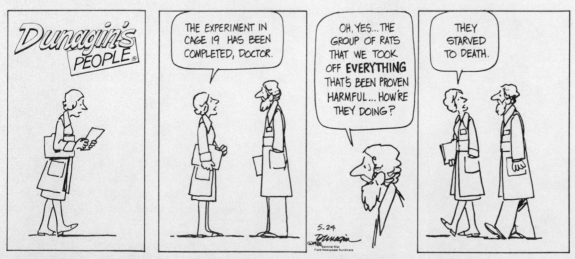

DUNAGIN'S PEOPLE by Ralph Dunagin © 1981 Field Enterprises, Inc. Courtesy of Field Newspaper Syndicate.

397

paranoia (para-NOY-uh): excessive or irrational suspiciousness and distrustfulness; unjustified fear.

para = beyond

nous = mind.

additive: a substance not normally consumed as a food by itself but added to food either intentionally or by accident.

intentional food additive: an additive intentionally added to food, such as nutrients or colors.

indirect (incidental) additive: an additive unintentionally added to a food by an accident of contamination, such as packaging materials or chemicals used during processing.

substances have been challenged as unsafe, including salt, sugar, xylitol, caffeine, MSG (monosodium glutamate), and all synthetic colors and flavors.[1] People wonder what they might be consuming now that will be banned in the future, and what harm it may be doing.

A public paranoia has thus developed that has destroyed many consumers' confidence in the safety of the food supply. This is doubly ironic. The public's mistrust has stemmed from the presence in foods of substances that were put there to make the foods safer, more attractive, or in other ways beneficial to consumers. And the banning of some of these substances has resulted from the requirement that they be tested, that the tests be closely monitored, and that the whole process be open to public view.

Before getting into some of the down-to-earth facts about additives, it is important to make a distinction and to offer a perspective. Harmful substances do occur in foods. Sometimes they are even put there intentionally, by people who haven't realized the potential harm they may cause. But a greater danger by far comes from harmful substances that get into foods accidentally by way of contamination with disease-causing microorganisms or with unwanted substances from packaging, processing materials, or environmental pollution. In other words, the term *additive* is too loose. We should distinguish between *intentional additives*, put there on purpose after a rational decision-making process, and *incidental* or *indirect additives*, which find their way into foods by accident.

This Highlight is about intentional additives, and comes to a not very alarming conclusion. The next Highlight (Highlight 11) is about contamination of foods and shows where some serious hazards may exist. To get a balanced picture of the safety of the food supply, you should read them both.

Terminology

To begin at the beginning, then, intentional food additives are substances put into foods to give them some desirable characteristic: color, flavor, texture, stability, or resistance to spoilage. Some additives are nutrients added to foods to increase their nutritional value, such as vitamin C added to fruit drinks or potassium iodide added to salt. The most common ones, roughly in order of the quantities used, are listed in the accompanying Miniglossary. In addition, there are numerous additives used in still smaller quantities for miscellaneous other purposes.

Regulations Governing Additives

The agency charged with the responsibility of deciding what additives shall be in foods is the Food and Drug Administration (FDA). FDA's authority over additives hinges primarily on their safety. The procedure a manufacturer has to go through to get permission to put a new additive in food puts the burden on him to prove the additive is safe, and may take

1   E. M. Foster, How safe are our foods? *Nutrition Reviews/Supplement*, January 1982, pp. 28–34.

Miniglossary of Intentional Food Additives

emulsifiers, **stabilizers**, **thickeners**: to give texture, smoothness, or other desired consistencies.

nutrients: to improve nutritive value.

flavoring agents: to add or enhance flavor.

leavening (neutralizing) agents: to control acidity or alkalinity.

preservatives, **antioxidants**, **sequestrants**, **antimyotic agents**: to prevent spoilage, rancidity of fats, and microbial growth.

coloring agents: to increase attractiveness.

bleaches: to whiten foods such as flour and cheese and to speed up the maturing of cheese.

humectants, **anticaking agents**: to retain moisture in some foods and to keep others (such as salts and powders) free-flowing.

---

several years. First he has to test it chemically to satisfy the FDA that:

- It is effective (it does what it is supposed to do).
- It can be detected and measured in the final food product.

Then he has to feed it in large doses to animals and prove that:

- It is safe (it causes no cancer, birth defects, or other injury).

The manufacturer can't do just any animal tests. The doses are specified; two kinds of animals (usually rodents and dogs) must be used; and the time periods must be long. Finally, the manufacturer must submit all his test results to FDA.[2]

FDA responds to the manufacturer's petition by announcing a public hearing. Consumers are invited to participate at these hearings, where experts present testimony for and against the acceptance of the additive for the proposed uses. Thus the consumer's rights and responsibilities are written into the provisions for deeming additives safe.

If FDA approves the additive's use, that doesn't mean the manufacturer can add it in any amount to any food. On the contrary: FDA writes a regulation stating in what amounts, and in what foods, the additive may be used. No additives are permanently approved; all are periodically reviewed.

Many substances were exempted from complying with this procedure at the time the law came into being, because there were no known hazards in their use. These substances, some 700 in all, were put on the GRAS list. However, any time substantial scientific evidence or public outcry has questionned the safety of any of the substances on the GRAS list, a special reevaluation has been made. Meanwhile, the entire GRAS list has been systematically and intensively reevaluated, and all substances about which

GRAS (generally recognized as safe) list: a list of food additives, established by the Food and Drug Administration (FDA), that had long been in use and were believed safe. The list is subject to revision as new facts become known.

2   P. Lehman, More than you ever thought you would know about food additives, *FDA Consumer*, April 1979 (reprint).

carcinogen (car-SIN-oh-jen): a cancer-causing agent.

carcino = cancer

gen = to produce).

Delaney Clause: a clause in the Food Additive Amendment to the Food, Drug, and Cosmetic Act that states that no substance that is known to cause cancer in animals or humans at any dose level shall be added to foods in any amount.

saccharine, **cyclamate**, **aspartame**: see Miniglossary in Chapter 2.

nitrite: a salt added to food to prevent botulism. **Nitrosamines** (nigh-TROHS-uh-meens) are derivatives of nitrites that may be formed in the stomach when nitrites combine with amines; and nitrosamines are carcinogenic.

botulism (BOTT-you-lism): a form of food poisoning caused by **botulinum toxin**, a toxin produced by bacteria that grow in meat.

any legitimate question was raised have been removed or reclassified. A set of 2,100 flavoring agents is similarly being reviewed, as well as some 200 coloring agents.[3]

One of the criteria an additive must meet to be placed on the GRAS list is that it must not have been found to be a carcinogen in any test on animals or humans. The Delaney Clause (a part of the law on additives) is uncompromising in addressing carcinogens in food and drugs and has been under fire in recent years for being too strict. This brings us to the questions of what laws are appropriate in regulating food additives, and what changes should be made.

The Delaney Clause is criticized because it does not allow for the different effects on the body of varying dose levels of an additive. For example, when the artificial sweetener cyclamate was banned in 1969, it was estimated that a human would have to drink, each day, at least 138 12-ounce bottles of soft drinks containing cyclamates to ingest an amount of cyclamate comparable to the quantity given animals in the tests that caused the ban.[4] The FDA was criticized for banning the use of cyclamates, but under the law it had no alternative. The Delaney Clause does not give FDA the right to make a judgment on dose levels of carcinogens or on the applicability of animal research to humans or even on the reproducibility of an experiment.

At present, a similar controversy centers on saccharin. Some animal tests have suggested that saccharin may be a weak carcinogen; thus it had to be automatically banned. But while consumers were grateful in 1969 when cyclamate was banned, they were upset and resentful in 1977 at the proposed banning of saccharin, the only familiar artificial sweetener remaining on the market. To satisfy both the law and the consumers, Congress passed the ban and then suspended it; as of 1983 saccharin was still being sold, but with a warning label: "Use of this product may be hazardous to your health. This product contains saccharin which has been determined to cause cancer in laboratory animals."

Nitrites, which are added to smoked meats such as hot dogs and cold cuts, have suffered a similar fate. A test on rats, published in 1978, suggested they caused cancer, and again an automatic ban had to be invoked. But the case of nitrites had a new twist. They are not added to meats just for flavor or eye appeal. They prevent bacterial spoilage, and in particular, the growth of the deadly bacterial species that produces botulinum toxin, the most potent biological poison known. An amount as tiny as a single crystal of salt can kill a person within an hour, and in survivors, troublesome after-effects linger for months. If nitrites were banned, the risk to users of these products would be intolerable; no other preservative was known that could do nitrite's job; and the only alternative seemed to be to take all smoked meats off the market.

The ban on nitrite was therefore suspended, pending further investigation. Not long after, the experiment connecting nitrites to cancer was heavily criticized, and its validity is doubtful. The risk to users of products

3 Lehman, 1979.

4 R. D. Middlekauf, Legalities concerning food additives, *Food Technology* 28 (May 1974): 42–49.

containing nitrites is probably slight in comparison to other risks, but consumers have been shaken by the alarms raised and are more inclined to be mistrustful of *all* additives as a result.

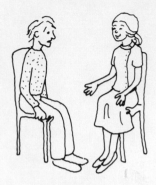

Nitrates, Nitrites, Nitrosamines

Q: What are the risks associated with these additives?

A: Wait a minute. You've asked the question wrong. These compounds aren't additives. Nitrates and nitrites are all salts that contain the nitrate or nitrite ions. Nitrosamines are compounds in which the nitrite ion has combined with an amine. All these compounds occur naturally in the environment; nitrates are used as fertilizer and are present in the water supply, and nitrites are present in high concentrations in many vegetables. Nitrites also form naturally in saliva and digestive juices. But it's true that nitrates and nitrites are *used* as additives.

Q: OK, so what are the risks associated with their use?

A: Well, again, whether they are added to food or present there naturally, or present in drinking water, the risks are the same. There is a chance that nitrates may cause cancer (we don't know for sure yet), and nitrosamines are known to do so. The main problem is that nitrates may be converted to nitrites, and nitrites to nitrosamines, during cooking or in the stomach.

Q: Nitrosamines *do* cause cancer, you say. Are nitrosamines ever added to foods?

A: No, never.

Q: How serious is the risk of cancer from nitrates and nitrites added to food?

A: That's a hard question to answer. It is not known for sure whether nitrosamines do form in the stomach when you eat nitrates and nitrites in foods. And it's not known whether they cause cancer in humans. They do, in animals.

Q: Can I avoid using nitrites if I want to?

A: Not very easily. FDA has estimated that they are present in 7 percent of our food supply. You could avoid using all products to which they are *added*—bacon, hot dogs, ham, processed poultry, fish, and meat—but even if you became a strict vegetarian, you'd get them from your own saliva and intestinal juices and from the vegetables you ate.

Q: How do the amounts in vegetables compare with those in meats?

A: Well, bacon is permitted to have 120 parts per million (ppm) of nitrite as sold in the store. Other meats can have 200 ppm, but most have less than 50. Smoked fish can have 500 ppm nitrate and 200 ppm nitrite. Some vegetables contain up to 3,000 ppm nitrates, and even drinking water sometimes has several hundred ppm. The average person probably gets about 200 micrograms a day from vegetables, 2,000-odd from cured meats, and some 8,000 from his own saliva.[5]

Q: So I have to avoid all processed meats and—oh, dear, which vegetables must I exclude from my diet?

A: Wait a minute, I didn't suggest you do any such thing. Remember, every move you make in life involves some risk, and every food can be toxic if taken in excess. I suggest you adopt a strategy of minimizing the risks.

Q: How can I minimize the risks?

A: Well, first of all, remember, variety ensures dilution. I mean, whenever you switch from food to food, you are diluting whatever's in one food with what's in the other. So eat *some* processed meats, but don't eat them all the time. And don't give up any vegetables; they're all good; you need them in your diet for many positive reasons.

Q: OK, the meat I'll choose to have occasionally is bacon; that's my favorite. How can I minimize the risks associated with bacon?

A: Good question. There are at least three things you can do. First, always consume a vitamin C source at the same meals, like orange juice or lettuce and tomatoes. Vitamin C is thought to prevent the formation of nitrosamines in the stomach. Second, don't fry the bacon too crispy. When it starts to burn, that's when the nitrosamines may be being formed. And third, don't re-use the bacon fat, because that's where they tend to be concentrated.

Q: Well, thanks for all the answers. I feel a little better informed. I wish I could say I feel reassured, too, but I don't. In fact I feel nervous about everything I eat these days.

A: I know how you feel. It takes a while to get comfortable with the idea of living with a certain amount of risk. I hope it won't be long before you feel OK about it.

Another additive, which had much of the public alarmed during the late 1970s, was yellow no. 5 (tartrazine), a color additive that in occasional rare instances causes an allergic reaction in people who are also allergic to aspirin. Tartrazine was for a while blamed for causing many (some people said most) cases of hyperactivity in children, and a special diet (the Feingold diet), composed entirely of additive-free foods, was recommended for these children. By 1980 it was clear that the majority of cases of hyperactivity are not caused by tartrazine or other additives, but legislation is now in force requiring that tartrazine must be mentioned on all labels of foods that contain it so that consumers can avoid it if they wish.

5   R. J. Hickey and R. G. Clelland, Hazardous food additives: Nitrite and saliva? (correspondence), *New England Journal of Medicine* 298 (1978): 1036.

The Public's Fears about Additives

Another reason for the public's sometimes unreasonable fear of additives is a generalized fear of anything "chemical" or "synthetic." Many deadly poisons are "natural" substances found in foods or produced by living organisms (consider mushrooms). Contrary to the public's suspicions, it is the processing of food and the introduction of additives that removes toxic substances, prevents the growth of dangerous microorganisms, and makes the food safe for our use. Foods are made of chemicals anyway, as Table 10–1 demonstrates. It has been argued that the food industry has not only the right but also the responsibility to educate the public about the safety of food additives. From this point of view, a food packager who advertises "no additives" is not doing the public a favor. By implying that there is something wrong with additives, he is exploiting the public's emotionalism rather than helping educate.[6]

TABLE H10–1 These chemicals are found naturally in foods. No additives are present! Chemical listings are not necessarily complete.

Toast and coffee cake
Gluten
Amino acids
Amylose
Starches
Dextrins
Sucrose
Pentosans
Hexosans
Triglycerides
Monoglycerides and
diglycerides
Sodium chloride
Phosphorus
Calcium
Iron
Thiamin (vitamin B_1)
Riboflavin
(vitamin B_2)
Niacin
Pantothenic acid
Vitamin D
Methyl ethyl ketone
Acetic acid
Propionic acid
Butyric acid
Valeric acid
Caproic acid
Acetone
Diacetyl
Maltol
Ethyl acetate
Ethyl lactate

Scrambled eggs
Ovalbumin
Conalbumin

Ovomucoid
Mucin
Globulins
Amino acids
Lipovitellin
Livetin
Cholesterol
Lecithin
Choline
Lipids (fats)
Fatty acids
Lutein
Zeaxanthine
Vitamin A
Biotin
Pantothenic acid
Riboflavin
(vitamin B_2)
Thiamin (vitamin B_1)
Niacin
Pyridoxine
(vitamin B_6)
Folic acid (folacin)
Cyanocobalamin
(vitamin B_{12})
Sodium chloride
Iron
Calcium
Phosphorus

Chilled cantaloupe
Starches
Cellulose
Pectin
Fructose
Sucrose
Glucose

Malic acid
Citric acid
Succinic acid
Anisyl propionate
Amyl acetate
Ascorbic acid
(vitamin C)
B-carotene
(vitamin A)
Riboflavin
(vitamin B_2)
Thiamin (vitamin B_1)
Niacin
Phosphorus
Potassium

Coffee
Caffeine
Methanol
Ethanol
Butanol
Methylbutanol
Acetaldehyde
Methyl formate
Dimethyl sulfide
Propionaldehyde
Pyridine
Acetic acid
Furfural
Furfuryl alcohol
Acetone
Methyl acetate
Furan
Methylfuran
Diacetyl
Isoprene
Guaiacol

Hydrogen sulfide

Tea
Caffeine
Tannin
Butanol
Isoamyl alcohol
Hexanol
Phenyl ethyl alcohol
Benzyl alcohol
Geraniol
Quercetin
3-galloyl epicatechin
3-galloyl
epigallocatechin

Sugar-cured ham
Myosin
Actomyosin
Myoglobin
Collagen
Elastin
Amino acids
Creatine
Lipids (fats)
Linoleic acid
Oleic acid
Lecithin
Cholesterol
Sucrose
Glucose
Pyroligneous acid
Phosphorus
Thiamin (vitamin B_1)
Riboflavin
(vitamin B_2)
Niacin

Cyanocobalamin
(vitamin B_{12})
Pyridoxine
(vitamin B_6)
Sodium chloride
Iron
Magnesium
Potassium

Cinnamon apple chips
Pectin
Hemicellulose
Starches
Sucrose
Glucose
Fructose
Malic acid
Lactic acid
Citric acid
Succinic acid
Ascorbic acid
(vitamin C)
B-carotene
(vitamin A)
Cinnamyl alcohol
Cinnamic aldehyde
Potassium
Phosphorus
Acetaldehyde
Amyl formate
Amyl acetate
Amyl caproate
Geraniol

Source: Kindly supplied by the Chemical Manufacturers Association.

6   M. J. Sheridan and E. M. Whelan, "Consumerism" and the American food industry, *ACSH News and Views* 1 (April 1980): 1, 14–15.

People who sell foods, like people who sell anything, may be inclined to take advantage of their customers in unfair ways, as we have often said before. A realistic (not necessarily cynical) view of this tendency helps protect you, the consumer, from being "taken." Take a close look, sometime, at the foods that claim to contain "no additives, no preservatives." Are they beneficial, nutritious foods? How do they resist spoilage—or do they? Do they contain large amounts of salt? (Salt is really an additive too, but not commonly thought of as one. In fact it is a very effective preservative—but is it preferable to other preservatives in terms of its effects on human health?) What is the motivation behind the claim on the label? Is the intention to reveal to you the unadorned truth about the contents of the package? Or is it trying to imply a health-promoting property that is really not unique to the food in the package—with or without additives? When a label says "no additives," ask yourself: "So what?"

Caution

Another reason the public has become scared about what's in foods is—ironically—because chemists are so much better at their jobs than they used to be, and the analytical techniques they use are so much more powerful than in the past. Where once they would say there were no detectable levels of a substance in food "down to one part per million," now they have ways of detecting the same substance at one part per *billion*. This makes it seem as if new substances are appearing in our foods while in fact they may have been there all the time but are only now being seen. And the concentrations are so extremely low as to be insignificant. It is ironic, too, that the removal of substances from the GRAS list, which has improved the safety of those permitted, so alarmed the public that the effect seems to have been to make them mistrustful of the entire process. But the main reason for exaggerated alarm about additives is the public's failure to understand the difference between toxicity and hazard.

Toxicity versus Hazard

"Toxicity—the capacity of a chemical substance to harm living organisms—is a general property of matter; hazard is the capacity of a chemical to produce injury under conditions of use. All substances are potentially toxic, but are hazardous only if consumed in sufficiently large quantities."[7]

People often fail to understand the distinction between toxicity and hazard, and so become overly afraid of dangers that are real, but small

toxicity: the ability of a substance to harm living organisms. All substances are toxic if high enough concentrations are used. See also *hazard*.

hazard: state of danger; used to refer to any circumstance in which toxicity is possible under normal conditions of use. See also *toxicity*.

7 F. M. Strong, Toxicants occurring naturally in foods, in *Nutrition Reviews' Present Knowledge in Nutrition*, 4th ed. (Washington, D.C.: Nutrition Foundation, 1976), pp. 516–527.

enough to ignore. For example: if you eat a bucketful of sand, it can kill you. (Anything—even water—is toxic if you take enough of it.) But this doesn't mean you should be afraid to eat a sandwich at the beach because it might have one grain of sand in it. (In contrast, though, you had *better* be afraid to eat spoiled meat that might contain botulinum toxin, because an amount as small as a grain of sand could kill several adults.) The question to ask is, "Is it dangerous like sand or water— where there's no chance I'll get enough to hurt me? Or is it dangerous like botulinum toxin—where the amount I actually consume can hurt me?" Food additives, if they are dangerous at all, are dangerous like water or sand. They are allowed in foods only with a wide margin of safety.

Caution

This distinction is readily accepted in other areas—such as air travel: "We fly in airplanes because they are 'safe,' but 'safe' is defined by the low number of deaths per million passenger miles, not the total absence of risk."[8] When chemicals are involved, however, there seems to be an added scare factor.

To see food additives in the correct perspective, it is necessary to understand the concept of margin of safety. Most additives that involve risk are allowed in foods only at levels 100 times below those at which the risk is still known to be zero; their margin of safety is 1/100. Experiments to determine the extent of risk involve feeding test animals the substance at different concentrations throughout their lifetimes. The additive is then permitted in foods at 1/100 the level that can be fed under these conditions without causing any harmful effect whatever. In many foods, naturally occurring substances appear at levels that bring their margin of safety closer to 1/10. Even nutrients, as you have seen, involve risks at high dosage levels. The margin of safety for vitamins A and D is 1/25 to 1/40; it may be less than 1/10 in infants.[9] For some trace elements, it is about ⅕. People consume common table salt daily in amounts only three to five times less than those that cause serious toxicity.[10]

The margin of safety concept also applies to nutrients when they are used as additives. Iodine has been added to salt to prevent iodine deficiency, but it has had to be added with care because it is a deadly poison in excess. Similarly, iron has been added to refined bread and other grains (enrichment), and has doubtless helped prevent many cases of iron-deficiency anemia in women and children who are prone to that disease. But the addition of too much iron could put men (who usually have enough) at risk for iron overload. The margin of safety for iron, too, is not so generous, and the upper limit has to be remembered.

margin of safety: as used when speaking of food additives, a zone between the concentration normally used and that at which a hazard exists. For common table salt, for example, the margin of safety is ⅕ (five times the concentration normally used would be hazardous).

8   A. M. Schmidt, Food and drug law: A 200-year perspective, *Nutrition Today* 10, no. 4 (1975): 29–32.

9   J. M. Coon, Natural food toxicants: A perspective, in *Nutrition Reviews' Present Knowledge*, 1976, pp. 528–546.

10   Strong, 1976.

All the additives just named are in foods for a reason. They offer benefits, in comparison with which the risks are deemed either small enough to ignore or worth taking. When the benefit to be gained from an additive is small, as in the case of color additives that only enhance the appearance of foods but do not improve their health value or safety, then the risks may be deemed not worth taking. Only 31 of a possible 200 color additives are now approved for use by FDA.

It is also the manufacturers' responsibility not to use more of an additive than they have to, to get the needed effect. The case of nitrites, where higher dose levels could conceivably be associated with a risk, is an obvious example. Additives should also *not* be used:

- To disguise faulty or inferior products.
- To deceive the consumer.
- Where they significantly destroy nutrients.
- Where their effects can be achieved by economical, sound manufacturing processes.[11]

Additives in Perspective

All that has been said so far has been reassuring. The use of additives in the food supply seems to be justified, in many cases, by the benefits we gain from them; the risks associated with their use are small. All intentional additives are, and will doubtless continue to be, closely regulated and monitored. Furthermore, in many cases, combinations of intentional additives are no more harmful than these additives used singly, and may even be beneficial. Giving further reassurance, the FAO/WHO Expert Committee on Food Additives has concluded that "an increase in the number of food additives on a permitted list does not imply an over-all increase in the [total amount of] additives used; the different additives are largely used as alternatives...there is *less* likelihood of long exposure, or of high or cumulative dose levels being attained if a wide range of substances is available for use."[12]

Finally, it should be noted that the safety of food additives is not first, or even third, on FDA's list of priority concerns; it is sixth. In order of concern, hazards within the FDA's areas of responsibility are:

- Food-borne infection, which is increasing because of large-scale operations and multiple transfers involving handling.
- Nutrition, which requires close attention as more and more artificially constituted foods appear on the market.
- Environmental contaminants, which are increasing yearly in number and concentration and whose consequences are difficult to foresee and forestall.

11 The use of chemicals in food production, processing, storage and distribution, *Nutrition Reviews* 31 (1973): 191–198.

12 Coon, 1976; emphasis added.

● Naturally occurring toxicants in foods, which occur randomly in arbitrary levels and constitute a hazard whenever people turn to consuming single foods either by choice (fad diets) or by necessity (famine).

● Pesticide residues.

● Intentional food additives, listed last "because so much is known about them, and all are now, and surely will continue to be, well regulated."[13]

The top item on this list is food poisoning, a real and frequent hazard to people who consume food that has been contaminated by toxic microorganisms during processing, packaging, transport, storage, or preparation in the home.

Deaths from food-borne infection can occur whenever batches of contaminated foods escape detection and are distributed. Close monitoring of processing, preparation, and distribution of food is extraordinarily effective, but individual consumers must be vigilant and knowledgeable in order to protect themselves against occasional hazards. Batch numbering makes it possible to recall all food items from a contaminated batch through public announcements on TV and radio. In the kitchen, the consumer must obey the rules of proper preparation and storage of foods to avoid the dangers of food poisoning (see note at end of Highlight).

Second on the above list is nutrition, the subject to which this entire book is addressed; third is contamination, the subject of the next Highlight. Fourth is naturally occurring toxicants in foods, a much more serious and real hazard than most consumers realize. This deserves a paragraph of attention.

Many commonly used plants and plant products contain naturally occurring toxicants. Mushrooms were mentioned earlier as a familiar example; but did you know a number of common foods have been observed to cause toxic effects?

● Cabbage, mustard, and other plants contain goitrogens, which can enlarge the thyroid gland.

● Potatoes contain solanine, a powerful inhibitor of nerve impulses; the margin of safety, assuming ordinary consumption of potatoes, is 1/10.

● Spinach and rhubarb contain oxalates, tolerable as usually consumed; but one normal serving of rhubarb contains ⅕ the toxic dose for humans.[14]

● Honey can be a host to the botulinum organism and can accumulate enough toxin to kill an infant.[15]

There are 700 other examples of plants that—as used—have caused serious illnesses or deaths in the Western hemisphere.[16] At the same time, there has been no case of a death or illness caused by an additive as used at legally

13   Schmidt, 1975.

14   Middlekauf, 1974.

15   I. B. Vyhmeister, What about honey? *Life and Health*, August 1980, pp. 5–7; R. W. Miller, Honey: Making sure it's pure, *FDA Consumer* 13 (September 1979): 12–13.

16   A. Brynjolfsson, Food irradiation and nutrition, *Professional Nutritionist*, Fall 1979, pp. 7–10.

permitted levels in food.[17] A well known environmental scientist has said, "One can predict that if the standards used to test manmade chemicals were applied to 'natural' foods, fully half of the human food supply would have to be banned."[18]

The fifth item on the list of FDA's hazards is pesticide residues, another issue touched on in the next Highlight, and sometimes a serious problem. In view of all this, the subject of this Highlight, FDA's sixth problem, would seem to have been given enough space here.

In summary, then, the ideas presented have been:

● All foods are composed of chemicals, even if they have no additives in them.

● Additives that might be toxic do not constitute a hazard at the concentrations used.

● Additives are allowed in foods only because they confer a benefit in comparison to which the risk, if any, is insignificant.

● The presence of several additives in foods is not more hazardous than the presence of any one of them.

● If rank-ordered among the problems related to the food supply, the risk from additives falls last below a number of more significant factors.

People who are concerned about the levels of various additives and pollutants in the food supply would be well advised to eat as wide a variety of foods as possible so as to dilute the amount of any one substance. "The wider the variety of food intake, the greater the number of different chemical substances consumed, and the less is the chance that any one chemical will reach a hazardous level in the diet."[19]

NOTE: The section on "Additives" in Appendix J offers many additional readings. *The Instructor's Manual* includes a supplementary lecture, "Foods in the Home," which explains how to prevent food poisoning.

17   M. W. Pariza, Food safety from the eye of a hurricane, *Professional Nutritionist*, Fall 1979, pp. 11–14.

18   R. Dubos, The intellectual basis of nutrition science and practice, paper presented at the NIH conference on the Biomedical and Behavioral Basis of Clinical Nutrition, June 19, 1978, in Bethesda, Maryland, and reprinted in *Nutrition Today*, July/August 1979, pp. 31–34.

19   Coon, 1976.

CHAPTER 11
The Trace Minerals

CONTENTS

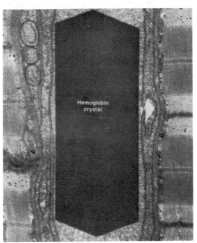

The red pigment of the blood cells is the protein hemoglobin, which contains iron. Hemoglobin is normally dispersed in the cell fluid, but here, due to an accident in preparation, the hemoglobin has crystallized, showing how abundant it is in the red blood cell. The cell is flanked by the walls of a capillary.

"Although erythrocytes occupy less than fifty percent of the volume of the blood fluid, they can absorb seventy-five times more oxygen than can possibly be dissolved in the plasma itself."

"[Hemoglobin] must be a tricky substance," said Mr. Tompkins thoughtfully.

GEORGE GAMOW and
MARTYNAS YCAS,
Mr. Tompkins inside Himself

If you could remove all of the trace minerals from your body, you would have only a bit of dust, hardly enough to fill a teaspoon. You would also die instantly. Although present in tiny quantities, each of the trace minerals performs some vital role for which no substitute will do. A deficiency of any of them may be fatal, and an excess of many is equally deadly. Remarkably, the way you eat and the way your body handles these minerals enables you to maintain a supply that is just sufficient for health and below the toxic level.

Laboratory techniques developed in the past few decades have enabled scientists to detect the minute quantities of trace minerals in living cells for the first time. Study of the "new" trace elements, using animals, is one of the most active areas of research in nutrition today. An obstacle to determining the precise role of a trace element lies in the nearly impossible task of providing an experimental diet devoid of that element. Even the dust in the air or the residue left on laboratory equipment by the rinsing water may contaminate the feed enough to prevent a deficiency. Thus research in this area is limited to the study of small laboratory animals, which can be fed highly refined, purified diets in an atmosphere free of all contamination.

The best-known trace elements—iron, iodine, and zinc—have been so thoroughly studied that we can describe many of their roles with certainty. Government authorities have established recommended daily intakes for these three. For six others, the Committee on RDA published tentative ranges for safe and adequate daily intakes for the first time in 1980. Five others are known to be essential nutrients, but the amounts needed are so tiny that they have not yet been measured. Many others are presently under study to determine whether they too perform indispensable roles in the body.

Whole books have been published just on the trace minerals. In selecting the information to present in this chapter we have chosen to give most attention to those that are likely to have the greatest impact on your health. Iron, for example, is often deficient in the diets of people the world over, and an iron deficiency profoundly hurts the quality of life. Iodine is easy to obtain in adequate amounts, but simple ignorance can precipitate a deficiency, with tragic and irreversible consequences. Until recently, zinc deficiencies were unheard of, but now we know they are present in many of the world's people. New knowledge of equal importance is coming to light about many of the other trace elements. An acquaintance with the few facts presented in this chapter should enable you to select a diet composed of protective foods that will ensure adequacy for all the essential nutrients.

Protective foods: see Chapter 1.

Iron

Iron is a problem nutrient for millions of people. If you want to plan and consume a diet adequate in iron, you must be well informed.

Iron in the Body

Iron is found in every cell, not only of the human body but of all living things, both plant and animal. It occurs in many vital proteins, including those involved in cell respiration and DNA synthesis, and is part of many major enzymes.

Most of the iron in the body is a component of the proteins hemoglobin and myoglobin. Both these proteins carry oxygen and release it. Hemoglobin is the oxygen carrier in the red blood cells, and myoglobin is the oxygen carrier in the muscle cells. Myoglobin has a greater holding capacity for oxygen and so serves as a reservoir; its presence in the muscle cells seems to draw oxygen into them. The muscle cells use this oxygen as the receiver for used-up carbon and hydrogen atoms flowing down the glucose-to-energy pathway. These atoms combine to make carbon dioxide and water, the final waste products of metabolism. Thus oxygen keeps the energy-yielding pathway open so that the muscles can remain active. As the

hemoglobin: the oxygen-carrying protein of the red blood cells.

hemo = blood

globin = globular protein

myoglobin: the oxygen-carrying protein of the muscle cells.

myo = muscle

muscles use up and excrete their oxygen (combined with carbons and hydrogens), the red blood cells shuttle between muscles and lungs to maintain fresh supplies.

The average red blood cell lives about four months. When it has aged and is no longer useful, it is removed from the blood by the spleen and liver cells, which take it apart and prepare many of the degradation products for excretion. The liver saves its iron, however, and attaches it to a protein carrier, which returns it to the bone marrow. The bone marrow, in turn, constantly produces new red blood cells. Thus, although red blood cells are born, live, and die within a four-month cycle, the iron in the body is recycled through each new generation. Only tiny amounts of iron are lost, principally in urine, sweat, shed skin, and (if bleeding occurs), in blood.

About 80 percent of the iron in the body is in the blood, so iron losses are greatest whenever blood is lost. For this reason, "women need more iron," as a well-known television commercial proclaims. Menstruation incurs losses that make a woman's iron needs nearly twice as great as a man's, but anyone who loses blood loses iron.

To help obtain iron, the body provides special proteins to absorb it from food and carry it to the liver, bone marrow, and other blood-manufacturing sites. Iron absorbed through the intestinal cells from food is captured by a blood protein, transferrin, that carries it to tissues throughout the body. Each tissue takes up the amount of iron that it needs. The bone marrow and liver take large quantities, other tissues take less. In a pregnant woman, the placenta is avid for iron, delivering large quantities to the fetus even if this means depriving the mother's tissues of iron. Should there be a surplus, special storage proteins in the bone marrow and other organs store it.

Iron clearly is the body's gold, a precious mineral to be hoarded and closely guarded. The number of special provisions for its handling show how vital it is. At the receiving end, in the intestines, another provision shows this even more clearly. Normally only about 10 percent of dietary iron is absorbed. But if the body's supply is diminished or if the need increases for any reason, absorption increases. More transferrin (the carrier that picks up iron from the intestines) is produced so that more than the usual amount of iron can be absorbed. Figure 11–1 shows how iron is absorbed and Figure 11–2 shows its routes in the body.

If absorption cannot compensate for a reduced supply and stores are used up, the red cells become depleted. Then anemia sets in. The most common tests for iron deficiency are measures of the number and size of the red blood cells and of their hemoglobin contents. But before these levels fall, at the very beginning of an iron deficiency, the transferrin concentration *rises*. A sensitive test that will detect a developing iron deficiency before it is full-blown measures the amount of transferrin in the blood and the amount of iron it is carrying.

For women only: you are often told that you need more iron, yet you may often have had your blood cell count or hemoglobin level pronounced normal. Does this mean that you don't need more iron? Not necessarily.

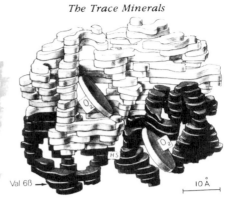

Val 6β ⟶   10 Å

Model of hemoglobin. The hundred-odd stacked planes represent the contours of the coiled protein chains. The flat discs represent hemes, to which oxygen binds.

Source: Courtesy of Dr. M. F. Perutz.

transferrin (trans-FURR-in): the body's iron-carrying protein.

Iron can also lodge in the mucosal cells and end up being excreted from the body. See *mucosal block*, a few pages further on.

The storage proteins are **ferritin** (FAIR-i-tin) and **hemosiderin** (heem-oh-SID-er-in).

Technically, this method is known as measuring the **total iron-binding capacity (TIBC)** and the **transferrin saturation**.

FIGURE 11–1 **Iron absorption**. The figure shows how iron absorption responds to the body's need. TH11-1

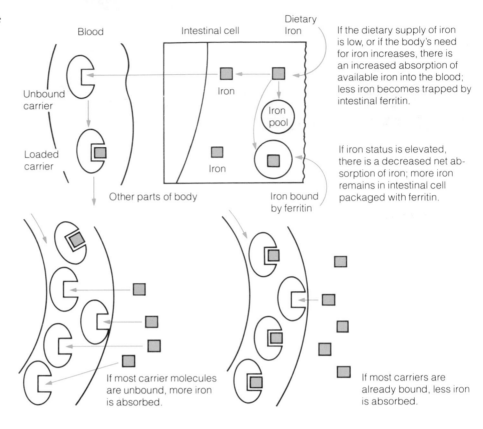

The difference between you and the men you know is a difference in your body stores of iron, which doesn't show up in these tests. Most men eat more food than women do, because they are bigger, and so their iron intakes are higher. Besides, women menstruate, and so their iron losses are greater. These two factors—lower intakes and higher losses—may put you much closer to the borderline of deficiency. Even though you may never have been diagnosed as iron-deficient, you are likely to be deficiency-prone. Should you lose blood for any reason (even by giving a blood donation) or become pregnant (so that your blood volume would need to increase), you would need to pay special attention to your diet in an effort to maintain your iron stores. The information about iron in foods, which appears later in this chapter, is especially important to you.

Caution

Iron-Deficiency Anemia

If iron stores are exhausted, the body cannot make enough hemoglobin to fill its new red blood cells. Without enough hemoglobin, the cells are small. Since hemoglobin is the bright red pigment of the blood, the skin of

FIGURE 11-2 **Iron routes in the body.**
TH11-2

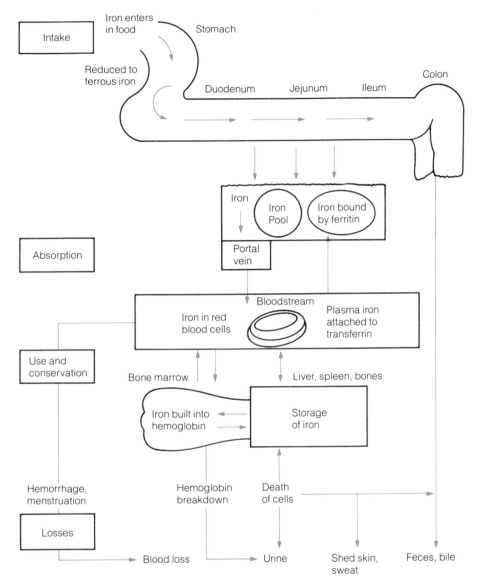

a fair person who is anemic may become noticeably pale. A sample of iron-deficient blood examined under the microscope shows smaller cells that are a lighter red than normal (Figure 11-3). The undersized cells can't carry enough oxygen from the lungs to the tissues, so energy release in the cells is hindered. Every cell of the body feels this effect; the result is fatigue, weakness, headaches, and apathy.

Long before the mass of the red blood cells is affected, however, a developing iron deficiency may affect other body tissues, including the brain. As researchers have become better acquainted with iron, they have learned that it plays roles in the brain not earlier appreciated. For example, iron works with an enzyme that helps to make neurotransmitters, the substances that carry messages from one nerve cell to another. Children

In a dark-skinned person, this symptom can be observed by looking in the corner of the eye. The eye lining, normally pink, will be very pale, even white.

Iron-deficiency anemia is a **micro-cytic** (my-cro-SIT-ic) **hypochromic** (high-po-KROME-ic) **anemia**.

micro = small

cytic = cells

hypo = too little

chrom = color

FIGURE 11–3 **Normal and anemic cells.**

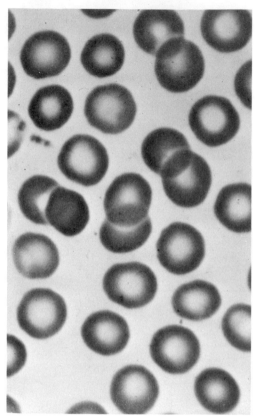

Normal blood cells.

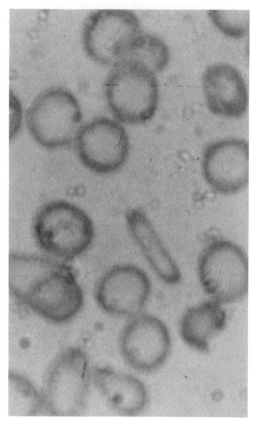

Blood cells in iron-deficiency anemia.

deprived of iron show some psychological disturbances, such as hyperactivity, decreased attentiveness, and even reduced IQ (see note at end of chapter). These symptoms are among the first to appear when the body's iron level begins to fall and among the first to disappear when iron intake is increased again.[1]

A curious symptom seen in some iron-deficient subjects is an appetite for ice, clay, paste, and other nonnutritious substances. Such people have been known to eat as many as eight trays of ice in a day, for example. This behavior has been observed for years, especially in women and children of low-income groups who are deficient in either iron or zinc, and has been given the name *pica*. Pica clears up dramatically within days after iron is given, long before the red blood cells respond.

Muscle tissue, too, is sensitive to depletion of iron stores. By the time the stores are exhausted, work capacity begins to be profoundly affected. One study has shown this especially clearly. As women's hemoglobin levels fell from normal to half of normal, their work capacity declined in proportion. At the lowest level they were unable to do much work at all (Figure 11–4).

pica (PIE-ka): a craving for nonfood substances. Also known as **geophagia** (gee-oh-FAY-gee-uh) when referring to clay-eating.

picus = woodpecker or magpie

geo = earth

phagein = to eat

1   R. L. Leibel, Behavioral and biochemical correlates of iron deficiency: A review, *Journal of the American Dietetic Association* 71 (1977): 399–404; E. Pollitt and R. L. Leibel, Iron deficiency and behavior, *Journal of Pediatrics* 88 (1976): 372–381.

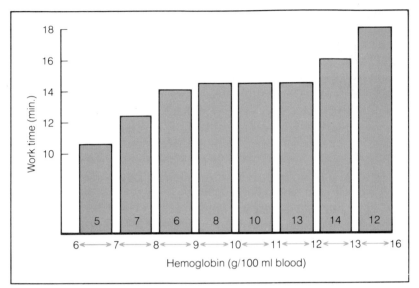

FIGURE 11-4 **Maximum treadmill work time in women with different hemoglobin levels.** The numbers within the bars show how many women were tested at each level. The chart shows that the lower a woman's hemoglobin level is, the less muscular work she can perform.

Source: Adapted from G. W. Gardner and coauthors, Physical work capacity and metabolic stress in subjects with iron deficiency anemia, *American Journal of Clinical Nutrition* 30 (1977): 910–917. Courtesy of the authors and publisher.

Many of the symptoms described here are easily mistaken for "mental" symptoms. A restless child who fails to pay attention in class might be thought contrary. An apathetic homemaker who has let her housework pile up might be thought lazy. But the possibility is real that both these persons' problems are nutritional.

No responsible nutritionist would ever claim that all mental problems are caused by nutrient deficiencies. But poor nutrition is always a possible cause or contributor to problems like these. When you are seeking the solution to a behavioral problem it makes sense to check the adequacy of the diet and to have a routine physical examination before undertaking more expensive and involved diagnostic and treatment options.

Caution

It is conventional to measure the body's iron status by measuring the amount of hemoglobin (in grams per 100 milliliters of blood). The normal level is considered 14 to 15 grams per 100 milliliters for adult men, 13 to 14 for women. Yet many people who have values lower than this have no obvious symptoms. U.S. blacks have average values about half a gram lower than these; it is not known whether this is a genetically determined characteristic or is due to insufficient iron intakes. Some women have no symptoms of anemia—at least as measured by the performance of mental tasks—at levels as low as 10 or even 8 grams.[2] Doubtless people vary; one man may feel miserable with a hemoglobin level of 12 grams; another may feel no effects at a drastically low level of, say, 6 grams: "Who, me? Anemic?"[3] Still,

2 P. C. Elwood and D. Hughes, Clinical trial of iron therapy on psychomotor function in anaemic women, *British Medical Journal* 3 (1970): 254–255.

3 W. H. Crosby, Current concepts in nutrition: Who needs iron? *New England Journal of Medicine* 297 (1977): 543–545.

Norms for children:

Ages 2–5:   11 g/100 ml.
Ages 6–12:   11.5 g/100 ml.

Note that hemoglobin is measured in grams per 100 milliliters, but we often just use the number alone in speaking of it: "Hemoglobin, 14."

secondary nutrient deficiency: one caused indirectly—not by inadequate intake but by the deficiency of another nutrient, interference with absorption, disease, or other causes.

such symptoms as fatigue, weakness, and the like are often seen at levels not much below the standards.

When hemoglobin begins to fall, it is a sign that a long period of depletion of body stores has already occurred. In view of this fact and in light of the behavioral effects of mild iron deficiency in children, it seems reasonable to try to achieve and maintain "normal" hemoglobin levels for the general population: 14 to 15 for men, 13 to 14 for women. Values much below these represent a real hazard to health and to the quality of life.

A low hemoglobin level may represent a dietary iron deficiency, and if it does, the doctor may prescribe iron supplements. But the cause of an iron deficiency may be something else. For example, a vitamin B_6 deficiency can indirectly cause anemia, because vitamin B_6 is required to make the iron-containing portion of the hemoglobin molecule. A vitamin E deficiency can cause anemia by making the red blood cell membranes so fragile that the cells lose their hemoglobin. A folacin deficiency can cause it, because this vitamin is used in making new red blood cells to replace the old ones as they die. A vitamin B_{12} deficiency can cause it, because folacin can't work without B_{12}. A vitamin C deficiency can cause it by reducing the absorption of iron. Vitamin A, too, is involved in the making of red blood cells, and some people's low hemoglobin levels can be corrected only by administering vitamin A.[4] Then there's the mineral copper (see later in this chapter).

Feeling fatigued, weak, and apathetic is a sign that something is wrong but does not indicate that you should take iron supplements. It indicates that (you guessed it!) you should consult your doctor. The doctor herself must use all her knowledge to diagnose correctly the primary cause of a secondary anemia; you don't have a chance at making this kind of diagnosis. In fact, taking iron supplements may be the worst possible thing you could do, because they may mask a serious medical condition, such as hidden bleeding from cancer or an ulcer. Once again —the caution deserves repeating—don't self-diagnose.

However, the role of all these nutrients in making and maintaining red blood cells dictates a preventive measure—eat right! A study of over 200 older adults in Boston provides evidence to support this recommendation. These people all had moderately low hemoglobin levels (below 13) to begin with. Two-thirds were given iron-fortified foods; the other third received the same foods without added iron. At the end of the study, *all* had higher hemoglobin levels. Food made the difference with or without added iron.[5]

Caution

4   R. E. Hodges and coauthors, Hematopoietic studies in vitamin A deficiency, *American Journal of Clinical Nutrition* 31 (1978): 876–885.

5   S. N. Gershoff, O. A. Brusis, H. V. Nino, and A. M. Huber, Studies of the elderly in Boston: I. The effects of iron fortification on moderately anemic people, *American Journal of Clinical Nutrition* 30 (1977): 226–234.

By these criteria, iron-deficiency anemia is a major health problem in both the United States and Canada and even more so in the rest of the world. It is especially common in older infants, children, women of childbearing age, and people in low-income and minority groups. The incidence of iron-deficiency anemia in these groups ranges from 10 to over 50 percent. It tends to cluster with indicators of low socioeconomic status, such as family instability, little money spent on food, little attention given to children.[6] But no segment of society is free of iron-deficiency anemia, and these groups are not the only ones affected. For example, 1 out of every 20 Canadian men is at moderate risk (hemoglobin 12 to 14), and 1 out of every 100 is at high risk (hemoglobin below 12).[7] Moreover, some subjects with normal hemoglobins are iron deficient by more sensitive tests.

Iron Overload

Iron toxicity is rare but not unknown. The body protects itself against absorbing too much iron by setting up a "block" in the intestinal cells. Proteins trap extra absorbed iron and hold it until it can be shed from the body when the mucosal cells are shed. The average life of an intestinal cell is only three days; so this method promptly removes excess iron from the system. Still, the mucosal block can be overwhelmed, and iron overload is the result.

Two kinds of iron overload are known. One is caused by a hereditary defect, the other by ingesting too much iron. Tissue damage, especially to the liver, occurs in both, and infections are likely because bacteria thrive in iron-rich blood. Tissue damage is most severe in those who also drink large quantities of alcohol, because alcohol not only damages the liver but also increases the absorption of ferric iron. Certain wines (especially red wines) contain substantial amounts of iron; so the overconsumption of wine is particularly risky. Detection of iron overload is best accomplished by measuring the serum ferritin level, which reflects the body's total iron stores.

Iron overload is more common in men than in women. An argument against the fortification of foods with iron to protect women is that it might put more men at risk of overload. Indeed, there is some evidence from Sweden, where foods are generously fortified with iron, that this measure has increased the incidence of iron overload in men. It is too bad that a measure meant to promote the health of one sex might put the other at risk.

The ingestion of massive amounts of iron can cause sudden death. The second most common cause (after aspirin) of accidental poisoning in small children is ingestion of iron supplements or vitamins with iron. As few as 6 to 12 tablets have caused death in a child.[8] A child suspected of iron

mucosal block to iron absorption: the provision of binding proteins (ferritin and a transferrin-like protein) in the mucosal cells to capture and hold unneeded iron to be shed with the cells.

iron overload: toxicity from iron overdose.

hemochromatosis (heem-oh-crome-a-TOCE-iss): iron overload characterized by deposits of iron-containing pigment in many tissues, with tissue damage. Hemochromatosis is a hereditary defect in iron metabolism.

hemosiderosis (heem-oh-sid-er-OH-sis): iron overload characterized by excessive iron deposits in hemosiderin, the normal iron-storage protein.

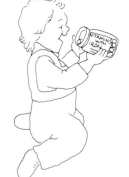

6   D. M. Czajka-Narins, T. B. Haddy, and D. J. Kallen, Nutrition and social correlates in iron deficiency anemia, *American Journal of Clinical Nutrition* 31 (1978): 955–960.

7   Z. I. Sabry, J. A. Campbell, M. E. Campbell, and A. L. Forbes, Nutrition Canada, *Nutrition Today*, January/February 1974, pp. 5–13.

8   Committee on Safety, Toxicity, and Misuse of Vitamins and Trace Minerals, National Nutrition Consortium, *Vitamin-Mineral Safety, Toxicity, and Misuse* (Chicago: American Dietetic Association, 1978).

poisoning should be rushed to the hospital to have his stomach pumped; 30 minutes may make a crucial difference.

Iron in Foods

The usual Western mixed diet provides only about 5 to 6 milligrams of iron in every 1,000 kcalories. The recommended daily intake for an adult man is 10 milligrams, and most men require more than 2,000 kcalories; so a man can easily meet his iron needs without special effort. The recommendation for a woman, however, is 14 to 18 milligrams per day. Because women typically consume fewer than 2,000 kcalories per day, they understandably have trouble achieving this intake. A woman who wants to meet her iron needs from foods must increase the iron-to-kcalorie ratio of her diet so that she will receive about double the average amount of iron—at least 10 milligrams per 1,000 kcalories. This means she must emphasize the most iron-rich foods in every food group.

Several factors influence the absorption of iron significantly enough so that they have to be considered by anyone who wants to know how much iron a person really gets from a meal. A system of calculating the iron absorbed from a meal has been worked out by Dr. E. R. Monsen and her coworkers; an example of the Monsen system is provided in this chapter's Self-Study (in Appendix Q).

The average amount of iron absorbed is 10 percent, but up to 40 percent of the iron in meat, fish, poultry, and soybeans may be absorbed. Less than 10 percent of the iron in eggs, whole grains, nuts, and dried beans is absorbed. At the bottom of the list is spinach; only 2 percent of its iron is absorbed. The iron from iron supplements, too, is absorbed at a rate of only about 2 percent. Vitamin C eaten with any iron source doubles or triples the amount of iron absorbed (except heme iron). The listing of common foods in Table 11–1 does not take this variability into account, but even so, meat, fish, and poultry are at the top. Obviously, then, a woman who includes some meat in everyday meal planning will get a head start toward meeting her iron needs, especially if she makes periodic use of liver and other organ meats.

Foods in the milk group are notoriously poor iron sources, as poor in iron as they are rich in calcium. Although these foods are an indispensable part of the diet, they should not be overemphasized. In considering the grain foods, remember that iron is one of the enrichment nutrients. Whole-grain or enriched breads and cereals—not refined, unenriched pastry products—are the best choices, and the more of them you eat, the more iron you receive. Finally, among other plant foods, the legume family, the dark greens, and dried fruits are the most iron rich. A set of guidelines, then, for planning an iron-rich diet:

● *Milk and cheese.* Don't overdo foods from the milk group (but don't omit them either; you need them for calcium). Drink skim milk to free kcalories to be invested in iron-rich foods.
● *Meat.* Use liver and other organ meats frequently, perhaps every week or two. Meat, fish, and poultry are excellent iron sources.

Recommended intakes of iron:

Men:	10 mg/day.
Women (Canada):	14 mg/day.
Women (U.S.):	18 mg/day.

How recommended daily intake for iron is calculated (for example, for an adolescent girl):

Losses from urine and shed skin:	0.5 to 1.0 mg
Losses through menstruation (about 15 mg total averaged over 30 days):	0.5 mg
Net for growth:	0.5 mg
Average daily need (total):	1.5 to 2.0 mg

Only 10 percent of ingested iron is absorbed, so this girl must ingest 15 to 20 mg per day.

About 40 percent of the iron in meat, fish, and poultry is bound into molecules of **heme** (HEEM), the iron-holding part of the hemoglobin and myoglobin proteins (Appendix C shows heme's structure). Heme iron is much more absorbable (23 percent) than nonheme iron. Meat, fish, and poultry also contain a factor ("MFP factor") other than heme that promotes the absorption of iron, even of the iron from other foods eaten at the same time as the meat. The way in which vitamin C assists in iron absorption is fully described in Chapter 8.

Overconsumption of milk is a common cause of iron deficiency in children; the resulting anemia is known as **milk anemia**.

TABLE 11–1 **Iron—Average Amounts in Groups of Foods** TH11-3

	Iron (mg)
Milk and Milk Products	
1 c milk or 1 oz cheese	-0-
Meat and Legumes	
3 oz fish steaks, salmon, or tuna	1.0
3 oz shrimp or sardines	2.5
3 oz liver,[a] raw clams, or oysters	6.0
3 oz other meat or poultry	2.0
1 egg	1.0
¾ c legumes, cooked[b]	3.0
4 oz soybean curd (tofu)	2.5
Fruits and Vegetables	
1 portion or piece fruit[c]	0.5
1 portion or piece dried fruit[b,d]	1.5
1 c iron-rich vegetables[e]	2.0
½ c other vegetables[b]	0.5
Grains	
1 slice bread or 1 portion any enriched or whole-grain product, including cakes and cookies[b]	0.5
1 portion fortified cereal[b]	(read label)
1 piece pie[f] or pizza pie	1.0
Other	
1 tbsp fat or oil	-0-
1 tbsp sugar or 1 candy	-0-
1 portion nuts or seeds (1 fat exchange)[b,g]	0.5
1 oz any chocolate candy	0.5
1 tbsp molasses (blackstrap only)[b]	3.0
1 c soup[b,h]	1.0
1 tbsp brewer's yeast	1.5
1 tbsp wheat germ	0.5
3½ oz table wine	0.5

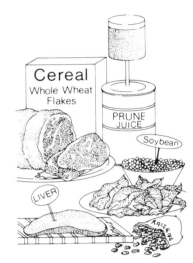

Foods rich in iron.

According to the values in the table, a person following the modified four food group plan would obtain:

2 c milk	-0- mg
2 (3-oz) portions meat, fish, or poultry	4.0
2 (¾ c) portions legumes	6.0
1 c iron-rich vegetable	2.0
½ c other vegetable and 2 portions fruit	1.5
4 portions enriched or whole grains	2.0
Total (compare the U.S. RDA of 18 mg)	15.5 mg

For a guarantee of adequacy, any additional foods selected should also be foundation foods such as soups, enriched or whole grains, and additional iron-rich fruits and vegetables. To boost iron intake, eat liver, raw clams, or oysters once every week or two, and use a tablespoon of brewer's yeast in cooking daily.

This table was made by consulting Appendix H, averaging the iron amounts in standard portions of the commonly used foods in each category, and rounding off each average to the nearest 0.5 mg. (Thus, 0 doesn't mean no iron, but rather, less than 0.3 mg.) Values agree approximately with the USDA table, Nutrients furnished by servings of foods, *Essentials of an Adequate Diet*, Bulletin no. 160, 1956. For more details, consult Appendix H.

[a] Liver or other organ meat such as heart.

[b] Absorption is poor compared with that of iron in meat. Eat meat and/or a vitamin C-rich food at the same meal.

[c] The highest value is 1.0 mg for ⅔ c strawberries or blueberries or a 4 by 4 inch wedge watermelon.

[d] ¼ c dried apricots, dates, dried peaches, prunes, or raisins.

[e] Dark green leafy vegetables, any variety including broccoli; asparagus; fresh lima beans; mung bean sprouts, raw or cooked; blackeyed peas; brussels sprouts; corn; green peas; winter squash; tomato juice; mixed frozen vegetables.

[f] 0.5 mg from the crust, 0.5 mg for the fruit.

[g] 45 kcalories of nuts (1 fat exchange): the average of 10 varieties of nuts is 0.3 mg. 45 kcalories of pumpkin seeds or squash kernels have 0.9 mg.

[h] Values range from about 0.5 to 1.5 mg. Cream soups are the lowest; beans soups, the highest.

● *Meat substitutes.* Don't forget legumes. A cup of peas or beans can supply up to 5 milligrams of iron.

● *Breads and cereals.* Use only whole-grain, enriched, and fortified products.

● *Vegetables.* The dark-green leafy vegetables are rich in iron. Eat vitamin C–rich vegetables often to enhance absorption of the iron from foods eaten with them.

● *Fruits.* Dried fruits like raisins, apricots, peaches, and prunes are high in iron. Eat vitamin C–rich fruits often with iron-containing foods.

Table 11–2 shows iron in foods compared to their kcalorie amounts and reveals that, for the person with a limited kcalorie allowance, some foods are much better choices than others.

TABLE 11–2 **Iron—Average Amounts in Groups of Foods**

	Iron/kCalories (mg/1,000 kcal)		Iron/kCalories (mg/1,000 kcal)
Milk and Milk Products		*Grains*	
Milk	0.7	Bread	
Cheddar cheese	1.7	white (enriched)	8.6
		raisin	9.2
Meat and Legumes		whole wheat	12.3
Chicken, broiled	12.5	Cereal	
Chicken, fried	8.1	oatmeal	10.8
Clams, oysters	80.0	fortified wheat cereal, plain	10.9
Eggs	12.5	fortified wheat cereal, sweet	4.3
Frankfurter	4.7	Chocolate cake with icing	4.3
Garbanzo beans (chickpeas)	20.0	Granola bar	7.1
Ground beef, lean	16.2	Popcorn	8.0
Lima beans	22.7	Rice (white, enriched)	8.0
Liver (beef), fried	38.5		
Sirloin steak (with fat)	7.6	*Other*	
Tuna	9.4	Almonds	8.0
		Brewer's yeast	56.0
Fruits and Vegetables		Fat or oil	0.0
Apple	5.0	Peanut butter	3.2
Blueberries	16.7	Minestrone soup	9.5
Broccoli	30.3	Sugar	0.0
Carrots	16.7		
Oranges	7.7		
Orange juice	4.5		
Potatoes	7.6		
Raisins	12.1		
Spinach	100.0		
Strawberries	27.2		
Tomatoes	24.0		
Watermelon	19.1		

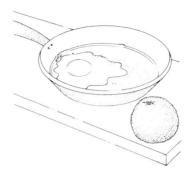

Knowledgeable cooking and menu planning can enhance the amount of iron delivered by your diet. The iron content of 100 grams of spaghetti sauce simmered in a glass dish is 3 milligrams, but it's 87 milligrams when the sauce is cooked in an iron skillet. Even in the short time it takes to scramble eggs, you can triple their iron content by cooking them in an iron pan. Admittedly, the absorption of this iron is poor, but every little bit helps. Therefore, an additional suggestion is:

● Cook with iron skillets whenever possible.

Even after taking all these precautions, a woman may not accumulate enough storage iron to prepare her for the increased demands of pregnancy and childbirth. In 1974 the Committee on RDA acknowledged for the first time that pregnant women might need supplemental iron. The Canadian Dietary Standard also includes this statement. However, since the iron from supplements is far less well absorbed than that from food, the doses have to be as high as 50 milligrams per day. Absorption of iron from supplements is improved when they are taken with meat or with vitamin C–rich foods or juices.

The use of fortified foods is another option. Some breakfast cereals boast that they contain 100 percent of the recommended daily intake of iron. These may indeed boost the day's iron intakes, even though absorption of their iron is poor. A number of proposals have been made for further fortification. Canada has considered adding iron to milk;[9] other ideas are to add it to coffee, to junk foods, even to salt. At present, 25 percent of all the iron consumed in the United States derives from fortified foods. A proposal to increase the iron level in enriched bread above that now prescribed by FDA regulations has been defeated. Ultimately, it is up to the consumer herself to see that she gets enough iron.

enrichment: the addition of iron, thiamin, riboflavin, and niacin to refined grain products to restore approximately their original contents.

fortification: the addition of nutrients to a food—but not necessarily the nutrients that were originally found there.

Zinc

Ten years ago, zinc was hardly known as a nutrient to the man on the street. In 1974, it appeared in the RDA tables for the first time, and today it is often added to vitamin-mineral supplements. Research on zinc has expanded to hundreds of articles.

Zinc in the Body

Zinc appears in every body tissue but is distributed unevenly. The adult human body contains 2 to 3 grams of zinc. The highest concentrations are in the eye, liver, kidney, muscle, skin, bones, and male reproductive organs. Zinc is tightly tied up in tissues such as the skin, hair, and bones and so is unavailable to the rest of the body except when tissue or bone breaks down. Zinc must therefore be provided relatively regularly in the diet.

9   D. Rosenfield, Nutritional optimization of new foods (commentary), *Journal of the American Dietetic Association* 72 (1978): 475–477.

cofactor: a mineral element that works with an enzyme, facilitating the enzyme's action.

The small molecule that assists in zinc absorption is known as the **zinc-binding ligand** (LYE-gand) **(ZBL)**.

The binding protein for zinc is a sulfur-rich protein known as **metallothionein** (meh-TAL-oh-THIGH-oh-neen).

metallo = containing a metal

thio = containing sulfur

ein = a protein

Zinc supports several physiological functions. Most importantly, there are now over 70 known enzymes which require zinc as a cofactor. Zinc occurs at the active site, maintains the structural integrity of the protein, and may also facilitate the enzyme's catalytic activity by lowering the amount of energy necessary to get it started.

Zinc works with proteins in every corner of the body. It is necessary for normal metabolism of protein, carbohydrate, fat, and alcohol. It is associated with the hormone insulin in the pancreas. It is involved in the synthesis of DNA and RNA, cell replication, immune reactions, the cells' production and disposal of carbon dioxide, utilization of vitamin A, taste perception, wound healing, the making of sperm, and the development of the fetus.

Absorption of zinc is known to occur in the upper intestine, but a complete description of this process has not yet been derived from research. Zinc is evidently pulled (by active transport) into cells even when its concentration is higher inside them than outside. Absorption is aided by a small molecule, whose exact nature is disputed.[10]

After zinc has entered a cell lining the intestine, it may become involved in the metabolic functions of the cell itself or pass through the far side of the cell into the portal blood. The absorbed zinc may also become trapped within the cell by a special binding protein similar to the one described earlier for iron.[11]

As for iron, a homeostatic mechanism seems to be at work to regulate the amount of zinc entering the body. Extra zinc (or iron) is held within the intestinal cell and only the amount needed is released into the bloodstream. The zinc status of the individual influences the percentage of zinc absorbed from the diet; if more is needed, more is absorbed. Cells are shed daily from the intestinal lining and are excreted in the feces; they carry the zinc they have retained out of the body with them. Figure 11–5 shows how zinc absorption is controlled.

Figure 11–6 shows the probable body pathways for zinc. Zinc circulating within the body is taken up by liver cells and is bound to a protein inside them (liver metallothionein). The amount bound depends on the amount of circulating zinc. Zinc circulates in the body until the concentration in and around liver cells reaches a certain threshold. Then any additional zinc is packaged with liver metallothionein.

While traveling in the bloodstream, zinc is transported by proteins. Plasma proteins such as albumin, transferrin, and others may bind significant amounts of zinc.[12] The significance of the involvement of either trans-

10   Researchers working to define this ligand have proposed that it may be a prostaglandin, citric acid, or picolinic acid. M. K. Song and N. F. Adham, Role of prostaglandin E_2 in zinc absorption in the rat, *American Journal of Physiology* 234 (1978): E99–E105; L. S. Hurley, B. Lonnerdal, and A. G. Stanislowski, Zinc citrate, human milk and acrodermatitis enteropathica, *Lancet* 1 (1979): 667–678; G. W. Evans and E. C. Johnson, Effect of iron, vitamin B_6 and picolinic acid on zinc absorption in the rat, *Journal of Nutrition* 111 (1981): 68–75.

11   R. J. Cousins, Regulation of zinc absorption: Role of intracellular ligands, *American Journal of Clinical Nutrition* 32 (1979): 339–345.

12   Cousins, 1979; G. W. Evans, Transferrin function in zinc absorption and transport, *Proceedings of the Society for Biology and Medicine* 151 (1976): 775–778.

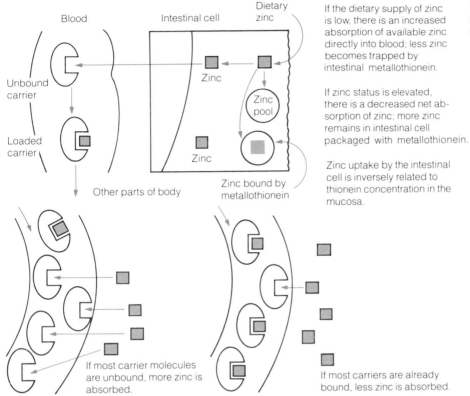

FIGURE 11-5 **Zinc absorption**. The figure shows how zinc absorption responds to the body's need. TH11-1

If the dietary supply of zinc is low, there is an increased absorption of available zinc directly into blood; less zinc becomes trapped by intestinal metallothionein.

If zinc status is elevated, there is a decreased net absorption of zinc; more zinc remains in intestinal cell packaged with metallothionein.

Zinc uptake by the intestinal cell is inversely related to thionein concentration in the mucosa.

Blood Intestinal cell Dietary zinc

Unbound carrier

Zinc

Zinc pool

Loaded carrier

Zinc

Other parts of body

Zinc bound by metallothionein

If most carrier molecules are unbound, more zinc is absorbed.

If most carriers are already bound, less zinc is absorbed.

ferrin or albumin with zinc transport is complex. Anything that leads to a decrease in plasma albumin—for example, pregnancy or malnutrition—would lower plasma zinc levels as well. Anything that binds transferrin might also hinder zinc absorption. In normal individuals, transferrin is usually less than 50 percent saturated with iron, but in cases of iron overload, it is more saturated. Iron excess thus leaves too few binding sites available, thereby causing an impairment of zinc absorption.

An interesting phenomenon in zinc nutriture is the cycling of zinc in the body. The intestine actually receives two doses of zinc with each meal—one from ingested foods and the other from the zinc–rich pancreatic secretions. Thus even zinc that has already entered the body is rescreened periodically by the intestine and can be refused entry or tied up in intestinal cells on any of its times around.

Excretion of zinc occurs primarily by way of the feces, which contain both unabsorbed zinc and zinc from the pancreatic juices. Some zinc is also lost in the urine. Alcohol abuse increases urinary losses of zinc. An increase in muscle catabolism, as in fasting, injury, or surgery, also incurs urinary losses of zinc. Free dietary amino acids such as histidine or cysteine can bind zinc, and thus cause losses. People who take supplements of amino acids to help their health may therefore actually be harming it by interfering with their zinc absorption.

Caution

FIGURE 11–6 **Zinc routes in the body.**

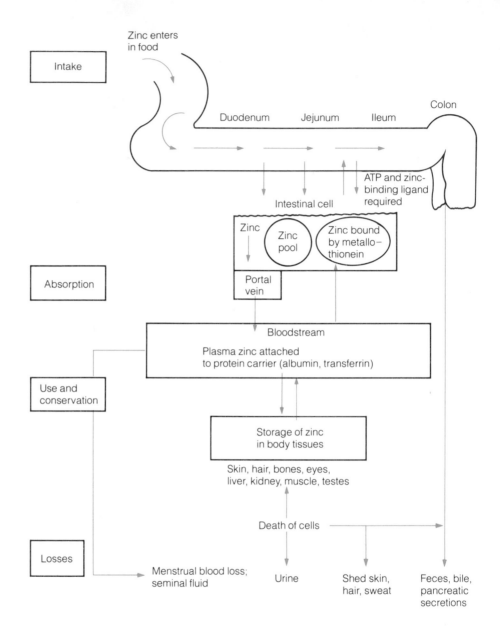

Other losses of zinc occur in sweat, hair, menstrual blood, seminal fluid, and human milk. Studies of all these losses added together have enabled researchers to estimate the human requirement for zinc.

Zinc Deficiency and Toxicity

A deficiency of zinc in humans was first reported in the 1960s from studies with growing children and adolescent males in Egypt, Iran, and Turkey. The native diets were typically low in animal protein and high in whole grains and beans; consequently they were high in fiber and phytates. The zinc deficiency was marked by dwarfism or severe growth retardation and

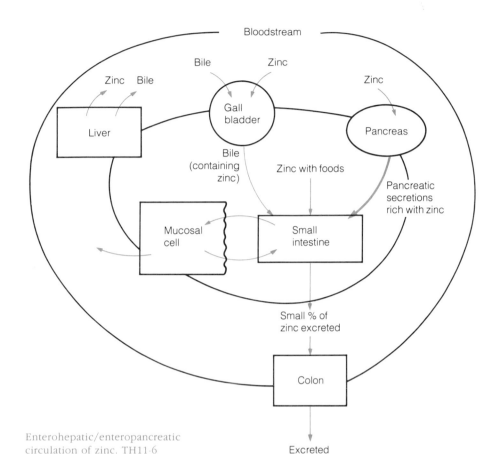

Enterohepatic/enteropancreatic
circulation of zinc. TH11-6

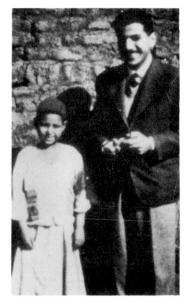

The Egyptian boy in this picture is seventeen years old but is only four feet tall, like a seven-year-old in the United States. His genitalia are like those of a six-year-old. The retardation is ascribed to zinc deficiency.

Source: Reproduced with permission of *Nutrition Today* magazine, P.O. Box 1829, Annapolis, Maryland, 21404, March 1968.

arrested sexual maturation—symptoms that were responsive to zinc supplementation. (A detailed list of symptoms of zinc deficiency is presented in Table 11–3.) Conditions other than diet which contribute to development of zinc deficiency include loss of blood due to parasitic infections, climates which increase sweat losses, and clay eating.

Since the reports of the 1960s, cases of zinc deficiency have been discovered closer to home, in U.S. schoolchildren.[13] A number of Denver children had low hair zinc levels, poor growth, poor appetite, and decreased taste sensitivity. The children were described as "picky eaters" and ate less than an ounce of meat per day. A recommendation from these observations might be that when poor growth is accompanied by poor appetite, the pediatrician should evaluate the child's zinc status.

Reports of the role of zinc in wound healing are controversial. It appears that in individuals with normal zinc status, zinc has no effect on wound healing. Healing appears to be delayed, however, in persons with zinc deficiency. Zinc is known to be required in collagen synthesis, and the skin is rich in zinc.

Clay eating (pica or geophagia) occurs among the poor in rural areas of the middle East, and has also been noted in the rural South in the United States. The clay acts to bind zinc (as well as iron) by attracting these positively charged ions, making them unabsorbable in the intestine.

13 K. M. Hambidge, C. Hambidge, M. Jacobs, and J. D. Baum, Low levels of zinc in hair, anorexia, poor growth, and hypogeusia in children, *Pediatric Research* 6 (1972): 868–874.

TABLE 11–3 **Zinc Deficiency**

DISEASE	AREA AFFECTED	MAIN EFFECTS
(No name)	Blood	Tendency to atherosclerosis; elevated ammonia levels; decreased alkaline phosphatase; decreased insulin concentration
	Bones	Growth retardation; abnormal collagen synthesis
	Cells (all)	Decreased DNA synthesis; impaired cell division and protein synthesis
	Digestive system	Lowered taste and smell acuity; weight loss; delayed glucose absorption
	Eyes	Abnormal adaptation to darkness
	Glandular system	Delayed onset of puberty; small gonads in males; decreased synthesis and release of testosterone; abnormal glucose tolerance; decreased synthesis of adrenocortical hormones
	Immune system	Altered skin test responses; reduced cell number in lymph tissue; thymus atrophy; decreased number of antibody-forming cells; altered white blood cell counts; increased susceptibility to infection
	Liver	Enlargement
	Nervous system	Anorexia (poor appetite); mental lethargy; irritability
	Reproductive system	Impaired reproductive function (rats); low sperm counts; fetal alcohol syndrome
	Skin	Generalized hair loss; lesions; rough, dry appearance; slow healing of wounds and burns
	Spleen	Enlargement
Acrodermatitis enteropathica (rare inherited disease)	Bones	Retarded growth
	Digestive system	Chronic diarrhea; malabsorption
	Eyes	Inflammation in the corners of the eyes (conjunctivitis); hypersensitivity to light (photophobia); scars on the cornea (corneal opacities)
	Glandular system	Small gonads in males
	Immune system	Frequent infections simultaneous with other diseases
	Nervous system	Emotional disorders; irritability; tremors; inability to coordinate muscular movements (cerebellar ataxia)
	Skin	Loss of hair (alopecia); dermatitis of extremities and of oral, anal, and genital areas, with pus

An intriguing example of the many nutrient-nutrient interactions in human nutrition is the case of zinc and vitamin A. Zinc is required for the synthesis of retinol-binding protein, RBP. RBP, in turn, is necessary for mobilization of vitamin A from the liver. A zinc deficiency may therefore cause an apparent vitamin A deficiency, because plasma levels of vitamin A will remain low even though there is plenty of vitamin A stored in the liver.

Zinc deficiency in humans appears to be related to abnormal rod function and impaired visual adaptation to darkness. Zinc is necessary for the reaction that produces the active form of vitamin A (retinal) necessary to form rhodopsin, the rods' visual pigment.

Zinc is a relatively nontoxic element. However, it can be toxic if consumed in large enough quantities. Accidental consumption of high levels of zinc may cause vomiting, diarrhea, fever, exhaustion, and a host of other symptoms (see Table 11–4).[14] Large doses can even be fatal.

Toxicity from ingestion of zinc could occur from misuse of supplements. Also, acidic foods or drinks which have been allowed to stand for long periods of time in galvanized containers may contain toxic levels of this trace mineral. Remember, too, that a large amount of one trace element may induce a deficiency of another. Such is the relationship between zinc and copper. Excess zinc intake may also interfere with the intestinal absorption of calcium, due to competition between the two elements for common intestinal binding sites.

galvanized: term referring to metal containers that have been treated with a zinc-containing coating to prevent rust.

By now, you can guess what populations might be at risk for developing inadequate zinc status. Primarily, they are people who are growing—infants, children, teenagers, and pregnant women. Pregnant teenagers are at particular risk, because they need zinc for their own ongoing growth as well as for the developing fetus. Persons on limited food intakes, such as those on weight control regimens, may also be at risk. A warning to those following very-low-kcalorie or starvation diets—they cause not only a low zinc intake but also a loss of zinc from body tissues being broken down as a source of energy. The elderly may also have limited food intakes due to socioeconomic factors. Hospital patients with decreased appetite or receiving improperly formulated tube feedings are also at risk. Certain drug therapies may also interfere with zinc absorption.

The diets of vegetarians, especially pregnant vegetarians, who consume large amounts of fiber, phytate, and dairy foods or low levels of protein

TABLE 11–4 **Zinc Toxicity**

AREA AFFECTED	MAIN EFFECTS
Blood	Anemia; reduced hemoglobin production
Bone	Growth depression
Digestive system	Diarrhea; vomiting; decreased calcium and copper absorption
Immune system	Fever; elevated white blood cell count
Kidney	Renal failure
Muscle	Muscular pain and incoordination
Nervous system	Nausea; exhaustion; dizziness; drowsiness
Reproductive system	Reproductive failure

14   M. A. Brown and coauthors, Food poisoning involving zinc contamination, *Archives of Environmental Health* 8 (1964): 657–660; Questions doctors ask, *Nutrition and the MD*, October 1978.

Recommended intake of zinc:

Adults (U.S.):	15 mg/day.
Men (Canada):	10 mg/day.
Women (Canada):	9 mg/day.

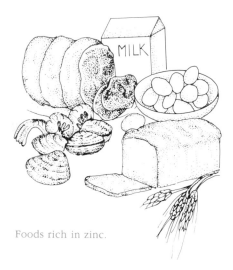

Foods rich in zinc.

Phytate or phytic acid (see Chapter 2) is a storage compound found in plant seeds. Phytic acid is concentrated in the husks of grains, legumes, and seeds, and is capable of binding zinc in an insoluble complex in the intestine. Phytate binds not only zinc but also other positive ions such as calcium, magnesium, copper, and iron.

need to be scrutinized for possible zinc deficiency. Populations dependent on food staples or cultural foods high in phytate and fiber content need to be evaluated as well for zinc status.

Zinc in Foods

The daily recommended intake of zinc is about 10 to 15 milligrams. This figure assumes that 40 percent of dietary zinc is available to the body, although, as we shall see later, this is not always the case. The RDA for all age groups are given inside the front cover. Requirements for infants and children are relatively high due to the role of zinc in normal growth and development.

Table 11–5 shows average zinc amounts in groups of foods. An average 1,500-kcalorie diet provides about 6.3 milligrams of zinc per day, or about 40 percent of the RDA.[15] Zinc is highest in foods of high protein content, such as shellfish (especially oysters), meats, and liver. As a rule of thumb, two ordinary servings a day of animal protein will provide most of the zinc a healthy person needs. Milk, eggs, and whole-grain products are good sources of zinc if large quantities are eaten. For the infant, breast milk is a good source of zinc, which is easier to absorb from human milk than from cow's milk. Vegetables, fresh or canned, vary in zinc content depending on the soil in which they are grown. The zinc content of cooking water varies from region to region as well.

Besides the zinc content of foods, many dietary factors affect the absorption of zinc. The refining of grains lowers their zinc content. Galvanized cooking pots, in earlier times, contributed zinc to foods, especially to acid foods, but with the increased use of stainless steel and plastic utensils to prepare and store food, this source of zinc is no longer significant.

Factors interfering with the availability of zinc for absorption include phytic acid, calcium, phosphorus, and fiber. Complexes with phytate become even more insoluble in the presence of calcium and phosphorus, as when people consume dairy foods. Calcium facilitates the binding of both zinc and copper to phytic acid. Zinc also forms insoluble complexes with some plant fibers. Therefore, a high-fiber diet may lead to a deficiency of zinc, especially if zinc is already in short supply.

Both phytic acid and fiber are prevalent in plant foods. As you might suspect, then, concern about the bioavailability of dietary zinc is increasing as more and more persons tend toward vegetarianism and higher fiber intakes. The plant foods highest in zinc, such as peanuts, cooked dried beans, and wheat germ, may not be able to nourish the body as effectively as animal foods because of their phytate and fiber content. Foods need to be selected carefully, not only for mineral content but also for mineral availability, so that vegetarian and high-fiber diets will supply the essential minerals in sufficient quantities to meet people's metabolic needs.

15   J. M. Holden, W. R. Wolf, and W. Mertz, Zinc and copper in self-selected diets, *Journal of the American Dietetic Association* 75 (1979): 23–28.

TABLE 11–5 **Zinc—Average Amounts in Groups of Foods** TH11-7

	Zinc (mg)
Milk and Milk Products	
1 c milk, 1 oz cheese, or 1 c cottage cheese[a]	1.0
1 c soy milk	0.5
Meat and Legumes	
3 oz fish or chicken	1.0
3 oz shrimp or clams	1.5
1 egg	0.5
3 oz crabmeat	3.0
3 oz oysters	8.0
3 oz meat (including beef and liver)	4.0
1½ frankfurters or 3 slices bologna (3 oz)	1.5
¾ c legumes, cooked [b]	2.0
Fruits and Vegetables	
1 portion or piece fruit[c]	-0-
1 c zinc-rich vegetable[d]	1.5
½ c other vegetable	0.5
Grains	
1 slice white (enriched) bread or refined cereal[e]	-0-
1 slice whole-grain bread or 1 portion whole-grain cereal[e,f]	0.5
1 piece cake or pie	0.5
Other	
1 tbsp fat or oil or 2 tbsp cream	-0-
1 tbsp sugar or 1 candy[g]	-0-
1 portion nuts or seeds (45 kcalories)[h]	0.5
1 c soup[i]	1.0
1 tbsp brewer's yeast	0.5

According to the values in the table, a person following the modified four food group plan would obtain:

2 c milk	2.0 mg
2 (3-oz) portions red meat, fish, or chicken	5.0
2 (¾ c) portions legumes	4.0
4 portions fruits and vegetables	1.0
4 portions whole-grain (not enriched) products	2.0
Total (compare the U.S. RDA of 15 mg):	14.0 mg

Without legumes and whole-grain vegetables, the zinc intake could be as low as 8 mg. To boost zinc intakes, eat oysters occasionally, and red meat about 3 or so times a week.

[a] 1 c milk, milk beverage, milk-based pudding or custard, kefir, buttermilk. 1 c soft-serve ice cream, chocolate milk, or skim milk yogurt with added milk solids has 2.0 mg. 1 c ricotta cheese has 3.0 mg.

[b] Canned beans with meat added generally have more zinc.

[c] Dried fruits and avocados appear from Appendix H to have more zinc, but when reduced to single 40-kcalorie portions, they have insignificant zinc.

[d] 1 c mung bean sprouts, turnip greens (raw, cooked), spinach (fresh cooked or canned), sauerkraut, or green peas (canned or frozen, cooked).

[e] Phytic acid is present in seeds of many plants. Cereal grains are the major contributor of phytic acid in the diet. Phytate decreases the bioavailability of zinc from these foods.

[f] Zinc is one of the nutrients not added back to refined bread when it is enriched, therefore the distinction has to be made between enriched and whole-grain bread.

[g] 1 oz of candy-coated nuts or chocolate syrup has about 0.5 mg.

[h] 45 kcalories of nuts (1 fat exchange). The average for 12 varieties of nuts is 0.3 mg zinc. 45 kcalories of pumpkin, squash, sesame, or sunflower seeds have 0.4 mg zinc.

[i] Values range from 0.2 to 3.0 mg. Beef soup, clam chowder, split pea soup, and bean soup with pork are the highest; tomato soup is the lowest.

Whole-grain breads and cereals contain zinc, but they also contain phytate and fiber. Refined breads and cereals are stripped of their phytate and fiber, but they also contain less zinc. Which is a better zinc source—the whole grain or the refined product? The answer has to do with the numbers of molecules of zinc and zinc-binder present in the grain. If 100 molecules of zinc are present together with 50 zinc-binding molecules, then 50 of the zinc molecules may be bound but the other 50 will be available for absorption. Whole grains contain phytate and fiber, yes, but they contain relatively more zinc, enough so that the excess zinc is greater per serving of whole-grain bread than the amount available from a comparable serving of refined bread. Thus even though whole grains do contain some bound, unavailable zinc, they are still preferred to refined products as a zinc source. Food research in the future will ask, not how much zinc or how much zinc binder is present in a food but how much zinc relative to the amount of binder—or better still, how much available zinc.

This example illustrates a principle that may well have occurred to you many times as you read earlier chapters. Nutrition "facts" are often more complicated than they may seem at first. You might remember this the next time someone tries to sell you something on the basis of an oversimplified statement. Always ask, "Is he telling the whole story?"

Caution

The process of baking bread usually includes the step of yeast fermentation. Enzymes produced by yeasts destroy phytate, thus helping make the zinc available for absorption. It is thought to be beneficial, when making whole-grain breads, to extend this period of fermentation.

In Middle Eastern countries where zinc deficiency has been reported, a common food staple is unleavened whole-grain breads. Without the fermentation process, the zinc availability from these breads is poor. The World Health Organization has suggested that intake recommendations for zinc be on a sliding scale based on the estimated biological availability of the mineral from various regional diets.[16]

The presence of competing ions—cadmium, lead, mercury, arsenic, copper, and calcium—also influences zinc status. The reverse is also true; in fact, in the future, zinc may be used to compete with metals such as lead to reduce their toxicity. With regards to copper, a high zinc intake is known to produce symptoms of copper deficiency such as anemia. The significance of toxic metals in our food supply is the subject of Highlight 11.

Iodine

Iodine occurs in the body in an infinitesimally small quantity, but its principal role in human nutrition is well known and the amount needed is

16   *Trace Elements in Human Nutrition*, Technical report series no. 532 (Geneva: WHO, 1973), pp. 9–15.

well established. Iodine is part of the thyroid hormones, which regulate body temperature, metabolic rate, reproduction, growth, the making of blood cells, nerve and muscle function, and more. The hormones enter every cell of the body to control the rate at which the cells use oxygen. This is the same as saying that thyroxin controls the rate at which energy is released.

Iodine must be available for thyroid hormones to be synthesized. The amount in the diet is variable and generally reflects the amount present in the soil in which plants are grown or on which animals graze. Iodine is plentiful in the ocean, so seafood is a dependable source. In the United States, in areas where the soil is iodine-poor (most notably the Plains states), the use of iodized salt has largely wiped out the iodine deficiency that once was widespread.

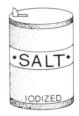

People sometimes wonder whether sea salt, made by drying ocean water, is preferable to purified sodium chloride for use in the salt shaker. Sea salt does contain trace minerals, but it loses its iodine during the drying process. Thus, in a region where goiter is a risk, iodized sodium chloride is the salt to choose.

Caution

When the iodine level of the blood is low, the cells of the thyroid gland enlarge in an attempt to trap as many particles of iodine as possible. If the gland enlarges until it is visible (Figure 11–7), it is called a simple goiter.

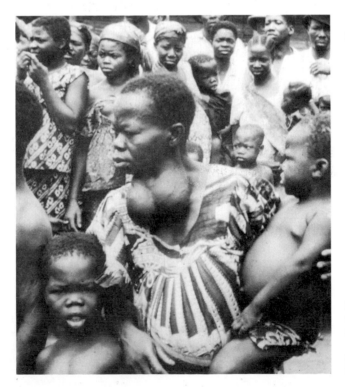

FIGURE 11–7 **Goiter**.

Source: Courtesy of FAO.

goiter (GOY-ter): an iodine-deficiency disease. Goiter caused by iodine deficiency is **simple goiter**.

goitrogen: a thyroid antagonist found in food; causes **toxic goiter**.

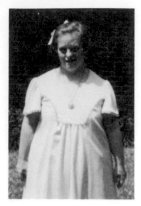

Laura Drake, age 38, a cretin.

cretinism (CREE-tin-ism): an iodine-deficiency disease characterized by mental and physical retardation.

The RDA for iodine: 150 μg.

Canadian *Dietary Standard:* 140–150 μg for men; 100–110 μg for women.

Goiter is estimated to affect 200 million people the world over. In all but 4 percent of these cases the cause is iodine deficiency. As for the 4 percent (8 million), they have goiter because they overconsume plants of the cabbage family and others that contain an antithyroid substance whose effect is not counteracted by dietary iodine.[17] The goitrogens present in plants serve as a reminder that food additives may not be such great offenders as some natural components of foods (see Highlight 10).

In addition to causing sluggishness and weight gain, an iodine deficiency may have serious effects on the development of an infant in the uterus. Severe thyroid undersecretion during pregnancy causes the extreme and irreversible mental and physical retardation known as cretinism. A cretin has an IQ as low as 20 and a face and body with many abnormalities. Much of the mental retardation associated with cretinism can be averted by early diagnosis and treatment.

The iodization of salt in the Plains states eliminated the widespread misery caused by goiter and cretinism in the local people during the 1930s. Once these scourges had disappeared, a new generation of children grew up who never saw the problem and so had no appreciation of its importance. Rejecting iodized salt out of ignorance, they allowed iodine deficiencies to creep back into their lives. Hopefully, now, education is keeping them informed of the need to continue using iodized salt.

The recommended intake of iodine for adults is 100 to 150 micrograms a day, a miniscule amount. Like chlorine, iodine is a deadly poison in large amounts, but the iodide ion, which occurs in foods, is far less toxic, and traces of it are indispensable to life. The need for iodine is easily met by consuming seafood, vegetables grown in iodine-rich soil, and (in iodine-poor areas) iodized salt. In the United States, you have to read the label to find out whether salt is iodized; in Canada all table salt is iodized.

Excessive intakes of iodine can also cause an enlargement of the thyroid gland resembling goiter, which in infants can be so severe as to block the airways and cause suffocation. A dramatic increase in iodine intakes in the United States concerns observers. Average consumption rose from 150 micrograms per day in 1960 to over 450 in 1970, and reached an all-time high of over 800 in 1974; since then it has declined somewhat but still is several times the RDA. The toxic level at which detectable harm results is thought to be over 2,000 micrograms per day for an adult, only a few times higher than current average consumption levels.[18]

Most of the excess iodine seems to be coming from iodates—dough conditioners used in the baking industry—and from milk produced by cows exposed to iodine-containing medications and disinfectants. Now that the problem has been identified, both industries have reduced their use of these compounds, but the sudden emergence of this problem points to a need for continued surveillance of the food supply.

17   F. M. Strong, Toxicants occurring naturally in foods, in *Nutrition Reviews' Present Knowledge in Nutrition,* 4th ed. (Washington, D.C.: Nutrition Foundation, 1976), pp. 516–527.

18   F. Taylor, Iodine—going from hypo to hyper, *FDA Consumer,* April 1981, pp. 15–18.

Copper

The body contains about 75 to 100 milligrams of copper, which performs several vital roles. It is a part of several enzymes. As a catalyst in the formation of hemoglobin, it helps to make red blood cells. It is involved in the manufacture of collagen and the healing of wounds, and it helps to maintain the sheath around nerve fibers. Most of what is known about copper comes from animal research, which has provided clues about its possible roles in humans. Copper's critical roles seem to have to do with helping iron shift back and forth between its +2 and +3 states. This means that copper is needed in many of the reactions related to respiration and the release of energy.

Copper deficiency is rare but not unknown. It has been seen in children with kwashiorkor and with iron-deficiency anemia and can severely disturb growth and metabolism. Excess zinc interferes with copper absorption and can cause deficiency.

Estimated safe and adequate daily dietary intake of copper (adults): 2–3 mg.

The best food sources of copper include grains, shellfish, organ meats, legumes, dried fruits, fresh fruits, and vegetables—a long list showing that copper is available from almost all foods. About a third of the copper taken in food is absorbed, and the rest is eliminated in the feces.

Manganese

The human body contains a tiny 20 milligrams of manganese, mostly in the bones and glands. Still, this represents billions on billions of molecules. Animal studies suggest that manganese cooperates with many enzymes, helping to facilitate dozens of different metabolic processes. Manganese deficiency in animals deranges many systems, including the bones, reproduction, the nervous system, and fat metabolism.

Deficiencies of manganese have not been seen in humans, but toxicity may be severe. Miners who inhale large quantities of manganese dust on the job over prolonged periods show many of the symptoms of a brain disease, with frightening abnormalities of appearance and behavior. "Facial expression is mask-like, the voice monotonous; and intention-tremor, muscle rigidity and spastic gait appear."[19]

Estimated safe and adequate daily dietary intake of manganese (adults): 2.5–5.0 mg.

The example of manganese underlines the fact that toxicity of the trace elements occurs at a level not far above the estimated requirement. Thus it is as important not to overdose as it is to have an adequate intake. The Committee on RDA underscores this point by adding the special warning to its trace-mineral table "not to exceed the upper end of the range

19   T. K. Li and B. L. Vallee, Trace elements, section B: The biochemical and nutritional role of trace elements, in *Modern Nutrition in Health and Disease*, 5th ed., ed. R. S. Goodhart and M. E. Shils (Philadelphia: Lea and Febiger, 1973), pp. 372–399.

of recommended intakes." The National Nutrition Consortium, too, worries that, now that more trace minerals are known, they will be added to vitamin-mineral pills, making toxic overdoses more likely. The FDA is not permitted to enforce limits on the amounts of trace minerals added to supplements; so this is an area in which the consumer himself has to be careful. Beware of supplements containing trace minerals. It is safer to consume a diet that provides foods from a variety of sources than to try to put together, without causing toxicity, a combination of pills that will meet all your needs.

Caution

Fluoride

The outer two layers of the teeth, enamel and dentin, are composed largely of calcium compounds, including hydroxyapatite and fluorapatite.

hydroxyapatite (high-droxy-APP-uh-tite): the major calcium-containing crystal of bones and teeth.

fluorapatite (floor-APP-uh-tite): the stabilized form of bone and tooth crystal, in which fluoride has replaced the hydroxy groups of hydroxyapatite.

Only a trace of fluoride occurs in the human body, but studies have demonstrated that where diets are high in fluoride, the crystalline deposits in bones and teeth are larger and more perfectly formed. When bones and teeth become calcified, first a crystal called hydroxyapatite is formed from calcium and phosphorus. Then fluoride replaces the hydroxy (OH) portions of the crystal, rendering it insoluble in water and resistant to decay.

Drinking water is the usual source of fluoride, although fish and tea may supply substantial amounts. Where fluoride is lacking in the water supply, the incidence of dental decay is very high. Dental problems can cause a multitude of health problems, affecting the whole body. Fluoridation of community water where needed, to raise its fluoride concentration to one part per million (1 ppm), is thus an important public health measure. Fluoridation of community water is presently practiced in more than 5,000 communities across the United States, and about 100 million people are drinking it (see Figure 11–8).

FIGURE 11–8 **Fluoridation in the United States.**

Source: D. P. DePaola and M. C. Alfano, Diet and oral health, *Nutrition Today*, May/June 1977, pp. 6–11, 29–32. Courtesy of the authors and of *Nutrition Today* magazine, 703 Giddings Avenue, Suite 6, Annapolis, MD 21401, copyright May/June 1977.

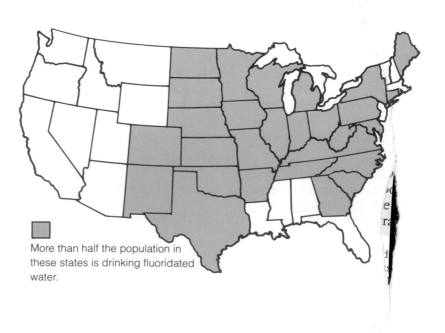

More than half the population in these states is drinking fluoridated water.

In some communities the natural fluoride concentration in water is high, 2 to 8 ppm, and children's teeth develop with mottled enamel (Figure 11-9). This condition, called fluorosis, may not be harmful (in fact, these children's teeth may be extraordinarily decay-resistant), but violates the prejudice that teeth "should" be white. Fluorosis does not occur in communities where fluoride is added to the water supply.

Not only does fluoride protect children's teeth from decay, but it makes the bones of older people resistant to adult bone loss (osteoporosis). Fluoride is also required for growth in animals and is an essential nutrient for humans; in fact, the continuous presence of fluoride in body fluids is desirable. Luckily, all normal diets include fluoride. It is toxic in excess, but toxicity symptoms appear only after chronic intakes of 20 to 80 milligrams a day over many years. The amount consumed from fluoridated water is typically about 1 milligram a day. Despite its value, violent disagreement often surrounds the introduction of fluoride to a community.

People whose water supplies do not contain adequate fluoride need to find alternative means of protecting their children's teeth. The best temporary solution seems to be to use fluoride toothpastes and/or to have children obtain a fluoride treatment of the surface of their teeth every year. Fluoride tablets are also available. For infants there are vitamin drops with fluoride in them, but their effectiveness is limited.

fluorosis (fleur-OH-sis): mottling of the tooth enamel; due to ingestion of too much fluoride during tooth development.

osis = too much

Osteoporosis: see p. 387.

Estimated safe and adequate daily dietary intake of fluoride (adults): 1.5–4.0 mg.

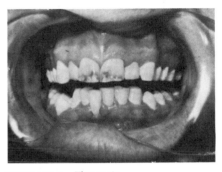

FIGURE 11–9 **Fluorosis.**

Source: Courtesy of H. Kaplan and V. P. Rabbach.

Chromium

Experiments on animals have shown that chromium works closely with the hormone insulin, facilitating the uptake of glucose into cells and the release of energy from it. When chromium is lacking, the effectiveness of insulin is severely impaired, and a diabetes-like condition results.

Like iron, chromium can have two different charges. The +3 ion seems to be the most effective in living systems. It also occurs in association with several different complexes in foods. The one that is best absorbed and most active is a small organic compound named the glucose tolerance factor (GTF). This compound has been purified from brewer's yeast and pork kidney and is believed to be present in many other foods. It may be that when more is known, the GTF, rather than chromium, will be dubbed an essential nutrient and classed among the vitamins.

Depleted tissue concentrations of chromium in human beings have been linked to adult-onset diabetes and growth failure in children with protein-kcalorie malnutrition. Chromium has also been shown to remedy impaired carbohydrate metabolism in several groups of older people in the United States.

GTF (glucose tolerance factor): a small organic compound containing chromium.

Estimated safe and adequate daily dietary intake of chromium (adults): 0.05–0.20 mg.

Selenium

Selenium is a trace element that functions as part of an enzyme. The enzyme acts as an antioxidant and can substitute for vitamin E in some of that vitamin's antioxidant activities.

selenium (se-LEEN-ee-um)

The enzyme of which selenium is a part is glutathione peroxidase, which destroys oxidative compounds that could otherwise oxidize other compounds in the cell.

The heart disease caused by selenium deficiency is named **Keshan disease**, for one of the provinces of China where it was studied.

Estimated safe and adequate daily dietary intake of selenium (adults): 0.05–0.20 mg.

Selenium deficiency affects the heart. A severe deficiency can cause heart failure; a chronic, mild deficiency enlarges the heart and impairs its function. In some parts of China, selenium deficiency affects hundreds of thousands of children; not until the 1970s, however, was the cause of their heart trouble confirmed and remedied with selenium supplements. The conclusive study of over 36,000 subjects was published in 1980.[20]

The region of China in which Keshan disease is prevalent is a region where the soil and foods are selenium-poor. In other parts of the world, selenium-poor soil has been found to correlate with certain kinds of cancer. The question whether selenium protects against cancer has stimulated research with both animal and human subjects, and it seems possible that dietary selenium adequacy may be one of the many health factors that defend against cancer. Results of research to date have not been clear, however. For example, an attempt was made to show a relationship between blood selenium and breast cancer incidence in women in a selenium-poor area in Oregon, but no such relationship was found. The authors were forced to conclude that there was "no justification at this time for the use of selenium supplements by the people living in this low selenium area."[21]

High doses of selenium are toxic, causing loss of hair and nails, lesions of the skin and nervous system, and possibly damage to the teeth. An outbreak of selenium poisoning arose in China in the 1960s when a local rice crop failed and inhabitants of five villages consumed vegetables from a region where selenium-rich coal contaminated the soil in which the vegetables were grown. Some 50 percent of the villagers became seriously ill before the cause was discovered.[22]

Molybdenum

molybdenum (mo-LIB-duh-num)

metalloenzyme: an enzyme that contains one or more minerals as part of its structure.

Estimated safe and adequate daily dietary intake of molybdenum (adults): 0.15–0.50 mg.

Finally, molybdenum has also been recognized as an important mineral in human and animal physiology. It functions as a working part of several metalloenzymes, some of which are giant proteins. One, for example, contains two atoms of molybdenum and eight of iron. Deficiencies of molybdenum are unknown in animals and humans, because the amounts needed are miniscule—as little as 0.1 part per million parts of body tissue. Excess molybdenum causes toxicity in animals, but this effect has not been seen in humans.

20   M. H. N. Golden, Trace elements in human nutrition, *Human Nutrition: Clinical Nutrition* 36C (1982): 185–202.

21   T. D. Schultz and J. E. Leklem, Selenium status of vegetarians, nonvegetarians, and hormone-dependent cancer subjects, *American Journal of Clinical Nutrition* 37 (1983): 114–118.

22   G. Yang, S. Wang, R. Zhou, and S. Sun, Endemic selenium intoxication of humans in China, *American Journal of Clinical Nutrition* 37 (1983): 872–881.

Other Trace Minerals

None of the trace minerals has been known for very long, and some are extremely recent newcomers. Nickel is now recognized as important for the health of many body tissues; deficiencies harm the liver and other organs. Silicon is known to be involved in bone calcification, at least in animals. Tin is necessary for growth in animals and probably in humans. Vanadium, too, is necessary for growth and bone development and also for normal reproduction; human intakes of vanadium may be close to the minimum needed for health. Cobalt is recognized as the mineral in the large vitamin B_{12} molecule; the alternative name for vitamin B_{12}, cobalamin, reflects the presence of cobalt. In the future we may discover that many other trace minerals also play key roles: silver, mercury, lead, barium, cadmium. Even arsenic—famous as the poisonous instrument of death in many murder mysteries and known to be a carcinogen—may turn out to be an essential nutrient in tiny quantities.

As research on the trace minerals continues, many interactions between them are also coming to light. An excess of one may cause a deficiency of another. (A slight manganese overload, for example, may aggravate an iron deficiency.) A deficiency of one may open the way for another to cause a toxic reaction. (Iron deficiency, for example, makes the body much more susceptible than normal to lead poisoning.) Good food sources of one are poor food sources of another; and factors that cooperate with some trace elements oppose others. (Vitamin C, for example, enhances the absorption of iron and depresses that of copper.[23]) The continuous outpouring of new information about the trace minerals is a sign that we have much more to learn.

The intricate vitamin B_{12} molecule contains one atom of cobalt.

Summing Up

Iron is found principally in the red blood cells, where it comprises part of the oxygen-carrier protein hemoglobin. When red blood cells die and are dismantled in the liver, the iron is retrieved and transported by iron-carrier proteins back to bone marrow, where new red blood cells are synthesized. There is no route of excretion for iron; losses are small except when blood is lost, as in menstruation or hemorrhage. Thus women's needs for iron are ordinarily greater than men's.

Iron-deficiency anemia, one of the world's most widespread malnutrition problems, is most common in women and children. Food sources of iron for women must be chosen carefully if even two-thirds of the recommended intake is to be met within a kcalorie allowance that is not excessive. The enrichment or fortification of foods somewhat improves women's iron intakes, but may produce iron overload in men. Addition of an iron supplement to the diet may be advisable for some women.

23   W. Mertz, The essential trace elements, *Science* 213 (1981): 1332–1338.

Foods relatively rich in iron include liver and other organ meats, soybeans, dried beans and legumes, red meats, and dark-green vegetables. Other significant contributors are enriched breads and cereals, eggs, and dried fruits. Iron is better absorbed from meats and soybeans than from other foods, and its absorption is enhanced if vitamin C is eaten at the same meal. Milk and milk products are notable for their lack of iron.

Zinc appears in every body tissue and supports several physiological functions, including normal growth and sexual development. As with iron, a homeostatic mechanism may regulate the amount of zinc absorbed by the body. Deficiencies of zinc have been observed in some children in the United States as well as in the Middle East. The richest food sources of zinc include shellfish, meat, and liver. Milk, eggs, and whole-grain products are also good sources. When estimating the amount of zinc in a diet, one must take into account all of the factors which affect its availability.

Iodine forms part of the thyroid hormones; deficiency may cause goiter, slowed metabolism, and cretinism. The use of iodized salt protects against deficiency. Copper is important for red blood cell formation, collagen synthesis, and central nervous system function. Manganese aids many body enzymes, but its safe range is narrow, with toxicity causing a severe brain-disease syndrome in humans. The fluoride ion combines with calcium and phosphorus to stabilize the crystalline structure of bones and teeth. In communities where the water contains fluoride, dental caries and osteoporosis are less prevalent than in communities where the water supply is low in fluoride. Chromium, as part of the glucose tolerance factor, works with insulin in promoting glucose uptake into cells and normal carbohydrate metabolism. Chromium deficiency is believed to be responsible for some cases of adult-onset diabetes and to cause growth failure in children with protein-kcalorie malnutrition. Selenium acts as cofactor for an antioxidant enzyme. A severe deficiency can cause heart failure. Selenium-poor soil may correlate with certain kinds of cancer. Molybdenum functions as a part of several enzyme systems. Other trace minerals with known physiological roles include nickel, silicon, tin, vanadium, and cobalt. Many other trace minerals are under investigation.

NOTE: Appendix J suggests books and papers that contain additional readings on the trace minerals; see "Books" and "Minerals." The Self-Study for this chapter in Appendix Q shows you how to:

● Estimate and evaluate your iron and zinc intakes.
● Compute your iron absorption from a meal of your choosing.
● Study your favorite foods as sources of iron.
● Check your iodine intake.
● Check your county's water supply for fluoride.

The *Instructor's Manual* includes an extra transparency/handout master demonstrating how to calculate iron absorption from foods. TH11-4

HIGHLIGHT 11
Contaminants in Foods

In regard to acute illness, man's food supply probably is safer today than at any time in recorded history . . . . [At the same time], unexpected hazards might arise from unfortunate combinations of circumstances in which only man is at fault or in which nature plays a role over which man has no control . . . .

J. M. COON and J. C. AYRES

Highlight 10 dealt with intentional food additives and concluded that as a hazard to consumers, they were greatly overrated. This Highlight deals with *indirect* additives—things that get into food by mistake—and concludes that they are a matter for real concern. Intentional additives are sixth and last on FDA's priority list of areas of concern; contaminants are third on that same list (see pp. 406–407), even when food poisoning and pesticide residues are set aside and considered separately.

indirect additive: a substance that can get into food not through intentional introduction but as a result of contact with the food during growing, processing, packaging, storing, or some other stage before the food is consumed.

What are contaminants, and why are they considered so dangerous? A few examples will help to answer this question.

In 1953 a number of people in Minamata, Japan, became ill with a disease no one had seen before. By 1960, 121 cases had been reported, including 23 in infants. Mortality was high; 46 died, and in the survivors the symptoms were ugly: "progressive blindness, deafness, incoordination, and intellectual deterioration."[1] The cause was ultimately revealed to be methylmercury contamination of fish from the bay these people lived on. The infants who contracted the disease had not eaten any fish but their mothers had, and even though the mothers exhibited no symptoms during their pregnancies, the poison had been affecting their unborn babies. Manufacturing plants in the region were discharging mercury into the waters of the bay, the mercury was turning to methylmercury on leaving the factories, and the fish in the bay were accumulating this poison in their bodies. Some of the families who were affected were eating fish from the bay every day.[2]

In 1910, Dr. Alice Hamilton of the United States began documenting her observations of the toxicity to humans of another environmentally derived heavy metal, lead. Factory workers intoxicated with lead poisoning experienced a wide variety of symptoms, she said, including anemia, constipa-

heavy metal: any of a number of mineral ions such as mercury and lead, so called because they are of relatively high atomic weight. Many heavy metals are poisonous.

1   W. A. Krehl, Mercury, the slippery metal, *Nutrition Today*, November/December 1972, pp. 4–15.
2   Krehl, 1972.

439

organic halogen: an organic compound containing one or more atoms of a **halogen**—fluorine, chlorine, iodine, or bromine.

tion, loss of appetite, abnormal kidney function, jaundice due to liver damage, "wrist drop" (loss of muscular control of the hand), irritability, drowsiness, stupor, and coma. Mothers exposed to lead more often had abortions and stillbirths, and their children were more often sick.[3] Lead also finds its way into food, as will be shown below.

In 1973, in Michigan, half a ton of polybrominated biphenyl (PBB), a toxic chemical, was accidentally mixed into some livestock feed that was distributed throughout the state. The chemical found its way into millions of animals and then into humans. The seriousness of the accident began to come to light when dairy farmers reported their cows going dry, aborting their calves, and developing abnormal growths on their hooves. Although more than 30,000 cattle, sheep, and swine and more than a million chickens were destroyed, effects on people were not prevented. By 1982 it was estimated that 97 percent of Michigan's residents had become contaminated with PBB. Nervous system aberrations and alterations in the liver and immune systems were among the effects in exposed farm residents.[4]

Mercury and lead are both heavy metals and PBB is an organic halogen. These two classes of chemicals are among the most toxic and widespread in our environment. A list of the chemical contaminants of greatest concern in foods is presented in Table H11–1.

On first studying this subject, a reader is likely to want the question answered, "How serious is all this—how dangerous is it for *me*?" Yet no one who has pursued the subject realistically expects to have that question answered in any simple way. It may be a negligible problem in your particular area today, but tomorrow it may become a severe one if there is a major spill or other accident. A general answer, then, is that the hazard is probably small, because we are generally well protected, but that in the event of an accident the risk of toxicity can suddenly become very great. (See Highlight 10 for the meaning of *hazard* as opposed to *toxicity*.)

The number of contaminants we could discuss here, and the amount of information available about them, is far beyond our scope. Instead of dealing superficially with all of them, our choice is to illustrate some principles by discussing only two contaminants in depth: lead and DDT.

TABLE H11–1 **Chemical Contaminants of Concern in Foods, U.S. 1970–1980**

HEAVY METALS	HALOGENATED COMPOUNDS	OTHERS
Lead	Chlorine	Asbestos
Mercury	Iodine	Dioxins
Cadmium	Vinyl chloride	Acrilonitrile
Selenium	Ethylene dichloride	Lysinoalanine
Arsenic	Trichloroethylene	Diethylstilbestrol
	Polychlorinated biphenyls (PCBs)	Heat induced mutagens
	Polybrominated biphenyls (PBBs)	Antibiotics (in animal feed)

Source: E. M. Foster, How safe are our foods? *Nutrition Reviews/Supplement*, January 1982, pp. 28–34.

3   M. A. Wessel and A. Dominski, Our children's daily lead, *American Scientist* 65 (1977): 294–298.

4   97% of Michigan population contaminated by 1973 spill, *Tallahassee Democrat*, 16 April 1982.

You can then apply the principles to your study of the others at another time.

Lead

Lead is a metal ion with two positive charges, similar in some ways to nutrient minerals like iron, calcium, and zinc. In fact, it competes with them for some of the slots they normally occupy in the body, but then is unable to fulfill their roles. Thus it interferes with many of the body's systems. The most vulnerable tissues are the nervous system, kidney, and bone marrow. Lead is readily transferred across the placenta and its most severe effects on the fetus are on the developing nervous system. Absorption of lead is five to eight times greater in children than it is in adults, and it tends to stay in their bodies.[5]

This brings us to the first of several points to be made about contamination. A factor in the potential harmfulness of a contaminant is the extent to which it lingers in the body. A few particles of sand or some glass beads (Chapter 5) don't even stay in the body long enough to worry about, and interact with it not at all. If a contaminant enters the system and then is rapidly metabolized to some harmless compound, then its ingestion may not give cause for concern. (Vitamin C seems to fall into the category of rapidly metabolized drugs, and this accounts for its relative lack of toxicity in most people.) If the contaminant is rapidly and preferentially excreted, then, too, it may be possible for the body to survive a brief exposure time. But if it enters the body, interacts with the body's systems, is not metabolized or excreted, and fools the cells' protein machinery into accepting it as part of their structure, then it is dangerous. Additional doses will be piled on top of the first ones and it will accumulate. All these things are true of lead and that's why it's so deadly.

Organic halogens like PBB are, as the term *organic* says, molecules like vitamin C that could in theory be metabolized and disposed of—but their deadliness is related to the same factors that make lead so dangerous. They are resistant to metabolism either inside the body (by the body's enzymes) or outside (by microorganisms), and furthermore they accumulate from one species to the next, with a consequent build-up in the food chain (Figure H11–1).

The anemia caused by lead poisoning is the result of many effects lead has on blood. Besides competing with iron for absorption, lead interferes with several enzymes that synthesize heme, the iron-containing portion of hemoglobin. Lead also deranges the structure of the red blood cell membrane, making it leaky and fragile. Lead interacts with white blood cells, too, impairing their ability to fight infection, and it also binds to antibodies, thereby reducing the body's resistance to disease.[6]

5   Metabolism of vitamin D in lead poisoning, *Nutrition Reviews* 39 (1981): 372–373.

6   Wessel and Dominski, 1977; Nutritional influences on lead absorption in man, *Nutrition Reviews* 39 (1981): 363–365; D. Pincus and C. V. Saccar, Lead poisoning, *American Family Physician* 19 (1979): 120–124.

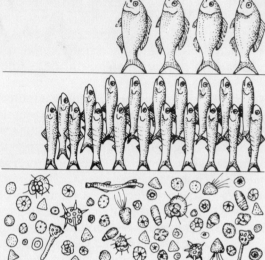

Level 4
a 150-pound person

Level 3
a hundred pounds of fish

Level 2
a few tons of plant-eating fish

Level 1
several tons of
producer organisms

FIGURE H11–1 **How a food chain works.**
A person whose principal animal protein
source is fish may consume about 100
pounds of fish in a year. These fish will,
in turn, have consumed a few tons of
plant-eating fish in the course of their
lifetimes. The plant eaters, in their lifetimes, will have consumed several tons of
photosynthetic producer organisms.

The concern about persistent contaminants is implicit in this pyramid. Assuming 100 percent retention of the
contaminant at each level (an oversimplification), a person, being at the top of
the food chain, could ingest in a year the
amount of contaminant that had accumulated in several tons of producer organisms. TH11-8

Lead has many other known molecular effects, but these few are enough
to illustrate several characteristics of heavy metals. For one thing, all heavy
metals act in some of the same ways. If you reread the description of the
symptoms of mercury poisoning in Minamata, you can imagine how they,
too, arise from interference by mercury with proteins that are trying to do
their jobs. Cadmium, another major environmental contaminant, has similar effects, and the interference of arsenic with respiratory proteins is well
known.

You can also see from these examples how interconnected nutrition is
with the effects of contaminants. There is more to that story, however,
because specific nutrients interact with heavy metals in specific ways. For
instance, total food intake; fat intake; and calcium, iron, and zinc intakes
are known to alter animals' (and probably humans') susceptibility to lead
toxicity. Examples:

● A diet low in calcium permits greater amounts of lead to accumulate in
the body, probably by permitting more lead to be absorbed.
● Iron deficiency, even mild iron deficiency, permits greater lead intoxication. Iron deficiency in a nursing female makes her milk's lead content
higher.

● Zinc status affects both tissue accumulation of lead and sensitivity to its effects.[7]

● The absorption of lead is greatest when the stomach is empty.[8]

The interaction of nutrients with contaminants like lead raises an important point. When an agency is charged with setting the "maximum permissible level" of an environmental contaminant, it sets about testing animals to see what levels bring about detectable ill effects. Usually these animals are being fed the standard laboratory chow—a very nutritious diet—and the only thing varied is their exposure to the contaminant. Healthy, well-nourished animals are likely to have considerably greater resistance to toxicity than they would if they were sick or malnourished. Yet the people to whom the results are applied may be neither healthy nor well nourished. This fact must be remembered when the limits are set.

Caution

In 1981, 535,000 U.S. children aged six months to five years were screened and 22,000 were found to have symptoms caused by lead toxicity, reflecting a prevalent national health problem. In the same screening, an almost equal number of children—23,000—were found to need treatment for iron deficiency, a long-familiar, widespread public health problem. Thus, lead toxicity ranks with iron deficiency in prevalence and severity and is more than just a theoretical hazard; 1 out of every 50 children in rural areas and more than 1 out of every 10 inner city children are affected with lead poisoning.[9]

A popular new "therapy" to prevent or relieve "poisoning" by heavy metals is "chelation therapy," in which you ingest a chelating agent and expect it to capture poisons and remove them from your body. You may remember from Chapter 8 that vitamin C helps iron to be absorbed into the body by chelating it; the principle of chelation therapy is to use an agent that is not absorbable but will carry ions such as lead (Pb^{++}) and mercury (Hg^{++}) out of the body with the feces.

chelation: see p. 296.

The agent most often used is EDTA, ethylene diamine tetraacetic acid, a nonspecific chelating agent that grabs cations (that is, ions with positive charges). EDTA is a small molecule. Unlike proteins, it can't distin-

7   K. R. Mahaffey, Nutritional factors in lead poisoning, *Nutrition Reviews* 39 (1981): 353–362.

8   M. B. Rabinowitz, J. D. Kopple, and G. W. Wetherill, Effect of food intake and fasting on gastrointestinal lead absorption in humans, *American Journal of Clinical Nutrition* 33 (1980): 1784–1788.

9   Update: Childhood lead poisoning, *Journal of the American Dietetic Association* 80 (1982): 592, 594.

guish ions you might want to absorb such as calcium (Ca++), iron (Fe++), magnesium (Mg++), and copper (Cu++) from those you might want not to absorb such as lead (Pb++), or mercury (Hg++). When you undergo a "therapy" such as EDTA chelation therapy, you do so at your own risk.

Caution

DDT

DDT has aroused concerns typical of those held by consumers about organic insecticides and pesticides in general. DDT is the oldest of the modern insecticides, and has been much studied. It is soluble in fat, and so finds its way into the fat or oil depots of animals or plants. Corn is often sprayed with DDT, so corn oil may contain it; animals fed the corn will then accumulate DDT in their body fat, including the fat of milk and dairy products. Human consumers of corn oil margarine, milk, or dairy products then receive it in their turn—and nursing mothers may then pass it on in their breast milk to their babies. No actual harm to human infants has been documented, but the concentrations of DDT in human milk have often been found to be two or more times higher than the maximum permitted in cows' milk, and it is not known what long-term effects might occur. DDT is known to impair the structure of the material from which birds' eggshells are made, and is partly to blame for the decline of several bird species, including the great bald eagle, the U.S. national emblem.

Opponents of the use of DDT have been very emotional at times: "Every time [the infant] sucks the swollen breasts he gets more DDT than is allowed in cow's milk at the supermarket. Be objective? Forget it. Objective is for fence posts. How can you be objective in the face of a global insanity that is DDT?"[10] However, others have countered by offering information that makes the DDT contamination of human milk seem less serious than it might at first appear to be.

The point made by those who say "Don't panic" is very important to an understanding of the whole issue of contamination of food with anything potentially harmful to health: that the *amount* of contamination makes all the difference. If it is low enough, then it can be tolerated without ill effects. In the case of DDT, it has been argued that the amount is, indeed, low enough. According to Dr. Thomas Jukes of the Medical Physics Division of the Donner Laboratory at the University of California, Berkeley, the comparison between breast milk and cow's milk DDT levels makes breast milk look bad because the cow's milk level is extremely low: "'Zero tolerance' has been the policy with respect to additives in milk. . . . More than ten years ago, it was evident that the entire stocks of canned milk in the United States gave positive tests for DDT. It was, therefore, necessary to

10   Ed Chaney, information director of National Wildlife Federation, quoted by T. H. Jukes, Fact and fancy in nutrition and food science, *Journal of the American Dietetic Association* 59 (1971), reprinted in T. P. Labuza, *The Nutrition Crisis: A Reader* (St. Paul, Minn.: West, 1975), pp. 456–473.

face facts, and two choices were available: to ban cows' milk from interstate commerce or to set a tolerance limit."[11] A tolerance limit was therefore set 140 times lower than the level permitted in most agricultural products.

Table H11–2 shows that the highest amount a baby would receive from breast milk containing this much DDT would be less than 1/25 as much as people have been seen to tolerate for years without ill effects. Even if infants were *ten times* more susceptible than adults (and this is highly unlikely), no ill effects could be expected. In all likelihood, infants are more resistant, not more sensitive, than adults to DDT.[12]

Before reaching any conclusions about the acceptability of any amount of DDT in any food, one would have to sift through much more information and make many judgments. *No conclusion has been reached here*, but a point has been made. If it is impossible to have "zero" contamination of food products with toxic substances, this is not necessarily a disaster. Testing can show where to draw the line below which doses are acceptable.

DDT can serve as an example of another point, also. Unlike the heavy metals and the persistent halogens, DDT is metabolized in the body, although slowly. It therefore accumulates less rapidly in tissues and builds up less rapidly in the food chain. However, its being metabolized offers a new concern. The question has to be asked, what does this contaminant get metabolized *to*? What are the effects of its metabolites in the body? (You may recall from Highlight 10 the case of nitrites, which may be metabolized to nitrosamines, which may in turn cause cancer.) In mice, DDT is metabolized to DDE, which is a carcinogen.[13] However, this metabolic pathway does not exist in other animals, and DDT has never caused cancer in human beings, even in those who have received DDT for many years at

TABLE H11–2 **Effects of DDT at Various Dose Levels**

DOSE	EFFECTS
A dose of 1/2 mg/kg/day	Observed to be tolerated by volunteers for 21 months and by workers for 6½ years
1/2 that dose	Tolerated by workers 19 years
1/25 that dose	The highest amount received by infants from breast milk[a]
1/62 that dose	The amount Native Americans were receiving in 1964 from food, and from their houses, which were sprayed.
1/200 that dose	The amount the general population of the U.S. was receiving, 1953–1954
1/1,250 that dose	The amount the U.S. population was receiving 20 years later

Source: Adapted from WHO statement, January 22, 1971, as quoted by T. H. Jukes, Fact and fancy in nutrition and food science, *Journal of the American Dietetic Association* 59 (1971): 203–211.
[a] Assuming the newborn baby would drink 1⅓ pints of milk per day.

11   Jukes, 1971.

12   Jukes, 1971.

13   D. V. Parke, Toxic chemicals in food, *Journal of the Forensic Science Society* 16 (1977): 189–196.

BHT (butylated hydroxytoluene)
(BYOO-til-ate-ed high-DROX-ee-TAHL-you-een): this and its relative
BHA (butylated hydroxyanisole)
(high-DROX-ee-ANN-is-ole) are antioxidants commonly used in bread and other baked products.

high levels.[14] Obviously, the question is important in each case of a metabolizable contaminant.

It should be noted that sometimes a substance can turn out to be beneficial, not harmful, because of the pathway it follows in the body. For example, the intentional additive BHT, often used as an antioxidant in breads, aroused consumers' fears some years ago on the grounds that it might cause cancer. But among the many tests that were performed on BHT and other additives were several showing that animals fed large amounts of these substances developed less cancer when exposed to carcinogens and lived *longer* than controls. These antioxidants apparently protect from cancer in two ways. They prevent carcinogens from binding to DNA, and they induce the liver to produce enzymes that destroy carcinogens. The effects occur at a concentration similar to that used for the additives in bread.[15]

DDT is like lead and probably all other contaminants in that its toxicity depends on the nutritional state of the animal exposed to it. It depresses liver stores of vitamin A in rats—when they are raised on a particular diet that is deficient in the amino acid methionine (soybeans).[16] It accumulates in body fat, and this leads to some effects that might surprise the observer unaware of the principles of nutrition and metabolism. As long as the animal is well fed, the DDT is tucked away (sequestered) in the body's fat. But if the animal is deprived of food, its body fat starts breaking down, the DDT is mobilized, and it produces blood concentrations potentially toxic to the central nervous system.[17]

No generalizations can be made as to what specific effects a particular contaminant will have on a particular nutrient in a given species. Similarly, no general statement can be made as to which kind of nutrient imbalance in the diet might most severely handicap an animal or a human in its efforts to resist a pesticide's effect. However, a generalization can be made. Not 100 percent of the time, but more often than not, an adequate diet and optimal health help to protect against the toxicity of food contaminants and other environmental pollutants.

By this token, it should be repeated, when animal tests are analyzed to determine what levels of a contaminant are acceptable, the analysis should be made with an awareness of the type of diet the test animals were receiving. It cannot be assumed that a dose level that can easily be resisted by healthy, well-nourished animals or people will also be acceptable for their weaker counterparts. Be careful to remember that

14   T. H. Jukes, How safe is our food supply? *Archives of Internal Medicine* 138 (1978): 772–774.

15   L. W. Wattenberg, Inhibitors of carcinogenesis, in *Carcinogens: Identification and Mechanisms of Action*, ed. A. C. Griffin and C. R. Shaw (New York: Raven Press, 1978), pp. 229–316.

16   R. A. Shakman, Nutritional influences on the toxicity of environmental pollutants: A review, *Archives of Environmental Health* 28 (1974): 105–113.

17   Shakman, 1974.

the toxicity of a substance always depends on the previous diet of the test animal or person.

This principle applies generally to actions taken by policymakers and it is taken into account in the margin-of-safety allowances made in setting permissible levels of contamination. But the principle also applies to each individual person. If you want to be well protected against possible exposure to toxic environmental contaminants in the future, you should look to your own nutritional health today. If you want your children to be protected, you should make sure that they receive an adequate and varied diet.

Caution

Perspective on Contaminants in Foods

It was said at the start that the hazard from contamination of food is probably small, and that the risk to individuals is from accidental gross contamination. However, this statement needs qualification. For one thing, lead toxicity is known to be a serious problem in U.S. children today. As for other contaminants, no one knows to what extent the total burden of contaminants accumulating in the environment may be reaching levels that constitute a hazard to human beings. No one knows whether some individuals may be susceptible today to contamination levels already present in some areas. Another unknown factor is the question of interaction among contaminants. A substance that poses no threat by itself may, in combination with others, present significant danger; an example is the chlorine in drinking water, mentioned in Chapter 10. Another unknown is the time factor. Many of the substances of concern have been around for only a short time. What are the effects of prolonged exposure to them? Contaminants are sometimes hard to identify; sometimes it is not even known that they are present; and so they are hard to regulate. There is no systematic procedure for monitoring or controlling their presence in food except in individual cases.[18] It will take vigilance and determination to detect these substances and control them appropriately. Among the qualifications the people who do this will have to have is an in-depth understanding of nutrition.

NOTE: Appendix J suggests additional readings; see "Contaminants."

18   S. M. Oace, Diet and cancer, *Journal of Nutrition Education* 10 (1978): 106–108.

CHAPTER 12

Nutrition Status, Food Choices, and Diet Planning

CONTENTS

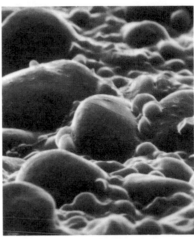

People seldom realize that the foods they eat are often as complex in structure as their own bodies' tissues. Shown here is a sample of dough; the large spheres are starch granules covered by a film of gluten (protein).

Food does not become nutrition until it passes the lips.

RONALD M. DEUTSCH

All the nutrients have been presented and discussed, the food sources of each are known, and the human needs for them have been described. Now, how do you go about determining whether individuals or groups are receiving the nutrients they need? And if they are not, what food choices do they need to change? Then, how do you set about improving the diet while honoring their food preferences? This chapter addresses these questions.

Nutrition Assessment

To learn whether a person's nutrient needs are being met, the dietitian or other health professional performs a nutrition assessment. To give all the details of such a procedure would go far beyond the scope of this book (whole graduate

449

courses are taught in the subject, and hundreds of pages of reading are required). However, any student of nutrition should know the basics of a proper nutrition assessment procedure, for two reasons.

For one thing, competent medical care includes attention to nutrition. The doctor should employ a person skilled in nutrition assessment techniques or refer all patients to such a person, to make sure their nutritional health is sound, while the health care organization (hospital or other) should make nutrition assessment a routine part of its workup on every patient so that nutrition handicaps will not hinder the response to medical treatment and the recovery from illness.

Second, because nutrition is such a popular subject today ("everybody's doing it"), fraudulent practices are even more abundant in this area than they have been in the past (and they have always been rampant). The knowledgeable consumer needs to know what procedures he or she can expect in a nutrition assessment, and what kinds of information they can yield.

For these reasons, this chapter begins with a brief summary of nutrition assessment techniques. Appendix E extends the information here with a compilation of standards, charts, and other forms commonly used in assessment.

Nutrition assessment involves making an inventory of nutrition assets and liabilities as determined by four techniques:

- History taking.
- Anthropometric measures.
- Physical examination.
- Biochemical analysis (clinical or lab tests).

Each of these involves collecting data by a number of means and interpreting the findings in relation to the total picture.

Historical Data

A person's history reveals many clues about his present nutrition status. The person making a nutrition assessment explores the history of the subject from a number of different angles: medical, social, and drug history, as well as diet. Table 12–1 lists the historical information that might indicate poor nutrition status, and Form 12–1 shows how such information might be collected. As you can see, many circumstances of a person's life, including the environment he lives in, his cooking facilities, previous illnesses, persons he associates with, and others, have an impact on his nutrition status and provide the assessor with clues to likely problems.

Medical and social histories are often obtained in a nutrition assessment by reference to charts already filled out by the attending physician, nurse, or other worker. The drug history has seldom already been taken in a way that is useful to the nutrition assessor and therefore often requires special attention. Hundreds of drugs interact with nutrients, creating the possibility of imbalances or deficiencies, and they should not be overlooked in assessing a person's nutrition status. Appendix E supplies a form that elicits the necessary information about drugs.

TABLE 12–1 **Risk Factors for Poor Nutrition Status**

MEDICAL HISTORY

Recent major illness	Alcoholism	Hyperlipidemia
Recent major surgery	Cancer	Hypertension
Surgery of the GI tract	Ciculatory problems	Mental retardation
Overweight	Liver disease	Multiple pregnancies[a]
Underweight	Lung disease	Neurologic disorders
Recent weight loss or gain	Kidney disease	Pancreatic insufficiency
Anorexia	Diabetes	Paralysis
Nausea	Heart disease	Physical disability
Vomiting	Heavy smoking	Radiation therapy
Diarrhea	Hormonal imbalance	Teenage pregnancies[a]

DIET HISTORY	SOCIAL/ECONOMIC HISTORY
Chewing or swallowing difficulties (including poorly fitted dentures, dental caries, and missing teeth)	Inadequate food budget
	Inadequate food preparation facilities
Inadequate food intake	Inadequate food storage facilities
Restricted or fad diets	Elderly
Frequently eating out	Living (eating) alone
No intake for 10 or more days	Poor education
Intravenous fluids (other than total parenteral nutrition) for 10 or more days	

DRUG HISTORY[b]

Antibiotics	Catabolic steroids
Anticancer agents	Oral contraceptives
Anticonvulsants	Vitamin and other nutrient preparations
Antihypertensive agents	

[a] See also Risk Factors for Poor Nutrition Status in Pregnancy, Chapter 13.

[b] See also Drug History Form in Appendix E.

As for the diet history, there are several means of obtaining food intake data, including the 24-hour recall, the usual intake record, the food frequency checklist, and the food diary. Great skill is necessary to obtain accurate food intake data. The dietitian trained in these techniques often uses food models and measuring devices to help clients identify serving sizes of food consumed.

The most commonly used method of obtaining food intake data is the 24-hour recall. To use this method one asks the person to recount everything eaten or drunk in the past 24 hours or for the previous day. (Form 12–2 shows a typical 24-hour recall form.) Seldom does this method give enough accurate information about an individual's food intake to be valid, however. It is more often used in nutrition surveys to obtain estimates of the typical food intakes of large numbers of people in given populations.

An advantage of the 24-hour recall is that it is easy to obtain. It is also less frustrating to elicit information from the past 24 hours than to require a person to estimate his intake over a long period of time. However, the previous day's intake may not be the usual intake; the subject may be unable to estimate the amounts of food eaten; the subject may conceal facts

FORM 12–1 **History**

Name _____   Today's date _____
Address _____   Age _____
_____   Sex _____
_____   Phone _____
Date of last medical checkup _____   Height _____
Reason for coming in _____   Weight _____
_____   Usual Weight _____

PERSONAL DATA

1. Last grade of school completed _____ Still in school? _____
2. Are you employed? _____ Occupation _____
3. Does someone else live at your home? _____ Who? _____
4. Do you smoke in any way? _____ How much? _____
5. Have you recently lost or gained more than 10 lb? _____ If yes, please explain how _____
6. Are you pregnant? _____ How many months? _____
7. How many pregnancies have you carried to term? _____
8. Are your menstrual periods normal? _____ If not, please explain _____
9. Have you been told that you have: (check any that apply)
   Diabetes _____ High blood pressure _____ Hardening of the arteries _____
   Lung disease _____ Kidney disease _____ Liver disease _____ Ulcers _____
   Cancer _____ Other _____
10. Do you eat at regular times each day? _____ How many times per day? _____
11. Do you usually eat snacks? _____ When? _____
12. Where do you usually eat your meal?
    Morning _____ Noon _____ Night _____
    With whom?
    Morning _____ Noon _____ Night _____
13. Would you say your appetite is good? _____ Fair? _____ Poor? _____
    If poor, please explain _____
14. What foods do you particularly dislike? _____
15. Are there foods you don't eat for other reasons? _____
16. Do you have any difficulty eating? _____
17. How would you describe your feelings about food? _____
    _____
18. Who prepares your meals? _____
19. Are you, or is any member of your family, on a special diet? _____
    If yes, who and what kind? _____
20. Do you drink alcohol? _____ How many drinks per day? _____
    Do you ever drink alcohol excessively? _____ How often? _____
21. Do you take any kind of medication, either prescribed by a doctor or over-the-counter, for any condition?[a] _____
22. How would you describe your exercise habits?
    Kind of exercise _____ How intense? _____
    How long at a time? _____ How often? _____
23. Are there any other facts about your lifestyle that you think might be related to your nutritional health? _____ Explain _____

[a] If the answer is yes, turn to Drug History Form (Appendix E).

about what she ate; and as a result, sometimes the information gathered in a 24-hour recall is totally meaningless as a reflection of a person's usual intake.

Another method is to obtain a "usual intake pattern." An inquiry on usual intake might begin with "What is the first thing you usually eat or drink

FORM 12–2 **Food Intake Record (used to obtain either a 24-hour recall or a usual intake pattern)**

Name and address _____ Date _____

_____

_____

Did you take a vitamin/mineral supplement? _____

If yes, what kind? _____ Dose _____

Please record the amount and type of foods and beverages consumed today. [Or: Please record the amount and type of foods and beverages you typically consume each day.]

FOOD	AMOUNT (c, tbsp, or piece)	DESCRIPTION
	(etc.)	

during the day?" Similar questions follow until a typical intake pattern is obtained. This method is similar to the 24-hour recall and can be recorded on the same form (Form 12–2). A skilled and patient interviewer can obtain much useful information from it. For a person whose intake varies widely from day to day, however, it may be hard to answer the questions, and in such a case the data obtained may be useless in estimating nutrient intake. However, the usual intake method is often useful to verify food intake when the past 24 hours have been atypical.

Another approach is to use a food frequency checklist. The purpose of this record is to ascertain how often an individual eats a specific type of food per day, week, month, or year. Subjects are asked to state how often they eat a certain food or food type, and a long list of foods is used to cover all possibilities. The information obtained can help pinpoint nutrients that may be excessive or deficient in the diet. If used in conjunction with the usual intake or 24-hour recall, the food frequency record permits double-checking the accuracy of the information obtained. Form 12–3 is a food frequency checklist.

Still another alternative is the food diary. (An example is provided in Form 12–4.) Completion of a diary often helps to determine factors associated with food intake (time of day, place eaten, mood, others present). The person keeping the diary is instructed to write down the required information immediately after eating. A food diary works well with cooperative people but requires considerable time and effort on their part.

The advantages of the food diary are several:

● The diary keeper must assume an active role.
● The person may for the first time begin to see and understand his own food habits.
● The assessor obtains an accurate picture of the diary keeper's lifestyle and factors that affect his food intake.

FORM 12–3 **Food Frequency Checklist**

The following information will help us to understand your regular eating habits so that we may offer you the best service possible. If you have any doubt about some items, be sure to underestimate the "goodness" of your habits rather than to overestimate.

1. How many times *per week* do you eat the following foods? Circle the appropriate number:

PER WEEK

Poultry	0 <1 1 2 3 4 5 6 7 8 9 >9 _____
Fish	0 <1 1 2 3 4 5 6 7 8 9 >9 _____
Hot dogs	0 <1 1 2 3 4 5 6 7 8 9 >9 _____
Bacon	0 <1 1 2 3 4 5 6 7 8 9 >9 _____
Lunch meat	0 <1 1 2 3 4 5 6 7 8 9 >9 _____
Sausage	0 <1 1 2 3 4 5 6 7 8 9 >9 _____
Pork or ham	0 <1 1 2 3 4 5 6 7 8 9 >9 _____
Salt pork	0 <1 1 2 3 4 5 6 7 8 9 >9 _____
Liver	0 <1 1 2 3 4 5 6 7 8 9 >9 _____
Beef or veal	0 <1 1 2 3 4 5 6 7 8 9 >9 _____
Other meats (which?) _____	0 <1 1 2 3 4 5 6 7 8 9 >9 _____
Eggs	0 <1 1 2 3 4 5 6 7 8 9 >9 _____
Fast foods	0 <1 1 2 3 4 5 6 7 8 9 >9 _____

2. How many times *per day* do you eat the following foods? Circle the appropriate number:

PER DAY

Bread, toast, rolls, muffins	0 <1 1 2 3 4 5 6 7 8 9 >9 _____
Milk (including on cereal)	0 <1 1 2 3 4 5 6 7 8 9 >9 _____
Yogurt or tofu	0 <1 1 2 3 4 5 6 7 8 9 >9 _____
Cheese or cheese dishes	0 <1 1 2 3 4 5 6 7 8 9 >9 _____
Sugar, jam, jelly, syrup, honey	0 <1 1 2 3 4 5 6 7 8 9 >9 _____
Butter or margarine	0 <1 1 2 3 4 5 6 7 8 9 >9 _____

3. How many times *per week* do you eat the following foods? Circle the appropriate number:

PER WEEK

Fruit or fruit juice	0 <1 1 2 3 4 5 6 7 8 9 >9 _____
Vegetables other than potato	0 <1 1 2 3 4 5 6 7 8 9 >9 _____
Potatoes and other starchy vegetables	0 <1 1 2 3 4 5 6 7 8 9 >9 _____
Salads or raw vegetables	0 <1 1 2 3 4 5 6 7 8 9 >9 _____
Cereal (which kind?) _____	0 <1 1 2 3 4 5 6 7 8 9 >9 _____
Pancakes or waffles	0 <1 1 2 3 4 5 6 7 8 9 >9 _____
Rice or other cooked grains	0 <1 1 2 3 4 5 6 7 8 9 >9 _____
Noodles (macaroni, spaghetti)	0 <1 1 2 3 4 5 6 7 8 9 >9 _____
Crackers or pretzels	0 <1 1 2 3 4 5 6 7 8 9 >9 _____
Sweet rolls or doughnuts	0 <1 1 2 3 4 5 6 7 8 9 >9 _____
Cooked dry beans or peas	0 <1 1 2 3 4 5 6 7 8 9 >9 _____
Peanut butter or nuts	0 <1 1 2 3 4 5 6 7 8 9 >9 _____
Milk or milk products	0 <1 1 2 3 4 5 6 7 8 9 >9 _____
T.V. dinners, pot pies, other prepared meals	0 <1 1 2 3 4 5 6 7 8 9 >9 _____
Sweet bakery goods (cake, cookies)	0 <1 1 2 3 4 5 6 7 8 9 >9 _____
Snack foods (potato or corn chips)	0 <1 1 2 3 4 5 6 7 8 9 >9 _____
Candy	0 <1 1 2 3 4 5 6 7 8 9 >9 _____
Soft drinks (which?) _____	0 <1 1 2 3 4 5 6 7 8 9 >9 _____
Coffee or tea	0 <1 1 2 3 4 5 6 7 8 9 >9 _____
Frozen sweets (which?) _____	0 <1 1 2 3 4 5 6 7 8 9 >9 _____
Instant meals, such as breakfast bars or diet meal beverages (which?) _____	0 <1 1 2 3 4 5 6 7 8 9 >9 _____
Wine	0 <1 1 2 3 4 5 6 7 8 9 >9 _____
Beer	0 <1 1 2 3 4 5 6 7 8 9 >9 _____
Whiskey, vodka, rum, etc	0 <1 1 2 3 4 5 6 7 8 9 >9 _____

FORM 12-3 **(continued)**

4. What specific kinds of the following foods do you eat most often? Include the name of the food; whether it is fresh, canned, or frozen; and how it is prepared.
   Fruits and fruit juices _____
   Vegetables _____
   Milk and milk products _____
   Meats _____
   Breads and cereals _____
   Desserts _____
   Snack foods _____

5. Please list the names of any liquid, powder, or pill form of vitamin or mineral product you take, and state how often you take it. Please list also any diet supplement you use (such as protein milkshakes or brewer's yeast), how much you use, and how often you use it. _____

6. Is there anything else we should know about your food/nutrient intake? _____
   _____

For these reasons food diaries are particularly useful in outpatient counseling for such nutrition problems as weight reduction or food allergy. The major disadvantages stem from poor compliance in recording the data and conscious or unconscious changes in eating habits that may occur while the diary is being kept.

After food intake data have been collected, they are used to determine nutrient intake, if appropriate. Comparison with standards such as the RDA or the Canadian *Dietary Standard* is the next step. The comparison is made either by estimating or by actually computing the amount of each nutrient obtained from each food on a typical day or in the recall.

This book provides two ways of estimating nutrient intakes from a diet history. One way is to use the tables in Chapters 8 through 11 to obtain rough estimates of the intakes of the vitamins thiamin, riboflavin, folacin, vitamin B$_6$, vitamin C, and vitamin A and the minerals calcium, iron, and zinc.

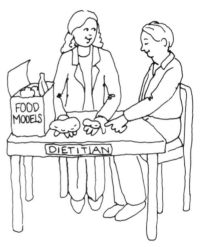

The dietitian uses food models in taking a diet history, so that the client will be able to report serving sizes accurately.

FORM 12-4 **Food Diary**

			Name _____		
			Date _____		
TIME	PLACE	WITH WHOM	EMOTIONAL STATE	HUNGRY OR NOT HUNGRY	FOOD EATEN (AMOUNT)
			(etc.)		

The other way is to look up every food in the table of food composition (Appendix H) and to add up manually the nutrients obtained; or to use a computer program that does the same thing automatically. This is an informative but time-consuming exercise, even when it is done with the help of a computer. It tends to imply an accuracy greater than can actually be obtained from data as uncertain as those that provide the starting information. Foods vary. Not all 200-gram tomatoes contain exactly 1.3 mg of niacin. Nutrient contents of foods are averages. Furthermore, the professionals who make up the tables assume that the foods are stored and prepared in a way that minimizes losses of vitamins.

Even more significantly, the person who reports eating "a serving" of greens may not know the difference between a quarter-cup and two whole cups; only trained individuals can accurately estimate serving sizes. Thus there are many possible sources of error in comparing nutrient intakes with nutrient needs in this way. Most history-takers learn to use shortcut systems to obtain rough estimates of nutrient intakes and then use the calculation method to pin down any suspected nutrient deficiencies or imbalances.

Once an estimate of nutrient intakes has been obtained by means of a diet history, it has to be combined with other sources of information to confirm or eliminate the possibility of suspected nutrition problems. The assessor must constantly remember that a sufficient intake of a nutrient does not guarantee adequate nutrient status for an individual. The individual's needs may be high; or his absorption, utilization, or excretion of the nutrient may be abnormal, so that even though he doesn't have a primary nutrient deficiency, he may have a secondary one.

primary deficiency: a nutrient deficiency caused directly by lack of that nutrient in the diet.

secondary deficiency: a deficiency caused by the body's inability to digest, absorb, or utilize a nutrient in the normal fashion, or by excess destruction or excretion of the nutrient.

Anthropometric Measures

Anthropometrics are physical measurements that reflect growth and development. The measurements taken on an individual are compared with standards specific for sex and age. Those standards, in turn, are derived from measurements taken on large numbers of people of the same race and geographic location as those being measured.

Height and weight are well recognized anthropometrics. Others include fatfold measurements and various measures of lean tissue. Some are used in specific situations. In infancy, a head circumference measurement may be useful. In liver disease, a measurement of abdominal girth may be informative. Anthropometrics are particularly useful when they are measured at intervals over time.

Anthropometric measures can be easy to take, and little equipment is required. However, their accuracy and value are limited by the skills of the measurer. Mastering the correct techniques takes time, and plenty of practice is needed before an assessor can use them reliably. Furthermore, significant changes in measurements are slow to occur in adults. When changes do occur in adults, they represent prolonged alterations in nutrient intake.

Among the standards used for anthropometric measures are several already presented. A table of average weights for height such as the one on the inside back cover is often used as a standard for individual people's

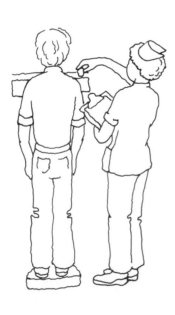

weight. To make the use of such a height-weight table meaningful, the assessor refers to a table of frame sizes such as the one based on elbow breadth (p. 233) or the one that compares wrist circumference to height (Appendix E). The table of average weights for height may not be useful in cases where a person has weighed much more or much less than the average all his life; to assess such a person's weight status it may be more informative to compare his weight, not with a supposed "ideal" body weight (IBW), but with his usual body weight (UBW); or to ask the person in a dietary interview, "Have you noticed a change in weight recently?"

The nutrition status of people suspected of being overnourished or undernourished with respect to protein and kcalories can be assessed anthropometrically. The triceps fatfold measurement, as used in assessing obesity, was mentioned in Chapter 7. To assess undernutrition, one uses not only weight for height and fatfold thickness but also measurements of the body's skeletal muscle and other lean tissue (visceral protein). Table 12–2 shows that different compartments are depleted, depending on whether the person has kwashiorkor (from protein deficiency), marasmus (from kcalorie deficiency), or a mixture of the two. The triceps fatfold measure provides an estimate of body fat. The midarm circumference (MAC) provides an index of the arm's total area; and an arithmetical calculation subtracts the fat from the total area, leaving an estimate of the lean tissue in the arm—the mid-arm muscle circumference (MAMC). The MAMC reflects the body's total skeletal muscle mass. Table 12–2 shows how these measures are used to help distinguish among different types of protein-kcalorie malnutrition (PCM) in malnourished hospital patients; standards for fatfold thickness, MAC, and MAMC are given in Appendix E together with a nomogram for deriving the MAMC. In conjunction with these; several lab tests are also used (see below).

Anthropometric measures are also used to assess growth in children and weight gain in pregnant women. The relevant tables and charts are in Appendix E.

TABLE 12–2 **Anthropometric and Biochemical Measures Used to Assess PCM**

	BODY COMPARTMENT MEASURED		
MEASURE	*Body Fat*	*Skeletal Muscle*	*Visceral Protein*
Anthropometrics			
Weight[a]	x	x	
Triceps skinfold[b]	x		
Midarm circumference[b]	x	x	
Midarm muscle circumference[b]		x	
Lab tests			
Serum albumin[b]			x
Serum transferrin[b]			x
Total lymphocyte count			x
Creatinine-height index[c]		x	

[a] A standard table of weight for height appears on the inside back cover.

[b] Standards for evaluation of these measures are in Appendix E.

[c] The amount of creatinine excreted is thought to reflect total skeletal mass. It therefore should be proportional to height. If creatinine excreted (for a person of a given height) is low, this reflects depleted skeletal muscle. Appendix E presents standards.

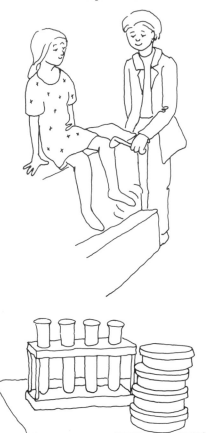

Physical Examination

Clues to a person's nutrition status can be identified by examining the person for physical signs of malnutrition. However, many of the signs are nonspecific: they can be associated with nutrient deficiencies but may be totally unrelated to nutrition. Physical findings can only be interpreted in light of other assessment findings.

Physical signs of malnutrition appear most rapidly in parts of the body where cells are being replaced at a high rate, such as in the hair, skin, and gastrointestinal tract. Chapters 8 to 11 presented many tables of symptoms of vitamin and mineral deficiencies and toxicities indicating the many tissues and organs that would reflect signs of malnutrition. Table 12–3 summarizes the signs of vitamin/mineral malnutrition, organized nutrient by nutrient, as well as the biochemical tests (next section) used to confirm them. A table in Appendix E presents the same information organized body system by body system.

Biochemical (Lab) Tests

Biochemical or clinical lab tests help to determine what is really happening inside the body. Blood and urine samples are most often used to directly measure nutrients or metabolites that are affected by poor nutrition. Biochemical measurements often can be used to detect subclinical malnutrition.

The lab tests most commonly used in hospitals today for nutrition assessment help uncover PCM. These include tests for serum albumin levels, serum transferrin levels, total lymphocyte count, and creatinine excretion. Used together with the anthropometric measures already mentioned (Table 12–2), these lab tests help differentiate among different types of PCM:

serum albumin: the chief blood protein used to assess protein nutrition status.

serum transferrin: an iron-carrying protein in the blood. The concentration of this protein *increases* if the person's iron stores are depleted (p. 411); it decreases in protein malnutrition.

total lymphocyte count: a count of white blood cells, a measure of immune function, which may or may not reflect nutrition status.

creatinine excretion: an indicator of lean body mass. Creatinine is a waste product produced by active muscle.

● *Marasmus:* somatic protein and fat severely depleted. Indicators: low %IBW or %UBW; fatfold thickness; MAC; MAMC; and creatinine-height index.

● *Kwashiorkor:* visceral protein severely depleted. Indicators: low total lymphocyte count, serum albumin, serum transferrin.

● *Kwashiorkor-marasmus mix:* both body compartments depleted. Indicators: all (Table 12–2).

Standards for determining the severity of depletion of serum albumin, transferrin, total lymphocyte count, and creatinine-height index are in Appendix E.

Not only blood and urine tests but also skin tests may be used to assess nutrition status in the hospital. Various forms of PCM have been associated with depression of the immune system. The total number of lymphocytes (white blood cells that defend against infection) appears to decrease as protein depletion occurs; and this is why the total lymphocyte count is an index useful in nutrition assessment. Another test of the immune function is antigen skin testing. Organisms (usually three to four kinds) to which most people are immune are injected just under the skin. After 48 hours the sites of the injections are inspected for raised, hardened areas. These will

TABLE 12–3 **Selected Physical Findings and Laboratory Tests Useful for Assessing Some Vitamin and Mineral Deficiencies**

VITAMINS	PHYSICAL FINDINGS ASSOCIATED WITH DEFICIENCY/TOXICITY[a]	LABORATORY TESTS USED FOR ASSESSMENT
Vitamin A	Triangular gray spots on eye; dryness of eye membranes and skin; night blindness; softening of the cornea; plugging of hair follicles with keratin; diarrhea; infections; bone pain; dental decay; nerve damage; anemia (Toxicity: bone abnormalities; joint pain; bleeding; slowed clotting time; stopping of menstruation; loss of appetite; headache; nausea; loss of hair; brittle nails; enlarged liver; jaundice)	Serum vitamin A Serum carotene
Thiamin	Loss of ankle and knee jerks; calf muscle pain; edema; wasting; mental confusion; weakness; peripheral paralysis; enlarged heart; cardiac failure	Urinary thiamin Thiamin load test Erythrocyte (red blood cell) transketolase
Riboflavin	Dermatitis around lips and nostrils; cracking at corners of mouth; reddening of eyes; magenta-colored tongue; hypersensitivity to light	Urinary riboflavin Erythrocyte glutathione reductase Riboflavin load test
Niacin	Bilateral symmetrical dermatitis; swollen, smooth, edematous tongue; mental confusion; irritability; diarrhea	Urinary N-methylnicotinamide Urinary 2-pyridone
Vitamin B₆	Dermatitis; cracking of corners of mouth; smooth, red tongue; irritation of sweat glands; abnormal brainwave pattern; convulsions	Tryptophan load test Urinary B₆ Blood transaminase Blood B₆
Folacin	Smooth, swollen tongue with cracking; diarrhea; macrocytic anemia	Erythrocyte folate Urinary formiminoglutamic acid Serum folate
Vitamin B₁₂	Smooth, swollen tongue; heightened sensitivity of skin; loss of sensation in fingers and toes; macrocytic anemia	Serum B₁₂ B₁₂ isotope methods Urinary methylmalonic acid Schilling test
Vitamin C	Swollen, spongy, bleeding gums; petechiae; poor wound healing; heart degeneration; rough skin; pain in joints; anemia; depression (Toxicity: nausea, cramps, diarrhea)	Serum vitamin C Urinary vitamin C Vitamin C load test
Vitamin D	Bowing of legs; beading of ribs; knock knees, wrist enlargement; retarded growth; poor tooth formation; protruding abdomen; muscle spasms (Toxicity: loss of appetite; headache; thirst; irritability; stones in soft tissues)	Serum 25-hydroxycholecalciferol Serum alkaline phosphatase Serum calcium and phosphorus
Vitamin E	Edema in infants; hemolysis (Toxicity: impaired blood clotting, GI distress)	Hydrogen peroxide hemolysis test Plasma tocopherol
Vitamin K	*Bruising; slowed clotting time*	Prothrombin time

(continued)

somatic protein: the protein of voluntary muscles.

soma = body

visceral (VISS-er-ul) **protein:** the protein of the internal organs.

viscera = internal organs

antigen skin testing: a test of the immune system's competence, in which an antigen is applied to the skin. A reaction means the immune system is working normally.

TABLE 12–3 (continued)

MINERALS	PHYSICAL FINDINGS ASSOCIATED WITH DEFICIENCY/TOXICITY[a]	LABORATORY TESTS USED FOR ASSESSMENT
Calcium	Rickets; seizures; osteoporosis; osteomalacia	Serum calcium
Potassium	Muscle weakness (Toxicity: abnormal heart action)	Serum potassium
Magnesium	Tetany (extreme muscle contraction); muscle weakness; hallucinations	Serum magnesium
Iron	Pale nail beds, eye membranes, and palmar creases; fatigue; weakness; headaches; shortened attention span (Toxicity: infections; iron deposits in tissues)	Hemoglobin Hematocrit Iron binding capacity Serum ferritin
Iodine	Enlarged thyroid gland; sluggishness; weight gain	Serum protein-bound iodine Urinary iodine Radioiodine uptake
Zinc	Skin rash; hair loss; growth retardation; loss of taste and smell; weight loss; night blindness; infections; liver enlargement; apathy; irritability; slow wound healing (Toxicity: anemia; diarrhea; fever; pain; nausea; exhaustion)	Serum or plasma zinc Hair zinc concentration

[a] A table organized body system by body system appears in Appendix E.

be apparent in well-nourished persons; but in malnourished persons, they will not appear or will be very small, because the body is unable to resist the antigens.

Many factors other than nutrition can interfere with the immune response, and the value of skin testing as an index of nutrition status has been questioned. No studies to date have considered all the factors that might affect skin test results. Among known factors are age, certain allergies, and certain drug regimens.

Besides helping to assess PCM, laboratory testing can help assess nutrition status with respect to vitamins and minerals. The tests most often used are listed in Table 12–3 by each nutrient. As is true throughout the nutrition assessment procedure, the assessor must use caution in interpreting results of tests like these. Vitamin and mineral levels present in the blood may reflect disease processes, abnormal hormone levels, or other aberrations rather than dietary intake. Even if they reflect dietary intake, they may be affected by what the person has been eating recently, and may not give a true picture of the state of the person's nutrient stores; this sometimes makes it difficult to detect a subclinical deficiency. Furthermore, many nutrients interact. The assessor has to keep in mind that an abnormal lab value for one nutrient may reflect abnormal status with respect to other nutrients.

subclinical deficiency: see pp. 26, 45.

Nutrition Assessment Completed

Once the assessor has accumulated all the puzzle pieces available from the many types of data, she assembles them into a complete picture. All these pieces are needed to make sense of a person's nutrition status. The ultimate diagnosis is appropriately tentative and is confirmed only after careful remedial steps have been taken and have been shown to successfully alleviate the observed problems.

The procedure just described is a far cry from the kind of experience the man on the street may encounter when he walks into a "nutrition clinic" and is offered a "nutrition assessment" by a "nutritionist." People today are easily led to believe that computers or "hair analysis" will accurately determine their nutrition status. They do not understand all the processes involved in doing such tests but they see that the "experts" seem to know a lot and that the systems being used are very complicated, and so they think there must be some validity to the "results."

It is important to realize that while computers are invaluable for doing rapid calculations on valid data that have been assembled with care, they turn out utterly meaningless nonsense when used to process data that are meaningless at the start. ("Garbage in, garbage out.") Hopefully, anyone who has read this far in this book is aware that there are many nutrients for which we do not yet have accurate food composition data. For example, no one knows how much chromium is in the typical apple or orange. No one knows how much molybdenum is in a potato or a T-bone steak. No one can tell you for sure how much vitamin B_6 or B_{12} or fiber you have eaten even if you provide a detailed and painstaking record of every food that you have consumed over the last seven days. The food composition data for these and other nutrients are not yet complete enough to be used in this way. A computer program based on data such as those in Appendix H, which have been assembled with knowledge and care from well-tested lab-derived measurements of the nutrients in foods, can provide a serviceable approximation of a person's nutrient intakes if used appropriately. But a computer program that uses assigned values for nutrients that have not been as carefully studied, or a program that has been assembled hastily and carelessly, cannot compute nutrient intakes accurately. Such a program is a fraud.

Similarly you may have noticed that hair analysis was not mentioned as one of the clinical tests from which nutrition status information is obtained. Hair analyses are still in the experimental stage. They are being studied to determine what their validity and usefulness may be. One way in which we can use hairs for nutrition assessment is to pull them out and measure the size or protein content of the roots. This provides a clue to protein nutrition status, because hair roots diminish in size and protein content early in a developing protein deficiency. However, the minerals in the shaft of the hair are not known to reflect accurately the body's total content of minerals, except in the case of some toxic metal contaminants and possibly zinc—and then only for

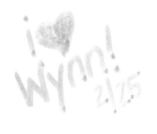

populations, not individuals. Hair analysis is a valuable method in research and shows promise as an assessment tool if the problems can be worked out, but at present it is not suitable for use in individual nutrition assessments. In several instances, hair contents of minerals have been demonstrated *not* to reflect body content in any consistent way.[1] Too many confounding variables interfere: air and water pollution, shampoos and dyes, water hardness, and many others.

We have singled out computer analysis and hair analysis as two practices that are being used by unscrupulous practitioners to elicit belief and extract money from an unsuspecting public. However, there are many other examples. The rule for the cautious consumer should be to stay skeptical. The fact that you do not understand, or haven't heard of, the method a "nutritionist" is using to test your nutrition status may not be a reflection on your limited knowledge. The test may simply be a fraud.

Caution

How Well Do We Eat?

Interest in the nutrition status of our people dates from before World War II, when a food-consumption survey suggested that as many as a third of the population might be poorly fed. Programs to correct nutrition problems have been evolving ever since. Significant among the early ones were:

● Enrichment of bread and cereal products. In those states that have enrichment legislation, refined bread and grain products must have iron, thiamin, riboflavin, and niacin added to make them comparable to whole-grain products in their contents of those nutrients.

● The National School Lunch Program. The school lunch makes available to public school children (in those districts that have adopted it) lunches that supply at least one-third of the RDA for all of the nutrients.

● Iodization of salt. In areas where the soil is iodine-poor, this is an important public health measure.

During the 1940s, 1950s, and 1960s, many surveys of the U.S. population were conducted. Nutrients found lacking in subgroups of the population were the minerals calcium and iron; the B vitamins thiamin and riboflavin; vitamin A; and occasionally vitamin C. Most vulnerable to nutrient deficiencies were girls, women, and elderly men; but no group was without some cases of iron deficiency. Other nutrients now known to be important—vitamin B$_6$, folacin, magnesium, and zinc, for example—were not studied in the early surveys.

---

1   R. S. Gibson, B. M. Anderson, and C. A. Scythes, Regional differences in hair zinc concentrations: A possible effect of water hardness, *American Journal of Clinical Nutrition* 37 (1983): 37–42; K. M. Hambidge, Hair analyses: Worthless for vitamins, limited for minerals, *American Journal of Clinical Nutrition* 36 (1982): 943–949.

During the 1970s, public awareness of the nutrition status of U.S. citizens reached a new high. The Senate's Poverty Subcommittee and the Select Committee on Nutrition and Human Needs held hearings, widely broadcast on national television, that projected a picture of the poor family unable to feed its children. Hunger and malnutrition in the United States became a controversy and a political issue, disclaimed by some who said the findings were exaggerated, and singled out by others who considered them a scandal and a national disgrace. The findings that generated the controversy arose from the Ten-State Survey, conducted in the late 1960s (1968–1970).

The Ten-State (National Nutrition) Survey

The ten states surveyed were California, Kentucky, Louisiana, Massachusetts, Michigan, South Carolina, Texas, Washington, New York, and West Virginia—chosen to represent geographic, ethnic, economic, and other features of the whole United States. Over 60,000 people were included.

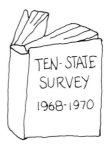

Not only food intake but also other indicators of nutrition status were used: clinical tests using blood and urine samples, physical examinations, anthropometric measures, and medical histories. Interviews were conducted, to gain insight into conditions likely to precipitate nutrient deficiencies or to have been caused by them. The subjects' educational levels and financial status were determined, and information about foods available to them was collected. The results were reported in relation to age, sex, ethnic background, and location (whether the person resided in a low-income or high-income state). The findings from such a survey might be slightly different today, but the kinds of information collected would be the same.

The physical examinations revealed few severe deficiencies—a good sign, indicating that nutrition knowledge and food intakes had improved enough to eliminate most of the worst cases of undernutrition seen in earlier years. Deficiencies were present, however, and it was clear that low-income and uneducated people had poorer nutrition in every respect, although wealthy, well-educated people could also have poor nutrition. Iron nutrition was still a problem in all groups, especially among blacks; vitamin A nutrition status was a major concern especially among teenagers and Spanish Americans. Riboflavin deficiency appeared to be a potential problem, especially among blacks, Spanish Americans, and young people of all ethnic groups. Iodized salt clearly had remained an important part of the diet in the north-central states; iodine deficiencies were not seen. Protein deficiency was not widespread but was seen more often in the poor than in the well-to-do. Pregnant women and those who were breastfeeding their babies had lower protein intakes and lower blood levels of protein than most other groups.

Indicators of nutrient deficiencies tended to cluster together. A person deficient in iron was likely to lack vitamin A as well, for example. Generally, blacks and Spanish Americans had a higher prevalence of multiple deficiencies; a higher prevalence also occurred in the low-income states. An important finding was that in families where the homemaker had completed fewer years of school, there were more multiple low values in the family members. Importantly, too, trends seen among the children were also seen in adults in the same families.

Anthropometric measures revealed that people with higher incomes had greater height, weight, fatness, skeletal weight, and other indicators of earlier and greater physical development. Blacks were taller than whites and were more advanced in skeletal and dental development, reflecting their genetic endowment. Obesity was more prominent in adult women, especially in black women.

Sugar intakes were high in most groups, and high sugar intakes were often seen together with dental decay, especially in adolescents. Low income accompanied dental decay in all groups.

Overall, several groups were found in need of help regarding their nutrition: obese people, blacks, Spanish and Mexican Americans, adolescents, and low-income families. The nutrients of greatest concern were iron, vitamin A, and riboflavin, with protein being a problem for pregnant and lactating women. Many nutrients were not studied, including vitamin B_6, folacin, magnesium, and zinc.

The Ten-State Survey provided a disturbing answer to the question "How well do U.S. citizens eat?" Clearly, not as well as might be expected in the most prosperous nation in the world. The identification of vulnerable groups confirmed the need for programs of many kinds to decrease the risk and incidence of nutrient deficiencies, and for continued surveillance of the U.S. population's nutrition status.

Nutrition Canada

Canada conducted a major survey of its people during the early 1970s. Over 19,000 people of all ages and all economic levels had medical, dental, and anthropometric examinations and a dietary interview; most also provided blood and urine samples for analysis. Among the findings were:

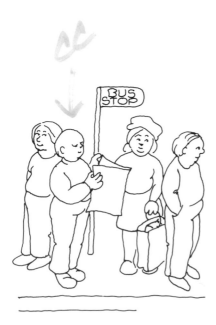

● The highest incidence of problems with nutrition status was found in lower-income middle-aged women and older men.
● A negative effect of low economic status on blood levels of certain nutrients, especially vitamin C and folacin, was seen.
● Evidence of iron-deficiency anemia in young and middle-aged women and elderly men was discovered.
● Evidence of low thiamin levels in adolescents and middle-aged adults was found.
● Considerable obesity was seen, especially in middle-aged adults.

The full report to the Canadian government appeared in 1974, and led to the establishment of priorities for government action to improve the nutrition status of Canadians. These included improved food-supply monitoring, consumer education programs, nutrition education for professionals, and continued surveillance of the nutritional health of the Canadian people.[2] The Canadian effort was praised by a critic who saw it as a model of "how to do a nutrition survey."[3]

The HANES and the Nationwide Food Consumption Survey

At about the same time (1971–1974), the U.S. National Center for Health Statistics conducted a study of over 20,000 people at 65 sampling sites in the United States. This study, known as the HANES (Health and Nutrition Examination Survey), avoided the bias of which the Ten-State Survey was accused by adjusting for the effects of oversampling among vulnerable groups. Careful efforts were also made to evaluate protein and kcalorie intakes in relation to height, sex, and age on an individual basis.[4]

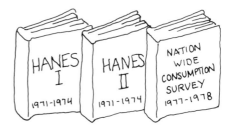

The investigators studied intakes of the same seven nutrients as previously, and niacin and kcalories in addition. Nutrient deficiencies were found only for protein, calcium, vitamin A, and iron. As expected, these were more extensive among people below the poverty line than among those above and generally more extensive in blacks than in whites. In particular:

- Protein intakes were low for low-income adolescents, women, and older men and for middle- and upper-income black women, older black men, and older white women.
- Calcium intakes were low for adult black women of all income groups.
- Vitamin A intakes were low for low-income white adolescents and young adult women and for adolescent black girls of all income groups.
- Iron intakes were low for all women and for infant boys regardless of income.[5]

HANES II, undertaken in 1977 as a follow-up to HANES, was designed to collect biochemical and other data, with an emphasis on determining whether the physical condition of the subjects studied reflected the nutrient intakes found earlier. Particularly, the investigators wondered whether the test results would reflect the extensive low iron intakes known to exist in the population. As of 1981, with funding becoming increasingly limited for analysis of the data, the results were just becoming available, and indeed, low blood and urine values were found:

2   Z. I. Sabry, J. A. Campbell, M. E. Campbell, and A. L. Forbes, Nutrition Canada, *Nutrition Today*, January/February 1974, pp. 5–13.

3   C. F. Enloe, Jr., How to do a nutrition survey (editorial), *Nutrition Today*, January/February 1974, p. 14.

4   S. Abraham, M. D. Carroll, C. M. Dresser, and C. L. Johnson, Dietary intake of persons 1–74 years of age in the United States, *Advance data from Vital and Health Statistics of the National Center for Health Statistics*, vol. 6, publication no. (HRA) 77–1250 (Rockville, Md.: U.S. Department of Health, Education, and Welfare, Public Health Service, Health Resources Administration, March 30, 1977).

5   P. Gunby, Federal agencies view food habit surveys (Medical News), *Journal of the American Medical Association* 244 (1980): 1536.

- For protein and vitamin A, in less than 3 percent of subjects.
- For thiamin, in 14 percent of white and 29 percent of black subjects.
- For riboflavin, in 3 percent of white and 8 percent of black subjects.
- For iron, by three measures, in 5 to 15 percent of white and 18 to 27 percent of black subjects.

Not everyone with low intakes of a nutrient had low lab values, and the investigators suggested that those with low intakes were "at risk" for malnutrition.[6]

In measuring the heights and weights of people, the HANES researchers observed that there is a continuing trend toward higher amounts of body fat among fatter Americans.[7] It has long been known that improved nutrition, and especially adequate intakes of protein, could alter the average height of a population over several generations. (A well-known example is the case of the Japanese, whose children after World War II grew taller than their parents thanks to the availability of more meat, as described in Chapter 14.) However, the trend toward higher weights in Americans reflects overnutrition, not "good" nutrition.

Trends in growth seen over years or generations and accounted for by changes in diet are known as **secular** trends. See Chapter 14.

Caution has to be exercised in interpreting the HANES study. As the researchers themselves pointed out, "High mean intakes can mask the fact that a substantial proportion of individuals within a group may have usual nutrient intakes far below the recommended dietary allowances."[8] In other words, severe deficiencies in individuals can be missed. On the other hand, findings based on a single day's intake—as the HANES findings were —can overestimate the extent of undernutrition. A critic notes: "All of us eat less than our usual intake half of the time. If we had an ideal survey of an ideal population [it] would still show 50 percent below standard over any relatively short period of time."[9] These two limitations of the HANES tend to cancel each other out. The survey's principal usefulness is in identifying the population subgroups most at risk of deficiency and the nutrients most in need of attention.

Further study is needed. In particular, the choice of indicator nutrients should be reexamined. Inadequate intakes may be more prevalent for vitamin B_6, zinc, magnesium, and folacin than for many of the nutrients usually covered in earlier surveys.[10]

Considerable savings in the cost of surveys could be achieved if the number of indicators could be reduced without loss of valuable information. A retrospective analysis of the Ten-State Survey data shows that this

6   G. R. Kerr and coauthors, Relationships between dietary and biochemical measures of nutritional status in HANES I data, *American Journal of Clinical Nutrition* 34 (1981): 294–307.

7   C. E. Cronk and A. F. Roche, Race- and sex-specific reference data for triceps and subscapular skinfolds and weight/stature, *American Journal of Clinical Nutrition* 35 (1982): 347–354.

8   Abraham and coauthors, 1977.

9   D. M. Hegsted, Energy needs and energy utilization, in *Nutrition Reviews' Present Knowledge in Nutrition*, 4th ed. (Washington, D.C.: Nutrition Foundation, 1976), pp. 1–9.

10   H. A. Guthrie and C. M. Guthrie, Factor analysis of nutritional status data from Ten State Nutrition Survey, *American Journal of Clinical Nutrition* 29 (1976): 1238–1241.

could be done, but that folacin should be included in any survey.[11] Folacin deficiency is probably the most common vitamin deficiency of all.[12]

Following HANES, another survey—the Nationwide Food Consumption Survey—was conducted in 1977–1978, to see how much and what kind of food people were eating at home and outside the home. Both surveys confirmed a dawning suspicion: that in spite of widespread obesity, people are not eating large amounts of kcalories. Although they are fat and getting fatter, their food consumption appears to be quite modest. This must mean that they are extraordinarily inactive. The average woman consuming the foods typically available to her, who stays within the kcalorie allowance that will maintain her weight, will fail to obtain RDA amounts of several nutrients.[13] Figure 12–1 compares the energy intakes found with those recommended.

The Nationwide Food Consumption Survey, like the Ten-State Survey, showed dietary adequacy related to income. Table 12–4 shows the results for six nutrients. People with lower incomes had lower intakes of five of them. Since 19 million people in the United States are now living at or below the poverty line, these nutrition problems are quite widespread.

Table 12–4 makes it appear that the people surveyed were most seriously underconsuming vitamin B_6, but it has to be remembered that people who are getting by on minimal amounts of protein need less vitamin B_6 to process that protein; so real deficiency problems may not be as widespread as they appear to be. The same can be said for the other nutrients. Although a person consuming only two-thirds of the RDA for a nutrient is clearly closer to the "at risk" line, he still may not be actually deficient. Where that line is, exactly, we do not know. An impression of the possible areas of concern, however, can be gained from Table 12–4.

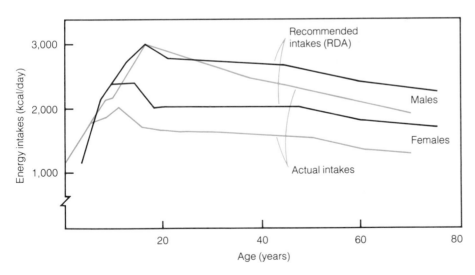

FIGURE 12–1 **Energy intakes found in the HANES survey, compared with the recommended intakes.**

Source: D. M. Hegsted, Agricultural potentials, in *Plasma Lipids: Optimal Levels for Health*, American Health Foundation (New York: Academic Press, 1980): pp. 143–153; Table 1, p. 144.

11   Hegsted, 1976.

12   C. L. Krumdieck, Folic acid, in *Nutrition Reviews' Present Knowledge*, 1976, pp. 175–190.

13   Implications from a recent Nationwide Food Consumption Survey, *Journal of the American Dietetic Association* 77 (1980): 473.

TABLE 12–4   **Persons with Nutrient Intakes at or below 70% of RDA**[a]

NUTRIENT	INCOME TO $6,000	INCOME $6,000 TO $9,999	INCOME $10,000 TO $15,999	INCOME $16,000 AND OVER
Vitamin A	36%	33%	32%	29%
Vitamin B$_6$[b]	59%	51%	49%	48%
Vitamin C	30%	29%	27%	23%
Calcium	49%	43%	39%	39%
Iron	29%	31%	33%	33%
Magnesium	48%	40%	36%	35%

[a] Data represent percentage of persons in each income group with intakes at or below 70% of RDA. Example: 36% of all those surveyed whose incomes were at or below $6,000 per year had vitamin A intakes below 70% of the RDA.

[b] Vitamin B$_6$ intakes may not be as deficient as they appear. People who get along on minimal protein intakes need less than the RDA of vitamin B$_6$ to handle the amount of protein they consume.

Source: USDA Nationwide Food Consumption Survey, 1977–1978.

Folacin and zinc intakes were not assessed in the Nationwide Food Consumption Survey; insufficient data are available on food contents of these nutrients and on the factors in food that affect their assimilation and use by the body. When further research makes it possible to include these two nutrients in a survey, it will be highly desirable to do so, because deficiencies of both nutrients are suspected in our population.

The survey data were analyzed not only with respect to nutrient intakes but also—in light of the U.S. *Dietary Goals* (Chapter 1)—with respect to sodium, fat, sugar, and cholesterol intakes. Sodium intakes were impossible to determine (how can a person report accurately the amount of salt he pours from the salt shaker?) but the following findings were of interest:

● Very few of those surveyed had fat intakes below 30 percent of kcalories (as suggested by the U.S. *Dietary Goals*).
● Sugar constituted 10 to 15 percent of the kcalorie intakes of most children. (The *Goals* recommend that it not exceed 10 percent.)
● Cholesterol intakes ranged up to 450–500 milligrams in boys and men. (The *Goals* suggest 300 milligrams as an upper limit.)

The health significance of these findings is uncertain, but they provide a base of information about our people's food choices that was not available before.

The Nationwide Food Consumption Survey also revealed that, as one reviewer said, all Americans seem to be eating "from a common table." In other words, most people are eating similar kinds and amounts of food. Probably, therefore, guidelines stated in terms of these foods would benefit everyone.

In offering nutrition guidelines to individuals and groups, dietitians, nutrition educators, and other health professionals have most often used the Four Food Group Plan, already described. A movement is now afoot to improve on that plan, perhaps replacing it with several plans, each suitable for a different subgroup of the population.

The many surveys recently conducted have yielded enough information so that it is possible to ask the research questions "What food consumption patterns do people actually follow?"[14] and "Which of these food patterns are found in the groups with the best nutrition status?"[15] From the answers to these questions, more specific guidelines may develop, tailored to people's specific nutrient needs and based on the patterns they already follow. The "average" man, for example, would be advised to eat more vegetables, fruits, beans, and nuts; more cereal and pasta; more bread and bakery products; less meat, fish, and poultry; and fewer eggs.

Meanwhile, what can you do about your own nutrition status? Knowing as much as you do about the nutrients you need and about the foods that supply them, you still have to work out a way to combine those foods into a healthful eating plan, and tailor that eating plan to your individual or family lifestyle. How can you integrate all that you know into a way of life in which meals yield up all the benefits you want from them: social enjoyment, sensory pleasure, ease of preparation, economy, *and* good health?

Eating is not, after all, just a matter of delivering nutrients to the body. Nor do people choose foods solely for their nutrient contributions. Food choices are irrational, to a great extent, and very resistant to change. Before undertaking diet planning, the planner must understand the dynamics of food choices, because she must honor people's food preferences when attempting to alter or influence their eating habits.

Food Choices

Among the reasons why you chose the foods you ate today may be any of the following:

- Personal preference (I like them).
- Habit or tradition (they are familiar; I always eat them).
- Social pressure (they were offered; I couldn't refuse).
- Availability (there were no others to choose from).
- Convenience (I was too rushed to prepare anything else).
- Economy (they were within my means).
- Nutritional value (I thought they were good for me).

Of these seven possible reasons, only one has to do with nutrition directly. Even people who pride themselves on obtaining good nutritional value in their meals will admit that the other six factors listed here also influence their food choices. Such being the case, it would be unrealistic to approach diet planning without taking all these factors into account. The only diet plan that will work is one that is in harmony with a person's preferences, social life, habits, environment, economic status, and lifestyle. No matter how nutritious a meal is, it cannot benefit a person's health until it is eaten.

14   F. J. Cronin, S. M. Krebs-Smith, B. W. Wyse, and L. Light, Characterizing food usage by demographic variables, *Journal of the American Dietetic Association* 81 (1982): 661–673.

15   H. S. Schwerin and coauthors, Food eating patterns and health—a reexamination of the Ten-State and HANES I surveys, *American Journal of Clinical Nutrition* 34 (1981): 568–580.

Personal Preference, Habit, Tradition

Why do we like certain foods? One reason, of course, is our preferences for certain tastes, and two of these preferences are widely shared: the tastes for sugar and salt. The taste sensors probably helped early humans to distinguish between edible and toxic substances, while their enjoyment encouraged them to eat large amounts to keep them alive until they found more food. Once, the tasty flavors of sugar and salt were available only from whole, natural foods; so they promoted behavior that benefitted health. The sweet and salty tastes helped people identify life-giving fruits, vegetables, and grains; the liking for the salty taste also ensured that they would consume sufficient quantities of the two important minerals, sodium and chloride. Today, now that sugar and salt are available in pure form, our instinctive liking for them can lead us to overconsume foods to which they have been added—sometimes to the point of doing ourselves harm. Only nutrition education can counter this tendency.

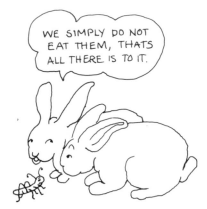

WE SIMPLY DO NOT EAT THEM, THATS ALL THERE IS TO IT.

Instinctive liking is one kind, but there are other kinds of liking—some of them almost as deep-seated and often as powerful. You like foods with which you have happy associations—those you eat in the midst of a warm family gathering at traditional holiday times, those someone who loved you gave you as a child, or those eaten by people you admire. By the same token, intense dislike—strong enough to be unalterable—can be attached to foods that you ate when you were sick, or that were forced on you when you weren't hungry, or that are eaten by people you don't respect. Your parents may have taught you to like and dislike certain foods for reasons of their own like these, without even being aware of the reasons. In fact, a parent may say to a child, "Eat that, it's good for you," without realizing that his great-grandparents told their children the same thing, and that what is being passed on is not necessarily wisdom, but generations of family custom.

Social Pressure

Social pressure is a powerful influence on food behavior. How can you refuse when your friends are going out for pizza and beer (or ice cream, or donuts)? Such pressure operates in all circles and across cultural lines. It is considered rude not to accept food or drink being shared by a group or offered by a host; you are not a member of the social gathering until you do. In today's world, where food is abundant, people are hard-pressed to find polite ways of refusing food that, in their self-interest, they must refuse. Many yield, if not to the temptation of the food itself, then to the pressure of social obligation.

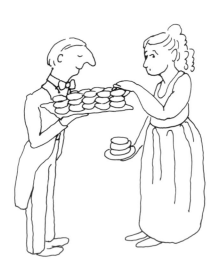

Availability, Convenience, Economy

We live in an era when we can choose our foods from among thousands of items on the supermarket shelf.[16] They have come from all over the world,

---

16 Parts of the following discussion are adapted from E. M. N. Hamilton and E. N. Whitney, *The problem of food choices,* in *Nutrition: Concepts and Controversies* (St. Paul, Minn.: West, 1979), pp. 7–8.

thanks to the efficiency of modern transportation systems. Modern techniques of processing and preserving foods permit long-term storage; many food items can sit on the shelf for years and still be safe to use. Fast-freezing methods now preserve the freshness of the harvest. Even after long trips in refrigerated trucks, extended time in the freezer section of the grocery store, and more time in your own freezer, spring and summer favorites like strawberries and corn on the cob can be enjoyed in the dead of winter. The cost of this luxury has been kept down by the increased productivity of our farmers. With effective pesticides and fertilizers, farmers have been able to increase their yields so that they not only feed the growing population at home but also keep the United States and Canada among the few remaining exporters of food in the world.

Not only is an abundance of foods available, but many have been made convenient in ways our grandparents never dreamed of—frozen meals, soup mixes, breakfast bars, total nutrition powders. Many foods have also been suited to our tastes by the addition of sugar and salt. These new foods have not been with us long enough to have stood the test of time. As they replace traditional foods, we will need to know to what extent they offer the nutrients we need.

The abundant, low-cost, and constant food supply has not been an unmixed blessing. Artificial fertilizers, mechanization of the farm, and burgeoning transportation needs have put serious drains on our energy supply. Also, to support our growing population, more and more farmland is being covered with concrete highways and with cities that depend on those highways for their food. Pesticides and fertilizers run off into our streams and lakes, polluting the water supply and contaminating the food chain. Among the factors affecting our food choices in the future, two questions must become increasingly important: "How much energy was required to produce this food?" and "How did the production of this food affect the environment?" Up to today, these questions have had little or no bearing on people's food choices.

Nutritional Value

People are more nutrition-conscious today than ever before. While the many factors discussed above influence everyone's food choices, the perceived nutritional value of food also has weight. But people often do not know how to choose among the many delicious, affordable foods available. The next section offers a summary that may be helpful.

Diet Planning

There is no such thing as "the perfect diet." And even if one person could devise "the perfect diet" for himself, it would not be suitable for the next person. Planners have to consider many factors in designing diets—all of those just mentioned, and many more. They also have many different foods to deal with, and there may be no overlap at all between the foods acceptable to a person of one nationality and those preferred by another. To complicate the task further, foods are not so simple as they once were. A hundred years ago, wherever you might have looked in the Western world, you would have found people eating the same basic types of foods—milk and dairy products, legumes, nuts, meats, vegetables, fruits, grains. But now we have to contend with TV dinners, vegeburgers, instant fruit drinks, engineered foods of all descriptions. The guidelines once offered in the past don't seem to apply to those foods. How does the Four Food Group Plan classify a vegeburger?

It can be done. It is still useful to think in terms of food groups for a start. Having reviewed the information about them from all the previous chapters, we can then add in the new foods with increased awareness and understanding of their place and value. The next few paragraphs review the suggestions offered so far, and then put the new foods in their places. (Remember that in the chapters these suggestions were surrounded by discussion of pros and cons. They are only suggestions, not "rules.")

See Chapter 2 for details.

Carbohydrate: Select foods high in complex carbohydrate, both starch and fiber (*grains, seeds, tubers, legumes, starchy vegetables*), and in naturally occurring sugars (*fruits, vegetables*). Avoid the overuse of concentrated sweets (*sugar, honey, cola beverages, cakes, candies,* and the like).

See Chapter 3.

Fat: Be moderate in the use of fat-rich foods (*meats, nuts*) and pure fats (*butter, margarine, oils*), and balance your saturated fat intake with an approximately equal amount of polyunsaturated fat.

See Chapter 4.

Protein: Obtain adequate but not excessive amounts of protein, making sure to get high-quality protein from at least one source (*meats, fish, poultry, eggs, cheese, milk*). Or, combine protein-containing foods so as to get high-quality protein from the combination (*grains* and *legumes*).

The vegetarian's strategy of combining foods to maximize protein quality is known as **mutual supplementation** or the use of **complementary proteins.** See note at end of chapter.

kCalories: Control kcalories so that the energy you take in from food equals the energy you expend for daily activities. If you are overweight, reduce kcalorie intake and increase activity in order to lose weight gradually.

See Chapters 6 and 7.

Alcohol (contributes kcalories, so is included here): Use in moderation, if at all.

See Chapters 8–11.

Vitamins and minerals: Choose foods that will supply ample amounts of all the essential vitamins and minerals, being careful to include a good vitamin A source (a serving of *dark-green or deep-orange vegetable or fruit*) at least every other day; a good vitamin C source (a serving of *citrus fruit or the equivalent*) every day; and a good calcium source (2 to 3 cups of *milk or the equivalent*) every day. Because vitamins and minerals—especially trace minerals—are lost when foods are refined or otherwise processed, emphasize *unrefined, unprocessed foods* in diet planning.

See Chapter 10.

Salt (sodium): Be moderate in its use, and if you have hypertension in your family, avoid sodium-rich foods and substitute potassium-rich foods (*whole, fresh fruits and vegetables*).

See Chapter 11.

Iodine: In areas where the soil is poor in iodine, be sure to use *iodized salt.*

Fluoride: Be aware whether the water supply in your area is fluoridated or contains 1 ppm or more fluoride naturally. If it lacks fluoride, follow your dentist's advice regarding toothpaste or fluoride applications to protect your family's teeth from decay.

See Chapter 11.

All these principles are familiar by now, as is the time-honored plan usually used as a guideline to abide by them: the Four Food Group Plan or its modified version that includes legumes. But the menu planner of today has to answer many questions:

● "Casseroles and soups don't fit in the Four Food Group Plan, but they are nutritious, aren't they?"
● "I like to eat Italian-style; is pizza (or lasagna or spaghetti and meatballs) good for you?"
● "I eat in restaurants all the time, usually fast-food places. When I do cook at home it's TV dinners or instant meals. Am I dying a slow death from malnutrition?"
● "I don't eat meat, fish, or poultry. How can I make my diet adequate?"

All these different kinds of people can assure themselves of good nutrition by learning a few facts about foods.

To answer the first two questions very briefly: Any combination of conventional foods can be fitted into the food groups with a little thought. A cup of vegetable soup, for example, could be considered to be roughly a serving of vegetables (ignore the broth as if it were mostly water). A cup of cream soup prepared with milk is nearly equal to a cup of milk. A slice of pizza could be counted roughly as a slice of bread and 1 fat (the dough) with the equivalent in calcium and protein of a cup of milk (if it's thickly coated with cheese) and a portion of vegetables (if it has, say, a half-cup or more of tomato and other vegetable topping on it). Basically, you simply use your common sense and your knowledge of what went into each dish.

No matter what country's cuisine you like, a little inspection will show that the custom of that country has evolved a balance of foods that meets people's nutrient needs. In Italy, the milk group is often represented by cheese; meats are included as such; the grains appear as pasta; and the vegetables are similar to those of North America. In China (to give one more example), the milk group is not apparent (Chinese adults don't use milk); rather, liberal uses of soybeans and soybean curd supply the needed calcium. Meats, again, appear as such; the grain is almost invariably rice; and there is an abundance of fruits and vegetables.

This short discussion should serve to answer the first two questions and illustrate the point that there is no one right diet, that many different ways of combining conventional foods can produce adequacy and balance. But the third question is more difficult to answer. What about the new foods?

Coping with the New Foods

The understandings won from learning to read labels can help you to mix and match new and traditional foods to your advantage. Dr. Daniel Rosenfield, director of nutrition affairs at Miles Laboratories, points out that even an imitation food, while inferior to conventional foods by a legal definition, might have desirably lower levels of some components and might be nutritionally superior.[17]

Many people fear that the new foods are inferior, however. Some are so put off by them that they try to avoid them altogether. Most use them with mixed feelings; the pleasure of the really delightful taste sensations sometimes offered is tainted with anxiety and guilt. (Some don't even think about it, of course.) Whatever your feelings on the subject, the chances are that you can't escape the new foods altogether. They are part of modern life, and in many ways a desirable part. They are easy to store and prepare, they save a tremendous amount of time and effort, and they are often tasty. Formulated foods used in school lunches are acceptable to children, who waste less of them, and they are lower in cost than conventional foods.[18] They have won wide acceptance in institutional settings as well as by homemakers and individual consumers, and their use is on the rise.[19] Rather than trying to avoid them altogether, it makes sense to learn to use them to your advantage.

Not all are of equal value. A substitute for hamburger made from textured soy protein, soy flour, wheat germ, and artificial flavors and colors may be lower in fat, higher in fiber, and equal in protein quality to a hamburger— that is, superior for some purposes. On the other hand, a TV dinner may cost twice as much as, and provide fewer nutrients than, the same meal prepared from the raw materials at home; and a fast-food meal may be three times as expensive as its home-made equivalent. The habitual use of a fortified breakfast cereal may prevent iron deficiency in a woman whose kcalorie intake is low; but the use of toasted, jam-filled, unenriched pastries for breakfast by her children may dilute the nutrients in their day's menus. (Highlight 2 defined *empty-kcalorie foods* and showed their nutrient contributions in a table.)

A strategy for dealing with the new foods is based on several principles. First, ask yourself how often you eat the food in question. The more often you use a food product, the more impact it will have on your diet, and the more important it is to be aware of the contributions it is, or isn't, making.

Second, consider a food's nutrient contributions in the context of the other foods in your diet. For example, the lack of vitamin C in the potato chips you eat is of no concern to you if you drink plenty of fruit juice, especially citrus juice, every day. But if you are relying on a food as a staple, to provide the nutrients usually contributed by a class of similar foods—for example, if you are regularly using a meat substitute in place of meat or soy milk instead of milk—then you owe it to yourself to be sure that the substitute provides the same nutrients the missing food would provide and

17   D. Rosenfield, Nutritional optimization of new foods (commentary), *Journal of the American Dietetic Association* 72 (1978): 475–477.

18   M. K. Head and R. J. Weeks, Conventional vs. formulated foods in school lunches: 2. Cost of food served, eaten, and wasted, *Journal of the American Dietetic Association* 71 (1977): 629–632.

19   C. P. Greecher and B. Shannon, Impact of fast food meals on nutrient intake of two groups, *Journal of the American Dietetic Association* 70 (1977): 368–372; Fast food expansion predicted (new items), *Journal of the American Dietetic Association* 70 (1977): 372.

is of high quality. (A cup of soy milk contributes only 20 milligrams of calcium whereas a cup of cow's milk contributes almost 300 milligrams.)

Third, keep the kcalories in mind. No matter how attractive, if a food you often use donates more kcalories than you can afford to consume, you have a hard fact to face up to. The concept of nutrient density is useful in this connection, and an exercise in Appendix Q is devoted to it.

nutrient density: see p. 12.

Finally, put the spotlight on yourself. No matter how nutritious the food you eat, it cannot compensate for other flaws in your lifestyle. A balanced, health-oriented approach to life including adequate rest, some exercise, and adequate time for meals at appropriate intervals will pay off in dividends no selection of foods by itself can offer you. Within such a context, common sense should help you to avoid unnecessary extremes. It is probably true that you should try to include foods that contribute vitamin C in every day's meals. On the other hand, the idea that you should always eat farm-fresh foods, sitting down, with a placemat under your plate and a linen napkin in your lap, reflects a set of values that you may or may not wish to call your own. Drinking your breakfast or bringing home your family's dinner in a bucket can be part of a satisfactory nutrition picture and of a lifestyle that you find comfortable and acceptable. For ourselves, it seems appropriate to draw the line where adequate, balanced, and safe nutrition is achieved and to be open-minded about all other options.

We have come a long way from the introduction of the term *nutrient* in Chapter 1 to the conclusion of this section on diet planning. Readers who have followed the path through all its turnings should consider themselves well grounded in the basics of nutrition. To apply these basics to individuals requires still another framework of knowledge: the framework supplied by facts about people's changing nutrition concerns at different ages and stages of life. The next chapters are devoted to nutrition through the life cycle, from conception to old age.

Summing Up

To learn whether an individual's nutrient needs are being met, the dietitian or other health professional performs a nutrition assessment, which involves several methods. Information is gathered on the person's medical, social, diet, and drug history. Anthropometric measurements provide an indirect assessment of skeletal muscle and body fat. A physical exam identifies possible clinical signs of malnutrition; and biochemical measurements confirm it and detect subclinical malnutrition. The above methods are also used to furnish information on the nutrition status of whole populations.

Programs designed to meet nutritional needs identified by early surveys include the enrichment of breads and cereals, the National School Lunch Program, and the iodization of salt. Recent surveys have identified other problems. The Ten State Survey of 1968–1970 showed that groups in need of nutritional help were blacks, Spanish and Mexican Americans, adolescents, and low-income groups. A problem of great magnitude was obesity. Among the nutrients studied, those of greatest concern were iron, vitamin A, and riboflavin. Protein was a problem for pregnant and lactating women. Many nutrients (including vitamins B₆ and folacin, zinc, and magnesium) were not evaluated.

A later survey, the HANES, identified infants, adolescents, and women of childbearing years as most at risk and the nutrient iron as being low enough in the U.S. diet to be a major public health concern.

Following HANES, the Nationwide Food Consumption Survey was conducted to see how much and what kinds of food people were eating at home and outside the home. There is general agreement that both U.S. and Canadian consumers need to eat more complex carbohydrates and less fat, sugar, and salt than they have been eating in recent years.

To combine foods into a healthy eating plan, a person's food preferences, social life, habits, environment, economic status, and lifestyle must be taken into account. The diet planner must remember that food cannot benefit a person's health until it is eaten.

Diet planners today are encouraged to emphasize the use of complex carbohydrates; high-quality protein; whole, fresh fruits (including citrus fruits) and vegetables (including dark green vegetables); and unrefined grain products; to be moderate in their use of fat, salt, sugar, and alcohol; and to check on the availability of iodine and fluoride in their food and water supplies. In using the Four Food Group Plan, they are encouraged to be flexible, including mixed dishes such as soups and casseroles, foods from other countries, and new foods, with an awareness of their nutritional quality. Many different personal styles are compatible with good nutritional health.

NOTE: References in Appendix J relevant to this chapter's topics are included under "Assessment of Nutrition Status," "Surveys," and "Food Choices."

The Self-Study for this chapter shows you how to:

● Evaluate the nutrient density of foods you like.
● Review your diet and critique its adequacy in light of all you have learned from this book.
● Single out the food choices you make that contribute most to your nutritional health, and those that contribute least; identify desirable changes that would be acceptable to you.

The *Instructor's Manual* includes an extra transparency/handout master on Federal Assistance Programs (TH12-1) and another demonstrating a technique for visualizing the nutrient density of foods (TH12-2). It also includes two supplementary lectures, "Diet Planning for the Vegetarian," and "Foods in the Home."

HIGHLIGHT 12

The New Foods and Nutrition Labeling

[If a] shopper is thoughtful, . . . [he] scratches his head. How much thiamin, he asks himself, is 0.09 mg?

RONALD M. DEUTSCH

The nutrition scene in the United States and Canada is changing fast. New in the picture since the 1940s are all kinds of foods: fast foods, convenience foods, fabricated foods, engineered foods. All of these are prepared by people other than ourselves, and there are more of them all the time.

According to one estimate, about half of all meals, whether consumed in restaurants, fast-food places, or at home, are now prepared outside the home. Among the trends creating the demand for these foods is the recruitment of women into the work force. The number of working mothers has more than doubled in the past two decades. Only 10 percent of all people in this country eat lunch at home even once a week, except on weekends. Thus reliance on the new foods, which are easy to store and carry along and quick to prepare, is greater than it has ever been before. But people who use these foods daily may be inclined to wonder what sort of nutrient contributions they make.

Those who oppose and fear this trend say that the new foods are "empty-kcalorie foods," "junk foods," and that often—because their labels claim large amounts of vitamins and minerals—they are fraudulently called nutritious. Others applaud the new technology, which represents the achievements of thousands of laboratory-trained food scientists. Before getting into the pros and cons of this issue, it is helpful to define some of the terms (see Miniglossary).

The fast foods are those prepared in quick-order restaurants, such as the hamburger stands and fried-chicken places that line our nation's main streets and highways. Convenience foods are those prepared at home from foods that have already been cooked or otherwise processed before reaching the market. They include:

- Cold breakfast cereals, to which you add milk and sugar.
- Powdered drinks, to which you add water and ice.
- Preprepared meals and desserts, to which you add water or milk and then stir, cook, and serve hot or cold.
- Canned foods that you open, heat if desired, and serve.

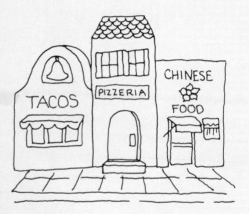

The complete nutrient contents of typical fast foods are shown in Appendix N.

Miniglossary of Food Types

convenience food: a food prepared or packaged in such a way that it is easy to cook and serve at home.

empty-kcalorie food: a popular term used to denote foods that contain no nutrients, only kcalories. Actually, almost all foods contain some nutrients. Therefore most nutritionists prefer to say "food of low nutrient density." A table on p. 79 makes clear the meaning of empty kcalories.

engineered food: a food subject to a complex technical process, such as extraction of certain components.

fabricated food: a food put together from highly processed ingredients, such as substitute-meat-burgers made from textured vegetable protein.

fast food: food prepared quickly in a fast-food restaurant such as a hamburger stand or fried-chicken place.

imitation food: a food nutritionally inferior to the food it imitates. This term must by law appear on the label of a food if it contains 10 percent less of the U.S. RDA of an essential nutrient than the food it imitates.

junk food: a popular term used to denote foods that are "bad" for one—for example, foods high in salt, sugar, or fat content.

natural food: an unprocessed food; a term often mistakenly used as synonymous with "good for you."

nutritious food: a food with high nutrient density.

processed food: any food subjected to a process such as enrichment, refining, fortification, alteration of texture, mixing, or cooking.

● Frozen foods such as frozen vegetables, concentrated juices, and TV dinners.

All of these convenience foods are processed foods—cooked, frozen, freeze-dried, or the like. Some are natural foods, in the sense that they are prepared from farm-grown animal or plant foods (for example, concentrated orange juice, frozen vegetables, bread made from whole-wheat flour). Others are engineered foods, or fabricated foods, made entirely from ingredients purified and mixed in laboratories (for example, drinks composed of sugar, additives, colors, and vitamins). Fabricated foods may be called *imitation foods*, a term whose use on labels now has precise legal limits.

The terms *junk food* and *empty-kcalorie food* may be applied to any food by a person who feels that it has little or no nutritional value. Snack foods found in convenience stores are most often deemed junk, especially if they contain large amounts of sugar, fat, or salt. *Empty-kcalorie food* is a less emotion-laden term, referring to foods of low nutrient density. The user of these terms often contrasts them with *health foods* and *organic foods*—but these terms may also be misleading.

Finally, there are enriched and fortified foods. You may remember that *enrichment* traditionally refers to addition of four nutrients (iron, thiamin, riboflavin, and niacin) to refined grain, from which they have been lost in

More about "health foods" and "organic foods"—Highlight 1A.

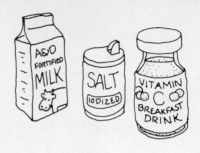

processing, in the approximate amounts in which they were originally present (double, in the case of riboflavin). *Fortification* refers to the addition of any nutrient to a food, even one that may not have been there originally, and may involve adding nutrients in amounts well above those found naturally in a food. A fortified breakfast cereal may have such large quantities of nutrients added that one serving provides 100 percent of the U.S. RDA for all of them. Other examples of fortified foods are

● Salt to which iodine is added.
● Milk to which vitamins A and D are added.
● An orange-colored drink composed mostly of sugar to which vitamin C is added.

The canny consumer will realize that the word *fortified* sometimes conveys an emptiness of other nutrients. Fruit *juice* is more nutritious than fortified fruit *drink*, even though the drink may be higher in vitamin C content.

To understand the issue, recall that the nutrients that have to be listed on labels that make nutrition claims are only a few of the essential nutrients and are in no way more important than the unlisted ones. Their appearance on the label makes the food look more nutritious than it really is—because they may be the *only* nutrients present. This problem has been a theme throughout this book, from the first comparison made between an orange and a vitamin C pill. Many authorities have expressed concern about it.

A desirable solution may be to relieve consumers of the burden of reading details on labels by allowing certain foods to state that they are nutritious. To accomplish this, the designers of legislation will have to define the term *nutritious* very carefully. As you might expect, proposals make use of the concept of nutrient density.

The object is to distinguish between nourishing foods—those that provide some nutrients besides kcalories—and *nutritious foods*, a term that requires a very precise definition. To identify a nutritious food, you have to consider two questions:

● How much of the nutrients does a serving of this food supply in relation to my need?
● How many kcalories does a serving supply in relation to my need?

If the food supplies half your daily allowance for a vitamin and at the same time only one-tenth of your daily allowance for kcalories, then it is a very good source of that vitamin. You could obtain a substantial quantity of the vitamin from it, at a low kcalorie cost. A Self-Study in Appendix Q offers practice estimating nutrient density.

The new foods have made it more important than ever for consumers to be able to read food labels, and to read between the lines. The rest of this Highlight offers the basic information you need in order to become an informed reader of food labels.

Claims and Information on Labels

First of all, according to law, all labels must state:

Food, Drug, and Cosmetic Act, 1938.

● The common name of the product.

- The name and address of the manufacturer, packer, or distributor.
- The net contents in terms of weight, measure, or count.
- The ingredients listed in descending order of predominance by weight.

This information has to be prominently displayed, and must be expressed in ordinary words. That's all there is to the required label—but if you know how to read the front and side of a package you're already a step ahead of the naive buyer. This is particularly true in regard to the ingredient list. Whatever is listed first is what the package contains the largest amount of. Consider the following ingredient lists:

- An orange powder that contains "Sugar, citric acid, orange flavor..." versus a juice can that contains "Water, tomato concentrate, concentrated juices of carrots, celery...."
- A cereal that contains "Puffed milled corn, sugar, corn syrup, molasses, salt..." versus one that contains "100% rolled oats."
- A canned fruit that contains nothing but "Apples, water."

If you read the label, you know what you're getting, and what the main ingredient is. Figure H12–1 demonstrates the reading of a label.

Labels often tell you more than the minimum, however. If a nutrient is added to a food (for example, vitamin D to a breakfast drink), or if an advertising claim is made (for example, that orange juice is a good source of vitamin C), then the package must provide an information panel that complies *fully* with the nutrition labeling requirements. Without a complete information panel, nutrition claims could deceive the consumer about the true nutritional value of a food.

Several types of claims may not be made on labels:

1 That a food is effective as a treatment for a disease.
2 That a balanced diet of ordinary foods cannot supply adequate amounts of nutrients (excepting the iron requirements of infants, children, and pregnant or lactating women).
3 That the soil on which food is grown may be responsible for deficiencies in quality.
4 That storage, transportation, processing, or cooking of a food may be responsible for deficiencies in its quality.
5 That a food has particular dietary qualities when such qualities have not been shown to be significant in human nutrition.
6 That a natural vitamin is superior to a synthetic vitamin.

The nutrition labeling section of the law then states that, if any nutrition information or claim is made on the label of a food package, it must conform to the following format under the heading "Nutrition Information":

- Serving or portion size.
- Servings or portions per container.
- kCalorie content per serving.
- Protein grams per serving.
- Carbohydrate grams per serving.
- Fat grams per serving.

Fair Packaging Labeling Act, 1966.

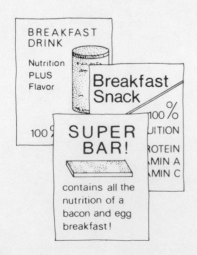

Labels making nutrition claims.

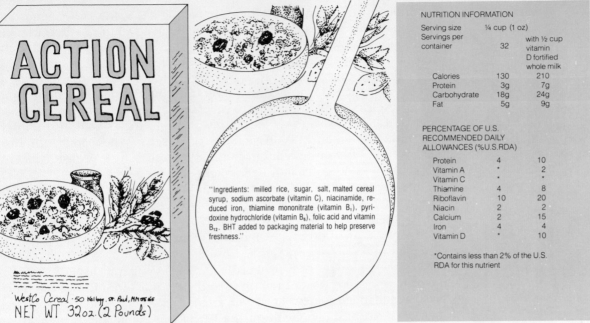

NUTRITION INFORMATION		
Serving size	¼ cup (1 oz)	
Servings per container	32	with ½ cup vitamin D fortified whole milk
Calories	130	210
Protein	3g	7g
Carbohydrate	18g	24g
Fat	5g	9g

PERCENTAGE OF U.S. RECOMMENDED DAILY ALLOWANCES (%U.S.RDA)		
Protein	4	10
Vitamin A	*	2
Vitamin C	*	*
Thiamine	4	8
Riboflavin	10	20
Niacin	2	2
Calcium	2	15
Iron	4	4
Vitamin D	*	10

*Contains less than 2% of the U.S. RDA for this nutrient

"Ingredients: milled rice, sugar, salt, malted cereal syrup, sodium ascorbate (vitamin C), niacinamide, reduced iron, thiamine mononitrate (vitamin B_1), pyridoxine hydrochloride (vitamin B_6), folic acid and vitamin B_{12}. BHT added to packaging material to help preserve freshness."

WestCo Cereal · 50 Kellog, St. Paul, MN 55165
NET WT 32 oz. (2 Pounds)

1 The front of the package must always tell you the product name, the name and address of the company, and the weight or measure; and it may list the ingredients.

2 The ingredient list on the front or side panel names the ingredients in order of predominance. Only products with standards of identity have no ingredient list.

3 The nutrition information panel tells you the nutrients in a serving. Now all you have to know is how to read "percent of U.S. RDA" (see text).

FIGURE H12–1 If you know how to read the front and side of a package, you're a step ahead.

● Protein, vitamins, and minerals as percentages of the U.S. RDA. (No claim may be made that a food is a significant source of a nutrient unless it provides at least 10 percent of the U.S. RDA of that nutrient in a serving.)

The side panel of the cereal box shown in Figure 12–1 provides all this information. To understand fully the meaning of this part of the label, you must be able to interpret statements about vitamins and minerals made in terms of the U.S. RDA, which is not quite the same as the RDA.

The U.S. RDA

The U.S. RDA table is shown on the inside *back* cover. It was derived mostly from the RDA tables of 1968 in order to set standards for labeling. The RDA tables (see inside *front* cover) give different recommendations for each age group. But the designers of the U.S. RDA decided to use one recommended amount for each nutrient—typically, whichever was the highest of the regular RDAs. (They did not use the RDAs for pregnant and lactating women, though, because they are too high for a general standard). Thus, in picking a U.S. RDA for iron, the decision makers chose the RDA of 18 milligrams—the one for women and teenagers—because it is

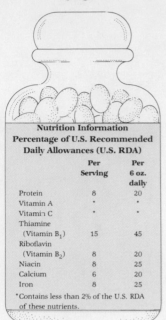

Nutrition Information Percentage of U.S. Recommended Daily Allowances (U.S. RDA)		
	Per Serving	Per 6 oz. daily
Protein	8	20
Vitamin A	*	*
Vitamin C	*	*
Thiamine (Vitamin B$_1$)	15	45
Riboflavin (Vitamin B$_2$)	8	20
Niacin	8	25
Calcium	6	20
Iron	8	25

*Contains less than 2% of the U.S. RDA of these nutrients.

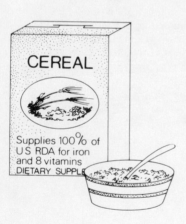

CEREAL

Supplies 100% of US RDA for iron and 8 vitamins
DIETARY SUPPLE

higher than that for any other group. In setting a U.S. RDA for magnesium they chose 400 milligrams—the RDA of males aged 15 to 18—because it is the highest RDA for any age group. Exceptions to this rule were made for some nutrients such as calcium and phosphorus—set a little lower than the very highest because needs vary so widely—and for four nutrients that did not appear in the RDA tables of 1968: biotin, pantothenic acid, copper, and zinc. These were already known to be essential for human beings, and so tentative U.S. RDAs were set for them so manufacturers could list them if they wished. Regular RDAs have since been set for these four nutrients; they are not different enough from the 1968 estimates to cause concern, and so the U.S. RDA has not been changed.

The U.S. RDA table includes two values for protein. If the protein is of high quality, less is needed, and the U.S. RDA is 45 grams. If it is of lower quality, then the U.S. RDA is 65 grams. This rule enables the consumer to "buy protein" in appropriate amounts, without having to understand the concept of protein quality.

In the years since 1968, when the U.S. RDA was published, the RDA tables have been revised three times and the values for most of the nutrients have changed somewhat. However, the U.S. RDA has not been revised, for several reasons. For one thing, the 1968 RDAs are generally higher than the later versions, but they are safe to consume. The most likely mistake the public will make is to think of them as maximum amounts ("I must get *up to* 100 percent of the U.S. RDA")—so it's better to let them be a little high than a little low.

Also, it would cost the industry and therefore the consumer a lot of money to re-label all the food packages now ready for distribution. A third reason is the confusion that would result for foods labeled as either enriched or fortified. When nutrients are inserted in foods at levels higher than 50 percent of the U.S. RDA, the foods have to be labeled as supplements. If the U.S. RDA were lowered to agree with the 1980 RDA, some enriched and fortified foods would end up as supplements and then would have to comply with further regulations and definitions.

With this understanding of the U.S. RDA, you can extract a lot of information from a nutrition label. If you just want to know generally what amounts of nutrients are in the package, the percent of U.S. RDA will tell you that without your having to do any calculating. If you read, for example, that a serving of breakfast cereal provides "Vitamin A—25 percent," then you can be sure it provides at least a quarter of *your* vitamin A allowance for a day (unless you are pregnant or lactating). If you want to know exactly how many units of vitamin A are in a serving, you can look at the U.S. RDA table, find out that the U.S. RDA is 1,000 RE, and figure that 25 percent of that is 250 RE. For the nutrients included in the RDA tables, then, all the information is there that most consumers might want.

Labeling laws also require that any food labeled *low in calories* must state the absolute number of kcalories per serving and must contain no more than 40 per serving. Any food calling itself a *reduced calorie food* must be at least a third lower in kcalories than the food it most closely resembles and must carry a nutrition label. Furthermore, wherever additives are listed on labels, their functions must be stated.

The information just presented helps you with ordinary foods labeled "fish" or "beans," and with foods that present information panels like breakfast cereals. But what about foods that simply say "TV dinner" or "macaroni and cheese"?

Nutrients in Convenience Foods

The FDA has devised nutritional quality guidelines for the nutrient contents of many kinds of convenience foods: frozen dinners; breakfast cereals; meal replacements; noncarbonated, vitamin C–fortified fruit-type or vegetable-type beverages; and main dishes such as pizza or macaroni and cheese. If a product complies with the nutritional quality guidelines, it may carry on its label the statement that it "provides nutrients in amounts appropriate for this class of food as determined by the U.S. government." For example, frozen dinners must contain one or more sources of protein from meat, poultry, fish, cheese, or eggs, and these must make up at least 70 percent of the total protein; they must include one or more vegetables or vegetable mixtures other than potatoes, rice, or cereal-based products; and they must have a certain minimum nutrient level for each 100 kcalories, as shown in Table H12–1.

What if the label says nothing more than a name, such as *mayonnaise*? For some items the law provides standards of identity and excuses manufacturers from the requirement of listing ingredients. Standards of identity exist for such foods as bread and mayonnaise—common foods that at one time were often prepared at home, so that the basic recipe was understood by almost everyone. Certain ingredients must be present in a specific percentage before the food may use the standard name. Any product like mayonnaise, for example, may use that name on the label only if it contains 65 percent by weight of vegetable oil, either vinegar or lemon juice, and egg yolk. The FDA does not have the authority to require that ingredients be listed for these foods, but it urges manufacturers to give the consumer more detailed information, and many manufacturers do so voluntarily.

HM. HAS 25% OF U.S. RDA FOR ALL THESE NUTRIENTS. GIVES ME AT LEAST A FOURTH OF MY NEEDS FOR A DAY.

If it delivers 25 percent of the U.S. RDA for a nutrient, then it almost certainly delivers at least 25 percent of *your* RDA for that nutrient. (For your RDA, see inside front cover. For U.S. RDA, see inside back cover.)

The vitamin A RDA for women is 800 RE; for men, 1,000 RE. For this one nutrient you then have to calculate further, using the factors 1 RE = 3.3 IU from animal foods or 1 RE = 10 IU from plant foods, before comparing with food composition tables.

TABLE H12–1 **Required Nutrient Content of Highly Processed Foods Such as Frozen Dinners**

NUTRIENT	REQUIRED IN EACH 100 kCALORIES OF FOOD	REQUIRED IN THE TOTAL PACKAGE
Protein, g	4.60	16.0
Vitamin A, IU	150.00	520.0
Thiamin, mg	0.05	0.2
Riboflavin, mg	0.06	0.2
Niacin, mg	0.99	3.4
Pantothenic acid, mg	0.32	1.1
Vitamin B_6, mg	0.15	0.5
Vitamin B_{12}, μg	0.33	1.1
Iron, mg	0.62	2.2

Source: M. Stephenson, Making food labels more informative, *FDA Consumer* 9, no. 8 (1975): 13–17.

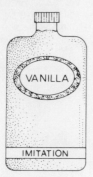

Imitation Foods

Another class of foods that concerns consumers is made up of inferior foods developed in imitation of, and as substitutes for, familiar foods. A section of the law requires that, if a food is an imitation of a traditional food, this fact must be stated on its label. With the new food technology, however, many imitation food products on the market may very well be superior to traditional foods; it is misleading to the consumer to imply that they are inferior. For this reason, the regulation now requires that the word *imitation* must be used on the label only if the product is "a substitute for and resembles another food but is nutritionally inferior to the food imitated.... Nutritional inferiority is defined as a reduction in the content of an essential vitamin or mineral or of protein that amounts to 10 percent or more of the U.S. RDA."

Thus if you read *imitation* on a label, you may conclude that the food is a poor imitation nutritionally. This may be of no consequence when the food is an incidental item in your diet, like vanilla, because you do not depend on vanilla for any nutrients. But if it's a fruit drink that you drink daily, and if you usually include no other items from the fruit and vegetable group in your diet, then the label may alert you to a needed change.

Up to this point you have learned you can tell from a food label:

- What the ingredients are.
- Whether anything has been added.
- The number of kcalories.

Often, you can also tell:

- The amount of protein, fat, and carbohydrate, and of the vitamins and minerals listed in the RDA tables.

You also have a feel for the nutrient contributions made by processed and convenience foods and by imitation foods. But the discerning reader may still ask, "Is this enough information? What else do I need to know?" The questions are worthwhile, because nutrition-minded people are still concerned about several aspects of food labeling.

Misleading Labels

As they presently appear, food labels provide useful information. But labels can be improved further. The law still allows loopholes through which can slip certain kinds of misleading claims. You might be interested in trying your skill at selecting from the following the two claims that are misleading even though true (all three claims are true):

1 A label says one serving of food provides 35 times as much iron as an 8-ounce glass of whole milk.
2 A label says a fortified product contains "more vitamin C than fresh orange juice."
3 A label says a brand of instant nonfat dry milk has "all the calcium, protein, B vitamins of whole milk."[1]

1   L. Schwartzberg, C. George, and M. C. Phillips, Issues in food advertising: The nutrition educator's viewpoint, *Journal of Nutrition Education* 9 (1977): 60–63.

Check the bottom of the page for the answers.[2] Two other ways a consumer might be led off the track are shown in the following examples:

4 A label claims that an artificially constituted food or dietary supplement contains all the vitamins and minerals known to be essential in human nutrition, in amounts equal to the U.S. RDA wherever this has been established. This implies a completeness that may be overestimated. A critic points out that "we really do not know everything that should be included in artificially constituted foods."[3]

5 A breakfast bar or snack food label gives nutrition information showing that the protein, fat, carbohydrate, and certain vitamin and mineral contents are the same as those found in a breakfast of milk, egg, toast, and orange juice. This fails to mention that the carbohydrate is sugar (versus the complex carbohydrate in toast), that the fat is saturated fat (versus the oil the egg might have been fried in), or that there is considerable salt in the food. Proposals under consideration for new labeling laws would require listing added sugar and salt in a prominent place on the label.

Consumers are putting pressure on legislatures to provide labeling laws that will make such misleading claims illegal.

Sugar and Salt

Another problem still to be resolved in nutrition labeling has to do with the amounts of sugar and salt in foods. Consumers want, and are entitled to, this information, but food producers are concerned that the labels not put them at an unfair disadvantage; so the exact requirements for labeling still have to be worked out. What should be called "sugar," for example: all monosaccharides and disaccharides, including those found naturally in the food? or all added sugars, including honey, corn syrup, and the like? or only added sucrose? How should sugar contents be listed? If in grams per serving, then the amount of sugar in a cola beverage will be seen to be more than that in a serving of sugar-coated cereal; but if sugar is stated as a percentage, then the amount in the cereal will appear very high, because it isn't diluted by water.

As for salt, should it be listed as salt, or as sodium? Should just the added salt or sodium be listed, or should that occurring naturally in the food be included? If the sodium occurring naturally in the food is included, how much expense should the manufacturer sustain in trying to make sure the amounts listed are accurate? Sodium content varies from one shipment of produce to the next. While no official decision has been made, all the major companies have voluntarily started sodium labeling in line with current practices (in milligrams per serving).

Regulations proposed by FDA, if approved, may ease the consumer's task in sizing up the sodium amounts in foods. The regulations define the

2 1. True but misleading, because milk is recognized as a poor source of iron. 2. True but misleading, because orange juice contains so many *other* nutrients by virtue of being a natural food. 3. True and responsible.

3 A. M. Schmidt, Food and drug law: A 200-year perspective, *Nutrition Today* 10, no. 4 (1975): 29–32.

conditions under which manufacturers may use the terms *sodium free, low sodium, reduced sodium,* and *moderately low sodium* on product labels. Basically, the regulations define how much sodium per serving a product could contain when certain claims were made on its label. A label could say, for example, "This product contains 25 percent less sodium than our regular product." FDA would also permit use of the terms *unsalted, without salt added,* and *no salt added* when no salt had been added during the processing of the food and when the product was a substitute for another food normally processed with salt. In these cases, sodium content would also have to be listed.

FDA also recommends that potassium content be listed in nutrition labeling. This is because people with kidney and other diseases who must control their sodium intake also must control their potassium intake, and because potassium often is used in place of sodium by people who must reduce their sodium intake to help treat high blood pressure and related health problems.[4]

Whatever decisions are finally made, the labels that include the kind of information described above will benefit consumers who wish to limit their intakes of these substances. It isn't enough to stop using the sugar bowl and the salt shaker, because only about one-third of your total intake of these additives is sprinkled on foods by you. The other two-thirds is added during processing. That's why they were called *additives* above. Highlight 10 raises and tries to answer some of the important questions people ask about additives.

NOTE: Appendix J provides further reading; see "Food Labels."

---

4   The last four paragraphs are paraphrased from *HHS News*, 15 June 1982, a newsletter from the Department of Health and Human Services.

CHAPTER 13
Mother and Infant

CONTENTS

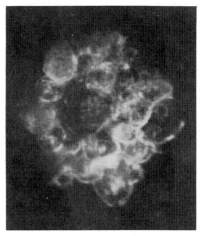

All that is needed to form a new human being is a single, fertilized egg cell containing instructions (in DNA) to make proteins. The rest will follow. This is a human embryo, three days old; the single egg cell has divided five times, producing 32 cells.

The Chinese . . . credit a child with the age of one year on the day of its birth . . . to recognize all the growth and development that has already occurred since the time of conception.

LINDA FERRILL ANNIS

We normally think of nutrition as affecting us here and now. You feel good this afternoon because you ate a good breakfast this morning; your friend feels sleepy because she had a sweet dessert after lunch. But the effects of nutrition also extend over years. The woman who is expecting a baby and the health professional advising such a woman will be strongly motivated to attend to her nutrition needs if they understand how critical the nutrients are to the normal course of events in prenatal development.

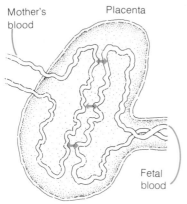

Mother's blood   Placenta

Fetal blood

placenta (pla-SEN-tuh): the organ inside the uterus in which the mother's and fetus's circulatory systems intertwine and in which exchange of materials between maternal and fetal blood takes place. The fetus receives nutrients and oxygen across the placenta; the mother's blood picks up carbon dioxide and other waste materials to be excreted via her lungs and kidneys.

implantation: the stage of development in which the fertilized egg embeds itself in the wall of the uterus and begins to develop, during the first two weeks after conception.

critical period: a finite period during development in which certain events may occur that will have irreversible, determining effects on later developmental stages. A critical period is usually a period of cell division in a body organ.

embryo (EM-bree-oh): the developing infant during its second to eighth week after conception. Before the second week, it is called an **ovum** (OH-vum) or **zygote** (ZYE-goat).

Pregnancy: the Impact of Nutrition on the Future

The only way nutrients can reach the developing infant in the uterus is through the mother's bloodstream. To convey these nutrients, the mother grows a whole new organ, the placenta, a sort of cushion in which the mother's and baby's blood vessels intertwine and exchange materials—nutrients and oxygen going into the baby's system, wastes leaving it to be excreted by the mother. If the mother's nutrient stores are inadequate early in pregnancy, then the early development of her infant will be adversely affected. No matter how well the mother eats later, her unborn baby will not receive optimum nourishment. The infant will be born small and may be unable to attain the full size and health that would otherwise have been possible. After getting such a poor start on life, a girl child may be ill equipped, in her turn, to store sufficient nutrients and so may also bear a poorly developed infant. Thus the poor nutrition of a woman during her early pregnancy can theoretically have an impact on the health of her *grandchild* even after that child has become an *adult*.

Such effects are impossible to demonstrate directly in people, nor would researchers want to experiment on pregnant mothers to see what caused stunting of the body or the brain in their children. But because the questions are important, many of them have been pursued through research using animals. We have every reason to believe that most findings from the animal experiments are applicable to human beings. Some have been inadvertently confirmed in human beings through accidents of history. Hospital records were maintained during the sieges of Holland and Leningrad in World War II, when women were starving before or during their pregnancies. These records showed that poor nutrition *prior* to pregnancy caused more birth defects and stillbirths than poor nutrition during pregnancy.

Critical Periods

Conditions in the uterus at the time of conception determine whether the fertilized egg will successfully implant itself in the uterine wall and begin development as it should. During the two weeks following fertilization, in the implantation stage, the egg cell divides into many cells, and these cells sort themselves into three layers. Very little growth in size takes place at this time; it is a critical period that precedes growth. Adverse influences at this time lead to failure to implant or to other disturbances so severe as to cause loss of the fertilized egg, possibly even before the woman knows she is pregnant. Many drugs affect the earliest intrauterine events and later cross the placenta freely. Most health professionals agree that, if possible, a potential mother should take no drugs at all, not even aspirin. Nutrition should be, and should have been, continuously optimal.

The next five weeks, the period of embryonic development, register astonishing physical changes (see Figure 13–1). From the outermost layer

FIGURE 13-1 **Stages of embryonic development.**

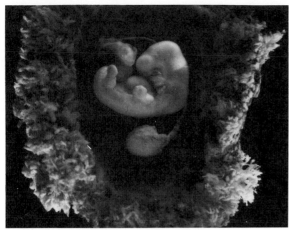

Six-week-old fetus attached to the placenta. At this time the fetus is less than half an inch long.

Source: Courtesy of Professor Emil Ludwig.

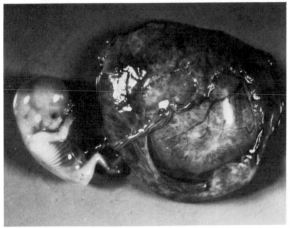

Ten-week-old fetus attached to the placenta. The blood vessels in the umbilical cord are clearly visible.

Source: Courtesy of Dr. Landrum B. Shettles and Dr. Roberts Rugh.

Eight-week-old fetus, showing development of the skeleton. The other tissues were treated so as to be transparent.

Source: Courtesy of Dr. Roberts Rugh and Dr. Landrum B. Shettles.

of cells, the nervous system and skin begin to develop; from the middle layer, the muscles and internal organ systems; and from the innermost layer, the glands and linings of the digestive, respiratory, and excretory systems. At eight weeks, the 3-centimeter-long embryo has a complete central nervous system, a beating heart, a fully formed digestive system, and the beginnings of facial features. Already, an embryonic tail has formed and almost completely disappeared again, and the fingers and toes are well defined.

The growth of each organ and tissue type has its own characteristic pattern and timing. In the fetus, for example, the heart and brain are well developed at 16 weeks, even though the lungs are still nonfunctional 10 weeks later. During the first year after birth, the brain doubles in weight, but it increases only about 20 percent thereafter. In contrast, the muscles will be more than 30 times heavier at maturity than at birth.

Each organ and tissue, then, has its own unique periods of intensive growth. Each organ needs the growth nutrients most during its own inten-

The brain and central nervous system are first to reach maturity.

Stages in organ growth:

1 **hyperplasia** (high-per-PLAY-zee-uh): an increase in cell number.
2 simultaneous hyperplasia and **hypertrophy** (high-PER-tro-fee): hyperplasia accompanied by an increase in cell size.
3 hypertrophy (except for the liver).

The brain also goes through a fourth period, multiplication of cell contacts, which depends on both nutrition and social stimulation (learning).

TABLE 13-1 **Overall Weight Gain During Pregnancy**

DEVELOPMENT	WEIGHT GAIN (lb)
Infant at birth	7½
Placenta	1
Increase in mother's blood volume to supply placenta	4
Increase in size of mother's uterus and muscles to support it	2½
Increase in size of mother's breasts	3
Fluid to surround infant in amniotic sac	2
Mother's fat stores	4
Total	24

sive growth period. Thus, a nutrient deficiency during one stage of development might affect the heart and at another might affect the developing limbs.

The cells of a single developing organ also follow a schedule unique to them. Each organ has its own specific time for cell division. This time may not be obvious, because it often precedes the period of growth in size. An interesting case is that of the brain. During development of the fetal brain, there is an early period when the cells are increasing dramatically in *number*. Each time a cell divides, it produces two that are half its size. These two do not grow but divide again, producing four cells that are still smaller. During this time of rapid cell division, the size of the brain hardly changes at all. Later, the cells begin to grow and also continue dividing, so that their *size* and *number* increase simultaneously. It is during these first two periods that the total number of cells to be found in the brain is determined for life. Later still, cell division ceases; thereafter, the total number of cells is fixed, but the cells continue to increase in *size*. During this last period, the brain's growth in size is obvious. The development of almost every organ in the body follows a similar pattern, but the timing is different for each.

The third period, during which increase in size is taking place, is the time when the most intensive growth appears to be going on. But actually, the most important events are already over. This fact has important implications for nutrition. The period of cell division is a critical period, critical in the sense that the cell division taking place during that time can occur at only that time and at no other. Whatever nutrients and other environmental conditions are needed in this period must be supplied on time if the organ is to reach its full potential. If cell division and the final cell number achieved are limited during a critical period, recovery is impossible. Thus, early malnutrition can have irreversible effects, although they may not become fully apparent until the person reaches maturity.

The effect of malnutrition during critical periods is seen in the shorter height of people who were undernourished in their early years; in the delayed sexual development of those undernourished during early adolescence; in the poor dental health of children whose mothers were malnourished during pregnancy; and in the smaller brain cell number of children who have suffered from episodes of marasmus. The irreversibility of these effects is obvious when abundant, nourishing food fed after the critical time fails to remedy the growth deficit. Among the many Korean orphans adopted by U.S. families after the Korean War, for example, several years of catch-up growth occurred but did not completely make up for the effects of early malnutrition.

An area of active recent research points strongly to the probability that malnutrition in the prenatal and early postnatal periods also affects learning ability and behavior. Much of the severe mental retardation seen in developed countries such as the United States is of unknown cause, but many cases are thought to be due to protein deficiency during pregnancy. Clearly, then, it is most critical to provide the best nutrition at early stages of life.

Fetal Growth

The last seven months of pregnancy, the fetal period, bring about a tremendous increase in the size of the fetus. Intensive periods of cell division occur in organ after organ.

Meanwhile, the mother's body has been undergoing changes. As already mentioned, she has grown the placenta, which transfers nutrients and oxygen to the fetus and carbon dioxide and other wastes to the mother's bloodstream for excretion by way of her lungs and kidneys. The amniotic sac has filled with fluid to cushion the infant. The mother's uterus and its supporting muscles have increased greatly in size, her breasts have changed and grown in preparation for lactation, and her blood volume has increased by half to accommodate the added load of materials to be carried. The normal gain in weight of mother and child during pregnancy amounts to about 25 to 30 pounds (see Table 13–1).

A mother's physiology changes so much during pregnancy that a naive observer might think that she is ill. She develops an apparent anemia, she may have edema, and her glucose tolerance changes as if she were diabetic. These and other changes are normal for her altered state, however.

The "physiological anemia of pregnancy" results from the great increase in the mother's blood volume. The red blood cells do not increase as much as the blood fluid, so the number of cells per milliliter is low compared with the nonpregnant state. Values for protein, iron, folacin, and other nutrients are correspondingly lowered, while other values rise (cholesterol and fat-soluble vitamins are examples). The clinician who assesses a pregnant woman's nutrition status therefore uses a set of standards specific for pregnancy (see "Pregnancy," in Appendix J).

The edema of pregnancy is also "physiological" (that is, expected and normal)—provided that it is not accompanied by indicators of kidney disease such as high blood pressure or protein in the urine. This normal edema results from the raised secretion of the hormone estrogen toward the end of pregnancy, which helps to ready the uterus for delivery.

The altered glucose tolerance of pregnancy is normal, too, but an untrained observer could easily confuse it with diabetes. These examples are intended to caution the reader who is unfamiliar with the special standards applicable to pregnancy not to jump to conclusions regarding out-of-line lab test values. The treatment of truly abnormal conditions is the subject of a later section ("Troubleshooting").

Nutrient Needs

Nutrient needs during periods of intensive growth are greater than at any other time and are greater for certain nutrients than for others, as shown in Figure 13–2. A study of the figure reveals some of the key needs.

One of the smallest increases apparent is in kcalories; an increase of only 15 percent (mostly in the latter half of pregnancy) is recommended, but many individual women may need much more. In each case, enough kcalories are needed to spare protein for its all-important tissue-building work. A recommended average intake is 40 kcalories per kilogram of body

fetus (FEET-us): the developing infant from the eighth week after conception until its birth.

uterus (YOO-ter-us): the womb, the muscular organ within which the infant develops before birth.

amniotic sac (am-nee-OTT-ic): the "bag of waters" in the uterus, in which the fetus floats.

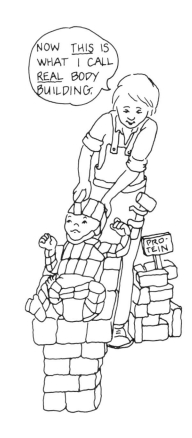

Recommended energy intake: 40 kcal/kg (18 kcal/lb).

Minimum energy intake: 36 kcal/kg (17 kcal/lb).

For a 120-lb woman, this represents at least 2,000 kcal and preferably 2,200 kcal/day.

Recommended protein intake: 75–100 g/day.

Recommended carbohydrate intake: about 50% of energy intake. In a 2,000 kcal/day intake, this represents 1,000 kcal of carbohydrate, or about 250 g. Four cups of milk a day will contribute about 50 g carbohydrate. An apple provides 10 g carbohydrate, and a slice of bread provides 15 g, so this recommendation implies generous intakes of fruit and bread exchanges.

Foods containing folacin:
Green, leafy vegetables.
Legumes.
Liver.
Orange juice and cantaloupe.
Other vegetables.
Whole wheat products.

Foods containing calcium:
Four cups of milk a day will supply 1.2 g calcium. For other food sources, see Chapter 10. The milk should be fortified with vitamin D; if it is not, a vitamin D supplement may be needed.

Ordinarily, a hemoglobin level below 13 g/100 ml is considered low for a woman (see Chapter 11). In pregnancy, values of 12 g are not unusual, and 11 g is where the line defining "too low" is often drawn.

Food sources of iron:
Liver, oysters.
Red meat, fish, other meat.
Dried fruits.
Legumes (dried beans, peas, limas).
Dark green vegetables.

weight, and energy intake should never fall below 36 kcalories per kilogram. The increased need for protein is more dramatic—from about 56 grams to about 75 grams per day or more—and generous amounts of carbohydrate are needed to spare the protein. There is no harm in a pregnant woman's taking up to 100 grams of protein or even more; in fact, if she has been poorly nourished prior to pregnancy, this may be an ideal intake.

The extraordinary need for folacin in the pregnant woman is due to the great increase in her blood volume. Folacin-deficiency anemia is more often seen in pregnant women than even iron-deficiency anemia, and it is often advisable for the physician to prescribe folacin as a supplement.[1] As you might expect, the vitamin needed in the next highest amount is the B vitamin that assists folacin in the manufacture of red blood cells—vitamin B_{12}.

Among the minerals, those involved in building the skeleton—calcium, phosphorus, and magnesium—are in great demand during pregnancy, and increases of about 50 percent are recommended. Intestinal absorption of calcium doubles early in pregnancy, and the mineral is stored in the mother's bones. Later, as the fetal bones begin to calcify, there is a dramatic shift of calcium across the placenta, and the mother's bone stores are drawn upon. Most mothers' intakes have to be increased well above their prepregnancy intakes. If the mother's intake is less than 1.2 grams per day, she will pay by losing more calcium from her bones than she has stored for this purpose.[2]

The body conserves iron even more than usual during pregnancy. Menstruation, which is normally the major route of excretion of iron, ceases; and absorption of iron increases up to threefold. (The blood protein responsible for iron absorption, transferrin, increases.) An additional adjustment is accomplished by the hormones of pregnancy, which act to raise the concentration of iron in the blood, by either increasing absorption still further, or mobilizing iron from its storage places in the bone marrow and internal organs, or both. Thus, a woman *theoretically* needs no more iron during pregnancy than she has needed all along, and the RDA for iron in pregnancy is not higher than for the nonpregnant woman. However, so few women enter pregnancy with adequate stores that the theoretical case hardly ever applies. Most women, even in the United States and Canada, have minimal iron stores; and the demands of pregnancy deplete them to the deficiency point. Even if a woman makes it to the end of pregnancy without falling into frank anemia, she may bleed excessively at delivery—hence the advisability of a prescribed iron supplement to boost her stores. At birth, a baby is supposed to have enough stored iron to last three to six months; this iron must also come from the mother's iron stores. It is considered advisable for almost all pregnant women to take an iron supplement throughout pregnancy and for two to three months after delivery.[3]

1   L. B. Bailey, C. S. Mahan, and D. Dimperio, Folacin and iron status in low-income pregnant adolescents and mature women, *American Journal of Clinical Nutrition* 33 (1980): 1997–2001; V. Herbert, The vitamin craze, *Archives of Internal Medicine* 140 (1980): 173–176.

2   R. Kumar, W. R. Cohen, and F. H. Epstein, Vitamin D and calcium hormones in pregnancy, *New England Journal of Medicine* 302 (1980): 1143–1145.

3   Committee on Dietary Allowances, *Recommended Dietary Allowances*, 9th ed. (Washington, D.C.: National Academy of Sciences, 1980), p. 138.

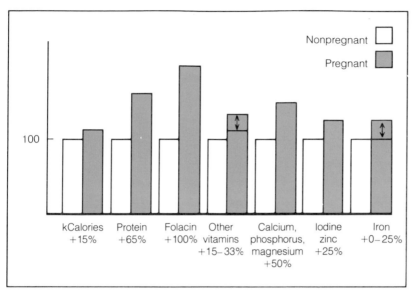

FIGURE 13–2 **Comparison of the nutrient needs of nonpregnant and pregnant women (over 23 years old).** The non-pregnant woman's needs are set at 100 percent, the pregnant woman's needs shown as increases over 100 percent. The pregnant woman's iron needs cannot be met by ordinary diets, and she may need to take an iron supplement.

Source: Calculated from the RDA table, inside front cover.

Eating Pattern and Weight Gain

If the woman's dietary pattern is already adequate at the start of pregnancy, it can be adjusted to meet changing nutrient needs. The nutrients needing the greatest increase are protein, calcium, phosphorus, magnesium, and folacin; so the foods selected for emphasis should normally be those in the milk, meat, and vegetable categories.

Because kcalorie needs increase less than nutrient needs, the pregnant woman must select foods of high nutrient density. For most women, appropriate choices include foods like skim milk, cottage cheese, lean meats, eggs, liver, dark-green vegetables, and whole-grain breads and cereals. For vitamin C, she should either increase the size of her one serving of a vitamin C–rich food, such as citrus fruit or broccoli, or add a second, fair vitamin C source, such as tomatoes. A suggested food pattern is shown in Table 13–2.

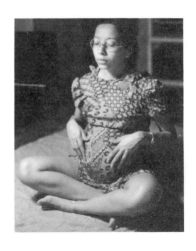

The pregnant woman must gain weight. Ideally, she will have begun her pregnancy at the appropriate weight for her height and will gain about 25 pounds, most of it in the second half of pregnancy. The ideal pattern is thought to be about 2 to 4 pounds during the first three months and a pound per week thereafter. The teenager needs to gain more. A woman who is underweight to begin with should gain more—perhaps 30 pounds —and a woman who is obese at the start of pregnancy could perhaps gain less but still should gain between 16 and 24 pounds.[4]

4   Maternal weight gain and the outcome of pregnancy, *Nutrition Reviews* 37 (1979): 318–321; California Department of Health, as cited in Nutrition and the pregnant obese woman, *Nutrition and the MD*, January 1978. Appendix E presents a weight-gain grid for use in evaluating the pregnant woman's progress, and cites a reference suggesting different patterns for underweight, normal weight, and overweight women.

TABLE 13–2 **Daily Food Guide for Pregnant or Lactating Women**

	NUMBER OF SERVINGS		
FOOD	*Nonpregnant woman*	*Pregnant woman*	*Lactating woman*
Protein foods			
Animal (2-oz serving)	2	2	2
Vegetable (at least one serving of legumes)	2	2	2
Milk and milk products	2	4	5
Enriched or whole-grain breads and cereals	4	4	4
Vitamin C–rich fruits and vegetables	1	1	1
Dark-green vegetables	1	1	1
Other fruits and vegetables	1	1	1

Source: California Department of Health, as cited in Nutrition and the pregnant obese woman, *Nutrition and the MD,* January 1978.

Twenty-five pounds for a normal-weight woman sounds like a lot, but if you look again at the components of the pregnant woman's weight gain (Table 13–1), you will see that she needs all these pounds—from nutritious kcalories—to provide for the growth of her placenta, uterus, blood, and breasts, as well as for a strong 7½-pound baby. There is little place in her diet, however, for the empty kcalories of sugar, fat, and alcohol, which provide no nutrients to support the growth of these tissues and only contribute to excessive fat accumulation. Much of the weight she gains is lost at delivery; the remainder is generally lost within a few weeks or months, as her blood volume returns to normal and she loses the fluids she has accumulated.

If a woman has gained more than the expected amount of weight early in pregnancy, she should not try to diet in the last weeks. Women have been known to gain up to 60 pounds in pregnancy without ill effects. (A *sudden* large weight gain, however, is a danger signal that may indicate the onset of toxemia; see "Troubleshooting.")

The underweight woman should try to gain weight before she becomes pregnant, to maximize her chance of having a healthy baby. But all women should be attending to their nutrition before they become pregnant. If nutrient supplementation is needed, the family-planning period is a good time to get it started.

If the mother does not gain the full amount of weight recommended, she may give birth to an underweight baby. To the uninitiated, this may seem like no catastrophe, and in some instances it is not. A small mother may give birth to a small, normal, alert, and healthy baby. Nothing is wrong with that. On the other hand, a low-birthweight baby may be a malnourished baby, one who is more likely to get sick. Such a baby also is likely to be unable to do its job of obtaining nourishment by sucking and to win its mother's attention by energetic, vigorous cries and other healthy behavior. It can therefore become an apathetic, neglected baby; and this compounds the original malnutrition problem. Such a baby's sickliness is often called "failure to thrive." Thus, for many reasons, babies of normal weight are usually more healthy.

Nutritionists seeking to find a measure by which they can evaluate the outcome of pregnancy have found that birthweight is the most potent single indicator of the infant's future health status. A low-birthweight baby, defined as one that weighs less than 5½ pounds (2,500 grams), has a statistically greater chance of contracting diseases and of dying early in life. Its birth is more likely to be complicated by problems during delivery than that of a normal baby (defined as weighing a minimum of 6½ pounds, or 3,000 grams).

About one in every 15 infants born in the United States is a low-birthweight baby, and about a quarter of them die within the first month of life. Worldwide, it is estimated that one-sixth of all live babies are of low birthweight; more than nine out of ten of these are born in the developing countries. Most of them are not premature but are full-term babies; they are small because of malnutrition. The impact of this malnutrition is further seen in the fact that nutritional deficiency, coupled with low birthweight, is the underlying or associated cause of more than half of all the deaths of children under five years old.[5]

Low birthweight is often associated with mental retardation, probably by way of deprivation of nutrients and oxygen to the developing brain. It is estimated that about half of all cases of mental retardation worldwide could be eliminated by improved maternal and infant care programs.

Practices to Avoid

The potential impact of harmful practices during pregnancy cannot be overestimated. Smoking restricts the blood supply to the growing fetus and so limits the delivery of nutrients and removal of wastes. It stunts growth, thus increasing the risk of retarded development and complications at birth. Drugs taken during pregnancy can cause grotesque malformations.

Dieting, even for short periods, is hazardous. Low-carbohydrate diets or fasts that cause ketosis deprive the growing brain of needed glucose and cause congenital deformity. Most serious may be the invisible effects. For example, carbohydrate metabolism may be rendered permanently defective, or the infant's brain may be permanently damaged.[6]

The consequences of protein deprivation can be severe. This has been observed most frequently in the underdeveloped countries, but it has also been seen among food faddists who adopted an untested vegetarian diet.

low birthweight (LBW): a birthweight of 5½ lb (2,500 g) or less, used as a predictor of poor health in the newborn and as a probable indicator of poor nutrition status of the mother during and/or before pregnancy. Normal birthweight is 6½ lb (3,000 g) or more. Low-birthweight infants are of two different types. Some are **premature**; they are born early and are the right size for their gestational age. Others have suffered growth failure in the uterus; they may or may not be born early but they are **small for gestational age (small for date)**.

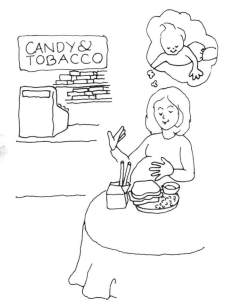

5   A. Petros-Barvazian and M. Béhar, Low birth weight: What should be done to deal with this global problem? *WHO Chronicle* 32 (June 1978): 231–232; *New Trends and Approaches in the Delivery of Maternal and Child Care in Health Services* (sixth report of the WHO Expert Committee on Maternal and Child Health), as cited in *Journal of the American Dietetic Association* 71 (1977): 357.

6   R. M. Pitkin, ed., Nutrition in pregnancy, *Dietetic Currents, Ross Timesaver,* January/February 1977; C. S. Mahan, Revolution in obstetrics: Pregnancy nutrition, *Journal of the Florida Medical Association*, April 1979, pp. 367–372.

fetal alcohol syndrome: the cluster of symptoms seen in an infant or child whose mother consumed excess alcohol during her pregnancy; includes mental and physical retardation with facial and other body deformities.

A table of the caffeine amounts in beverages and medications is provided in Chapter 15.

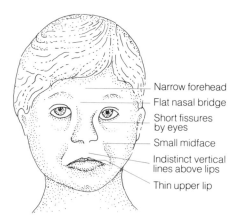

Narrow forehead
Flat nasal bridge
Short fissures by eyes
Small midface
Indistinct vertical lines above lips
Thin upper lip

These facial traits reflect fetal alcohol syndrome, caused by drinking early in pregnancy. Brain damage and irreversible mental and physical retardation accompany these surface features.

Their children's height and head circumference were markedly and irreversibly diminished. Iron deficiency during pregnancy in animals has been seen to give rise to offspring whose brain cells could never store the needed iron thereafter.[7]

Most importantly, excessive alcohol consumption can cause irreversible brain damage and mental and physical retardation in the fetus (fetal alcohol syndrome). The damage can occur with as few as two drinks a day, and its most severe impact is likely to be in the first month, before the woman even is sure she is pregnant. About 1 in every 750 children born in the United States is a victim of this preventable damage.[8]

Excessive caffeine consumption (more than 8 cups of coffee a day) has also been thought to cause complications in delivery, but a recent review of the evidence suggests this may have been a false alarm. One or two cups of coffee or tea a day or the equivalent are well within safe limits. Some question exists about the overuse of saccharin, too, and even sugar. A general guideline can be offered: don't feel obligated to avoid these substances altogether, but use them and all others in moderation.

Troubleshooting

To avoid the most common problems encountered during pregnancy, some additional measures are helpful. Diabetes is a condition that can make pregnancy more difficult than usual, and sometimes the onset of diabetes occurs when a woman is pregnant. To make sure women with this complication get medical help, it is recommended that all pregnant women be screened for diabetes at about the sixth month. Thereafter, at every checkup, a woman's urine should be tested for ketones. Ketonuria may be a clue to diabetes or may indicate the starvation ketosis of ill-advised dieting, a warning sign that permanent brain damage to the fetus may ensue.

It has been mentioned that a certain degree of edema is to be expected in late pregnancy, but in a poorly nourished woman, it is often part of the larger cluster of symptoms known as toxemia, a condition involving high blood pressure and kidney problems that requires medical attention. Toxemia causes thousands of infant deaths every year, and babies born of toxemic mothers are likely to have retarded growth, lung problems, and other, even more severe birth defects.

Research has shown that toxemia is most common in low-income mothers and pregnant teenagers; often poor nutrition contributes to it. Lack of protein, kcalories, calcium, and/or salt may be involved. Adequate calcium is thought to have a direct effect in preventing high blood pressure.[9] To avert toxemia, a pregnant woman should obtain ample protein-rich foods, both meat and milk, in her diet, and even her salt needs are

7   R. L. Leibel, Behavioral and biochemical correlations of iron deficiency: A review, *Journal of the American Dietetic Association* 71 (1977): 399–404.

8   K. K. Sulik, M. C. Johnston, and M. A. Webb, Fetal alcohol syndrome: Embryogenesis in a mouse model, *Science* 214 (1981): 936–938.

9   J. M. Belizan and J. Villar, The relationship between calcium intake and edema-, protein-uria-, and hypertension-gestosis: An hypothesis, *American Journal of Clinical Nutrition* 33 (1980): 2202–2210.

higher than usual. This doesn't mean that she should add any salt; the increased need is normally met by the increased food intake. But she shouldn't severely restrict the salt in her diet, either, unless she has a medical condition that makes it necessary to do so. Even after toxemia has set in, it is likely that salt intake should not be reduced, and diuretics (to cause sodium excretion) may be harmful.[10] Good nutrition and rest are the cornerstones of treatment.

Imagine a course of events that goes like this: A pregnant woman notices some puffiness and swelling of her ankles. She consults an advisor who doesn't recognize this as the normal edema of pregnancy and who thinks it is a sign of toxemia setting in. The advisor recommends salt restriction, which is necessary for the edema of severe renal disease or congestive heart failure; but the change in diet imposed on this woman is inappropriate and gradually causes real malnutrition. After two months of taking this precaution, the woman has *true* toxemia.

The message in this story is, of course, not to take advice from anyone who lacks medical or nutrition knowledge. Consult a doctor about medical conditions; consult a qualified nutrition professional (R.D.) on nutrition. Better still, consult both. And, as has been said many times before, don't self-diagnose.

Caution

toxemia (tox-EEM-ee-uh): a cluster of symptoms seen in pregnancy, including edema and often hypertension and kidney complications (*tox* = poison; *emia* = in the blood). A variety of terms are associated with toxemia. Most common is **eclampsia**; its symptoms include convulsions and coma, associated with high blood pressure, edema, and protein in the urine. Eclampsia may be preceeded by **preeclampsia**, from mild to severe. High blood pressure may also exist throughout pregnancy without toxemia's developing.

The normal edema of pregnancy responds to gravity; blood pools in the ankles. The edema of toxemia is a generalized edema. The distinction helps with diagnosis.

Two anemias are common in pregnancy: iron-deficiency anemia and folacin-deficiency anemia. Both can be missed, for reasons related to the physiology of pregnancy. Iron-deficiency anemia must be diagnosed against the background of the physiological anemia already mentioned. Folacin-deficiency anemia causes nausea (among many symptoms), which can easily be overlooked because the woman thinks it is just morning sickness. It is important to detect and correct—or, better, to prevent—both anemias; both iron and folacin supplements are often prescribed as a precautionary measure.

The nausea of "morning" sickness (actually any time) seems unavoidable, because it arises from the hormonal changes taking place early in pregnancy, but it can often be alleviated. A strategy some expectant mothers have found effective in quelling nausea is to start the day with a few sips of water and a few nibbles of a soda cracker or other bland carbohydrate food, to get something in their stomachs before getting out of bed. Carbonated beverages may also help.

Another problem sometimes seen in pregnancy is vitamin B_6 deficiency, which may in some cases cause depression. Depression can, of course, have other causes, however; so its presence is not necessarily an indication that a nutrition problem is present.

Later, as the hormones of pregnancy alter her muscle tone and the thriving infant crowds her intestinal organs, an expectant mother may complain

Most severe risk factors for malnutrition in pregnancy:

Age 15 or under.

Unwanted pregnancy.

Many pregnancies close together.

History of poor outcomes.

Poverty.

Food faddism.

Heavy smoking.

Drug addiction.

Alcohol abuse.

Chronic disease requiring special diet.

More than 15% underweight.

More than 15% overweight.

These factors at the start of pregnancy indicate that poor nutrition is very likely to be present and to affect the pregnancy adversely.

10   Simple test helps to identify women at risk for toxemia of pregnancy (Medical News), *Journal of the American Medical Association* 237 (1977): 1541–1542.

of constipation. A high-fiber diet and a plentiful water intake will help to relieve this condition. Laxatives should be used only if the doctor orders them, and the type of laxative should be determined by the doctor.

Calcification of the baby teeth begins in the fifth month after conception; for this and for the bones, fluoride may be needed. The woman in a county without fluoridated water may need a prescription for a supplement that includes fluoride.

What a lot for a woman to remember! And this is only the briefest summary of the nutrient needs in pregnancy. With all of this to worry about, can a woman relax and enjoy expecting her baby?

Pregnancy for many women is a time of adjustment to major changes. The woman who is expecting to bear a baby is a growing person in more ways than one. Not only physically, but also emotionally, her needs are changing. If it is her first baby, she senses that her lifestyle will have to change as she takes on the new responsibility of caring for a child. Ideally, she will be encouraged to develop this sense of responsibility by caring for herself during pregnancy. The expectant mother needs support in thinking of herself as a thoroughly worthwhile and important person with a new and challenging task that she can and will perform well. She is also, as a young adult, still working out her relationship with her mate, and he and she both know that the coming of a first baby will affect that relationship profoundly. There is a need for sensitive communication and understanding on both parts in this time of transition.

Women's cravings during pregnancy do not seem to reflect real physiological needs. Yet women going through this major experience should not be laughed at, and the validity of their feelings should be recognized. If a woman wakes her husband at 2 o'clock in the morning and begs him to go to the nearest all-night grocery to buy her some pickles and chocolate sauce, it is probably not because she lacks a combination of nutrients uniquely supplied by these foods. She is expressing a need, however, as real and as important as her need for nutrients—for support, understanding, and love.

Preparing for Breastfeeding

Toward the end of her pregnancy, a woman who plans to breastfeed her baby should begin to prepare. No elaborate or expensive procedures are necessary; but breastfeeding in humans involves many behaviors and attitudes that require learning, and it usually goes more smoothly for the mother who prepares than for the one who expects it to happen automatically. More is involved than can be discussed in detail here; it is recommended that she read at least one of the many handbooks available to breastfeeding mothers (see Appendix J). Talking with women who have breastfed their babies successfully is also helpful, as is having a family and medical team support system.

As far as possible, the mother should discuss her plans in advance with the members of that support system, whoever they may be—her husband, her mother, her other children, the doctor, the midwife, a nurse. Ideally, there will be classes that she and her husband can attend together before

A pregnant woman may crave and eat clay, ice, cornstarch, and other non-nutritious substances. This is **pica** (recall Chapter 11) and reflects a need for iron or zinc. The behavior is not adaptive, however; the substances she craves do not deliver the nutrients she needs.

the baby is born. Before the birth time, if possible, she should acquire two or more nursing bras—the kind that give good support and that have drop-flaps so that either breast can be freed for nursing. Also, if her nipples are tender, she should prepare them so that they will become tougher. One book says that human nipples tend to be "overprotected" by the clothing we wear and can be toughened by the following means:

● Stop using soap on the breasts for the last three months of pregnancy so that the skin's own protective secretions can make the nipple area strong and resistant to irritation.
● Let the nipples rub against the outer clothing (wear the nursing bra open or cut holes in an older bra for each nipple) so that they will be chafed.

A woman with flat or inverted nipples may want to manipulate her breasts by hand to help correct this condition or obtain a nipple shield that will help the nipple evert.

Breastfeeding

If a mother chooses to breastfeed, her nutrient supplies will continue to support the infant's development as well as her own even after birth. Adequate nutrition of the mother makes a highly significant contribution to successful lactation; without it, lactation is likely to falter or fail. She should continue to eat high-quality foods to the end of her pregnancy, not attempt to restrict her weight gain unduly, and plan to enjoy ample food and fluid at frequent intervals after she has given birth and until lactation is established. At birth, more learning is necessary (see "How to Breastfeed" and "Troubleshooting"), but a few more words about nutrition of the mother are in order first.

Nutrient Needs

A nursing mother produces 30 ounces of milk a day, on the average, with wide variations possible. At 20 kcalories per ounce, this milk output amounts to 600 kcalories per day. In addition, energy is needed to produce this milk; so the energy allowance for a lactating woman is a generous 750 kcalories per day above her ordinary need. The RDA table suggests that 500 kcalories come from added food, and the rest from the stores of fat her body accumulated during pregnancy for that purpose. Calcium, phosphorus, magnesium, and protein needs continue to be high, as these nutrients are secreted into the milk for the baby. Little iron is secreted in milk; so no increase in iron intake is needed, provided, of course, that the mother's iron nutrition has been good all along. The folacin requirement is lower in lactation than in pregnancy, because the mother's blood volume declines.

Eating Pattern

Logically, because the mother is making milk, she needs to consume something that resembles it in composition. The obvious choice is cow's milk.

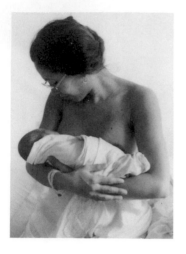

The nursing mother who can't drink milk needs to find nutritionally similar substitutes such as cheese or calcium-fortified soy milk. As before, nutritious foods should make up the remainder of the needed kcalorie increase. Because breast milk is a fluid, the mother's fluid intake should be liberal; a busy new mother often forgets this.

The question is often raised whether a mother's milk may lack a nutrient if she is not getting enough in her diet. The answer differs from one nutrient to the next, but in general the effect of nutritional deprivation of the mother is to reduce the quantity, not the quality, of her milk. For the energy nutrients and most vitamins and minerals, the milk has a constant composition. If one nutrient is in short supply, correspondingly less milk will be produced, but it still will have the proper composition. The mother's diet may make her blood cholesterol higher or lower to some extent but seems not to affect her breast milk cholesterol. For some of the water-soluble vitamins and trace minerals, the composition may be more variable, but most evidence seems to indicate that for these ingredients, too, the breast milk concentrations are constant. Even the taking of a vitamin-mineral supplement seems not to raise nutrient concentrations in the breast milk of an otherwise well-nourished mother. It is best to avoid "megadoses" of vitamins or other nutrients, of course. And to repeat: water is the major ingredient of milk, and a nursing mother's fluid intake should be ample.

The period of lactation is the natural time for a woman to lose the extra body fat she accumulated during pregnancy. If her choice of foods is judicious, a kcalorie deficit and a gradual loss of weight (1 pound per week) can easily be supported without any effect on her milk output. Fat can only be mobilized slowly, however, and too large a kcalorie deficit will inhibit lactation. On the other hand, if a mother does not breastfeed, she may not as easily lose the fat she gained during pregnancy.

Advantages of Breastfeeding

During the first two or three days of lactation, the breasts produce colostrum, a premilk substance whose antibody content is even higher than that of the milk that comes later. Both colostrum and breast milk are sterile as they leave the breast, and the baby cannot contract a bacterial infection from them even if his mother has one. Both contain active white blood cells in the same concentration as in the mother's blood to devour enemy agents such as bacteria and viruses. Thus, colostrum and breast milk protect infants just as modern medicine (vaccinations) and technology (sanitary water supplies) are intended to protect people.

Breast milk is also tailor-made to meet the nutrient needs of the human infant. It offers its carbohydrate as lactose; its fat as a mixture with a generous proportion of the essential fatty acid, linoleic acid; and its protein largely as lactalbumin, a protein the human infant can easily digest. Its vitamin contents are ample. Even vitamin C, for which milk is not normally a good source, is supplied generously by breast milk.

As for minerals, the calcium-to-phosphorus ratio (2-to-1) is ideal for the absorption of calcium, and both of these minerals and magnesium are

colostrum (co-LAHS-trum): a milk-like secretion from the breast, rich in protective factors, present during the first day or so after delivery, before milk appears.

lactalbumin (lact-AL-byoo-min): the chief protein in human breast milk, as opposed to **casein** (CAY-seen), the chief protein of cow's milk.

present in amounts appropriate for the rate of growth expected in a human infant. Breast milk is also low in sodium. In addition, it contains factors that favor absorption of the iron it contains. On the average, 49 percent of the iron is absorbed from breast milk, as compared with only 4 percent from fortified formula.[11] Zinc, too, is better absorbed from breast milk, which contains a zinc-binding protein necessary for absorption of zinc by the newborn.[12]

Powerful agents against bacterial infection also occur in breast milk. Among them is lactoferrin, an iron-grabbing compound, which keeps bacteria from getting the iron they need to grow on, helps absorb iron into the infant's bloodstream, and also works directly to kill some bacteria.[13]

Breast milk also contains antibodies, although not as many as colostrum. These antibodies protect specifically against the intestinal diseases most likely to threaten the infant's life. Entering the infant's body with the milk, these antibodies inactivate bacteria within the digestive tract, where they would otherwise cause harm. Some of the antibodies also "leak" into the bloodstream, because the infant's immature digestive tract cannot completely exclude whole proteins. These antibodies provide additional protection against such diseases as polio. Breast milk also contains a factor (the bifidus factor) that favors the growth of the "friendly" bacteria *Lactobacillus bifidus* in the infant's digestive tract, so that other, harmful bacteria cannot grow there. Another factor present in breast milk stimulates the development of the infant's GI tract.[14]

As this is written, other factors are still being identified and characterized, including:

● Several enzymes.[15]
● A factor that enhances the infant's absorption of folacin.[16]
● Several hormones, including thyroid hormone and prostaglandins.[17]
● Lipids (in addition to antibodies and white blood cells) that protect the infant against infection.[18]

lactoferrin (lak-toe-FERR-in): a factor in breast milk that binds iron and keeps it from supporting the growth of the infant's intestinal bacteria.

bifidus (BIFF-id-us, by-FEED-us) **factor**: a factor in breast milk that favors the growth, in the infant's intestinal tract, of the "friendly" bacteria *Lactobacillus* (lack-toh-ba-SILL-us) *bifidus*, so that other, less desirable intestinal inhabitants will not flourish.

11 J. A. McMillan, S. A. Landaw, and F. A. Oski, Iron sufficiency in breast-fed infants and the availability of iron from human milk, *Pediatrics* 58 (1976): 686–691.

12 Acrodermatitis enteropathica, zinc, and human milk, *Nutrition Reviews* 36 (1978): 241–242.

13 R. R. Arnold, M. F. Cole, and J. R. McGhee, A bactericidal effect for human lactoferrin, *Science* 197 (1977): 263–265; Probable role of lactoferrin in the transport of iron across the intestinal brush border, *Nutrition Reviews* 38 (1980): 256–257.

14 M. Winick, Infant nutrition: Formula or breast feeding? *Professional Nutritionist*, Spring 1980, pp. 1–3.

15 These enzymes include RNAse, lipoprotein lipase, and lysozyme, among others. K. M. Shahani, A. J. Kwan, and B. A. Friend, Role and significance of enzymes in human milk, *American Journal of Clinical Nutrition* 33 (1980): 1861–1868.

16 N. Colman, N. Hettiarachchy, and V. Herbert, Detection of a milk factor that facilitates folate uptake by intestinal cells, *Science* 211 (1981): 1427–1429.

17 Thyroid hormones in human milk, *Nutrition Reviews* 37 (1979): 140–141; Prostaglandins in human milk, *Nutrition Reviews* 39 (1981): 302–303.

18 J. J. Kabara, Lipids as host-resistance factors of human milk, *Nutrition Reviews* 38 (1980): 65–73.

● A morphine-like compound, perhaps transmitted from food the mother has eaten, for which there are corresponding receptors in the infant's brain.[19]

Much remains to be learned about the composition and characteristics of human milk, but clearly it is a very special substance.

In addition, there are indications that breastfeeding provides other benefits:

● It is less likely to produce an obese child.
● It promotes better tooth and jaw alignment.
● It protects against allergy development during the vulnerable first few weeks.
● It favors optimum bonding between mother and child.

It may have other advantages, too; some studies suggest that mothers who breastfeed are less likely to develop breast cancer and to form unwanted clots in the bloodstream after delivery. A woman who wants to breastfeed can derive justification and satisfaction from all these advantages.

Advantages of Formula Feeding

The substitution of formula feeding for breastfeeding involves copying nature as closely as possible. A comparison of the nutrient composition of human and cow's milk shows that they differ. Cow's milk is significantly higher in protein, calcium, and phosphorus, for example, to support the calf's faster growth rate. But a formula can be prepared from cow's milk that does not differ significantly from human milk in these respects; the formula makers first dilute the milk and then add carbohydrate and nutrients to make it nutritionally comparable to human milk.

The antibodies in cow's milk do not protect the human baby from disease (they protect the calf from cattle diseases), but the high level of preventive medical care (vaccinations) and public health measures achieved in the developed countries, especially in the United States and Canada, make these considerations less important than they were in the past. Safety and sanitation can be achieved with either mode of feeding by the educated mother whose water supply is reliable.

Like the breastfeeding mother, the one who feeds formula should be supported in her choice. Bearing and nurturing a baby involves much more than merely pouring nutrients in, in whatever form. The mother who offers formula to her baby has valid reasons for making her choice, and her feelings should be honored. She and the baby can benefit in many ways from the supportive approval of those around them.

One of the major advantages of formula feeding is that gained by the mother whose attempts at breastfeeding have met with frustration. If she truly doesn't want to breastfeed or, worse, if she earnestly does want to and can't, continuing to try is an agonizing course, as hard on the baby as on the mother. When the mother finally accepts the necessity of formula feeding and weans the baby to the bottle, a period of anguish for both may be followed by the onset of peace and the first real opportunity to develop the

Lactose is the sugar of milk, but sometimes sucrose is added to formula because it is sweeter and less expensive. On the assumption that formula should copy breast milk as closely as possible, the sugar added should be lactose.

19   E. Hazum and coauthors, Morphine in cow and human milk: Could dietary morphine constitute a ligand for specific morphine (mu) receptors? *Science* 213 (1981): 1010–1012.

all-important mother-child love. Other advantages:

● The mother can be sure the baby is getting enough milk; there is no limit to the supply.

● She can offer the same closeness, warmth, and stimulation during feedings as the breastfeeding mother does.

● Other family members can get close to the baby and develop a warm relationship in feeding sessions.

● The mother will be free, sooner, to give time to her other children or to contribute to the family's income by returning to work.

The attendant who is asked to advise on breastfeeding versus bottle-feeding should remember the advantages of both. In fact, when addressing any audience, you should remember that some members of that audience will be women who bottle-fed their babies. To praise breastfeeding out of proportion or without qualification can only make them feel guilty or angry.

Many mothers choose to breastfeed at first but wean within the first one to six months. This is a nice compromise. Even a few weeks of breastfeeding will significantly reduce the likelihood of the baby's developing an allergy to cow's milk, and this advantage alone is important if such an allergy is likely. Furthermore, the baby gets the immunological protection and all the special advantages of breastfeeding during the most critical first few weeks or months. Then the mother can choose to shift to the bottle and can know she has already given the baby those benefits. But it is imperative that she wean the baby onto *formula*, not onto plain milk of any kind—whole, lowfat, or skim. Only formula contains enough iron (to name but one of many, many factors) to support normal development in the baby's first year.

When Breastfeeding Is Preferred

It has been stated that a woman should be free to choose the mode of feeding she prefers. This implies that the two modes of feeding are equally beneficial to the infant. However, if the infant is premature, if the family is poor, or if other factors act to the baby's disadvantage, then breastfeeding becomes the preferred choice.

Some authorities feel that a premature baby should be fed breast milk even if the mother can't nurse. That is, if the baby is being kept sealed away in an incubator in the intensive care unit, the mother should milk herself with her hands or a breast pump and carry the milk to the intensive care unit to be fed to the baby. Her own milk is thought to be better for the baby than that of a full-term mother, because it is of a composition better suited to a premature infant's needs. Breastfeeding manuals show how to use manual massage or breast pumps to obtain milk.

Some communities maintain breast milk "banks"—storage and delivery facilities for breast milk. Mothers who have milk to spare donate it to the bank; others can purchase it when it is needed. Success and safety in milk banking requires use of aseptic technique by the donor and prompt freezing of the milk. Breast milk normally contains bacteria and viruses from the mother's skin and nipple ducts—acceptable for her own baby but not for someone else's. Freezing is necessary to prevent spoilage while preserving the milk's antibodies and other protective factors, which would be

aseptic technique: the technique of working in a sterile fashion—that is, in an area free of all bacteria, and kept free of contamination.

a = without

sepsis = infection

504

bonding: the forming of a bond between mother and infant. A critical event in bonding, thought to be mediated by chemical messengers in breast milk, occurs in the first 45 minutes after birth, so this is an especially important time for mother and infant to be close, if possible. However, emotional bonding is facilitated by many other events and behaviors of mother and infant during the early months and years.

We're calling the baby *he* most of the time, because we have to call the mother *she*. But we like girl babies too.

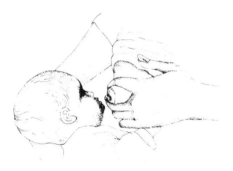

Gently squeeze the areola between two fingers to insert the nipple far enough into the baby's mouth.

areola (a-REE-uh-luh): the colored halo around the nipple. Beneath the areola lie the ducts that bring milk from the mammary glands. Pumping action on the areola promotes flow of milk from the glands through the ducts.

The hormone that promotes milk production is **prolactin**; the one that initiates let-down is **oxytocin**.

rooting reflex: the reflex that makes a newborn turn towards whichever cheek is touched and search for the nipple.

destroyed by pasteurization. The current recommendation is that a premature or ill baby's own mother collect, freeze, and transport her milk daily to the hospital and that banked milk only be used temporarily, if there is no better alternative. Breast milk can be stored safely in the freezer for up to six months, provided that it stays solidly frozen (below 0° F).[20]

A premature baby receiving breast milk may be given a supplement of special formula for premature infants, depending on the philosophy of the clinic responsible for its care. Babies not receiving breast milk can be successfully nourished on this formula alone and even on total parenteral nutrition (nutrients delivered directly into a central vein).

How to Breastfeed

The most important pointers for the breastfeeding mother are presented in list form here, to save space. To help carry them out, the team present at the baby's birth will ideally provide the necessary support. Thereafter, whoever attends the mother should make sure she learns these things. A home visit after a week or ten days is advisable for followup.

1 At the moment of birth, the healthy, full-term infant starts to breathe on its own and within moments makes sucking motions showing readiness to feed. Within the first 30 minutes the sucking reflex is especially strong; nursing the baby right away will get breastfeeding off to a good start. The first 45 minutes are also a critical period for bonding, the formation of a physical and emotional tie between mother and infant that will persist throughout infancy.

If the mother can't nurse right away (if she is sedated), the newborn should wait. He doesn't need the nutrients; he needs the appropriate first impression. Do *not* give him a bottle, for he can develop an attachment to it and then resist the breast later.

2 Beginning at the first feeding, the mother should learn how to *relax* and position herself so that she and the baby will both be comfortable and so that the baby can drink without having his breathing obstructed. She needs to learn how to squeeze the areola between two fingers so that she can slip enough of it into the baby's mouth to promote good pumping action. She also needs to learn how to make the baby let go—don't pull! Break the suction by slipping a finger between his gums or holding his nose for a second.

3 The infant's sucking is the stimulus for the release of a hormone that promotes the making of more milk. Therefore, if the infant is hungry he should be allowed to suck longer; this will ensure a greater milk supply at the next nursing. The same hormone promotes the contraction of the uterus, so that it stops bleeding and returns to normal size as quickly as possible after birth—another reason to put the baby to the breast immediately after birth, if possible.

4 The rooting reflex makes the infant turn his mouth towards whichever side of his face is touched. If you want the infant to nurse, you should not touch his other cheek, or he will turn his head away from the nipple toward your hand. Touch his cheek with the nipple so that he will turn and take the breast.

20   Questions readers ask, *Nutrition and the MD*, December 1981.

5 The let-down, or milk-ejection, reflex makes the milk flow. At first, the stimulus for let-down is the baby's actual sucking. Later, when the reflex is well established, the sound of the baby's crying may be enough to trigger it. You can tell it is working when, while the mother is nursing the baby on one breast, milk drips from the other. Let-down has to occur for the baby to obtain milk easily; if it is slow, the baby may struggle and tire before getting enough. The mother must learn to relax and go with the let-down reflex; it may take several weeks for this habit to become established. A glass of water before nursing can help; some people recommend a moderate drink of beer or wine for the late afternoon feeding, when the mother may be tense.

6 The draught reflex, which occurs later during a nursing session, draws milk from the hindmost milk-producing glands of the breast after the foremilk has been released. The mother can feel this as a tingly sensation within the breast. The baby should be allowed and encouraged to nurse after the draught has begun, so that he will get enough milk. If feeding is interrupted after the draught reflex has occurred, it may not occur again for some time and the baby may not get enough milk. Hindmilk is richer in fat than foremilk and so provides satiety after the baby has sucked enough to satisfy his sucking need.

7 The sucking and swallowing reflexes work together so that the baby's tongue and jaw pump milk from the breast and the swallow follows. The nipple has to rest well back on the baby's tongue, and his lips and gums have to be pressing on the areola if he is to stimulate milk release successfully and then swallow the milk.

8 Although the baby can suck half the milk from the breast within two minutes and 80 to 90 percent of it within four minutes, he should continue sucking for ten minutes or more on one breast. The sucking itself, as well as the removal of milk from the breast, is believed to stimulate lactation. After he has put in his ten minutes or so—his share of the work—the baby can be given the other breast to finish satisfying his hunger. Nursing sessions should normally start on alternate breasts, so that each breast is emptied regularly. When the baby seems to be full, hold him upright to let him expel any swallowed air (burping), and then given him another chance to nurse.

9 For the first ten days, even if everything is going smoothly at home, the nursing mother should ideally have enough help and support so that she can rest in bed for several hours a day. Real rest and a plentiful fluid intake are indispensable to successful lactation.

10 Demand feedings, no fewer than six a day, are most likely to promote optimal milk production and infant growth. The infant should be encouraged to nurse; or the milk should be manually pumped out at intervals to keep the supply going. A mother who nurses her baby even 12 times a day during the first two weeks will ensure that supply keeps up with demand and will gain enough practice to maintain successful lactation easily later on. The midnight feeding should not be skipped, even if the baby is inclined to sleep through it. If the mother feels that she is spending immense amounts of time breastfeeding, she should remind herself that the bottle-feeding mother is spending as much or more time washing bottles, sterilizing formula, and feeding her baby. Breastfeeding will not

let-down reflex: the reflex that forces milk to the front of the breast when the infant begins to nurse.

draught reflex (DRAFT reflex): the reflex that moves the hindmilk toward the nipple after the infant has drawn off the foremilk.

satiety (sat-EYE-uh-tee): a feeling of fullness or satisfaction from eating or drinking.

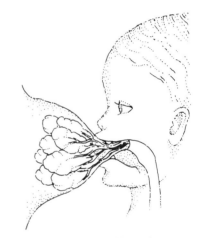

The baby's gums are milking the mammary glands by pressing on the milk ducts; the milk is squirting into the baby's throat.

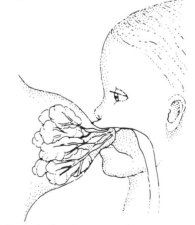

This baby hasn't got an adequate grasp on the nipple and will not get enough milk.

engorgement: overfilling of the breasts with milk so that they become swollen and hard.

You can tell if a nipple is inverted by pressing the areola between two fingers. An inverted nipple folds inward toward the breast. Pushing the areola toward the chest wall (manually or with a shield) everts the nipple.

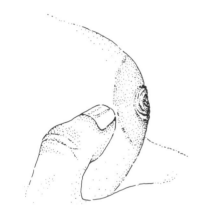

Inverted nipple.

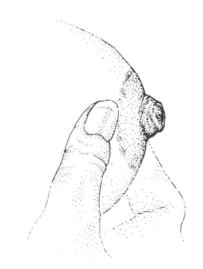

Normal nipple.

continue to be so time consuming for more than a very few weeks. Remember the advantages; remember that this time will pass; and enjoy it while it lasts.

11 Mothers often want to know if they can skip an occasional feeding, substituting a bottle of formula. To be sure not to suppress lactation, the mother should express the amount of milk the baby would drink, even if she doesn't expect to use it; that way, the breast gets the message to keep on producing that much milk. The mother who is confident that lactation is well established, however, may not bother to do this, and will experience no noticeable diminution of the supply.

A mother who wants to skip one or two feedings daily—for example, if she goes to work outside the home—can substitute formula for those feedings and continue to breastfeed morning and evening. She will probably find that her milk is not adequate to restore the missed feedings easily (for example, on weekends), but that she and her baby can continue to enjoy the morning and evening feedings for as long as desired.

Troubleshooting

Solutions can be found for almost all the problems that arise in connection with breastfeeding. Breastfeeding manuals give many further details beyond those listed below.

1 Sore nipples should be treated kindly, but nursing can continue even if the nipples are bleeding. Air and sunlight between feedings will help to heal them. Getting the let-down reflex going smoothly helps a lot, because then the baby doesn't have to suck hard on the nipple. Nurse on the less-sore breast first; when the milk lets down, switch to the sore one and position the baby to minimize the pain; then, when most of the fast-flowing, early milk from that breast is gone, switch back and let the baby satisfy the sucking need on the other breast.

2 Engorgement can make the breasts so full and hard that the baby can't get his mouth around the nipple. Pump out some of the milk, use a nipple shield, and/or massage or warm the breasts to help let-down get started. They will get smaller and softer, while still producing ample milk, after the first several days of lactation.

3 An inverted nipple can be managed similarly. A nipple shield can be used to press around the nipple and make it poke out so the baby can get hold of it.

4 An undrained sinus can make a hard, uncomfortable lump in the breast. Massage the lump while the baby is nursing, to move the milk toward the nipple where it will join the main supply.

5 Supplemental water can be offered if the baby seems to be thirsty after a long feed, but offering sugar-water or other supplemental feedings in the first few weeks is ill advised. Infants fed sweetened water in the first few months tend to have a greater preference for sweets later in infancy.[21] Also,

21 G. K. Beauchamp, Ontogenesis of taste preferences (paper presented at the fifth congress of the International Organization for the Study of Human Development, Campione, Italy, May 1980), cited in G. K. Beauchamp, M. Bertino, and M. Moran, Sodium regulation: Sensory aspects, *Journal of the American Dietetic Association* 80 (1982): 40–45.

sweetened water carries kcalories, which should come to the infant only from the breast. The full extent of the baby's demand should be communicated to the mother's body by way of sucking, so that the milk supply will increase to meet it.

6 Infection of a breast is best managed by *continuing to breastfeed*. By drawing off the milk, the infant helps to relieve pressure in the infected area; he does not become infected because the infection is between the milk-producing glands, not inside them.

7 The baby who seems to be up all night crying for milk and asleep much of the day *may* be getting less milk by day and may therefore be hungry at night. In any case, to rectify the situation, the *mother* should relax and nap during the day, too. (To do this, she must have support, or must be willing to let all but the indispensable chores wait until another day or week.) This way, she'll have more milk during the day and can gradually get the baby turned around. By six weeks, these problems will probably be ironed out.

8 If the mother wants to prevent a next pregnancy, she will need to make a decision about contraception while breastfeeding. The hormones of lactation to some extent inhibit ovulation; so long as a woman is breastfeeding intensively and has not resumed menstruation, she probably has natural protection against pregnancy. The hormones in *oral* contraceptives can inhibit lactation, and so the use of a barrier contraceptive method is preferred at least for the first six months. A decision tree designed by a physician to minimize the overlap of oral contraceptive use with natural protection and limit the risk of accidental pregnancy is shown in Figure 13–3.

Infection of a breast is **mastitis**.

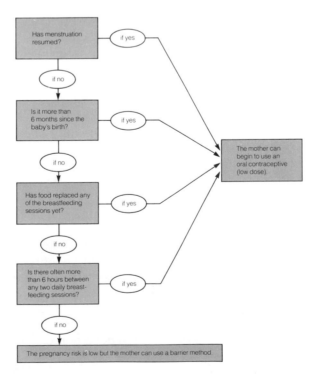

FIGURE 13–3 **Decision tree for contraception during lactation.**

Source: Adapted from M. H. Labbock, Breastfeeding and contraception (letter to the editor), *New England Journal of Medicine* 308 (1983): 51.

9 Most importantly, if the baby is irritable and wakeful, the mother may fear that her milk supply is inadequate. The baby's small bowel movements may suggest to her that he is not getting enough milk, but she can be reassured that there is little indigestible material in breast milk and therefore little waste. Worrying itself can inhibit lactation. She should be reassured that bottle-fed babies cry, too, and that her own ability to calm down, relax, and let her fears go will help more than any amount of anxiety. However, if she really wants to wean the baby, she can be supported in that choice and congratulated on having nursed for as long as she did. Even feeding for only a few days, so that the baby gets the benefit of the protective factors in colostrum, makes a contribution to the baby's health and development in which the mother can take pride.

When Not to Breastfeed

If a woman has a communicable disease that could threaten the infant's health so that they have to be separated, then of course she cannot breastfeed. Similarly, if she must take medication that is secreted in breast milk and that is known to affect the infant, she must not breastfeed. Drug addicts, including alcohol abusers, are capable of taking such high doses that their infants can become addicts by way of breast milk; in these cases, too, breastfeeding is contraindicated.

Most prescription drugs, however, do not reach nursing infants in sufficiently large quantities to affect them adversely. Moderate use of alcohol and moderate smoking are compatible with breastfeeding. Coffee drinking is fine, in moderation, as is the eating of foods such as garlic and spices. A particular food may affect the baby's liking for the mother's milk; this is a matter that requires individual detective work. If a woman has an ordinary cold, she can go on nursing without worry. The infant will catch it from her anyway, if he is susceptible, and he may be less susceptible thanks to immunologic protection than a bottle-fed baby would be.

A woman sometimes hesitates to breastfeed because she has heard that environmental contaminants such as DDT may enter her milk and harm her baby. DDT has been reported in the milk of mothers at higher concentrations than are allowed in cow's milk. The significance of these findings is hard to evaluate, and the decision whether to breastfeed on this basis might best be made after consultation with a physician or dietitian familiar with the local circumstances.

For more about DDT and PCBs, turn to Highlight 11.

Another environmental contaminant that has caused concern is the PCBs, which are found in rivers and waterways polluted by industry. An episode of accidental PCB consumption by pregnant women in Japan arose when they consumed contaminated cooking oil; later they gave birth to abnormally small babies whose skin was unusually dark for a while. PCBs are stored in body fat and remain in the body; they are excreted only in the fat of breast milk.

According to the Committee on Environmental Hazards of the American Academy of Pediatrics, women need not fear contamination of their breast milk with PCBs unless they have eaten large amounts of fish caught in PCB-contaminated rivers such as the Saint Lawrence Seaway or have been directly exposed because of their occupations. Should a woman have any question about PCBs in her breast milk, she should ask the advice of the local state health department.[22]

How to Feed Formula

These pointers are important to all mothers—both those who choose to feed formula from the start, and those who will need to substitute occasional bottles of formula for breast milk.

1 The choice of formula is usually not critical. Any brand that meets the AAP standards[23] is fine for most babies. For the allergic or ill baby, or for one with an inborn error, however, special formulas are necessary (see Figure 13–4).

2 The mother who chooses not to breastfeed may experience some discomfort as her own milk dries up. An injection of estrogen or a large dose of

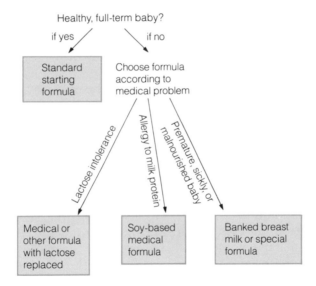

FIGURE 13–4 **Choosing a formula.**

Source: E. N. Whitney and C. B. Cataldo, Highlight 15: Choosing formulas and milk substitutes, in *Understanding Normal and Clinical Nutrition* (St. Paul, Minn.: West, 1983), pp. 559-568.

22   Committee on Environmental Hazards, Academy of Pediatrics, PCBs in breast milk, *Pediatrics* 62 (1978): 407.

23   The AAP (American Association of Pediatrics) standards are available in Committee on Nutrition, American Academy of Pediatrics, Commentary on breast feeding and infant formulas, including proposed standards for formulas, in *Pediatric Nutrition Handbook* (Evanston, Ill.: American Academy of Pediatrics, 1979), pp. 119–138. Choices of formulas were discussed in E. N. Whitney and C. B. Cataldo, Highlight 15: Choosing Formulas and Milk Substitutes, in *Understanding Normal and Clinical Nutrition* (St. Paul, Minn.: West, 1983), pp. 559–568.

vitamin B$_6$ may be used to hasten the process. (Vitamin B$_6$ is needed in food, of course, but megadoses can be used to suppress lactation.[24])

3 Formula today in the United States and Canada is often bought premixed and sterile in cans from the store and is easy to feed in disposable bottle liners. But the mother who mixes or bottles her own must learn the rules of safe formula preparation and administration. Until the baby is strong and clearly resistant to infection (at two to three months), formula should be prepared with great care, with safe, pure water and fresh, refrigerated, or canned ingredients. It has to be sterilized and kept sterile until it is presented to the baby. (These rules can be relaxed if the total environment is clean and the water supply is pure. Then all that is necessary is to wash bottle and nipples well with soapy water and rinse them thoroughly before preparing a fresh batch of formula.) If half a bottle is left after a feeding, it should be resterilized immediately if it is to be used again; this shouldn't be a regular practice, however, because nutrient losses are incurred by high temperature treatment. Unsterile formula should never stand at room temperature.

The mother should be trained in formula preparation by an experienced person and should be observed and guided at least once as she goes through the steps herself. The less well educated, economically well off, and experienced she is, and the less strong and healthy her baby is, the more important are these safeguards. In poor areas, especially where a sanitary water supply is not dependable, these rules and training are crucial.

4 Formula can be offered warm or cold. The baby may prefer warm formula if accustomed to it, but no harm is done by feeding it cold unless it is refused.

5 Close contact during feeding is important. Infant and mother should both be comfortable and relaxed, and the infant should be positioned so that he can drink easily. His head should be higher than his body so that he will be drinking "downhill." The nipple hole should be large enough to allow one swallow of milk to flow each time the baby sucks; if it is too small, it should be enlarged; and if it is too large, it should be replaced. Check the nipple to make sure the formula is flowing. The bottle should be tilted so that the nipple is full of formula, not air, while the baby is sucking.

6 When the baby stops drinking, he should be sat or held upright and patted on the back to help him bring up any bubbles of air he may have swallowed. Then after he has burped, offer him more formula. But don't try to force him to finish the bottle; like making children clean their plates, this promotes obesity.

7 The feeding schedule can vary but best promotes development if adjusted to the baby's expressed hunger needs at first, within reason. Some babies need to feed much more frequently than others. Remember that a dehydrated baby (feverish, hot) may be thirsty for water, which can be offered in place of formula if the baby cries soon after a feeding.

8 Sterilized formula can be replaced by regular, clean, fresh formula and

Formula preparation:

Liquid concentrate (inexpensive, relatively easy)—mix with equal part water.

Powdered formula (cheapest, lightest for travel)—read label directions.

Ready-to-feed (easiest, most expensive)—pour directly into clean bottles.

Evaporated milk—ask nutritionist or nurse; use *both* vitamins and iron in addition.

Whole milk—do not use.

24 "Large doses" means over 200 milligrams pyridoxine, 100 times the RDA. M. D. Foukas, An antilactogenic effect of pyridoxine, *Journal of Obstetrics and Gynecology, British Commonwealth* 80 (1973): 718–720; R. G. Marcus, Suppression of lactation with high doses of pyridoxine, *South Africa Medical Journal* 49 (1975): 2155–2156.

then by milk as the baby grows older. Some authorities say the switch to milk can be made at six months, others say to wait until a year. The pediatrician should be consulted in each individual case.

9 Babies love their bottles; the sucking provides needed stimulation as well as nutrients. They should never be allowed to sleep with them, however, because of the potential damage to developing teeth. The bedtime bottle may be the most cherished, but it should be firmly removed. At weaning time (some time around nine months or so, when the baby can sit up and begin to manage a cup), one of the daily bottles at a time can be taken away and replaced by milk in a drinking cup. The last bottle may be the one at bedtime, and this could be given up at about a year at the discretion of the parents and pediatrician.

10 Most importantly (to repeat), hold the baby as closely and lovingly as a breastfeeding mother does. Much more occurs during a feeding than the mere transfer of nutrients into the baby's body. The human warmth and stimulation delivered with the formula do as much as the formula itself to promote normal, healthy development.

Vitamin-Mineral Supplements for the Infant

It is unnecessary to give vitamin-mineral supplements to a newborn infant. If he is breastfed, breast milk and his own internal stores will meet most of his nutrient needs until he is well into the second half of his first year, and then the introduction of intelligently chosen juices and foods will keep up with his changing requirements. The only exceptions to this statement have to do with vitamin D, fluoride, and possibly iron.

Breast milk does not provide enough vitamin D, and the infant who has little exposure to sunlight is at risk of developing rickets. People often wonder how much sunlight it takes to prevent deficiency. So many variables are involved that no single answer to this question is possible. Among the relevant factors are:

- Latitude (how far from the sun).
- Season (winter versus summer).
- Area of skin exposed (winter versus summer clothes).
- Color of skin (light versus dark).
- City versus country (smog filters out the vitamin D-producing ultraviolet rays of the sun).

A light-skinned baby with just a diaper on in strong summer sun and clear air might make enough vitamin D in a few minutes to meet his daily need. A dark-skinned baby wrapped up for cold weather in a smoggy city might not make enough even if he was outside for several hours.[25] For most babies in

25   At particular risk are inner-city black Muslim infants who are breastfed. Not all milks are kind, *Nutrition and the MD*, May 1980; W. F. Loomis, Skin-pigment regulation of vitamin-D biosynthesis in man, *Science* 157 (1967): 501–506; R. M. Neer, The evolutionary significance of vitamin D, skin pigment, and ultraviolet light, *American Journal of Physical Anthropology* 43 (1975): 409–416.

most circumstances, some exposure of a small amount of skin to the sun at midday each day would provide a protective dose of vitamin D.[26]

Also, the fluoride contents of breast milk may be somewhat unreliable.[27] The baby's pediatrician is likely to be well informed on this matter and to prescribe appropriate supplementation. As for iron, it may be desirable to begin iron supplements for the breastfed infant at about four months.[28]

If the baby is formula-fed, the makeup of the formula determines what further supplementation may be necessary. Vitamins A and D, vitamin C, and fluoride are needed if the formula is not fortified with them. Again, the pediatrician is the expert to consult on local needs. Table 13–3 shows what supplements are needed as the transitions are made from breastfeeding to formula, and formula to milk.

Nutrition of the Infant

A baby grows faster during the first year than ever again, as Figure 13–5 shows. The growth of infants and children directly reflects their nutritional

TABLE 13–3 **Transitions in Milk Feeding**

BEFORE 6 MONTHS	AFTER 6 MONTHS	AFTER 1 YEAR

Breast-fed infant should receive:
  Breast milk.
  Vitamin D.
  Fluoride and iron at pediatrician's discretion.
 	
Formula-fed infant should receive:
  Vitamins A and D in formula or separately.
  Vitamin C in formula or separately.
  Fluoride at pediatrician's discretion.
 	
If weaning from breast milk before 6 months, wean to formula as above.
 	
Wait to wean from formula until at least 6 months.
	If weaning from breast milk after 6 months, wean to formula or whole cow's milk with supplementation.
	
	Whole cow's milk (may be fresh or evaporated) should be supplemented with:
	  Vitamins A and D if not fortified.
	  Iron and/or iron-fortified cereals.
	  Vitamin C or C–rich foods or juices.
	  Fluoride at pediatrician's discretion.
		When all four food groups are eaten daily, whole or low-fat cow's milk is acceptable.
		
		Continue checking diet for vitamin C, iron, and all nutrients.
		
		Continue fluoride supplements if necessary.

Source: Adapted from recommendations made in *Pediatrics* 62 (1978): 733 and *Nutrition and the MD*, March 1980.

26   P. M. Fleiss, J. Gordon, and J. Douglass, The vitamin D activity of milk (letter to the editor), *Nutrition Reviews* 40 (1982): 286.

27   J. C. Gallagher and B. L. Riggs, Nutrition and bone disease, *New England Journal of Medicine* 298 (1978): 193–195.

28   Dr. James C. Penrod, pediatrician, of Tallahassee, Florida (personal communication, June 1983).

FIGURE 13–5 **Weight gain of human infants (boys) in the first five years**.

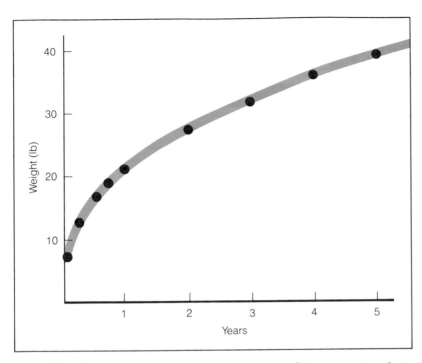

well-being and is the most important parameter used in assessing their nutrition status. The birthweight doubles in four months, from 7 to 14 pounds, and another 7 pounds is added in the next eight months. (If a ten-year-old child were to do this, the child's weight would increase from 70 to 210 pounds in a single year.) By the end of the first year, the growth rate has slowed down, and the weight gained between the first and second birthdays amounts to only about 5 pounds. This tremendous growth is a composite of the differing growth patterns of all the internal organs. The generalization that many critical periods occur early still holds true.

Changes in body organs during the first year affect the baby's readiness to accept solid foods. At first, all he can do is suck (and he can do that powerfully), but he can only swallow liquids that are well back in his throat. Later (at two months or so) he can move his tongue against his palate to swallow semisolid food. Still later, the first teeth erupt, but it is not until sometime during the second year that a baby can begin to handle chewy food. The stomach and intestines are immature at first; they can digest milk sugar (lactose) but can't manufacture significant quantities of the starch-digesting enzyme, amylase, until somewhat later and so cannot digest starch until about three months, with some variation depending on the individual baby.

The baby's kidneys are unable to concentrate waste efficiently, so a baby must excrete relatively more water than an adult to carry off a comparable amount of waste. This means that dehydration, which can be dangerous, can occur more easily in an infant than in an adult. Because infants can communicate their needs only by crying, it is important to remember that they may be crying for fluid. A baby's metabolism is fast, so his energy needs are high.

Baby's metabolism:
Heart rate: 120–140 beats/min.
Respiration rate: 20/min.

Adult's metabolism:
Heart rate: 70–80 beats/min.
Respiration rate: 12–14/min.

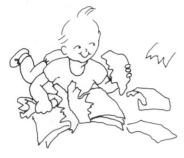

kCalories saved by slower growth are spent in greatly increased activity.

Nutrient Needs

The rapid growth and metabolism of the infant demand ample supplies of the growth and energy nutrients. Babies, because they are small, need smaller total amounts of these nutrients than adults do; but as a percentage of body weight, babies need over twice as much of most nutrients. Figure 13–6 compares a three-month-old baby's needs with those of an adult man; as you can see, some of the differences are extraordinary. After three months, energy needs continue to increase even though the growth rate slows down. As a baby nears the first birthday, the kcalories saved by slower growth are spent in greatly increased activity. (Babies are now known to require fewer kcalories in the middle of their first year than was believed in the past, and new recommendations were being made as of 1981.[29])

Iron is the nutrient hardest to provide for infants, because it doesn't occur in adequate amounts in milk (except breast milk or iron-fortified formula). One U.S. survey showed in 1979 that by the end of the first year more than 70 percent of infants were receiving less than the RDA for iron, and almost half of them were receiving less than two-thirds of the RDA, a bottom line for adequacy. Iron was the nutrient most needing attention in infant nutrition.[30]

FIGURE 13–6 **Comparison of the nutrient needs of three-month-old infants with those of adult males (23 years old and up) per pound of body weight.** The adult male's needs are set at 100 percent.

Source: Calculated from the RDA table, inside front cover.

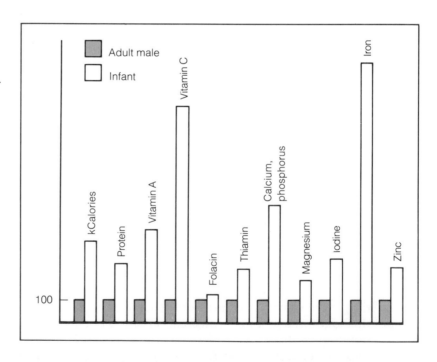

29 Part of the significance of the infant's lower energy needs at six months is that breastfeeding will be seen to be more adequate when measured against them. R. G. Whitehead, A critical analysis of measured food energy intakes during infancy and early childhood in comparison with current international recommendations, *Journal of Human Nutrition* 35 (1981): 339–348.

30 G. H. Johnson, G. A. Purvis, and R. D. Wallace, What nutrients do our infants really get? *Nutrition Today*, July/August 1981, pp. 4–10, 23–26.

First Foods

The timing for adding solid foods to a baby's diet depends on several factors. If the baby is breastfed, additions to the diet can probably wait until about six months, but not later. Babies not fed solid foods in the second half of the first year suffer delayed growth.[31] If the baby is formula-fed, a reasonable pattern for adding foods to the diet is as shown in Table 13–4. Solids should not be introduced too early, because infants are more likely to develop allergies to them in the early months.[32] But all babies are different, and the program of additions should depend on the individual baby, not on any rigid schedule.

The addition of foods to a baby's diet should be governed by three considerations: the baby's nutrient needs, the baby's physical readiness to handle different forms of foods, and the need to detect and control allergic reactions. With respect to nutrient needs, nutrients needed early, especially by the formula-fed baby, are iron and vitamin C. Juices and fruits that contain vitamin C are usually among the first foods introduced. A baby's stored iron supply from before birth runs out after the birthweight doubles, so formula with iron; iron-fortified cereals; and later, meat are recommended.

It has been suggested that the early introduction of sweet fruits to babies' diets might favor their developing a preference for sweets and lessen their liking for vegetables introduced later. To prevent this, the order should perhaps be changed: vegetables first, fruits later. This practice now has a wide following.

A term used by many authorities to mean supplemental or weaning foods is **beikost** (BYE-cost).

TABLE 13–4 **First Foods for the Formula-Fed Baby**

AGE (MONTHS)	ADDITION
0–1	Supplement (depending on what's in formula)
1–2	Diluted orange juice (for vitamin C)
4–6	Iron-fortified rice cereal followed by other cereals (for iron; baby can swallow and can digest starch now)[a]
5–7	Strained vegetables and/or fruits and their juices, one by one
6–8	Protein foods (cheese, yogurt, cooked beans, meat, fish, chicken, egg yolk)
9	Finely chopped meat (baby can chew now), toast, teething crackers (for emerging teeth)
10–12	Whole egg (allergies less likely now)

[a] Later you can change cereals, but don't forget to keep on using the iron-fortified varieties. According to *Nutrition and the MD,* April 1981, the iron in cereal specially prepared for babies is so bioavailable that 3 level tablespoons a day is all they need.
Source: Adapted from the 1979 *Recommendations for Infant Feeding Practices of the California Department of Health Services* as presented in Current infant feeding practices, *Nutrition and the MD,* January 1980.

31   M. Winick, Infant nutrition: Formula or breast feeding? *Professional Nutritionist,* Spring 1980, pp. 1–3.

32   L. A. Barness, Feeding children, *Journal of the Florida Medical Association,* April 1979, pp. 443–448.

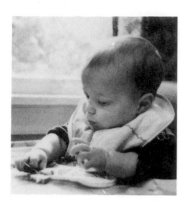

Physical readiness develops in many small steps. For example, the ability to swallow solid food develops at around four to six months, and experience with solid food at that time helps to develop swallowing ability by desensitizing the gag reflex. Later still, a baby can sit up, can handle finger foods, and is teething; then hard crackers and other hard finger foods should be introduced. These promote the development of manual dexterity and control of the jaw muscles.

Some parents want to feed solids at an earlier age, on the theory that "stuffing the baby" at bedtime will make him (or her) more likely to sleep through the night. There is no proof for this theory. On the average, babies start to sleep through the night at about the same age, regardless of when solid foods are introduced.[33]

New foods should be introduced singly so that allergies can be detected. For example, when cereals are introduced, try rice cereal first for several days; it causes allergy least often. Try wheat cereal last; it is the most common offender. If a cereal causes an allergic reaction (irritability, misery), discontinue its use before going on to the next food. About nine times out of ten, the allergy won't be evident immediately but will manifest itself in vague symptoms occurring up to five days after the offending food is eaten, so it isn't easy to detect.

About one out of every four people may have an allergy of one kind or another, and about half of these allergies are caused by foods—most commonly, milk, wheat, egg (whites), corn, and pork.[34] If parents detect allergies in their infant's early life, they can spare the whole family much grief.

As for the choice of foods, baby foods commercially prepared in the United States and Canada are generally safe, nutritious, and of high quality. In response to consumer demand, baby food companies have removed much of the added salt and sugar their products contained in the past, and baby foods also contain few or no additives.[35] They generally have high nutrient density, except for mixed dinners (which contain little meat) and desserts (which are heavily sweetened). An alternative for the parent who wants the baby to have family foods is to "blenderize" a small portion of the table food at each meal. This necessitates cooking without salt, though. Foods adults prepare for themselves often contain much more salt than even commercial baby foods. The adults can salt their own food after the baby's portion has been taken. And babies should never be fed canned vegetables; not only is the sodium content too high but also the risk of lead contamination is present.[36] It is also important to take precautions against

33　By three months, 74 percent are sleeping through the night whether or not they are receiving solid food. L. L. Clark and V. A. Beal, Age at introduction of solid foods to infants in Manitoba, *Journal of the Canadian Dietetic Association* 42 (1981): 72–78.

34　J. C. Breneman, Food allergy, *Contemporary Nutrition* 4 (March 1979).

35　Gerber Products Company, Why we put what we put in Gerber baby foods (advertisement), *Nutrition Today*, September/October 1973, p. 24; and J. C. Suerth (chairman of the board, Gerber Products Company), Letter to the editor, *Nutrition Today*, May/June 1977, pp. 34–35. According to *Nutrition and the MD*, January 1980, there was no more sugar in Beechnut foods and much less in Heinz than formerly.

36　C. M. Kerr, Jr., K. S. Reisinger, and F. W. Plankey, Sodium concentration of home-made baby foods, *Pediatrics* 62 (1978): 331–335; Questions readers ask, *Nutrition and the MD*, May 1980.

food poisoning and to avoid the use of vegetables in which nitrites are likely to form—notably, home-prepared carrots, beets, and spinach.[37] Honey should never be fed to infants because of the risk of botulism.

At a year of age, the obvious food to supply most of the nutrients the baby needs is still milk; 2 to 3½ cups a day are now sufficient. More milk than this would displace foods necessary to provide iron and would cause the iron-deficiency anemia known as milk anemia. The other foods—meat, iron-fortified cereal, enriched or whole-grain bread, fruit, and vegetables— should be supplied in variety and in amounts sufficient to round out total kcalorie needs. The one-year-old should be sitting at the table and eating the foods everyone else eats. A meal plan that meets these requirements for the one-year-old is shown in Table 13–5.

Looking Ahead

The first year of a baby's life is the time to lay the foundation for future health. From the nutrition standpoint, the relevant problems most common in later years are obesity and dental disease. Prevention of obesity should also help prevent the development of the obesity-related diseases—atherosclerosis, diabetes, and cancer.

Infant obesity should be avoided. Probably the most important single measure to undertake during the first year is to encourage eating habits that will support continued normal weight as the child grows. Primarily, this means introducing nutritious foods in an inviting way; not forcing the baby to finish the bottle or the baby food jar; avoiding concentrated sweets and empty kcalorie foods; and encouraging vigorous physical activity.

To discourage development of the behaviors and attitudes that plague the obese, parents should avoid teaching babies to seek food as a reward, to expect food as comfort for unhappiness, or to associate food deprivation with punishment. If they cry for thirst, they should be given water, not milk or juice. Babies seem to have no internal "kcalorie counter," and they stop eating when their stomachs are full, so low-kcalorie foods will satisfy as long as they provide bulk.

Beyond these recommendations, some thought is being given to the idea that infants should be started on a "prudent diet" like that recommended for heart patients: restrict fat, increase the ratio of polyunsaturated to saturated fat, and reduce cholesterol intake. Such a diet has been tried with infants up to three years of age. It seems to have done them no harm, while lowering their serum cholesterol.[38] However, this kind of program is only experimental. Babies need the kcalories and fat of normal milk, and most experts agree that they should be fed whole or at least low-fat—not skim— milk until after they are a year old. The only exception might be the seriously obese baby, who should perhaps be started on a prudent diet as early as three months of age.[39] Tampering with the amount of protein in

milk anemia: iron-deficiency anemia caused by drinking so much milk that iron-rich foods are displaced from the diet.

TABLE 13–5 **Meal Plan for a One-Year-Old**

BREAKFAST	SNACK
1 c milk	½ c milk
3 tbsp cereal	Teething crackers
2–3 tbsp strained fruit	
Teething crackers	

LUNCH	SUPPER
1 c milk	1 c milk
2–3 tbsp vegetables	1 egg
Chopped meat	2 tbsp cereal or potato
2–3 tbsp pudding	2–3 tbsp cooked fruit
	Teething crackers

Babies develop sensitivity to their own satiety (see p. 238) at about ten months, another example of developmental readiness.

For more about the prudent diet, turn to Highlight 3.

37   C. A. Thomson and I. S. Sheremate, Current issues in infant feeding, *Journal of the Canadian Dietetic Association* 39 (July 1978): 189–194.

38   G. Friedman and S. J. Goldberg, An evaluation of the safety of a low-saturated-fat, low-cholesterol diet beginning in infancy, *Pediatrics* 58 (1976): 655–657.

39   The prudent diet in pediatric practice, *Nutrition and the MD*, November 1979.

a baby's diet could be especially undesirable, because altered amounts of protein affect the baby's body composition, with unpredictable consequences.[40]

Normal dental development is promoted by the same strategies as those outlined above: supplying nutritious foods, avoiding sweets, and discouraging association of food with reward or comfort. In addition, the practice of giving a baby a bottle as a pacifier is strongly discouraged by dentists on the grounds that sucking for long periods of time pushes the normal jawline out of shape and causes the bucktooth profile: protruding upper and receding lower teeth. Further, prolonged sucking on a bottle of milk or juice bathes the upper teeth in a carbohydrate-rich fluid that favors the growth of decay-producing bacteria. Babies permitted to do this are sometimes seen with their upper teeth decayed all the way to the gum line. A photograph of this effect appears on p. 83.

Mealtimes

The wise parent of a one-year-old offers nutrition and love together. Both promote growth. It is literally true that "feeding with love" produces better growth in both weight and height of children than feeding the same food in an emotionally negative climate.[41] It also promotes better brain development. The formation of nerve-to-nerve connections in the brain depends both on nutrients and on environmental stimulation.[42]

The person feeding a one-year-old has to be aware that this is a period in the child's life when exploring and experimenting are normal and desirable behaviors. The child is developing a sense of autonomy that, if allowed to flower, will provide the foundation for later confidence and effectiveness as an individual. The child's impulses, if consistently denied, can turn to shame and self-doubt. In light of the developmental and nutritional needs of one-year-olds, and in the face of their often contrary and willful behavior, a few feeding guidelines may be helpful. Following are several problem situations with suggestions for handling them.

● He stands and plays at the table instead of eating. Don't let him. This is unacceptable behavior and should be firmly discouraged. Put him down and let him wait until the next feeding to eat again. Be consistent and firm, not punitive. If he is really hungry, he will soon learn to sit still while eating. A baby's appetite is less keen at a year than at eight months, and his kcalorie needs are relatively lower. A one-year-old will get enough to eat if he lets his own hunger be his guide.

● She wants to poke her fingers into her food. Let her. She has much to learn from feeling the texture of her food. When she knows all about it, she'll naturally graduate to the use of a spoon.

40   L. E. Holt, Jr., Protein economy in the growing child, *Postgraduate Medicine* 27 (1960): 783–798.

41   E. M. Widdowson, Mental contentment and physical growth, *Lancet* 1 (1951): 1316–1318.

42   J. Cravioto, Nutrition, stimulation, mental development and learning, *Nutrition Today*, September/October 1981, pp. 4–8, 10–15.

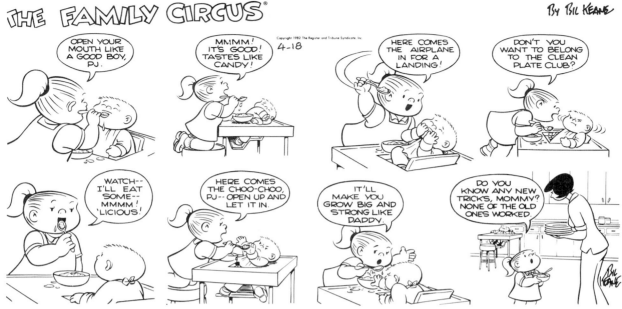

A one-year-old feels like eating less.

● He wants to manage the spoon himself but can't handle it. Let him try. As he masters it, withdraw gradually until he is feeding himself competently. This is the age at which a baby can learn to feed himself and is most strongly motivated to do so. He will spill, of course, but he'll grow out of it soon enough.

● She refuses food that her mother knows is good for her. This way of demonstrating autonomy, one of the few available to the one-year-old, is most satisfying. Don't force. It is in the one- to two-year-old stage that most of the feeding problems develop that can last throughout life. As long as she is getting enough milk and is offered a variety of nutritious foods to choose from, she will gradually acquire a taste for different foods—provided that she feels she is making the choice. This year is the most important year of a child's life in establishing future food preferences. If a baby refuses milk, an alternative source of the bone- and muscle-building nutrients it supplies must be provided. Milk-based puddings, custards, and cheese are often successful substitutes. For the baby who is allergic to milk, soy milk and other formulas are available.

● He prefers sweets—candy and sugary confections—to foods containing more nutrients. Human beings of all races and cultures have a natural inborn preference for sweet-tasting foods. Limit them strictly. There is no room in a baby's daily 1,000 kcalories for the kcalories from sweets, except occasionally. The meal plan shown before provides more than 500 kcalories from milk; one or two servings of each of the other types of food provide the other 500. If a candy bar were substituted for any of these foods, the baby would lose out on valuable nutrients; if it were added daily, he would gradually become obese.

Summing Up

Growth is a major factor influencing the nutritional needs of developing infants and children. The growth rate is fastest during prenatal life and the first year. Growth patterns for different organs vary. Most are characterized by critical periods, during which cells divide and nutrition has greater importance than usual. Psychological growth accompanies and facilitates physical growth.

During pregnancy, changes in both mothers' and infants' bodies necessitate increased intakes of the growth nutrients. A pregnant woman should gain about 25 to 30 pounds from foods of high nutrient density. Malnutrition during pregnancy affects the developing fetus; low-birthweight babies often fail to thrive. Alcohol, smoking, drugs, dieting, and unbalanced nutrient intakes of all kinds should be avoided for the duration of pregnancy. Protein and ample kcalories are especially important. Fluid intake should be liberal and salt normally should not be restricted.

The breastfeeding mother needs additional kcalories from foods of high nutrient density and a generous fluid intake. The rapidly growing newborn infant requires milk, preferably breast milk, which provides the needed nutrients in quantities suitable to support the infant's growth. Advantages of breast milk over formula, especially in underdeveloped countries, are that it protects the infant against disease and that it is sanitary, economical, and premixed to the correct proportions. To avoid allergy, all susceptible infants should be breastfed at first, even in developed countries.

Formula feeding matches breastfeeding as closely as possible. The mother should be supported and assisted with whichever mode of feeding she selects. The health professional can greatly benefit the health of both mother and infant by learning what information the mother needs and offering that information in usable terms.

Additions to a baby's diet are selected according to the baby's changing nutrient needs and readiness to handle new foods. Among the first nutrients needed in amounts beyond those provided by milk are iron and vitamin C. By a year of age, a baby can be eating foods from all four food groups. Normal weight gain, tooth development, and health can be promoted by feeding a balanced diet, avoiding empty-kcalorie foods, and encouraging infants to learn to like foods from all four food groups. The first year of life is the most important for setting future food habits.

NOTE: Appendix J suggests further reading; see "Pregnancy, Lactation, and Infancy."

CHAPTER 14
Child and Teen

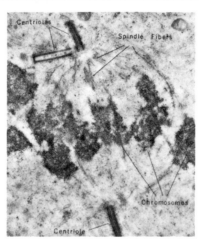

Healthy growth . . . is dependent on an adequate and continuous supply of energy, protein, and other nutrients to all cells of the body so that they may divide and increase in size to reach their maximum potential.

ETHEL AUSTIN MARTIN and
VIRGINIA A. BEAL

Growth requires that cells duplicate all their materials and copy their DNA instructions so each daughter will have a set; and then portion out the two sets to the two daughters. This dividing cell is sorting out its genetic material so that one complete copy will be delivered to each daughter cell. Many kcalories and nutrients are needed to support cell division.

The years of life described in this chapter are often called "the growing years," although, as we have seen, the year before birth and the first year after it may be the most growing years of all. Still, there is more to come. From age one to twenty or thereabouts, height more than triples, and weight increases up to eightfold or tenfold. Optimal nutrition permits development to realize its full potential.

Secular Trends in Nutrition

Not everyone—indeed, not every population—enjoys the benefits of optimal nutrition. Observations of populations during times of change in their foodways have demonstrated that altered nutrition profoundly affects the timing and extent of their young people's maturation.

These effects, which can be seen over time measured in years, are known as **secular trends** in nutrition.

saecula = age

Bones of the hand or wrist can be used as an indicator of skeletal maturity. Here, eight developing bony centers are shown. They are markedly more fully mineralized in one child's hand than in the other, although both children are six.

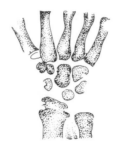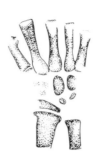

menarche (MEN-ark): the age at which the first menstrual period occurs.

mens = menstruation

arche = beginning

Skeletal maturity can be measured by x-raying the 31 bones of the hand and wrist to see how completely formed they are. It can also be measured by timing the fusion of the **epiphyses** (eh-PIFF-uh-sees) to the shafts of the long bones. The epiphyses, the end segments of long bones, contain a thin area of active bone growth. This growth eventually stops, after which no significant growth in height can occur—only a slight elongation of the trunk.

epi = on

phyein = to grow

Among the variables affected are age at menarche, skeletal maturity, and ultimate height achieved. Changes in these variables within a population depend on many factors, but nutrition is thought to be highly significant among them. Others are improvements in medical care and sanitation, which help to prevent disease. These indicators of bettered socioeconomic status together permit children to mature faster and more fully than their parents may have done. Conversely, socioeconomic setbacks such as natural disasters or wars limit the growth and maturation rates of young people.

Ultimately, when all environmental conditions are ideal, the full genetic potential of a people can be realized, but until then it is impossible to know what that potential may be. In 1840 it might have been thought, for example, that women were supposed to have their first periods at 15 years of age. Their great-granddaughters, in 1930, however, had their first periods at 12 to 13 years of age. This secular trend, a decrease in the mean age at menarche of one-third year per decade from 1840 to 1930, paralleled the accumulation of many economic advantages in our society and ceased in 1930—presumably because the limits of genetic possibility had then been reached.

Height, too, increases with improvement in socioeconomic conditions, but the limit has been reached, at least for the middle and upper classes in Western Europe and North America. The ultimate height achieved is also reached at an earlier age today than it was 100 years ago. Today, most females arrive at their full height by the age of 16 or 17, and males by 18 or 19, whereas 50 years ago both sexes reached their full height at 26 years. Figure 14–1 shows that the average heights of ten-year-olds in the United States increased 10 percent from 1870 to 1970—not because they were growing 10 percent taller, but because they had accomplished 10 percent more of their total growth by that age. In the 1960s, ten-year-olds in India and the United Arab Republic were as tall as ten-year-olds in the United States were around the turn of the century, reflecting the fact that conditions in India and the U.A.R. are not as conducive to rapid growth and early development as conditions here.

All of this is not to say that all humans "should" attain the same heights at the same ages or at maturity. Different races have different genetic potentials. Some are smaller, some taller, because they have inherited different genes for height. Several U.S. surveys have shown that blacks mature earlier

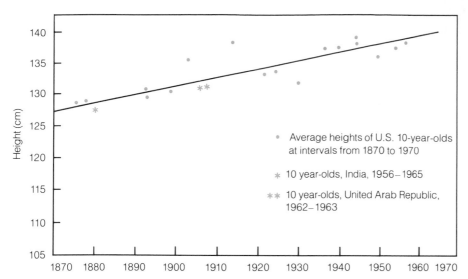

FIGURE 14-1 Children mature earlier today than 100 years ago. The figure shows that ten-year-olds in 1970 were about 140 cm tall, whereas 100 years earlier they were under 130 cm. Indian and Arab children in the 1960s were as tall as U.S. children had been at the turn of the century.

Source: P. V. V. Hamill, F. E. Johnston, and S. Lemeshow, *Height and Weight of Children: Socioeconomic Status, United States*, Vital and Health Statistics series 11, no. 119, DHEW publication no. (HSM) 73-1601 (Washington, D.C.: Government Printing Office, 1972). Data for Indian and U.A.R. children from E. A. Martin and V. A. Beal, *Roberts' Nutrition Work with Children*, 4th ed. (Chicago: University of Chicago Press, 1978), p. 88.

and grow taller than whites, all else (including income) being equal. But the example of the Japanese shows that we cannot attribute differences in physical development to differing genetic heritages until we have ruled out the possibility of environmental influences, including differences in adequacy and steady supply of food.

In the case of the Japanese, the adverse effects of times of deprivation as well as the benefits of improved nutrition have both been demonstrated in secular trends within this century. The heights of children at each age have steadily increased since 1900, probably mostly as a result of increased protein intakes—except during the Second World War, when food deprivation was severe. The effects are shown in Figure 14-2.

The rest of this chapter describes the growth and development of individuals—in the context of an advanced, industrialized society in which even the poor, compared with those of other countries, are not much poorer than the middle class. In other countries, poverty is so much more extreme that many parents' expectations for the physical and mental development of their children cannot realistically be so high as they are here.

Early and Middle Childhood

Nutrient needs change steadily throughout life and vary from individual to individual, depending on the rate of growth, the sex, the previous nutrition and health history, and many other factors. This section takes a general look at preschool and school-age children's needs, and later sections are devoted to the special concerns of teenagers.

After the age of one, a child's growth rate slows, but the body continues

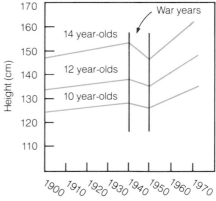

FIGURE 14-2 **Effect of the war years on heights of Japanese boys**. The faster the boys were growing, the more severely they were affected. The figure also shows that boys at each age were taller in 1970 than boys of those ages were in 1900— believed to be an effect of improved protein nutrition. (The same effects were seen in girls.)

Source: Adapted from E. A. Martin and V. A. Beal, *Roberts' Nutrition Work with Children*, 4th ed. (Chicago: University of Chicago Press, 1978), p. 147, as adapted in turn from Helen S. Mitchell.

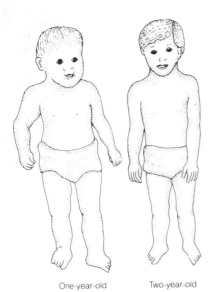

One-year-old   Two-year-old

One-year-old and two-year-old shown as same height for comparison of body shape.

to change dramatically. At one, babies have just learned to stand and toddle; by two, they can take long strides with solid confidence and are learning to run, jump, and climb. The internal change that makes these new accomplishments possible is the accumulation of a larger mass and greater density of bone and muscle tissue. The changes are obvious in the margin figure. The two-year-old has lost much of his baby fat; his muscles (especially in the back, buttocks, and legs) have firmed and strengthened, and his leg bones have lengthened and increased in density.

Thereafter, the same trend—lengthening of the long bones and an increase in musculature—continues, unevenly and more slowly, until adolescence. Growth comes in spurts; a six-year-old child may wear the same pair of shoes for a year, then need new shoes twice in the next four months.

Just before adolescence, the growth patterns of girls and boys begin to become distinct. In girls, fat becomes a larger percentage of the total body weight, and in boys the lean body mass—muscle and bone—becomes much greater. Around this time, growth in height may seem to stop altogether for a while. This is the calm before the storm.

Nutrition Needs and Feeding

A one-year-old child needs perhaps 1,000 kcalories a day; a three-year-old needs only 300 to 500 kcalories more. Appetite decreases markedly around the age of one year, in line with the great reduction in growth rate. Thereafter, the appetite fluctuates; a child will need and demand much more food during periods of rapid growth than during slow periods. The nutrients protein and calcium continue to need emphasis, and the food best suited to supply them continues to be milk.

The preadolescent period is the last one in which parental food choices have much influence. As children gather their forces for the adolescent growth spurt, they are accumulating stores of nutrients that will be needed in the coming years. When they take off on that growth spurt, there will be a period during which their nutrient intakes, especially of calcium, cannot meet the demands of rapidly growing bones. Then they will draw on these nutrient stores. The denser their bones are before this occurs, the better prepared they will be.

The gradually increasing needs for all nutrients during the growing years are evident from the RDA table and the Canadian Dietary Standard, which list separate averages for each span of three years. To provide these nutrients, the Four Food Group Plan recommends the following for growing children:

- 3 cups or 4 ¾-cup servings of milk or milk products.
- 1 egg and 2 servings of other meat or meat substitutes.
- 4 or more servings of fruits and vegetables.
- 4 or more servings of breads and cereals.

For meat, fruits, and vegetables, a serving is loosely defined as 1 tablespoon per year. Thus, at four years of age, a serving of any of these foods would be 4 tablespoons (¼ cup). Because the serving sizes adjust as the child grows older, these recommendations are good from age two to the teen years. Table 14–1 shows details of diet patterns based on this plan.

TABLE 14–1 **Children's Daily Food Pattern for Good Nutrition**

FOOD GROUP	REQUIRED SERVINGS PER DAY	AVERAGE SIZE OF SERVING		
		1 to 3 Years	*4 to 5 Years*	*6 to 12 Years*
Milk and cheese (1 oz cheese = 1 c milk)	4	½ to ¾ c	¾ c	¾ to 1 c
Meat group (protein foods)	3, more permitted			
Eggs		1	1	1
Lean meat, fish, poultry, legumes (liver once a week)		2 tbsp	4 tbsp	2 to 4 oz
Peanut butter		0 to 1 tbsp	2 tbsp	2 to 3 tbsp
Fruits and vegetables	4, more recommended			
Vitamin C source (citrus fruits, berries, tomato, cabbage, cantaloupe)	1 or more	⅓ to ½ c	½ c	1 medium orange
Vitamin A source (green or yellow fruits and vegetables)	1 or more	2 to 3 tbsp	4 tbsp	¼ to ⅓ c
Other vegetables (including potato) and	2	2 to 3 tbsp	4 tbsp (¼ c)	⅓ to ½ c
Other fruits (apple, banana)		¼ to ⅓ c	½ c	1 medium piece
Cereals (whole-grain or enriched)	4, more recommended			
Bread, buns, pizza		½ to 1 slice	1½ slices	1 to 2 slices
Ready-to-eat cereals		½ to ¾ oz	1 oz	1 oz
Cooked grains (cereals, macaroni, grits, rice)		¼ to ⅓ c	½ c	½ to ¾ c
	OPTIONAL			
Fats and sugars	These high-kcalorie foods may be included in limited amounts only in addition to the required servings of nutritious foods.			
Butter, margarine, mayonnaise, oils	Maximum	1 tbsp	1 tbsp	2 tbsp
Desserts and sweets: 100-kcalorie portions as follows:		1 to 1½ portions	1½ portions	3 portions
⅓ cup pudding or ice cream				
2-3 cookies, 1 oz cake				
1⅓ oz pie, 2 tbsp jelly, jam, honey, sugar				

Source: Adapted from B. B. Alford and M. L. Bogle, *Nutrition During the Life Cycle* (New Jersey: Prentice-Hall, Inc., 1982), pp. 60–61.

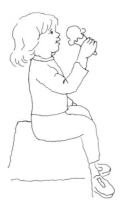

Calcium and riboflavin in a delicious form.

After the crucial first year, there is still much a parent can do to foster the development of healthy eating habits. The goal is to teach children to like nutritious foods in all four categories.

Experimentation with children's food patterns shows that candy, cola, and other concentrated sweets must be limited in a child's diet if the needed nutrients are to be supplied. If such foods are permitted in large quantities, there are only two possible outcomes: nutrient deficiencies and/or obesity. The child can't be trusted to choose nutritious foods on the basis of taste alone; the preference for sweets is innate.[1] On the other hand, an active child can enjoy the higher-kcalorie nutritious foods in each category; ice cream or pudding in the milk group, cake and cookies (whole-grain or enriched only, however) in the bread group. These foods, made from milk and grain, carry valuable nutrients and encourage a child to learn, appropriately, that eating is fun.

Children sometimes seem to lose their appetites for a while; this is nothing to worry about. The perfection of appetite regulation in children of normal weight guarantees that their kcalorie intakes will be right for each stage of growth. As long as the kcalories they do consume are from nutritious foods, they are well provided for. (One caution, however: wandering school-age children may be spending pocket money at the nearby candy store.) An overzealous mother, unaware that her one-year-old is supposed to slow down, may begin a lifelong conflict over food by trying to force more food on the child than the child feels like eating.

Nutrition at School

While parents are doing what they can to establish favorable eating behavior during the transition from infancy to childhood, other factors are entering the picture. At five or so, the child goes to school and encounters foods prepared and served by outsiders. The U.S. government funds several programs to provide nutritious, high-quality meals for children at school. School lunches are designed to meet certain requirements. They must include specified servings of milk, protein-rich food (meat, cheese, eggs, legumes, or peanut butter), vegetables, fruits, bread or other grain foods, and butter or margarine. The design is intended to provide at least a third of the RDA for each of the nutrients. The school lunch pattern was split into several patterns in 1980 to provide for the needs of different ages better than it had done in the past (see Table 14–2).

Parents rely on the school lunch program to meet a significant part of their children's nutrient needs on school days, but children don't always like what they are served. In response to children's differing needs and tastes, the school lunch program has been attempting to do better at feeding children both what they want and what will nourish them. The trend is:

● To increase the variety of offerings and allow children to choose what they are served.

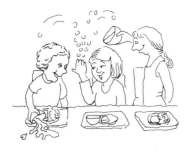

1   R. B. Choate, *Selling cavities—U.S. style* (address presented at the American Dental Association annual meeting, 11 October 1977). According to the speaker, the taste for sweetness already exists in the fetus, peaks at 14 years, and is more marked in blacks than in whites.

TABLE 14–2 **School Lunch Patterns for Different Ages**

	PRESCHOOL		GRADES		
	Ages 1–2	*Ages 3–4*	*K–3*	*4–12*	*7–12*
Meat or meat alternate					
One serving					
Lean meat, poultry, or fish	1 oz	1½ oz	1½ oz	2 oz	3 oz
Cheese	1 oz	1½ oz	1½ oz	2 oz	3 oz
Large egg(s)	1	1½	1½	2	3
Cooked dry beans or peas	½ c	¾ c	¾ c	1 c	1½ c
Peanut butter	2 tbsp	3 tbsp	3 tbsp	4 tbsp	6 tbsp
Vegetable and/or fruit					
Two or more servings, both to total	½ c	½ c	½ c	¾ c	¾ c
Bread or bread alternate					
Servings[a]	5 per week	8 per week	8 per week	8 per week	10 per week
Milk					
A serving of fluid milk	¾ c	¾ c	1 c	1 c	1 c

Source: From School lunch patterns: Ready, set, go! *School Food Service Journal* 34 (August 1980), p. 31.
[a] A serving is 1 slice of whole-grain or enriched bread; a whole-grain or enriched biscuit, roll, muffin, etc.; ½ c cooked pasta or other cereal grain such as bulgur or grits.

● To vary portion sizes, so that little children may take little servings.
● To involve students (in secondary schools) in the planning of menus.
● To improve the scheduling of lunches so that children can eat when they are hungry and can have enough time to eat well.

A step toward making the lunches more consistent with today's ideals of healthful food has been to drop the requirement for whole milk and to offer low-fat or skim milk instead. Another alteration has been to eliminate the requirement that butter or margarine be served. To help the schools economize, the program no longer requires that children be served every item, but permits them to select what they will eat, so that there will be less plate waste.

Coincident with the school lunch program is a program of nutrition education and training (NET program) in all the public schools. Originally allocated 50 cents per year per child, this program was cut in 1980 to 9 cents per child, but is reported to be still going strong because program administrators are highly motivated and have been ingenious and creative in accomplishing the program's highest-priority objectives.[2]

One way in which children can learn a lot, sometimes with only small expense to the school, is to take field trips to nearby facilities where nutrition and food operations are going on. Some possible places to visit are listed in the margin.

Children can learn from:
Bakeries
Mills
Dairy farms
Milk bottling plants
Farmers' markets
Vegetable farms and fields
Food processing plants
Fast-food places
Institutional kitchens
Supermarkets
Convenience stores
Neighborhood gardens
Natural food stores
Food salvage banks

2   H. R. Armstrong and D. B. Root, Managing a lean NET program, *Community Nutritionist* 2 (1983): 8–10.

At the very least, children can go to the depots where the school food comes in and to the kitchens where it is prepared; and teachers who themselves know something about nutrition can then use the questions that come up as opportunities to do some teaching. Children growing up today need not only to be fed well in the interest of their growth and development, but to learn enough about nutrition to become able to make adaptive food choices when the choices become theirs to make.

Television and Vending Machines

For the most part, children learn nutrition from parents or teachers who know very little about it. Meanwhile, they hear a great deal about foods from the television set. Many authorities are concerned that television commercials may have a less-than-desirable impact. It is estimated that the average child sees more than 10,000 commercials a year, of which many more than half are for sugary foods. Hundreds of millions of dollars are spent in the effort to sell these foods to children.[3] Most of the concern centers on the issue of sugar. You may recall that not all the public disapproval of sugar is based on scientific findings. However, there is widespread agreement on one point: sticky, sugary foods left in the teeth provide an ideal environment for the growth of mouth bacteria and the formation of cavities. No regulations to prevent the promotion of sticky, sugary foods are in force, however.

It thus remains up to us to determine which food commercials we will believe and which we will not. Dentists, especially, have the obligation to educate their patients individually as long as misleading claims continue to appear on national television. A model eating plan that favors dental health is shown in Table 14–3.

TABLE 14–3 **Eating Habits to Favor Good Dental Health**

FOOD GROUP	FOODS TO EAT	FOODS TO AVOID
Milk and milk products	Milk Cheese Plain yogurt	All dairy products with added sugar
Fruit	Fresh fruit Water-packed canned fruit	Dried fruit Sugar-packed canned fruit Jams and jellies
Juice	Unsweetened	Sweetened
Vegetables	Most vegetables	Candied sweet potatoes Glazed carrots
Grains	Most grain products	Grain products with added sugar

Notice that granola bars are among the "bad guys" singled out by dentists. They are a grain food, but so sticky that dentists consider them akin to candy bars. Similarly, dentists see fruit yogurt as the equivalent of ice cream.
Source: L. P. DiOrio, What should we eat? A dentist's perspective (address presented at the American Dental Association annual meeting, 11 October 1977).

3   Choate, 1977.

Television is not the only environmental force affecting children's food choices. Another is vending machines, especially in schools. The American Dental Association (ADA) has established a National Task Force for the Prohibition of the Sale of Confections (sticky, sugary foods) in Schools and has resolved that the task force should seek changes in the School Lunch Act to eliminate the sale of confections as snacks in schools.[4] Such efforts by the ADA have so far met with little success, and most progress has been made by way of individual, voluntary initiatives. An experiment in six Canadian schools, for example, showed that children would choose more nutritious snacks if they were offered side by side with the sugary foods. When apples were made available in vending machines, there was a 27 percent reduction in the selection of chocolate bars. When milk was made available, soft-drink use dropped by 42 percent.[5]

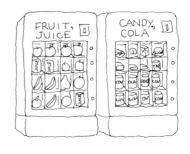

Soft drinks contain not only sugar but also caffeine, which is a matter of some concern to pediatricians. A cup of hot chocolate or a 12-ounce cola beverage may contain as much as 50 milligrams of caffeine; two or more such beverages are equivalent in the body of a 60-pound child to the caffeine in eight cups of coffee for a 175-pound man.[6] Chocolate bars also contribute caffeine. Children and young adults who are troubled by irregular heartbeats or difficulty in sleeping may need to control their caffeine consumption. (A table of caffeine contents of beverages and medications appears in the next chapter.) As long as such undeniably attractive temptations as cola beverages and candy bars surround children, barriers against their abuse have to be provided by parents and other concerned adults and by teaching the children themselves.

Looking Ahead

In children, as in infants, eating habits help determine whether development takes place in a positive or negative direction. To avoid obesity, the preschool child should be trained to "eat thin." Mealtimes should be relaxed and leisurely. Children should learn to eat slowly, pause and enjoy their table companions, and stop eating when they are full. The "clean your plate" dictum should be stamped out for all time, and in its place parents who wish to avoid waste should learn to serve smaller portions or teach their children to serve themselves as much as they truly want to eat. Physical activity should be encouraged on a daily basis to promote strong skeletal and muscular development and to establish habits that will undergird good health throughout life.

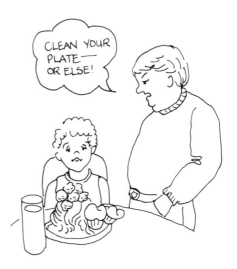

4   N. L. Shory, School confection sale bans: What can the dental profession do? (address presented at the American Dental Association annual meeting, 11 October 1977).

5   L. Crawford, Junk food in our schools? A look at student spending in school vending machines and concessions, *Journal of the Canadian Dietetic Association* 38 (July 1977): 193. Abstract cited in *Journal of the American Dietetic Association* 71 (1977): 572. See also San Jose: Moving more nutritious lunches, *Institutions/Volume Feeding Magazine*, 1 August 1977, pp. 42–43; and E. Ott, Quieting our detractors' voices, *Food Management* 14 (1979): 25–26.

6   Some constructive ways to improve your diet, *Consumers' Research Magazine*, October 1976, p. 62.

The child who has already become obese needs careful handling. As in pregnancy, weight loss may easily have a harmful effect on growth. J. L. Knittle, who has worked with obese children, recommends that they be fed so as to maintain a constant weight while they grow. The object is to restrict the multiplication of fat cells while promoting normal lean body development. Thus the child can "grow out of his obesity."[7]

Of all nutritional disorders other than obesity found in U.S. children, the most common is iron-deficiency anemia. It is most prevalent in low-birthweight infants, babies from six months to two years of age, and children and adolescents from low-income families.[8]

Dr. S. J. Fomon, pediatrician and specialist in children's nutrition, recommends supplementing the diet of infants to ensure an iron intake of 7 milligrams a day and modifying their food intakes as they grow older so that they will receive 5.5 milligrams of iron or more per 1,000 kcalories. To achieve this latter goal, milk must not be overemphasized in the diet, because it is a poor iron source; dairy products should be consumed only in the amounts needed to ensure adequate calcium and riboflavin intakes. If skim or low-fat milk is used instead of whole milk, there will be kcalories left for investment in such iron-rich foods as lean meats, fish, poultry, eggs, and legumes. Grain products should be whole-grain or enriched only, and children should learn to avoid bakery goods unfortified with iron, candies, and soft drinks.[9]

Cardiovascular disease is another condition to prevent, and many experts seem to agree that early childhood is the time to put practices into effect that until recently were recommended only for adults. Snacking on high-fat, high-sugar, and high-salt foods should be discouraged, because it sets a pattern that favors the development of atherosclerosis and hypertension. Instead, recommendations like those of the *Dietary Guidelines*, emphasizing foods with a high nutrient density, should be followed.

The *Guidelines* might also help to prevent or retard the onset of diabetes in children who have the genetic tendency toward it. Those who have been studying the effect of nutrition on cancer have suggested that children should follow a "prudent diet," since evidence is increasing that "appropriate biological control in terms of fat and cholesterol may be set early in life."[10] The prudent diet was originally developed for heart patients, but its outlines are the same as those recommended by nutritionists interested in the prevention of cancer.

Not everyone agrees that all children should be placed on diets strictly limited in sugar, salt, and fat and high in fruits, vegetables, and whole-grain cereals. However, even those who do not go this far recommend that children be screened early with an eye to determining what conditions

The prudent diet is described on p. 119.

7   J. L. Knittle, Obesity in childhood: A problem in adipose tissue development, *Journal of Pediatrics* 81 (December 1972): 1048–1059.

8   S. J. Fomon, T. A. Anderson, H. Y. W. Stephen, and E. E. Ziegler, *Nutritional Disorders of Children: Prevention, Screening, and Followup*, DHEW publication no. (HSA) 76–5612 (Washington, D.C.: Government Printing Office, 1976), p. 100.

9   Fomon and coauthors, 1976, p. 116.

10   E. L. Wynder, The dietary environment and cancer, *Journal of the American Dietetic Association* 71 (1977): 385–392.

each of them might be likely to develop and then paying appropriate attention to diet in each special case. (Figure 14–3 outlines the screening process.) Thus, the child of a parent with high blood pressure should be raised on a diet relatively low in salt; the child of a diabetic parent should avoid sugar and be encouraged to eat foods high in complex carbohydrate; and the child of a parent with coronary artery disease should eat foods low in fat, especially saturated fat, and possibly cholesterol. In all these situations, the greatest success is likely to be achieved if the whole family, and not just the child, follows the recommended dietary guidelines.

Poor dental health is another preventable condition. The measures recommended for its prevention center around two objectives. First, adequate nutrition is needed to help the mouth and teeth develop properly. This means providing an adequate diet, especially in terms of protein; calcium; vitamins A, C, and D; and fluoride. Where local water supplies are not fluoridated, direct application of fluoride to the teeth at intervals may be necessary. Second, it is important to restrict the supply of carbohydrate foods to the bacteria that cause tooth decay. This means brushing the teeth or washing the mouth after meals (especially meals high in carbohydrate), avoiding snacks that contain sticky carbohydrate, and dislodging persistent particles with dental floss or other devices.

FIGURE 14–3 **Nutritional screening of children.**

Source: From S. J. Fomon, T. A. Anderson, H. Y. W. Stephen, and E. E. Ziegler, *Nutritional Disorders of Children: Prevention, Screening, and Followup*, DHEW publication no. (HSA) 76–5612 (Washington, D.C.: Government Printing Office, 1976), inside front cover.

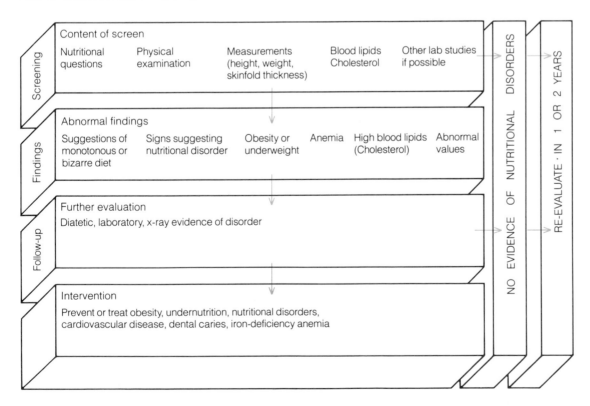

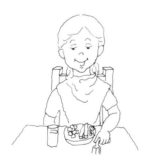

Mealtimes with Children

It is desirable for children to learn to like nutritious foods in all of the food groups. With one exception, this liking usually develops naturally. The exception is vegetables, which young children frequently dislike and refuse. Even a tiny serving of spinach, cooked carrots, or squash may elicit an expression that registers the utmost in negative feelings (as well as great pride in the ability to make an ugly face). Since most youngsters need to eat more vegetables, the next few paragraphs are addressed to this problem.

Do you remember how you felt when first offered a cup of vegetable soup, a serving of runny spinach, or a pile of peas and carrots? If the soup burned your tongue, it may have been years before you were willing to try it again. As for the spinach, it was suspiciously murky looking. (Who could tell what might be lurking in that dark, ugly liquid?) The peas and carrots troubled your sense of order. Before you could eat them, you felt compelled to sort the peas onto one side of the plate and the carrots onto the other. Then you had to separate, into a reject pile, all those that got mashed in the process or contaminated with gravy from the mashed potatoes. Only then might you be willing to eat the intact, clean peas and carrots one by one—perhaps with your fingers, since the peas, especially, kept rolling off the fork.

Why children respond in this way to foods that look "off" or "messy" to them is a matter for conjecture. Parents need only be aware that this is how many children feel and then honor those feelings. Children prefer vegetables that are slightly undercooked and crunchy, bright in color, served separately, and easy to eat. They should be warm, not hot, because a child's mouth is much more sensitive than an adult's. The flavor should be mild (a child has more taste buds), and smooth foods such as mashed potatoes or pea soup should have no lumps in them (a child wonders, with some disgust, what the lumps might be). Irrational as the fear of strangeness may seem, the parent must realize that it is practically universal among children and may even have a built-in biological basis.

Little children like to eat at little tables and to be served little portions of food. They also love to eat with other children and have been observed to stay at the table longer and eat much more when in the company of their peers. A bright, unhurried atmosphere free of conflict is also conducive to good appetite. Parents who serve the food in a relaxed and casual manner, without anxiety, provide the emotional climate in which a child's negative emotions will be minimized.

Ideally, each meal is preceded, not followed, by the activity the child looks forward to the most. In a number of schools, it has been discovered that children eat a much better lunch if recess occurs before, rather than after, the meal. With recess after, they are likely to hurry out to play, leaving food on their plates that they were hungry for and would otherwise have eaten. Before sitting down to eat, small children should be helped to clean themselves thoroughly, washing their hands and faces so that they can enjoy their meal with "that clean feeling."[11]

---

11 We are indebted for many of these suggestions to Dr. Joyce Williams, coauthor (with M. Smith) of *Middle Childhood: Behavior and Development* (New York: Macmillan, 1974).

Many little children, both boys and girls, enjoy helping in the kitchen. Their participation provides many opportunities to encourage good food habits. Vegetables are pretty, especially when fresh, and provide opportunities to learn about color, about growing things and their seeds, about shapes and textures—all of which are fascinating to young children. Measuring, stirring, decorating, cutting, and arranging vegetables are skills even a very small child can practice with enjoyment and pride.

When introducing new foods at the table, parents are advised to offer them one at a time—and only a small amount at first. Whenever possible, the new food should be presented at the beginning of the meal, when the child is hungry. If the child is cross, irritable, or feeling sick, don't insist but withdraw the new food and try it again a few days later. Remember, parents have inclinations and dislikes to which they feel entitled; children should be accorded the same privilege. Never make an issue of food acceptance; a power struggle almost invariably results in a confirmed pattern of resistance and a permanently closed mind on the child's part.

The key word, at one year, is *trust*; the parental behavior best suited to promote it is affectionate holding. At two years, the word is *autonomy*; parents should allow children to help make family choices, including sometimes giving them the right to say their favorite word (NO!)—at the same time, of course, sensibly preventing the child from dominating the family. At four, when the development of *initiative* is their proudest achievement, children can be encouraged to participate in the planning and preparation of meals. At each age, food can be given and enjoyed in the context of encouraging emotional as well as physical growth. If the beginnings are right, children will grow without the kind of conflict and confusion over food that can lead to nutritional problems.

At every age, there is a negative counterpart—distrust, shame, guilt, inferiority—to the desired development. These, too, can be promoted by unaware parents, even if they have the best of intentions. Mealtimes can be nightmarish for the child who is struggling with these issues. If, as she sits down to the table, she is confronted with a barrage of accusations—"Susie, your hands are filthy...your report card...and clean your plate! Your mother cooked that food"—mealtimes may be unbearable. Her stomach may recoil, because her body as well as her mind reacts to stress of this kind.

In the interest of promoting both a positive self-concept and a positive attitude toward good food, it is important for parents to help their children remember that they are good kids. What they *do* may sometimes be unacceptable; but what they *are*, on the inside, is normal, healthy, growing, fine human beings.

The Teen Years

Teenagers are not fed; they eat. For the first time in their lives, they assume responsibility for their own food intakes. At the same time, they are intensely involved in day-to-day life with their peers and preparation for their future lives as adults. Social pressures thrust choices at them: to drink or not to drink, to smoke or not to smoke, to develop their bodies to meet sometimes extreme ideals of slimness or athletic prowess. Few become interested in foods and nutrition except as part of the effort to define themselves by way of vegetarianism, crash dieting, or other efforts. The next few sections emphasize the factors that affect their health for good or for ill and the information they need to develop and maintain food habits conducive to good health throughout adulthood.

Growth and Nutrient Needs

The adolescent growth spurt begins in girls at 10 or 11 and reaches its peak at 12, being completed at about 15. In boys, it begins at 12 or 13 and peaks at 14, ending at about 19. This intensive growth period brings not only a dramatic increase in height but hormonal changes that profoundly affect every organ of the body (including the brain) and that culminate in the emergence of physically mature adults within two or three years. The same nutrition principles apply to this period as to the growth periods previously discussed. The growth nutrients are needed in increased quantities, and there is an added need for iron, caused by the onset of menstruation in girls and by the great increase in lean body mass in boys. These changes, which are taking place in nearly adult-size people, may increase total nutrient needs at adolescence more than at any other time in life. A rapidly growing, active boy of 15 may need 4,000 kcalories or more a day just to maintain his weight.

At the same time, an inactive girl of the same age, whose growth is nearly at a standstill, may need fewer than 2,000 kcalories if she is to avoid becoming obese. Thus, there is tremendous variation in the nutrient needs of adolescents.

There is also tremendous variation in the rates and patterns of their growth. Growth charts used for children cannot be used any longer when the signs of puberty begin to appear. The only way to be sure a teenager is growing normally is to compare his or her height and weight with previous measures taken at intervals and note whether reasonably smooth progress is being made. A teenager who wants to know what he or she should weigh should be reassured that any of a wide range of weights is considered normal at this time in life. The rule of thumb on the inside back cover can be modified for teenage girls down to age 18 (see margin) and considered a weight to aim at; but weights well in excess of these are normal, too. Teenage boys can be told that when they have finished growing, they should expect to weigh what the adult charts show, but that while they are growing it is not unusual for their weights to be quite different from the adult standards.

Teenagers as a group do have nutritional problems, however. Nearly every nutrient can be found lacking in one or another group: iron in girls, kcalories in young men (especially blacks), vitamin A in girls (especially Mexican- and Spanish-Americans), calcium, riboflavin, vitamin C, even protein. The insidious problem of obesity becomes more apparent, mostly

Rule of thumb for teen girls:

For 5 ft, consider 100 lb a reasonable weight.

For each inch over 5 ft, add 5 lb.

For each year under 25 (down to 18), subtract 1 lb.

For men, see inside back cover.

in girls, especially in black girls. Serious nutrient deficiencies often arise in pregnant teenage girls.

Eating Patterns

Teenagers come and go as they choose and eat what they want when they have time. With a multitude of after-school, social, and job activities, they almost inevitably fall into irregular eating habits. The adult becomes a gatekeeper, controlling the availability but not the consumption of food in the teenager's environment. The adult can't nag, scold, or pressure teenagers into eating as they should, because teens typically turn a deaf ear to coercion and often to persuasion. To "feed" effectively, the gatekeeper must make every effort to allow these young people independence while providing a physical environment that favors healthy development and an emotional climate that encourages adaptive choices.

In the home, a wise maneuver is to provide access to nutritious and economical energy foods low in sugar and fat and discouraging to tooth decay. The snacker—and a well-established characteristic of teenagers is that they are snackers—who finds only nutritious foods around the house is well provided for.

Inevitably, teenagers will do a lot of eating away from home. There, as well as at home, their nutritional welfare can be favored or hindered by the choices they make. A lunch of a hamburger, a chocolate shake, and french fries supplies nutrients in the amounts shown in Table 14-4, at a kcalorie cost of 780. Except for vitamin A, these are substantial percentages of recommended intakes at a kcalorie cost many teenagers can afford. Depending on how they adjust their breakfast and dinner choices, teenagers may meet their nutritional needs more than adequately with this sort of lunch. They need only select fruits and vegetables (for vitamins A and C), good fiber sources, and more good iron sources at their other meals.

On the average, about a fourth of teenagers' total daily kcalorie intake comes from snacks. Their irregular schedules may worry adults who think they are feeding themselves poorly, but usually the kcalories they eat are far from empty. They receive substantial amounts of protein, thiamin, riboflavin, vitamin B₆, iron, magnesium, zinc, and even calcium (if they snack on dairy products). The nutrients they most often fail to obtain are vitamin A and folacin. Protein usually need not be stressed, but some teenagers should be encouraged to recognize and consume more dairy products, for calcium, and more good vitamin A and folacin sources. (Wherever vitamin A is lacking, folacin is too, because both are found in green vegetables.)

The teenager's iron needs are a special problem, caused by several factors. Two already mentioned are the teenager's burgeoning iron need and the lack of iron in traditional snack foods. Other factors are the overemphasis on dairy products by some teenagers, vegetarianism, and the low contribution made by fast foods to iron intakes. A National Academy of Sciences committee, writing on this special problem, finds it doubtful that long-term administration of iron tablets is practical and advises against the measure of fortifying snacks and other foods with iron. Instead, the com-

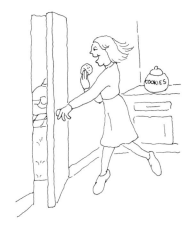

For the nutritive value of selected fast foods, see Appendix N.

TABLE 14-4 **Nutrients in a Hamburger, Chocolate Shake, and Fries**

NUTRIENT	PERCENTAGE OF NEED
Protein	42%
Calcium	47%
Iron	21%
Vitamin A	3%
Thiamin	25%
Riboflavin	57%
Vitamin C	21%

Source: Calculated from the RDA for a teenage male.

mittee recommends that physicians and clinics screen all teenagers for low levels of iron in the blood. Their report stresses the fact that the best dietary source of absorbable iron is meats of all varieties, a point that should in turn be stressed in the nutrition education of teenagers.[12] No doubt they should learn as well to enjoy iron-rich plant foods such as legumes and whole grains. A later section addresses the problem of teaching teens about nutrition.

Anorexia Nervosa and Bulimia

A concern of teenagers, especially girls, is dieting to maintain a slim and beautiful figure. To accomplish this, many go on fad diets that are neither safe nor effective. The matters of obesity, overweight, and fad diets have been fully discussed elsewhere (see Chapters 6 and 7) but two special problems should be mentioned here: anorexia nervosa and bulimia.

Anorexia nervosa is an extreme preoccupation with weight loss that seriously endangers the health and even the life of the dieter. Although no two persons with anorexia nervosa are alike, certain features are considered typical of the condition. The anorexic is almost always female and in her mid-teens. She is usually from an educated, middle-class, success-oriented, weight-conscious family that is proud of her and is surprised to see her develop a problem. She strives to achieve and chooses weight loss as one means of becoming successful herself. Being highly competitive and perfectionistic, she carries the weight-loss effort to an extreme: she will have the slimmest, most perfect body of anyone in her high school class.

So far this description probably fits many young women you know; but unlike most of them, this girl develops anorexia nervosa. When she has lost weight to well below the average for her height and is no longer slim but too slim, she still doesn't stop. Weight loss has become an obsession, she is afraid of losing control, and she allows her self-imposed starvation regimen to rule her life. At this point, according to Dr. Hilde Bruch, an authority who has studied and worked with anorexics, starvation has begun to affect her physiology, thinking patterns, and personality, and physical symptoms are emerging. Although they are the symptoms of starvation, the girl sees them as desirable and prides herself on holding out against her extreme hunger.

Among the physical symptoms are:

- Wasting of the whole body, including muscle tissue.
- Arresting of sexual development and stopping of menstruation.
- Drying and yellowing of the skin, from an accumulation of stored carotene released from body fat.
- Loss of health and texture of hair.
- Pain on touch.

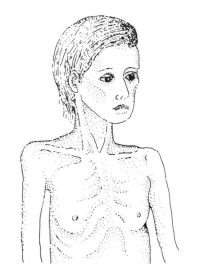

Anorexia nervosa.

Source: Copied from a woodcut accompanying Sir William Gull, Anorexia nervosa, *Lancet* 1 (1888).

anorexia nervosa: literally, "nervous lack of appetite," a disorder (usually seen in teenage girls) involving self-starvation to the extreme.

---

12   Committee on Nutrition of the Mother and Preschool Child, Food and Nutrition Board, National Academy of Sciences, *Iron Nutriture in Adolescence*, DHEW publication no. (HSA) 77–5100 (Washington, D.C.: Government Printing Office, 1977).

- Lowered blood pressure and metabolic rate.
- Anemia.
- Severe sleep disturbance.[13]

There may also be abnormal secretion of the antidiuretic hormone, which affects thought processes as well as water excretion, and makes it hard to break out of the abnormal mental state.[14]

Simultaneously, a set of bizarre mental symptoms develop in the anorexic, including an inability to see herself as others see her (she still sees herself as too fat), a preoccupation with death, a frantic pursuit of physical fitness by means of stringent exercise routines, and a manipulative way of dealing with her parents and family such that they make her the center of attention. Diet has become so all-engrossing, now, that she may be quite isolated socially except from friends who stick by her and worry about her without knowing how to help.

By this time, the anorexic has reached an absolute minimum body weight (65 to 70 pounds for a woman of average height) and is on the verge of incurring permanent brain damage and chronic invalidism or death.

Before 1950, the condition was very rare (1 in 2,000) and only 1 out of 4 such girls could be expected to recover. By 1970, the incidence was increasing and the success rate in treatment was closer to 3 out of 4. During the 1970s, anorexia nervosa became still more widespread and familiar to doctors and therapists. Treatment was further improved to the point where success could be expected more often; still, 1 in 5 anorexics die.

Dr. Bruch describes the treatment of the anorexic as a three-stage process. First, normal nutrition must be restored, by tube-feeding directly into the stomach if necessary. As she begins to return to normal weight, family interactions have to be dealt with. With progress in these two areas, she can begin to be taught some new understanding and clear up some of her misconceptions about nutrition.[15]

Anorexia nervosa is a disease of the developed countries, and becomes more prevalent as wealth increases. Its victims seem to be reacting to the cultural values that emphasize fashion and material success over personal actualization and self-esteem. Whatever its cause, it serves as but one of many possible examples of the ways teenagers feel pressured and the ways they react to those pressures.

Another reaction is bulimia, periodic binge eating alternating with intervals of dieting or self-starvation. Bulimia was officially recognized only in 1980, although it had existed long before that. The binge eater typically ingests a large amount of food in an episode she or he feels is uncontrollable. The binge may last from minutes to hours and usually takes place in private. The foods chosen are usually sweet or starchy, require little chewing, and are high in kcalories. The binge ends when it would hurt to eat any

Right now I weigh 58 lbs., which isn't too bad for 5'2", though I want to lose a few more pounds—my hips are still fat. Lately I've got it down to no breakfast, a can of mushrooms for lunch, and a can of wax beans for dinner with lots of iced tea. I reward myself with a big, green apple at the end of the day, if I've stuck to The Plan. A. CISEAUX

bulimia, bulimarexia: binge eating (literally, eating like an ox). Known popularly as "pigging out" or "blind munchies." When followed by self-induced vomiting or the taking of laxatives, this form of eating behavior has been called the **binge-purge syndrome.**

buli = ox

orex = mouth

13 H. Bruch, Anorexia nervosa, *Nutrition Today,* September/October 1978, pp. 14–18.

14 P. W. Gold, W. Kaye, G. L. Robertson, and M. Ebert, Abnormalities in plasma and cerebrospinal-fluid arginine vasopressin in patients with anorexia nervosa, *New England Journal of Medicine* 308 (1983): 1117–1123.

15 Bruch, 1978.

more or when the person goes to sleep, induces vomiting, or is interrupted.[16]

Since 1980, bulimia has attracted much attention in the media, especially the variety in which the person binges and then vomits or takes laxatives to undo the "damage." A handful of professional articles have appeared on the subject, doubtless to be followed by many more.[17] It is not yet clear whether bulimic eaters are psychologically disturbed; they may simply be compensating for going to the extreme of self-imposed starvation by swinging to the other extreme of overeating. This is a not-surprising mode of behavior in a society that imposes an unrealistically thin ideal, especially on girls. As many as two or three out of every five women in some subgroups of society may be bulimic for some part of their lives (for example, dancers, who are often told they must weigh considerably *less* than the already-thin "ideal weight").

Although binge eating is seldom life-threatening, at the extreme it can be physically damaging, causing lacerations of the stomach, irritation of the esophagus (in those who vomit frequently), and malnutrition (in the vomiters and laxative-takers). It is highly desirable that binge eaters should learn to see food, and themselves, in a more positive light and should come to accept a realistic weight goal for themselves. Further thoughts on this problem are offered in Highlight 7.

The Pregnant Teenage Girl

A special case is that of the pregnant teenage girl. Even if she were not pregnant, she would be hard put to meet her own nutrient needs at this time of maximal growth. Nourishing the baby doubles her burden. Figure 14–4 shows that her needs for many nutrients double, although her kcalorie allowance increases by only a few percent. In the case of a girl who begins pregnancy with inadequate nutrient stores or who lacks the education, resources, and support she needs, these problems are compounded.

The complications of pregnancy were discussed in Chapter 13, where it was shown that the consequences of poor nutrition are acute and long-lasting. Sickness is common in pregnant teenagers, with toxemia occurring in about one out of every five girls under the age of 15. If one pregnancy is followed by another, "the conditions are established for a rapid and irreversible slide from simple toxemia to [kidney] damage and hypertensive heart disease."[18]

Teenage pregnancy has become common. About one out of every five babies is born to a mother under 19 years of age, and more than a tenth of these mothers are 15 or younger.[19] Emphasis on preparing young girls for

16   R. L. Pyle, J. E. Mitchell, and E. D. Eckert, Bulimia: A report of 34 cases, *Journal of Clinical Psychiatry* 42 (1981): 60–64.

17   For example, Pyle, Mitchell, and Eckert, 1981; also J. Wardle and H. Beinart, Binge eating: A theoretical review, *British Journal of Clinical Psychology* 20 (1981): 97–109.

18   B. S. Worthington, Nutritional needs of the pregnant adolescent, in *Nutrition in Pregnancy and Lactation*, ed. B. S. Worthington, J. Vermeersch, and S. R. Williams (St. Louis: Mosby, 1977), pp. 119–132.

19   Worthington, 1977.

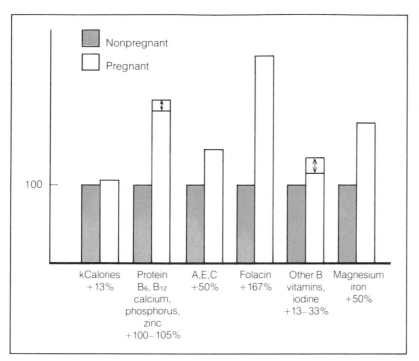

FIGURE 14–4 **Comparison of the nutrient needs of a 10-year-old girl with those of a pregnant 15-year-old girl.** We calculated these values by adding the difference between the RDA for a 10-year-old and a 14-year-old to the difference between the RDA for a 14-year-old and a pregnant woman (see inside front cover).

future pregnancy is needed in public schools and public health programs. Faced with her parents' and classmates' often insensitive reactions, a pregnant girl is likely to wind up alone, with little or no money to buy food and no motivation to seek prenatal care. She urgently needs programs addressed to all her problems, including medical attention, nutrition guidance, emotional support, and continued schooling. A model program for giving nutrition help to teenage mothers, among others, is the WIC (Women's, Infants', and Children's) program, a federally funded program that provides nutrition information and low-cost nutritious foods to low-income pregnant women and their children.

Alcohol and Drugs

The teen years bring exposure to factors not encountered before. Some complicate the nutrition picture: use and abuse of alcohol, prolonged use of prescription medications, drug use (and abuse), use of caffeine, use of oral contraceptives, and many more. Because alcohol is by far the most widely used of all drugs in the United States, it receives emphasis here.

In the mid-teens comes a choice point: whether to drink alcohol or to abstain. A 1975 study showed that more than half of all seventh-graders nationwide had tried alcohol at least once within the previous year; nine-tenths of all high school seniors had had experience with alcohol.[20]

20   Young people and alcohol, *Alcohol Health and Research World*, DHEW publication no. (ADM) 75–157 (Washington, D.C.: Government Printing Office, Summer 1975), pp. 2–10.

The year between the ages of 13 and 14 seems to mark the decision point for most white teenagers; and the year between 15 and 16 is critical for blacks. Another transition stage occurs between the ages of 17 and 18, when infrequent drinkers apparently make a decision either to abstain or to drink more heavily. The highest proportion of heavy drinkers by ethnic group is found in Native American youth (16.5 percent), followed by Orientals (13.5) and Spanish (10.9). For whites, the proportion is 10.7 percent, and for blacks, 5.7 percent. Those receiving high grades in school are less likely to become alcohol drinkers; the heavy drinkers characteristically spend more time with peers who also drink.[21]

By the time students get to college, alcohol abuse is frequent and considered part of normal college life. About 90 percent of all college students use alcohol, and heavy drinking is common, with a third or more of all students getting drunk more than once a month.[22] Only a few college students are alcoholics, but 5 to 10 percent will experience serious complications as a result of drinking, and 1 in 12 will go on to become an adult problem drinker or an alcoholic.[23] Among adults in the United States, about 100 million drink, and 9 million are estimated to be alcoholics.

The nutrition implications of alcohol use and the consequences of its abuse were described in Highlight 8A. To sum them all up, alcohol is an empty-kcalorie beverage and can displace needed nutrients from the diet while simultaneously altering metabolism so that even good nutrition cannot normalize it. Those who are unable to use alcohol with moderation must abstain completely from its use if they are to maintain good health.

Many myths and misconceptions comprise the public's picture of alcohol use, and teenagers often cherish wrong beliefs that lead them to alcohol abuse and addiction if they are susceptible. Being susceptible to alcohol addiction, like being potentially diabetic, is probably an inherited trait and is therefore nothing to be ashamed of. The teenager, however, is apt to be exposed to peer pressure that favors everyone's drinking, and those who can't do so safely are in an unfortunate predicament.

Among mistaken beliefs especially common among teenagers is the notion that a beer drinker can never become an addict. On the contrary, because beer contains alcohol, it is just as capable of contributing to alcoholism as is wine or "hard" liquor (whiskey, gin, vodka, and the like). It is not the beverage but the constitution of the consumer that determines whether he or she will become addicted to alcohol.

Some beer drinkers maintain that beer has some redeeming features. It makes people drunk less quickly, and it provides valuable nutrients. True, because the alcohol in beer is diluted, it will reach the bloodstream more slowly from the stomach than the same amount of alcohol taken straight.

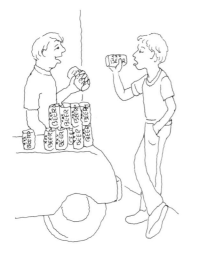

21   Drinking motivations: Habits of youth illuminated by national survey results, *NIAAA Information and Feature Service* 18, DHEW publication no. (ADM) 75–151 (Washington, D.C.: Government Printing Office, 26 November 1975).

22   D. P. Kraft, College students and alcohol: The 50 + 12 project, *Alcohol Health and Research World*, DHEW publication no. (ADM) 76–157 (Washington, D.C.: Government Printing Office, Summer 1976), pp. 10–14.

23   G. Globetti, as quoted in *Alcohol Health and Research World*, Summer 1975.

But the carbonation in beer stimulates the stomach, hastening the entry of alcohol into the intestine, where it will immediately be absorbed. As for the nutrient content of beer, an adult male would have to drink at least a six-pack of 12-ounce cans to meet one day's niacin needs and nine six-packs to meet one day's protein needs.

Some young people choose to abstain from alcohol consumption because they know or suspect they are prone to an alcohol problem. Others make the same choice for other reasons. Such people have a hard time in some social settings, because drinking is often not only accepted but even demanded. It is hoped that this discussion will have shown why it is desirable not to pressure other persons to drink. Considerate hosts or social groups will welcome the nondrinker and provide nonalcoholic beverages for his or her enjoyment just as they would provide nonmeat food for a guest who is a vegetarian.

Not only alcohol but also many medicines affect the body's need for and use of nutrients. Prescription medications can affect nutrition status by:

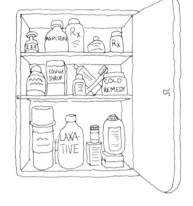

- Increasing or decreasing appetite.
- Causing nausea, vomiting, or an altered sense of taste.
- Inhibiting the synthesis of nutrients.
- Reducing the absorption or increasing the excretion of nutrients.
- Altering the transport, use, or storage of nutrients.

Foods and nutrients can also affect the drugs in the body. The interactions between drugs and nutrition status comprise such a big subject that whole books have been written about them (see Appendix J).

The special case of the person taking oral contraceptives deserves a moment's attention. The Pill alters blood levels of several nutrients, raising some (vitamin A and iron) and lowering others (B vitamins and vitamin C). Women often wonder what vitamin supplements they should take while on the Pill. The answer seems to be "None. You are risking nutrient deficiencies only if your diet is grossly inadequate, especially in folacin. And if it is, you need diet counseling more than you need a vitamin pill."[24]

Like alcohol, marihuana also has characteristic effects on the body, and like alcohol, it has not been shown to have many pronounced harmful effects even with long-term use, unless the use is very heavy (five to six cigarettes a day for six months). The active ingredients are rapidly and completely (90 percent) absorbed from the lungs.[25] Then, being fat soluble, they are packaged in protein (possibly in lipoproteins[26]) before being transported by the blood to the various body tissues. They are processed by many tissues (not just by the liver), and they persist for several days in body fat, being excreted over a period of a week or more after the smoking of a single cigarette.[27]

Smoking a marihuana cigarette has characteristic effects on hearing,

marihuana: alternative spelling, **marijuana**

24   D. A. Roe, Drugs, diet and nutrition, *Contemporary Nutrition* 3 (June 1978).

25   L. J. King, J. D. Teale, and V. Marks, Biochemical aspects of cannabis, in *Cannabis and Health*, ed. J. D. Graham (New York : Academic Press, 1976).

26   L. E. Hollister, Marihuana in man: Three years later, *Science* 172 (1971): 21–29.

27   King and coauthors, 1976; Hollister, 1971.

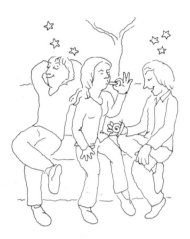

THC is **tetrahydrocannabinol**, the primary active ingredient of marihuana.

touch, taste, and smell and on perceptions of time, space, and the body; it also produces changes in mental sensations and alterations in the nature of sleep. Among the taste changes apparently induced is a great enjoyment of eating, especially of sweets ("the munchies"), but it is not known how this effect occurs.[28] The drug apparently does not change the blood glucose level.[29] Investigators speculate that the so-called hunger induced by marihuana is actually a social effect caused by the suggestibility of the group in which it is smoked.[30] Prolonged use of the drug does not seem to bring about a weight gain; in one small sample, regular users (30 smokers) were observed to weigh less than comparable nonsmokers by about 7 pounds.[31]

Many young people in the United States have turned to marihuana as an alternative to alcohol. The number of individuals using it at least once a day had grown from half a million in 1971 to over 3 million before 1980.[32] There is much disagreement about the desirability of this trend, and despite much current research, little is known about the possible risks of regular smoking.

It has become clear, however, that even in "socially acceptable" concentrations, the drug brings about a deterioration in some aspects of driving performance.[33] Another effect widely agreed on is that it causes alterations in heart action, including rapid and sometimes irregular heartbeat.[34] It also reduces the body's immune response and, in young men, reduces the sex hormone level and sperm count after a lag period of about six weeks. Reporting on this effect, an investigator points out that marihuana "is much like other drugs, such as tobacco and liquor, in that the greatest potential hazard exists for those who abuse it.... There is still no convincing evidence that casual, infrequent use of marihuana produces any ill effects."[35]

The potency of marihuana preparations reaching this country has been increasing. Before 1970, most marihuana used in the United States was a very weak domestic variety with an average THC content of about 0.2 percent. During the 1970s, users shifted to a Mexican variety (about 1.5 percent THC), then to Jamaican and Colombian marihuana (3 to 4 percent). The present trend is toward even higher concentrations. Users looking for a greater "high" then sometimes shift to hashish oil, a much more

28   E. L. Abel, Effects of marihuana on the solution of anagrams, memory and appetite, *Nature* 231 (1971): 260–261; C. T. Tart, Marijuana intoxication: Common experiences, *Nature* 226 (1970): 701–704.

29   L. E. Hollister, Hunger and appetite after single doses of marihuana, alcohol, and dextroamphetamine, *Clinical Pharmacology and Therapeutics* 12 (1971): 44–49; J. D. P. Graham and D. M. F. Li, The pharmacology of cannabis and cannabinoids, in *Cannabis and Health*, 1976.

30   Hollister, 1971.

31   Marijuana: Truth on health problems, *Science News*, 22 February 1975, p. 117.

32   T. H. Maugh, II, Marihuana: New support for immune and reproductive hazards, *Science* 190 (1975): 865–867.

33   Graham and Li, 1976; Pot update: Possible motor effects, *Science News*, 4 February 1978, p. 71.

34   Graham and Li, 1976.

35   Infrequent use might be defined as three cigarettes a week or less. Maugh, 1975.

concentrated form of the active drug (about 40 to 50 percent THC and up to 90 percent), at which point the risks probably increase dramatically.[36]

Most investigators agree that, with moderate use, the hazards of marihuana smoking are few and small. However, it should be remembered that, because possession and use of the drug is not legal, no controls are exerted by any agency, such as the FDA, on the content of preparations sold as marihuana. There is a significant hazard associated with the possibility that they may be contaminated with pesticides or that they may contain "hard" (addictive) drugs such as heroin, concealed in them by pushers to create a demand for a product they can sell for greater profits. Also, when marihuana use escalates into the use of other drugs, the nutrition and health effects become pronounced, as the next paragraph illustrates.

Alcohol and marihuana have received most of the attention here, but other drugs deserve a mention for their effects on nutrition. Among the drugs in most common use today are heroin, morphine, LSD, PCP, and cocaine. Users of these drugs face multiple nutrition problems:

- They spend their money for drugs rather than for food.
- They lose interest in food during "high" periods.
- Some drugs (for example, amphetamines) induce at least a temporary depression of appetite.
- Their lifestyle lacks the regularity and routine that would promote good eating habits.
- They often have hepatitis, a liver disease transmitted from person to person by the use of contaminated needles, which causes taste changes and loss of appetite.
- They often depend on alcohol, especially when withdrawing from drug use.
- They often become ill with infectious diseases that increase their need for nutrients.

During their withdrawal from drugs, one of the most important aspects of treatment is to identify and correct these nutrition problems while teaching and supporting adaptive eating habits.[37]

hepatitis (hep-uh-TIGHT-us): a severe viral liver disease transmitted from person to person either through contaminated water or (as in the case of drug addicts) by way of contaminated needles.

Teenagers' Food Choices

The teen years are well known as a time of rebellion. This rebellion extends to foods as well as to all other aspects of lifestyle. The choice of what to eat is up to teenagers themselves. Access points already mentioned include the refrigerator, the school lunch, and vending machines, but other than controlling the contents of these, adults can expect to have little impact on the nutrient intakes of adolescents—especially by such conventional means as education. Still, most young adults in this country are well fed, for reasons perceptively stated by Dr. Ruth M. Leverton: they get hungry; they like to eat; they want energy, vigor, and the means to compete

---

36 Maugh, 1975.

37 R. T. Frankle and G. Christakis, eds., Some nutritional aspects of "hard" drug addiction, *Dietetic Currents, Ross Timesaver* 2 (July/August 1975).

and excel in whatever they do; and they have many good habits, which are just as hard to break as the bad ones.[38]

Nutrition educators who wish to reach the teenager and young adult with nutrition information must find out and pay attention to two factors: why they sometimes are poorly nourished or develop poor food habits and what means of communicating reaches them effectively.

The young person with poor food habits and a negative attitude toward food is likely to have at least one of the following characteristics:

● He thinks nutrition means eating what you don't like because it's good for you.
● She has been criticized for her eating pattern but feels fine and sees no ill effects.
● He is uninterested in food, and it plays a negligible role in his very busy life.
● The people she is most likely to listen to are not knowledgeable about nutrition.[39]

The parent or teacher concerned about a teenager's food habits should be aware of what teenagers feel about themselves (some reflection into your own past may recall painful memories in this connection). They crave acceptance, especially from their peers. They need to fit in. In many cases they are greatly dissatisfied with themselves. One of the most important aspects of their image is the body image. Young men want larger biceps, shoulders, chest, and forearms; young women want smaller hips, thighs, and waists.[40] One study of U.S. teenagers revealed that 59 percent of the young men wanted to gain weight, although only 25 percent actually needed to do so. Similarly, 70 percent of the girls wanted to lose weight, but no more than about 15 percent were obese.[41] (Chapter 7 offers help with both objectives.) Words to the effect that "you look fine as you are" fall on deaf ears. (The same can be said of adults in some cases, up to the age of about 99.) To be conveyed effectively, nutrition information can be sold as part of a package that will bring about these desired changes. Fortunately, it happens to be true that nutrient-dense, low-kcalorie foods favor the development of strong biceps in men and a trim figure in women.

When the young person who is the target of your campaign possesses and cherishes nutrition misinformation, one of the first questions to ask is whether the practice is beneficial, neutral, or harmful. Opposing a loved ideal is more likely to polarize than to convert the opposition. A practice such as vegetarianism, dieting, or consuming a "muscle-building diet" can be encouraged—with modifications—rather than condemned. Only the most hazardous nutrition practices should be singled out for attention; silence is an option about the others.

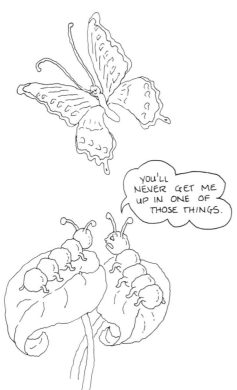

YOU'LL NEVER GET ME UP IN ONE OF THOSE THINGS.

38   R. M. Leverton, The paradox of teen-age nutrition, *Journal of the American Dietetic Association* 53 (1968): 13–16.

39   Leverton, 1968.

40   B. Lucas, Nutrition and the adolescent, in P. Pipes, *Nutrition in Infancy and Childhood*, 2nd ed. (St. Louis: Mosby, 1981), pp. 179–204.

41   Lucas, 1981.

One of the most effective ways to teach nutrition is by example. When nutrition teachers are moralists who fail to practice what they preach, their words fall on deaf ears. The coach and gym teacher, the friendly young French teacher, the admired city recreation director—those who enthusiastically maintain their own health—can have a great impact on teenagers. Remember, this is the period of identity formation, the time of seeking and emulating models.

When communicating nutrition information, above all be sure that you have it straight. We make fools of ourselves when we (for example) admonish our students to follow restrictive patterns when their own choices are already as good as ours or better. There may be no harm in using candy bars to meet part of the kcalorie allowance of an active young adult. It may not be necessary to drink milk if calcium, vitamin D, and riboflavin needs are being met by cheese or other food sources. Satisfactory diets can be designed on a great variety of foundations. It is the nutrient content and balance of foods, not the specific foods consumed, that make the difference between "good" and "bad" diets.

Much of the work of "teaching" nutrition can be delegated to teenagers themselves. Those who are interested and motivated can be guided to reliable sources and allowed to indulge their own desire to benefit their friends and classmates. Among the best materials prepared to teach teenagers the importance of good nutrition are those made by teenagers themselves.

Finally, remember that teenagers have the right to make their own decisions—even if they are ones you violently disagree with. You can set up the environment so that the foods available are those you favor, and you can stand by with reliable nutrition information and advice, but you will have to leave the rest to them. Ultimately, they make the choices.

Summing Up

After the age of one, a child's growth rate slows, and with it, the appetite. However, all essential nutrients continue to be needed in adequate amounts from foods with a high nutrient density. Milk remains important but should not exceed three servings a day for preteens, because it is a poor source of iron and vitamin C.

When children go to school, their nutrition needs are partly met by school lunch programs. Another influential factor in the lives of children is television, with many advertisements for sugary foods; another is vending machines, which often limit choices to foods of low quality. Dentists and other health professionals are concerned that the advertisement and availability of sugary foods should be controlled; there may also be a need to control some children's caffeine consumption from cola beverages and cocoa products.

Sound nutrition practices may prevent future health problems to some extent—among them, obesity, iron-deficiency anemia, cardiovascular disease, and diabetes. Screening for these conditions helps early detection.

Good dental health can be promoted by avoiding sticky, sugary foods and adopting healthy eating habits as well as brushing and flossing teeth regularly.

It is desirable for children to learn to like nutritious foods in all the food groups. This liking seems to come naturally except, in some children, the liking for vegetables. The person who feeds the child must be aware of the child's psychological and emotional development. With wise handling, children can learn eating habits that will continue to promote their good health and well-being after they have become adults.

The teen years mark the transition from a time when children eat what they are fed to a time when they choose for themselves what to eat. Nutrition education becomes important as a means of encouraging healthy food habits. Teenagers' snacking patterns and lifestyles predispose them to certain nutrient inadequacies, notably a lack of iron, but teenagers vary so widely that generalizations are difficult. Screening for problems is one way to detect them early.

A special problem in the teen years is anorexia nervosa, self-imposed starvation. An anorexic may diet to only 65 to 70 pounds and may need extremely careful treatment by knowledgeable professionals to recover. A related problem is bulimia, or binge eating, which may be followed by self-induced vomiting or other "purging" strategies. Both anorexia nervosa and bulimia appear to be related to our society's overemphasis on extreme thinness as an ideal weight.

Special problems that may arise in the teen years and affect nutrition include pregnancy, alcohol, and drug use. The pregnant teenage girl, whose nutrient needs are higher than those of any other person, needs medical attention, nutrition guidance, and emotional support. Alcohol use is common among teenagers, and 90 percent of U.S. college students use alcohol. One out of 20 is likely to become an alcohol abuser. Beer, as well as hard liquor, can be abused and can lead to alcoholism.

Prolonged use of prescription drugs may affect appetite, nutrient metabolism, and other aspects of the body's handling of nutrients. Drugs also interact with one another and with alcohol, causing nutrition problems. Awareness of this and attention to diet planning provides safeguards against health hazards. Marihuana has characteristic effects on taste and appetite, but the long-term effects of heavy use are not well understood. Users of other drugs may suffer profound health damage, and an important part of the rehabilitation process is the identification and correction of nutrition problems.

Teenagers and adults make their own choices. The nutrition educator is advised to be aware of the sources of their motivation and to convey important information in a way that honors their individuality.

NOTE: Appendix J suggests further reading; See "Children and Teenagers." Two optional lectures in the *Instructor's Manual* explore the relationships between nutrition and children's behavior, including the effects of allergies, additives, nutrient deficiencies, and sugar.

CHAPTER 15
The Later Years

CONTENTS

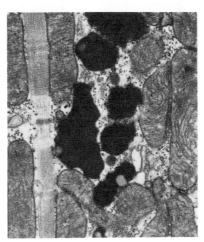

As cells grow old, the "aging pigment," lipofuscin, accumulates. Shown here is a heart muscle fiber (the striped strand at left) surrounded by many mitochondria. The dark, disorganized bodies are lipofuscin.

After the attainment of middle age, the body becomes more and more subject to the diseases resulting from the regime followed during the first half . . . . Nevertheless, the importance of the diet during the latter half of life must be of nearly the same order as during the first half.

CLIVE McCAY

One out of every nine U.S. citizens is above 65 years of age, and the percentage is increasing. This fact is evident everywhere. Retirement villages are springing up, especially in the warmer climates. Senior citizen centers are being established for congregate meals and leisure activities. Older adults can be heard on political matters at "silver-haired legislatures." The newspapers tell us the social security fund is nearing bankruptcy because many who were contributors are now retired and receiving payments from the fund. Civic and church organizations note that there is a preponderance of gray hair in their audiences. The data from recent census reports confirm these observations (see Figure 15–1).

Older people cherish their independence. Contrary to the popular view, only 5 percent live in nursing homes.[1] Most live in the community, either alone or with nonrelatives, thus remaining independent. As we will see, this very independence fosters nutrition problems.

1   M. Chou, Selling to older Americans, *Cereal Foods World* 26 (1981): 633.

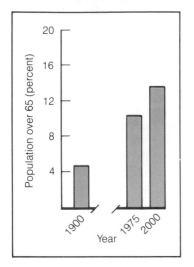

FIGURE 15–1 **Census findings**. One out of every nine citizens in the United States is above 65 years of age, and the percentage is increasing.

Of the 6 million elderly who live alone, 1.3 million are men and 4.7 million, women.[2] Most are in reasonably good health and have enough money to support themselves, if not in luxury, at least not in poverty. When we look around us and see the great needs of some people, we sometimes overlook those who are enjoying their later years. They have leisure to pursue some of their favorite activities and are unencumbered for the first time in their lives by family responsibilities. These facts contradict the popular belief that older people are all poor, lonely, and ill. They are not; they are as individual as all other age segments. Grouping them into a stereotype is a disservice to everyone, especially to young adults who might project into their futures a depressing view of old age. Just as only a few teenagers are reckless drivers, only a minority of older people have the "typical problems" attributed to them. Aunt Charlotte at 77 jets every winter to Europe to enjoy the social life of Paris; Uncle James at 84 is out early every morning in his vegetable garden hoeing his cabbages; and it is only Grandma Sadie who at 82 is lonely, withdrawn, ill, and forgetful, a problem to her family. Two-thirds of the elderly are relatively free of major problems.

However, the one-third who live at or below the poverty line deserve our attention. The average income of all older *single* people in the United States is $75 a week. Of aged black women, nearly half have a yearly income of under $1,000.[3] Clearly, these people need help in many areas, one of them being nutrition.

In exploring nutrition for the older adult, it will be necessary to remember statistics like these but also to recognize the wide range of individual situations represented in these statistics. It will be helpful to keep three questions in mind:

● What can I do now to prepare myself for the time when I will be an older adult?

● What can I do when I am older (or now that I am older) to keep myself healthy and vigorous so I will enjoy these years?

● How can I, as a relative or a health professional, help those who are in need?

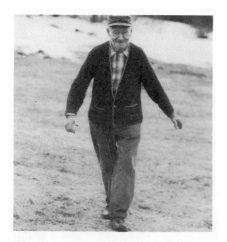

Theories on Aging

The "increased life span" of people in the twentieth century is not a reality. Most people are not now living much beyond the limit of threescore years and ten mentioned in the Bible. In fact, in the last 25 years there has been no increase in life expectancy for people who are already 20 or older in spite of our miracle drugs and huge medical bills.[4] Since the beginning of

2   U.S. Bureau of the Census, Money income in 1975 of families and persons in the United States, in *Current Population Reports*, Series P-60, no. 101, (Washington, D.C.: Government Printing Office, 1976).

3   U.S. Bureau of the Census, 1976.

4   J. Mayer, Aging and nutrition, *Geriatrics* 29, no. 5 (1974): 57–59.

the nineteenth century, as mortality from bacterial diseases has been brought under control by modern medicine, deaths from other causes have increased, so that the total life expectancy (for any individual) has remained at about 70 years. It is only the average length of life (for the population) that has increased. This has come about because more infants are surviving to adulthood, and so there are fewer infant deaths to bring the average down. Thus it seems that something built into the human organism (we call it aging) cuts off life at a rather fixed point in time.

Natural selection has not operated in favor of genes that promote longevity. However, the human race, with its superior brain, can collect and store information that helps keep individuals alive after they have reproduced. In today's world, older people may contribute accumulated experience and wisdom to the benefit of society long after they have passed their reproductive years and the time when they would contribute genes.

We humans have not comprehended what is involved in the aging process, nor have we figured out how to prevent or postpone it. Even our definitions of the process are vague, and research has been scarce. Current interest in the aging process is increasing, due in large part to the rising numbers of older people and the impact they are having on our social and governmental institutions, but answers are still few and far between.

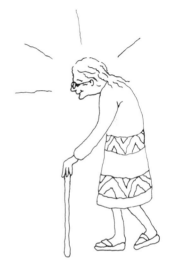

If age is venerated, people will claim to be old.

It has been hoped that we might discover an extremely long-lived race of people and then learn from them the secrets of long life. One scientist traveled far and wide in search of such people, and for a while thought that he had found them in two different geographical areas, because many people in these areas claimed to have lived for over 100 years. Further study revealed, however, that the age range in these populations was similar to that in others, only these people exaggerated their age because in their societies age was venerated. The elderly people in these societies were healthy, primarily because they lived a physically active life, but they were not remarkably long-lived. The moral of this story seems to be that people will always lie about their age, but not always in the same direction.

Caution

Aging of Cells

Cells seem to undergo a built-in (genetic) aging process and also to age in response to outside (environmental) forces. Environmental stresses that promote aging include extremes of heat and cold, disease, lack of nutrients, the wear and tear of hard physical labor, and the lack of stimulation caused by disuse (for example, of the muscle cells in the legs of a cripple who can't exercise). But even in the most pleasant and supportive of environments, inevitable changes take place in the structure and function of the body's cells.

All theories of aging have one element in common. They agree that at some point the cells become incapable of replenishing their constituents.

In a complex organism such as the human body, the cells are interdependent. When some cells die and their function is lost, other cells dependent on the first ones suffer and also eventually die. Thus whole systems are affected.

A second common element seems to be that aging cells are programmed to stop reproducing once a certain stage of development has been reached. Cells have different timetables for reproduction, but each type of cell seems to come to a natural end somehow. For example, red blood cells undergo division only as long as they are in the marrow of the long bones. When they are mature, they move out of the marrow to perform their function in the bloodstream. In the blood, they no longer reproduce; they work for four months and then die.

The brain cells are also programmed to stop reproducing, but they all stop within the first two years of life. Thus, at about 14 months of age, the human organism already has all the brain cells it will ever have. Many of them maintain themselves without further cell division, for about 70 years. Thousands die daily, but the daily loss is not noticeable because so many cells remain. The accumulated loss over a lifetime is felt only in the slowing of reflexes and in garbled messages' going to other organs. It seems strange that the human species should have evolved such a magnificent instrument for receiving, storing, interpreting, and retrieving information and yet not have evolved a method of repairing it. Some scientists view this evolutionary mishap as a "self-destruct" mechanism for the human body.

Some cells seem never to die but only to reproduce. However, even in optimal conditions, the cells of a multicellular organism seem unable to go on dividing forever. About 50 to 55 replications seems to be the maximum for human cells.

A third factor in the aging process seems to be that, with the passage of time, cells become cluttered with debris—partially completed proteins and oxidized lipids that are never totally dismantled. This intracellular "sludge" interferes with the efficiency of operations within the cells. The lipid material that accumulates in the cells is known as the pigment of old age.

The aging pigment is **lipofuscin** (lip-oh-FEW-sin).

lipo = lipid

fuscus = brownish-gray

Another factor may be that cells lose their ability to interpret the DNA genetic code words and so make their proteins incorrectly. As reduced amounts of protein or wrong proteins are produced, cell and organ functions that depend on those proteins also falter. Organs elsewhere in the body may also be adversely affected. A theory somewhat allied to this one is that through some environmental stress, such as radiation, the DNA code itself may become altered. This, too, would lead to the production of wrong proteins.

If wrong proteins are produced for any reason, another theory states, the body's immune system will react to them as if they were foreign proteins from outside and will produce antibodies to counteract them. Complexes then form between the antibodies and these proteins and accumulate in and among cells as useless debris. This autoimmune theory may account in part for the accumulation of deposits in joints, which causes arthritis.

Finally, another theory of aging suggests that cosmic rays bombard molecules in the cells and split them into highly reactive compounds known as free radicals. These free radicals then bind rigidly to other cellular molecules by way of disulfide bridges. This disrupts the informational content of important molecules and so impairs their function. As in other cases, the cells in which this occurs, as well as others that depend on them, then die. (Some investigators have suggested that the formation of free radicals might be retarded by the taking of vitamin E supplements.)

An analogy may help to show how all these processes work together to cause aging. A shipbuilding firm must have an office, where the plans and specifications for all the various boats are kept, and a warehouse, where the materials to carry out these orders are stored. There must also be a site where the actual construction takes place. When an order is received for a particular boat to be constructed, the plans on file are duplicated for a working copy, and messengers are sent to bring the materials to the construction site. By following the instructions, workers then build the boat.

If, through years of heavy use, the warehouse becomes cluttered and disorganized, then it will become increasingly difficult to fill the orders efficiently. (This parallels the theory that, with age, the cell fluid becomes cluttered with debris.) If some of the messengers take the wrong orders from the files or bring the wrong materials, this too will cause production to slow down or cease. (This parallels the cells' loss of ability to read the genetic code words.) With rain or fire damage to the files themselves, some of the specifications will become unavailable or illegible (like the cellular DNA's becoming altered by cosmic ray bombardment). Should one worker be instructed to burn the trash, he might lazily leave behind marred instructions or parts (as in the autoimmune theory). Vandalism (free radicals) might do further damage. With inefficient management of the warehouse, there might be delays in getting supplies. (For the cell, the nutrients might not be present in the blood because they were not taken in, or there might be a breakdown in the ability of the intestinal cells to absorb the nutrients.) Finally, the warehouse might have been set up for a limited order—its destruction, once it had produced a certain number of boats, might have been planned from the beginning. (This represents the idea that cells are programmed to self-destruct after a certain number of generations.) None of the theories of cellular aging are more than theories, but they suggest explanations for the aging of organs described in the next section.

For a picture of the disulfide bridges in insulin, a protein molecule, see p. 127. Free radical formation is explained in Appendix B.

Aging of Organs

The aging of cells is reflected by changes in the organs they are a part of. The most visible changes take place in the skin. As people age, wrinkles increase, partly because of a loss of the fat that underlies the skin and partly because of a loss of elasticity. The scars that have accumulated from many small cuts roughen the texture of the skin. Exposure to sun, wind, and cold hasten the drying process and contribute to wrinkling. The hair disappears also, particularly from the head and face of males.

Another obvious and traumatic change, in the digestive system, is painful deterioration of the gums and subsequent loss of teeth. According to the Ten State Survey, gum disease exists in 90 percent of the population by age

65 to 74.[5] In addition, the senses of taste and smell diminish, which reduces the pleasure of eating.

In other parts of the digestive system, secretion by the stomach of hydrochloric acid and enzymes decreases with age, as does the secretion of digestive juices by the pancreas and small intestine. The GI tract muscles weaken with reduced use, so that pressure in the large intestine causes the outpocketings of diverticulosis. With reduced strength and motility of intestinal muscles, constipation becomes a problem.

The liver is somewhat different. Liver cells regenerate themselves throughout life, so with normal aging, the loss of liver cells is not a major problem. However, even with good nutrition, fat gradually infiltrates the liver, reducing its work output. The response of the liver to moderate blood glucose levels is not appreciably altered with age, but the response to a large glucose load is reduced. There may be two reasons for this. First, the pancreas cells may be less responsive to high blood glucose levels, so that it takes more glucose to make them respond by producing insulin. Second, the body's cells become resistant to insulin, so that it takes more to make them respond.

As the heart and blood vessels age, the volume of blood that the heart can pump decreases. The arteries lose their elasticity. The amount of blood going into the networks of capillaries in the various organs decreases. Fat deposits form in the walls of the arteries, and calcium salts invade these deposits, making them hard and inflexible. Because all organs and tissues depend on the circulation of nutrients and oxygen, degenerative changes in the cardiovascular system critically affect all other systems.

The decrease in blood flow through the kidneys makes them gradually less efficient at their task of removing nitrogen and other wastes from the blood and maintaining the correct amounts of salts, glucose, and other valuable nutrients in the body fluids. As the heart pumps less blood into the capillary trees of the kidneys, the capillary trees diminish in size, causing some kidney cells to be deprived of their nutrient and oxygen supply. Cells formerly fed by these capillaries then die. Since both the heart rate and the volume of blood pumped into the kidneys depend on the muscular activity of the person, this degenerative process can be retarded by regular exercising.

The ability of the brain to direct the activities of the body decreases during aging. The older adult compensates for this somewhat, with learning gained from experience, but the nerve cells are not replaceable; so any damage by accident permanently diminishes mental ability. This is probably the greatest cause of unhappiness among older people and their relatives, because it decreases the ability to enjoy life. Visual impairment, hearing loss, loss of the senses of smell and taste, and loss of the sense of balance are all evidence of impaired nerve cell function.

The body's systems lose their ability to function at different rates and to different extents. In a lifetime, nerve conduction velocity appears to be

As the heart pumps less blood into an organ, the capillary trees within that organ recede, leaving some of the cells without nourishment. Exercise promotes maintenance and even growth of capillaries.

5   *Ten-State Nutrition Survey, 1968–1970*, DHEW publication no. (HSM) 72–8130–8133 (Atlanta, Ga.: Center for Disease Control, 1972).

affected least and lung function most, with other functions between the extremes:

- Nerve conduction velocity and cellular enzyme activities decline about 15 percent.
- Cardiac index falls 30 percent.
- Vital capacity and renal blood flow decrease by 50 percent.
- Maximum breathing capacity, maximum work rate, and maximun oxygen uptake fall by 60 to 70 percent.[6]

Aging of the Skeleton

Like the body's other organ systems, the skeletal system is subject to change with the passage of time. Bone is a structure composed of salts of calcium, phosphorus, and other minerals. Bone-building and bone-dismantling cells are constantly working on this structure, remodeling it to adjust to the body's changing needs.

After 40, bone loss becomes more rapid than bone-building. Bone loss occurs in both sexes, although it is four times more prevalent in women than in men after 50, and no one knows for sure what the causes are. The result, however, is osteoporosis—thinning and weakening of the bones so severe as to produce fractures in as many as one out of every three people over 65.[7] A hip fracture caused by osteoporosis may not be a clean break but a shattering of the bone into fragments that can't be readily reassembled. Repair can then only be accomplished by replacing the bone or joint with an artificial substitute.

Among the factors suspected of causing or contributing to osteoporosis are:

- A too-low intake, reduced absorption, or increased excretion of calcium.
- Hormonal changes.
- Reduced physical activity.

The person who wants to prevent or retard the process of bone loss should be aware of all these factors.

A too-low calcium intake is, of course, any intake that does not completely compensate for total calcium losses. But how much calcium is enough to ensure balance? Special populations have been known to maintain balance on as little as 200 milligrams of calcium a day (the adult RDA is 800), but for most men, the minimum intake appears to be above 400 milligrams, and for women after menopause, it is about 1,000 or even more.[8] High-fiber diets impair calcium absorption, and high intakes of protein promote urinary excretion. In the light of several research findings confirming the high calcium need of older women, several authorities

cardiac index: the cardiac output per square meter of body surface area.
cardiac output: the quantity of blood pumped by the left ventricle into the aorta each minute. Cardiac output is responsible for transport of substances to and from the tissues; it changes markedly with body size.

vital capacity: the maximum volume of air that can be inhaled into or exhaled from the lungs.

The many factors affecting the body's handling of calcium are discussed in Chapter 10.

6   D. M. Watkin, The physiology of aging, *American Journal of Clinical Nutrition* 36 (Supplement, October 1982): 750–758.

7   L. Lutwak, Symposium on osteoporosis: Nutritional aspects of osteoporosis, *Journal of the American Geriatrics Society* 17 (1969): 115–119.

8   J. C. Gallagher and B. L. Riggs, Nutrition and bone disease, *New England Journal of Medicine* 298 (1978): 193–195.

were by 1980 recommending that they maintain a daily intake of 1 to 1½ grams of calcium, the amount available from 5 cups of milk a day.[9]

The second factor named above is hormonal changes. The reduction of estrogen secretion in women after menopause is known to accelerate bone loss. Estrogen replacement therapy may help prevent bone loss but cannot strengthen bones already weakened. Other hormones are implicated in bone loss, and knowledge now being gathered may lead some day to effective therapy, but for the present the facts all point one way. It is better to prevent than to attempt to restore bone loss.[10]

The third factor, physical exercise, deserves strong emphasis. Bones lose material at a dramatic rate when they are inactive or immobilized. One prominent investigator considers it urgent to "educate middle-aged people to manage their lives to prevent. . .thinning of bone tissue"—meaning, primarily, to maintain regular physical activity.[11] Evidence is accumulating that bone loss can indeed be slowed, prevented, or even reversed by physical exercise.[12]

Perhaps the factors that promote or prevent the development of osteoporosis can be traced back to the growing years at the beginning of life. The higher the density of the bones at maturity, the more bone can be lost before osteoporosis becomes debilitating (see Figure 15-2). Heredity also plays some part. Men have denser bones than women, and Mediterranean, Latin American, and African populations have denser bones than Northern European and Asian peoples. Adequate intakes of both calcium and fluoride throughout life doubtless protect against osteoporosis; the condition is not usually seen in a person who has had a consistently high calcium intake. In fact, people with osteoporosis give a lifelong history of exceptionally low calcium intakes.[13]

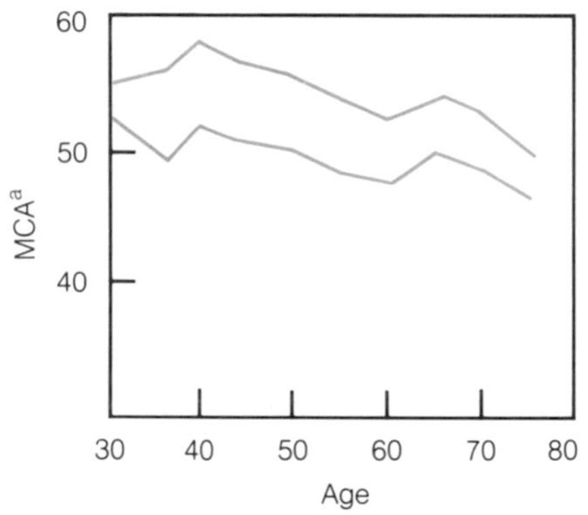

No one of middle age or over can, however, revisit her childhood, obtain the calcium and other nutrients she needs to build bone, and exercise them into place. Because "you can't learn younger," it is important for the person embarking on the later years to plan positively to obtain the needed nutrients and schedule physical workouts as part of a regular routine.

Arthritis, a painful swelling of the joints, is another problem that troubles many people as they grow older. During movement, the bones must rub against each other at the joints. The ends are protected from wear by cartilage and by small sacs of fluid that act as a lubricant. With age, the ends of the bone become pitted or eroded as a result of wear. The cause of arthritis is unknown, but it affects millions around the world and is a major problem of the elderly.

FIGURE 15-2 **Loss of bone mass after age 40 in two groups of males.** The group that reached a peak near 60 MCA at age 40 still had as much bone mass at age 75 as the other group had at its peak.

[a]MCA: metacarpal cortical area, an indicator of bone mass.
Source: Adapted from R. P. Heaney and coauthors, Calcium nutrition and bone health in the elderly, *American Journal of Clinical Nutrition* 36 (Supplement, November 1982): 986–1013.

9   Gallagher and Riggs, 1978; G. D. Whedon, Osteoporosis (editorial), *New England Journal of Medicine* 305 (1981): 397–399; R. P. Heaney, Premenopausal prophylactic calcium supplementation: Questions and answers, *Journal of the American Medical Association* 245 (1981): 1362.

10   J. L. Marx, Osteoporosis: New help for thinning bones, *Science* 207 (1980): 628–630.

11   Marx, 1980.

12   J. F. Aloia, Exercise and skeletal health, *Journal of the American Geriatrics Society* 29 (1981): 104–107.

13   Lutwak, 1969.

People with arthritis can often fall prey to the enticements of quack remedies, including diet "cures." Two or three new popular books on diet for arthritis come out every year, urging that arthritis sufferers eat no meat, or drink no milk, or eat all their food raw, or eat only "natural" food, or avoid all additives, or—who knows what will be next? Actually no known diet prevents, relieves, or cures arthritis, but as long as people keep buying the books that make these claims, the law of supply and demand dictates that such books will keep coming out.

Recently, a true, positive finding has been reported that links diet to arthritis. The researchers surveyed the diets of 36 people with arthritis and found them marginal with respect to several essential nutrients. They singled out vitamin E and zinc as the most significant of these, because these two nutrients are important to normal function of the body's immune system, and an abnormal immune response may be a contributor to arthritis. Although no final conclusions can be reached, as yet, they find it "prudent to advise patients to maintain sound nutritional practices in accordance with contemporary standards"—that is, to make efforts to obtain adequate, balanced diets.[14] This is an undramatic conclusion, perhaps, but it is honest, good advice.

Caution

The process of aging can be retarded by maintaining a strong cardiovascular and respiratory system. Exercise, regular and active enough to increase the heartbeat and respiration rate, is one of the keys to good health in the later years. An added benefit of exercise, as you already know, is to prevent the atrophy of all muscles (not only the heart), which would take place with inactivity. A good flow of blood requires a strong heartbeat and strongly flexing muscles to press expelled lymph back into the bloodstream for recirculation. Many older persons believe that they can't participate in strenuous exercise, but studies have shown that they can do more than they think they can. Even modest endurance training can improve cardiovascular and respiratory function and promote good muscle tone while controlling the accumulation of body fat.[15] The older person who has never worked out hard before may be encouraged to learn that the trainability of older people does not depend on their physical prowess in their youth. Also, their increase in muscle strength during training is not due to the improvement in their muscles but to the improvement in the nervous system which results from the increased blood flow to the brain engendered by the exercise.[16]

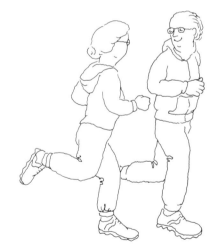

14   B. Kowsari and coauthors, Assessment of the diet of patients with rheumatoid arthritis and osteoarthritis, *Journal of the American Dietetic Association* 82 (1983): 657–659.

15   K. H. Sidney, R. J. Shephard, and J. E. Harrison, Endurance training and body composition of the elderly, *American Journal of Clinical Nutrition* 30 (1977): 326–333.

16   H. A. DeVries, Physiological effects of an exercise training regimen upon men aged 52 to 88, *Journal of Gerontology* 25 (1970): 325–336.

Nutrition Implications of Aging

Good health habits, including good nutrition throughout life, are the best guarantee of healthy and enjoyable later years. Many of the nutrient needs of the elderly are the same as for younger persons, but some special considerations deserve emphasis. As you read the following discussions about particular elements of the diet, remember that older adults who overemphasize one food group to the exclusion of others are most at risk nutritionally. The familiar maxim holds true throughout the life cycle—that the best dietary guideline is to eat a balanced and varied selection of foods.

kCalories

Energy needs decrease with advancing age. For one thing, the number of active cells in each organ decreases, bringing about a reduction in the body's overall metabolic rate. For another, older people are less active physically (although they need not be). In 1980, for the first time, the RDA tables presented recommended energy intakes for the older set; these recommendations reflect an estimated reduction of about 5 percent per decade in energy output. The variation is great, so the ranges are wide (see Appendix O), but average figures for people 75 and older are 2,050 kcalories per day for the man and 1,600 for the woman. Table 15–1 shows food patterns that would supply amounts of kcalories a little lower than the RDA tables show. Because overweight is well recognized as a shortener of the life span, these seem to be life-sustaining recommendations.

Protein-kcalorie malnutrition is common in older people and often goes unnoticed. An observer, seeing the wasted muscle, weakness, and sometimes swelling of protein deficiency, may think, "That person looks old," when in fact he should recognize the symptoms of PCM. Older people who have been trying to lose weight or eating monotonous or bizarre diets are most likely to be affected.[17]

Protein foods should contribute about 12 to 20 percent of the kcalories in the older person's diet. Fats should provide no more than 30 percent, and the remainder should come from complex carbohydrates.[18] On such a limited kcalorie allowance, all foods must be nutrient dense. There is little leeway for such empty-kcalorie foods as sugar, sweets, fats, oils, or alcohol.

One side of the energy budget is for kcalories to be taken in, and the other side is for the expenditure of those kcalories. Increase in activity, as already mentioned, should be emphasized for any person interested in maintaining good health in the later years. People responsible for the care of older adults should encourage more activity of all kinds and shorter recuperation periods in bed following illnesses.

17   S. R. Gambert and A. R. Guansing, Protein-calorie malnutrition in the elderly, *Journal of the American Geriatrics Society* 28 (1980): 272–275.

18   D. B. Rao, Problems of nutrition in the aged, *Journal of the American Geriatrics Society* 21 (1973): 362–367.

TABLE 15-1   **Eating Patterns to Supply the Recommended kCalorie Amounts for Older People (Exchange System)**

	NUMBER OF EXCHANGES	
EXCHANGE LIST	*Woman (1,500 kcal)*	*Man (2,000 kcal)*
Milk (skim)	4	4
Vegetable	2	3
Fruit	4	6
Bread	5	9
Meat (lean)	6	7
Fat	6	8

You may have heard of some experiments in which young rats, just weaned, were fed diets extremely restricted in kcalories for a short period early in life and then lived much longer than their age-mates who had enjoyed ample kcalories from an early age throughout life. The first of these experiments were performed long ago, but recent reviews of them have inspired articles in the popular press with titles like "EAT LESS—LIVE LONGER."

True, the life spans of rats were lengthened by drastic restrictions of their food intakes during the time when they would normally be growing. In one experiment, for example, animals allowed to eat freely lived to an average 656 days while those whose feed was restricted lived to an average 949 days. The experiments were interesting because it was possible to study growth retardation of various organ systems, and to speculate on the cause of the increased length of life of some of the animals—a delay in the onset of certain diseases, for example. But the experiments did *not* suggest any direct applications to human nutrition. One thing often overlooked in discussing them is the disadvantages incurred in the animals given restricted feedings.

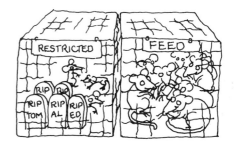

For example, half of the restricted animals died *very* early (before 300 days). The average length of life was long because the few survivors lived a very long time. Also, the restriction was very severe: "even the shortest period of food restriction in this study was comparable to restriction of the food intake of a human infant kept in an isolated environment for 20 to 25 years to an amount that would permit the infant to grow during that time to about the size of a one-year-old child."[19] Furthermore, the restricted animals that survived were retarded and malformed in a number of ways.

Old people, then, need not conclude on the basis of this evidence that their parents should have starved them when they were younger. Moderation in kcalorie intake is desirable, of course, but extreme starvation, like any extreme, is hardly worth the price.

Caution

19   A. E. Harper, Nutrition, aging, and longevity, *American Journal of Clinical Nutrition* 36 (Supplement, October 1982): 737–749.

Protein

The need for essential amino acids is the same for older adults as it is for younger adults. However, the older person needs to get these essential nutrients from less food; so care should be taken that the protein is of high quality. The protein should also be protected from being used for energy by the inclusion of complex carbohydrates in the diet.

It has been shown that, for older persons living at home, milk or its equivalent in cheese is one of the foods most often omitted from the diet. Another protein food, meat, is often omitted because it is difficult to chew; in one study, only those with excellent teeth had a high protein intake. Both milk and meat may also be omitted because of difficulties with purchasing and storage. Low hemoglobin levels have been shown to correlate with protein (as well as iron) content of the diet,[20] and may be the cause of the fatigue and apathy so often mentioned as a problem by older persons. The National Academy of Sciences' National Research Council (NAS/NRC) recommends that older persons consume 12 percent of their kcalories as protein, which works out to an amount slightly above the RDA for most people. Food patterns that restrict fat and offer abundant carbohydrate of necessity often supply up to 20 percent of the kcalories as protein.

Fat

For many reasons, fat should be limited in the older person's diet. Cutting fat helps cut kcalories (recall that fat delivers two and a half times as many kcalories as the other energy nutrients) and may also help retard the development of atherosclerosis. On the limited kcalorie allowance recommended for older adults, it would be difficult to obtain the many vitamins and minerals that come from foods rich in protein and complex carbohydrates if too much of the energy came from the relatively empty kcalories of fat. Moreover, high fat intakes can interfere with calcium absorption, promoting osteoporosis.

On the other hand, if fat kcalories are restricted too greatly, the fat-soluble vitamins and essential fatty acids may be deficient. An appropriate lower limit might be 20 percent of the kcalories from fat. Of those, about half should perhaps be from polyunsaturated fat to contribute the essential fatty acids and to displace the saturated fat thought to contribute to high levels of cholesterol in the blood.

Carbohydrate

Emphasis in the older person's diet should be on securing a wide variety of complex carbohydrate foods to provide the vitamins and minerals they contain. Older people often omit fruits and vegetables from their diets. It is not known whether this is due to earlier consumption patterns or to their finding fruits and vegetables too expensive or too difficult to store and prepare. Any educational campaign conducted to improve the diets of the elderly should emphasize the great amount of essential nutrients, miner-

20   A. F. Morgan, Nutrition of the aging, *Gerontologist* 2 (1962): 77–84.

als, and fiber contributed by complex carbohydrate foods. Programs such as those serving congregate meals to older people can furnish bags so that the participants can take home the fruit that was served for dessert, as a way of encouraging the use of fruit.

Vitamins

Many of the problems seen in the elderly may result from decreased vitamin intakes. Vitamin deficiency is likely unless great care is taken to include foods from each of the food groups. Studies have shown that the one food group omitted most often by the elderly is the vegetable group. About 18 percent of older people are reported to eat no vegetables at all. Fruit is lacking in many diets, and 34 percent in one study reported never eating fruit.[21] Some men and women do not eat whole-grain breads and cereals, and so lose a significant source of many B vitamins and several minerals. Vitamin D deficiency is possible in older people who are homebound or who live in smoggy cities; some authorities suggest that the RDA for vitamin D for older people should be set at 15 to 20 micrograms per day, rather than at the present 10 micrograms.[22] The destruction of vitamin E by heat processing and oxidation is well known, and the processed and convenience foods so often used by the elderly and by nursing homes are thought to contribute to a vitamin E deficiency if their use continues over several years.[23] These statistics have somber implications for the health of older persons.

Not only the omission of certain food groups but also other conditions contribute to vitamin deficiency in the elderly. As mentioned, many are housebound (or hospital-bound) and thus are deprived of the vitamin D they would get from sunshine on their skin. Many do not drink milk. Many take laxatives regularly, and this causes such a rapid transit time through the intestine that many vitamins do not get absorbed. The use of mineral oil as a laxative especially robs the person of the fat-soluble vitamins. Some drugs regularly taken by older adults cause vitamin deficiencies. For example, some antibiotics kill intestinal bacteria that produce vitamin K; and the anticonvulsant drugs used in the treatment of epilepsy produce a folacin deficiency.

The recommended intakes for many of the vitamins are thought by some nutritionists to be too low for the over-65 group. They recommend supplements, particularly for the water-soluble vitamins, because toxicity from large amounts does not pose a great threat. However, other nutritionists feel that recommending vitamin supplements is a "cop-out" laying the elderly open to exploitation by quacks. Money is better spent, they say, on food of higher quality. The older person would probably be wise to follow

21   J. Pelcovits, Nutrition to meet the human needs of older Americans, *Journal of the American Dietetic Association* 60 (1972): 297–300.

22   A. M. Parfitt and coauthors, Vitamin D and bone health in the elderly, *American Journal of Clinical Nutrition* 36 (Supplement, November 1982): 1014–1031.

23   H. H. Koehler, H. C. Lee, and M. Jacobson, Tocopherols in canned entrees and vended sandwiches, *Journal of the American Dietetic Association* 70 (1977): 616–620.

the rule of thumb that if the kcalorie intake is below about the 1,500 level, then a vitamin-mineral supplement is recommended—not a megavitamin, but just a once-daily type supplement. This means that many older persons, all except those who are so active that their kcalorie allowance has remained high, should take this precaution.

Minerals

Iron-deficiency anemia is not as common in older adults as has been believed in the past, but it still occurs in some, especially in those with low kcalorie intakes.[24] Low blood hemoglobin can result from a diet low in protein, as already mentioned; but diets low in iron are also common. Heavy reliance on a "tea and toast" diet is cited as a double risk in this connection; what little iron the toast provides is poorly absorbable, while the tannins in tea inhibit iron absorption. (Actually, something in coffee inhibits iron absorption, too, though we don't know yet what it is.[25]) But any diet that is low in kcalories and lacks color (and therefore lacks iron-containing red meats as well as fruits and vegetables rich in vitamin C to aid in iron absorption) suggests risk of iron deficiency.

Aside from diet, other factors in many older people's lives increase the likelihood of iron deficiency:

● Chronic blood loss from ulcers, hemorrhoids, or other disease conditions.
● Poor iron absorption due to reduced stomach acid secretion.
● Antacid use, which interferes with iron absorption.
● Use of medicines that cause blood loss, including arthritis medicines, anticoagulants, and aspirin.

The person counseling an older client on health and nutrition should not forget to ask about these possibilities.

Zinc deficiencies are probably common in older people. They may affect several functions. Most often associated with zinc deficiencies are loss of taste and slowed wound healing. Loss of taste, however, is often not responsive to zinc supplementation, and it may often arise from some other factor associated with aging. When wounds—for example, bed sores in the sick—are slow to heal, however, a zinc deficiency should be suspected, as these often do respond to zinc therapy.

Another mineral often lacking in older people's diets is calcium, the need for which increases with advancing age. Bone loss occurs insidiously, and may be alarmingly extensive and severe before a person realizes there is any problem at all. The recommendation that an older adult ingest the equivalent of 5 cups of milk a day is difficult to meet, especially for the person who is unaccustomed to using much milk at all. However, there are many alternative strategies for obtaining the needed calcium. If fresh milk

24   S. R. Lynch, C. A. Finch, E. R. Monsen, and J. D. Cook, Iron status of elderly Americans, *American Journal of Clinical Nutrition* 36 (Supplement, November 1982): 1032–1045.

25   T. A. Morck, S. R. Lynch, and J. D. Cook, Inhibition of food iron absorption by coffee, *American Journal of Clinical Nutrition* 37 (1983): 416–420.

causes flatulence (gas), as some older people report, then cheese should be included. Dry skim milk can be incorporated into many foods. Soup stock made from bones can be used daily. These and other strategies are offered in the next section ("Practical Pointers").

The use of medications impairs calcium absorption severely. So does the use of alcohol. Older people who use both are especially prone to calcium deficiency.

Salt, which contains the mineral sodium, should be curtailed in the older person's diet—not only by those with hypertension, congestive heart failure, or cirrhosis of the liver, but by all older people. Salt is conducive to the retention of fluid, which results in raised blood pressure. Convenience foods and processed foods are high in sodium content and are widely used by older persons living alone, thus making it difficult for them to restrict their salt intake. Wherever possible, fresh foods should be eaten instead.

To obtain the needed minerals, the older person should follow the same recommendation as for vitamins. Every food group—milk and milk products, meat and meat alternatives, fruits and vegetables, and grains—should be represented in the diet every day.

Fiber

The fiber recommendations for the general population should be stressed to older citizens as well: increase the use of fruits, vegetables, and whole-grain cereals. The fiber content of these food groups is important to the health of the muscles of the intestinal tract. If there is bulk for these muscles to work against, constipation is less likely and it is less necessary to resort to the use of laxatives. In addition, some fibers (except wheat bran) bind cholesterol and carry it out of the body.

Fiber is discussed in more detail in Chapter 2.

Water

The elderly need to be reminded to drink fluids, because they are likely to be somewhat insensitive to their own thirst signals. They should drink 6 to 8 glasses a day, enough to bring their urine output to about 1,500 milliliters (6 cups) per day. A large percentage of foster home operators note that one of the biggest problems with their elderly clients is getting them to use more water and fruit juices.

Caffeine

Older people often find they cannot tolerate caffeine as well as they could when they were younger. Caffeine is a true stimulant drug, increasing the respiration rate, heart rate, blood pressure, and secretion of the stress and other hormones. Its "wake-up" effect is maximal within an hour after the dose. In moderate amounts (50 to 200 milligrams a day), caffeine seems to be relatively harmless.

Caffeine is not addictive, but it is habit-forming, and the body adapts to its use to some extent. A dose greater than what the body is adapted to

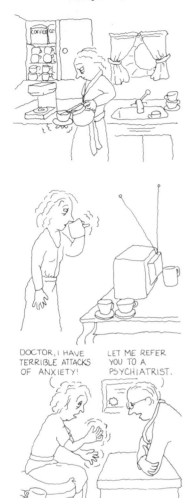

DOCTOR, I HAVE TERRIBLE ATTACKS OF ANXIETY!

LET ME REFER YOU TO A PSYCHIATRIST.

causes jitteriness, nervousness, and intestinal discomfort. Sudden abstinence from the drug after long use, even if use has been moderate, causes a characteristic withdrawal reaction; the most frequently observed symptom is a headache. If a person has adapted to a much higher dose level than 50 to 200 milligrams (see Table 15–2), then dropping back to this level may cause the same withdrawal reaction.

An overdose of caffeine produces actions in the body that are indistinguishable from those of an anxiety attack. People who drink between 8 and 15 cups of coffee a day, for example, have been known to seek help from doctors for complaints such as dizziness, agitation, restlessness, recurring headaches, and sleep difficulties. Before prescribing a tranquilizer, the doctor would do well to inquire about the caffeine consumption of such patients.

A large dose of caffeine can also cause extra heartbeats and is believed to have caused heart attacks in people whose hearts were already damaged by degenerative disease. However, neither caffeine nor its vehicle, coffee, can be considered a risk factor for the development of atherosclerosis. Still, moderation in the use of caffeine-containing foods and beverages is advisable for all ages, and older people should be alert to the need to reduce their customary doses.

Alcohol

A recent estimate sets the incidence of alcoholism in people over 60 in our society at 2 to 10 percent. Alcohol use has its most profound effects on the vitamins thiamin and folacin and on the minerals calcium and zinc, but it affects nearly every nutrient to some extent. Where it is a problem in elderly people it must be recognized before it can be dealt with.

Practical Pointers

All of the objectives outlined for the older person's diet may seem worthwhile, but they may be hard to achieve, especially for the person living alone who has difficulty buying groceries and preparing meals. Packages of meat and vegetables are often prewrapped in quantities suitable for a family of four or more, and even a head of lettuce can perish before one person can use it all. A large package of meat is often a good buy, but defrosting it enough to get a portion from it for dinner is time-consuming; futhermore, the rest tends to thaw, too. Small packets get "lost" in the freezer and ruined by freezer burn. For the person who has little or no freezer space, the problem of storage is further compounded. Following is a collection of ideas gathered from single people who are doing a good job of solving these problems and getting nourishing food:

● Buy only three pieces of each kind of fresh fruit: a ripe one, a medium one, and a green one. Eat the first right away and the second soon, and let the last one ripen on your windowsill.
● Buy the small cans of vegetables even though they are more expensive.

Remember, it is also expensive to buy a regular-size can and let the unused portion spoil in the refrigerator.

● Buy only what you will use. Don't be timid about asking the grocer to break open a package of wrapped meat or fresh vegetables.

● Think up a variety of ways to use a vegetable when you must buy it in a quantity larger than you can use. For example, you can divide a head of cauliflower into thirds. Cook one third and eat it as a hot vegetable. Put the other two thirds into a vinegar and oil marinade for use as an appetizer or in a salad. You can keep half a package of frozen vegetables with other vegetables to be used in soup or stew.

● Make mixtures, using what you have on hand. A thick stew prepared from leftover green beans, carrots, cauliflower, broccoli, and any meat, with some added onion, pepper, celery, and potatoes, makes a complete and balanced meal—except for milk. But see the uses of powdered milk that follow: you could add some to your stew.

● Buy fresh milk in the size best suited for you. If your grocer doesn't carry pints or half-pints, try a nearby service station or convenience store.

● Buy a half-dozen eggs at a time. The carton of a dozen can usually be broken in half. However, eggs keep for long periods in the refrigerator and are such a good source of high-quality protein that you will probably use a dozen before they lose their freshness.

● Set aside a place in your kitchen for rows of glass jars containing shelf staple items that you can't buy in single-serving quantities—rice, tapioca, lentils or other dry beans, flour, cornmeal, dry skim milk, macaroni, cereal, or coconut, to name only a few possibilities. Place each jar, tightly sealed, in the freezer for one night to kill any eggs or contaminants before storing it on the shelf. Then the jars will keep the bugs out of the foods indefinitely. They make an attractive display and will remind you of possibilities for variety in your menus. Cut the directions-for-use label from the package and store it in the jar.

● Learn to use dry skim milk. It is the greatest convenience food there is. Not only does it offer much more calcium than any other food, it also is fortified with vitamins A and D. Dry milk can be stored on the shelf for several months at room temperature. It can be mixed with water to make fluid milk in as small a quantity as you like—but once it is mixed, it will sour just like fresh milk. One person says he keeps a jar of dry skim milk next to his stove and "dumps it into everything": hamburgers, gravies, soups, casseroles, sauces, even beverages such as iced coffee. The taste is negligible, but five "dumpings" of a heaping tablespoon each would be the equivalent of a cup of fresh milk. Ask a friend who is a member of Weight Watchers to give you some recipes for delicious milkshakes and ice cream using dry skim milk. Their recipes are for single servings.

● Make soup stock from leftover pork and chicken bones soaked in vinegar. The bones release their calcium into the acid medium, and the vinegar boils off when the stock is boiled. One *tablespoon* of such stock may contain over 100 milligrams of calcium.[26] Then cook something in this

TABLE 15–2 **Caffeine Sources**

SOURCE	CAFFEINE (mg)
Brewed coffee (1 c)	85
Instant coffee (1 c)	60
Brewed black tea (1 c)	50
Brewed green tea (1 c)	30
Instant tea (1 c)	30
Decaffeinated coffee (1 c)	3
Cola beverage (12 oz)	32–65
Aspirin compound (pill containing aspirin, phenacetin, and caffeine)	32
Cope, Midol, etc.	32
Excedrin, Anacin (tablet)	60
Pre-Mens	66
Many cold preparations	30
Many stimulants	100
Cocoa (1 c)	6–42
No Doz (tablet) or Vivarin	100–200

Source: Adapted from "Food allergy," *Nutrition and the MD*, July 1978; and P. E. Stephenson, Physiologic and psychotropic effects of caffeine on man, *Journal of the American Dietetic Association* 71 (1977): 240–247.

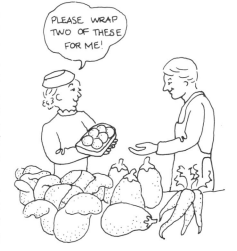

PLEASE WRAP TWO OF THESE FOR ME!

26   A. Rosanoff and D. H. Calloway, Calcium source in Indochinese immigrants (correspondence), *New England Journal of Medicine* 306 (1982): 239–240.

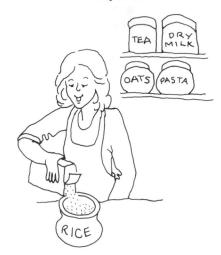

stock every day: vegetables, rice, stew—and of course, make soups with it.

● Cook for several meals at a time. For example, boil three potatoes with skins. Eat one hot with margarine and chives. When the others have cooled, use one to make a potato-cheese casserole ready to be put into the oven for the next evening's meal. Slice the third one into a covered bowl and pour over it the juice from pickles. The pickled potato will keep several days in the refrigerator and can be used in a salad.

● Experiment with stir-fried foods. Use a frying pan if you don't have a wok. Ask your Chinese friends for some recipes. A variety of vegetables and meat can be enjoyed this way; inexpensive vegetables such as cabbage and celery are delicious when crisp-cooked in a little oil with soy or lemon added. Cooked, leftover vegetables can be dropped in at the last minute. There are frozen mixtures of Chinese or Polynesian vegetables available in the larger grocery stores. Bonus: Only one pan to wash.

● Depending on your freezer space, make double or even six times as much as you need of a dish that takes time to prepare: a casserole, vegetable pie, or meatloaf. Save the little aluminum trays from frozen foods and store the extra servings, labeled, in the trays in the freezer. Be sure to date these so you will use the oldest first. Somehow, the work seems worthwhile when you prepare several meals at once.

● Learn to connect food with socializing. Cook for yourself with the idea that you are also preparing for guests you might want to invite. Or turn this suggestion around: invite guests and make enough food so that you will have some left for yourself at a later meal. These suggestions came from a young widow and an 86-year-old widow. The young widow, after her husband's death, purposely cooked generous amounts so she could make her own frozen dinners from the leftovers. With a wide variety of these on hand, she feels free to invite one or another of her single friends on the spur of the moment to "Come over and share my frozen dinners with me tonight." She says she devised this method of managing her food out of the need to manage her "five o'clock loneliness." The 86-year-old widow invites guests for dinner every Sunday, because "it is no fun to cook for one," and she, too, loves having the leftovers.

● Buy a loaf of bread and immediately store half, well wrapped, in the freezer. The freezer keeps it fresher than the refrigerator.

● If you have space in your freezing compartment, buy frozen vegetables in the very large bags rather than in the small cartons. You can take out the exact amount you need and close the bag tightly with a rubber band. If you return the package quickly to the freezer each time, the vegetables will stay fresh for a long time.

● If you have ample freezing space, you can buy large packages of meat such as pork chops, ground meat, or chicken when they are on special sale. Immediately divide the package into individual servings. Wrap in aluminum foil, not freezer paper: the foil can become the liner for the pan in which you bake or broil the meat, thus saving work over the sink. Don't label these individually, but put them all in a brown bag marked "hamburger" or "chicken thighs" or whatever the meat is, along with the date. The bag is easy to locate in the freezer, and you'll know when your supply is running low.

Although these suggestions will help the older person with the mechanics of food preparation and storage, they meet only a part of the need. Loneliness, too, needs to be dealt with if single life in the later years is to be enjoyed. Even for nutrition's sake, it is important to attend to this problem.

Mealtimes Alone

The concept of old age as being a time of losses is a depressing one, certainly unpleasant to consider. But it is realistic and needs to be faced. Many people who arrive at this time of life don't comprehend the universality of the aging experience. They have made no mental preparations for it. Then, when faced with some of the normal experiences of later life—the children's wanting to be independent from the parents, for example—they turn inward for the explanation and conclude that there must be something wrong with them. Depression follows such reasoning and compounds the distress of the original problem.

Losses can occur in several areas. Old friends are lost whey they die or move away; offspring move away also and are too busy to write; there is loss of income on retirement and loss of status in the community. There is loss of control of the environment, such as finding that the home that was to be a haven in retirement now sits in the middle of a high-crime area so that one can no longer walk the streets or visit with neighbors. Familiar shops and fruit stands, where a person knows the owner and is known by them, may close. The aging person develops a feeling of deep loneliness as the familiar environment constantly shifts. But what place, you may well ask, does such a discussion have in a book on nutrition?

Many authorities believe that malnutrition among the elderly is most often due to loneliness. For the 6 million adults over 65 who live alone, the pressing need seems to be for companionship first, then for food. Without companionship, appetite decreases. The association of food with human companionship is built into our genes, and our very first experience with food was combined with human body contact. The social life of the adult is built around food. Most invitations into adults' homes are accompanied by an offer of food or drink. We must admit that feeding is, for human beings, as much a social and psychological event as a biological one.

Having spent a lifetime internalizing the concept of food as part of a social activity, the older adult, alone all day every day, must exert a wrenching effort to place enough importance on the nutrient content of food to prepare it and to eat it alone. Purchasing, storing, and preparing food, as well as cleaning the kitchen, take a tremendous amount of energy. The lonely, depressed person, looking at the task, may forget about the body's needs and say, "What's the use?"

Dr. Jack Weinberg, professor of psychiatry at the University of Illinois, wrote perceptively of this problem:

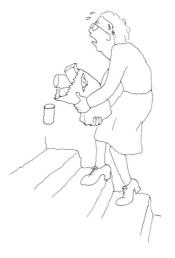

> In our efforts to provide the aged with a proper diet, we often fail to perceive it is not *what* the older person eats but *with whom* that will be the deciding factor in proper care for him. The oft-repeated complaint of the older patient that he has little incentive to prepare food for only himself is not merely a

statement of fact but also a rebuke to the questioner for failing to perceive his isolation and aloneness and to realize that food...for one's self lacks the condiment of another's presence which can transform the simplest fare to the ceremonial act with all its shared meaning.[27]

The lack of social interaction is no respecter of income. It is equally important in the lives of the financially secure and in the lives of the poverty-stricken. Newspapers occasionally carry stories of wealthy older persons' being discovered in their mansions, alone and without food. The stories are newsworthy because people wonder why such victims did not ask for help or make arrangements for someone to take care of them—after all, they had plenty of money. The reason is simple. Apathy evolves from loneliness; apathy is expressed in inaction. A victim may sit for long hours in a chair without the energy even to lift her arms. There is no energy to eat, even when food is just a phone call away. Without adequate food, nutrient deficiencies develop that increase the apathy and depression and eventually result in mental confusion. The downward spiral continues, unless intervention by neighbors or friends breaks it at some point.

Let's look at what happens when a person receives too little food. In the first place, the body can't tell why it is receiving too few nutrients or kcalories. The situation is the same for a child dying in a famine in Bangladesh as for a wealthy solitary person who is depressed and refusing food. The B vitamins and vitamin C are quickly depleted because they are needed daily. If they are not restored, mental confusion that resembles senility will be manifest and may even progress to hallucinations and insanity.

If protein foods, protected by complex carbohydrates, are insufficient, then enzymes to digest food and antibodies to protect against infection cannot be synthesized. When iron and vitamin C are absent, the protein hemoglobin cannot be made for the delivery of oxygen, so the feeling of weakness and tiredness grows. With tiredness from lack of food added to apathy from loneliness, there is even less energy with which to make the effort to secure nourishment. If the confusion of vitamin deficiency is diagnosed as senility, the elderly person may be wrongly confined to a nursing home.

The story is told of a woman who took her mother-in-law to live with her while the older woman waited for a place in a nursing home. The mother-in-law had exhibited the classic signs of senility—mental confusion, inability to make decisions, forgetting to perform important tasks such as turning off a stove burner—so the family had decided she needed institutional care. After several weeks in the daughter-in-law's home—eating good meals and enjoying social stimulation—she became her old self again and returned to her home. This story has been repeated with many variations and serves to remind us to seek a careful medical diagnosis before concluding that a person is senile and needs institutional care. What harm could there be in first trying good, balanced meals served with plenty of tender, loving care?

Lonely people:
Become apathetic.
Have no energy to seek food.
Become tired.
Become more apathetic.
Don't reach out to others.
Become more lonely.
Do not eat.
Become malnourished.
Become mentally confused.
Become more isolated.
Become more lonely.

The symptoms of B-vitamin deficiencies are listed in Chapter 8, Table 8-2.

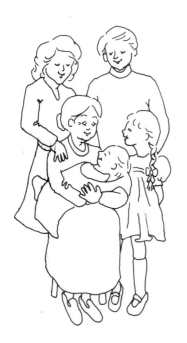

27   J. Weinberg, Psychologic implications of the nutritional needs of the elderly, *Journal of the American Dietetic Association* 60 (1972): 293–296.

Money and Other Worries

To add anxiety to their problems, most retired persons have a loss of real income that occurs because the retirement check is fixed while all other expenses are increasing. This has a direct effect on the amount of money spent on food, because food (and clothing) purchases are among the few flexible items in the budget. Costs of shelter, utilities, and medical care must be paid and then the amount left over stretched to cover food and other needs.

Forced to practice economy, the older person usually first eliminates so-called "luxury" items such as fresh fruit, vegetables, and milk. In some cases, transportation to and from the market is both expensive and difficult, so that use is made of a nearby convenience store. The foods offered there are limited in variety and are, for the most part, more expensive than the same items in the larger markets. The amount of food that can be purchased is thus curtailed even further, and eating, which should be a pleasure, becomes another reminder of reduced status.

Sometimes older persons fall prey to food fads and fallacies. Led by false claims to believe that health can be improved, aging forestalled, and illness cured by magical food and nutrient preparations, they spend money needlessly on fraudulent health-food products, thus depleting their already limited funds.

Two programs are helpful with older people's money problems, although they are not designed specifically for older people but for the poor of all ages. The Food Stamp program enables people who qualify to obtain stamps with which to buy food. The Supplemental Security Income (SSI) program is aimed at directly improving the financial plight of the very poor, by increasing a person's or family's income to the defined poverty level. This sometimes helps older people retain their independence.

A self-help effort aimed at enabling older people on limited incomes to buy good food for less money is the establishment of food banks in several areas. A food bank project buys industry's "irregulars"—products that have been mislabeled, underweighted, redesigned, or mispackaged and would ordinarily therefore be thrown away. Nothing is wrong with this food, the industry can credit it as a donation, and the buyer (often a food-preparing site) can buy the food for a small handling fee (10 cents a pound) and make it available for a greatly reduced price. A 1981 observation on this effort was: "This kind of activity becomes even more important as we begin to realize that we're not going to get any additional federal money in the future. We have to find other ways to provide the same services."[28]

Besides loneliness, loss, and limited income, the older person faces an increased likelihood of illness and invalidism. Poor dental health, mental illness, and chronic alcoholism are other problems prevalent among the elderly. In light of all these problems and of the increasing numbers of

28   C. Schuster, Feeding at life's end, *Food Management* 16 (December 1981): 41, 68–71, 76.

people in the older age group, it is not surprising that at least a few individuals and agencies are concerned enough to ask what can be done to help.

Assistance Programs

In recent years, we have come to recognize that the responsibility for support in old age cannot be left entirely to the individual. Two programs arising from this awareness have already been mentioned (the Food Stamp and Supplemental Security Income programs). The first venture into help for older persons grew out of the experiences of the depression years of the 1930s. The Social Security Act was put into effect in 1935. Under this act, employees and employers pay into a fund from which the employee collects benefits at retirement.

A second major political move to benefit the elderly was the Older Americans Act of 1965. Title III C (formerly title VII) of this act is an amendment, "Nutrition Program for the Elderly," which was signed into law by President Nixon in 1972. The major goals of this amendment are to provide:

Social Security

- Low-cost nutritious meals.
- Opportunity for social interaction.
- Auxiliary nutrition, homemaker education, and shopping assistance.
- Counseling and referral to other social and rehabilitative services.
- Transportation services.

Title III C

The nutrition program of Title III C is based on the belief that people living alone are apt to be poorly nourished. If their nutrition status could be improved, they might avoid medical problems, continue living in communities of their own choice, and stay out of institutions. The program was not designed as charity, but during its first years it was found that 80 percent of the participants had incomes less than $200 a month and 34 percent had incomes under $100 a month.[29]

Meals on Wheels

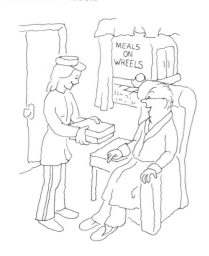

Sites chosen for congregate meals under this program must be accessible to most of the target population. Church or school facilities are often used when they are conveniently located. Providing transportation increases the cost of meals by 20 to 30 percent, but it often is indispensable to the existence of a project. Some projects have been successful in recruiting volunteers to help with the transportation. Volunteers may also deliver meals to those who are homebound either permanently or temporarily; these efforts are known as Meals on Wheels. By 1980 there were several hundred Meals on Wheels programs in the United States.

Every effort is made to persuade the elderly person to come to the congregate meal site. The social atmosphere at the sites is as valuable as the nutrition. One participant was heard to remark, "It is better to come to

29   Pelcovits, 1972.

the congregate meal and eat at a table with others, even if no one speaks to me, than it is to sit at home and stare at a wall while I eat."[30]

Independence is rated high by those over 65, and is usually equated with staying in the home where they have lived many years. But this aloneness may not be a wise choice from a nutrition standpoint. There are alternatives that would enhance elderly people's health without threatening their independence. One alternative is covenant living, a lifestyle in which a number of congenial people, wishing to live in a family group but having no families of their own, agree to live together. Another way of gaining sociability while remaining independent is for several older persons to remain in their own homes but meet together regularly for meals, each one taking a turn at preparing the food. Socializing encourages a better food intake, and the one who prepares the food has leftovers to enjoy the next day. Some of the participants in the congregate meal programs have formed what they call "diners' clubs" and go to restaurants in a group on the days when the congregate meal is not served. This kind of arrangement among friends helps improve the dietary intake of many older persons.

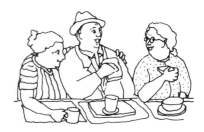

Another alternative is to move into a retirement community. Some are very expensive, but some have a rule that no one who has an income above a certain moderate amount is eligible. Foster home care has proven to be another alternative for people who need some supportive care but do not need medical supervision.

Churches and synagogues are ideal organizations to help with the problems of the elderly for a number of reasons: (1) they have neighborhood facilities that lie idle a good portion of the week; (2) they are "caring" organizations; (3) they have a target population, either among their own members or in their neighborhoods; and (4) they have a reservoir of volunteers to help cut down on labor costs. Many religious organizations have taken the lead in establishing retirement and nursing homes. However, these facilities are very expensive and usually necessitate the residents' leaving their own communities, which means leaving behind the people who care about them. In addition, a nursing home is a medical solution to what, in many cases, is a social problem.[31]

For people who need constant medical care, nursing homes provide a less expensive facility than hospitals, however. Nursing homes are patterned after hospitals in their approach to their clients. Sometimes this is detrimental to clients' attitudes toward themselves and their future. However, for some, especially the crippled, paralyzed, or bedridden, the nursing home offers a valuable service. There has been a great deal of unfavorable publicity of some substandard homes, which makes many older people frightened at the prospect of having to enter one. But investigation by relatives can identify a home that provides the kind of service the individual needs.

The relative inquiring into nursing homes should ask the director or dietitian some questions about the food service. Is a choice given the

30   J. Pelcovits, Nutrition for older Americans, *Journal of the American Dietetic Association* 58 (1971): 17–21.

31   R. L. Kane and R. A. Kane, Care of the aged: Old problems in need of new solutions, *Science* 200 (1978): 913–919.

resident in the selection of food? How often are the menus repeated (is the cycle monotonous)? How often are fresh fruits and vegetables served? Is the food fresh and tasty when served? Is a plate check conducted regularly, at least once a week, to discover what the resident is consuming? Does the staff keep track of each person's weight? Is there good communication between the nursing staff and the dietitian so that the dietitian will know if someone is not eating? Is the resident encouraged and helped to go to the dining room to eat so that some socializing will occur? What is the environment like in which the residents eat? Does someone help those who can't manage feeding themselves? Are minced meats offered to those who have problems with their dentures? Are religious dietary restrictions honored? How high a proportion of the foods are prepackaged? (No guide can be given for what proportion is desirable, but it should be remembered that processed foods are low in vitamin content and high in salt.) Other questions that the investigator will want to ask have to do with the general atmosphere of the nursing home, in recognition of the effect of social climate on a person's appetite. A nursing home that views residents as persons, not as patients, gets a mark in its favor.

In the nursing home, the dietitian, nutritionist, or nurse responsible for the residents' care should keep in mind the special needs associated with their time in life. The average age of a nursing home resident is 81, and many have problems that can affect nutrition status:

- At least one chronic disease.
- Constipation or incontinence.
- Confusion due to change in environment.
- Poor eyesight or hearing.
- Ill-fitting or missing dentures.
- Inability to feed themselves because of arthritis or stroke.
- Psychological problems, especially depression.
- Anorexia and loss of interest in eating.
- Lack of opportunity to socialize at mealtimes.
- Long-established food preferences.
- Slowed reactions (seeing, holding utensils, chewing, swallowing).[32]

On admission, their nutrition status should be assessed immediately, and the person responsible for their nutrition care should make every effort to rectify any problems promptly. Thereafter they should be reassessed at regular, frequent intervals and adjustments made as needed.

Opinions differ on the philosophy to adopt for nursing home menus. A multitude of different special diets is difficult and expensive to manage, and one authority recommends a "liberalized geriatric diet" for most cases, rather than modified diets. Based on the assumption that older people "should have the right to choose the food they eat," this general, liberal approach provides in one package the key characteristics of several special diets:

32 E. Luros, A rational approach to geriatric nutrition, *Dietetic Currents, Ross Timesaver* 8 (November–December 1981).

● 1,500 to 2,000 kcalories per day, mostly from nutrient-dense foods, with simple desserts not too high in kcalories.
● Minimal salt used in preparation.
● 65 to 70 grams protein per day from 2 cups milk and 4 to 6 ounces meat or alternate.
● At least 6 milligrams iron per day (the RDA for older people is 10 milligrams per day).
● Generous amounts of natural fiber and fluid intake of 64 ounces per day.[33]

Further modifications can be made for people with severe disease conditions.

Preparing for the Later Years

The programs just described can do much to help older people adjust to their changing circumstances, but the very best help we could give our elderly citizens would be a change of attitude. As a nation, we value the future more than the present, putting off enjoying today so that tomorrow we will have money or prestige or time to have fun. The elderly feel this loss of future. The present is their time for leisure and enjoyment, but they have no experience in the use of leisure time.

Our culture also values the doers, those concerned with action and achievement. The Spanish mother may enjoy her child because he is sitting in her lap and laughing in her face; however, the Anglo-American mother is more likely preoccupied with how well her child is preparing for tomorrow. The elderly are aware of the status given those who are doing something and of the disrespect given those who lead a contemplative life in retirement.

It would take a near miracle to change the attitude of a nation, but there is a change in attitude that individual persons can make toward themselves as they age. Preparation for this period should of course include financial planning, but other lifelong habits should be developed as well. Each adult needs to learn to reach out to others, to forestall the loneliness that will otherwise ensue. Each needs to learn some skills or activities that can continue into the later years—volunteer work with organizations, reading, games, hobbies, or intellectual pursuits—which will give meaning to the days. Each needs to develop the habit of adjusting to change, especially when it comes without consent, so that it will not be seen as a loss of control over life. The goal is to arrive at maturity with as healthy a mind and body as it is possible to have, and this means cultivating good nutrition status and maintaining a program of daily exercise.

Preparation for the later years begins early in life, both psychologically and nutritionally. Everyone knows older people who have gathered around themselves many contacts—through relatives, church, synagogue, or fraternal orders—and have not allowed themselves to drift into isolation.

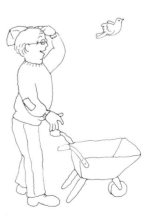

33   Luros, 1981.

Upon analysis, you will see that their favorable environment came through a lifetime of effort. They spent their entire lives reaching out to others and practicing the art of weaving themselves into other people's lives. Likewise, a lifetime of effort is required for good nutrition status in the later years. A person who has eaten a wide variety of foods, has stayed trim, and has remained physically active will be most able to withstand the assaults of change.

Summing Up

In the United States, 11 percent of the population is over 65, amounting to over 30 million people. Many live alone, and only a few are in nursing homes; their lifestyles are diverse, and fewer than half are poor.

Health of the elderly can be improved and prolonged by good nutrition, although aging is a natural process and in some ways cannot be prevented. Life still ends at about 70 for most people; the increase in the number of older people seen in U.S. census reports does not reflect an increase in life expectancy but an increase in the number of people surviving the early years and so living to about 70.

Aging of cells may occur for any of several reasons. They may accumulate debris; they may lose the ability to read the genetic code words that specify their functions; they may make wrong proteins, to which the body reacts by producing antibodies; or they may be programmed to divide a definite number of times before they die. Cellular aging is reflected in such familiar phenomena as wrinkling of the skin, loss of digestive functions, loss of responsiveness to changes such as increased blood glucose, loss of elasticity of blood vessels, and loss of function of the kidneys. The brain and nervous system lose cells, and those that remain slow down in reaction time. To some extent people can slow these changes by maintaining a strong cardiovascular and respiratory system through regular exercise. Adult bone loss (osteoporosis) is least likely in those whose bones were dense at maturity, thanks to good mineral and vitamin nutrition in the early years; some calcium loss does occur in aging, however. Continued ample calcium intakes and physical activity are two important factors retarding bone loss.

Nutrition requirements of the older person are for fewer kcalories, increased protein, reduced fat, sufficient complex carbohydrates, sufficient vitamins and minerals (especially vitamin C, iron, and calcium), adequate water intake, and ample fiber from fruits, vegetables, and whole grains. Caffeine consumption should be somewhat curtailed. Meals should be regular and, as far as possible, prepared from fresh ingredients. The enjoyment of food is enhanced if loneliness—a major problem of older people living alone—can be alleviated. Eating with others often restores the appetite and health that may seem to be failing due to degenerative disease.

Having enough money is basic to coping with the nutrition problems of the later years. Government programs designed to help by providing money, either directly or for food, include Social Security, the Food Stamp program, the Supplemental Security Income program, and Title III C of the Older Americans Act, which includes both congregate meals and Meals on Wheels. Alternatives to institutional care are desirable to preserve the older person's independence; among the possibilities are covenant living, diners' clubs, retirement communities, and foster home care. When a nursing home is chosen, its food service should be examined for characteristics that will facilitate good nutrition and appetite.

Old age need not be a time of despair, isolation, and ill health. Preparation for enjoyable later years should include financial planning, the establishment of lasting social contacts, the learning of skills and activities that can be pursued into later life, the maintenance of a program of regular physical activity, and the cultivation of healthy nutrition status throughout life.

NOTE: Appendix J suggests further reading; see "Older Adults."

APPENDIX A
Books Not Recommended

The following list was compiled from several sources, two of which deserve special mention. The Chicago Nutrition Association has for many years been reviewing books on food and nutrition and providing information about them to the public in its *Nutrition References and Book Reviews* (the fifth edition was published in 1981). The 1981 edition lists a total of 288 books, presenting a one-paragraph review of each one not previously reviewed so that you can see why, in the association's judgment, the book was identified as "recommended" or "not recommended." The association has bestowed its approval on most of the books it has reviewed, listing 187 of them as follows:

Recommended—70.

Recommended for special purposes—82.

Recommended for advanced reading—35.

It has given qualified approval to a few, and its reviews explain why:

Recommended with reservations—27.

It has identified a minority as:

Not recommended—74.

Again, its reviews explain why. They also provide a "how to choose a book" section for evaluating other nutrition references you may come across.

The association's reviews provide valuable assistance to busy professionals who can't afford the time to read and assess all the new books appearing monthly in the field. All books marked here with an asterisk (*) have been on the association's "not recommended" lists; many of the books it recommends are named in Appendix J. *Nutrition References and Book Reviews* is available for $5 a copy (11 copies or more, quantity price); consult Appendix J for the address.

The American Council on Science and Health, since 1979, has been performing a similar service. *ACSH News and Views* is published every two months and carries several thoughtful reviews of new books on health in each

issue. Consumers Union, which publishes *Consumer Reports*, and the Nutrition Foundation, which publishes *Nutrition Reviews*, also serve the public by sifting valid from misleading nutrition information. Books reviewed by these reviewers are identified by numbered footnotes.

We have selected for inclusion in this appendix books that have received negative reviews from at least one of the sources named above. Inclusion here does not, however, necessarily mean that we dislike these books or think they are badly written. We have many of them in our own libraries; some offer good ideas and inspiration; and some are very well written indeed—but they do not provide reliably valid nutrition information. Many of the claims they make are groundless and much of the advice they offer is unfounded and even downright dangerous.

For books we recommend to provide the core of a professional library, turn to Appendix J.

Abrahamson, E. M., and Pezet, A. W. *Body, Mind & Sugar.*[1]

Adams, C. *Eat Well Diet Book.**

Adams, R. *Miracle Medicine Foods.**

Air Force Diet.[2]

Alexander, D. D. *Arthritis and Common Sense.**

Altman, N. *Eating for Life—a Book about Vegetarianism.**

Anchell, M. *How I Lost 36,000 Pounds.**

Arnow, I. *Food Power: A Doctor's Guide to Commonsense Nutrition.**

Ashley, R., and Duggal, H. *Dictionary of Nutrition.**

Atkins, R. *Dr. Atkins' Diet Revolution.**

1   This book was reviewed by Consumers Union and found to contain misleading information as reported in: *Health Quackery* (New York: Consumers Union, 1980).
2   This book was reviewed and found to contain misinformation as reported in: *Nutrition Reviews, Special Supplement on Misinformation and Food Faddism*, July 1974.

A

Atkins, R. *Dr. Atkins' Nutrition Breakthrough.*[3]

Bailey, H. *Your Key to a Healthy Heart.**

Barnes, B., and Barnes, C. *Solved: Riddle of Heart Attacks.**

Bassler, T., and Burger, R. *Whole Life Diet.**

Blaine, T. R. *Goodbye Allergies.*[4]

Blaine, T. R. *Mental Health Through Nutrition.**

Boody, S., and Clausen, M. *High-Energy, Low-Budget, Weight-Loss Diet.**

Breneman, J. *Basics of Food Allergy.**

Cantor, A. J. *Dr. Cantor's Longevity Diet.**

Cantor, A. J. *How to Lose Weight the Doctor's Way.**

Carey, R. L., Vyhmeister, I. B., and Hudson, J. S. *Common-Sense Nutrition.**

Carkin, G. *Today's Manna.**

Clark, L. *Be Slim and Healthy (How to Have a Trimmer Body the Natural Way).**

Clark, L. *Stay Young Longer.**

Cooper, J., and Hagen, P. *Dr. Cooper's Fabulous Fructose Diet.**

Cousins, N. *Anatomy of an Illness: Reflections on Healing and Regeneration.*[5]

Cummings, B. *Stay Young and Vital.**

Davis, A. *Let's Cook It Right.**[6]

Davis, A. *Let's Eat Right to Keep Fit.**

Davis, A. *Let's Get Well.**

Davis, A. *Let's Have Healthy Children.**

Davis, A. *Vitality through Planned Nutrition.**

Davis, A. *You Can Stay Well.**

Dean, M. *Complete Gourmet Nutrition Cookbook.**

DeGroot, R. *How I Reduced with the Rockefeller Diet.**

Dong, C. M., and Banks, J. *Arthritis Cookbook.*[7]

Dufty, W. *Sugar Blues.*

Edelstein, B. *Woman Doctor's Diet for Women.**

Eiteljorg, S. *Sweet Way to Diet.**

Elwood, C. *Feel Like a Million.**

Feingold, B., and Feingold, H. *Feingold Cookbook for Hyperactive Children.**

Ferguson, J., and Taylor, C. *A Change for Heart.**

Fiore, E. L. *Low Carbohydrate Diet.**

Fredericks, C. *Carlton Fredericks Cookbook for Good Nutrition.**[8]

Fredericks, C. *Eat, Live and be Merry.**

Fredericks, C. *Eat Well, Get Well, Stay Well.*[9]

Fredericks, C. *Food Facts and Fallacies.**

Fredericks, C. *Low Blood Sugar and You.**

Fredericks, C. *New and Complete Nutrition Handbook.**

Fredericks, C. *Nutrition: Your Key to Good Health.**

Fredericks, C. *Psycho-Nutrition.**

Fredericks, C., and Bailey, H. *Food Facts and Fallacies.**

Friedman, M., and Rosenman, R. *Type A Behavior and Your Heart.**

Glass, J. *Live to Be 180.**

Harvey, W. *On Corpulence in Relation to Disease.*[10]

Hatfield, A., and Stanton, P. *Right! It's Fun to Eat: How to Help Your Child Eat Cookbook and Guide to Better Nutrition.**

Hauser, G. *Be Happier, Be Healthier.**

Hauser, G. *Look Younger, Live Longer.**

Hauser, G. *Mirror, Mirror on the Wall.**

Hauser, G. *New Diet Does It.**

Hauser, G. *New Guide to Intelligent Reducing.**

Health Quarterly[11]

Hunter, B. *Great Nutrition Robbery.**

Hunter, B. *Natural Food Cookbook.**

Hunter, K. *Health Foods and Herbs.**

Hurd, F. J., and Hurd, R. *Ten Talents.**

Jacobson, M. *Eaters Digest: Consumer's Factbook of Food Additives.**

Jacobson, M., and Center for Science in the Public Interest. *Nutrition Scoreboard: Your Guide to Better Eating.**

Jameson, G., and Williams, E. *Drinking Man's Diet.*[12]

3   F. J. Stare and V. Aronson, Book review, *ACSH News and Views*, November/December 1981, pp. 6–7.
4   *Health Quackery*, 1980.
5   T. Smith, Book review, *ACSH News and Views*, April 1980, p. 7.
6   Can you spot quackery? *Indianapolis News*, 3 March 1982, as reprinted in *ACSH Media Update*, Fall 1982, p. 30.
7   *Health Quackery*, 1980.

8   Can you spot quackery? 1982.
9   M. A. Cassese and F. J. Stare, Book review, *ACSH News and Views*, January/February 1981, pp. 7, 10.
10   *Nutrition Reviews, Special Supplement*, 1974.
11   Can you spot quackery? 1982.
12   *Health Quackery*, 1980.

Jarvis, D. C. *Folk Medicine—a Vermont Doctor's Guide to Good Health.**

Kaplan, R., Saltzman, B., Ecker, L., and Williams, P. *Wholly Alive.**

Kirschnerr, H. E. *Life Food Juices.**

Kloss, J. *Back to Eden.**

Kordel, L. *Cook Right—Live Longer.**

Kordel, L. *Eat and Grow Younger.**

Kordel, L. *Eat Your Troubles Away.**

Kordel, L. *Live to Enjoy the Money you Make.**

Lasky, M. *Complete Junk Food Book.**

Lederman, M. *Slim Gourmet or the Joys of Eating.**

Leinwoll, S. *Low Cholesterol, Lower Calorie French Cooking.**

Leonard, J. N., Hofer J. L., and Pritikin, N. *Live Longer Now.*

Levitt, E. *Wonderful World of Natural-Food Cookery.**

Levy, J., and Bach-y-Rita, P. *Vitamins: Their Use and Abuse.**

Lewis, C. *Nutrition, Nutritional Considerations for the Elderly.**

Linn, R., and Stuart, S. L. *Last Chance Diet.*

Living Better: Recipes for a Healthy Heart.

MacKarness, R. *Eat Fat and Grow Slim.**

Maislen, R., Kadish, T., and Lerner, N. *Eat, Think and Be Thinner the Weigh of Life Way.**

Malone, F. *Bees Don't Get Arthritis.*[13]

Martin, C. G. *How to Live to Be 100.*

Mazel, J. *Beverly Hills Diet.*[14]

Miller, S., and Miller, J. *Food for Thought.**

Mulhauser, R. *More Vitamins and Minerals with Fewer Calories.**

Munro, D. C. *Man Alive—You're Half Dead.**

Murray, F. *Program Your Heart for Health.**

*National Health Federation Bulletin.** [15]

Newbold, H. *Vitamin C against Cancer.**

Newton, M. *New Life Cook Book: Based on the Health and Nutritional Philosophy of the Edgar Cayce Readings.**

Null, G. *Body Pollution.* Now retitled: *How to Get Rid of the Poisons in Your Body.**

Null, G., and Null, S. *Complete Handbook of Nutrition.**

*Nutrition Almanac.**

O'Brian, L. H. *Forget About Calories.**

Oski, F., and Bell, J. *Don't Drink Your Milk!**

Passwater, R. *Easy No-Flab Diet.**

Patrick, L. *How to Eat Well and Live Longer.**

Pauling, L. *Vitamin C and the Common Cold.*

Pearson, D., and Shaw, S. *Life Extension: A Practical Scientific Approach.*[16]

Pelstring, L., and Hauck, J. *Food to Improve Your Health.**

Petrie, S., and Stone, R. *Fat Destroyer Foods: Magic Metabolic Diet.**

Pfeiffer, C. *Zinc and Other Micro-Nutrients.**

Philpott, W., and Kalita, D. K., *Brain Allergies: The Psychonutrient Connection.*[17]

Pim, L. *Invisible Additives.*[18]

*Prevention Magazine.** [19]

Pritikin, N., and McGrady, P. *Pritikin Program for Diet and Exercise.**

Reuben, D. *Everything You Always Wanted to Know About Nutrition.** [20]

Righter, C. *Your Astrological Guide to Health and Diet.**

Rodale, J. I. *Complete Book of Food and Nutrition.**

Rodale, J. I. *Complete Book of Vitamins.**

Rodale, J. I. *Happy People Rarely Get Cancer.*[21]

Rodale, J. I. *How to Grow Vegetables and Fruits by the Organic Method.**

Rodale, J. I. *Live to Eighty, Feel Like Forty.**

Rodale, J. I. *My Own Technique of Eating for Health.**

Rodale, J. I. *Our Poisoned Earth.**

Rodale, J. I. *Prostate.*[22]

Rodale Press.[23]

13   *Health Quackery*, 1980.
14   E. McDowell, Behind the best sellers, *New York Times*, 23 August 1981, as reprinted in *ACSH Media Update*, Fall 1981, p. 26.
15   Can you spot quackery? 1982.
16   J. Hancock, Book review, *Journal of Nutrition Education* 15 (1983): pp. 36–37.
17   B. McPherrin, Book review, *ACSH News and Views*, May/June 1981, pp. 7, 10.
18   D. Roll, Book review, *ACSH News and Views*, May/June 1982, p. 14.
19   Can you spot quackery? 1982.
20   Can you spot quackery? 1982.
21   *Nutrition Reviews, Special Supplement*, 1974.
22   *Nutrition Reviews, Special Supplement*, 1974.
23   Can you spot quackery? 1982.

A

Ronsard, N. *Cellulite—Those Lumps, Bumps and Bulges You Couldn't Lose Before.**

Rose, I. F. *Faith, Love and Seaweed.**

Rosenberger, A. *Eat Your Way to Better Health.**

Rosenvold, L., and Rosenvold, D. *Nutrition for Life.**

Roth, J. *Cooking for the Hyperactive Child.**

Roth, J. *Food/Depression Connection.**

Roty, J., and Philips, N. N. *Bio-Organics: Your Food and Your Health.**

Schiff, M. *Doctor Schiff's Miracle Weight Loss Guide.**

Schneour, E. *Malnourished Mind.**

Shefferman, M. *Food for Longer Living.**

Sheinkin, D., Schachter, M., and Hutton, R. *Food Connection.**

Simmons, R. *Never Say Diet Book.*

Smith, L. *Feed Your Kids Right.*[24]

Solomon, N. *Truth about Weight Control.**

Stillman, I. M., and Baker, S. S. *Doctor's Quick Inches-Off Diet.**

Stillman, I. M., and Baker, S. S. *Doctor's Quick Teenage Diet.**

Stillman, I. M., and Baker, S. S. *Doctor's Quick Weight Loss Diet.**

Stone, I. *Healing Factor, "Vitamin C" against Disease.**

Taller, H. *Calories Don't Count.**

Tarnower, H., and Baker, S. *Complete Scarsdale Medical Diet.**

Tobe, J. H. *"No-Cook" Book.**

Toms, A. *Eat Drink and Be Healthy—the Joy of Eating Natural Foods.**

Top, J. D. *You Don't Have to Be Sick.**

Turchetti, R., and Morella, J. *New Age Nutrition.**

Verrett, J., and Carper, J. *Eating May Be Hazardous to Your Health: The Case against Food Additives.**

Vitamin E for Ailing and Healthy Hearts.[25]

Vitamin E: Key to Sexual Satisfaction.[26]

Vitamin E: Your Key to a Healthy Heart.[27]

Wade, C. *Arthritis, Nutrition and Natural Therapy.*[28]

Walczak, M. *Nutrition—Applied Personally.**

Watson, G. *Nutrition and Your Mind.**

West, R. *Stop Dieting! Start Losing!**

West, R. *Teen-age Diet Book.**

Williams, R. *Nutrition against Disease.**

Williams, R. *Nutrition in a Nutshell.**

Williams, R. *Wonderful World within You: Your Inner Nutritional Environment.**

Wilson, M. *Double Your Energy and Live without Fatigue.**

Winter, R. *A Consumer's Dictionary of Food Additives.**

Wood, H. C. *Overfed but Under-Nourished—Nutritional Aspects of Health and Disease.**

Yntema, S. *Vegetarian Baby.*

Yudkin, J. *Sweet and Dangerous.**

24   Can you spot quackery? 1982; M. Kroger, Book review, *ACSH News and Views*, February 1980, p. 6.

25   *Health Quackery*, 1980.
26   *Health Quackery*, 1980.
27   *Health Quackery*, 1980.
28   *Health Quackery*, 1980.

APPENDIX B
Basic Chemistry Concepts

CONTENTS

This appendix is intended to provide the background in basic chemistry that you need to understand the nutrition concepts presented in this book.

Chemistry is the branch of natural science that is concerned with the description and classification of matter, with the changes that matter undergoes, and with the energy associated with these changes. **Matter** is anything that takes up space and has mass. **Energy** is the ability to do work.

Matter: The Properties of Atoms

Every substance has characteristics or properties that distinguish it from all other substances and thus give it a unique identity. These properties are both physical and chemical. The physical properties include such characteristics as color, taste, texture, and odor, as well as the temperatures at which a substance changes its state (changes from a solid to a liquid or from a liquid to a gas) and the weight of a unit volume (its density). The chemical properties of a substance have to do with how it reacts with other substances or responds to a change in its environment so that new substances with different sets of properties are produced.

A physical change is one that does not change a substance's chemical composition. For example, when ice changes to liquid water and to steam, two hydrogen atoms and one oxygen atom remain bound together in all three states. However, a chemical change does occur if an electric current is passed through water. The water disappears, and two different substances are formed: hydrogen gas, which is flammable, and oxygen gas, which supports life. Chemical changes are also referred to as **chemical reactions**.

Substances: Elements and Compounds

Molecules are the smallest particles of a substance that retain all the properties of that substance. If the molecules of a substance are composed of atoms that are all alike, the substance is an **element**. If the molecules are composed of two or more different kinds of atoms, the substance is a **compound**.

Just over 100 elements are known, and these are listed in Table B–1. A familiar example is hydrogen, whose molecules are composed only of hydrogen atoms linked together in pairs (H_2). On the other hand, over a million compounds are known. An example is the sugar glucose. Each of its molecules is composed of 6 carbon, 6 oxygen, and 12 hydrogen atoms linked together in a specific arrangement (as described in Chapter 2).

The Nature of Atoms

Atoms themselves are made of smaller particles. The atomic nucleus contains **protons** (positively charged particles); and **electrons** (negatively charged particles) surround the nucleus. Because opposite charges attract, the number of protons ($+$) in the nucleus of an atom determines the number of electrons ($-$) around it. The positive charge on a proton is equal to the negative charge on an electron, so

TABLE B-1   **Chemical Symbols for the Elements**

NUMBER OF PROTONS (ATOMIC NUMBER)	ELEMENT	NUMBER OF ELECTRONS IN OUTER SHELL	NUMBER OF PROTONS (ATOMIC NUMBER)	ELEMENT	NUMBER OF ELECTRONS IN OUTER SHELL
1	Hydrogen (H)	1	52	Tellurium (Te)	6
2	Helium (He)	2	53	Iodine (I)	7
3	Lithium (Li)	1	54	Xenon (Xe)	8
4	Beryllium (Be)	2	55	Cesium (Cs)	1
5	Boron (B)	3	56	Barium (Ba)	2
6	Carbon (C)	4	57	Lanthanum (La)	2
7	Nitrogen (N)	5	58	Cerium (Ce)	2
8	Oxygen (O)	6	59	Praseodymium (Pr)	2
9	Fluorine (F)	7	60	Neodymium (Nd)	2
10	Neon (Ne)	8	61	Promethium (Pm)	2
11	Sodium (Na)	1	62	Samarium (Sm)	2
12	Magnesium (Mg)	2	63	Europium (Eu)	2
13	Aluminum (Al)	3	64	Gadolinium (Gd)	2
14	Silicon (Si)	4	65	Terbium (Tb)	2
15	Phosphorus (P)	5	66	Dysprosium (Dy)	2
16	Sulfur (S)	6	67	Holmium (Ho)	2
17	Chlorine (Cl)	7	68	Erbium (Er)	2
18	Argon (Ar)	8	69	Thulium (Tm)	2
19	Potassium (K)	1	70	Ytterbium (Yb)	2
20	Calcium (Ca)	2	71	Lutetium (Lu)	2
21	Scandium (Sc)	2	72	Hafnium (Hf)	2
22	Titanium (Ti)	2	73	Tantalum (Ta)	2
23	Vanadium (V)	2	74	Tungsten (W)	2
24	Chromium (Cr)	1	75	Rhenium (Re)	2
25	Manganese (Mn)	2	76	Osmium (Os)	2
26	Iron (Fe)	2	77	Iridium (Ir)	2
27	Cobalt (Co)	2	78	Platinum (Pt)	1
28	Nickel (Ni)	2	79	Gold (Au)	1
29	Copper (Cu)	1	80	Mercury (Hg)	2
30	Zinc (Zn)	2	81	Thallium (Tl)	3
31	Gallium (Ga)	3	82	Lead (Pb)	4
32	Germanium (Ge)	4	83	Bismuth (Bi)	5
33	Arsenic (As)	5	84	Polonium (Po)	6
34	Selenium (Se)	6	85	Astatine (At)	7
35	Bromine (Br)	7	86	Radon (Rn)	8
36	Krypton (Kr)	8	87	Francium (Fr)	1
37	Rubidium (Rb)	1	88	Radium (Ra)	2
38	Strontium (Sr)	2	89	Actinium (Ac)	2
39	Yttrium (Y)	2	90	Thorium (Th)	2
40	Zirconium (Zr)	2	91	Protactinium (Pa)	2
41	Niobium (Nb)	1	92	Uranium (U)	2
42	Molybdenum (Mo)	1	93	Neptunium (Np)	2
43	Technetium (Tc)	1	94	Plutonium (Pu)	2
44	Ruthenium (Ru)	1	95	Americium (Am)	2
45	Rhodium (Rh)	1	96	Curium (Cm)	2
46	Palladium (Pd)	—	97	Berkelium (Bk)	2
47	Silver (Ag)	1	98	Californium (Cf)	2
48	Cadmium (Cd)	2	99	Einsteinium (Es)	2
49	Indium (In)	3	100	Fermium (Fm)	2
50	Tin (Sn)	4	101	Mendelevium (Md)	2
51	Antimony (Sb)	5	102	Nobelium (No)	2

that the charges cancel each other out and leave the atom neutral.

The nucleus may also include **neutrons**, subatomic particles that have no charge. Protons and neutrons are of equal mass, and together they give an atom its weight. Electrons are of negligible mass but represent the atom's chemical energy.

Each type of atom has a characteristic number of protons in its nucleus. The hydrogen atom (symbol H) is the simplest of all. It possesses a single proton, with a single electron associated with it:

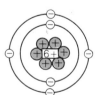

electron

proton

Hydrogen atom (H), atomic number 1.

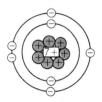

Nitrogen atom (N), atomic number 7.

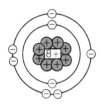

Oxygen atom (O), atomic number 8.

In these and all diagrams of atoms that follow, only the protons and electrons are shown. The neutrons, which contribute only to atomic weight, not to charge, are omitted.

Just as hydrogen always has one proton, helium always has two, lithium three, and so on. The **atomic number** of each type of atom represents the number of protons it contains. The atomic number never changes; it gives the atom its identity. The atomic numbers for the known elements are listed in Table B–1.

All atoms except hydrogen also have neutrons in their nuclei, and these contribute to their atomic weight. Helium, for example, has two neutrons in its nucleus in addition to its two protons, for a total of four nuclear particles and an atomic weight of 4. However, only the two protons are charged, and these determine the number of electrons the atom has. The number of electrons determines how the atom will chemically react with other atoms. Hence the atomic number, not the weight, is what gives an atom its chemical nature.

Besides hydrogen, the atoms most common in living things are carbon (C), nitrogen (N), and oxygen (O), whose atomic numbers are 6, 7, and 8 respectively. Their structures are more complicated than that of hydrogen. Each possesses a number of electrons equal to the number of protons in its nucleus. These electrons have two energy levels, symbolized in the following diagrams as two orbits, or shells:

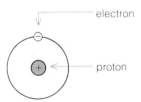

Carbon atom (C), atomic number 6.

The shells closest to the nucleus are occupied by electrons of lesser energy. Thus the two electrons in the first shells of carbon, nitrogen, and oxygen have less energy than the electrons in their second, or outer, shells. Also, the first shell can hold only two electrons; when it is full, it is in a very stable energy state, or a state of lowest energy.

The most important structural feature of an atom for determining its chemical behavior is the number of electrons in its outer shell. The first shell is full when it is occupied by two electrons; so an atom with three protons has a filled first shell. Its third electron possesses greater energy and has a greater probability of being farther from the nucleus. In other words, the third electron is not so tightly bound as the first two and has a high probability of flying off to join other substances in chemical reactions. As a matter of fact, lithium, atomic number 3, is just such a highly reactive element.

The second shell is completely full when it has eight electrons. A substance that has a full outer shell tends to enter into no chemical reactions. Atomic number 10, neon, is a chemically inert substance, because its outer shell is complete. Fluorine, atomic number 9, has a great tendency to draw an electron from other substances to complete its outer shell and thus is highly reactive. Carbon has a half-full outer shell, which helps explain its great versatility; it can combine with other elements in a great variety of ways to form a large number of compounds.

Atoms seek to reach a state of maximum stability or of lowest energy in the same way that a ball will roll down a hill until it reaches the lowest place. An atom achieves a state of maximum stability by two means:

B

● By having a filled outer shell (occupied by the maximum number of electrons it can hold).
● By being electrically neutral.

In order to achieve this stability, an atom may become bonded to other atoms.

Chemical Bonding

Atoms often complete their outer shells by sharing electrons with other atoms. In order to complete its outer shell, a carbon atom requires four electrons. A hydrogen atom requires one. Thus when a carbon atom shares electrons with four hydrogen atoms, each completes its outer shell:

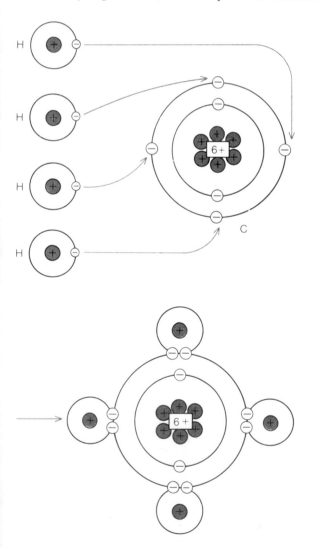

Methane molecule. The **chemical formula** for methane is CH_4. (Note that with the sharing of electrons, every atom has a filled outer shell.)

This electron sharing binds the atoms together and satisfies the conditions of maximum stability for the molecule. The outer shell of each atom is complete, since hydrogen effectively has the required two electrons in its first and outer shell and carbon has eight electrons in its second and outer shell; and the molecule is electrically neutral, with a total of ten protons and ten electrons.

Bonds that involve the sharing of electrons, like the bond between carbon and hydrogen, are the most stable kind of association that atoms can form with one another. They are sometimes called **covalent bonds**, and the resulting combinations of atoms are called molecules. A single pair of shared electrons forms a **single bond**. A simplified way to represent a single bond is with a single line. Thus the structure of methane could be represented like this (ignoring the inner-shell electrons, which do not participate in bonding):

```
      H
      |
  H — C — H
      |
      H            Methane (chemical structure).
```

Similarly, one nitrogen atom and three hydrogen atoms can share electrons to form one molecule of ammonia:

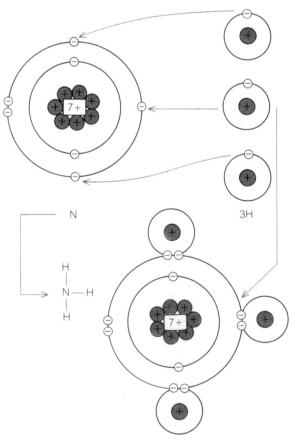

Ammonia molecule (NH_3). Count the electrons in each atom's outer shell.

One oxygen atom may be bonded to two hydrogen atoms to form one molecule of water:

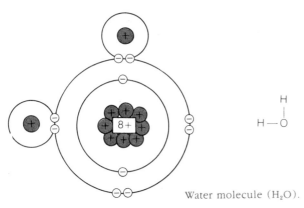

Water molecule (H_2O).

When two oxygen atoms form a molecule of oxygen, they must share two pairs of electrons. This **double bond** may be represented as two single lines:

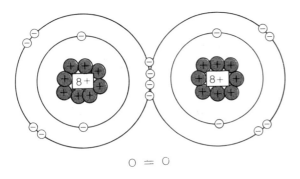

$$O = O$$

Oxygen molecule (O_2).

Small atoms form the tightest, most stable bonds. H, O, N, and C are the smallest atoms capable of forming one, two, three, and four electron-pair bonds (respectively). This fact is the basis for the simple statement in Chapter 2 that when you draw compounds containing these atoms, hydrogen must always have one, oxygen two, nitrogen three, and carbon four lines radiating to other atoms.

$$H- \quad -O- \quad \overset{|}{\underset{|}{N}}- \quad -\overset{|}{\underset{|}{C}}-$$

The stability of the associations between these small atoms and the versatility with which they can combine make them very common in living things. Interestingly, all cells, whether they come from animals, plants, or bacteria, contain the same elements in very nearly the same proportions.[1] The atomic elements found in living things are shown in Table B-2.

1   V. Rodwell, Appendix: Organic chemistry (a brief review), in *Review of Physiological Chemistry*, ed. H. Harper (Los Altos, Calif.: Lange Medical Publications, 1971), p. 499.

TABLE B-2   **Elemental Composition of Living Cells**

ELEMENT	CHEMICAL SYMBOL	COMPOSITION BY WEIGHT (%)
Oxygen	O	65
Carbon	C	18
Hydrogen	H	10
Nitrogen	N	3
Calcium	Ca	1.5
Phosphorus	P	1.0
Sulfur	S	0.25
Sodium	Na	0.15
Magnesium	Mg	0.05
TOTAL		99.30[a]

[a] The remaining 0.70% by weight is contributed by the trace elements: copper (Cu), zinc (Zn), selenium (Se), molybdenum (Mo), fluorine (F), chlorine (Cl), iodine (I), manganese (Mn), cobalt (Co), iron (Fe). There are also variable traces of some of the following in cells: lithium (Li), strontium (Sr), aluminum (Al), silicon (Si), lead (Pb), vanadium (V), arsenic (As), bromium (Br), and others.

Formation of Ions

An atom such as sodium (Na, atomic number 11) is more likely to lose an electron than to share electrons. Sodium possesses a filled inner shell of two electrons and a filled second shell of eight; there is only one electron in its outermost shell:

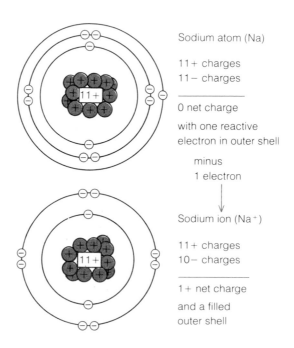

Sodium atom (Na)

11+ charges
11− charges
_____
0 net charge

with one reactive electron in outer shell

minus
1 electron
↓

Sodium ion (Na$^+$)

11+ charges
10− charges
_____
1+ net charge

and a filled outer shell

If sodium loses this electron, it satisfies one condition for stability: a filled outer shell (now its second shell counts as the outer shell). However, it is not electrically neutral. It has 11 protons (positive) and only 10 electrons (negative). It therefore is positively charged. Such a structure is called an **ion**—an atom or molecule that has lost or gained one or more electrons and so is electrically charged.

An atom such as chlorine (Cl, atomic number 17) is likely to gain an electron for a similar reason. It possesses filled inner shells of two and eight electrons and has seven electrons in its outermost shell. Gaining one electron makes its outer shell complete and thus makes it a negatively charged ion:

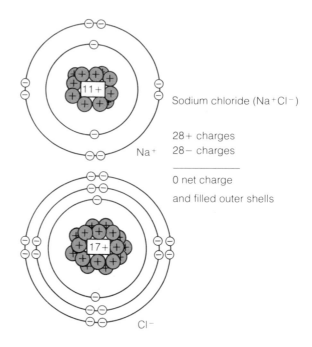

Sodium chloride (Na$^+$Cl$^-$)

28+ charges
28− charges
_____
0 net charge
and filled outer shells

Na$^+$

Cl$^-$

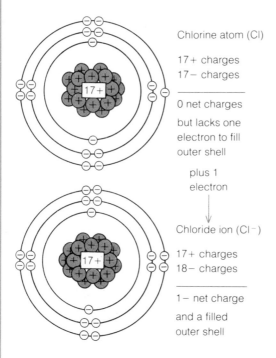

Chlorine atom (Cl)

17+ charges
17− charges
_____
0 net charges

but lacks one electron to fill outer shell

plus 1 electron

↓

Chloride ion (Cl$^-$)

17+ charges
18− charges
_____
1− net charge

and a filled outer shell

With all its electrons, sodium is a shiny, highly reactive metal; chlorine is the poisonous greenish-yellow gas that was used in World War I. But after they have transferred electrons, they form the harmless white salt familiar to you as table salt, or sodium chloride (Na$^+$Cl$^-$). The dramatic difference illustrates how profoundly the electron arrangement can influence the nature of a substance. The wide distribution of salt in nature attests to the stability of the union between the ions. Each meets the other's needs (a good marriage).

When dry, salt exists as crystals; its ions are stacked very regularly into a lattice, with positive and negative ions alternating in a sort of three-dimensional checkerboard structure. In water, however, the salt quickly dissolves, and its ions separate from each other, forming an electrolyte solution in which they move about freely. Covalently bonded molecules do not dissociate like this in water solution. Molecules and ion pairs (salts) behave very differently in many ways.

An ion can also be a group of atoms bound together in such a way that the group has a charge and enters into reactions as a single unit. Many such groups are active in the fluids of the body. The bicarbonate ion is composed of five atoms—one H, one C, and three Os—and has a net charge of −1 (HCO_3^-). Another important ion of this type is a phosphate ion with one H, one P, and four Os, and a net charge of −2 (HPO_4^{-2}).

A positively charged ion such as a sodium ion (Na$^+$) is a **cation**; a negatively charged ion such as a chloride ion (Cl$^-$) is an **anion**. Cations and anions attract one another to form **salts**:

Whereas many elements have only one configuration in the outer shell and thus only one way to bond with other elements, some elements have the possibility of varied configurations. Iron is such an element. Under some conditions iron loses two electrons, and under other circumstances it loses three. If iron loses two electrons, it then has a net charge of +2, and we call it ferrous iron. If it donates three electrons to another atom, it becomes the +3 ion, or ferric iron.

(Note: It is important to remember that a positive charge on an ion means that negative charges—electrons—have been lost and not that positive charges have been added. If you could add two protons to an iron atom, they would go to the nucleus, adding 2 to its atomic number. Then it would no longer be iron, atomic number 26, but nickel, atomic number 28—and it would gain two more electrons to balance its positive charges.)

$$Fe^{++} \qquad\qquad Fe^{+++}$$

Ferrous iron (Fe^{++})
(had 2 outer-shell
electrons but has
lost them)

26+ charges
24– charges
_____

2+ net charge

Ferric iron (Fe^{+++})
(had 3 outer-shell
electrons but has
lost them)

26+ charges
23– charges
_____

3+ net charge

Water, Acids, and Bases

The water molecule is electrically neutral, having equal numbers of protons and electrons. However, if the hydrogen atom is to share its one electron with oxygen, that electron must spend most of its time near the large positively charged oxygen nucleus on the oxygen side of the hydrogen atom. This leaves the positive proton (nucleus of the hydrogen atom) exposed on the outer part of the water molecule. We know, too, that the two hydrogens both bond toward the same side of the oxygen. These two ideas explain the fact that water molecules are **polar**: they have regions of more positive and more negative charge.

Polar molecules like water are drawn to one another by the attractive forces between the positive polar areas of one and the negative poles of another. These attractive forces, sometimes known as polar or **hydrogen bonds**, occur among many molecules and also within the different parts of single large molecules. Although very weak in comparison with covalent bonds, polar bonds may occur in such abundance

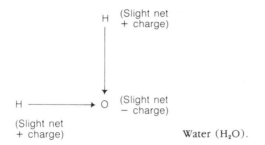

Water (H_2O).

The arrows on the diagram of the polar molecule show displacement of electrons toward the O nucleus; so the negative region is near the O, the positive region near the Hs.

that they become exceedingly important in determining the structure of such large molecules as proteins and DNA.

Water molecules have a slight tendency to ionize, separating into positive and negative ions. In any given amount of pure water, a small but constant number of these ions is present, and the number of positive ions exactly equals the number of negative ions.

An **acid** is a substance that releases H^+ ions (protons) in water solution. Hydrochloric acid (HCl) is such a substance, because it dissociates in water solution into H^+ and Cl^- ions. Acetic acid is also an acid, because it ionizes in water to acetate ions and free H^+:

$$H-\overset{\overset{\displaystyle H}{|}}{\underset{\underset{\displaystyle H}{|}}{C}}-\overset{\overset{\displaystyle O}{\|}}{C}-O-H \longrightarrow H-\overset{\overset{\displaystyle H}{|}}{\underset{\underset{\displaystyle H}{|}}{C}}-\overset{\overset{\displaystyle O}{\|}}{C}-O^- \quad + \quad H^+$$

Acetic acid dissociates into an acetate ion and a hydrogen ion.

The more H^+ ions free in a water solution, the stronger the acid.

Chemists define degrees of acidity by means of the **pH scale**. The pH scale runs from 0 to 14. A pH of 1 is extremely acidic, 7 is neutral, and 13 is very basic. There is a tenfold difference between points on this scale. A solution with pH 3, for example, has *ten times* as many H^+ ions as a solution with pH 4. At pH 7, the concentrations of free H^+ and OH^- are exactly the same—1/10,000,000 moles per liter (10^{-7} moles per liter).[2] At pH 4, the concentration of free H^+ ions is 1/10,000 (10^{-4}) moles per liter. This is a higher concentration of H^+ ions, and the solution is therefore acidic.

A **base** is a substance that can soak up or combine with H^+ ions, thus reducing the acidity of a solution. The com-

2   A mole is a certain number (about 6×10^{23}) of molecules. The pH of a solution is defined as the negative logarithm of the hydrogen ion concentration of the solution. Thus if the concentration is 10^{-2} (moles per liter), the pH is 2; if 10^{-8}, the pH is 8; and so on.

B

pound ammonia is such a substance. The ammonia molecule has two electrons that are not shared with any other atom; a hydrogen ion (H^+) is just a naked proton with no shell of electrons at all. Thus the proton readily combines with the ammonia molecule to form an ammonium ion and so is withdrawn from the solution as a free proton and no longer contributes to its acidity. Many compounds containing nitrogen are important bases in living systems. Acids and bases neutralize each other to produce substances that are neither acid nor base.

$$\begin{array}{ccc}
\quad H & & \quad H \\
\quad | & & \quad | \\
\mathbf{:} N - H & + \quad H^+ \longrightarrow \quad H - N^+ - H \\
\quad | & & \quad | \\
\quad H & & \quad H
\end{array}$$

Ammonia captures a hydrogen ion from water.

The two dots here represent the two electrons not shared with another atom. These are ordinarily not shown in chemical structure drawings. Compare this with the earlier diagram of an ammonia molecule.

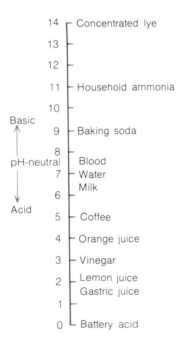

The pH scale.

Note: Each step is ten times as concentrated in base (1/10 as much acid, than H^+) as the one below it.

Chemical Reactions

A chemical reaction, or chemical change, results in the disappearance of substances and the formation of new ones. Almost all such reactions involve a change in the bonding of atoms. Old bonds are broken, and new ones are formed. The nuclei of atoms are never involved in chemical reactions—only their outer-shell electrons. At the end of a reaction there is always the same number of atoms of each type as there was at the beginning. For example, two hydrogen molecules can react with one oxygen molecule to form two water molecules. In this reaction two substances (hydrogen and oxygen) disappear, and a new one (water) is formed, but at the end of the reaction there are still four H atoms and two O atoms, just as there were at the beginning. The only difference is in how they are linked.

Hydrogen and oxygen react to form water:

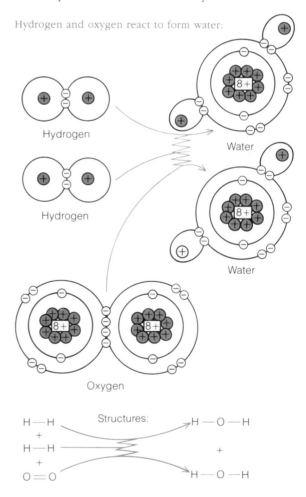

Formulas: $2\,H_2 \ + \ O_2 \longrightarrow 2\,H_2O$

In many instances chemical reactions involve not the relinking of molecules but the exchanging of electrons or protons among them. In such reactions, the molecule that gains one or more electrons (or loses one or more protons) is said to be reduced; the molecule that loses electrons (or gains protons) is oxidized. Oxidation and reduction take place simultaneously, because an electron or proton that is lost by one molecule is accepted by another. The addition of an atom of oxygen is also oxidation, because oxygen (with six electrons) accepts two electrons in becoming bonded. **Oxidation**, then, is loss of electrons, gain of protons, or addition of oxygen (with six electrons); **reduction** is the opposite—gain of electrons, loss of protons, or loss of oxygen. The addition of hydrogen atoms to oxygen to form water can thus be described as the reduction of oxygen—or the oxidation of hydrogen.

If a reaction results in a net increase in the energy of a compound, it is called an **endergonic**, or "uphill," reaction (energy, *erg*, is added into, *endo*, the compound). An example is the chief result of photosynthesis, the making of sugar in a plant from carbon dioxide and water using the energy of sunlight. Conversely, the oxidation of sugar to carbon dioxide and water is an **exergonic**, or "downhill," reaction, because the end products have less energy than the starting products. Oftentimes, but not always, reduction reactions are endergonic, resulting in an increase in the energy of the products. Oxidation reactions often, but not always, are exergonic.

Chemical reactions tend to occur spontaneously if the end products are in a lower energy state (are more stable) than the reacting compounds were. These reactions often give off energy in the form of heat as they occur. The generation of heat by wood burning in a fireplace and the maintenance of human body warmth both depend on energy-yielding chemical reactions. These downhill reactions occur easily, although they may require some activation energy to get them started, just as a ball requires a push to get started rolling downhill.

Uphill reactions, in which the products contain more energy than the reacting compounds started with, do not occur until an energy source is provided. An example of such an energy source is the sunlight used in photosynthesis, where carbon dioxide and water (low-energy compounds) are combined to form the sugar glucose (a higher-energy compound). Another example is the use of the energy in glucose to combine two low-energy compounds in the body into the high-energy compound ATP. The energy in ATP may be used to power many other energy-requiring, uphill reactions. Clearly, any of many different molecules can be used as a temporary storage place for energy.

Neither downhill nor uphill reactions occur until some-

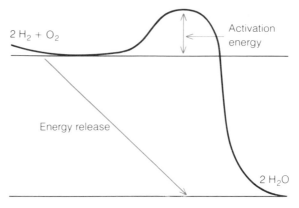

Start of reaction → End of reaction

Reactants → Products

$2 H_2 + O_2 → 2 H_2O$

Energy Change as Reaction Occurs

thing sets them off (activation) or until a path is provided for them to follow. The body uses enzymes as a means of providing paths and controlling chemical reactions (see Chapter 4). By controlling the availability and the action of its enzymes, the body can "decide" which chemical reactions to prevent and which to promote.

Formation of Free Radicals

Normally, when a chemical reaction takes place, bonds break and reform with some redistribution of atoms and rearrangement of bonds to form new, stable compounds. Normally, bonds don't split in such a way as to leave a molecule with an odd, unpaired electron. However, weak bonds can split this way, and when they do, **free radicals** are formed. Free radicals are highly unstable and quickly react with other compounds, forming more free radicals in a chain reaction.

A physical event such as the arrival of an energy-carrying particle of light or other radiation starts the process by breaking a weak bond so that free radicals are formed. A cascade may ensue in which many highly reactive radicals are generated, resulting finally in the disruption of a living structure such as a cell membrane.

```
H — O — O — H                              H — O•    +    •O — H
      or              Heat or light              or
R — O — O — H        ――――――――――→         R — O•    +    •O — H
```

Hydrogen peroxide   Two free radicals
or any hydroperoxide
(R is any carbon
chain with appropriate
numbers of Hs.)

Free radicals are formed. The dots represent single electrons that are available for sharing (the atom also needs another electron to fill its outer shell).

```
                 H                                    H
                 |                                    |
H — O•   +    H — C — H    ――――――→    H — O — H   +   H — C•
                 |                                    |
                 H                                    H

                or                                   or

              R — H                                  R•
```

Free radical   Compound with   New stable   Free radical
                  weak bond (perhaps   compound
                  an unsaturated   (water or
                  fatty acid)   an alcohol)

The free radical attacks a weak bond in a biological compound, disrupting it and forming a new stable molecule and another free radical. This can attack another biological compound, and so on.

Destruction of biological compounds by free radicals.

Oxidation of some compounds can be induced by air at room temperature in the presence of light. Such reactions are thought to take place through the formation of compounds called peroxides:

```
H — O — O — H    Hydrogen peroxide

R — O — O — H    Hydroperoxides (R is any
                 carbon chain with
                 appropriate numbers
                 of Hs.)

R — O — O — R    Peroxide                  Peroxides.
```

Some peroxides readily disintegrate into free radicals, initiating chain reactions like those just described.

Free radicals are of special interest in nutrition because the antioxidant properties of vitamin E are thought to protect against their destructive effects. Vitamin E on the surface of the lungs reacts with (and is destroyed by) free radicals, thus preventing them from reaching underlying cells and oxidizing the lipids in their membranes.

APPENDIX C
Biochemical Structures

CONTENTS

The diagrams of nutrients presented here are meant to enhance your understanding of the most important organic molecules in the human diet. The names used are those agreed on by the American Institute of Nutrition and other scientific organizations in 1976.[1] Following the diagrams of nutrients are sections on the major metabolic pathways mentioned in Chapter 6—glycolysis, the TCA cycle, and the electron transport chain.

Carbohydrates

Monosaccharides

Glucose (alpha form). The ring would be at right angles to the plane of the paper. The bonds directed upward are above the plane; those directed downward are below the plane. This molecule is considered an alpha form because the OH carbon 1 points downward.

Glucose (beta form). The OH points upward.

Fructose, galactose: see Chapter 2.

1   Nomenclature policy: Generic descriptors and trivial names for vitamins and related compounds, *Journal of Nutrition* 112 (1982): 7–14; Nomenclature policy: Abbreviated designations of amino acids, in the same journal, p. 15.

Disaccharides

Maltose.

Lactose (alpha form). The zigzag link between galactose and glucose permits us to show both sugars "right side up." A truer representation of the molecules would show one of them upside down so that the link between them would be similar to that in maltose.

Sucrose.

Polysaccharides

As described in Chapter 2, starch, glycogen, and cellulose are all long chains of glucose molecules covalently linked together.

Amylose

Amylopectin

Starch. Two kinds of covalent linkages occur between glucose molecules in starch, giving rise to two kinds of chains. Amylose is composed of straight chains, with carbon 1 of one glucose linked to carbon 4 of the next. Amylopectin is made up of straight chains like amylose but has occasional branches arising where the carbon 6 of a glucose is also linked to the carbon 1 of another glucose. (See the rules for simplified chemical structures on p. 54.)

Glycogen: like amylopectin but with longer chains and many more branches.

Cellulose. Some of the linkages in cellulose are beta linkages like those in lactose. Another way to depict this molecule would be to draw the second glucose unit upside down.

Lipids

Saturated Fatty Acids Found in Natural Fats

SATURATED FATTY ACID	CHEMICAL FORMULA	SOURCE
Butyric	C_3H_7COOH	Butter fat
Caproic	$C_5H_{11}COOH$	Butter fat
Caprylic	$C_7H_{15}COOH$	Coconut oil
Capric	$C_9H_{19}COOH$	Palm oil
Lauric	$C_{11}H_{23}COOH$	Coconut oil
Myristic[a]	$C_{13}H_{27}COOH$	Nutmeg oil, animal fat (butter)
Palmitic[a]	$C_{15}H_{31}COOH$	Animal and vegetable fat
Stearic[a]	$C_{17}H_{35}COOH$	Animal and vegetable fat
Arachidic	$C_{19}H_{39}COOH$	Peanut oil

[a] Most common saturated fatty acids.

Palmitic acid.

Stearic acid.

Unsaturated Fatty Acids Found in Natural Fats

UNSATURATED FATTY ACID	CHEMICAL FORMULA	POSITION OF DOUBLE BONDS	SOURCE
Palmitoleic	$C_{15}H_{29}COOH$	C9-C10	Butter fat
Oleic	$C_{17}H_{33}COOH$	C9-C10	Olive oil
Linoleic	$C_{17}H_{31}COOH$	C9-C10 C12-C13	Linseed oil
Linolenic	$C_{17}H_{29}COOH$	C9-C10 C12-C13 C15-C16	Linseed oil
Arachidonic	$C_{19}H_{31}COOH$	C5-C6 C8-C9 C11-C12 C14-C15	Lecithin

Palmitoleic acid.

Oleic acid.

Linoleic acid.

Linolenic acid.

Arachidonic acid.

Proteins: Amino Acids[2]

The common amino acids may be classified into the seven groups listed below. Amino acids marked with an asterisk (*) are essential, because human beings cannot synthesize them.

1 With aliphatic side chains, which consist of hydrogen and carbon atoms (hydrocarbons).

$$CH_3-\overset{\overset{\displaystyle H}{|}}{C}-\overset{\overset{\displaystyle O}{\|}}{C}-OH$$
$$\underset{NH_2}{|}$$

Alanine (Ala).

Valine* (Val).

Leucine* (Leu).

Glycine (Gly).

Isoleucine* (Ile).

2   A discussion of the designated abbreviations for the common amino acids presented here is found in: Nomenclature policy: Abbreviated designations of amino acids, 1982.

C

2 With hydroxylic (OH) side chains.

HO—CH₂—C(H)—C(O)—OH, NH₂
Serine (Ser).

CH₃—CH—C(H)—C(O)—OH, OH NH₂
Threonine* (Thr).

3 With side chains containing acidic groups or their amides, which contain the group NH₂.

HO—C(O)—CH₂—C(H)—C(O)—OH, NH₂
Aspartic acid (Asp).

HO—C(O)—CH₂—CH₂—C(H)—C(O)—OH, NH₂
Glutamic acid (Glu).

NH₂—C(O)—CH₂—C(H)—C(O)—OH, NH₂
Asparagine (Asn).

NH₂—C(O)—CH₂—CH₂—C(H)—C(O)—OH, NH₂
Glutamine (Gln).

4 With basic side chains.

NH₂—CH₂—CH₂—CH₂—CH₂—C(H)—C(O)—OH, NH₂
Lysine* (Lys).

NH₂—C(NH)—NH—CH₂—CH₂—C(H)—C(O)—OH, NH₂
Arginine (Arg).

4 With basic side chains.

H—C=C—CH₂—C(H)—C(O)—OH, N—C—N—H, C—H, NH₂
Histidine (His).

NH₂—CH₂—CH₂—CH₂—C(H)—C(O)—OH, NH₂
Ornithine (Orn).

5 With aromatic side chains, which are characterized by the presence of at least one cyclical (ring) structure.

—CH₂—C(H)—C(O)—OH, NH₂
Phenylalanine* (Phe).

HO—...—CH₂—C(H)—C(O)—OH, NH₂
Tyrosine (Tyr).

—CH₂—C(H)—C(O)—OH, NH₂
Tryptophan* (Trp).

6 With side chains containing sulfur atoms.

HS—CH₂—C(H)—C(O)—OH, NH₂
Cysteine (Cys).

7 Amino acids.

Cystine (Cys·Cys).

Methionine* (Met).

Proline (Pro).[3]

3   Proline has the same H₂N·C·COOH structure as the other amino acids, but its amino group has given up a hydrogen to form a ring, as shown.

Vitamins and Coenzymes

Vitamin A: retinol.

Vitamin A: retinal.

C

Vitamin A: beta-carotene.

Thiamin hydrochloride. Chloride ions (Cl⁻) are shown nearby because two of the nitrogens in this compound have donated their spare outer-shell electrons to bond with positively charged ions (see Appendix B). Thus the whole molecule is positively charged (+2) and will attract two negatively charged ions (Cl⁻) into its vicinity. When crystallized out of water solution, this complex precipitates as the salt thiamin hydrochloride. This chemical name usually appears on vitamin bottles containing thiamin.

Thiamin pyrophosphate (TPP). TPP is a coenzyme that includes the thiamin molecule as part of its structure.

Riboflavin. This molecule is a part of two coenzymes—flavin mononucleotide (FMN) and flavin adenine dinucleotide (FAD).

Flavin mononucleotide (FMN).

C

Flavin adenine dinucleotide (FAD).

Niacin (nicotinic acid and nicotinamide). These molecules are a part of two coenzymes—nicotinamide adenine dinucleotide (NAD$^+$) and nicotinamide adenine dinucleotide phosphate (NADP$^+$).

Nicotinamide adenine dinucleotide (NAD$^+$) and nicotinamide adenine dinucleotide phosphate (NADP$^+$). NAD has also been called coenzyme I and DPN; NADP has been called coenzyme II and TPN. NADP has the same structure as NAD but with a phosphate group attached at the dagger (†).

Reduced NAD$^+$ (NADH). When NAD$^+$ is reduced, by the addition of H$^+$ and two electrons, it becomes the coenzyme NADH. (The dots on the Hs entering this reaction represent electrons—see Appendix B.)

C

Vitamin B$_6$ is a general name for three compounds—pyridoxine, pyridoxal, and pyridoxamine. Pyridoxal phosphate and pyridoxamine phosphate are the coenzymes necessary for transamination and other important processes.

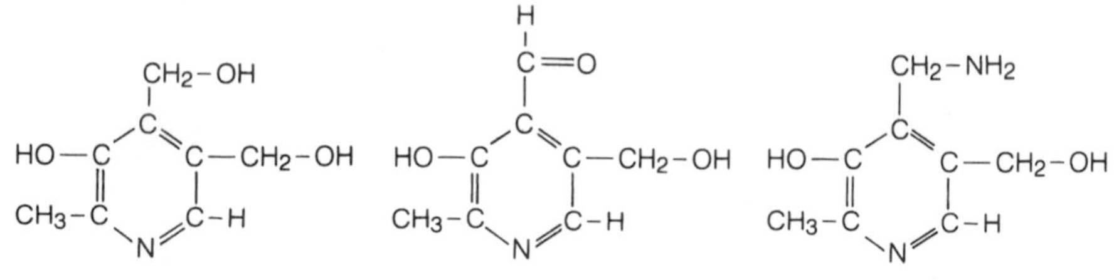

Pyridoxine

Pyridoxal

Pyridoxamine

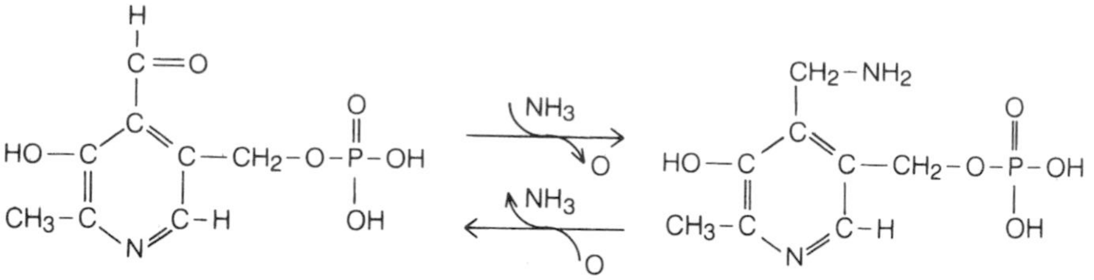

Pyridoxal phosphate

Pyridoxamine phosphate

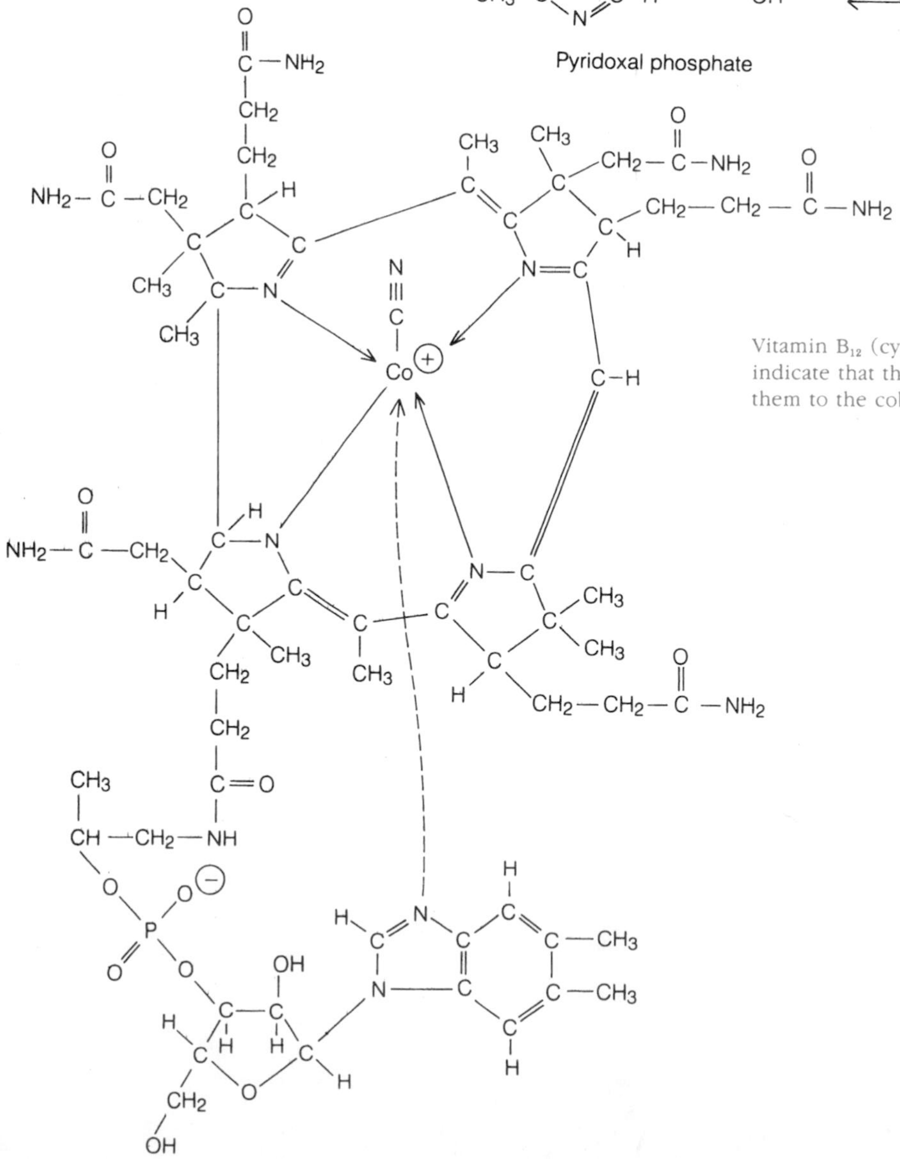

Vitamin B$_{12}$ (cyanocobalamin). The arrows in this diagram indicate that the spare electron pairs on the nitrogens attract them to the cobalt.

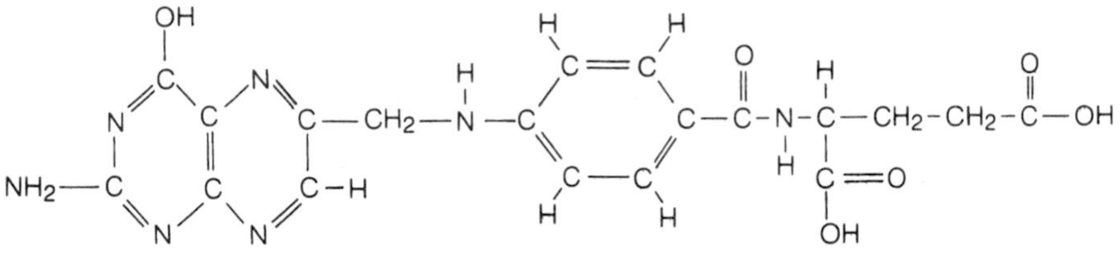

Folacin (folic acid).[4]

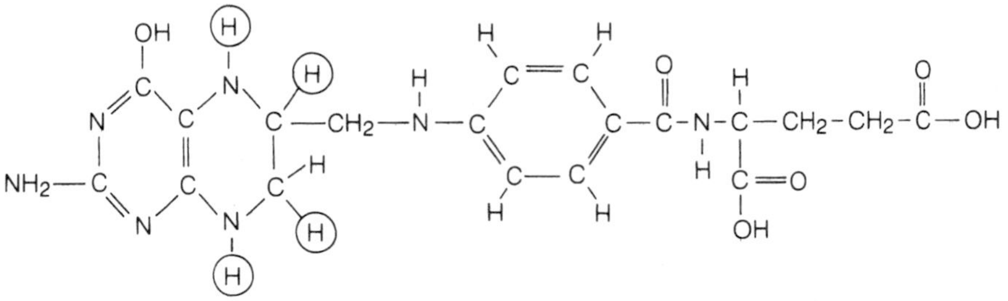

Tetrahydrofolic acid, the active coenzyme form of folacin. (The four hydrogens added to folacin are circled.)

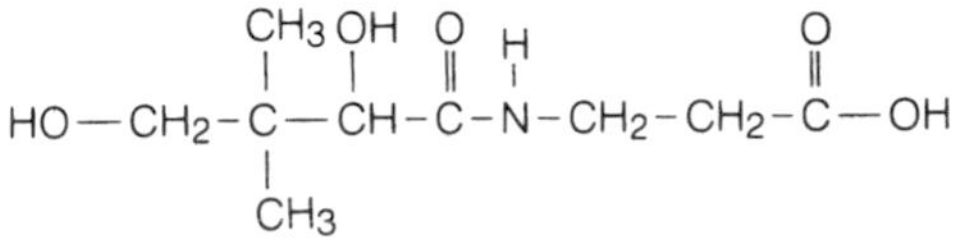

Pantothenic acid

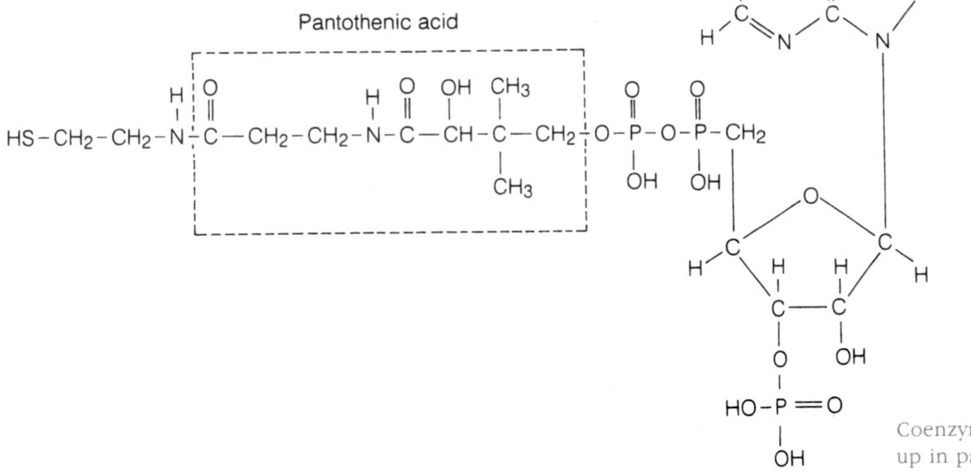

Coenzyme A (CoA). This molecule is made up in part of pantothenic acid.

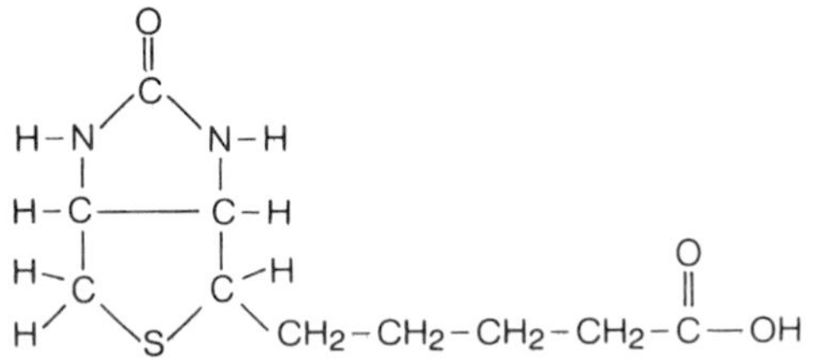

Biotin.

4   The term *folacin* is to be used as the generic descriptor for folic acid and related compounds. For further discussion, see: Nomenclature policy: Generic descriptors and trivial names for vitamins and related compounds, 1982.

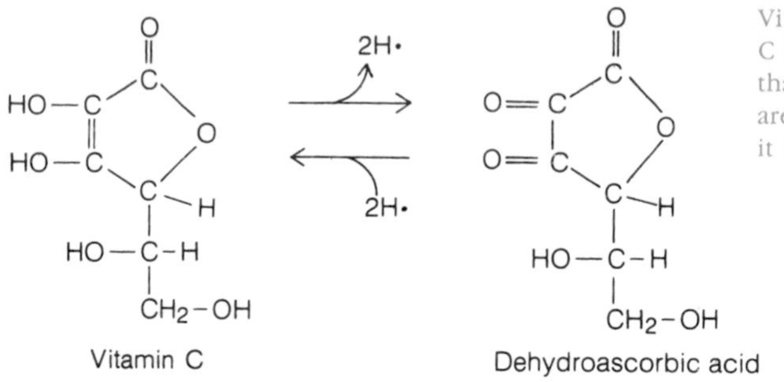

C

Vitamin C

Dehydroascorbic acid

Vitamin C (ascorbic acid).[5] The oxidized form of vitamin C is dehydroascorbic acid. (The dots on the Hs indicate that two hydrogen atoms, complete with their electrons, are lost when ascorbic acid is oxidized and gained when it is reduced again.)

Active vitamin D and its precursors, beginning with 7-dehydrocholesterol. (The carbon atoms at which changes occur are numbered.) Compare the structure of 7-dehydrocholesterol with that of cholesterol, p. 101.

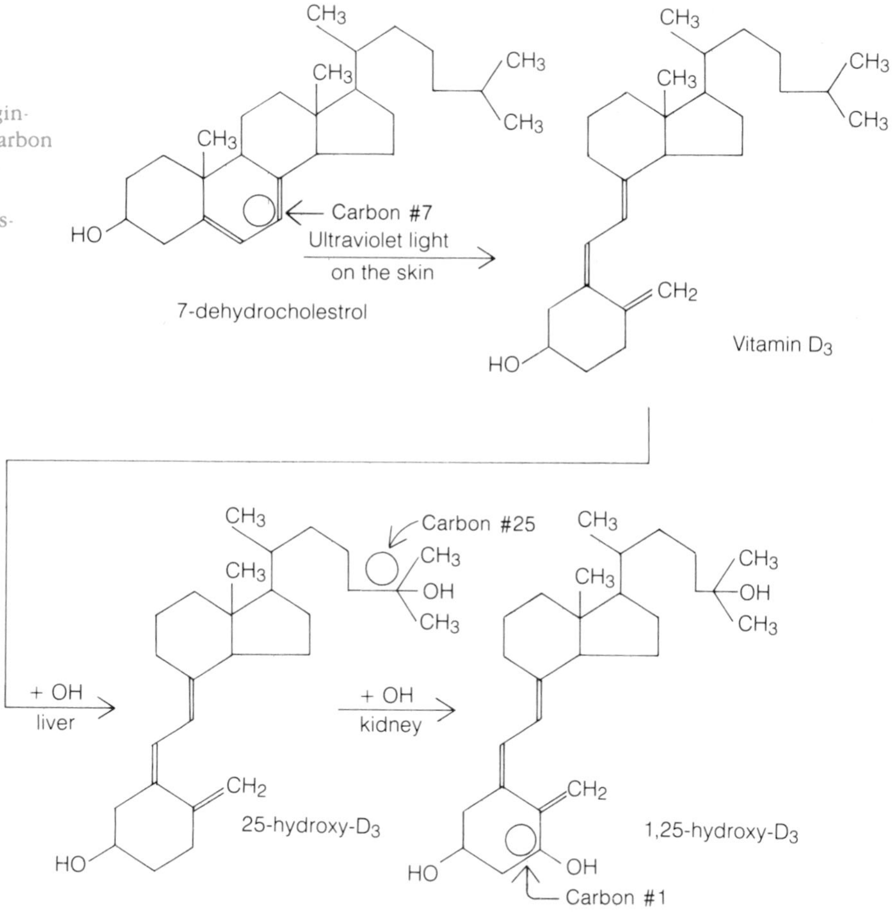

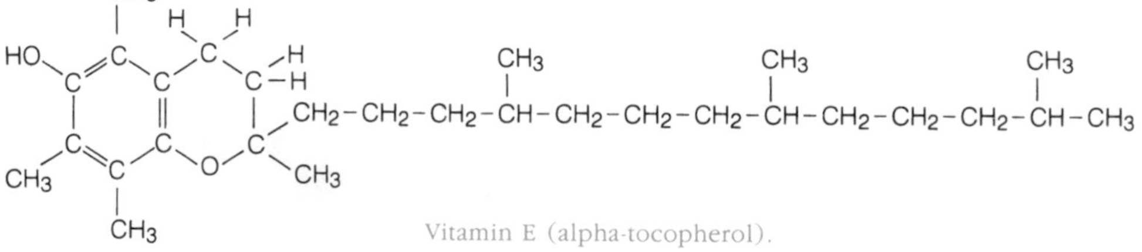

7-dehydrocholestrol

← Carbon #7
Ultraviolet light on the skin →

Vitamin D₃

Carbon #25

+ OH liver →

25-hydroxy-D₃

+ OH kidney →

1,25-hydroxy-D₃

Carbon #1

Vitamin E (alpha-tocopherol).

5   The term *vitamin C* should be used for all compounds with the biological activity of ascorbic acid. See: Nomenclature policy: Generic descriptors and trivial names for vitamins and related compounds, 1982.

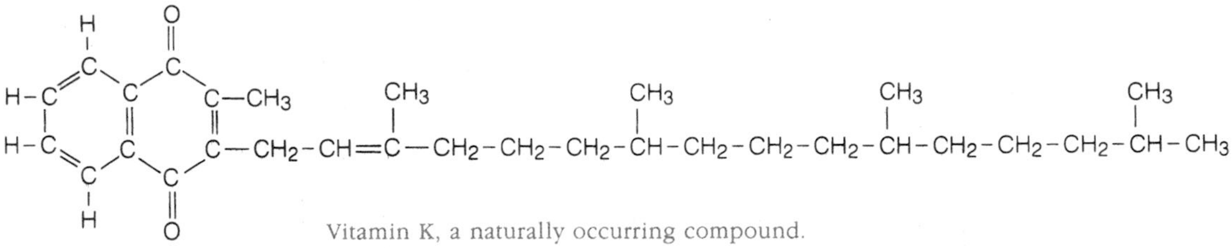

C

Vitamin K, a naturally occurring compound.

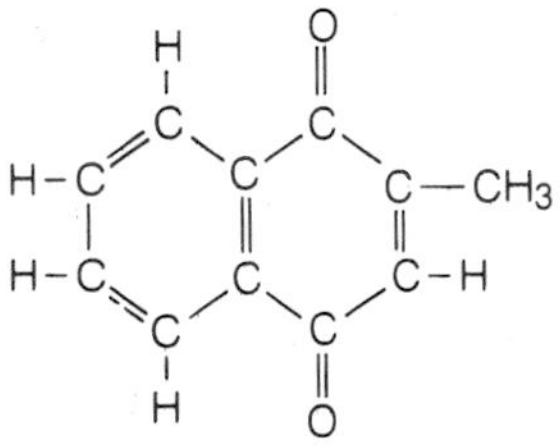

Menadione, a synthetic compound that exhibits vitamin K activity.

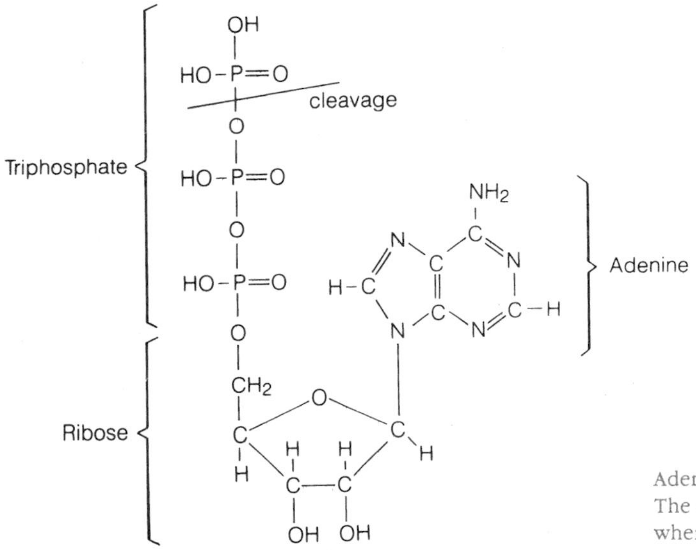

Triphosphate

Ribose

Adenine

Adenosine triphosphate (ATP), the energy carrier. The cleavage point marks the bond that is broken when ATP splits to become ADP + P.

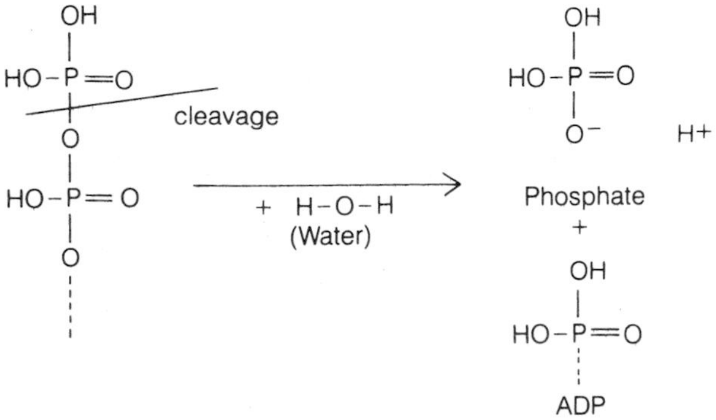

Phosphate
+

ADP

Adenosine diphosphate (ADP).

Glycolysis

Figure C-1 depicts the events of glycolysis. First, glucose must be given some activation energy before it can proceed toward the release of its own energy, just as a log must be given some heat from twigs and paper before it will burn spontaneously. This activation of glucose is accomplished in a coupled reaction with ATP. (A **coupled reaction** is a chemical event in which an enzyme complex catalyzes two reactions simultaneously. It often involves the breakdown of one compound to two and the synthesis of another from two.)

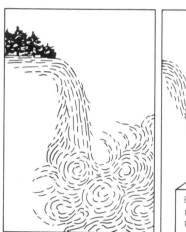

Energy of falling water dissipated without doing work.

Energy of falling water coupled to the turning of a series of water wheels.

Analogy for a coupled reaction.

Breakdown of glucose is coupled to making of ATP
or
Breakdown of ATP is coupled to activation of glucose (making glucose-P).

In the process of activation, a phosphate is attached to the carbon that chemists call number 6. The product is called, logically enough, glucose-6-phosphate. In the next step, glucose-6-phosphate is rearranged by an enzyme, and a phosphate is added in another coupled reaction with ATP. The product this time is fructose-1,6-diphosphate. At this point the six-carbon sugar has been activated. It has a phosphate group on its first and sixth carbons and enough

energy to break apart. Two ATPs have been used to accomplish this.

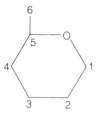

This is the way chemists number the carbons in a glucose molecule

(From this point to the production of pyruvate we will use letters in place of compound names. The names are in Figure C-1, for those who wish to know them.)

When fructose-1,6-diphosphate breaks in half, the two three-carbon compounds (A and A′) are not identical. Each has a phosphate group attached, but only one converts directly to pyruvate. The other compound converts easily to the first. (Compound A′ is usually ignored, except for its role as the point of entry for glycerol; we say that two molecules of compound A are derived from one glucose.)

In the step from compound A to compound B, enough energy is released to convert NAD^+ to $NADH + H^+$. Also, in the steps from B to C and from E to pyruvate, ATP is regenerated. Remember that there are effectively two molecules of compound A coming from glucose; therefore, four ATP molecules are generated. Two ATPs were needed to get the sequence started, so the net gain at this point is two ATPs and two molecules of $NADH + H^+$.

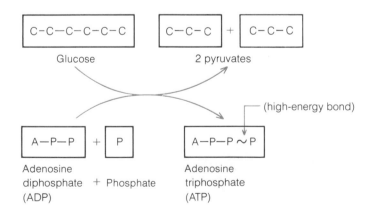

Breakdown of glucose is coupled to making of ATP simplified. Actually 2 ATP are used to activate glucose, and 4 ATP are gained in catabolism to 2 pyruvate. See Figure IM6-1.

So far, no oxygen has been used; the process has been anaerobic. But at this point, oxygen is needed. If oxygen is not immediately available, pyruvate converts to lactic acid, to soak up the hydrogens from the $NADH + H^+$ that was generated. Lactic acid accumulates until oxygen becomes available. However, in the energy path from glucose to carbon dioxide, this side step usually is not necessary. As you will see later, each $NADH + H^+$ moves to the electron transport chain to unload its hydrogens onto oxygen. The associated energy produces two ATPs, making the total yield eight ATPs for the process from glucose to pyruvate.

The TCA Cycle

The tricarboxylic acid, or TCA, cycle (Figure C–2) is the name given to the set of reactions involving oxygen and leading from acetyl CoA to carbon dioxide (and water). To link glycolysis to the TCA cycle, pyruvate is converted to acetyl CoA. This set of aerobic reactions is not restricted to the metabolism of carbohydrate. It also includes fat and protein. Any substance that can be converted to acetyl CoA directly, or indirectly through pyruvate, may enter the cycle.

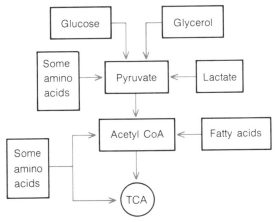

Any substance that can be converted to acetyl CoA either directly, or indirectly through pyruvate, may enter the TCA cycle.

The step from pyruvate to acetyl CoA is exceedingly complex. We have included only those substances that will help you understand the transfer of energy from the nutrients.

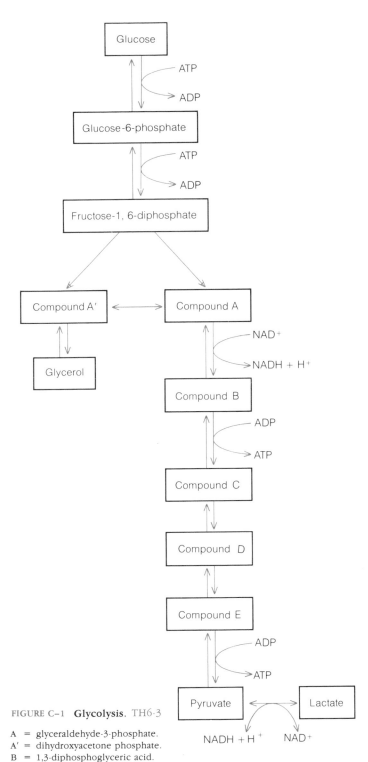

FIGURE C–1 **Glycolysis.** TH6-3

A = glyceraldehyde-3-phosphate.
A' = dihydroxyacetone phosphate.
B = 1,3-diphosphoglyceric acid.
C = 3-phosphoglyceric acid.
D = 2-phosphoglyceric acid.
E = phosphoenol pyruvic acid.

C

When pyruvate is in the presence of oxygen, it loses a carbon in the form of carbon dioxide, and CoA is attached. In the process, NAD^+ picks up two hydrogens with their associated energy, becoming $NADH + H^+$.

As the acetyl CoA breaks down to carbon dioxide and water, its energy is captured in ATP. Let's follow the steps by which this occurs (see Figure C–2):

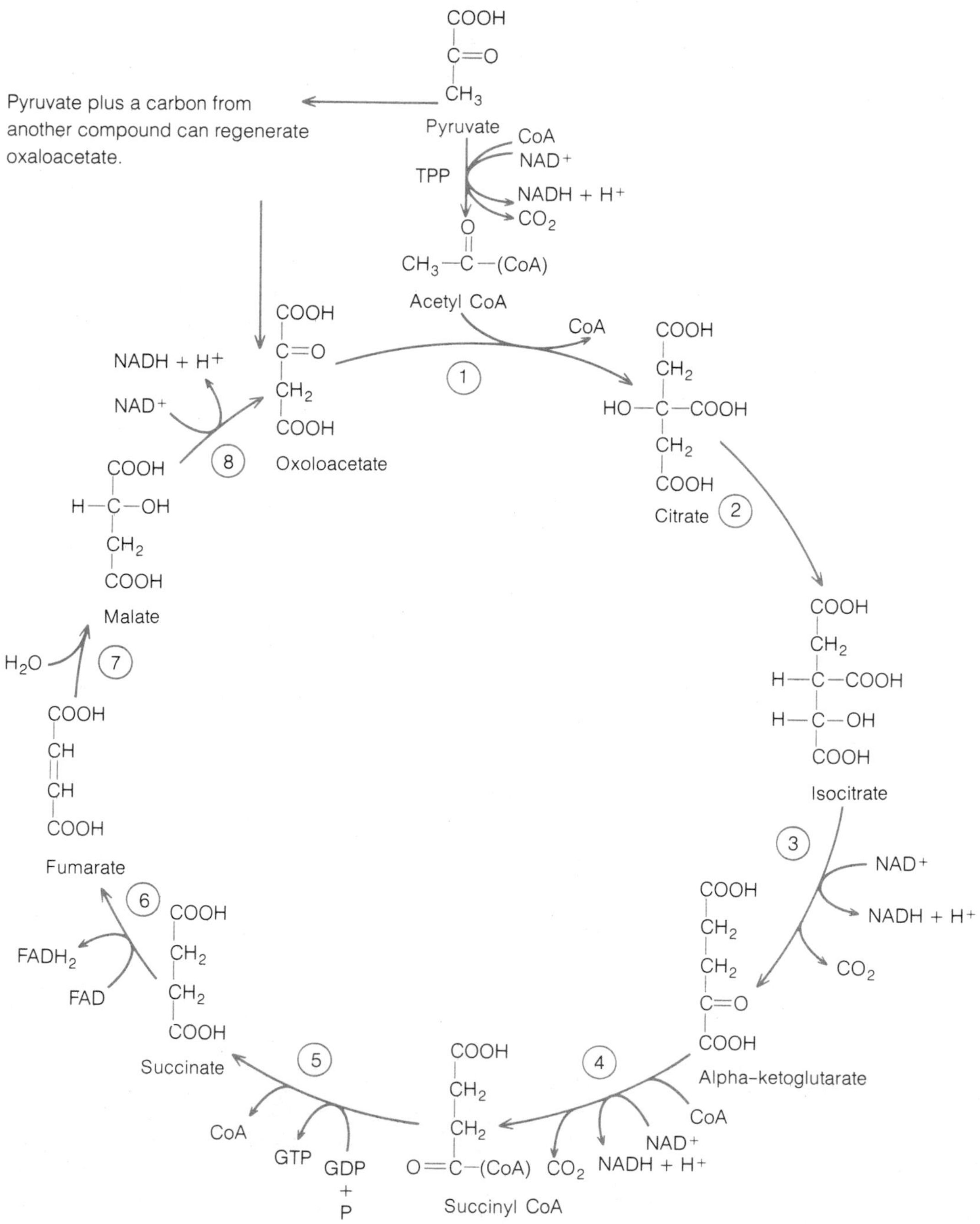

FIGURE C–2 **The TCA cycle.** TH6-4

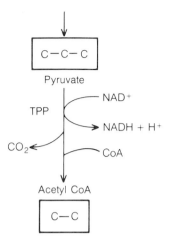

(TPP is a helper compound containing the B vitamin thiamin.)

The step from pyruvate to acetyl CoA.

1 Acetyl CoA combines with a four-carbon compound, oxaloacetate. The CoA comes off, and the product is a six-carbon compound, citrate.
2 The atoms of citrate are rearranged to form isocitrate.
3 Now NAD^+ reacts with isocitrate. Two Hs and two electrons are removed from the isocitrate. One H becomes attached to the NAD^+ with the two electrons; the other H is released as a free proton. Thus NAD^+ becomes NADH + H^+. *(Remember this NADH + H^+. It is carrying the Hs and the energy from the last reaction. But let's follow the carbons first.)* A carbon is removed and combined with oxygen, forming carbon dioxide (which diffuses away in the blood and is exhaled). What is left is the five-carbon compound alpha-ketoglutarate.
4 Now two compounds interact with alpha-ketoglutarate—a molecule of CoA and a molecule of NAD^+. In this complex reaction, a carbon is removed and combined with oxygen (forming carbon dioxide); two Hs are removed and go to NAD^+ (forming NADH + H^+); and the CoA is attached to the remaining four-carbon compound, forming succinyl CoA. *(Remember this NADH + H^+ also. You will see later what happens to it.)*
5 Now two molecules react with succinyl CoA—a molecule called GDP and one of phosphate (P). The CoA comes off, the GDP and P combine to form the high-energy compound GTP, and succinate remains. *(Remember this GTP.)*
6 In the next reaction, two Hs with their energy are removed from succinate and are transferred to a molecule called FAD (an electron-hydrogen receiver like NAD^+) to form $FADH_2$. The product that remains is fumarate. *(Remember this $FADH_2$.)*

7 Next a molecule of water is added to fumarate, forming malate.
8 A molecule of NAD^+ reacts with the malate; two Hs with their associated energy are removed from the malate and form NADH + H^+. The product that remains is the four-carbon compound oxaloacetate. *(Remember this NADH + H^+.)*

We are back where we started. The oxaloacetate formed in this process can combine with another molecule of acetyl CoA (step 1), and the cycle can begin again. (The whole scheme is shown in Figure C–2.)

So far, what you have seen is that two carbons are brought in with acetyl CoA and that two carbons end up in carbon dioxide. But where is the energy and the ATP we promised you?

Each time a pair of hydrogen atoms is removed from one of the compounds in the cycle, it carries a pair of electrons with it. This chemical bond energy is thus captured into the compound to which the Hs become attached. A review of the eight steps of the cycle shows that energy is thus transferred into other compounds in steps 3, 4, 6, and 8. In step 5, energy is harnessed to bind GDP and P together to form GTP. Thus the compounds NADH + H^+ (three molecules) $FADH_2$, and GTP are built with energy originally found in acetyl CoA. To see how this energy ends up in ATP, we must follow the electrons further. Let us take those attached to NAD^+ as an example.

The Electron Transport Chain

The six reactions described here are those of the **electron transport chain**. Since oxygen is required for these reactions and ADP and P are combined to form ATP in several of them (ADP is phosphorylated), they are also called **oxidative phosphorylation**.

An important concept to remember at this point is that an electron is not a fixed amount of energy. The electrons that bond the H to NAD^+ in NADH have a relatively large amount of energy. In the series of reactions that follow, they lose this energy in small amounts, until at the end they are attached (with Hs) to oxygen (O) to make water (H_2O). In some of the steps, the energy they lose is captured into ATP in coupled reactions.

In the first step of the electron transport chain, NADH reacts with a molecule called a flavoprotein, losing its electrons (and their Hs). The products are NAD^+ and reduced flavoprotein. A little energy is lost as heat in this reaction.

The flavoprotein passes on the electrons to a molecule called coenzyme Q. Again they lose some energy as heat,

C

but ADP and P participate in this reaction and gain much of the energy to bond together and form ATP. This is a coupled reaction: $ADP + P \rightarrow ATP$.

Coenzyme Q passes the electrons to cytochrome *b*. Again the electrons lose energy.

Cytochrome *b* passes the electrons to cytochrome *c* in a coupled reaction in which ATP is formed: $ADP + P \rightarrow ATP$.

Cytochrome *c* passes the electrons to cytochrome *a*.

Cytochrome *a* passes them (with their Hs) to an atom of oxygen (O), forming water (H_2O). This is a coupled reaction in which ATP is formed: $ADP + P \rightarrow ATP$.

The entire electron transport chain is diagrammed in Figure C-3. As you can see, each time NADH is oxidized (loses its electrons) by this means, the energy it loses is parceled out into three ATP molecules. When the electrons are passed on to water at the end, they have much less energy than they had to begin with. This completes the story of the electrons from NADH.

As for $FADH_2$, its electrons enter the electron transport chain at coenzyme Q. From coenzyme Q to water there are only two steps in which ATP is generated. Therefore, $FADH_2$ coming out of the TCA cycle yields just two ATP molecules.

One energy-receiving compound of the TCA cycle (GTP) does not enter the electron transport chain but gives its energy directly to ADP in a simple phosphorylation reaction, yielding one ATP.

It is now possible to draw up a balance sheet of glucose metabolism (see Table C-1). Glycolysis has yielded 4 NADH + H$^+$ and 4 ATP molecules and has spent 2 ATPs. The 2 acetyl CoAs going through the TCA cycle have yielded 6 NADH + H$^+$, 2 $FADH_2$, and 2 GTP molecules. After the NADH + H$^+$ and $FADH_2$ have gone through the electron transport chain, there are 34 ATPs. Added to these are the 4 ATPs from glycolysis and the 2 ATPs from GTP, making the total 40 ATPs generated from one molecule of glucose. After the expense of 2 ATPs is subtracted, there is a net gain of 38 ATPs.

The TCA cycle and the electron transport chain are the body's major means of capturing the energy from nutrients

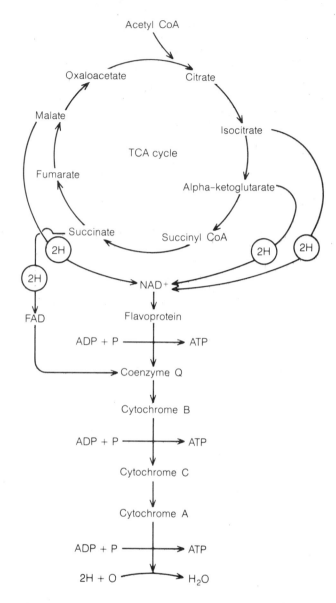

FIGURE C-3   **The electron transport chain.** TH6-5

TABLE C–1   **Balance Sheet for Glucose Metabolism**

	EXPEND-ITURES	INCOME
Glycolysis:		
1 glucose	2 ATP	4 ATP
1 fructose-1,6-diphosphate		2 NADH + H^+
2 pyruvate		2 NADH + H^+
TCA cycle:		
2 isocitrate		2 NADH + H^+
2 alpha-ketoglutarate		2 NADH + H^+
2 succinyl CoA		2 GTP
2 succinate		2 $FADH_2$
2 malate		2 NADH + H^+
Total ATPs collected:		
From glycolysis	2 ATP	4 ATP
From 10 NADH + H^+		30 ATP
From 2 GTP		2 ATP
From 2 $FADH_2$		4 ATP
Totals:	2 ATP	40 ATP
Balance on hand from 1 molecule glucose:		38 ATP

in ATP molecules. Other means, such as anaerobic glycolysis, contribute, but the aerobic processes are the most efficient. Biologists and chemists understand much more about these processes than has been presented here.

APPENDIX D
Measures of Protein Quality

CONTENTS

Some of the problems of determining protein quality were discussed in Chapter 4. This appendix amplifies that discussion for those who are interested.

Chemical Score

Two FAO/WHO reference scoring patterns for the eight essential amino acids are shown in Table D–1. To interpret the table for egg, read, "For every 3,060 units of essential amino acids, 340 must be isoleucine, 540 must be leucine," and so on. For the FAO/WHO pattern, read, "For every 2,250 units of essential amino acids, 250 must be isoleucine, 440 must be leucine," and so on.

To compare a test protein with one of these reference proteins (let's use egg for an example), the experimenter would first obtain a chemical analysis of the test protein's amino acids. Then, taking 3,060 units of the essential amino acids, he would compare the amount of each to the amount found in 3,060 units of essential amino acids in egg protein. For example, suppose the test protein contained (per 3,060 units) 360 units of isoleucine, 500 units of leucine, 350 of lysine, and for each of the other amino acids, more units than egg protein contains. The two amino acids that are low are leucine (500 as compared to 540 in egg) and lysine (350 versus 440 in egg). The ratio—amino acid in test protein divided by amino acid in egg—is 500/540 or about 0.93 for leucine and 350/440 or about 0.80 for lysine. Lysine is the limiting amino acid (lowest ratio compared to egg), so the test protein receives a chemical score of 80.

The advantages of chemical scoring are that it is simple and inexpensive, it identifies in one step the limiting amino acid, and it can be used to score mixtures of different proportions of two or more proteins mathematically without having to make them up and test them. Its chief weaknesses are that it fails to predict the digestibility of a protein, which may severely affect its quality; it relies on a chemical procedure in which certain amino acids may be destroyed, so that the pattern that is analyzed may lack accuracy; and it is blind to other features of the test protein, such as toxic materials, that would only be revealed by a test in living animals.

TABLE D–1 **FAO/WHO Reference Patterns**

ESSENTIAL AMINO ACIDS	WHOLE EGG	FAO/WHO PATTERN, 1973 *(mg amino acid per g nitrogen)*
Isoleucine	340	250
Leucine	540	440
Lysine	440	340
Methionine + cystine[a]	355	220
Phenylalanine + tyrosine[b]	580	380
Threonine	294	250
Tryptophan	106	60
Valine	410	310
TOTAL	3,060[c]	2,250

[a] Methionine is essential and is also used to make cystine. Thus the methionine requirement is lower if cystine is supplied.
[b] Phenylalanine is essential and is also used to make tyrosine if there is not enough of the latter. Thus the phenylalanine requirement is lower if tyrosine is also supplied.
[c] Rounded off.

Biological Value (BV)

In a test of biological value, two nitrogen-balance studies are done. In the first, no protein is fed, and nitrogen (N) excretion in the urine and feces is measured. It is assumed that N lost in the urine (called endogenous N) is the amount the body loses by filtration into the urine each day regardless of what protein is fed. The N lost in the feces (called metabolic N) is the amount the body invariably loses into the intestine each day. (To help you remember terms: endogenous N is "urinary N on a zero-protein diet"; metabolic N is "fecal N on a zero-protein diet.")

In the second experiment, an amount of protein slightly below the requirement is fed. Intake and losses are measured. BV is then derived with this formula:

$$BV = \frac{\text{Food N} - (\text{fecal N} - \text{metabolic N}) - (\text{urinary N} - \text{endogenous N})}{\text{Food N} - (\text{fecal N} - \text{metabolic N})} \times 100.$$

The denominator of this equation expresses the amount of nitrogen *absorbed*: food N minus fecal N (excluding the N the body would lose in the feces anyway, even without food). The numerator expresses the amount of N *retained* from the N absorbed: absorbed N (as in the denominator) minus the N excreted in the urine (excluding the N the body would lose in the urine anyway, even without food). Thus it can be more simply expressed:

$$BV = \frac{\text{N retained}}{\text{N absorbed}} \times 100.$$

This method has the advantage of being based on experiments with human beings (it can be done with animals too, of course) and of measuring actual nitrogen retention. But it is also cumbersome, expensive, and often impractical and is based on many assumptions that may not be valid. For example, the subjects used for testing may not be similar physiologically or in terms of their normal environment or typical food intake to those for whom the test protein may ultimately be used. For another example, the fact that protein is retained in the body does not necessarily mean that it is being well utilized. There is considerable protein turnover (synthesis and degradation) within every cell of the body, and there is much exchange among tissues. These processes are hidden from view when only N intake and output are measured.

Net Protein Utilization (NPU)

Like measurements of BV, NPU determinations involve two balance studies, one on zero and the other on submaximal nitrogen intake. The formula for NPU is:

$$NPU = \frac{\text{Food N} - (\text{fecal N} - \text{metabolic N}) - (\text{urinary N} - \text{endogenous N})}{\text{Food N}} \times 100.$$

The numerator is the same as for BV, but the denominator represents food N intake only—not absorbed N. More simply expressed:

$$NPU = \frac{\text{N retained}}{\text{N intake}}.$$

This method has advantages similar to those of BV determinations and is more frequently used, with animals employed as the test subjects. A drawback is that if a low NPU is obtained, the test results offer no help in distinguishing between two possible causes: a poor amino acid composition of the test protein or poor digestibility. There is also a limit to the extent to which animal test results can be assumed to be applicable to human beings, as with PER (below).

Protein Efficiency Ratio (PER)

This is the best-known procedure for evaluating protein quality and is used in the United States as the basis for regulations regarding food labeling and for the protein RDA. Young rats are fed a measured amount of protein and weighed periodically as they grow. PER is expressed as:

$$PER = \frac{\text{Weight gain (g)}}{\text{Protein intake (g)}}.$$

This method has the virtues of economy and simplicity but also has many drawbacks. The experiments are time consuming; the amino acid needs of rats are not the same as for human beings; and the amino acid needs for growth are not the same as for the maintenance of adult animals (growing animals need more lysine, for example).

All these methods and others have their uses, and some of their disadvantages balance one another out. One reviewer recommends that chemical scoring be relied on more heavily than it has been in the past and that the biological techniques be used to amplify and help interpret the findings from scoring.[1] The evaluation of protein quality remains a vitally important research area in a world where it is becoming more and more critical to provide nourishing food to millions who live on the edge of starvation.[2]

D

1   P. L. Pellett, Protein quality evaluation revisited, *Food Technology*, May 1978, pp. 60, 62, 64–66, 70–72, 74, 76, 78–79.
2   The interested reader will find additional useful information in Pellett, 1978; R. L. Pike and M. L. Brown, *Nutrition: An Integrated Approach*, 2nd ed. (New York: Wiley, 1975); and R. S. Goodhart and M. E. Shils, eds., *Modern Nutrition in Health and Disease*, 6th ed. (Philadelphia: Lea and Febiger, 1980).

To Explore Further
The critiques of the PER and other measures of protein quality in this reference are probably the best available:

● P. L. Pellett and V. R. Young, eds. *Nutritional Evaluation of Protein Foods*. Tokyo: United Nations University, 1980.

APPENDIX E
Assessment Standards and Tools

CONTENTS

Some assessment standards and tools appear elsewhere in this book. Listed here are all the items needed for the four components of nutrition assessment: diet histories, anthropometric measures, physical examination, and lab tests. Those that appear in this appendix are listed in **boldface type**.

History

To identify the risk factors for poor nutrition status in a history, use:

- Table 12–1—general.
- Unnumbered table, p. 496—risk factors in pregnancy.
- Form 12–1—form for collecting historical information.
- **Table E–1**—drug history questionnaire.

For diet history forms, use:

- Form 12–2—24-hour recall or usual intake record.
- Form 12–3—food frequency checklist.
- Form 12–4—food diary form.

Anthropometric Measures

Standards and tools useful with anthropometric measures include those for assessing weight and frame size:

- Table on inside back cover—average weights for heights.

- Table 7–1—frame size by elbow breadth measure.
- **Table E–2**—frame size by wrist circumference.
- **Table E–3**—degree of underweight as an indicator of malnutrition (PCM).

To assess body fat and lean compartments, use:

- **Table E–4**—triceps fatfold standards.
- **Table E–5**—midarm circumference (MAC) standards.
- **Figure E–1 (A and B)**—nomogram for using the above two measures to determine midarm muscle circumference (MAMC).
- **Table E–6**—midarm muscle circumference (MAMC) standards.
- Table 12–2—table used to interpret these measures (degree of depletion of body weight, triceps fatfold, and MAMC) as a reflection of the severity of malnutrition (PCM).

To assess growth in children, use:

- **Figure E–2 (A and B)**—length for age and weight for age in infants and children up to 3 years.
- **Figure E–3 (A and B)**—head circumference and weight for length in infants and children up to 3 years.
- **Figure E–4 (A and B)**—height for age and weight for age in children 2 to 18 years.
- **Figure E–5 (A and B)**—weight for height in children 2 to 18 years.

Note: to assess growth in infants and children using these four figures, follow these steps:

1 Select the appropriate chart based on age and sex. For example, for a 3-month-old female infant weighing 12 pounds with a length of 23 inches, you would use the chart for girls, birth to 36 months (Figure 2A).

E

2 Locate the child's age on bottom or top of chart (in our example, 3 months).

3 Locate the child's weight in pounds or kilograms on the lower left or right side of the chart (in our example, 12 pounds).

4 Mark the chart where the age and weight lines intersect. (In our example, this is just above the 50th percentile. Note where we marked the chart.)

5 To find the child's percentile for length or height and age, start by locating the child's age on the top of the chart and the length on the upper right or left side. Proceed as you did when you were comparing age and weight. (Note the mark on the chart for the baby in our example.)

Figures 2A and 2B are useful for comparing infants' length and weight gain to those of other babies in the same population. Use Figures 3A and 3B to determine the percentile of head circumference development, and for assessing weight for length.

Children's growth in height and weight may be compared with the standards in Figures 4A and 4B. Figures 5A and 5B omit the age factor when comparing the heights and weights of prepubescent children with the standards, and are useful for determining if weight is appropriate for height.

For assessing weight gain in a pregnant woman, use:

● **Figure E-6**—weight gain grid.[1]

Physical Examination

For assessment of findings from physical examination, use:

● Tables in Chapters 8, 9, 10, 11—list symptoms of deficiency and toxicity for nutrients.
● Table 12-3—summarizes symptoms by nutrient.
● **Table E-7**—lists symptoms by body system.

Clinical (Laboratory) Tests

For lab tests used in assessment:

● Table 12-2—lab tests used to assess PCM (including serum albumin, transferrin, and creatinine excretion).
● **Table E-8**—standards for interpretation of serum albumin and transferrin.
● **Table E-9**—creatinine excretion standards.[2]

Note about creatinine excretion: in Chapter 12 (Table 12-2), creatinine was described as a metabolite of energy breakdown in skeletal muscle. It is considered to be a reflection of the amount of skeletal muscle present in a person's body. Another useful aspect of the 24-hour creatinine output is that it can be used as a standard against which to compare the urinary output of the water-soluble vitamins involved in energy metabolism, such as riboflavin and thiamin. Creatinine is a reflection of actively metabolizing muscle tissue and is a value that remains relatively constant from day to day. Use Tables E-9A and E-9B as standards of 24-hour creatinine excretion for height and sex to calculate a person's creatinine height index (CHI).

---

1   The use of a single weight gain grid for pregnant women has been criticized. This reference suggests using different grids for women who are underweight, normal weight, and overweight at the start of their pregnancies: E. McCarthy, Report of a Montreal Diet Dispensary experience, *Journal of the Canadian Dietetic Association* 44 (1983): 71–75.

2   Limits on the accuracy and validity of creatinine excretion as an indicator of muscle mass are discussed in: S. B. Heymsfield and coauthors, Measurement of muscle mass in humans: Validity of the 24-hour urinary creatinine method, *American Journal of Clinical Nutrition* 37 (1983): 478–494.

TABLE E-1 **Drug History (Adult)**

1a. Do you have any health problems for which you are taking prescription medications at the present time? Yes _____ No _____
If yes:

Health problem	Proprietary name of drug	Generic name of drug	Dose	Frequency	Duration of intake

1b. Are you taking any other medication a doctor has prescribed (name or reason unknown)? Yes _____ No _____
If yes:

Description of drug	Dose	Frequency	Duration of intake

2a. Have you taken prescription medication for any of the health problems listed below within the past three months? Yes _____ No _____
If yes:

Health problem	Drug name	Duration of intake	When discontinued	Reason for stopping	Still taking[a]
Asthma					
Arthritis					
High blood pressure					
Fluid retention					
Infection (specify)					
Tuberculosis					
Malaria					
Psoriasis					
Colitis					
High cholesterol					
Parkinson's disease					
Liver disease					
Kidney disease					
Blood disease					
Bone disease					
Gout					
Blood clots					
Diabetes					
Other (specify)					

[a] Check (✔) if still taking.

2b. Have you taken any other medication within the past three months that a doctor has prescribed (name or reason unknown)? Yes _____ No _____
If yes:

Description	Dose	Frequency	Duration of intake

3a. Do you take medications, self-prescribed, for any of the complaints listed below? Yes _____ No _____
If yes:

Complaint	Constantly	Frequently	Occasionally
Constipation			
Indigestion			
Headache			
Nervousness			
Insomnia			
Pain			
Menstrual cramps			
Colds and sinus trouble			
Other (state)			

(continued)

TABLE E-1   (continued)

3b. If response to 3a is positive in one or more categories, what medication do you take to relieve these complaints, and how much do you need to gain relief?

Complaint	Drug	Dose	Frequency	Duration
Constipation				
Indigestion				
Headache				
Nervousness				
Insomnia				
Pain				
Menstrual cramps				
Colds and sinus trouble				
Other (state)				

4. Are you taking birth control pills now?   Yes _____   No _____

If yes:
Name:
Duration of intake:

Have you taken birth control pills within the past six months?   Yes _____   No _____

If yes:
Name:
Duration of intake:
Date discontinued:
Reason for stopping:

Source: Adapted from D. Roe, *Drug-Induced Nutritional Deficiencies* (Westport, Conn.: Avi Publishing Company, 1976), Table 4.2, pp. 106–108.

TABLE E-4   **Triceps Fatfold Percentiles (millimeters)**

	MALE					FEMALE				
Age	5th	25th	50th	75th	95th	5th	25th	50th	75th	95th
1–1.9	6	8	10	12	16	6	8	10	12	16
2–2.9	6	8	10	12	15	6	9	10	12	16
3–3.9	6	8	10	11	15	7	9	11	12	15
4–4.9	6	8	9	11	14	7	8	10	12	16
5–5.9	6	8	9	11	15	6	8	10	12	18
6–6.9	5	7	8	10	16	6	8	10	12	16
7–7.9	5	7	9	12	17	6	9	11	13	18
8–8.9	5	7	8	10	16	6	9	12	15	24
9–9.9	6	7	10	13	18	8	10	13	16	22
10–10.9	6	8	10	14	21	7	10	12	17	27
11–11.9	6	8	11	16	24	7	10	13	18	28
12–12.9	6	8	11	14	28	8	11	14	18	27
13–13.9	5	7	10	14	26	8	12	15	21	30
14–14.9	4	7	9	14	24	9	13	16	21	28
15–15.9	4	6	8	11	24	8	12	17	21	32
16–16.9	4	6	8	12	22	10	15	18	22	31
17–17.9	5	6	8	12	19	10	13	19	24	37
18–18.9	4	6	9	13	24	10	15	18	22	30
19–24.9	4	7	10	15	22	10	14	18	24	34
25–34.9	5	8	12	16	24	10	16	21	27	37
35–44.9	5	8	12	16	23	12	18	23	29	38
45–54.9	6	8	12	15	25	12	20	25	30	40
55–64.9	5	8	11	14	22	12	20	25	31	38
65–74.9	4	8	11	15	22	12	18	24	29	36

Source: Adapted from A. R. Frisancho, New norms of upper limb fat and muscle areas for assessment of nutritional status, *American Journal of Clinical Nutrition* 34 (1981): 2540–2545.

TABLE E-2 **Frame Size from Height-Wrist Circumference Ratios (r)**

	MALE r VALUES[a]	FEMALE r VALUES[a]
Small	>10.4	>11.0
Medium	9.6–10.4	10.1–11.0
Large	<9.6	<10.1

[a] $r = \dfrac{Height\ (cm)}{Wrist\ circumference\ (cm)^b}$

[b] The wrist is measured where it bends (distal to the styloid process), on the right arm.

TABLE E-3 **Weight as an Indicator of Malnutrition**

%IBW[a]	%UBW[b]	DEGREE OF UNDERNUTRITION
80–90%	85–95%	Mildly depleted
70–79%	75–84%	Moderately depleted
<70%	<75%	Severely depleted

[a] Percent ideal body weight.
[b] Percent usual body weight.
Source: Adapted from J. P. Grant, Patient selection, *Handbook of Total Parenteral Nutrition* (Philadelphia: Saunders, 1980), p. 11.

TABLE E-5 **Midarm Circumference (MAC) (centimeters)**

	MALE					FEMALE				
Age	5th	25th	50th	75th	95th	5th	25th	50th	75th	95th
1–1.9	14.2	15.0	15.9	17.0	18.3	13.8	14.8	15.6	16.4	17.7
2–2.9	14.1	15.3	16.2	17.0	18.5	14.2	15.2	16.0	16.7	18.4
3–3.9	15.0	16.0	16.7	17.5	19.0	14.3	15.8	16.7	17.5	18.9
4–4.9	14.9	16.2	17.1	18.0	19.2	14.9	16.0	16.9	17.7	19.1
5–5.9	15.3	16.7	17.5	18.5	20.4	15.3	16.5	17.5	18.5	21.1
6–6.9	15.5	16.7	17.9	18.8	22.8	15.6	17.0	17.6	18.7	21.1
7–7.9	16.2	17.7	18.7	20.1	23.0	16.4	17.4	18.3	19.9	23.1
8–8.9	16.2	17.7	19.0	20.2	24.5	16.8	18.3	19.5	21.4	26.1
9–9.9	17.5	18.7	20.0	21.7	25.7	17.8	19.4	21.1	22.4	26.0
10–10.9	18.1	19.6	21.0	23.1	27.4	17.4	19.3	21.0	22.8	26.5
11–11.9	18.6	20.2	22.3	24.4	28.0	18.5	20.8	22.4	24.8	30.3
12–12.9	19.3	21.4	23.2	25.4	30.3	19.4	21.6	23.7	25.6	29.4
13–13.9	19.4	22.8	24.7	26.3	30.1	20.2	22.3	24.3	27.1	33.8
14–14.9	22.0	23.7	25.3	28.3	32.3	21.4	23.7	25.2	27.2	32.2
15–15.9	22.2	24.4	26.4	28.4	32.0	20.8	23.9	25.4	27.9	32.2
16–16.9	24.4	26.2	27.8	30.3	34.3	21.8	24.1	25.8	28.3	33.4
17–17.9	24.6	26.7	28.5	30.8	34.7	22.0	24.1	26.4	29.5	35.0
18–18.9	24.5	27.6	29.7	32.1	37.9	22.2	24.1	25.8	28.1	32.5
19–24.9	26.2	28.8	30.8	33.1	37.2	21.1	24.7	26.5	29.0	34.5
25–34.9	27.1	30.0	31.9	34.2	37.5	23.3	25.6	27.7	30.4	36.8
35–44.9	27.8	30.5	32.6	34.5	37.4	24.1	26.7	29.0	31.7	37.8
45–54.9	26.7	30.1	32.2	34.2	37.6	24.2	27.4	29.9	32.8	38.4
55–64.9	25.8	29.6	31.7	33.6	36.9	24.3	28.0	30.3	33.5	38.5
65–74.9	24.8	28.5	30.7	32.5	35.5	24.0	27.4	29.9	32.6	37.3

Source: Adapted from A. R. Frisancho, New norms of upper limb fat and muscle areas for assessment of nutritional status, *American Journal of Clinical Nutrition* 34 (1981): 2540–2545.

E

TABLE E–6   **Midarm Muscle Circumference (MAMC) (centimeters)**

Age	MALE					FEMALE				
	5th	*25th*	*50th*	*75th*	*95th*	*5th*	*25th*	*50th*	*75th*	*95th*
1–1.9	11.0	11.9	12.7	13.5	14.7	10.5	11.7	12.4	13.9	14.3
2–2.9	11.1	12.2	13.0	14.0	15.0	11.1	11.9	12.6	13.3	14.7
3–3.9	11.7	13.1	13.7	14.3	15.3	11.3	12.4	13.2	14.0	15.2
4–4.9	12.3	13.3	14.1	14.8	15.9	11.5	12.8	13.6	14.4	15.7
5–5.9	12.8	14.0	14.7	15.4	16.9	12.5	13.4	14.2	15.1	16.5
6–6.9	13.1	14.2	15.1	16.1	17.7	13.0	13.8	14.5	15.4	17.1
7–7.9	13.7	15.1	16.0	16.8	19.0	12.9	14.2	15.1	16.0	17.6
8–8.9	14.0	15.4	16.2	17.0	18.7	13.8	15.1	16.0	17.1	19.4
9–9.9	15.1	16.1	17.0	18.3	20.2	14.7	15.8	16.7	18.0	19.8
10–10.9	15.6	16.6	18.0	19.1	22.1	14.8	15.9	17.0	18.0	19.7
11–11.9	15.9	17.3	18.3	19.5	23.0	15.0	17.1	18.1	19.6	22.3
12–12.9	16.7	18.2	19.5	21.0	24.1	16.2	18.0	19.1	20.1	22.0
13–13.9	17.2	19.6	21.1	22.6	24.5	16.9	18.3	19.8	21.1	24.0
14–14.9	18.9	21.2	22.3	24.0	26.4	17.4	19.0	20.1	21.6	24.7
15–15.9	19.9	21.8	23.7	25.4	27.2	17.5	18.9	20.2	21.5	24.4
16–16.9	21.3	23.4	24.9	26.9	29.6	17.0	19.0	20.2	21.6	24.9
17–17.9	22.4	24.5	25.8	27.3	31.2	17.5	19.4	20.5	22.1	25.7
18–18.9	22.6	25.2	26.4	28.3	32.4	17.4	19.1	20.2	21.5	24.5
19–24.9	23.8	25.7	27.3	28.9	32.1	17.9	19.5	20.7	22.1	24.9
25–34.9	24.3	26.4	27.9	29.8	32.6	18.3	19.9	21.2	22.8	26.4
35–44.9	24.7	26.9	28.6	30.2	32.7	18.6	20.5	21.8	23.6	27.2
45–54.9	23.9	26.5	28.1	30.0	32.6	18.7	20.6	22.0	23.8	27.4
55–64.9	23.6	26.0	27.8	29.5	32.0	18.7	20.9	22.5	24.4	28.0
65–74.9	22.3	25.1	26.8	28.4	30.6	18.5	20.8	22.5	24.4	27.9

Source: Adapted from A. R. Frisancho, New norms of upper limb fat and muscle areas for assessment of nutritional status, *American Journal of Clinical Nutrition* 34 (1981): 2540–2545.

TABLE E–7   **Physical Findings Associated with Various Nutrient Imbalances**

PHYSICAL FINDINGS	PROTEIN- kCALORIE	VITAMIN A	B VITAMINS	VITAMIN C	VITAMIN D	IRON	OTHER
Hair Dull, dry, sparse, readily plucked, lighter and darker bands (flag sign), depigmented	x						
Face Swollen	x						
Dark areas of skin over eyes and under cheeks, flaky skin around nose		x					
Pale		x				x	
Eyes Triangular, shiny gray spots on exposed portion of conjunctiva (mucous membrane lining eyelid)		x					
Dull, opaque, or dry cornea		x					
Softening of cornea, inner eyelids		x					

(continued)

TABLE E–7   **(continued)**

PHYSICAL FINDINGS	PROTEIN-kCALORIE	VITAMIN A	B VITAMINS	VITAMIN C	VITAMIN D	IRON	OTHER
Inner eyelids and whites dry and pigmented		x					
Cracked and red at corners			x				
Pale conjunctiva			x			x	
White ring around iris							Elevated blood lipids
Raised yellow spots on eye							Elevated blood lipids
Lips							
Bilateral redness, cracking, scaling, or scarring at corners of mouth			x				
Swollen, red lips with vertical cracks			x				
Tongue							
Swollen, magenta colored			x				
Smooth surface			x				
Atrophy of the surface structures			x				
Bright red, painful			x				
Teeth							
Caries							Excess sugar
Mottled enamel							Excess fluoride
Gums							
Bleeding, spongy, receding				x			
Glands							
Enlarged thyroid gland (located at front of neck)							Iodine
Enlarged parotid gland (located just below earlobes)	x						General undernutrition
Skin							
Depigmentation, patches of hyperpigmented skin that peels off (flaky-paint dermatosis)	x						
Dry, scaling, rough (skin may appear to have permanent goosebumps)		x					Essential fatty acids
Bilateral hyperpigmentation with redness and swelling on body areas exposed to sunlight; scrotal or vulval dermatosis			x				
Small red or purple skin hemorrhages				x			
Nails							
Spoon-shaped, brittle, ridged						x	
Pale nail beds						x	
Subcutaneous tissue							
Edematous (swollen)	x						
Decreased fat stores	x						
Excessive fat stores							Obesity

TABLE E-8   Relationship between
Degree of Undernutrition and Serum Proteins

DEGREE OF DEPLETION	INDICATOR	
	Albumin (g/100 ml)	*Transferrin (mg/100 ml)*
Mild	2.8–3.4	150–200
Moderate	2.1–2.7	100–149
Severe	<2.1	<100

TABLE E-9A   Creatinine Excretion Standards for Men

HEIGHT		SMALL FRAME		MEDIUM FRAME		LARGE FRAME	
in	*cm*	*Ideal weight (kg)*	*Creatinine (mg per 24 hr)*	*Ideal weight (kg)*	*Creatinine (mg per 24 hr)*	*Ideal weight (kg)*	*Creatinine (mg per 24 hr)*
61	154.9	52.7	1,212	56.1	1,290	60.7	1,396
62	157.5	54.1	1,244	57.7	1,327	62.0	1,426
63	160.0	55.4	1,274	59.1	1,359	63.6	1,463
64	162.5	56.8	1,306	60.4	1,389	65.2	1,500
65	165.1	58.4	1,343	62.0	1,426	66.8	1,536
66	167.6	60.2	1,385	63.9	1,470	68.9	1,585
67	170.2	62.0	1,426	65.9	1,516	71.1	1,635
68	172.7	63.9	1,470	67.7	1,557	72.9	1,677
69	175.3	65.9	1,516	69.5	1,598	74.8	1,720
70	177.8	67.7	1,557	71.6	1,647	76.8	1,766
71	180.3	69.5	1,599	73.6	1,693	79.1	1,819
72	182.9	71.4	1,642	75.7	1,741	81.1	1,865
73	185.4	73.4	1,688	77.7	1,787	83.4	1,918
74	187.9	75.2	1,730	80.0	1,846	85.7	1,971
75	190.5	77.0	1,771	82.3	1,893	87.7	2,017

TABLE E-9B   Creatinine Excretion Standards for Women

HEIGHT		SMALL FRAME		MEDIUM FRAME		LARGE FRAME	
in	*cm*	*Ideal weight (kg)*	*Creatinine (mg per 24 hr)*	*Ideal weight (kg)*	*Creatinine (mg per 24 hr)*	*Ideal weight (kg)*	*Creatinine (mg per 24 hr)*
56	142.2	43.2	778	46.1	830	50.7	913
57	144.8	44.3	797	47.3	851	51.8	932
58	147.3	45.4	817	48.6	875	53.2	958
59	149.8	46.8	842	50.0	900	54.5	981
60	152.4	48.2	868	51.4	925	55.9	1,006
61	154.9	49.5	891	52.7	949	57.3	1,031
62	157.5	50.9	916	54.3	977	58.9	1,060
63	160.0	52.3	941	55.9	1,006	60.6	1,091
64	162.5	53.9	970	57.9	1,042	62.5	1,125
65	165.1	55.7	1,003	59.8	1,076	64.3	1,157
66	167.6	57.5	1,035	61.6	1,109	66.1	1,190
67	170.2	59.3	1,067	63.4	1,141	67.9	1,222
68	172.7	61.4	1,105	65.2	1,174	70.0	1,260
69	175.2	63.2	1,138	67.0	1,206	72.0	1,296
70	177.8	65.0	1,170	68.9	1,240	74.1	1,334

Source: A. Grant, *Nutritional Assessment Guidelines*, 2nd ed., 1979 (available from P.O. Box 25057, Northgate Station, Seattle, WA 98125).

FIGURE E–1A   FIGURE E–1B

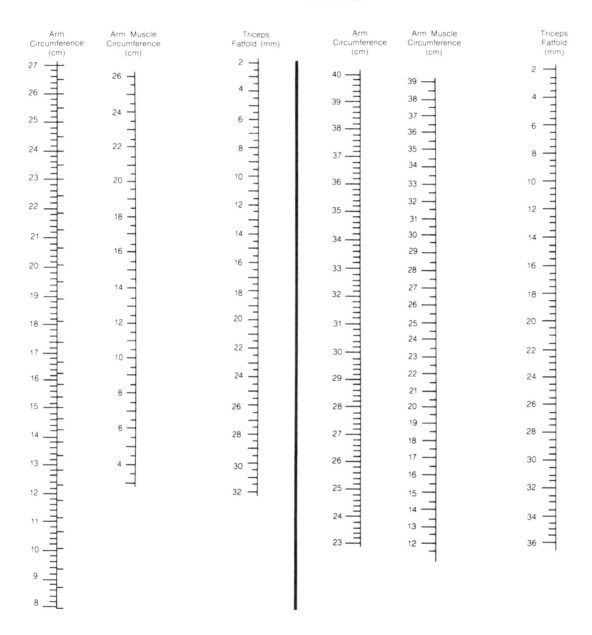

To obtain muscle circumference using either nomogram, lay ruler
between values of arm circumference and fatfold and read off muscle
circumference.

FIGURE E–1 **Nomograms for determination of midarm muscle circumference (MAMC).**

Source: Reproduced with permission from J. Gurney and D. Jelliffe, Arm anthropometry in nutritional assessment; nomogram for rapid calculation of muscle circumference and cross-sectional muscle and fat areas, *American Journal of Clinical Nutrition* 26 (1973): 912, as adapted by A. Grant, *Nutritional Assessment Guidelines*, 2nd ed., 1979 (available from P.O. Box 25057, Northgate Station, Seattle, WA 98125).

GIRLS: BIRTH TO 36 MONTHS
PHYSICAL GROWTH
NCHS PERCENTILES*

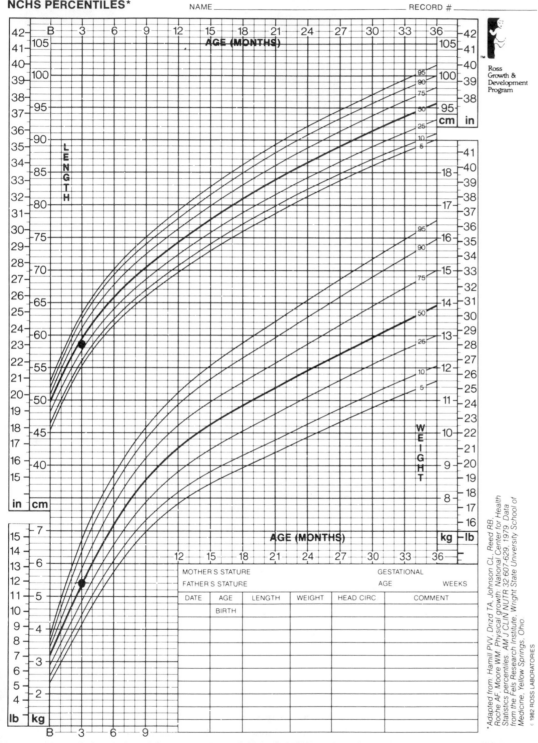

FIGURE E-2A Girls: Birth to 36 months physical growth NCHS percentiles—length and weight for age.

BOYS: BIRTH TO 36 MONTHS
PHYSICAL GROWTH
NCHS PERCENTILES*

NAME _____ RECORD # _____

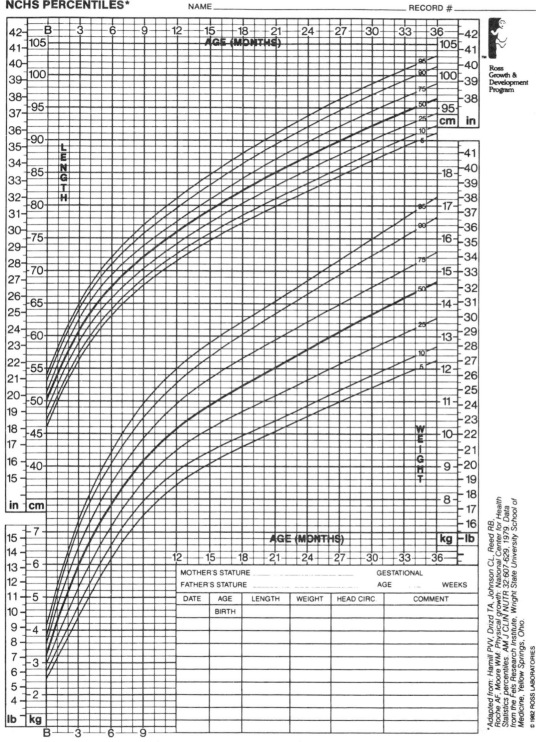

Ross
Growth &
Development
Program

*Adapted from: Hamill PVV, Drizd TA, Johnson CL, Reed RB, Roche AF, Moore WM. Physical growth: National Center for Health Statistics percentiles. AM J CLIN NUTR 32:607-629, 1979. Data from the Fels Research Institute, Wright State University School of Medicine, Yellow Springs, Ohio.
© 1982 ROSS LABORATORIES

| MOTHER'S STATURE | | GESTATIONAL | | | |
| FATHER'S STATURE | | AGE | | WEEKS | |

DATE	AGE	LENGTH	WEIGHT	HEAD CIRC	COMMENT
	BIRTH				

FIGURE E-2B   Boys: Birth to 36 months physical growth NCHS percentiles—length and weight for age.

GIRLS: BIRTH TO 36 MONTHS
PHYSICAL GROWTH
NCHS PERCENTILES*

NAME _____   RECORD # _____

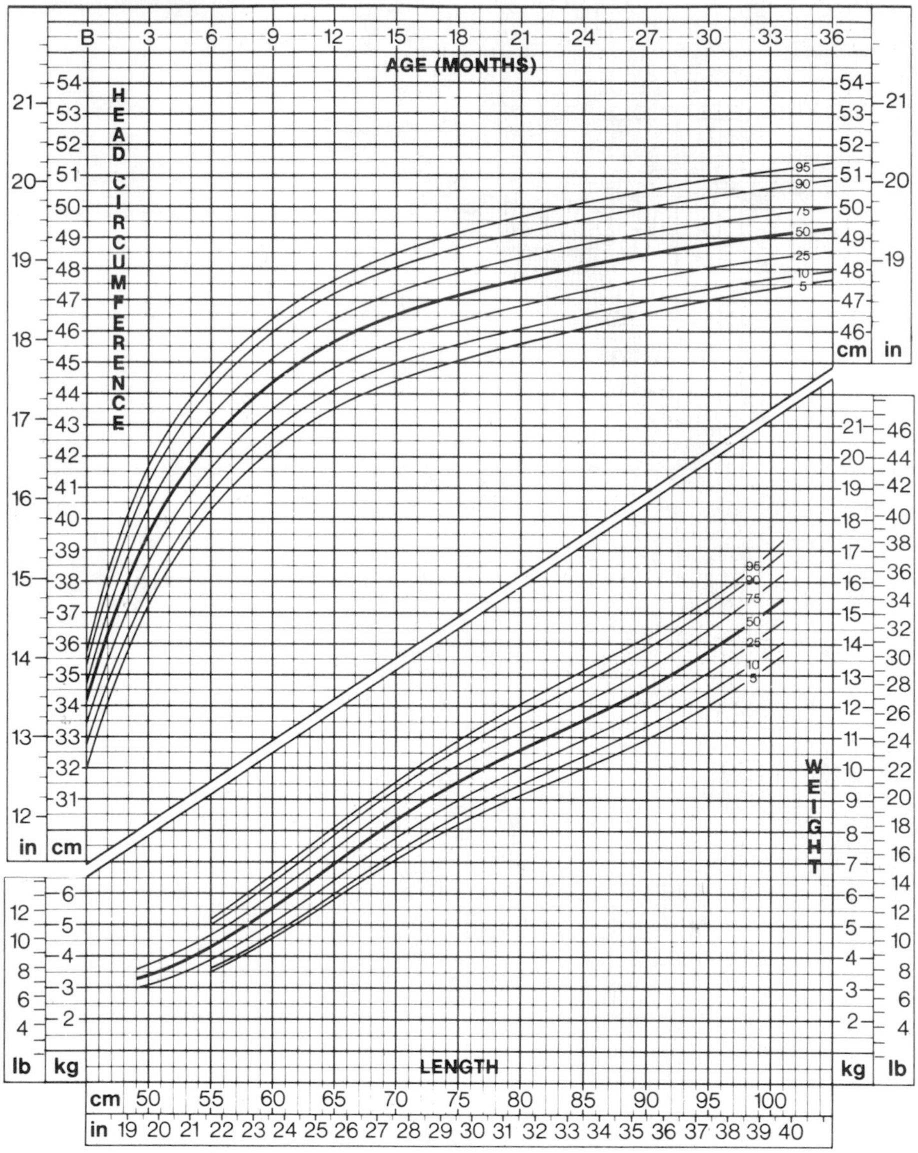

FIGURE E-3A   Girls: Birth to 36 months physical growth NCHS percentiles—head circumference for age and weight for length.

BOYS: BIRTH TO 36 MONTHS
PHYSICAL GROWTH
NCHS PERCENTILES*

NAME _____   RECORD # _____

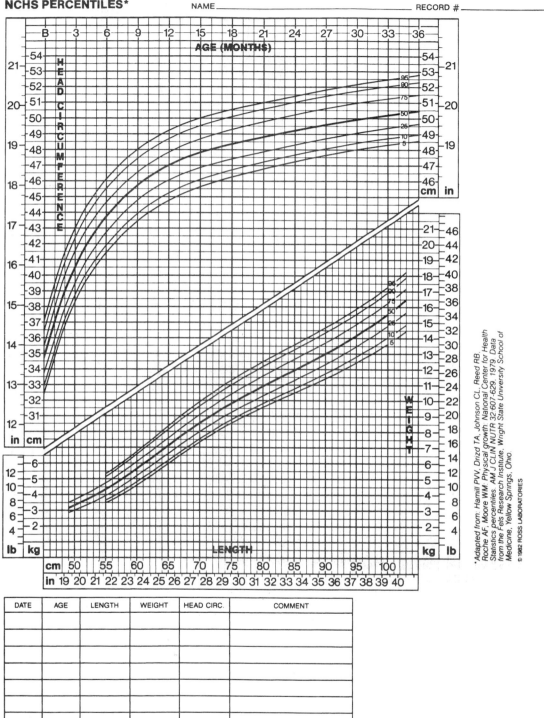

FIGURE E-3B   Boys: Birth to 36 months physical growth NCHS percentiles—head circumference for age and weight for length.

E

GIRLS: 2 TO 18 YEARS
PHYSICAL GROWTH
NCHS PERCENTILES*

NAME _____   RECORD # _____

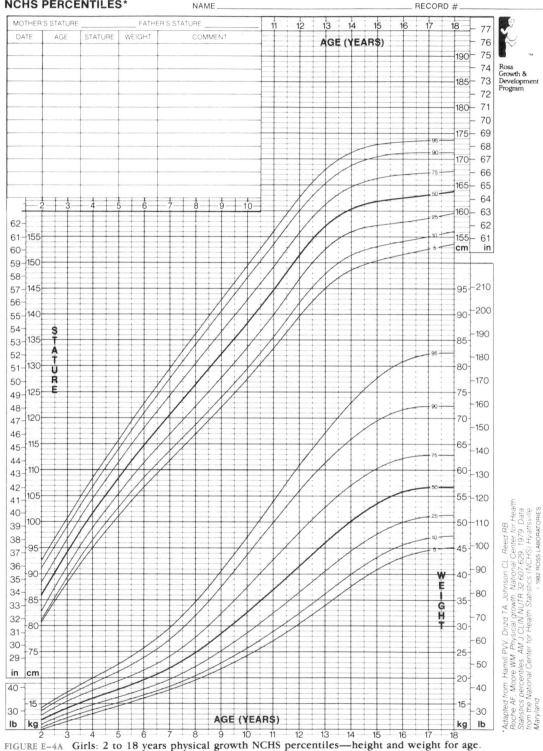

FIGURE E–4A   Girls: 2 to 18 years physical growth NCHS percentiles—height and weight for age.

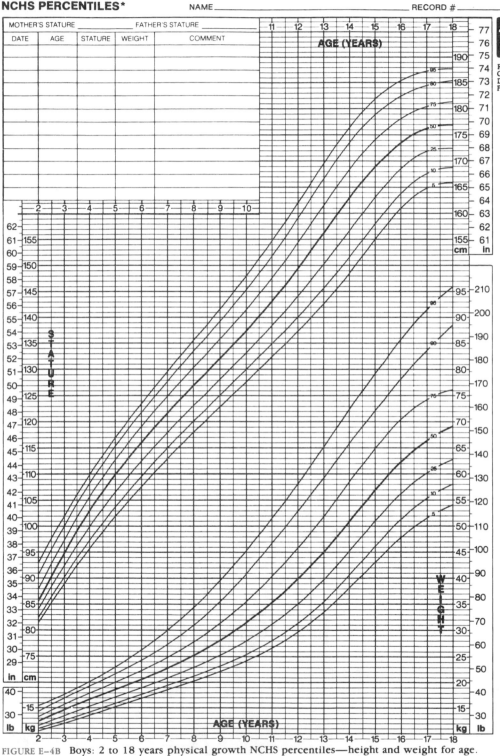

FIGURE E–4B Boys: 2 to 18 years physical growth NCHS percentiles—height and weight for age.

GIRLS: PREPUBESCENT
PHYSICAL GROWTH
NCHS PERCENTILES*

NAME _____ RECORD # _____

E

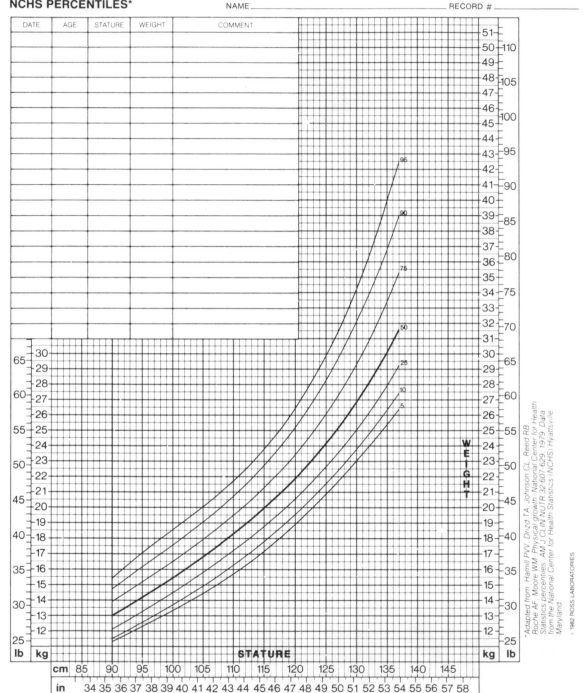

Adapted from Hamill PVV, Drizd TA, Johnson CL, Reed RB, Roche AF, Moore WM. Physical growth: National Center for Health Statistics percentiles. AM J CLIN NUTR 32 607-629 1979. Data from the National Center for Health Statistics (NCHS) Hyattsville, Maryland

c 1982 ROSS LABORATORIES

FIGURE E–5A Girls: Prepubescent physical growth NCHS percentiles—weight for height.

BOYS: PREPUBESCENT PHYSICAL GROWTH NCHS PERCENTILES*

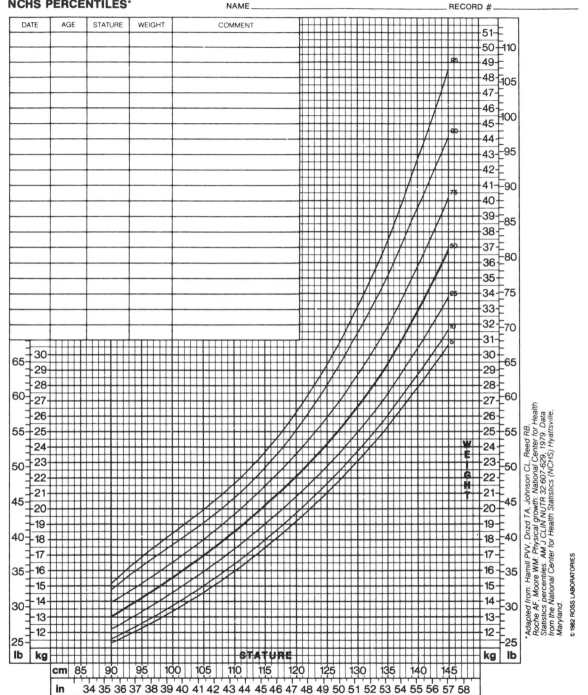

FIGURE E–5B   Boys: Prepubescent physical growth NCHS percentiles—weight for height.

E

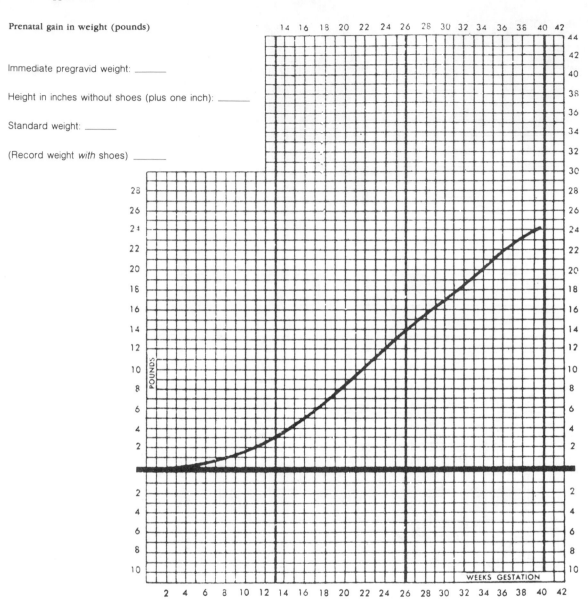

Prenatal gain in weight (pounds)

Immediate pregravid weight: _____

Height in inches without shoes (plus one inch): _____

Standard weight: _____

(Record weight *with* shoes) _____

FIGURE E-6 **Prenatal weight gain grid.**

APPENDIX F
Sugar in Foods

Table F–1 presents the amount of refined sugar in common foods measured in teaspoons. No one will be surprised to see that soft drinks contain a large quantity of refined sugar, but it may be a surprise to learn that sugar is added to dried fruits, hamburger buns, and other items.

You may know that 1 tablespoon is equal to 3 teaspoons and wonder how 4 to 6 teaspoons of sugar could be fitted into a tablespoon of jam or jelly. This is not an error. Dry sugar, being crystalline, takes up more space than sugar in water solution.

TABLE F–1 **Refined Sugar in Common Foods**

FOOD	PORTION SIZE	APPROXIMATE SUGAR CONTENT (tsp)[a]
Beverages		
Cola drinks	12 oz	9
Ginger ale	12 oz	7
Lemon soda	12 oz	11
Orange soda	12 oz	11½
Orangeade	8 oz	5
Root beer	10 oz	4½
Seven-Up	12 oz	9
Soda pop	8 oz	5
Soda water	8 oz	0
Sweet cider	1 c (8 oz)	4½
Tonic water	8 oz	5½

TABLE F–1 (continued)

FOOD	PORTION SIZE	APPROXIMATE SUGAR CONTENT (tsp)[a]
Jams and jellies		
Apple butter	1 tbsp	1
Jelly	1 tbsp	4–6
Orange marmalade	1 tbsp	4–6
Peach butter	1 tbsp	1
Strawberry jam	1 tbsp	4
Candies		
Milk chocolate bar (Hershey bar)	1½ oz	2½
Chewing gum	1 stick	½
Chocolate cream	1 piece	2
Chocolate mints	1 piece	2
Fudge	1 oz square	4½
Gum drop	1	2
Hard candy	4 oz	20
Lifesavers	1	⅓
Peanut brittle	1 oz	3½
Marshmallow	1	1½
Fruits and canned juices		
Raisins	½ c	4
Currants, dried	1 tbsp	4
Prunes, dried	3–4 medium	4
Apricots, dried	4–6 halves	4
Dates, dried	3–4 stoned	4½
Figs, dried	1½–2 small	4

F

TABLE F–1 **(continued)**

FOOD	PORTION SIZE	APPROXIMATE SUGAR CONTENT (tsp)[a]
Fruit cocktail	½ c	5
Rhubarb, stewed, sweetened	½ c	8
Canned apricots	4 halves and 1 tbsp syrup	3½
Applesauce, sweetened	½ c	2
Prunes, stewed, sweetened	4–5 medium and 2 tbsp juice	8
Canned peaches	2 halves and 1 tbsp syrup	3½
Fruit salad	½ c	3½
Fruit syrup	2 tbsp	2½
Orange juice	½ c	2
Pineapple juice, unsweetened	½ c	2⅗
Grape juice, commercial	½ c	3⅖
Canned fruit juices, sweetened	½ c	2
Breads and cereals		
White bread	1 slice	½
Cornflakes, Wheaties, Krispies, etc.	1 bowl and 1 tbsp sugar	4–8
Hamburger bun	1	3
Hot dog bun	1	3
Cakes and cookies		
Angel food cake	4 oz	7
Applesauce cake	4 oz	5½
Banana cake	2 oz	2
Cheesecake	4 oz	2
Chocolate cake, plain	4 oz	6
Chocolate cake, iced	4 oz	10
Coffeecake	4 oz	4½
Cupcake, iced	1	6
Fruitcake	4 oz	5
Jelly-roll	2 oz	2½
Orange cake	4 oz	4
Pound cake	4 oz	5
Sponge cake	1 oz	2
Strawberry shortcake	1 serving	4

TABLE F–1 **(continued)**

FOOD	PORTION SIZE	APPROXIMATE SUGAR CONTENT (tsp)[a]
Brownies, unfrosted	1 (¾ oz)	3
Molasses cookies	1	2
Chocolate cookies	1	1½
Fig newtons	1	5
Ginger snaps	1	3
Macaroons	1	6
Nut cookies	1	1½
Oatmeal cookies	1	2
Sugar cookies	1	1½
Chocolate eclair	1	7
Cream puff	1	2
Donut, plain	1	3
Donut, glazed	1	6
Snail	1 (4 oz)	4½
Dairy products		
Ice cream	⅓ pint (3½ oz)	3½
Ice cream bar	1 (depending on size)	1–7
Ice cream cone	1	3½
Eggnog, all milk	1 (8 oz)	4½
Ice cream soda	1	5
Cocoa, all milk	1 c (5 oz milk)	4
Ice cream sundae	1	7
Chocolate, all milk	1 c (5 oz milk)	6
Malted milk shake	1 (10 oz)	5
Sherbet	½ c	9
Yogurt,[b] sweetened fruit	1 c	9
Desserts		
Apple cobbler	½ c	3
Custard	½ c	2
French pastry	1 (4 oz)	5
Jello	½ c	4½
Apple pie	1 slice (average)	7
Junket	½ c	3
Berry pie	1 slice	10
Cherry pie	1 slice	10

TABLE F–1 **(continued)**

FOOD	PORTION SIZE	APPROXIMATE SUGAR CONTENT (tsp)[a]
Cream pie	1 slice	4
Custard pie	1 slice	10
Coconut pie	1 slice	10
Lemon pie	1 slice	7
Peach pie	1 slice	7
Pumpkin pie	1 slice	5
Raisin pie	1 slice	13
Rhubarb pie	1 slice	4
Banana pudding	½ c	2
Bread pudding	½ c	1½
Chocolate pudding	½ c	4
Plum pudding	½ c	4
Rice pudding	½ c	5
Tapioca pudding	½ c	3
Brown betty	½ c	3
Plain pastry	1 (4 oz)	3
Sugars and syrups		
Brown sugar	1 tbsp	3[c]
Granulated sugar	1 tbsp	3[c]
Corn syrup	1 tbsp	3[c]
Karo syrup	1 tbsp	3[c]
Honey	1 tbsp	3[c]
Molasses	1 tbsp	3½[c]
Chocolate sauce	1 tbsp	3½[c]
Wines		
Wine, medium rosé	3½ oz	¾
Wine, dry white	3½ oz	trace
Wine, medium sherry	3½ oz	1
Vermouth, dry	3½ oz	1½
Vermouth, sweet	3½ oz	4½

[a] Measured in teaspoon equivalents of granulated sugar.
[b] For the total carbohydrate content, add about 3% lactose. Value reflects only sucrose, glucose, and fructose.
[c] Actual sugar content.
Sources: All the values in this table were adapted from: Hidden sugars in foods (a three-page typescript), Department of Pedodontics, College of Dentistry, University of Iowa, Iowa City, Iowa, March 1974, developed by Arthur J. Nowak, D.M.D., professor, College of Dentistry, Department of Pedodontics, University of Iowa, and reprinted with his permission; D. A. T. Southgate, A. A. Paul, A. C. Dean, and A. A. Christie, Free sugars in foods, *Journal of Human Nutrition* 32 (1978): 335–347; and M. C. Martin-Villa, C. Vidal-Valverde, and E. Rojas-Hidalgo, Soluble sugars in soft drinks, *American Journal of Clinical Nutrition* 34 (1981): 2151–2153.

Table F–2 shows which brands of ready-to-eat cereals have the most and which have the least refined sugar. The percentages of sugar per cereal weight are arranged in rank order, from lowest to highest. The dentist who published most of this information suggested, tentatively, that to avoid promoting the development of dental decay, the consumer should choose cereals containing less than 20 percent refined sugar.

TABLE F–2 **Refined Sugar (Sucrose) in Breakfast Cereals**

CEREAL	SUCROSE (percent)
Less than 10 percent sucrose[a]	
Shredded Wheat, large biscuit	1.0
Shredded Wheat, spoon-size biscuit	1.3
Cheerios	2.2
Puffed Rice	2.4
Uncle Sam Cereal	2.4
Wheat Chex	2.6
Grape Nut Flakes	3.3
Puffed Wheat	3.5
Alpen	3.8
Post Toasties	4.1
Product 19	4.1
Corn Total	4.4
Special K	4.4
Wheaties	4.7
Corn Flakes, Kroger	5.1
Peanut Butter	5.2
Grape Nuts	6.6
Corn Flakes, Food Club	7.0
Crispy Rice	7.3
Corn Chex	7.5
Corn Flakes, Kellogg	7.8
Total	8.1
Rice Chex	8.5
Crisp Rice	8.8
Raisin Bran, Skinner	9.6
Concentrate	9.9
10 to 19 percent sucrose	
Rice Krispies, Kellogg	10.0
Raisin Bran, Kellogg	10.6
Buck Wheat	13.6
Life	14.5
Granola, with dates	14.5

F

TABLE F-2   (continued)

CEREAL	SUCROSE (percent)
Granola, with raisins	14.5
Sugar-Frosted Corn Flakes	15.6
40% Bran Flakes, Post	15.8
Team	15.9
Brown Sugar–Cinnamon Frosted Mini Wheats	16.0
40% Bran Flakes, Kellogg	16.2
Granola, plain	16.6
Quaker 100% Natural, with brown sugar and honey	18.2
100% Bran	18.4
20 to 29 percent sucrose	
All Bran	20.0
C.W. Post, plain	21.0
Heartland, coconut	21.2
Granola, with almonds and filberts	21.4
Quaker 100% Natural, with apples and cinnamon	21.9
Fortified Oat Flakes	22.2
Familia	22.4
Vita Crunch, regular	22.7
Heartland	23.1
Nature Valley Granola, with cinnamon and raisins	24.0
C.W. Post, with raisins	24.3
Super Sugar Chex	24.5
Heartland, with raisins	24.7
Quaker 100% Natural, with raisins and dates	25.0
Country Morning	25.8
Vita Crunch, with raisins	26.0
Vita Crunch, with almonds	26.5
Nature Valley Granola, with fruit and nuts	28.0
Sugar Frosted Flakes	29.0
30 to 39 percent sucrose	
Bran Buds	30.2
Sugar Sparkled Corn Flakes	32.2
Frosted Mini Wheats	33.6
Sugar Pops	37.8
40 to 49.5 percent sucrose	
Alpha Bits	40.3
Sir Grapefellow	40.7
Super Sugar Crisp	40.7

TABLE F-2   (continued)

CEREAL	SUCROSE (percent)
Cocoa Puffs	43.0
Cap'n Crunch	43.3
Crunch Berries	43.4
Kaboom	43.8
Frankenberry	44.0
Frosted Flakes	44.0
Count Chocula	44.2
Orange Quangeroos	44.7
Quisp	44.9
Boo Berry	45.7
Vanilly Crunch	45.8
Baron Von Redberry	45.8
Cocoa Krispies	45.9
Trix	46.6
Froot Loops	47.4
Honeycomb	48.8
Pink Panther	49.2
50 to 59 percent sucrose	
Cinnamon Crunch	50.3
Lucky Charms	50.4
Cocoa Pebbles	53.5
Apple Jacks	55.0
Fruity Pebbles	55.1
King Vitamin	58.5
More than 60 percent sucrose	
Sugar Smacks	61.3
Super Orange Crisp	68.0

[a] The glucose content of these cereals is less than 5 percent, except for Special K and Kellogg Corn Flakes (6.4 percent), Kellogg Raisin Bran (14.1 percent), and Heartland, with raisins (5.6 percent). Other sugars, such as fructose, were not analyzed.

Sources: B. W. Li and P. J. Schuhmann, Gas chromatographic analysis of sugars in granola cereals, *Journal of Food Science* 46 (1981): 425–427; I. L. Shannon, Sucrose and glucose in dry breakfast cereals, *Journal of Dentistry for Children,* September/October 1974, pp. 17–20. The reader who wants to pursue the subject further might find another article interesting: I. L. Shannon and W. B. Wescott, Sucrose and glucose concentrations of frequently ingested foods, *Journal of the Academy of General Dentistry,* May/June 1975, pp. 37–43. It presents sucrose and glucose contents for diet soft drinks (less than 0.1 percent); commercially available cheeses (less than 2 percent); fresh fruits and vegetables (from 0 to about 5 percent); commercially available luncheon meats (less than 1 percent for those analyzed); commercially available crackers and wafers (from about 1 to 10 percent, except for graham crackers, Cinnamon Treats, Cinnamon Crisp, and glazed Sesame Crisp, which contained from 10 to 30 percent); commercially available breads (less than 1 percent for those analyzed, except for old-fashioned cinnamon loaf); and commercially available snack foods (from 0 to 3 percent, except for Morton's Kandi-roos, which contained almost 50 percent sucrose). Dr. Shannon's data are used here with his permission and that of the publisher.

Sugar amounts in Country Morning, C.W. Post, Familia, Heartland, Nature Valley, Quaker Natural, and Vita Crunch were estimated from sugar amounts in dry weights of cereal, assuming the cereals were 5 percent water (in fact, 10 other cereals ranged from 2 to 8 percent water).

You may also be surprised to learn that sucrose is not only added to foods in processing but is also found as a natural ingredient in many common foods. Table F-3 lists a few of these foods.

TABLE F-3   **Free Sugars in Foods**

FOOD[a]	GLUCOSE (g/100 g edible portion)	FRUCTOSE (g/100 g edible portion)	SUCROSE (g/100 g edible portion)	TOTAL SUGARS (g/100 g edible portion)
Apples	1.5	6.0	3.0	10.5
Bananas	5.8	3.8	6.6	16.2
Grapes, white	7.6	7.4	0.5	15.5
Oranges	2.5	2.2	3.7	8.4
Peaches	1.0	1.1	6.6	8.7
Plums	4.3	2.0	4.9	11.2
Orange juice, unsweetened	3.4	2.8	2.3	8.5
Beans, red, kidney	—	—	3.0	3.0
Cabbage, white	1.7	1.6	0.4	3.7
Carrots	0.8	0.8	3.8	5.4
Sweet corn, on the cob	0.6	0.2	0.8	1.7
Tomatoes	1.1	1.2	0.1	2.4

[a] Raw unless otherwise noted.

Source: Adapted from D. A. T. Southgate, A. A. Paul, A. C. Dean, and A. A. Christie, Free sugars in foods, *Journal of Human Nutrition* 32 (1978): 335–347. This reference shows the breakdown into glucose, fructose, lactose, maltose, and sucrose for about 150 foods, including some unusual ones, such as rose-hip syrup.

F

APPENDIX G
Fats: Cholesterol and Fatty Acids

To adopt a "prudent diet," you are advised to control kcalories and salt intake; to avoid empty-kcalorie foods, especially those high in concentrated sugars; and to make sure that fat intake is kept in line. To manage fat consumption, three measures are recommended: (1) cut total fat; (2) reduce cholesterol intake; and (3) adjust the ratio of polyunsaturated to saturated fat so that it balances in favor of the polyunsaturates.

For the first objective, total fat intake can be calculated as suggested in the Self-Study for Chapter 3 (see Appendix Q).

For the second objective, cholesterol intake can be estimated using Table G-1 in this appendix. Most authorities suggest a cholesterol intake of 300 mg a day or less, although there is some disagreement about this recommendation (see Highlight 3).

As for the third objective, nutritionists tend to think in terms of the P:S ratio (the ratio of polyunsaturated to saturated fat). In general, according to present thinking, the higher the P:S ratio, the better. The P:S ratio of a day's food intake or menu can be calculated precisely using Table G-2. Use the linoleic acid column to compute "P" (polyunsaturated fat intake), and the saturated fat column to compute "S." (Ignore the oleic acid column; this represents monounsaturated fatty acids, which are not part of the P:S ratio.) The ratio is: total grams of "P" to total grams of "S" divided by a factor such that the smaller of the two numbers becomes 1. (Thus a P:S ratio of 10 grams "P" to 2 grams "S" becomes 5 to 1; a ratio of 10 grams "P" to 30 grams "S" becomes 1 to 3. These are expressed as "5:1" and "1:3" respectively.)

The fatty acid values of foods in Table G-2 are taken from USDA's Home and Garden Bulletin No. 72, *Nutritive Values of Foods*.[1] The item numbers are the same as those in

Appendix H. Some item numbers are missing because USDA provided no fatty acid values for these foods; in most cases, their fat content is insignificant anyway. Only a brief description identifies each food; the complete descriptions are in Appendix H.

Table G-3 is for the person who does not wish to go through the precise calculation of P:S ratio. It classifies common fat-containing foods as having high, medium, or low P:S ratios.

TABLE G-1 **Cholesterol Content of Foods**

FOOD	SERVING SIZE	CHOLESTEROL (mg)
Meat, fish, poultry		
Beef, cooked, lean, trimmed of separable fat	3 oz	77
Lamb, lean, cooked	3 oz	83
Pork, cooked, lean, trimmed	3 oz	77
Veal, cooked, lean	3 oz	86
Chicken, dark meat	3 oz	76
Chicken, light meat	3 oz	54
Turkey, dark meat	3 oz	86
Turkey, light meat	3 oz	65
Rabbit, domestic	3 oz	52
Variety meats		
liver (beef, calf, lamb), cooked	3 oz	372
chicken liver	3 oz	480
heart	3 oz	274
sweetbreads	3 oz	396
brain	3 oz	1,810
kidney	3 oz	690

1   C. Adams and M. Richardson, *Nutritive Value of Foods, Home and Garden Bulletin No. 72* (Washington, D.C.: Government Printing Office, 1981).

TABLE G–1   **(continued)**

FOOD	SERVING SIZE	CHOLESTEROL (mg)
Fish		
caviar (fish roe)	1 tbsp	48
cod	3 oz	72
haddock	3 oz	51
halibut	3 oz	51
flounder	3 oz	43
herring	3 oz	83
salmon, cooked	3 oz	40
trout	3 oz	47
tuna, packed in oil	3 oz	56
sardines	1 can (3¾ oz)	109
Shellfish		
abalone	3 oz	120
crab	3 oz	85
clams	3 oz	55
lobster	½ c	57
oysters	3 oz	40
scallops	½ c (scant)	45
shrimp	3 oz	96
Eggs		
Yolk	1 medium	240
White		0
Dairy products		
Milk, whole	1 c (8 oz)	34
Milk, low-fat (2%)	1 c	22
Milk, nonfat (skim)	1 c	5
Buttermilk	1 c	14
Yogurt, low-fat plain	1 c	17
Yogurt, low-fat flavored	1 c	14
Sour cream	1 tbsp	8
Whipped cream	1 tbsp	20
Half and half	1 tbsp	6
Ice milk	1 c	26
Ice cream	1 c	56
Butter	1 tsp	12
Cheese		
American	1 oz	26
Blue or roquefort	1 oz	25
Camembert	1 oz	28

TABLE G–1   **(continued)**

FOOD	SERVING SIZE	CHOLESTEROL (mg)
Cheddar, mild or sharp	1 oz	28
Cottage		
creamed (4% fat)	1 c	48
uncreamed	1 c	13
Cream cheese	1 tbsp	16
Mozzarella, low moisture, part skim	1 oz	18
Muenster	1 oz	25
Parmesan	1 oz	27
Ricotta, part skim	1 oz	14
Swiss	1 oz	28
Nondairy fats		
Lard or other animal fat	1 tsp	5
Margarine, all vegetable		0
Margarine, ⅔ animal fat, ⅓ vegetable fat	1 tsp	3

Source: Adapted from the booklet by the Greater Los Angeles Affiliate of the American Heart Association, *Consumers Guide to Fat: Cholesterol-Controlled Food Products* (Los Angeles: American Heart Association, 1978); and from E. N. Whitney and E. M. N. Hamilton, *Understanding Nutrition*, 1st ed. (St. Paul, Minn.: West, 1977), pp. 537–538.

TABLE G–2   **Fatty Acids in Foods**

FOOD AND MEASURE	SATURATED FAT (g)	OLEIC ACID (g)	LINOLEIC ACID (g)
Dairy Products			
Cheeses			
1. Blue (1 oz)	5.3	1.9	0.2
2. Camembert (1 wedge)	5.8	2.2	.3
3. Cheddar (1 oz)	6.1	2.1	.2
4. (1 cu in)	3.7	1.3	.1
5. (1 cup)	24.2	8.5	.7
6. Cottage, large curd (1 cup)	6.4	2.4	.2
7. Small curd (1 cup)	6.0	2.2	.2
8. 2% fat (1 cup)	2.8	1.0	.1
9. 1% fat (1 cup)	1.5	.5	.1
10. Dry, ½% fat (1 cup)	.4	.1	<.1
11. Cream (1 oz)	6.2	2.4	.2
12. Mozzarella, whole (1 oz)	4.4	1.7	.2

G

TABLE G-2 (continued)

FOOD AND MEASURE	SATUR-ATED FAT (g)	OLEIC ACID (g)	LINOLEIC ACID (g)
13. Skim (1 oz)	3.1	1.2	.1
14. Parmesan (1 cup)	19.1	7.7	.3
15. (1 tbsp)	1.0	.4	<.1
16. (1 oz)	5.4	2.2	.1
17. Provolone (1 oz)	4.8	1.7	.1
18. Ricotta, whole (1 cup)	20.4	7.1	.7
19. Skim (1 cup)	12.1	4.7	.5
21. Swiss (1 oz)	5.0	1.7	.2
22. American (process) (1 oz)	5.6	2.1	.2
23. Swiss (process) (1 oz)	4.5	1.7	.1
24. Cheese food, American (1 oz)	4.4	1.7	.1
25. Cheese spread, American (1 oz)	3.8	1.5	.1
Creams			
26. Half & half (1 cup)	17.3	7.0	.6
27. (1 tbsp)	1.1	.4	<.1
28. Coffee (1 cup)	28.8	11.7	1.0
29. (1 tbsp)	1.8	.7	.1
30. Whipping, light (1 cup)	46.2	18.3	1.5
31. (1 tbsp)	2.9	1.1	1.5
32. Heavy (1 cup)	54.8	22.2	2.0
33. (1 tbsp)	3.5	1.4	.1
34. Topping (1 cup)	8.3	3.4	.3
35. (1 tbsp)	.4	.2	<.1
36. Sour cream (1 cup)	30.0	12.1	1.1
37. (1 tbsp)	1.6	.6	.1
38. Frozen liquid creamer (1 cup)	22.8	.3	<.1
39. (1 tbsp)	1.4	<.1	0
40. Powdered creamer (1 cup)	30.6	.9	<.1
41. (1 tsp)	.7	<.1	0
42. Whipped topping, frozen (1 cup)	16.3	1.0	.2
43. (1 tbsp)	.9	.1	<.1
44. Whipped topping, mix (1 cup)	8.5	.6	.1
45. (1 tbsp)	.4	<.1	<.1
46. Whipped topping, pressurized (1 cup)	13.2	1.4	.2
47. (1 tbsp)	.8	.1	<.1
48. Imitation sour cream (1 cup)	31.2	4.4	1.1
49. (1 tbsp)	1.6	.2	.1
Milks, Milk Products			
50. Whole (1 cup)	5.1	2.1	.2
51. Lowfat, 2% (1 cup)	2.9	1.2	.1
52. Label claim normal protein (1 cup)	2.9	1.2	.1

TABLE G-2 (continued)

FOOD AND MEASURE	SATUR-ATED FAT (g)	OLEIC ACID (g)	LINOLEIC ACID (g)
53. Label claim high protein (1 cup)	3.0	1.2	.1
54. 1% fat (1 cup)	1.6	.7	.1
55. 1% fat normal protein (1 cup)	1.5	.6	.1
56. 1% fat high protein (1 cup)	1.8	.7	.1
57. Skim (1 cup)	.3	.1	<.1
58. Normal protein (1 cup)	0.4	0.1	<.1
59. High protein (1 cup)	.4	.1	<.1
60. Buttermilk (1 cup)	1.3	.5	<.1
61. Evaporated, whole (1 cup)	11.6	5.3	0.4
62. Skim (1 cup)	.3	.1	<.1
63. Sweetened, condensed (1 cup)	16.8	6.7	.7
64. Buttermilk, dried (1 cup)	4.3	1.7	.2
65. Nonfat, instant (1 envelope)	.4	.1	<.1
66. (1 cup)	.3	.1	<.1
67. Chocolate, whole (1 cup)	5.3	2.2	.2
68. 2% fat (1 cup)	3.1	1.3	.1
69. 1% fat (1 cup)	1.5	.7	.1
70. Eggnog (1 cup)	11.3	5.0	.6
71. Malted, chocolate (1 cup)	5.5	—	—
72. Natural (1 cup)	6.0	—	—
Ice Cream; Ice Milk			
73. Thick shake, chocolate (1 container)	5.0	2.0	.2
74. Vanilla (1 container)	5.9	2.4	.2
75. Ice cream, hard (½ gal)	71.3	28.8	2.6
76. (1 cup)	8.9	3.6	.3
77. (3 fl oz)	3.4	1.4	.1
78. Ice cream, soft (1 cup)	13.5	5.9	.6
79. Hard, rich (½ gal)	118.3	47.8	4.3
80. (1 cup)	14.7	6.0	.5
81. Ice milk, hard (½ gal)	28.1	11.3	1.0
82. (1 cup)	3.5	1.4	.1
83. Soft (1 cup)	2.9	1.2	0.1
84. Sherbet (½ gal)	19.0	7.7	.7
85. (1 cup)	2.4	1.0	.1
Puddings, Custards			
86. Custard, baked (1 cup)	6.8	5.4	.7
87. Pudding, homemade chocolate (1 cup)	7.6	3.3	.3

TABLE G–2 (continued)

TABLE G–2 (continued)

FOOD AND MEASURE	SATUR- ATED FAT (g)	OLEIC ACID (g)	LINOLEIC ACID (g)
88. Vanilla (1 cup)	6.2	2.5	.2
89. Tapioca (1 cup)	4.1	2.5	.5
90. From mix, cooked (1 cup)	4.3	2.6	.2
91. Instant, chocolate (1 cup)	3.6	2.2	.3
Yogurts			
92. Yogurt, fruit flavored (1 container)	1.8	.6	.1
93. Plain (1 container)	2.3	.8	.1
94. Nonfat milk (1 container)	.3	.1	<.1
95. Whole milk (1 container)	4.8	1.7	.1
Eggs			
96. Whole (1 egg)	1.7	2.0	.6
97. White (1 white)	0	0	0
98. Yolk (1 yolk)	1.7	2.1	.6
99. Fried (1 egg)	2.4	2.2	.6
100. Hard cooked (1 egg)	1.7	2.0	.6
101. Poached (1 egg)	1.7	2.0	.6
102. Scrambled egg or omelet (1 egg)	2.8	2.3	.6
Fats, Oils; Related Products			
103. Butter (1 stick)	57.3	23.1	2.1
104. (1 tbsp)	7.2	2.9	.3
105. (1 pat)	2.5	1.0	.1
106. Whipped (1 stick)	38.2	15.4	1.4
107. (1 tbsp)	4.7	1.9	.2
108. (1 pat)	1.9	.8	.1
109. Shortening (1 cup)	48.8	88.2	48.4
110. (1 tbsp)	3.2	5.7	3.1
111. Lard (1 cup)	81.0	83.8	20.5
112. (1 tbsp)	5.1	5.3	1.3
113. Margarine (1 stick)	16.7	42.9	24.9
114. (1 tbsp)	2.1	5.3	3.1
115. (1 pat)	.7	1.9	1.1
116. Soft (1 container)	32.5	71.5	65.4
117. (1 tbsp)	2.0	4.5	4.1
118. Whipped (1 stick)	11.2	28.7	16.7
119. (1 tbsp)	1.4	3.6	2.1
Oils			
120. Corn (1 cup)	27.7	53.6	125.1
121. (1 tbsp)	1.7	3.3	7.8
122. Olive (1 cup)	30.7	154.4	17.7
123. (1 tbsp)	1.9	9.7	1.1
124. Peanut (1 cup)	37.4	98.5	67.0
125. (1 tbsp)	2.3	6.2	4.2
126. Safflower (1 cup)	20.5	25.9	159.8
127. (1 tbsp)	1.3	1.6	10.0
128. Soybean (1 cup)	31.8	93.1	75.6
129. (1 tbsp)	2.0	5.8	4.7
130. Soybean-cottonseed (1 cup)	38.2	63.0	99.6
131. (1 tbsp)	2.4	3.9	6.2
Salad Dressings			
132. Blue cheese, regular (1 tbsp)	1.6	1.7	3.8
133. Low-kcalorie (1 tbsp)	.5	.3	<.1
134. French, regular (1 tbsp)	1.1	1.3	3.2
135. Low-kcalorie (1 tbsp)	.1	.1	.4
136. Italian, regular (1 tbsp)	1.6	1.9	4.7
137. Low-kcalorie (1 tbsp)	.1	.1	.4
138. Mayonnaise (1 tbsp)	2.0	2.4	5.6
139. Mayonnaise-type dressing, regular (1 tbsp)	1.1	1.4	3.2
140. Low-kcalorie (1 tbsp)	.4	.4	1.0
141. Tartar sauce (1 tbsp)	1.5	1.8	4.1
142. Thousand Island, regular (1 tbsp)	1.4	1.7	4.0
143. Low-kcalorie (1 tbsp)	.4	.4	1.0
144. Homemade, cooked (1 tbsp)	.5	.6	.3
Fish, Shellfish, Meat, Poultry, Related Products			
147. Clams, canned (3 oz)	0.2	<.1	<.1
148. Crabmeat, canned (1 cup)	.6	0.4	0.1
150. Haddock (3 oz)	1.4	2.2	1.2
151. Ocean perch (3 oz)	2.7	4.4	2.3
152. Oysters, raw (1 cup)	1.3	.2	.1
153. Salmon, canned (3 oz)	.9	.8	.1
154. Sardines, canned (3 oz)	3.0	2.5	.5
157. Shrimp, canned (3 oz)	.1	.1	<.1
158. Fried (3 oz)	2.3	3.7	2.0
159. Tuna, canned (3 oz)	1.7	1.7	.7
160. Salad (1 cup)	4.3	6.3	6.7
Meats			
161. Bacon (2 slices)	2.5	3.7	.7
162. Beef pot roast, regular (3 oz)	6.8	6.5	.4
163. Lean (3 oz)	2.1	1.8	.2
164. Ground beef, 10% fat (3 oz)	4.0	3.9	.3
165. 21% fat (2.9 oz)	7.0	6.7	.4

TABLE G–2 (continued)

FOOD AND MEASURE	SATURATED FAT (g)	OLEIC ACID (g)	LINOLEIC ACID (g)
166. Beef rib roast, regular (3 oz)	14.0	13.6	.8
167. Lean (1.8 oz)	3.0	2.5	.3
168. Beef round roast, regular (3 oz)	2.8	2.7	.2
169. Lean (2.8 oz)	1.2	1.0	0.1
170. Sirloin steak, regular (3 oz)	11.3	11.1	.6
171. Lean (2 oz)	1.8	1.6	.2
172. Braised round steak, regular (3 oz)	5.5	5.2	.4
173. Lean (2.4 oz)	1.7	1.5	.2
174. Corned beef, canned (3 oz)	4.9	4.5	.2
175. Corned beef hash, canned (1 cup)	11.9	10.9	.5
176. Chipped beef (2½ oz)	2.1	2.0	.1
177. Beef stew (1 cup)	4.9	4.5	.2
178. Beef pot pie (1 piece)	7.9	12.8	6.7
179. Chili, canned (1 cup)	7.5	6.8	.3
180. Chop suey, homemade (1 cup)	8.5	6.2	.7
181. Beef heart (3 oz)	1.5	1.1	.6
182. Lamb chop, broiled, regular (3.1 oz)	14.8	12.1	1.2
183. Lean (2 oz)	2.5	2.1	.2
184. Lamb leg, roasted, regular (3 oz)	7.3	6.0	.6
185. Lean (2.5 oz)	2.1	1.8	.2
186. Lamb shoulder roast, regular (3 oz)	10.8	8.8	.9
187. Lean (2.3 oz)	3.6	2.3	.2
188. Beef liver (3 oz)	2.5	3.5	.9
189. Ham (3 oz)	6.8	7.9	1.7
190. Sliced, packaged (1 oz)	1.7	2.0	.4
191. Canned lunchmeat (1 slice)	5.4	6.7	1.0
192. Pork chop, broiled, regular (2.7 oz)	8.9	10.4	2.2
193. Lean (2 oz)	3.1	3.6	.8
194. Pork roast, regular (3 oz)	8.7	10.2	2.2
195. Lean (2.4 oz)	3.5	4.1	.8
196. Pork shoulder, simmered, regular (3 oz)	9.3	10.9	2.3
197. Lean (2.2 oz)	2.2	2.6	.6
Sausages			
198. Bologna (1 oz)	3.0	3.4	.5
199. Braunschweiger (1 oz)	2.6	3.4	.8

TABLE G–2 (continued)

FOOD AND MEASURE	SATURATED FAT (g)	OLEIC ACID (g)	LINOLEIC ACID (g)
200. Brown and serve, link (1 link)	2.3	2.8	.7
201. Deviled ham, canned (1 tbsp)	1.5	1.8	.4
202. Frankfurter (1 frank)	5.6	6.5	1.2
204. Pork link (1 link)	2.1	2.4	.5
205. Salami, dry (1 slice)	1.6	1.6	.1
206. Cooked (1 slice)	3.1	3.0	.2
207. Vienna sausage, canned (1 sausage)	1.2	1.4	.2
208. Veal cutlet (3 oz)	4.0	3.4	.4
209. Veal rib roast (3 oz)	6.1	5.1	.6
210. Fried chicken, breast (2.8 oz)	1.4	1.8	1.1
211. Drumstick (1.3 oz)	1.1	1.3	.9
212. Broiled, ½ chicken (6.2 oz)	2.2	2.5	1.3
213. Canned chicken (3 oz)	3.2	3.8	2.0
214. Chicken a la king (1 cup)	2.7	14.3	3.3
215. Chicken and noodles (1 cup)	5.9	7.1	3.5
217. Chicken chow mein, homemade (1 cup)	2.4	3.4	3.1
218. Chicken pot pie, homemade (1 piece)	11.3	10.9	5.6
219. Roast turkey, dark (4 pieces)	2.1	1.5	1.5
220. Light (2 pieces)	.9	.6	.7
221. Mixed (1 cup)	2.5	1.7	1.8
222. (3 pieces)	1.5	1.0	1.1
Fruits and Fruit Products			
233. Avocado, California (1 avocado)	5.5	22.0	3.7
234. Florida (1 avocado)	6.7	15.7	5.3
Grain Products			
319. Bagel, egg (1 bagel)	0.5	0.9	0.8
320. Water (1 bagel)	.2	.4	.6
321. Barley, raw (1 cup)	.3	.2	.8
322. Biscuit, homemade (1 biscuit)	1.2	2.0	1.2
323. From mix (1 biscuit)	.6	1.1	.7
324. Breadcrumbs, dry (1 cup)	1.0	1.6	1.4
Breads			
325. Boston brown (1 slice)	.1	.2	.2
326. Cracked wheat (1 loaf)	2.2	3.0	3.9
327. (1 slice)	.1	.2	.2

TABLE G–2 **(continued)**

FOOD AND MEASURE	SATURATED FAT (g)	OLEIC ACID (g)	LINOLEIC ACID (g)
328. French or Vienna (1 loaf)	3.2	4.7	4.6
329. French (1 slice)	.2	.4	.4
330. Vienna (1 slice)	.2	.3	.3
331. Italian (1 loaf)	.6	.3	1.5
332. (1 slice)	<.1	<.1	<.1
333. Raisin (1 loaf)	3.0	4.7	3.9
334. (1 slice)	.2	.3	.2
335. Rye (1 loaf)	0.7	0.5	2.2
336. (1 slice)	<.1	<.1	<.1
337. Pumpernickel (1 loaf)	.7	.5	2.4
338. (1 slice)	.1	<.1	.2
339. White, soft crumb, regular loaf (1 loaf)	3.4	5.3	4.6
340. Slice (1 slice)	.2	.3	.3
341. Toasted (1 slice)	.2	.3	.3
342. Smaller slice (1 slice)	.2	.2	.2
343. Toasted (1 slice)	.2	.2	.2
344. White, soft crumb, large loaf (1 loaf)	5.2	7.9	6.9
345. Slice (1 slice)	.2	.3	.3
346. Toasted (1 slice)	.2	.3	.3
347. Smaller slice (1 slice)	.2	.3	.2
348. Toasted (1 slice)	.2	.3	.2
349. White bread cubes (1 cup)	.2	.3	.3
350. Crumbs (1 cup)	.3	.5	.5
351. White, firm crumb, regular loaf (1 loaf)	3.9	5.9	5.2
352. Slice (1 slice)	.2	.3	.3
353. Toasted (1 slice)	.2	.3	.3
354. White, firm crumb, large loaf (1 loaf)	7.7	11.8	10.4
355. Slice (1 slice)	.2	.3	.3
356. Toasted (1 slice)	.2	.3	.3
357. Whole-wheat, soft crumb (1 loaf)	2.2	2.9	4.2
358. Slice (1 slice)	.1	.2	.2
359. Toasted (1 slice)	.1	.2	.2
360. Whole-wheat, firm crumb (1 loaf)	2.5	3.3	4.9
361. Slice (1 slice)	.1	.2	.3
362. Toasted (1 slice)	.1	.2	.3
Breakfast cereals			
363. Grits, cooked, enriched (1 cup)	<.1	<.1	.1
364. Unenriched (1 cup)	<.1	<.1	.1
365. Farina, unenriched, cooked (1 cup)	<.1	<.1	.1

TABLE G–2 **(continued)**

FOOD AND MEASURE	SATURATED FAT (g)	OLEIC ACID (g)	LINOLEIC ACID (g)
366. Oatmeal, cooked (1 cup)	.4	.8	.9
Buckwheat			
383. Buckwheat flour (1 cup)	.2	.4	.4
Cakes			
387. Coffee cake (1 cake)	11.7	16.3	8.8
388. (1 piece)	2.0	2.7	1.5
389. Cupcakes, plain (1 cake)	.8	1.2	.7
390. With icing (1 cake)	2.0	1.6	.6
391. Devil's food layer (1 cake)	50.0	44.9	17.0
392. (1 piece)	3.1	2.8	1.1
393. Devil's food cupcake (1 cake)	1.6	1.4	.5
394. Gingerbread (1 cake)	9.7	16.6	10.0
395. (1 piece)	1.1	1.8	1.1
396. White (1 cake)	48.2	46.4	20.0
397. (1 piece)	3.0	2.9	1.2
398. Yellow (1 cake)	47.8	47.8	20.3
399. (1 piece)	3.0	3.0	1.3
400. Boston cream (1 cake)	23.0	30.1	15.2
401. (1 piece)	1.9	2.5	1.3
402. Fruitcake (1 cake)	14.4	33.5	14.8
403. (1 piece)	.5	1.1	.5
404. Sheetcake, plain (1 cake)	29.5	44.4	23.9
405. (1 piece)	3.3	4.9	2.6
406. Iced (1 cake)	42.2	49.5	24.4
407. (1 piece)	4.7	5.5	2.7
408. Pound cake (1 cake)	42.9	73.1	39.6
409. (1 piece)	2.5	4.3	2.3
410. Spongecake (1 cake)	13.1	15.8	5.7
411. (1 piece)	1.1	1.3	.5
Cookies, Bars			
412. Brownies, homemade (1 brownie)	1.5	3.0	1.2
413. From mix (1 brownie)	.9	1.4	1.3
414. Frozen (1 brownie)	2.0	2.2	.7
415. Chocolate chip cookies (4 cookies)	2.8	2.9	2.2
416. Homemade (4 cookies)	3.5	4.5	2.9
417. Fig bars (4 bars)	.8	1.2	.7
418. Gingersnaps (4 snaps)	.7	1.0	.6
419. Macaroons (2 cookies)			
420. Oatmeal with raisins (4 cookies)	2.0	3.3	2.0
421. Plain, refrigerated dough (4 cookies)	3.0	5.2	2.9

G

TABLE G–2 (continued)

FOOD AND MEASURE	SATUR-ATED FAT (g)	OLEIC ACID (g)	LINOLEIC ACID (g)
422. Sandwich (4 cookies)	2.2	3.9	2.2
Cornmeal			
424. Whole ground, unbolted (1 cup)	.5	1.0	2.5
425. Bolted (1 cup)	.5	.9	2.1
426. Degermed, enriched, dry (1 cup)	.2	.4	.9
427. Cooked (1 cup)	<.1	.1	.2
428. Unenriched, dry (1 cup)	.2	.4	.9
429. Cooked (1 cup)	<.1	.1	.2
Crackers, Pastries, Doughnuts			
430. Graham (2 crackers)	.3	.5	.3
432. Saltines (4 crackers)	.3	.5	.4
433. Danish (1 ring)	24.3	31.7	16.5
434. (1 pastry)	4.7	6.1	3.2
435. (1 oz)	2.0	2.7	1.4
436. Doughnuts, cake, plain (1 doughnut)	1.2	2.0	1.1
437. Raised, glazed (1 doughnut)	3.3	5.8	3.3
Macaroni, Muffins, Pancakes			
441. Macaroni and cheese, canned (1 cup)	4.2	3.1	1.4
442. Homemade (1 cup)	8.9	8.8	2.9
443. Muffins, homemade, blueberry (1 muffin)	1.1	1.4	.7
444. Bran (1 muffin)	1.2	1.4	.8
445. Corn (1 muffin)	1.2	1.6	.9
446. Plain (1 muffin)	1.0	1.7	1.0
447. Corn, from mix (1 muffin)	1.2	1.7	.9
450. Pancakes, buckwheat (1 pancake)	.8	.9	.4
451. Plain, home recipe (1 pancake)	.5	.8	.5
452. From mix (1 pancake)	.7	.7	.3
Pies, Popcorn, Pretzels			
453. Apple (1 pie)	27.0	44.5	25.2
454. (1 piece)	3.9	6.4	3.6
455. Banana cream (1 pie)	26.7	33.2	16.2
456. (1 piece)	3.8	4.7	2.3
457. Blueberry (1 pie)	24.8	43.7	25.1
458. (1 piece)	3.5	6.2	3.6
459. Cherry (1 pie)	28.2	45.0	25.3
460. (1 piece)	4.0	6.4	3.6
461. Custard (1 pie)	33.9	38.5	17.5
462. (1 piece)	4.8	5.5	2.5
463. Lemon meringue (1 pie)	26.1	33.8	16.4
464. (1 piece)	3.7	4.8	2.3

TABLE G–2 (continued)

FOOD AND MEASURE	SATUR-ATED FAT (g)	OLEIC ACID (g)	LINOLEIC ACID (g)
465. Mince (1 pie)	28.0	45.9	25.2
466. (1 piece)	4.0	6.6	3.6
467. Peach (1 pie)	24.8	43.7	25.1
468. (1 piece)	3.5	6.2	3.6
469. Pecan (1 pie)	27.8	101.0	44.2
470. (1 piece)	4.0	14.4	6.3
471. Pumpkin (1 pie)	37.4	37.5	16.6
472. (1 piece)	5.4	5.4	2.4
473. Pie crust, homemade (1 crust)	14.8	26.1	14.9
474. From mix (1 crust)	22.7	39.7	23.4
475. Pizza (1 piece)	1.7	1.5	0.6
476. Popcorn, plain (1 cup)	<.1	.1	.2
477. With oil and salt (1 cup)	1.5	.2	.2
478. Sugar coated (1 cup)	.5	.2	.4
482. Rice, instant, hot (1 cup)	<.1	<.1	<.1
483. Raw (1 cup)	.2	.2	.2
484. Cooked (1 cup)	.1	.1	.1
485. Rice, parboiled, raw (1 cup)	.2	.1	.2
486. Cooked (1 cup)	.1	.1	.1
Rolls, Spaghetti			
487. Brown and serve (1 roll)	.4	.7	.5
488. Cloverleaf or pan, commercial (1 roll)	.4	.6	.4
489. Frankfurter or hamburger (1 roll)	.5	.8	.6
490. Hard (1 roll)	.4	.6	.5
491. Hoagie or submarine (1 roll)	.9	1.4	1.4
492. Cloverleaf, homemade (1 roll)	.8	1.1	.7
495. Spaghetti, with sauce, homemade (1 cup)	2.0	5.4	.7
496. Canned (1 cup)	.5	.3	.4
497. With meatballs, homemade (1 cup)	3.3	6.3	.9
498. Canned (1 cup)	2.2	3.3	3.9
Waffles			
500. Waffle, homemade (1 waffle)	2.3	2.8	1.4
501. From mix (1 waffle)	2.8	2.9	1.2
Wheat Flours			
502. All-purpose, sifted (1 cup)	0.2	0.1	0.5
503. Unsifted (1 cup)	.2	.1	.5
504. Cake, sifted (1 cup)	.1	.1	.3

TABLE G–2 (continued)

FOOD AND MEASURE	SATUR-ATED FAT (g)	OLEIC ACID (g)	LINOLEIC ACID (g)
505. Self-rising, unsifted (1 cup)	.2	.1	.5
506. Whole-wheat, unenriched, stirred (1 cup)	.4	.2	1.0
Legumes (dry), Nuts, Seeds; Related Products			
507. Almonds, chopped (1 cup)	5.6	47.7	12.8
508. Slivered (1 cup)	5.0	42.2	11.3
512. Canned beans, with pork and tomato (1 cup)	2.4	2.8	.6
513. With pork and sweet sauce (1 cup)	4.3	5.0	1.1
517. Nuts, Brazil (1 oz)	4.8	6.2	7.1
518. Cashew (1 cup)	12.9	36.8	10.2
519. Coconut meat, fresh (1 piece)	14.0	.9	.3
520. (1 cup)	24.8	1.6	.5
521. Filberts (1 cup)	5.1	55.2	7.3
523. Peanuts, roasted in oil (1 cup)	13.7	33.0	20.7
524. Peanut butter (1 tbsp)	1.5	3.7	2.3
526. Pecans (1 cup)	7.2	50.5	20.0
527. Seeds, pumpkin (1 cup)	11.8	23.5	27.5
528. Sunflower (1 cup)	8.2	13.7	43.2
529. Walnuts, black, chopped (1 cup)	6.3	13.3	45.7
530. Ground fine (1 cup)	4.0	8.5	29.2
531. English (1 cup)	8.4	11.8	42.2
Sugars and Sweets			
533. Cake icing, coconut, cooked (1 cup)	11.0	.9	<.1
534. Chocolate, uncooked (1 cup)	23.4	11.7	1.0
535. Fudge, from mix (1 cup)	5.1	6.7	3.1
536. White, uncooked (1 cup)	12.7	5.1	.5
537. Caramels, plain or chocolate (1 oz)	1.6	1.1	.1
538. Milk chocolate (1 oz)	5.5	3.0	.3
539. Semisweet (1 cup)	36.2	19.8	1.7
540. Chocolate-covered peanuts (1 oz)	4.0	4.7	2.1
541. Fondant (1 oz)	.1	.3	.1
542. Fudge (1 oz)	1.3	1.4	.6
546. Cocoa powder, with dry milk (1 oz)	.5	.3	<.1

TABLE G–2 (continued)

FOOD AND MEASURE	SATUR-ATED FAT (g)	OLEIC ACID (g)	LINOLEIC ACID (g)
547. Without milk (1 oz)	.4	.2	<.1
553. Syrup, chocolate, thin (1 fl oz)	.5	.3	<.1
554. Fudge (1 fl oz)	3.1	1.6	.1
Vegetables and Vegetable Products			
648. Potatoes, french fries, cooked from raw (10 strips)	1.7	1.2	3.3
649. From frozen (10 strips)	1.1	.8	2.1
650. Hashbrowns, cooked from frozen (1 cup)	4.6	3.2	9.0
651. Mashed, cooked from raw (1 cup)	.7	.4	<.1
652. With milk added (1 cup)	5.6	2.3	0.2
653. From flakes (1 cup)	3.6	2.1	.2
654. Potato chips (10 chips)	2.1	1.4	4.0
655. Potato salad (1 cup)	2.0	2.7	1.3
668. Sweet potatoes, candied (1 piece)	2.0	.8	.1
Miscellaneous Items			
685. Barbecue sauce (1 cup)	2.2	4.3	10.0
697. Chocolate, baking (1 oz)	8.9	4.9	.4
701. Olives, green (4 olives)	.2	1.2	.1
702. Ripe (3 olives)	.2	1.2	.1
708. Soup, made with milk, cream of chicken (1 cup)	4.2	3.6	1.3
709. Cream of mushroom (1 cup)	5.4	2.9	4.6
710. Tomato (1 cup)	3.4	1.7	1.0
711. Soup, made with water, bean with pork (1 cup)	1.2	1.8	2.4
713. Beef noodle (1 cup)	.6	.7	.8
714. Clam chowder, Manhattan (1 cup)	.5	.4	1.3
715. Cream of chicken (1 cup)	1.6	2.3	1.1
716. Cream of mushroom (1 cup)	2.6	1.7	4.5
717. Minestrone (1 cup)	.7	.9	1.3
718. Split pea (1 cup)	1.1	1.2	.4
719. Tomato (1 cup)	.5	.5	1.0
723. Soup, dry, onion (1½ oz pkg)	1.1	2.3	1.0
728. White sauce (1 cup)	19.3	7.8	.8

G

TABLE G–3 **P:S Ratios of Foods**

RELATIVE P:S RATIO	FOODS
High (more than 2½ times as much polyunsaturated as saturated fat)	Almonds
	Corn oil
	Cottonseed oil
	Linseed oil
	Margarine, soft
	Mayonnaise (made with any of the oils in this group)
	Safflower oil
	Sesame oil
	Soybean oil
	Sunflower oil
	Walnuts
Medium-high (about twice as much polyunsaturated as saturated fat)	Chicken breast, skin, thigh
	Freshwater fish
	Peanut oil
	Semisolid margarines
Medium (about equal amounts of polyunsaturated and saturated fat)	Beef, heart and liver
	Chicken heart
	Hydrogenated or hardened vegetable oils
	Pecans
	Peanut butter
	Solid margarines
Low (about a tenth to a half as much polyunsaturated as saturated fat)	Chicken liver
	Lard
	Olive oil
	Palm oil
	Pork
	Veal
Very low (less than a tenth as much polyunsaturated as saturated fat)	Beef, both lean and fat
	Butter
	Coconut oil
	Egg yolk
	Milk and milk products
	Mutton, both lean and fat

G

APPENDIX H
*Table of Food Composition**

by D. D. Truesdell

This table of food composition is not the standard table found in most nutrition textbooks. It is an expanded version of USDA's *Home and Garden Bulletin No. 72* by C. F. Adams and M. Richardson,[1] to which are added the nutrient contents of many other foods people commonly eat. The choice of foods to add was based on a questionnaire distributed to over 300 users of this text. Responses indicated a great need for the composition of vegetarian foods, snack

*   This table was prepared under a grant from the West Publishing Company and is copyrighted, 1984. Data in the table for added vegetarian foods are from a published article in the *Journal of the American Dietetic Association*, also copyrighted, and used with the permission of the authors and the American Dietetic Association. Rights to the use of the data in this table must be obtained by writing to the West Publishing Company (address on back of copyright page), and the American Dietetic Association (address in Appendix J).

1   C. Adams and M. Richardson, *Nutritive Value of Foods, Home and Garden Bulletin No. 72* (Washington, D.C.: Government Printing Office, 1981). This bulletin, reporting the nutrient contents of 730 foods, can be purchased from the Government Printing Office (address in Appendix J) as a softcover booklet. However, this bulletin does not include the zinc and folacin contents of foods, the foods added in this appendix, or vitamin A in RE.

foods, Mexican-American foods, and Chinese-American foods. The foods most frequently requested are included; among them are a number of Chinese foods and the foods in the vegetarian exchange lists, whose nutrient contents were published in the *Journal of the American Dietetic Association*.[2] Folacin and zinc values for all foods appear for the first time, and the vitamin A values are in retinol equivalents (RE) rather than international units (IU), for the user's convenience in comparing them with recommended intakes.

Few fast foods are listed in this table, but references appear throughout to their location in Appendix N. The nutrient contents of many brand-name products—cookies, snack foods, cookie mixes, canned fruits, TV dinners, condiments, and so forth—are available from *Consumer Guide*.[3] The composition of Mexican foods can be estimated from the data provided in Appendix N for Taco Bell. The composition of a variety of foods used by various ethnic groups, not listed in this table, can be requested from USDA.[4]

A comprehensive compilation of food composition data is presently being published in installments by USDA's Consumer Nutrition Center as *Agriculture Handbooks 8-1, 8-2*, etc. It includes total folacin, vitamin A in IU and RE, and other vitamin and mineral information, as well as the amino acid, fatty acid, fiber, ash, and cholesterol contents of foods.[5]

The data used to create this table were from reliable sources: government publications such as *Agriculture Handbook No. 456*, *Agriculture Handbooks 8-1* through *8-9*, and private publications such as Pennington's *Dietary Nutrient Guide* and Pennington and Church's *Bowes and Church's Food Values of Portions Commonly Used*.[6] An extensive collection of refereed journal sources provided folacin and zinc values, and many of the values reported on legumes, grains, sprouts, seeds, and nuts. R. Matthews in personal correspondence from the Consumer Nutrition Center, USDA, provided many of the values not available elsewhere.[7] Occasionally, industry representatives provided the nutrient contents of their products (see table notes).

Estimates of nutrient amounts for the foods and nutrients added here include all possible adjustments in the interest of accuracy. Whenever water percentages were available, estimates of nutrient amounts were adjusted for water content. When no water was given, water percentage was assumed to be that shown in the table. Whenever a weight was not reported and could not be estimated from available data, the weight of a typical product is given. When estimates of nutrient amounts in cooked foods were derived from reported amounts in raw foods, published retention factors were applied.[8]

Nutrient amounts appear wherever values were missing in the USDA table or expressed by USDA as "—" or "trace."

2   Nutrient amounts in Chinese foods were kindly provided by Professor Stanley Winter of Golden West College, Huntington Beach, California, from his nutrient data bank. The exchange lists appear in *Supplement to Exchange Lists for Meal Planning, Vegetarian Cookery* (Washington, D.C.: The American Diabetes Association, 1978), available from the American Dietetic Association, Washington, D.C. Area Affiliate, 4405 East-West Highway, Suite 403, Bethesda, MD 20014. The nutrient amounts in the vegetarian foods were published in D. D. Truesdell, E. N. Whitney, and P. B. Acosta, Nutrients in vegetarian foods, *Journal of the American Dietetic Association* 84 (1984): 26-35, and are used with permission of the authors and the American Dietetic Association.

3   *Food: The Brand Name Game* (Skokie, Ill.: Consumer Guide, 1974).

4   *Composition of Foods Used by Ethnic Groups: Selected References to Sources of Data* can be requested from the Food and Diet Appraisal Group, Consumer and Food Economics Institute, U.S. Department of Agriculture, Agricultural Research Service, Hyattsville, MD 20782. For Japanese-American food equivalents, a reprint is available from the American Dietetic Association (address in Appendix J).

5   *Agriculture Handbooks No. 8-1* through *8-9* can be purchased from the Government Printing Office (address in Appendix J).

6   C. F. Adams, *Nutritive Value of American Foods in Common Units, Agriculture Handbook No. 456* (Washington, D.C.: Government Printing Office, 1975); L. P. Posati and M. L. Orr, *Composition of Foods: Dairy and Egg Products—Raw, Processed, Prepared, Agriculture Handbook No. 8-1*, rev. ed. (Washington, D.C.: Government Printing Office, 1976) and its sequels on poultry products, sausages, herbs and spices, soups, and other foods; J. A. T. Pennington, *Dietary Nutrient Guide Using Index Nutrients per Serving Size of Mini-List Foods*, pp. 74-113 (available from the Avi Publishing Company, Inc., P.O. Box 831, Westport, CT 06881), from which permission was granted to use the values that appear in this table; J. A. T. Pennington and H. N. Church, *Bowes and Church's Food Values of Portions Commonly Used*, 13th ed. (New York: Harper and Row, 1980), copyright © 1980 by Helen Nichols Church, B.S., and Jean A. T. Pennington, Ph.D., R.D., from which approximately 20 zinc values are reprinted by permission of Harper and Row.

7   R. H. Matthews, written and telephone correspondence, 1982-1983, Room 314, Federal Building, Consumer Nutrition Division (CND), Human Nutrition Information Service (HNIS), USDA, Hyattsville, MD 20782.

8   S. L. Garland, *Provisional Table on Percent Retention of Nutrients in Food Preparation*, 1982, Nutrient Data Research Group, CND, HNIS, USDA, Hyattsville, MD 20782.

However, the reader can easily tell which are USDA data and which are new. USDA data appear as unshaded numbers *without* parentheses, brackets, or "less than" (<) signs, and all USDA item numbers have been retained (item 613 in the original USDA table still appears as item 613). The new data appear in shaded columns (folacin and zinc) and shaded lines, and their item numbers all include the letter *x*. Where new values are present outside of shaded areas for USDA foods, they are in brackets or appear with "less than" (<) signs. USDA's footnotes also remain as numbered notes, as they were in the original table; an occasional number is missing that applied to columns no longer in the table. The new footnotes have superscript letters (a, b, c) and appear after the USDA notes at the end of the table.

Protein, Lipid, Carbohydrate, Fiber. Protein, total fat, and carbohydrate are included, but individual fatty acid analyses are not. Fatty acid and cholesterol data are presented separately, in Appendix G. Appendix F presents additional information on sucrose in foods, and Appendix K presents fiber contents of foods.

Minerals. Of the minerals in *Bulletin No. 72*, calcium and iron are included in this table, and zinc has been added. Sodium and potassium values are in Appendix I. Phosphorus has been excluded, due to lack of space. This nutrient is widely distributed in foods and deficiencies are unknown.

Folacin. Until recently, not enough data were available to permit accurate estimates of the folacin contents of foods. Data are still scanty, but where data are missing, the gaps are filled using folacin values for closely similar foods. Values are for total folacin, not free folacin; the rationale is that when folacin-containing foods are ingested, additional folacin is freed by enzyme (conjugase) activity in the GI tract. There are considerable differences in the bioavailability of folacin from different food sources, a fact that should be remembered when this table's values are used to estimate folacin intakes from foods.

Vitamin A. The conversion of vitamin A (IU) to vitamin A (RE) was accomplished as explained by the Committee on RDA: IU in animal foods and fortified foods were divided by 3.33; and IU in plant foods by 10.[9] For mixed foods, IU were divided by 5 to estimate RE values. Values in the unshaded

9   Food and Nutrition Board, Committee on Recommended Allowances, *Recommended Dietary Allowances*, 9th ed. (Washington, D.C.: National Academy of Sciences, 1980), pp. 56-57.

(USDA) parts of the vitamin A column, arrived at by dividing by 5, are in brackets.

Niacin. Niacin values are for preformed niacin and do not include additional niacin that may form in the body from tryptophan. See p. 283 for conversion information.

NOTE: To use this table with appropriate conservatism, the student should be aware of the variability of laboratory analyses, of nutrient availability, of individual foods, and many other factors. The nutrient values in Appendix H are taken from values derived by several investigators in various laboratories. The individual values reported are not absolute and do not necessarily reflect the nutrient amount that a person will receive after consumption. Different analytical techniques used in different laboratories, together with variety among the foods analyzed, give rise to differences in reported nutrient contents that are sometimes quite marked.

Even if the values in a table such as Appendix H were absolute, the actual amounts of nutrients in individual foods would vary because of many factors—foremost among them, different methods of processing, storing, and preparing foods. The availability of nutrients is also affected by the presence of other substances in the food they appear in, and in other foods eaten with them. Folacin bioavailability, for example, has been reported to range from 10 to 100 percent. Similarly, the minerals in foods, even foods rich in minerals, may be unavailable due to the presence of fiber, oxalates, and/or phytates. Zinc is better absorbed from white bread, but the amount in unleavened whole wheat bread is more than twice the amount in white bread, more than compensating for the impairment of its availability by other substances in whole wheat bread.

The table in Appendix H presents the amounts of nutrients in foods as analyzed, and does not take varying availability into account. However, the RDA do allow for this varying availability, and a student using Appendix H values who finds that his nutrient intakes compare favorably with the RDA (remembering, of course, that the RDA were designed for groups, not individuals) will in general not be misled by this finding. Still, the concept of varying availabilities is important and should be remembered by anyone working with these data. Further comments on the methodology used to enter data into Appendix H and references on these aspects of food composition data are in the *Instructor's Manual*, Appendix 2.

I gratefully acknowledge the authors' support and contributions to this table. Further information on the data is available on request. For information on the folacin and

H

zinc values and on the added foods, write to D. Truesdell; on the vitamin A values and on the values inserted to replace USDA's dashes (—), write to E. Whitney, both in care of the publisher.

H

TABLE H1 COMPOSITION OF FOODS
(For purposes of calculating, use "0" for "<1," "<1," etc. Where a range is given, use the midpoint.)

Item No. (A)	Foods, approximate measures, units, and weight (edible part unless footnotes indicate otherwise) (B)	Grams	Water (C) Per cent	Food energy (D) kCalories	Protein (E) Grams	Fat (F) Grams	Carbohydrate (G) Grams	Calcium (H) Milligrams	Iron (I) Milligrams	Zinc (J) Milligrams	Vitamin A (K) Retinol equivalents	Thiamin (L) Milligrams	Riboflavin (M) Milligrams	Niacin (N) Milligrams	Folacin (O) Micrograms	Vitamin C (P) Milligrams
	DAIRY PRODUCTS (CHEESE, CREAM, IMITATION CREAM, MILK; RELATED PRODUCTS)															
	Butter. See Fats, oils; related products, items 103-108.															
	Cheese:															
	Natural:															
1	Blue ... 1 oz	28	42	100	6	8	1	150	.1	.8	61	.01	.11	.3	10	0
1x	Brick ... 1 oz.	28	42	105	7	8	1	191	.1	.7	86	(0)	.10	(0)	6	0
2	Camembert (3 wedges per 4-oz container) ... 1 wedge	38	52	115	8	9	<1	147	.1	.9	106	.01	.19	.2	24	0
	Cheddar:															
3	Cut pieces ... 1 oz	28	37	115	7	9	<1	204	.2	.9	91	.01	.11	<.1	5	0
4	Cut pieces ... 1 cu in	17	37	70	4	6	<1	124	.1	.5	55	<.01	.06	<.1	3	0
5	Shredded ... 1 cup	113	37	455	28	37	1	815	.8	3.5	364	.03	.42	.1	21	0
	Cottage (curd not pressed down):															
	Creamed (cottage cheese, 4% fat):															
6	Large curd ... 1 cup	225	79	235	28	10	6	135	.3	.8	112	.05	.37	.3	27	<1
7	Small curd ... 1 cup	210	79	220	26	9	6	126	.3	.8	103	.04	.34	.3	26	<1
8	Low fat (2%) ... 1 cup	226	79	205	31	4	8	155	.4	1.0	48	.05	.42	.3	30	<1
9	Low fat (1%) ... 1 cup	226	82	165	28	2	6	138	.3	.9	24	.05	.37	.3	28	<1
10	Uncreamed (cottage cheese dry curd, less than ½% fat) ... 1 cup	145	80	125	25	1	3	46	.3	.7	12	.04	.21	.2	21	0
11	Cream ... 1 oz	28	54	100	2	10	1	23	.3	.2	121	<.01	.06	<.1	4	0
11x₄	Edam ... 1 oz.	28	42	101	7	8	0	207	.1	1.1	[72]	.01	.11	(0)	5	0
11x₄	Gorgonzola ... 1 oz.	28	39	111	7	9	0	149	[0.2]	[.6-1.6]	[103]	.01	.09	.2	9	0
11x₄	Gouda ... 1 oz.	28	42	101	7	8	1	198	.1	1.1	49	.01	.10	(0)	6	0
11x₄	Gruyere ... 1 oz.	28	34	117	9	9	0	287	[0.2]	[.6-1.6]	[105]	.02	.08	(0)	3	0
11x₄	Liederkranz ... 1 oz.	28	53	87	5	8	0	[110]	[0.2]	[.6-1.6]	[91]	[.01]	[.18]	.1	34	0
11x₄	Limburger ... 1 oz.	28	49	93	6	8	0	141	(0)	[.6-1.6]	[110]	.02	.14	.1	16	0
	Mozzarella, made with—															
12	Whole milk ... 1 oz	28	48	90	6	7	1	163	.1	.7	79	<.01	.08	<.1	2	0
13	Part skim milk ... 1 oz	28	49	80	8	5	1	207	.1	.9	55	<.01	.10	<.1	3	0
13x	Muenster ... 1 oz.	28	42	104	7	9	0	203	.1	.8	90	(0)	.09	(0)	3	0
	Parmesan, grated:															
14	Cup, not pressed down ... 1 cup	100	18	455	42	30	4	1,376	1.0	3.2	212	.05	.39	.3	8	0
15	Tablespoon ... 1 tbsp	5	18	25	2	2	<1	69	<.1	.2	12	<.01	.02	<.1	0	0
16	Ounce ... 1 oz	28	18	130	12	9	1	390	.3	.9	61	.01	.11	.1	2	0
17	Provolone ... 1 oz	28	41	100	7	8	1	214	.1	.9	70	.01	.09	<.1	3	0
	Ricotta, made with—															
18	Whole milk ... 1 cup	246	72	430	28	32	7	509	.9	2.9	367	.03	.48	.3	10	0

H

Parentheses ( ) indicate that no value was found in the literature for the nutrient in the food, but that a value was found for the same food in a slightly different form or prepared in a slightly different way (for example, the value for a raw vegetable, adjusted for nutrient retention, may appear in the place of the value for the cooked vegetable). Brackets [ ] in the shaded areas of the table indicate that the value for that particular food was not found; the value shown is based on a similar food (for folacin in blackberries, for example, the published value for folacin in blueberries is substituted). Brackets in the unshaded areas indicate that the number was substituted for USDA's "—." In these instances, the values were arrived at by reference to other literature sources for the same food or by calculation from recipes. "Less than" symbols (<) are substituted for some of USDA's "—" and "trace," where the available information indicated that the amount of the nutrient, although possibly detectable, was essentially zero. Where an amount of a nutrient was less than half the smallest number in a column (0.5, 0.05, or 0.005), it was rounded off to 0. For a few foods (from Truesdell, Whitney, and Acosta, 1984), ranges are shown wherever two or more published values differed by more than 20 percent.

TABLE H-1   COMPOSITION OF FOODS — Continued
(For purposes of calculating, use "0" for "<1," "<.1," etc. Where a range is given, use the midpoint.)

Item No. (A)	Foods, approximate measures, units, and weight (edible part unless footnotes indicate otherwise) (B)		Grams	Water (C) Percent	Food energy (D) kCalories	Protein (E) Grams	Fat (F) Grams	Carbohydrate (G) Grams	Calcium (H) Milligrams	Iron (I) Milligrams	Zinc (J) Milligrams	Vitamin A (K) Retinol equivalents	Thiamin (L) Milligrams	Riboflavin (M) Milligrams	Niacin (N) Milligrams	Folacin (O) Micrograms	Vitamin C (P) Milligrams
	DAIRY PRODUCTS (CHEESE, CREAM, IMITATION CREAM, MILK; RELATED PRODUCTS)—Con.																
	Cheese:																
	Natural:																
	Ricotta, made with—Continued																
19	Part skim milk	1 cup	246	74	340	28	19	13	669	1.1	3.3	321	.05	.46	.2	10	0
20	Romano	1 oz	28	31	110	9	8	1	302	[.1]	[.8]	48	[.01]	.11	<1	2	0
21	Swiss	1 oz	28	37	105	8	8	1	272	<.1	1.1	73	.01	.10	<.1	2	0
	Pasteurized process cheese:																
22	American	1 oz	28	39	105	6	9	<1	174	.1	.9	103	.01	.10	<.1	2	0
23	Swiss	1 oz	28	42	95	7	7	1	219	.2	1.0	70	<.01	.08	<.1	2	0
24	Pasteurized process cheese food, American.	1 oz	28	43	95	6	7	2	163	.2	.9	79	.01	.13	<.1	(2)	0
25	Pasteurized process cheese spread, American.	1 oz	28	48	80	5	6	2	159	.1	.7	67	.01	.12	<.1	2	0
	Cream, sweet:																
26	Half-and-half (cream and milk)	1 cup	242	81	315	7	28	10	254	.2	1.2	79	.08	.36	.2	6	2
27		1 tbsp	15	81	20	<1	2	1	16	<.1	<.1	6	.01	.02	<.1	<1	<1
28	Light, coffee, or table	1 cup	240	74	470	6	46	9	231	.1	.7	524	.08	.36	.1	6	2
29		1 tbsp	15	74	30	<1	3	1	14	<.1	0	33	<.01	.02	<.1	<1	<1
	Whipping, unwhipped (volume about double when whipped):																
30	Light	1 cup	239	64	700	5	74	7	166	.1	.6	815	.06	.30	.1	9	1
31		1 tbsp	15	64	45	<1	5	<1	10	<.1	0	52	<.01	.02	<.1	1	<1
32	Heavy	1 cup	238	58	820	5	88	7	154	.1	.6	1,061	.05	.26	.1	9	1
33		1 tbsp	15	58	80	<1	6	<1	10	<.1	0	67	<.01	.02	<.1	1	<1
34	Whipped topping, (pressurized)	1 cup	60	61	155	2	13	7	61	<.1	.2	167	.02	.04	<.1	[0]	0
35		1 tbsp	3	61	10	<1	1	<1	3	<.1	0	9	<.01	<.01	<.1	[0]	0
36	Cream, sour	1 cup	230	71	495	7	48	10	268	.1	.6	552	.08	.34	.2	25	2
37		1 tbsp	12	71	25	<1	3	1	14	<.1	0	27	<.01	.02	<.1	1	<1
	Cream products, imitation (made with vegetable fat):																
	Sweet:																
	Creamers:																
38	Liquid (frozen)	1 cup	245	77	335	2	24	28	23	.1	1.2	[1]22	0	0	0	[0]	0
39		1 tbsp	15	77	20	<1	1	2	1	<.1	<.1	[1]1	0	0	0	[0]	0
40	Powdered	1 cup	94	2	515	5	33	52	21	.1	.5	[1]9	0	[1].16	0	0	0
41		1 tsp	2	2	10	<1	1	1	<1	<.1	0	[1]<1	0	[1]<.01	0	0	0
	Whipped topping:																
42	Frozen	1 cup	75	50	240	1	19	17	5	.1	0	[1]65	0	0	0	0	0
43		1 tbsp	4	50	15	<1	1	1	<1	<.1	0	[1]3	0	0	0	0	0
44	Powdered, made with whole milk.	1 cup	80	67	150	3	10	13	72	<.1	.2	[1][58]	.02	.09	<.1	3	1
45		1 tbsp	4	67	10	<1	<1	1	4	<.1	0	[1][2]	<.01	<.01	<.1	0	<1
46	Pressurized	1 cup	70	60	185	1	16	11	4	<.1	0	[1]33	0	0	0	0	0
47		1 tbsp	4	60	10	<1	1	1	<1	<.1	0	[1]2	0	0	0	0	0
48	Sour dressing (imitation sour cream) made with nonfat dry milk.	1 cup	235	75	415	8	39	11	266	.1	.9	[1]2	.09	.38	.2	28	2
49		1 tbsp	12	75	20	<1	2	1	14	<.1	0	[1]<1	.01	.02	<.1	1	<1

(A)	(B)		Grams	(C)	(D)	(E)	(F)	(G)	(H)	(I)	(J)	(K)	(L)	(M)	(N)	(O)	(P)
	Ice cream. See Milk desserts, frozen (items 75-80).																
	Ice milk. See Milk desserts, frozen (items 81-83).																
	Milk:																
	Fluid:																
50	Whole (3.3% fat)	1 cup	244	88	150	8	8	11	291	.1	.7	[b]94	.09	.40	.2	12	2
	Lowfat (2%):																
51	No milk solids added	1 cup	244	89	120	8	5	12	297	.1	1.0	152	.10	.40	.2	12	2
	Milk solids added:																
52	Label claim less than 10 g of protein per cup.	1 cup	245	89	125	9	5	12	313	.1	.1	152	.10	.42	.2	13	2
53	Label claim 10 or more g of protein per cup (protein fortified).	1 cup	246	88	135	10	5	14	352	.1	1.1	152	.11	.48	.2	15	3
	Lowfat (1%):																
54	No milk solids added	1 cup	244	90	100	8	3	12	300	.1	1.0	152	.10	.41	.2	12	2
	Milk solids added:																
55	Label claim less than 10 g of protein per cup.	1 cup	245	90	105	9	2	12	313	.1	1.0	152	.10	.42	.2	13	2
56	Label claim 10 or more g of protein per cup (protein fortified).	1 cup	246	89	120	10	3	14	349	.1	1.1	152	.11	.47	.2	15	3
	Nonfat (skim):																
57	No milk solids added	1 cup	245	91	85	8	<1	12	302	.1	1.0	152	.09	.34	.2	13	2
	Milk solids added:																
58	Label claim less than 10 g of protein per cup.	1 cup	245	90	90	9	1	12	316	.1	1.0	152	.10	.43	.2	13	2
59	Label claim 10 or more g of protein per cup (protein fortified).	1 cup	246	89	100	10	1	14	352	.1	1.1	152	.11	.48	.2	15	3
60	Buttermilk	1 cup	245	90	100	8	2	12	285	.1	1.0	[b]24	.08	.38	.1	12	2
60x	Kefir[a]	1 cup	233	82	160	9	5	9	350	.5	.9	155	.45	.44	.3	20	6
	Canned:																
	Evaporated, unsweetened:																
61	Whole milk	1 cup	252	74	340	17	19	25	657	.5	1.9	[b]185	.12	.80	.5	20	5
62	Skim milk	1 cup	255	79	200	19	1	29	738	.7	2.3	[d]303	.11	.79	.4	22	3
63	Sweetened, condensed	1 cup	306	27	980	24	27	166	868	.6	2.9	[d]303	.28	1.27	.6	34	8
	Dried:																
64	Buttermilk	1 cup	120	3	465	41	7	59	1,421	.4	4.8	[b]79	.47	1.90	1.1	57	7
	Nonfat instant:																
65	Envelope, net wt., 3.2 oz[4]	1 envelope	91	4	325	32	1	47	1,120	.3	4.0	[e]655	.38	1.59	.8	45	5
66	Cup[7]	1 cup	68	4	245	24	<1	35	837	.2	3.0	[d]488	.28	1.19	.6	34	4
66x	Goat's milk	1 cup	244	88	163	8	10	11	315	.2	.9	(117)	.10	.27	.7	2	2
	Milk beverages (see also Appendix N, Fast Foods):																
	Chocolate milk (commercial):																
67	Regular	1 cup	250	82	210	8	8	26	280	.6	1.0	[b]91	.09	.41	.3	12	2
68	Lowfat (2%)	1 cup	250	84	180	8	5	26	284	.6	1.0	152	.10	.42	.3	12	2
69	Lowfat (1%)	1 cup	250	85	160	8	3	26	287	.6	1.0	152	.10	.40	.2	12	2
70	Eggnog (commercial)	1 cup	254	74	340	10	19	34	330	.5	1.2	270	.09	.48	.3	2	4

For notes, see end of table.

H

TABLE H-1 COMPOSITION OF FOODS — Continued
(For purposes of calculating, use "0" for "<1," "<1," etc. Where a range is given, use the midpoint.)

Item No. (A)	Foods, approximate measures, units, and weight (edible part unless footnotes indicate otherwise) (B)	Grams	Water (C) Percent	Food energy (D) kCalories	Protein (E) Grams	Fat (F) Grams	Carbohydrate (G) Grams	Calcium (H) Milligrams	Iron (I) Milligrams	Zinc (J) Milligrams	Vitamin A (K) Retinol equivalents	Thiamin (L) Milligrams	Riboflavin (M) Milligrams	Niacin (N) Milligrams	Folacin (O) Micrograms	Vitamin C (P) Milligrams
	DAIRY PRODUCTS (CHEESE, CREAM, IMITATION CREAM, MILK; RELATED PRODUCTS)—Con.															
	Milk beverages:—Continued															
	Malted milk, home-prepared with 1 cup of whole milk and 2 to 3 heaping tsp of malted milk powder (about ¾ oz):															
71	Chocolate ... 1 cup of milk plus ¾ oz of powder.	265	81	235	9	9	29	304	.5	1.1	100	.14	.43	.7	17	2
72	Natural ... 1 cup of milk plus ¾ oz of powder.	265	81	235	11	10	27	347	.3	1.1	115	.20	.54	1.3	22	2
	Shakes, thick:[a]															
73	Chocolate, container, net wt., 10.6 oz. ... 1 container	300	72	355	9	8	63	396	.9	1.4	79	.14	.67	.4	15	0
74	Vanilla, container, net wt., 11 oz. ... 1 container	313	74	350	12	9	56	457	.3	1.2	109	.09	.61	.5	21	0
	Milk desserts, frozen:															
	Ice cream:															
	Regular (about 11% fat):															
75	Hardened ... ½ gal	1,064	61	2,155	38	115	254	1,406	1.0	11.3	1,315	.42	2.63	1.1	22	6
76	... 1 cup	133	61	270	5	14	32	176	.1	1.4	164	.05	.33	.1	3	1
77	... 3-fl oz container	50	61	100	2	5	12	66	<.1	.5	61	.02	.12	.1	1	<1
78	Soft serve (frozen custard) ... 1 cup	173	60	375	7	23	38	236	.4	2.0	239	.08	.45	.2	9	1
79	Rich (about 16% fat), hardened. ... ½ gal	1,188	59	2,805	33	190	256	1,213	.8	9.7	2,181	.36	2.27	.9	19	5
80	... 1 cup	148	59	350	4	24	32	151	.1	1.2	273	.04	.28	.1	2	1
	Ice milk:															
81	Hardened (about 4.3% fat) ... ½ gal	1,048	69	1,470	41	45	232	1,409	1.5	4.4	518	.61	2.78	.9	24	6
82	Hardened (about 4.3% fat) ... 1 cup	131	69	185	5	6	29	176	.1	.6	64	.08	.35	.1	3	1
83	Soft serve (about 2.6% fat) ... 1 cup	175	70	225	8	5	38	274	.3	.9	55	.12	.54	.2	5	1
84	Sherbet (about 2% fat) ... ½ gal	1,542	66	2,160	17	31	469	827	2.5	10.6	448	.26	.71	1.0	111	31
85	... 1 cup	193	66	270	2	4	59	103	.3	1.3	58	.03	.09	.1	14	4
	Milk desserts, other:															
86	Custard, baked ... 1 cup	265	77	305	14	15	29	297	1.1	[b]1.2	282	.11	.50	.3	[b]27	1
	Puddings:															
	From home recipe:															
	Starch base:															
87	Chocolate ... 1 cup	260	66	385	8	12	67	250	1.3	[2.1]	118	.05	.36	.3	[10]	1
88	Vanilla (blancmange) ... 1 cup	255	76	285	9	10	41	298	<.1	[1.4]	124	.08	.41	.3	(19)	2
89	Tapioca cream ... 1 cup	165	72	220	8	8	28	173	.7	[b].7	145	.07	.30	.2	[b]15	2
	From mix (chocolate) and milk:															
90	Regular (cooked) ... 1 cup	260	70	320	9	8	59	265	.8	[1.4]	103	.05	.39	.3	[10]	2
91	Instant ... 1 cup	260	69	325	8	7	63	374	1.3	[1.4]	103	.08	.39	.3	[10]	2
	Milk substitutes:															
91x₁	Soy milk (unfortified) ... ½ cup	100	91	45	3	3	2	10	.4	.2	0	.28	.60	.2	28	0
91x₂	Soy powder, instant (Soy Quick)[c] ... 2 tbsp. or ½ oz.	14	[10]	50	7	0	5	40	1	[9]	10	.02	.34	.8	[24]	<1

(A)	(B)	(C)	(D)	(E)	(F)	(G)	(H)	(I)	(J)	(K)	(L)	(M)	(N)	(O)	(P)	
91x₈	Flavored with vanilla, coffee, or lemon[d] — 1 container, net wt, 8 oz	227	(89)	200	11	4	32	350	[.2]	1.2	30	.06	.34	[.3]	[25]	<1
	Yogurt:															
	With added milk solids:															
	Made with lowfat milk:															
92	Fruit-flavored[a] — 1 container, net wt, 8 oz	227	75	230	10	3	42	343	.2	1.5	[10]36	.08	.40	.2	19	1
93	Plain — 1 container, net wt, 8 oz	227	85	145	12	4	16	415	.2	1.3	[10]45	.10	.49	.3	17	2
94	Made with nonfat milk — 1 container, net wt, 8 oz	227	85	125	13	<1	17	452	.2	2.0	[10]6	.11	.53	.3	25	2
	Without added milk solids:															
95	Made with whole milk — 1 container, net wt, 8 oz	227	88	140	8	7	11	274	.1	1.3	85	.07	.32	.2	17	1
	EGGS															
	Eggs, large (24 oz per dozen):															
	Raw:															
96	Whole, without shell — 1 egg	50	75	80	6	6	1	28	1.0	.7	79	.04	.15	<.1	32	0
97	White — 1 white	33	88	15	3	<1	<1	4	<.1	0	0	<.01	.09	<.1	5	0
98	Yolk — 1 yolk	17	49	65	3	6	<1	26	.9	.6	94	.04	.07	<.1	26	0
	Cooked:															
99	Fried in butter — 1 egg	46	72	85	5	6	1	26	.9	.6	88	.03	.13	<.1	22	0
100	Hard-cooked, shell removed — 1 egg	50	75	80	6	6	1	28	1.0	.7	79	.04	.14	<.1	24	0
101	Poached — 1 egg	50	74	80	6	6	1	28	1.0	.7	79	.04	.13	<.1	24	0
102	Scrambled (milk added) in butter. Also omelet — 1 egg	64	76	95	6	7	1	47	.9	.7	94	.04	.16	<.1	22	0
	FATS, OILS; RELATED PRODUCTS															
	Butter:															
	Regular (1 brick or 4 sticks per lb):															
103	Stick (½ cup) — 1 stick	113	16	815	1	92	<1	27	.2	<.1	[11]1,052	.01	.04	<.1	3	0
104	Tablespoon (about ⅛ stick) — 1 tbsp	14	16	100	<1	12	<1	3	<.1	0	[11]130	<.01	<.01	<.1	0	0
105	Pat (1 in square, ⅓ in high; 90 per lb) — 1 pat	5	16	35	<1	4	<1	1	<.1	0	[11]45	<.01	<.01	<.1	0	0
	Whipped (6 sticks or two 8-oz containers per lb):															
106	Stick (½ cup) — 1 stick	76	16	540	1	61	<1	18	.1	(<.1)	[11]700	<.01	.03	<.1	2	0
107	Tablespoon (about ⅛ stick) — 1 tbsp	9	16	65	<1	8	<1	2	<.1	0	[11]88	<.01	<.01	<.1	0	0
108	Pat (1¼ in square, ⅓ in high; 120 per lb) — 1 pat	4	16	25	<1	3	<1	1	<.1	0	[11]36	0	<.01	<.1	0	0
109	Fats, cooking (vegetable shortenings) — 1 cup	200	0	1,770	0	200	0	0	0	(.1)	0	0	0	0	(2)	0
110	— 1 tbsp	13	0	110	0	13	0	0	0	(0)	[0]	0	0	0	(0)	0
	Lard:															
111	— 1 cup	205	0	1,850	0	205	0	0	0	.4	0	0	0	0	0	0
112	— 1 tbsp	13	0	115	0	13	0	0	0	0	0	0	0	0	0	0
	Margarine:															
	Regular (1 brick or 4 sticks per lb):															
113	Stick (½ cup) — 1 stick	113	16	815	1	92	<1	27	.2	.2	[12]1,136	.01	.04	<.1	1	0
114	Tablespoon (about ⅛ stick) — 1 tbsp	14	16	100	<1	12	<1	3	<.1	0	[12]142	<.01	<.01	<.1	0	0
115	Pat (1 in square, ⅓ in high; 90 per lb) — 1 pat	5	16	35	<1	4	<1	1	<.1	0	[12]52	<.01	<.01	<.1	0	0
116	Soft, two 8-oz containers per lb — 1 container	227	16	1,635	1	184	<1	53	.4	.5	[12]2,273	.08	.08	.1	2	0
117	— 1 tbsp	14	16	100	<1	12	<1	3	<.1	0	[12]142	<.01	<.01	<.1	0	0

H

For notes, see end of table.

H

TABLE H–1   COMPOSITION OF FOODS — Continued
(For purposes of calculating, use "0" for "<1," "<.1," etc. Where a range is given, use the midpoint.)

NUTRIENTS IN INDICATED QUANTITY

Item No. (A)	Foods, approximate measures, units, and weight (edible part unless footnotes indicate otherwise) (B)		Water (C) Percent	Food energy (D) kCalories	Protein (E) Grams	Fat (F) Grams	Carbohydrate (G) Grams	Calcium (H) Milligrams	Iron (I) Milligrams	Zinc (J) Milligrams	Vitamin A (K) Retinol equivalents	Thiamin (L) Milligrams	Riboflavin (M) Milligrams	Niacin (N) Milligrams	Folacin (O) Micrograms	Vitamin C (P) Milligrams
		Grams														
	FATS, OILS; RELATED PRODUCTS—Con.															
	Margarine:—Continued															
	Whipped (6 sticks per lb):															
118	Stick (½ cup) . . . . 1 stick	76	16	545	<1	61	<1	18	.1	.2	[12]758	<.01	.03	<.1	1	0
119	Tablespoon (about ⅛ stick) . 1 tbsp	9	16	70	<1	8	<1	2	<.1	0	[12]94	<.01	<.01	<.1	0	0
	Oils, salad or cooking:															
120	Corn . . . . 1 cup	218	0	1,925	0	218	0	0	0	(.4)	[<1]	0	0	0	[<1]	0
121	. . . . 1 tbsp	14	0	120	0	14	0	0	0	(0)	[0]	0	0	0	[0]	0
122	Olive . . . . 1 cup	216	0	1,910	0	216	0	0	0	.1	[<1]	0	0	0	<1	0
123	. . . . 1 tbsp	14	0	120	0	14	0	0	0	0	[0]	0	0	0	0	0
124	Peanut . . . . 1 cup	216	0	1,910	0	216	0	0	0	0	[<1]	0	0	0	[<1]	0
125	. . . . 1 tbsp	14	0	120	0	14	0	0	0	0	[0]	0	0	0	[0]	0
126	Safflower . . . . 1 cup	218	0	1,925	0	218	0	0	0	.4	[<1]	0	0	0	[0]	0
127	. . . . 1 tbsp	14	0	120	0	14	0	0	0	0	[0]	0	0	0	[0]	0
128	Soybean oil, hydrogenated (partially hardened). . . . . 1 cup	218	0	1,925	0	218	0	0	0	(.4)	[<1]	0	0	0	[<1]	0
129	. . . . 1 tbsp	14	0	120	0	14	0	0	0	(0)	[0]	0	0	0	[0]	0
130	Soybean-cottonseed oil blend, hydrogenated. . . . . . 1 cup	218	0	1,925	0	218	0	0	0	.4	[<1]	0	0	0	[<1]	0
131	. . . . 1 tbsp	14	0	120	0	14	0	0	0	0	[0]	0	0	0	[0]	0
	Salad dressings:															
	Commercial:															
	Blue cheese:															
132	Regular . . . . 1 tbsp	15	32	75	1	8	1	12	<.1	(.3)	9	<.01	.02	<.1	(8)	<1
133	Low kcalorie (5 kcal per tsp). . . . . 1 tbsp	16	84	10	<1	1	1	10	<.1	(.1)	9	<.01	.01	<.1	(3)	<1
	French:															
134	Regular . . . . 1 tbsp	16	39	65	<1	6	3	2	.1	0	[<1]	[<.01]	[<.01]	[<.1]	[0]	[<1]
135	Low kcalorie (5 kcal per tsp). . . . . 1 tbsp	16	77	15	<1	1	2	2	.1	0	[<1]	[<.01]	[<.01]	[<.1]	[<1]	[<1]
	Italian:															
136	Regular . . . . 1 tbsp	15	28	85	<1	9	1	2	<.1	0	<1	<.01	<.01	<.1	(0)	[<1]
137	Low kcalorie (2 kcal per tsp). . . . . 1 tbsp	15	90	10	<1	1	<1	<1	<.1	[0]	<1	<.01	<.01	<.1	<1	[<1]
138	Mayonnaise . . . . 1 tbsp	14	15	100	<1	11	<1	3	.1	0	12	<.01	.01	<.1	1	<1
	Mayonnaise type:															
139	Regular . . . . 1 tbsp	15	41	65	<1	6	2	2	<.1	[0]	9	<.01	<.01	<.1	<1	[<1]
140	Low kcalorie (8 kcal per tsp). . . . . 1 tbsp	16	81	20	<1	2	2	3	<.1	[0]	12	<.01	<.01	<.1	<1	[<1]
141	Tartar sauce, regular . . . 1 tbsp	14	34	75	<1	8	1	3	.1	(0)	9	<.01	<.01	<.1	(<1)	<1
	Thousand Island:															
142	Regular . . . . 1 tbsp	16	32	80	<1	8	2	2	.1	0	15	<.01	<.01	<.1	<1	<1
143	Low kcalorie (10 kcal per tsp). . . . . 1 tbsp	15	68	25	<1	2	2	2	.1	[0]	15	<.01	<.01	<.1	[<1]	<1
	From home recipe:															
144	Cooked type . . . . 1 tbsp	16	68	25	1	2	2	14	.1	[0]	24	.01	.03	<.1	[<1]	<1

H

FISH, SHELLFISH, MEAT, POULTRY; RELATED PRODUCTS

(A)	(B)	(C)	(D)	(E)	(F)	(G)	(H)	(I)	(J)	(K)	(L)	(M)	(N)	(O)	(P)
	Fish and shellfish (see also Appendix N, Fast Foods):														
145	Bluefish, baked with butter or margarine. 3 oz	68	135	22	4	0	25	.6	.9	12	.09	.08	1.6	4	[<1]
	Clams:														
146	Raw, meat only 3 oz	82	65	11	1	2	59	5.2	1.4	27	.08	.15	1.1	13	8
147	Canned, solids and liquid 3 oz	86	45	7	1	2	47	3.5	1.0	[19]	.01	.09	.9	9	[<1]
148	Crabmeat (white or king), canned, not pressed down. 1 cup	77	135	24	3	1	61	1.1	4.9	[33]	.11	.11	2.6	(27)	[<1]
149	Fish sticks, breaded, cooked, frozen (stick, 4 by 1 by ½ in). 1 fish stick or 1 oz	66	50	5	3	2	3	.1	.3	0	.01	.02	.5	6	[<1]
150	Haddock, breaded, fried[14] 3 oz	66	140	17	5	5	34	1.0	[.7]	[15]	.03	.06	2.7	(14)	2
151	Ocean perch, breaded, fried[14] 1 fillet	59	195	16	11	6	28	1.1	[.7]	[15]	.10	.10	1.6	8	[<1]
152	Oysters, raw, meat only (13-19 medium Selects) 1 cup	85	160	20	4	8	226	13.2	e22.0	224	.34	.43	6.0	24	[<1]
153	Salmon, pink, canned, solids and liquid. 3 oz	71	120	17	5	0	[18]167	.7	.8	18	.03	.16	6.8	17	[<1]
154	Sardines, Atlantic, canned in oil, drained solids. 3 oz	62	175	20	9	0	372	2.5	.9	58	.02	.17	4.6	14	[<1]
155	Scallops, frozen, breaded, fried, reheated. 6 scallops	60	175	16	8	9	[104]	[2.7]	1.3	[22]	[.05]	[.07]	[2.1]	14	[<1]
156	Shad, baked with butter or margarine, bacon. 3 oz	64	170	20	10	0	20	.5	.9	9	.11	.22	7.3	9	[<1]
	Shrimp:														
157	Canned meat 3 oz	70	100	21	1	1	98	2.6	1.8	15	.01	.03	1.5	13	[<1]
158	French fried[16] 3 oz	57	190	17	9	9	61	1.7	(1.7)	[22]	.03	.07	2.3	(8)	[<1]
	Tuna:														
159	Canned in oil, drained solids 3 oz	61	170	24	7	0	7	1.6	1.0	21	.04	.10	10.1	13	[<1]
159x	Canned in water, chunk style 3¼ oz. (1 small can)	70	117	26	<1	0	15	1.5	.4	(9)	(.04)	.09	12.2	15	(1)
160	Tuna salad[17] 1 cup	70	350	30	22	7	41	2.7	1.0	179	.08	.23	10.3	51	2
	Meat and meat products (see also Appendix N, Fast Foods):														
161	Bacon, (20 slices per lb, raw), broiled or fried, crisp. 2 slices	8	85	4	8	<1	2	.5	.2	0	.08	.05	.8	0	[<1]
	Beef,[18] cooked:														
	Cuts braised, simmered or pot roasted:														
162	Lean and fat (piece, 2½ by 2½ by ¾ in). 3 oz	53	245	23	16	0	10	2.9	4.9	9	.04	.18	3.6	3	[<1]
163	Lean only from item 162 2.5 oz	62	140	22	5	0	10	2.7	4.2	3	.04	.17	3.3	3	[<1]
	Ground beef, broiled:														
164	Lean with 10% fat 3 oz or patty 3 by ⅝ in	60	185	23	10	0	10	3.0	3.7	6	.08	.20	5.1	3	[<1]
165	Lean with 21% fat 2.9 oz or patty 3 by ⅝ in	54	235	20	17	0	9	2.6	3.6	9	.07	.17	4.4	3	[<1]
	Roast, oven cooked, no liquid added:														
	Relatively fat, such as rib:														
166	Lean and fat (2 pieces, 4⅛ by 2¼ by ¼ in). 3 oz	40	375	17	33	0	8	2.2	4.9	21	.05	.13	3.1	3	[<1]
167	Lean only from item 166 1.8 oz	57	125	14	7	0	6	1.8	3.2	3	.04	.11	2.6	2	[<1]

For notes, see end of table.

TABLE H-1 **COMPOSITION OF FOODS** — Continued
(For purposes of calculating, use "0" for "<1," "<.1," etc. **Where a range is given, use the midpoint.**)

Item No. (A)	Foods, approximate measures, units, and weight (edible part unless footnotes indicate otherwise) (B)		Grams	Water Per-cent (C)	Food energy kCal-ories (D)	Pro-tein Grams (E)	Fat Grams (F)	Carbo-hydrate Grams (G)	Calcium Milli-grams (H)	Iron Milli-grams (I)	Zinc Milli-grams (J)	Vitamin A Retinol equi-valents (K)	Thiamin Milli-grams (L)	Riboflavin Milli-grams (M)	Niacin Milli-grams (N)	Folacin Micro-grams (O)	Vitamin C Milli-grams (P)
	Meat and meat products:																
	Beef, cooked:—Continued																
	Relatively lean, such as heel of round:																
168	Lean and fat (2 pieces, 4⅛ by 2¼ by ¼ in).	3 oz	85	62	165	25	7	0	11	3.2	4.9	3	.06	.19	4.5	3	[<1]
169	Lean only from item 168.	2.8 oz	78	65	125	24	3	0	10	3.0	4.5	<1	.06	.18	4.3	3	[<1]
	Steak:																
	Relatively fat-sirloin, broiled:																
170	Lean and fat (piece, 2½ by 2½ by ¾ in).	3 oz	85	44	330	20	27	0	9	2.5	4.9	15	.05	.15	4.0	3	[<1]
171	Lean only from item 170.	2 oz	56	59	115	18	4	0	7	2.2	3.3	3	.05	.14	3.6	2	[<1]
	Relatively lean-round, braised:																
172	Lean and fat (piece, 4⅛ by 2¼ by ½ in).	3 oz	85	55	220	24	13	0	10	3.0	4.9	6	.07	.19	4.8	3	[<1]
173	Lean only from item 172.	2.4 oz	68	61	130	21	4	0	9	2.5	3.9	3	.05	.16	4.1	2	[<1]
	Beef, canned:																
174	Corned beef.	3 oz	85	59	185	22	10	0	17	3.7	(1.7)	[0]	.01	.20	2.9	[6]	[0]
175	Corned beef hash.	1 cup	220	67	400	19	25	24	29	4.4	f 4.4	[<1]	.02	.20	4.6	15	[0]
176	Beef, dried, chipped.	2½-oz jar	71	48	145	24	4	0	14	3.6	(4.1)	[0]	.05	.23	2.7	[3]	0
177	Beef and vegetable stew.	1 cup	245	82	220	16	11	15	29	2.9	3.2	[480]	.15	.17	4.7	27	17
178	Beef potpie (home recipe), baked[19] (piece, ⅓ of 9-in diam. pie).	1 piece	210	55	515	21	30	39	29	3.8	b[3.9]	[344]	.30	.30	5.5	b[39]	6
179	Chili con carne with beans, canned.	1 cup	255	72	340	19	16	31	82	4.3	f 4.1	[30]	.08	.18	3.3	41	[2]
180	Chop suey with beef and pork (home recipe).	1 cup	250	75	300	26	17	13	60	4.8	4.5	[120]	.28	.38	5.0	123	33
181	Heart, beef, lean, braised.	3 oz	85	61	160	27	5	1	5	5.0	(5.3)	6	.21	1.04	6.5	(6)	1
	Lamb, cooked:																
	Chop, rib (cut 3 per lb with bone), broiled:																
182	Lean and fat.	3.1 oz	89	43	360	18	32	0	8	1.0	4.1	[0]	.11	.19	4.1	3	[<1]
183	Lean only from item 182.	2 oz	57	60	120	16	6	0	6	1.1	2.7	[0]	.09	.15	3.4	2	[<1]
	Leg, roasted:																
184	Lean and fat (2 pieces, 4⅛ by 2¼ by ¼ in).	3 oz	85	54	235	22	16	0	9	1.4	3.7	[0]	.13	.23	4.7	2	[<1]
185	Lean only from item 184.	2.5 oz	71	62	130	20	5	0	9	1.4	3.0	[0]	.12	.21	4.4	2	[<1]
	Shoulder, roasted:																
186	Lean and fat (3 pieces, 2½ by 2½ by ¼ in).	3 oz	85	50	285	18	23	0	9	1.0	3.7	[0]	.11	.20	4.0	3	[<1]
187	Lean only from item 186.	2.3 oz	64	61	130	17	6	0	8	1.0	3.0	[0]	.10	.18	3.7	2	[<1]
188	Liver, beef, fried[20] (slice, 6½ by 2⅜ by ⅜ in).	3 oz	85	56	195	22	9	5	9	7.5	4.3	a 13,755	.22	3.56	14.0	123	23
	Pork, cured, cooked:																
189	Ham, light cure, lean and fat, roasted (2 pieces, 4⅛ by 2¼ by ¼ in).[22]	3 oz	85	54	245	18	19	0	8	2.2	3.4	0	.40	.15	3.1	9	[<1]

NUTRIENTS IN INDICATED QUANTITY

H

(A)	(B)			(C)	(D)	(E)	(F)	(G)	(H)	(I)	(J)	(K)	(L)	(M)	(N)	(O)	(P)
	Luncheon meat:																
190	Boiled ham, slice (8 per 8-oz pkg.).	1 oz	28	59	65	5	5	0	3	.8	1.1	0	.12	.04	.7	3	[<1]
	Canned, spiced or unspiced:																
191	Slice, approx. 3 by 2 by ½ in.	1 slice	60	55	175	9	15	1	5	1.3	2.4	0	.19	.13	1.8	2	[<1]
	Pork, fresh,[18] cooked:																
	Chop, loin (cut 3 per lb with bone), broiled:																
192	Lean and fat	2.7 oz	78	42	305	19	25	0	9	2.7	3.0	0	.75	.22	4.5	4	[<1]
193	Lean only from item 192	2 oz	56	53	150	17	9	0	7	2.2	2.1	0	.63	.18	3.8	2	[<1]
	Roast, oven cooked, no liquid added:																
194	Lean and fat (piece, 2½ by 2½ by ¾ in).	3 oz	85	46	310	21	24	0	9	2.7	5.3	0	.78	.22	4.8	3	[<1]
195	Lean only from item 194	2.4 oz	68	55	175	20	10	0	9	2.6	2.1	0	.73	.21	4.4	3	[<1]
	Shoulder cut, simmered:																
196	Lean and fat (3 pieces, 2½ by 2½ by ¼ in).	3 oz	85	46	320	20	26	0	9	2.6	2.6	0	.46	.21	4.1	4	[<1]
197	Lean only from item 196	2.2 oz	63	60	135	18	6	0	8	2.3	2.0	0	.42	.19	3.7	3	[<1]
	Sausages (see also Luncheon meat (items 190-191)):																
198	Bologna, slice (8 per 8-oz pkg.).	1 slice	28	56	85	3	8	<1	2	.5	.5	[0]	.05	.06	.7	1	[<1]
199	Braunschweiger, slice (6 per 6-oz pkg.).	1 slice	28	53	90	4	8	1	3	1.7	.8	561	.05	.41	2.3	[<1]	[<1]
200	Brown and serve (10-11 per 8-oz pkg.), browned.	1 link	17	40	70	3	6	<1	[<1]	[.3]	(.3)	[0]	[.10]	[.04]	[.5]	<1	[<1]
201	Deviled ham, canned	1 tbsp	13	51	45	2	4	0	1	.3	(.3)	0	.02	.01	.2	(<1)	[<1]
202	Frankfurter (8 per 1-lb pkg.), cooked (reheated).	1 frankfurter	56	57	170	7	15	1	3	.8	1.1	[0]	.08	.11	1.4	2	[<1]
203	Meat, potted (beef, chicken, turkey), canned.	1 tbsp	13	61	30	2	2	0	[<1]	[.3]	[.3]	[<1]	<.01	.03	.2	[<1]	[<1]
204	Pork link (16 per 1-lb pkg.), cooked.	1 link	13	35	60	2	6	<1	1	.3	.3	0	.10	.04	.5	0	[<1]
	Salami:																
205	Dry type, slice (12 per 4-oz pkg.).	1 slice	10	30	45	2	4	<1	1	.4	.3	[0]	.04	.03	.5	0	[<1]
206	Cooked type, slice (8 per 8-oz pkg.).	1 slice	28	51	90	5	7	<1	3	.7	.7	[0]	.07	.07	1.2	<1	[<1]
207	Vienna sausage (7 per 4-oz can).	1 sausage	16	63	40	2	3	<1	1	.3	.3	[0]	.01	.02	.4	<1	[<1]
	Veal, medium fat, cooked, bone removed:																
208	Cutlet (4⅛ by 2¼ by ½ in), braised or broiled.	3 oz	85	60	185	23	9	0	9	2.7	3.5	[0]	.06	.21	4.6	3	[<1]
209	Rib (2 pieces, 4⅛ by 2¼ by ¼ in), roasted.	3 oz	85	55	230	23	14	0	10	2.9	3.5	[0]	.11	.26	6.6	3	[<1]
	Poultry and poultry products (see also Appendix N, Fast Foods):																
	Chicken, cooked:																
210	Breast, fried,[23] bones removed, ½ breast (3.3 oz with bones).	2.8 oz	79	58	160	26	5	1	9	1.3	1.0	21	.04	.17	11.6	3	[<1]

For notes, see end of table.

TABLE H–1   COMPOSITION OF FOODS — Continued
(For purposes of calculating, use "0" for "<1," "<.1," etc. Where a range is given, use the midpoint.)

Item No. (A)	Foods, approximate measures, units, and weight (edible part unless footnotes indicate otherwise) (B)		Grams	Water (C) Percent	Food energy (D) kCalories	Protein (E) Grams	Fat (F) Grams	Carbohydrate (G) Grams	Calcium (H) Milligrams	Iron (I) Milligrams	Zinc (J) Milligrams	Vitamin A (K) Retinol equivalents	Thiamin (L) Milligrams	Riboflavin (M) Milligrams	Niacin (N) Milligrams	Folacin (O) Micrograms	Vitamin C (P) Milligrams
	Poultry and poultry products:																
	Chicken, cooked:[25]—Continued																
211	Drumstick, fried,[25] bones removed (2 oz with bones).	1.3 oz	38	55	90	12	4	<1	6	.9	1.0	15	.03	.15	2.7	3	[<1]
212	Half broiler, broiled, bones removed (10.4 oz with bones).	6.2 oz	176	71	240	42	7	0	16	3.0	2.2	48	.09	.34	15.5	7	[<1]
213	Chicken, canned, boneless	3 oz	85	65	170	18	10	0	18	1.3	1.0	61	.03	.11	3.7	5	3
214	Chicken a la king, cooked (home recipe).	1 cup	245	68	470	27	34	12	127	2.5	b[3.0]	[226]	.10	.42	5.4	b[11]	12
215	Chicken and noodles, cooked (home recipe).	1 cup	240	71	365	22	18	26	26	2.2	(2.8)	[86]	.05	.17	4.3	(5)	<1
	Chicken chow mein:																
216	Canned	1 cup	250	89	95	7	<1	18	45	1.3	b[1.3]	[30]	.05	.10	1.0	(12)	13
217	From home recipe	1 cup	250	78	255	31	10	10	58	2.5	b[2.5]	[56]	.08	.23	4.3	b[16]	10
218	Chicken potpie (home recipe), baked,[19] piece (⅓ of 9-in diam. pie).	1 piece	232	57	545	23	31	42	70	3.0	b[2.0]	[618]	.34	.31	5.5	b[29]	5
	Turkey, roasted, flesh without skin:																
219	Dark meat, piece, 2½ by 1⅝ by ¼ in.	4 pieces	85	61	175	26	7	0	[7]	2.0	3.5	[3]	.03	.20	3.6	8	[<1]
220	Light meat, piece, 4 by 2 by ¼ in.	2 pieces	85	62	150	28	3	0	[7]	1.0	1.7	[3]	.04	.12	9.4	5	[<1]
	Light and dark meat:																
221	Chopped or diced	1 cup	140	61	265	44	9	0	11	2.5	4.3	[5]	.07	.25	10.8	11	[<1]
222	Pieces (1 slice white meat, 4 by 2 by ¼ in with 2 slices dark meat, 2½ by 1⅝ by ¼ in).	3 pieces	85	61	160	27	5	0	7	1.5	2.6	[3]	.04	.15	6.5	7	[<1]
	FRUITS AND FRUIT PRODUCTS																
	Apples, raw, unpeeled, without cores:																
223	2¾-in diam. (about 3 per lb with cores).	1 apple	138	84	80	<1	1	20	10	.4	<.1	12	.04	.03	.1	4	6
224	3¼-in diam. (about 2 per lb with cores).	1 apple	212	84	125	<1	1	31	15	.6	<.1	19	.06	.04	.2	1	8
225	Applejuice, bottled or canned[24]	1 cup	248	88	120	<1	<1	30	15	1.5	<.1	[10]	.02	.05	.2	<1	35[2]
	Applesauce, canned:																
226	Sweetened	1 cup	255	76	230	1	<1	61	10	1.3	.1	10	.05	.03	.1	2	35[3]
227	Unsweetened	1 cup	244	89	100	<1	<1	26	10	1.2	.1	10	.05	.02	.1	1	35[2]
	Apricots:																
228	Raw, without pits (about 12 per lb with pits).	3 apricots	107	85	55	1	<1	14	18	.5	.3	289	.03	.04	.6	9	11
229	Canned in heavy sirup (halves and sirup).	1 cup	258	77	220	2	<1	57	28	.8	.3	449	.05	.05	1.0	4	10

NUTRIENTS IN INDICATED QUANTITY

(A)	(B)		(C)	(D)	(E)	(F)	(G)	(H)	(I)	(J)	(K)	(L)	(M)	(N)	(O)	(P)
	Dried:															
230	Uncooked (28 large or 37 medium halves per cup). 1 cup	130	25	340	7	1	86	87	7.2	1.0	1,417	.01	.21	4.3	13	16
231	Cooked, unsweetened, fruit and liquid. 1 cup	250	76	215	4	1	54	55	4.5	.7	750	.01	.13	2.5	0	8
232	Apricot nectar, canned. 1 cup	251	85	145	1	<1	37	23	.5	.2	238	.03	.03	.5	3	[35]36
	Avocados, raw, whole, without skins and seeds:															
233	California, mid- and late-winter (with skin and seed, 3⅛-in diam.; wt., 10 oz.) 1 avocado	216	74	370	5	37	13	22	1.3	.9	63	.24	.43	3.5	134	30
234	Florida, late summer and fall (with skin and seed, 3⅛-in diam.; wt., 1 lb.) 1 avocado	304	78	390	4	33	27	30	1.8	1.3	88	.33	.61	4.9	162	43
235	Banana without peel (about 2.6 per lb with peel). 1 banana	119	76	100	1	<1	26	10	.8	.2	23	.06	.07	.8	23	12
236	Banana flakes 1 tbsp	6	3	20	<1	<1	5	2	.2	<1	5	.01	.01	.2	[3]	<1
237	Blackberries, raw 1 cup	144	85	85	2	1	19	46	1.3	.4	29	.04	.06	.6	[9]	30
238	Blueberries, raw 1 cup	145	83	90	1	1	22	22	1.5	.2	15	.04	.09	.7	9	20
	Cantaloup. See Muskmelons (item 271).															
	Cherries:															
239	Sour (tart), red, pitted, canned, water pack. 1 cup	244	88	105	2	<1	26	37	.7	.2	166	.07	.05	.5	20	12
240	Sweet, raw, without pits and stems. 10 cherries	68	80	45	1	<1	12	15	.3	0	7	.03	.04	.3	3	7
	Cranberry apple juice drink. See item 696x5.															
241	Cranberry juice cocktail, bottled, sweetened. 1 cup	253	83	165	<1	<1	42	13	.8	<1	<1	.03	.03	.1	<1	[37]81
242	Cranberry sauce, sweetened, canned, strained. 1 cup	277	62	405	<1	1	104	17	.6	.1	6	.03	.03	.1	4	6
	Dates:															
243	Whole, without pits 10 dates	80	23	220	2	<1	58	47	2.4	.2	4	.07	.08	1.8	10	0
244	Chopped 1 cup	178	23	490	4	1	130	105	5.3	.5	9	.16	.18	3.9	22	0
244x	Figs, dried 3½ oz.	100	26	266	3	1	68	152	2.1	.5	13	.07	.09	.7	9	1
245	Fruit cocktail, canned, in heavy sirup. 1 cup	255	80	195	1	<1	50	23	1.0	.2	36	.05	.03	1.0	[5]	5
	Fruit punch drink. See item 696x4.															
	Grapefruit: Raw, medium, 3¾-in diam. (about 1 lb 1 oz):															
246	Pink or red ½ grapefruit with peel[25]	241	89	50	1	<1	13	20	.5	.2	54	.05	.02	.2	29	44
247	White ½ grapefruit with peel[25]	241	89	45	1	<1	12	19	.5	.2	1	.05	.02	.2	24	44
248	Canned, sections with sirup 1 cup	254	81	180	2	<1	45	33	.8	.2	3	.08	.05	.5	22	76
	Grapefruit juice:															
249	Raw, pink, red, or white 1 cup	246	90	95	1	<1	23	22	.5	.2	[28]	.10	.05	.5	26	93
	Canned, white:															
250	Unsweetened 1 cup	247	89	100	1	<1	24	20	1.0	.2	2	.07	.05	.5	26	84
251	Sweetened 1 cup	250	86	135	1	<1	32	20	1.0	.2	3	.08	.05	.5	26	78
	Frozen, concentrate, unsweetened:															
252	Undiluted, 6-fl oz can 1 can	207	62	300	4	1	72	70	.8	.8	6	.29	.12	1.4	53	286

For notes, see end of table.

H

TABLE H–1   COMPOSITION OF FOODS — Continued
(For purposes of calculating, use "0" for "<1," "<.1," etc. Where a range is given, use the midpoint.)

NUTRIENTS IN INDICATED QUANTITY

Item No. (A)	Foods, approximate measures, units, and weight (edible part unless footnotes indicate otherwise) (B)		Grams	Water Per-cent (C)	Food energy kCal-ories (D)	Pro-tein Grams (E)	Fat Grams (F)	Carbo-hydrate Grams (G)	Calcium Milli-grams (H)	Iron Milli-grams (I)	Zinc Milli-grams (J)	Vitamin A Retinol equi-valents (K)	Thiamin Milli-grams (L)	Ribo-flavin Milli-grams (M)	Niacin Milli-grams (N)	Folacin Micro-grams (O)	Vitamin C Milli-grams (P)
	FRUITS AND FRUIT PRODUCTS—Con.																
	Grapefruit juice:																
	Frozen, concentrate, unsweetened:—Continued																
253	Diluted with 3 parts water by volume.	1 cup	247	89	100	1	<1	24	25	.2	.1	2	.10	.04	.5	9	96
254	Dehydrated crystals, prepared with water (1 lb yields about 1 gal).	1 cup	247	90	100	1	<1	24	22	.2	.2	2	.10	.05	.5	26	91
	Grapes, European type (adherent skin), raw:																
255	Thompson Seedless	10 grapes	50	81	35	<1	<1	9	6	.2	0	5	.03	.02	.2	2	2
256	Tokay and Emperor, seeded types.	10 grapes[30]	60	81	40	<1	<1	10	7	.2	0	6	.03	.02	.2	2	2
	Grapejuice:																
257	Canned or bottled	1 cup	253	83	165	1	<1	42	28	.8	.1	[1]	.10	.05	.5	7	[33]<1
	Frozen concentrate, sweetened:																
258	Undiluted, 6-fl oz can		216	53	395	1	<1	100	22	.9	.6	4	.13	.22	1.5	19	[33]32
259	Diluted with 3 parts water by volume.	1 cup	250	86	135	1	<1	33	8	.3	.1	1	.05	.08	.5	3	[33]10
260	Grape drink, canned	1 cup	250	86	135	<1	<1	35	8	.3	(0)	[<1]	[33].03	[33].03	.3	(<1)	(33)
261	Lemon, raw, size 165, without peel and seeds (about 4 per lb with peels and seeds).	1 lemon	74	90	20	1	<1	6	19	.4	0	1	.03	.01	.1	8	39
	Lemon juice:																
262	Raw	1 cup	244	91	60	1	<1	20	17	.5	.1	5	.07	.02	.2	32	112
263	Canned, or bottled, unsweetened	1 cup	244	92	55	1	<1	19	17	.5	.2	5	.07	.02	.2	25	102
264	Frozen, single strength, unsweetened, 6-fl oz can.	1 can	183	92	40	1	<1	13	13	.5	<.1	4	.05	.02	.2	18	81
	Lemonade concentrate, frozen:																
265	Undiluted, 6-fl oz can	1 can	219	49	425	<1	<1	112	9	.4	(<.1)	4	.05	.06	.7	(12)	66
266	Diluted with 4⅓ parts water by volume.	1 cup	248	89	105	<1	<1	28	2	.1	0	1	.01	.02	.2	11	17
	Limeade concentrate, frozen:																
267	Undiluted, 6-fl oz can	1 can	218	50	410	<1	<1	108	11	.2	(<1)	<1	.02	.02	.2	(10)	26
268	Diluted with 4⅓ parts water by volume.	1 cup	247	89	100	<1	<1	27	3	<.1	(0)	<1	<.01	<.01	<.1	(2)	6
	Limejuice:																
269	Raw	1 cup	246	90	65	1	<1	22	22	.5	.1	2	.05	.02	.2	(32)	79
270	Canned, unsweetened	1 cup	246	90	65	1	<1	22	22	.5	.2	2	.05	.02	.2	20	52
	Muskmelons, raw, with rind, without seed cavity:																
271	Cantaloup, orange-fleshed (with rind and seed cavity, 5-in diam., 2⅓ lb).	½ melon with rind[88]	477	91	80	2	<1	20	38	1.1	.1	924	.11	.08	1.6	143	90
272	Honeydew (with rind and seed cavity, 6½-in diam., 5¼ lb).	1/10 melon with rind[88]	226	91	50	1	<1	11	21	.6	[<1]	6	.06	.04	.9	[68]	34

H

(A)	(B)	(C)	(D)	(E)	(F)	(G)	(H)	(I)	(J)	(K)	(L)	(M)	(N)	(O)	(P)
	Oranges, all commercial varieties, raw:														
273	Whole, 2⅝-in diam., without peel and seeds (about 2½ per lb with peel and seeds). 1 orange	131	65	1	<1	16	54	.5	.3	26	.13	.05	.5	60	66
274	Sections without membranes . . . 1 cup	180	90	2	<1	22	74	.7	.1	36	.18	.07	.7	55	90
	Orange juice:														
275	Raw, all varieties . . . . . . 1 cup	248	110	2	<1	26	27	.5	.1	50	.22	.07	1.0	136	124
276	Canned, unsweetened . . . . 1 cup	249	120	2	<1	28	25	1.0	.2	50	.17	.05	.7	(68)	100
	Frozen concentrate:														
277	Undiluted, 6-fl oz can . . . . 1 can	213	360	5	<1	87	75	.9	.4	162	.68	.11	2.8	331	360
278	Diluted with 3 parts water by volume. 1 cup	249	120	2	<1	29	25	.2	.1	54	.23	.03	.9	109	120
279	Dehydrated crystals, prepared with water (1 lb yields about 1 gal). 1 cup	248	115	1	<1	27	25	.5	.1	50	.20	.07	1.0	(45)	109
	Orange and grapefruit juice:														
	Frozen concentrate:														
280	Undiluted, 6-fl oz can . . . . 1 can	210	330	4	1	78	61	.8	(.5)	80	.48	.06	2.3	(330)	302
281	Diluted with 3 parts water by volume. 1 cup	248	110	1	<1	26	20	.2	.2	27	.15	.02	.7	(109)	102
282	Papayas, raw, ½-in cubes . . . . 1 cup	140	55	1	<1	14	28	.4	.1	245	.06	.06	.4	(3)	78
	Peaches:														
	Raw:														
283	Whole, 2½-in diam., peeled, pitted (about 4 per lb with peels and pits). 1 peach	100	40	1	<1	10	9	.5	.1	**133	.02	.05	1.0	3	7
284	Sliced . . . . 1 cup	170	65	1	<1	16	15	.9	.2	**226	.03	.09	1.7	6	12
	Canned, yellow-fleshed, solids and liquid (halves or slices):														
285	Sirup pack . . . . 1 cup	256	200	1	<1	51	10	.8	.2	110	.03	.05	1.5	8	8
286	Water pack . . . . 1 cup	244	75	1	<1	20	10	.7	.2	110	.02	.07	1.5	8	7
	Dried:														
287	Uncooked. . . . . 1 cup	160	420	5	1	109	77	9.6	.9	624	.02	.30	8.5	<1	29
288	Cooked, unsweetened, halves and juice. 1 cup	250	205	3	1	54	38	4.8	.5	305	.01	.15	3.8	<1	5
	Frozen, sliced, sweetened:														
289	10-oz container . . . . 1 container	284	250	1	<1	64	11	1.4	.1	185	.03	.11	2.0	(18)	#116
290	Cup . . . . 1 cup	250	220	1	<1	57	10	1.3	.1	163	.03	.10	1.8	(16)	#103
	Pears:														
	Raw, with skin, cored:														
291	Bartlett, 2½-in diam. (about 2½ per lb with cores and stems). 1 pear	164	100	1	1	25	13	.5	.2	3	.03	.07	.2	12	7
292	Bosc, 2½-in diam. (about 3 per lb with cores and stems). 1 pear	141	85	1	1	22	11	.4	.2	3	.03	.06	.1	10	6
293	D'Anjou, 3-in diam. (about 2 per lb with cores and stems). 1 pear	200	120	1	1	31	16	.6	.2	4	.04	.08	.2	15	8
294	Canned, solids and liquid, sirup pack, heavy (halves or slices). 1 cup	255	195	1	1	50	13	.5	.2	1	.03	.05	.3	0	3
	Pineapple:														
295	Raw, diced . . . . 1 cup	155	80	1	<1	21	26	.8	.1	11	.14	.05	.3	16	26

For notes, see end of table.

TABLE H-1   COMPOSITION OF FOODS — Continued
(For purposes of calculating, use "0" for "<1," "<.1," etc. Where a range is given, use the midpoint.)

											NUTRIENTS IN INDICATED QUANTITY						
Item No. (A)	Foods, approximate measures, units, and weight (edible part unless footnotes indicate otherwise) (B)	Grams	Water Percent (C)	Food energy kCalories (D)	Protein Grams (E)	Fat Grams (F)	Carbohydrate Grams (G)	Calcium Milligrams (H)	Iron Milligrams (I)	Zinc Milligrams (J)	Vitamin A Retinol equivalents (K)	Thiamin Milligrams (L)	Riboflavin Milligrams (M)	Niacin Milligrams (N)	Folacin Micrograms (O)	Vitamin C Milligrams (P)
	FRUITS AND FRUIT PRODUCTS—Con.															
	Pineapple:—Continued															
	Canned, heavy sirup pack, solids and liquid:															
296	Crushed, chunks, tidbits ... 1 cup	255	80	190	1	<1	49	28	.8	.3	13	.20	.05	.5	12	18
	Slices and liquid:															
297	Large ... 1 slice; 2¼ tbsp liquid	105	80	80	<1	<1	20	12	.3	<.1	5	.08	.02	.2	11	7
298	Medium ... 1 slice; 1¼ tbsp liquid	58	80	45	<1	<1	11	6	.2	<.1	3	.05	.01	.1	6	4
	Pineapple-grapefruit juice drink, pineapple-orange juice drink. See items 696x₃ and 696x₄.															
299	Pineapple juice, unsweetened, canned. ... 1 cup	250	86	140	1	<1	34	38	.8	.3	13	.13	.05	.5	58	[note]80
	Plums:															
	Raw, without pits:															
300	Japanese and hybrid (2⅛-in diam., about 6½ per lb with pits). ... 1 plum	66	87	30	<1	<1	8	8	.3	<1	16	.02	.02	.3	1	4
301	Prune-type (1½-in diam., about 15 per lb with pits). ... 1 plum	28	79	20	<1	<1	6	3	.1	0	8	.01	.01	.1	<1	1
	Canned, heavy sirup pack (Italian prunes), with pits and liquid:															
302	Cup ... 1 cup[M]	272	77	215	1	<1	56	23	2.3	.2	313	.05	.05	1.0	6	5
303	Portion ... 3 plums; 2¼ tbsp liquid[M]	140	77	110	1	<1	29	12	1.2	.1	161	.03	.03	.5	3	3
	Prunes, dried, "softenized," with pits:															
304	Uncooked ... 4 extra large or 5 large prunes.[M]	49	28	110	1	<1	29	22	1.7	.3	69	.04	.07	.7	2	1
305	Cooked, unsweetened, all sizes, fruit and liquid. ... 1 cup[M]	250	66	255	2	1	67	51	3.8	.6	159	.07	.15	1.5	<1	2
306	Prune juice, canned or bottled ... 1 cup	256	80	195	1	<1	49	36	1.8	.5	[113]	.03	.03	1.0	1	5
	Raisins, seedless:															
307	Cup, not pressed down ... 1 cup	145	18	420	4	<1	112	90	5.1	.5	3	.16	.12	.7	5	1
308	Packet, ½ oz (1½ tbsp) ... 1 packet	14	18	40	<1	<1	11	9	.5	0	<1	.02	.01	.1	<1	<1
	Raspberries, red:															
309	Raw, capped, whole ... 1 cup	123	84	70	1	1	17	27	1.1	.6	16	.04	.11	1.1	(19)	31
310	Frozen, sweetened, 10-oz container ... 1 container	284	74	280	2	1	70	37	1.7	.5	20	.06	.17	1.7	74	60
	Rhubarb, cooked, added sugar:															
311	From raw ... 1 cup	270	63	380	1	<1	97	211	1.6	.3	22	.05	.14	.8	14	16
312	From frozen, sweetened ... 1 cup	270	63	385	1	1	98	211	1.9	.2	19	.05	.11	.5	14	16
	Strawberries:															
313	Raw, whole berries, capped ... 1 cup	149	90	55	1	1	13	31	1.5	.2	9	.04	.10	.9	26	88
	Frozen, sweetened:															
314	Sliced, 10-oz container ... 1 container	284	71	310	1	1	79	40	2.0	.2	9	.06	.17	1.4	42	151
315	Whole, 1-lb container (about 1¾ cups). ... 1 container	454	76	415	2	1	107	59	2.7	.2	14	.09	.27	2.3	17	249
316	Tangerine, raw, 2⅜-in diam., size 176, without peel (about 4 per lb with peels and seeds). ... 1 tangerine	86	87	40	1	<1	10	34	.3	(.4)	36	.05	.02	.1	17	27

(A)		(B)		(C)	(D)	(E)	(F)	(G)	(H)	(I)	(J)	(K)	(L)	(M)	(N)	(O)	(P)
317	Tangerine juice, canned, sweetened.	1 cup	249	87	125	1	<1	30	44	.5	<.1	104	.15	.05	.2	[11]	54
318	Watermelon, raw, 4 by 8 in wedge with rind and seeds (1/16 of 32⅔-lb melon, 10 by 16 in).	1 wedge with rind and seeds[87]	926	93	110	2	1	27	30	2.1	.7	251	.13	.13	.9	20	30
	GRAIN PRODUCTS																
	Bagel, 3-in diam.:																
319	Egg	1 bagel	55	32	165	6	2	28	9	1.2	.5	10	.14	.10	1.2	13	0
320	Water	1 bagel	55	29	165	6	1	30	8	1.2	.5	0	.15	.11	1.4	13	0
321	Barley, pearled, light, uncooked	1 cup	200	11	700	16	2	158	32	4.0	3.1	0	.24	.10	6.2	40	0
	Biscuits, baking powder, 2-in diam. (enriched flour, vegetable shortening):																
322	From horne recipe[g]	1 biscuit	28	27	105	2	5	13	34	.4	.2	<1	.08	.08	.7	2	<1
323	From mix[g]	1 biscuit	28	29	90	2	3	15	19	.6	.2	<1	.09	.08	.8	2	<1
	Breadcrumbs (enriched):[88]																
324	Dry, grated[g]	1 cup	100	7	390	13	5	73	122	3.6	.4	<1	.35	.35	4.8	(39)	<1
	Soft. See White bread (items 349-350).																
	Breads:																
325	Boston brown bread, canned, slice, 3¼ by ½ in.[88]	1 slice	45	45	95	2	1	21	41	.9	(.3)	[89]0	.06	.04	.7	(12)	0
	Cracked-wheat bread (¾ enriched wheat flour, ¼ cracked wheat):[88,g]																
326	Loaf, 1 lb	1 loaf	454	35	1,195	39	10	236	399	9.5	4.5	<1	1.52	1.13	14.4	(222)	<1
327	Slice (18 per loaf)	1 slice	25	35	65	2	1	13	22	.5	.3	<1	.08	.06	.8	(12)	<1
	French or vienna bread, enriched:[88,g]																
328	Loaf: 1 lb	1 loaf	454	31	1,315	41	14	251	195	10.0	2.9	<1	1.80	1.10	15.0	168	<1
	Slice:																
329	French (5 by 2½ by 1 in)	1 slice	35	31	100	3	1	19	15	.8	.2	<1	.14	.08	1.2	[13]	<1
330	Vienna (4¾ by 4 by ½ in)	1 slice	25	31	75	2	1	14	11	.6	.2	<1	.10	.06	.8	[9]	<1
	French toast. See item 437x₁.																
	Italian bread, enriched:[g]																
331	Loaf, 1 lb	1 loaf	454	32	1,250	41	4	256	77	10.0	.2	0	1.80	1.10	15.0	(111)	0
332	Slice, 4½ by 3¼ by ¾ in	1 slice	30	32	85	3	<1	17	5	.7	<.1	0	.12	.07	1.0	(12)	0
332x	Pita bread (Arabic bread, Syrian bread).	½ of 2½-oz. loaf (1 pocket)	35	31	99	4	1	20	29	.9	.3	(0)	.27	.13	1.7	[9-21]	0
	Raisin bread, enriched:[88,g]																
333	Loaf, 1 lb	1 loaf	454	35	1,190	30	13	243	322	10.0	2.4	<1	1.70	1.07	10.7	[159]	<1
334	Slice (18 per loaf)	1 slice	25	35	65	2	1	13	18	.6	.1	<1	.09	.06	.6	[9]	<1
	Rye Bread:																
	American, light (⅔ enriched wheat flour, ⅓ rye flour):[g]																
335	Loaf, 1 lb	1 loaf	454	36	1,100	41	5	236	340	9.1	7.3	0	1.35	.98	12.9	104	0
336	Slice (4¾ by 3¾ by 7/16 in)	1 slice	25	36	60	2	<1	13	19	.5	.4	0	.07	.05	.7	6	0
	Pumpernickel (⅔ rye flour, ⅓ enriched wheat flour):[g]																
337	Loaf, 1 lb	1 loaf	454	34	1,115	41	5	241	381	11.8	5.0	0	1.30	.93	8.5	[222]	0
338	Slice (5 by 4 by ⅜ in)	1 slice	32	34	80	3	<1	17	27	.8	.4	0	.09	.07	.6	[16]	0

For notes, see end of table.

TABLE H-1 COMPOSITION OF FOODS — Continued
(For purposes of calculating, use "0" for "<1," "<.1," etc. Where a range is given, use the midpoint.)

Item No. (A)	Foods, approximate measures, units, and weight (edible part unless footnotes indicate otherwise) (B)	Grams	Water (C) Percent	Food energy (D) kCalories	Protein (E) Grams	Fat (F) Grams	Carbohydrate (G) Grams	Calcium (H) Milligrams	Iron (I) Milligrams	Zinc (J) Milligrams	Vitamin A (K) Retinol equivalents	Thiamin (L) Milligrams	Riboflavin (M) Milligrams	Niacin (N) Milligrams	Folacin (O) Micrograms	Vitamin C (P) Milligrams
	GRAIN PRODUCTS—Con.															
	Breads:—Continued															
	White bread, enriched:[aa]															
	Soft-crumb type:[g]															
339	Loaf, 1 lb . . . . 1 loaf	454	36	1,225	39	15	229	381	11.3	2.7	<1	1.80	1.10	15.0	178	<1
340	Slice (18 per loaf) . . . 1 slice	25	36	70	2	1	13	21	.6	.2	<1	.10	.06	.8	10	<1
341	Slice, toasted . . . 1 slice	22	25	70	2	1	13	21	.6	.2	<1	.08	.06	.8	9	<1
342	Slice (22 per loaf) . . . 1 slice	20	36	55	2	1	10	17	.5	.2	<1	.08	.05	.7	8	<1
343	Slice, toasted . . . 1 slice	17	25	55	2	1	10	17	.5	.2	<1	.06	.05	.7	7	<1
344	Loaf, 1½ lb . . . 1 loaf	680	36	1,835	59	22	343	571	17.0	4.0	<1	2.70	1.65	22.5	265	<1
345	Slice (24 per loaf) . . . 1 slice	28	36	75	2	1	14	24	.7	.2	<1	.11	.07	.9	11	<1
346	Slice, toasted . . . 1 slice	24	25	75	2	1	14	24	.7	.2	<1	.09	.07	.9	10	<1
347	Slice (28 per loaf) . . . 1 slice	24	36	65	2	1	12	20	.6	.1	<1	.10	.06	.8	9	<1
348	Slice, toasted . . . 1 slice	21	25	65	2	1	12	20	.6	.1	<1	.08	.06	.8	9	<1
349	Cubes . . . 1 cup	30	36	80	3	1	15	25	.8	.2	<1	.12	.07	1.0	12	<1
350	Crumbs . . . 1 cup	45	36	120	4	1	23	38	1.1	.2	<1	.18	.11	1.5	18	<1
	Firm-crumb type:[g]															
351	Loaf, 1 lb . . . 1 loaf	454	35	1,245	41	17	228	435	11.3	2.7	<1	1.80	1.10	15.0	177	<1
352	Slice (20 per loaf) . . . 1 slice	23	35	65	2	1	12	22	.6	.1	<1	.09	.06	.8	9	<1
353	Slice, toasted . . . 1 slice	20	24	65	2	1	12	22	.6	.2	<1	.07	.06	.8	8	<1
354	Loaf, 2 lb . . . 1 loaf	907	35	2,495	82	34	455	871	22.7	5.4	<1	3.60	2.20	30.0	354	<1
355	Slice (34 per loaf) . . . 1 slice	27	35	75	2	1	14	26	.7	.2	<1	.11	.06	.9	11	<1
356	Slice, toasted . . . 1 slice	23	24	75	2	1	14	26	.7	.2	<1	.09	.06	.9	10	<1
	Whole-wheat bread:															
	Soft-crumb type:[aa]															
357	Loaf, 1 lb . . . 1 loaf	454	36	1,095	41	12	224	381	13.6	7.0	<1	1.37	.45	12.7	263	<1
358	Slice (16 per loaf) . . . 1 slice	28	36	65	3	1	14	24	.8	.5	<1	.09	.03	.8	16	<1
359	Slice, toasted . . . 1 slice	24	24	65	3	1	14	24	.8	.4	<1	.07	.03	.8	14	<1
	Firm-crumb type:[aa]															
360	Loaf, 1 lb . . . 1 loaf	454	36	1,100	48	14	216	449	13.6	6.6	<1	1.17	.54	12.7	263	<1
361	Slice (18 per loaf) . . . 1 slice	25	36	60	3	1	12	25	.8	.4	<1	.06	.03	.7	15	<1
362	Slice, toasted . . . 1 slice	21	24	60	3	1	12	25	.8	.4	<1	.05	.03	.7	12	<1
	Breakfast cereals:															
	Hot type, cooked:															
	Corn (hominy) grits, degermed:															
363	Enriched . . . 1 cup	245	87	125	3	<1	27	2	.7	.2	[40]<1	.10	.07	1.0	3	0
364	Unenriched . . . 1 cup	245	87	125	3	<1	27	2	.2	.2	[g]<1	.05	.02	.5	3	0
365	Farina, quick-cooking, enriched.[g] . . . 1 cup	245	89	105	3	<1	22	147	(48)	.2	[h]0	.12	.07	1.0	5	0
366	Oatmeal or rolled oats . . . 1 cup	240	87	130	5	2	23	22	1.4	1.2	0	.19	.05	.2	10	0
367	Wheat, rolled . . . 1 cup	240	80	180	5	1	41	19	1.7	1.4	0	.17	.07	2.2	(26)	0
368	Wheat, whole-meal . . . 1 cup	245	88	110	4	1	23	17	1.2	1.2	0	.15	.05	1.5	26	0
	Ready-to-eat (see also Appendix F, Sugar):															
369	Bran flakes (40% bran), added sugar, salt, iron, vitamins. . . . 1 cup	35	3	105	4	1	28	19	5.6	1.2	467	.46	.52	6.2	[i]100	0
370	Bran flakes with raisins, added sugar, salt, iron, zinc, vitamins. . . . 1 cup	50	7	145	4	1	40	28	7.9	[i]5.1	[aa]667	(46)	(46)	(46)	[i]136	0

NUTRIENTS IN INDICATED QUANTITY

H

(A)	(B)		(C)	(D)	(E)	(F)	(G)	(H)	(I)	(J)	(K)	(L)	(M)	(N)	(O)	(P)
	Corn flakes:															
371	Plain, added sugar, salt, iron, vitamins.	1 cup	25	95	2	<1	21	(44)	(44)	<.1	(44)	(44)	(44)	(44)	j88	a13
372	Sugar-coated, added salt, iron, vitamins.	1 cup	40	155	2	<1	37	1	(44)	.1	533	.53	.60	7.1	141	a21
373	Corn, oat flour, puffed, added sugar, salt, iron, vitamins.	1 cup	20	80	2	1	16	4	5.7	k.2	267	.26	.30	3.5	[75]	11
374	Corn, shredded, added sugar, salt, iron, thiamin, niacin.	1 cup	25	95	2	<1	22	1	.6	l<.1	0	.33	.05	4.4	l88	13
374x	Granola, homemade.	1 oz or ¼ cup	28	138	4	8	16	18	1.1	1.0	1	.17	.07	.5	23	0
375	Oats, puffed, added sugar, salt, minerals, vitamins.	1 cup	25	100	3	1	19	44	4.0	m.6	333	.33	.38	4.4	m6	13
	Rice, puffed:															
376	Plain, added iron, thiamin, niacin.	1 cup	15	60	1	<1	13	3	.3	.1	0	.07	.01	.7	3	0
377	Presweetened, added salt, iron, vitamins.	1 cup	28	115	1	0	26	3	.3	.3	a378	(44)	(44)	(44)	6	a15
377x	Special K.	1 oz.	28	111	6	<1	21	8	4.5	3.7	375	.40	.40	5.0	100	15
378	Wheat flakes, added sugar, salt, iron, vitamins.	1 cup	30	105	3	<1	24	12	4.8	[.8]	400	.40	.45	5.3	9	16
	Wheat, puffed:															
379	Plain, added iron, thiamin, niacin.	1 cup	15	55	2	<1	12	4	.6	.4	0	.08	.03	1.2	5	0
380	Presweetened, added salt, iron, vitamins.	1 cup	38	140	3	<1	33	7	(44)	.9	509	.50	.57	6.7	12	a20
381	Wheat, shredded, plain.	1 oblong biscuit or ½ cup spoon-size biscuits.	25	90	2	1	20	11	.9	.6	0	.06	.03	1.1	13	0
382	Wheat germ, without salt and sugar, toasted.	1 tbsp	6	25	2	1	3	3	.5	1.0	1	.11	.05	.3	18	1
	Buckwheat flours:															
382x	Dark.	3 tbsp	18	61	2	1	13	6	.5	.5	(0)	.11	.03	.5	(8.30)	(0)
383	Light, sifted.	1 cup	98	340	6	1	78	11	1.0	2.6	0	.08	.04	.4	(101)	0
	Bulgur:															
384	Canned, seasoned.	1 cup	135	245	8	4	44	27	1.9	1.4	0	.08	.05	4.1	6	0
384x	Dry.	2 tbsp	21	75	2	0	16	6	.8	.5	(0)	.06	.03	1.0	2	(0)
384x₁	Cake, cheese, commercial.	1/6 cake	o(100)	302	5	19	29	56	.5	.4	76	.03	.13	.5	[18]	[5]
	Cake icings. See Sugars and Sweets (items 532-536).															
	Cakes made from cake mixes with enriched flour:[44]															
	Angelfood:															
385	Whole cake (9¾-in diam. tube cake).	1 cake	635	1,645	36	1	377	603	2.5	.6	0	.37	.95	3.6	[51]	0
386	Piece, 1/12 of cake.	1 piece	53	135	3	<1	32	50	.2	<.1	0	.03	.08	.3	[4]	0
	Coffeecake:															
387	Whole cake (7¾ by 5⅝ by 1¼ in).	1 cake	430	1,385	27	41	225	262	6.9	1.9	[138]	.82	.91	7.7	[133]	1
388	Piece, 1/6 of cake.	1 piece	72	230	5	7	38	44	1.2	.6	[24]	.14	.15	1.3	[22]	<1
	Cupcakes, made with egg, milk, 2½-in diam.:															
389	Without icing.	1 cupcake	25	90	1	3	14	40	.3	<.1	[8]	.05	.05	.4	(2)	<1
390	With chocolate icing.	1 cupcake	36	130	2	5	21	47	.4	(.5)	[12]	.05	.06	.4	(2)	<1

For notes, see end of table.

H

TABLE H–1   COMPOSITION OF FOODS — Continued
(For purposes of calculating, use "0" for "<1," "<1," etc. Where a range is given, use the midpoint.)

Item No. (A)	Foods, approximate measures, units, and weight (edible part unless footnotes indicate otherwise) (B)		Grams	Water Per-cent (C)	Food energy kCal-ories (D)	Pro-tein Grams (E)	Fat Grams (F)	Carbo-hydrate Grams (G)	Calcium Milli-grams (H)	Iron Milli-grams (I)	Zinc Milli-grams (J)	Vitamin A Retinol equi-valents (K)	Thiamin Milli-grams (L)	Ribo-flavin Milli-grams (M)	Niacin Milli-grams (N)	Folacin Micro-grams (O)	Vitamin C Milli-grams (P)
	GRAIN PRODUCTS—Con.																
	Cakes made from cake mixes with enriched flour:—Continued																
	Devil's food with chocolate icing:																
391	Whole, 2 layer cake (8- or 9-in diam.).	1 cake	1,107	24	3,755	49	136	645	653	16.6	6.6	[332]	1.06	1.65	10.1	77	1
392	Piece, 1/16 of cake	1 piece	69	24	235	3	8	40	41	1.0	.4	[20]	.07	.10	.6	5	<1
393	Cupcake, 2½-in diam.	1 cupcake	35	24	120	2	4	20	21	.5	.3	[10]	.03	.05	.3	4	<1
	Gingerbread:																
394	Whole cake (8-in square)	1 cake	570	37	1,575	18	39	291	513	8.6	2.3	<1	.84	1.00	7.4	38	<1
395	Piece, 1/9 of cake	1 piece	63	37	175	2	4	32	57	.9	.2	<1	.09	.11	.8	4	<1
	White, 2 layer with chocolate icing:																
396	Whole cake (8- or 9-in diam.)	1 cake	1,140	21	4,000	44	122	716	1,129	11.4	4.1	[136]	1.50	1.77	12.5	55	2
397	Piece, 1/16 of cake	1 piece	71	21	250	3	8	45	70	.7	.3	[8]	.09	.11	.8	4	<1
	Yellow, 2 layer with chocolate icing:																
398	Whole cake (8- or 9-in diam.)	1 cake	1,108	26	3,735	45	125	638	1,008	12.2	5.9	[310]	1.24	1.67	10.6	130	2
399	Piece, 1/16 of cake	1 piece	69	26	235	3	8	40	63	.8	.4	[20]	.08	.10	.7	8	<1
	Cakes made from home recipes using enriched flour:[c]																
	Boston cream pie with custard filling:																
400	Whole cake (8-in diam.)	1 cake	825	35	2,490	41	78	412	553	8.2	[3.4]	[346]	1.04	1.27	9.6	[45]	2
401	Piece, 1/12 of cake	1 piece	69	35	210	3	6	34	46	.7	[.3]	[28]	.09	.11	.8	[4]	<1
	Fruitcake, dark:																
402	Loaf, 1-lb (7½ by 2 by 1½ in)	1 loaf	454	18	1,720	22	69	271	327	11.8	[2.2]	54	.72	.73	4.9	[36]	2
403	Slice, 1/30 of loaf	1 slice	15	18	55	1	2	9	11	.4	[<.1]	2	.02	.02	.2	[1]	<1
	Plain, sheet cake:																
	Without icing:																
404	Whole cake (9-in square)	1 cake	777	25	2,830	35	108	434	497	8.5	2.7	[264]	1.21	1.40	10.2	54	2
405	Piece, 1/9 of cake	1 piece	86	25	315	4	12	48	55	.9	.4	[30]	.13	.15	1.1	[15]	<1
	With uncooked white icing:																
406	Whole cake (9-in square)	1 cake	1,096	21	4,020	37	129	694	548	8.2	[4.9]	[438]	1.22	1.47	10.2	[110]	2
407	Piece, 1/9 of cake	1 piece	121	21	445	4	14	77	61	.8	[.5]	[48]	.14	.16	1.1	[12]	<1
	Pound:[d]																
408	Loaf, 8½ by 3½ by 3¼ in	1 loaf	565	16	2,725	31	170	273	107	7.9	[2.2]	[282]	.90	.99	7.3	[44]	0
409	Slice, 1/17 of loaf	1 slice	33	16	160	2	10	16	6	.5	[.1]	[16]	.05	.06	.4	[2]	0
	Spongecake:																
410	Whole cake (9¾-in diam. tube cake).	1 cake	790	32	2,345	60	45	427	237	13.4	9.6	[712]	1.10	1.64	7.4	55	<1
411	Piece, 1/12 of cake	1 piece	66	32	195	5	4	36	20	1.1	.8	[60]	.09	.14	.6	15	<1
	Cookies made with enriched flour:[e,f,g]																
	Brownies with nuts:																
	Home prepared, 1¾ by 1¾ by ⅞ in:																
412	From home recipe	1 brownie	20	10	95	1	6	10	8	.4	[.3]	[8]	.04	.03	.2	[2]	<1
413	From commercial recipe	1 brownie	20	11	85	1	4	13	9	.4	[.3]	[4]	.03	.02	.2	[2]	<1

NUTRIENTS IN INDICATED QUANTITY

(A)	(B)	(C)	(D)	(E)	(F)	(G)	(H)	(I)	(J)	(K)	(L)	(M)	(N)	(O)	(P)
414	Frozen, with chocolate icing,[54] 1½ by 1¾ by ⅞ in. … 1 brownie	25	105	1	5	15	10	.4	[.4]	[10]	.03	.03	.2	[3]	<1
	Chocolate chip:														
415	Commercial, 2¼-in diam., ⅜ in thick. … 4 cookies	42	200	2	9	29	16	1.0	.4	[10]	.10	.17	.9	4	<1
416	From home recipe, 2⅓-in diam … 4 cookies	40	205	2	12	24	14	.8	.5	[8]	.06	.06	.5	5	<1
417	Fig Bars, square (1⅝ by 1⅝ by ⅜ in) or rectangular (1½ by 1¾ by ½ in). … 4 cookies	56	200	2	3	42	44	1.0	.4	[12]	.04	.14	.9	3	<1
418	Gingersnaps, 2-in diam., ¼ in thick. … 4 cookies	28	90	2	2	22	20	.7	.1	[4]	.08	.06	.7	2	0
419	Macaroons, 2¾-in diam., ¼ in thick. … 2 cookies	38	180	2	9	25	10	.3	[.2]	0	.02	.06	.2	[4]	0
420	Oatmeal with raisins, 2⅝-in diam., ¼ in thick. … 4 cookies	52	235	3	8	38	11	1.4	.3	[6]	.15	.10	1.0	[6]	<1
421	Plain, prepared from commercial chilled dough, 2½-in diam., ¼ in thick. … 4 cookies	48	240	2	12	31	17	.6	.2	[6]	.10	.08	.9	4	0
422	Sandwich type (chocolate or vanilla), 1¾-in diam., ⅜ in thick. … 4 cookies	40	200	2	9	28	10	.7	(.2)	0	.06	.10	.7	(1)	0
423	Vanilla wafers, 1¾-in diam., ¼ in thick. … 10 cookies	40	185	2	6	30	16	.6	.1	[10]	.10	.09	.8	[4]	0
	Cornmeal:														
424	Whole-ground, unbolted, dry form. … 1 cup	122	435	11	5	90	24	2.9	1.0	[54]62	.46	.13	2.4	29	0
425	Bolted (nearly whole-grain), dry form. … 1 cup	122	440	11	4	91	21	2.2	1.0	[54]59	.37	.10	2.3	29	0
	Degermed, enriched:[8]														
426	Dry form … 1 cup	138	500	11	2	108	8	4.0	1.1	[54]61	.61	.36	4.8	33	0
427	Cooked … 1 cup	240	120	3	<1	26	2	1.0	.1	[54]14	.14	.10	1.2	(5)	0
	Degermed, unenriched:														
428	Dry form … 1 cup	138	500	11	2	108	8	1.5	1.0	[54]61	.19	.07	1.4	33	0
429	Cooked … 1 cup	240	120	3	<1	26	2	.5	(.1)	[54]14	.05	.02	.2	(5)	0
	Crackers:[55]														
430	Graham, plain, 2½-in square … 2 crackers	14	55	1	1	10	6	.5	.1	0	.02	.08	.5	2	0
431	Rye wafers, whole-grain, 1⅞ by 3½ in. … 2 wafers	13	45	2	<1	10	7	.5	.4	0	.04	.03	.2	[8]	0
432	Saltines, made with enriched flour.[8] … 4 crackers or 1 packet	11	50	1	1	8	2	.5	<.1	0	.05	.05	.4	2	0
	Danish pastry (enriched flour), plain without fruit or nuts:[54][8]														
433	Packaged ring, 12 oz. … 1 ring	340	1,435	25	80	155	170	6.1	2.9	[210]	.97	1.01	8.6	[110]	<1
434	Round piece, about 4¼-in diam. by 1 in. … 1 pastry	65	275	5	15	30	33	1.2	.6	[40]	.18	.19	1.7	[21]	<1
435	Ounce … 1 oz	28	120	2	7	13	14	.5	.2	[18]	.08	.08	.7	[9]	<1
	Doughnuts, made with enriched flour:[56][8]														
436	Cake type, plain, 2½-in diam., 1 in high. … 1 doughnut	25	100	1	5	13	10	.4	.1	[4]	.05	.05	.4	2	<1
437	Yeast-leavened, glazed, 3¾-in diam., 1¼ in high. … 1 doughnut	50	205	3	11	22	16	.6	.2	[5]	.10	.10	.8	(11)	0

For notes, see end of table.

H

H

TABLE H-1 COMPOSITION OF FOODS — Continued
(For purposes of calculating, use "0" for "<1," "<1," etc. Where a range is given, use the midpoint.)

Item No. (A)	Foods, approximate measures, units, and weight (edible part unless footnotes indicate otherwise) (B)		Water (C) Per- cent	Food energy (D) kCal- ories	Pro- tein (E) Grams	Fat (F) Grams	Carbo- hydrate (G) Grams	Calcium (H) Milli- grams	Iron (I) Milli- grams	Zinc (J) Milli- grams	Vitamin A (K) Retinol equi- valents	Thiamin (L) Milli- grams	Ribo- flavin (M) Milli- grams	Niacin (N) Milli- grams	Folacin (O) Micro- grams	Vitamin C (P) Milli- grams
		Grams														
	GRAIN PRODUCTS—Con.															
	Flour. See Buckwheat flours (items 382x and 383), Carob flour (item 696x), Soybean flours (items 492x₈ and 492x₉), Wheat flours (items 502-506).															
437x₁	French toast, 1 slice	[35]	53	83	3	4	9	39	.7	.3	[6]	.07	.09	.6	9	0
437x₂	Granola bar, 1 small bar	28	4	127	3	5	19	17	.9	1.0	(1)	.08	.03	.2	(23)	(0)
	Macaroni, enriched, cooked (cut lengths, elbows, shells):8															
	Tender stage:															
438	Firm stage (hot), 1 cup	130	64	190	7	1	39	14	1.4	.7	0	.23	.13	1.8	[4]	0
439	Cold macaroni, 1 cup	105	73	115	4	<1	24	8	.9	.5	0	.15	.08	1.2	[2]	0
440	Hot macaroni, 1 cup	140	73	155	5	1	32	11	1.3	.7	0	.20	.11	1.5	[3]	0
	Macaroni (enriched) and cheese:8															
441	Canned⁵⁵, 1 cup	240	80	230	9	10	26	199	1.0	1.2	[52]	.12	.24	1.0	[7]	<1
442	From home recipe (served hot)⁵⁰, 1 cup	200	58	430	17	22	40	362	1.8	1.0	[172]	.20	.40	1.8	[12]	<1
442x	Millet, cooked, ½ cup	95	86	54	1	1	11	3	1.1	.4	(0)	.10	.06	.7	10	(0)
	Muffins made with enriched flour:⁵⁶g															
	From home recipe:															
443	Blueberry, 2⅜-in diam., 1½ in high, 1 muffin	40	39	110	3	4	17	34	.6	.2	[18]	.09	.10	.7	[17]	<1
444	Bran, 1 muffin	40	35	105	3	4	17	57	1.5	.9	[18]	.07	.10	1.7	17	<1
445	Corn (enriched degermed cornmeal and flour), 2⅜-in diam., 1½ in high.8, 1 muffin	40	33	125	3	4	19	42	.7	P.3	[*24]	.10	.10	.7	[5]	<1
446	Plain, 3-in diam., 1½ in high, 1 muffin	40	38	120	3	4	17	42	.6	P(.2)	[8]	.09	.12	.9	[5]	<1
	From mix, egg, milk:															
447	Corn, 2⅜-in diam., 1½ in high.⁵⁸, 1 muffin	40	30	130	3	4	20	96	.6	.3	[*20]	.08	.09	.7	[6]	<1
448	Noodles (egg noodles), enriched, cooked.8, 1 cup	160	71	200	7	2	37	16	1.4	1.0	[22]	.22	.13	1.9	[6]	0
449	Noodles, chow mein, canned.⁵⁸, 1 cup	45	1	220	6	11	26	[5]	[.9]	[.1]	[0]	[.05]	[.50]	[1.6]	[10]	[0]
450	Pancakes, (4-in diam.).⁵⁸, 1 cake	27	58	55	2	2	6	59	.4	[.4]	[12]	.04	.05	.2	[6]	<1
	Buckwheat, made from mix (with buckwheat and enriched flours), egg and milk added.8															
	Plain:															
451	Made from home recipe using enriched flour.8, 1 cake	27	50	60	2	2	9	27	.4	.2	[6]	.06	.07	.5	3	<1
452	Made from mix with enriched flour, egg and milk added.8, 1 cake	27	51	60	2	2	9	58	.3	.2	[14]	.04	.06	.2	3	<1
	Pies, piecrust made with enriched flour, vegetable shortening (9-in diam.):															
	(See also Appendix N, Fast Foods.)															
	Apple:															
453	Whole, 1 pie	945	48	2,420	21	105	360	76	6.6	1.6	28	1.06	.79	9.3	47	9
454	Sector, 1/7 of pie, 1 sector	135	48	345	3	15	51	11	.9	.2	4	.15	.11	1.3	7	2

NUTRIENTS IN INDICATED QUANTITY

(A)	(B)		(C)	(D)	(E)	(F)	(G)	(H)	(I)	(J)	(K)	(L)	(M)	(N)	(O)	(P)
	Banana cream:															
455	Whole	1 pie	910	54	2,010	41	85	279	601	7.3	[6.3]	[456]	.77	1.51	7.0	[79]	9
456	Sector, 1/7 of pie	1 sector	130	54	285	6	12	40	86	1.0	[.9]	[66]	.11	.22	1.0	[11]	1
	Blueberry:															
457	Whole	1 pie	945	51	2,285	23	102	330	104	9.5	0	28	1.03	.80	10.0	[93]	28
458	Sector, 1/7 of pie	1 sector	135	51	325	3	15	47	15	1.4	0	4	.15	.11	1.4	[13]	4
	Cherry:															
459	Whole	1 pie	945	47	2,465	25	107	363	132	6.6	.4	416	1.09	.84	9.8	[103]	<1
460	Sector, 1/7 of pie	1 sector	135	47	350	4	15	52	19	.9	<.1	59	.16	.12	1.4	[15]	<1
	Custard:															
461	Whole	1 pie	910	58	1,985	56	101	213	874	8.2	6.3	[418]	.79	1.92	5.6	b[79]	0
462	Sector, 1/7 of pie	1 sector	130	58	285	8	14	30	125	1.2	.9	[60]	.11	.27	.8	b[11]	0
	Lemon meringue:															
463	Whole	1 pie	840	47	2,140	31	86	317	118	6.7	2.4	[286]	.61	.84	5.2	76	25
464	Sector, 1/7 of pie	1 sector	120	47	305	4	12	45	17	1.0	.3	[40]	.09	.12	.7	11	4
	Mince:															
465	Whole	1 pie	945	43	2,560	24	109	389	265	13.3	[1.5]	[4]	.96	.86	9.8	[29]	9
466	Sector, 1/7 of pie	1 sector	135	43	365	3	16	56	38	1.9	[.2]	<1	.14	.12	1.4	[4]	1
	Peach:															
467	Whole	1 pie	945	48	2,410	24	101	361	95	8.5	.1	690	1.04	.97	14.0	[69]	28
468	Sector, 1/7 of pie	1 sector	135	48	345	3	14	52	14	1.2	.1	99	.15	.14	2.0	[10]	4
	Pecan:															
469	Whole	1 pie	825	20	3,450	42	189	423	388	25.6	[6.9]	[264]	1.80	.95	6.9	[77]	<1
470	Sector, 1/7 of pie	1 sector	118	20	495	6	27	61	55	3.7	[1.0]	[38]	.26	.14	1.0	[11]	<1
	Pumpkin:															
471	Whole	1 pie	910	59	1,920	36	102	223	464	7.3	[3.2]	[4,496]	.78	1.27	7.0	[95]	<1
472	Sector, 1/7 of pie	1 sector	130	59	275	5	15	32	66	1.0	[.5]	[642]	.11	.18	1.0	[14]	<1
473	Piecrust (home recipe) made with enriched flour and vegetable shortening, baked.[8]	1 pie shell, 9-in diam.	180	15	900	11	60	79	25	3.1	1.0	0	.47	.40	5.0	[32]	0
474	Piecrust mix with enriched flour and vegetable shortening, 10-oz pkg, prepared and baked.[8]	Piecrust for 2-crust pie, 9-in diam.	320	19	1,485	20	93	141	131	6.1	.9	0	1.07	.79	9.9	[57]	0
475	Pizza (cheese) baked, 4¾-in sector; ⅛ of 12-in diam. pie.[19]	1 sector	60	45	145	6	4	22	86	1.1	.7	[46]	.16	.18	1.6	22	4
	Popcorn, popped:															
476	Plain, large kernel	1 cup	6	4	25	1	<1	5	1	.2	.3	[9]	[<.01]	.01	.1	[3]	0
477	With oil (coconut) and salt added, large kernel	1 cup	9	3	40	1	2	5	1	.2	.3	[9]	[<.01]	.01	.2	[3]	0
478	Sugar coated	1 cup	35	4	135	2	1	30	2	.5	(.3)	[9]	[<.01]	.02	.4	[3]	0
	Pretzels, made with enriched flour:[8]															
479	Dutch, twisted, 2¾ by 2⅝ in	1 pretzel	16	5	60	2	1	12	4	.2	.2	0	.05	.04	.7	3	0
479x	Round	1 oz or 5 large	30	3	119	3	1	24	8	.6	.3	(0)	(.09)	(.08)	(1.3)	5	(0)
480	Thin, twisted, 3¼ by 2¼ by ¼ in	10 pretzels	60	5	235	6	3	46	13	.9	.6	0	.20	.15	2.5	10	0
481	Stick, 2¼ in long	10 pretzels	3	5	10	<1	<1	2	1	<1	0	0	.01	.01	.1	0	0
	Rice: White, enriched:[8]															
481x	Fried	1 cup	180	70	180	5	12	40	[34]	[1.8]	[1.2]	[44]	[.2]	[.06]	[1.7]	[21]	[3]
482	Instant	1 cup	165	73	180	4	<1	40	5	1.3	.4	0	.21	[58]	1.7	18	0
	Long grain:															
483	Raw	1 cup	185	12	670	12	1	149	44	5.4	1.7	0	.81	.06	6.5	18	0
484	Cooked, served hot	1 cup	205	73	225	4	<1	50	21	1.8	.8	0	.23	.02	2.1	23	0

For notes, see end of table.

H

TABLE H–1 COMPOSITION OF FOODS — Continued
(For purposes of calculating, use "0" for "<1," "<1." etc. Where a range is given, use the midpoint.)

Item No. (A)	Foods, approximate measures, units, and weight (edible part unless footnotes indicate otherwise) (B)	(weight) Grams	Water (C) Percent	Food energy (D) kCalories	Protein (E) Grams	Fat (F) Grams	Carbohydrate (G) Grams	Calcium (H) Milligrams	Iron (I) Milligrams	Zinc (J) Milligrams	Vitamin A (K) Retinol equivalents	Thiamin (L) Milligrams	Riboflavin (M) Milligrams	Niacin (N) Milligrams	Folacin (O) Micrograms	Vitamin C (P) Milligrams
	GRAIN PRODUCTS—Con.															
	Rice:															
	White, enriched:—Continued															
	Parboiled:															
485	Raw ... 1 cup	185	10	685	14	1	150	111	5.4	2.0	0	.81	.07	6.5	20	0
486	Cooked, served hot ... 1 cup	175	73	185	4	<1	41	33	1.4	.5	0	.19	.02	2.1	4	0
486x	Brown, cooked, long grain, hot ... ⅓ cup	65	70	77	2	0	17	8	.3	(.4-.7)	(0)	.06	.01	.9	3	(0)
486x₄	Wild, cooked ... ½ cup	[100]	76	92	4	0	19	5	1.1	1.2	(0)	.11	.16	1.6	35	(0)
	Rolls, enriched:**[8]															
	Commercial:															
487	Brown-and-serve (12 per 12-oz pkg.), browned. ... 1 roll	26	27	85	2	2	14	20	.5	.2	<1	.10	.06	.9	10	<1
488	Cloverleaf or pan, 2½-in diam., 2 in high. ... 1 roll	28	31	85	2	2	15	21	.5	.3	<1	.11	.07	.9	(11)	<1
489	Frankfurter and hamburger (8 per 11½-oz pkg.). ... 1 roll	40	31	120	3	2	21	30	.8	.2	<1	.16	.10	1.3	[15]	<1
490	Hard, 3¾-in diam., 2 in high. ... 1 roll	50	25	155	5	2	30	24	1.2	.6	<1	.20	.12	1.7	(30)	<1
491	Hoagie or submarine, 11½ by 3 by 2½ in. ... 1 roll	135	31	390	12	4	75	58	3.0	(.8)	<1	.54	.32	4.5	(80)	<1
	From home recipe:															
492	Cloverleaf, 2½-in diam., 2 in high. ... 1 roll	35	26	120	3	3	20	16	.7	(.3)	[6]	.12	.12	1.2	(13)	<1
492x₄	Rye flour, medium, sifted, spooned into cup. ... 3 tbsp.	17	11	58	2	0	12	(5)	.4	.2	(0)	.05	.02	.4	13	(0)
	Soybean flours:															
492x₄	Full fat, not stirred ... ¼ cup	21	8	90	8	4	7	42	1.8	(.3-1.0)	2	.18	.07	.5	67	0
492x₄	Full fat, stirred ... ¼ cup	18	8	74	6	4	5	35	1.5	(.3-.9)	2	.15	.06	.4	56	0
	Spaghetti, enriched, cooked:[8]															
493	Firm stage, "al dente," served hot. ... 1 cup	130	64	190	7	1	39	14	1.4	.3	0	.23	.13	1.8	[4]	0
494	Tender stage, served hot ... 1 cup	140	73	155	5	1	32	11	1.3	.4	0	.20	.11	1.5	(3)	0
	Spaghetti (enriched) in tomato sauce with cheese:[8]															
495	From home recipe ... 1 cup	250	77	260	9	9	37	80	2.3	(1.4)	[216]	.25	.18	2.3	(26)	13
496	Canned ... 1 cup	250	80	190	6	2	39	40	2.8	1.4	[186]	.35	.28	4.5	(26)	10
	Spaghetti (enriched) with meat balls and tomato sauce:[8]															
497	From home recipe ... 1 cup	248	70	330	19	12	39	124	3.7	f(2.3)	[318]	.25	.30	4.0	(26)	22
498	Canned ... 1 cup	250	78	260	12	10	29	53	3.3	f(2.3)	[200]	.15	.18	2.3	(26)	5
498x	Taco shells ... 1 shell	[20]	4	91	2	4	13	28	.5	.3	[29]	.06	.03	.3	[4]	0
499	Toaster pastries ... 1 pastry	50	12	200	3	6	36	**54	1.9	.3	[100]	.16	.17	2.1	40	(**)
499x	Tortillas ... 1 tortilla	[20]	46	45	1	1	9	28	.4	.3	[3]	.03	.02	.3	[4]	0
	Waffles, made with enriched flour, 7-in diam.:**[8]															
500	From home recipe ... 1 waffle	75	41	210	7	7	28	85	1.3	.7	[50]	.17	.23	1.4	14	<1
501	From mix, egg and milk added ... 1 waffle	75	42	205	7	8	27	179	1.0	.5	[34]	.14	.22	.9	2	<1
501x	Wheat berries, cooked ... ½ cup	50	86	28	(1)	0	6	3	.3	(.4-.5)	(0)	.04	.01	.4	6	(0)
	Wheat flours (see also Flour):															
	All-purpose or family flour, enriched:[8]															
502	Sifted, spooned ... 1 cup	115	12	420	12	1	88	18	3.3	.8	0	.74	.46	6.1	24	0

| NUTRIENTS IN INDICATED QUANTITY |

(A)	(B)		(C)	(D)	(E)	(F)	(G)	(H)	(I)	(J)	(K)	(L)	(M)	(N)	(O)	(P)
503	Unsifted, spooned	1 cup	125	455	13	1	95	20	3.6	.9	0	.80	.50	6.6	26	0
504	Cake or pastry flour, enriched, sifted, spooned.8	1 cup	96	350	7	1	76	16	2.8	.3	0	.61	.38	5.1	(20)	0
505	Self rising, enriched, unsifted, spooned.8	1 cup	125	440	12	1	93	331	3.6	(.9)	0	.80	.50	6.6	(26)	0
506	Whole-wheat, from hard wheats, stirred.	1 cup	120	400	16	2	85	49	4.0	2.9	0	.66	.14	5.2	65	0
506x	Wheat germ, toasted, without sugar	1 tbsp.	6	23	2	1	3	3	.5	.9	1	.11	.05	.3	20	1

LEGUMES (DRY), NUTS, SEEDS; RELATED PRODUCTS

Almonds, shelled:

(A)	(B)		(C)	(D)	(E)	(F)	(G)	(H)	(I)	(J)	(K)	(L)	(M)	(N)	(O)	(P)
507	Chopped (about 130 almonds)	1 cup	130	775	24	70	25	304	6.1	4.6	0	.31	1.20	4.6	125	<1
508	Slivered, not pressed down (about 115 almonds).	1 cup	115	690	21	62	22	269	5.4	4.1	0	.28	1.06	4.0	110	<1
508x₁	Whole, shelled	¼ cup	36	212	7	19	7	83	1.7	(.9-1.3)	0	.09	.33	1.3	34	(0)

Beans:
Mature seeds, dry, cooked, drained:

(A)	(B)		(C)	(D)	(E)	(F)	(G)	(H)	(I)	(J)	(K)	(L)	(M)	(N)	(O)	(P)
508x₂	Black beans (turtle beans)	½ cup	(100)	85	6	0	15	30	1.7	(.7-.8)	1	.09	.04	.4	49	(0)
508x₃	Broad beans (fava beans)	½ cup	[100]	119	7	2	19	35	1.5	.9	33	.09	.08	.7	104	0
508x₄	Garbanzo beans (chickpeas)	½ cup	85	145	8	2	25	47	2.9	1.5	[<1]	.09	.04	.4	42	0
509	Great Northern	1 cup	180	210	14	1	38	90	4.9	1.6	0	.25	.13	1.3	54	0
510	Pea (navy)	1 cup	190	225	15	1	40	95	5.1	1.7	0	.27	.13	1.3	129	0
510x	Pinto beans	½ cup	100	131	8	1	25	48	3.3	1.3	[1]	.25	.05	.4	(59, 106)	(0)

Canned, solids and liquid:
White with—

(A)	(B)		(C)	(D)	(E)	(F)	(G)	(H)	(I)	(J)	(K)	(L)	(M)	(N)	(O)	(P)
511	Frankfurters (sliced)	1 cup	255	365	19	18	32	94	4.8	(2.8)	33	.18	.15	3.3	[54, 61]	<1
512	Pork and tomato sauce	1 cup	255	310	16	7	48	138	4.6	[2.2]	33	.20	.08	1.5	(61)	5
513	Pork and sweet sauce	1 cup	255	385	16	12	54	161	5.9	[2.6]	[<1]	.15	.10	1.3	[61]	[<1]
514	Red kidney	1 cup	255	230	15	1	42	74	4.6	(2.3)	1	9.13	.10	1.5	[94]	[<1]
515	Lima, cooked, drained (see also items 569-570).	1 cup	190	260	16	1	49	55	5.9	2.2	[<1]	.25	.11	1.3	217	[<1]
516	Blackeye peas, dry, cooked (with residual cooking liquid). See also items 585-586.	1 cup	250	190	13	1	35	43	3.3	2.2	3	.40	.10	1.0	148	[<1]
517	Brazil nuts, shelled (6-8 large kernels).	1 oz	28	185	4	19	3	53	1.0	1.1	<1	.27	.03	.5	1	[<1]
518	Cashew nuts, roasted in oil	1 cup	140	785	24	64	41	53	5.3	7.2	14	.60	.35	2.5	95	<1
519	Coconut meat, fresh: Piece, about 2 by 2 by ½ in	1 piece	45	155	2	16	4	6	.8	.3	0	.02	.01	.2	9	1
520	Shredded or grated, not pressed down.	1 cup	80	275	3	28	8	10	14	.6	0	.04	.02	.4	16	2
521	Filberts (hazelnuts), chopped (about 80 kernels).	1 cup	115	730	14	72	19	240	3.9	2.4	[0]	.53	[.47]	1.0	83	<1
521x	Humous (hommous, hummus)	1 tbsp.	84	185	7	11	13	43	2.9	1.3	11	.16	.07	.8	37	8
522	Lentils, whole, cooked	1 cup	200	210	16	<1	39	50	4.2	2.0	4	.14	.12	1.2	64	4
522x	Miso (bean paste, fermented)	3 tbsp	50	102	6	3	14	34	1.8	3.3	0	.03	.07	.7	[22]	0
523	Peanuts, roasted in oil, salted (whole, halves, chopped).	1 cup	144	840	37	72	27	107	3.0	4.3	[<1]	.46	.19	24.8	153	0
524	Peanut butter	1 tbsp	16	95	4	8	3	9	.3	.5	[0]	.02	.02	2.4	13	0
525	Peas, split, dry, cooked	1 cup	200	230	16	1	42	22	3.4	1.7	8	.30	.18	1.8	14	[<1]

For notes, see end of table.

H

H

TABLE H–1 COMPOSITION OF FOODS — Continued
(For purposes of calculating, use "0" for "<1," "<1." etc. Where a range is given, use the midpoint.)

											NUTRIENTS IN INDICATED QUANTITY						
Item No. (A)	Foods, approximate measures, units, and weight (edible part unless footnotes indicate otherwise) (B)		Water (C)	Food energy (D)	Protein (E)	Fat (F)	Carbohydrate (G)	Calcium (H)	Iron (I)	Zinc (J)	Vitamin A (K) Retinol equivalents	Thiamin (L)	Riboflavin (M)	Niacin (N)	Folacin (O)	Vitamin C (P)
		Grams	Percent	kCalories	Grams	Grams	Grams	Milligrams	Milligrams	Milligrams		Milligrams	Milligrams	Milligrams	Micrograms	Milligrams
	LEGUMES (DRY), NUTS, SEEDS; RELATED PRODUCTS—Con.															
526	Pecans, chopped or pieces (about 120 large halves). 1 cup	118	3	810	11	84	17	86	2.8	4.2	15	1.01	.15	1.1	28	2
526x, 526x₄	Pignolia nuts (pinenuts). 6 tbsp	67	6	374	21	32	8	[91]	[3.6]	[1.3-3.4]	(0)	.43	[.40]	[1.5]	[16-71]	(0)
	Pistachios, shelled. ¼ cup	35	5	216	7	20	7	48	2.7	.8	8	.24	[.21]	.5	20	<1
527	Pumpkin and squash kernels, dry, hulled. 1 cup	140	4	775	41	65	21	71	15.7	[7.6]	10	.34	.27	3.4	[128]	[<1]
527x	Sesame seeds. dry, hulled. 4 tbsp	32	6	188	6	17	6	36	.8	1.9	[2-3]	.04	.04	1.6	32	0
	Soy products. See Milk substitutes (items 91x, and 91x₄,) Miso (item 522x), Soybean flours (items 492x₄ and 492x₄,), and Tofu (item 528x₄).															
528	Sunflower seeds, dry, hulled. 1 cup	145	5	810	35	69	29	174	10.3	7.9	7	2.84	.33	7.8	339	<1
528x,	Tahini (tahini butter). 1 tsp	7	3	45	1	4	1	7	.6	.3	(0)	.04	.02	.3	7	<0
528x₄	Tofu (soybean curd). 2½ by 2¾ by 1 in	120	r85	86	r9	5	3	r154	2.3	.9	0	.07	.04	.1	[55]	0
	Walnuts:															
	Black:															
529	Chopped or broken kernels. 1 cup	125	3	785	26	74	19	<1	7.5	2.9	38	.28	.14	.9	(83)	<1
530	Ground (finely). 1 cup	80	3	500	16	47	12	<1	4.8	1.8	24	.18	.09	.6	(53)	<1
531	Persian or English, chopped (about 60 halves). 1 cup	120	4	780	18	77	19	119	3.7	2.7	4	.40	.16	1.1	79	2
	SUGARS AND SWEETS															
	Cake icings:															
	Boiled, white:															
532	Plain. 1 cup	94	18	295	1	0	75	2	<.1	[.5]	0	<.01	.03	<.1	[0]	0
533	With coconut. 1 cup	166	15	605	3	13	124	10	.8	[.8]	0	.02	.07	.3	[8]	0
	Uncooked:															
534	Chocolate made with milk and butter. 1 cup	275	14	1,035	9	38	185	165	3.3	[1.3]	176	.06	.28	.6	[8]	1
535	Creamy fudge from mix and water. 1 cup	245	15	830	7	16	183	96	2.7	[1.1]	<1	.05	.20	.7	[7]	<1
536	White. 1 cup	319	11	1,200	2	21	260	48	<.1	(.2)	261	<.01	.06	<.1	[6]	<1
	Candy:															
537	Caramels, plain or chocolate. 1 oz	28	8	115	1	3	22	42	.4	[.1]	<1	.01	.05	.1	(0)	<1
	Chocolate:															
538	Milk, plain. 1 oz	28	1	145	2	9	16	65	.3	(.1)	24	.02	.10	.1	(0)	<1
539	Semisweet, small pieces (60 per oz). 1 cup or 6-oz pkg	170	1	860	7	61	97	51	4.4	(.7)	9	.02	.14	.9	[2]	0
540	Chocolate-coated peanuts. 1 oz	28	1	160	5	12	11	33	.4	(.8)	<1	.10	.05	2.1	(30)	<1
541	Fondant, uncoated (mints, candy corn, other). 1 oz	28	8	105	<1	1	25	4	.3	(.1)	0	<.01	<.01	<.1	(0)	0
542	Fudge, chocolate, plain. 1 oz	28	8	115	1	3	21	22	.3	(.1)	<1	.01	.03	.1	(3)	<1
543	Gum drops. 1 oz	28	12	100	<1	<1	25	2	.1	(0)	0	0	<.01	<.1	0	0
544	Hard. 1 oz	28	1	110	0	<1	28	6	.5	0	0	0	0	0	0	0
545	Marshmallows. 1 oz	28	17	90	1	<1	23	5	.5	0	0	0	<.01	<.1	0	0
	Carob. See item 696x₄.															

(A)	(B)		(C)	(D)	(E)	(F)	(G)	(H)	(I)	(J)	(K)	(L)	(M)	(N)	(O)	(P)
	Chocolate-flavored beverage powders (about 4 heaping tsp per oz):															
546	With nonfat dry milk	1 oz	28	2	100	5	1	20	167	.5	.3	3	.04	.21	.2	[6]	1
547	Without milk	1 oz	28	1	100	—	—	25	9	.6	.3	[<1]	.01	.03	.1	[0]	0
548	Honey, strained or extracted	1 tbsp	21	17	65	<1	0	17	1	.1	0	0	<.01	.01	.1	[3]	<1
549	Jams and preserves	1 tbsp	20	29	55	<1	<1	14	4	.2	0	<1	<.01	.01	<.1	(2)	<1
550	Jellies	1 packet	14	29	40	<1	<1	10	3	.1	(0)	<1	<.01	.01	<.1	(1)	<1
551		1 tbsp	18	29	50	<1	<1	13	4	.3	(0)	<1	<.01	.01	<.1	(2)	1
552		1 packet	14	29	40	<1	<1	10	3	.2	(0)	<1	<.01	<.01	<.1	(1)	1
	Sirups:																
	Chocolate-flavored sirup or topping:																
553	Thin type	1 fl oz or 2 tbsp	38	32	90	1	1	24	6	.6	.4	<1	.01	.03	.2	(2)	0
554	Fudge type	1 fl oz or 2 tbsp	38	25	125	2	5	20	48	.5	.4	[12]	.02	.08	.2	(2)	<1
	Molasses, cane:																
555	Light (first extraction)	1 tbsp	20	24	50	[<1]	[<1]	13	33	.9	(0)	[0]	.01	.01	<.1	3	[0]
556	Blackstrap (third extraction)	1 tbsp	20	24	45	[<1]	[<1]	11	137	3.2	(0)	[0]	.02	.04	.4	(3)	[0]
557	Sorghum	1 tbsp	21	23	55	[<1]	[<1]	14	35	2.6	(0)	[0]	[<.01]	.02	<.1	(4)	[0]
558	Table blends, chiefly corn, light and dark	1 tbsp	21	24	60	0	0	15	9	.8	0	0			0	(3)	0
	Sugars (see also Appendix F, sugar):																
559	Brown, pressed down	1 cup	220	2	820	0	0	212	187	7.5	0	0	.02	.07	.4	0	0
	White:																
560	Granulated	1 cup	200	1	770	0	0	199	0	.2		0	0	0	0	0	0
561		1 tbsp	12	1	45	0	0	12	0	<.1	.1	0	0	0	0	0	0
562		1 packet	6	1	23	0	0	6	0	<.1	0	0	0	0	0	0	0
563	Powdered, sifted, spooned into cup	1 cup	100	1	385	0	0	100	0	.1	0	0	0	0	0	0	0
	VEGETABLES AND VEGETABLE PRODUCTS																
	Asparagus, green:																
	Cooked, drained:																
	Cuts and tips, 1½- to 2-in lengths:																
564	From raw	1 cup	145	94	30	3	<1	5	30	.9	.7	131	.23	.26	2.0	142	38
565	From frozen	1 cup	180	93	40	6	<1	6	40	2.2	(1.0)	153	.25	.23	1.8	142	41
	Spears, ½-in. diam. at base:																
566	From raw	4 spears	60	94	10	1	<1	2	13	.4	(.3)	54	.10	.11	.8	(37)	16
567	From frozen	4 spears	60	92	15	2	<1	2	13	.7	(.3)	47	.10	.08	.7	47	16
568	Canned, spears, ½-in diam. at base	4 spears	80	93	15	2	<1	3	15	1.5	.4	64	.05	.08	.6	68	12
568x	Bamboo shoots, raw, cut into 1 inch long pieces	¾ cup	113	91	31	3	0	6	15	.6	[.3]	2	.17	.08	.7	[13-72]	5
	Beans:																
	Lima, immature seeds, frozen, cooked, drained (see also item 515):																
569	Thick-seeded types (Fordhooks)	1 cup	170	74	170	10	<1	32	34	2.9	(.7)	39	.12	.09	1.7	111	29
570	Thin-seeded types (baby limas)	1 cup	180	69	210	13	<1	40	63	4.7	(.8)	40	.16	.09	2.2	(117)	22

For notes, see end of table.

H

TABLE H-1 COMPOSITION OF FOODS — Continued
(For purposes of calculating, use "0" for "<1," "<.1," etc. Where a range is given, use the midpoint.)

Item No. (A)	Foods, approximate measures, units, and weight (edible part unless footnotes indicate otherwise) (B)		Grams	Water Per-cent (C)	Food energy kCal-ories (D)	Pro-tein Grams (E)	Fat Grams (F)	Carbo-hydrate Grams (G)	Calcium Milli-grams (H)	Iron Milli-grams (I)	Zinc Milli-grams (J)	Vitamin A Retinol equi-valents (K)	Thiamin Milli-grams (L)	Ribo-flavin Milli-grams (M)	Niacin Milli-grams (N)	Folacin Micro-grams (O)	Vitamin C Milli-grams (P)
	VEGETABLES AND VEGETABLE PRODUCTS—Con.																
	Beans:—Continued																
	Snap:																
	Green:																
	Cooked, drained:																
571	From raw (cuts and French style)	1 cup	125	92	30	2	<1	7	63	.8	.4	68	.09	.11	.6	50	15
	From frozen:																
572	Cuts	1 cup	135	92	35	2	<1	8	54	.9	(.3)	78	.09	.12	.5	43	7
573	French style	1 cup	130	92	35	2	<1	8	49	1.2	(.3)	69	.08	.10	.4	(30)	9
574	Canned, drained solids (cuts)	1 cup	135	92	30	2	<1	7	61	2.0	.3	63	.04	.07	.4	24	5
	Yellow or wax:																
	Cooked, drained:																
575	From raw (cuts and French style)	1 cup	125	93	30	2	<1	6	63	.8	[.4]	29	.09	.11	.6	[50]	16
576	From frozen (cuts)	1 cup	135	92	35	2	<1	8	47	.9	(.3)	14	.09	.11	.5	(32)	8
577	Canned, drained solids (cuts)	1 cup	135	92	30	2	<1	7	61	2.0	.2	14	.04	.07	.4	[24]	7
	Beans, mature. See Beans, dry (items 509-515) and Blackeye peas, dry (item 516).																
	Bean sprouts, raw:																
577x	Alfalfa	1 cup	[105]	93	27	3	0	3	23	.8	.7	16	.07	.13	.4	[12]	8
578	Mung	1 cup	105	89	35	4	<1	7	20	1.4	1.5	2	.14	.14	.8	sr[6]	20
578x	Soy	1 cup	105	86	48	7	2	6	50	1.1	.9	8	.24	.21	.8	[12]	14
	Bean sprouts, cooked, drained:																
579	Mung	1 cup	125	91	35	4	<1	7	21	1.1	(1.7)	3	.11	.13	.9	[12]	8
579x	Soy	1 cup	125	89	48	7	2	5	54	.9	.9	10	.20	.19	.9	[12]	5
	Beets:																
	Cooked, drained, peeled:																
580	Whole beets, 2 in diam.	2 beets	100	91	30	1	<1	7	14	.5	(<.1)	2	.03	.04	.3	78	6
581	Diced or sliced	1 cup	170	91	55	2	<1	12	24	.9	(<.1)	3	.05	.07	.5	133	10
	Canned, drained solids:																
582	Whole beets, small	1 cup	160	89	60	2	<1	14	30	1.1	.5	3	.02	.05	.2	46	5
583	Diced or sliced	1 cup	170	89	65	2	<1	15	32	1.2	.3	3	.02	.05	.2	49	5
584	Beet greens, leaves and stems, cooked, drained.	1 cup	145	94	25	2	<1	5	144	2.8	.6	740	.10	.22	.4	[171]	22
	Blackeye peas, immature seeds, cooked and drained (see also item 516):																
585	From raw	1 cup	165	72	180	13	1	30	40	3.5	2.0	58	.50	.18	2.3	170	28
586	From frozen	1 cup	170	66	220	15	1	40	43	4.8	2.4	29	.68	.19	2.4	240	15
	Broccoli:																
	Cooked, drained:																
	From raw:																
587	Stalk, medium size	1 stalk	180	91	45	6	1	8	158	1.4	.3	450	.16	.36	1.4	101	162
588	Stalks cut into ½-in pieces	1 cup	155	91	40	5	<1	7	136	1.2	.2	388	.14	.31	1.2	87	140
	From frozen:																
589	Stalk, 4½ to 5 in long	1 stalk	30	91	10	1	<1	1	12	.2	(<.1)	57	.02	.03	.2	18	22
590	Chopped	1 cup	185	92	50	5	1	9	100	1.3	(.3)	481	.11	.22	.9	111	105

NUTRIENTS IN INDICATED QUANTITY

H

(A)	(B)	(C)	(D)	(E)	(F)	(G)	(H)	(I)	(J)	(K)	(L)	(M)	(N)	(O)	(P)
590x	Raw, stalk, small . . . . ¼ lb	114	36	4	<1	7	117	1.3	(.3)	284	.11	.26	1.0	79	128
	Brussels sprouts, cooked, drained:														
591	From raw, 7-8 sprouts (1¼-to 1½-in diam.). . . . . 1 cup	155	55	7	1	10	50	1.7	.6	81	.12	.22	1.2	56	135
592	From frozen . . . . 1 cup	155	50	5	<1	10	33	1.2	(.6)	88	.12	.16	.9	136	126
	Cabbage:														
	Common varieties:														
	Raw:														
593	Coarsely shredded or sliced. 1 cup	70	15	1	<1	4	34	.3	.3	9	.04	.04	.2	46	33
594	Finely shredded or chopped. 1 cup	90	20	1	<1	5	44	.4	.4	12	.05	.05	.3	59	42
595	Cooked, drained . . . . . . 1 cup	145	30	2	<1	6	64	.4	.6	19	.06	.06	.4	26	48
596	Red, raw, coarsely shredded or sliced. 1 cup	70	20	1	<1	5	29	.6	(.3)	3	.06	.04	.3	24	43
597	Savoy, raw, coarsely shredded or sliced. 1 cup	70	15	2	<1	3	47	.6	(.3)	14	.04	.06	.2	(32)	39
598	Cabbage, celery (also called pe-tsai or wongbok), raw, 1-in pieces. 1 cup	75	10	1	<1	2	32	.5	(.3)	11	.04	.03	.5	62	19
599	Cabbage, white mustard (also called bokchoy or pakchoy), cooked, drained. 1 cup	170	25	2	<1	4	252	1.0	(.7)	527	.07	.14	1.2	(32)	26
	Carrots:														
	Raw, without crowns and tips, scraped:														
600	Whole, 7½ by 1⅛ in, or strips, 2½ to 3 in long. . . . . . 1 carrot or 18 strips	72	30	1	<1	7	27	.5	.3	793	.04	.04	.4	23	6
601	Grated . . . . 1 cup	110	45	1	<1	11	41	.8	.4	1,210	.07	.06	.7	35	9
602	Cooked (crosswise cuts), drained. 1 cup	155	50	1	<1	11	51	.9	.5	1,628	.08	.08	.8	37	9
	Canned:														
603	Sliced, drained solids . . . 1 cup	155	45	1	<1	10	47	1.1	.5	2,325	.03	.05	.6	9	3
604	Strained or junior (baby food) 1 oz (1¾ to 2 tbsp)	28	10	<1	<1	2	7	.1	0	369	.01	.01	.1	4	1
604x	Carrot juice . . . . ½ cup	[122]	49	1	<1	11	29	.6	.2	2,575	.10	.06	.5	5	10
	Cauliflower:														
605	Raw, chopped . . . . 1 cup	115	31	3	<1	6	29	1.3	.3	7	.13	.12	.8	63	90
	Cooked, drained:														
606	From raw (flower buds) . . . . 1 cup	125	30	3	<1	5	26	.9	(.2)	8	.11	.10	.8	43	69
607	From frozen (flowerets) . . . . 1 cup	180	30	3	<1	6	31	.9	(.3)	5	.07	.09	.7	68	74
	Celery, Pascal type, raw:														
608	Stalk, large outer, 8 by 1½ in, at root end. . . . . . 1 stalk	40	5	<1	<1	2	16	.1	<.1	11	.01	.01	.1	5	4
609	Pieces, diced . . . . 1 cup	120	20	1	<1	5	47	.4	.2	32	.04	.04	.4	14	11
	Collards, cooked, drained:														
610	From raw (leaves without stems) 1 cup	190	65	7	1	10	357	1.5	(.5)	1,482	.21	.38	2.3	[s]61	144
611	From frozen (chopped) . . . . 1 cup	170	50	5	1	10	299	1.7	(.4)	1,156	.10	.24	1.0	85	56
	Corn, sweet:														
	Cooked, drained:														
612	From raw, ear 5 by 1¾ in . . . . 1 ear[a]	140	70	2	1	16	2	.5	.6	[a]31	.09	.08	1.1	(50)	7
	From frozen:														
613	Ear, 5 in long . . . . 1 ear[a]	229	120	4	1	27	4	1.0	(.9)	[a]44	.18	.10	2.1	82	9
614	Kernels . . . . 1 cup	165	130	5	1	31	5	1.3	.7	[a]58	.15	.10	2.5	(59)	8
	Canned:														
615	Cream style . . . . 1 cup	256	210	5	2	51	8	1.5	1.3	[b]84	.08	.13	2.6	(100)	13
	Whole kernel:														
616	Vacuum pack . . . . 1 cup	210	175	5	1	43	6	1.1	(1.0)	[a]74	.06	.13	2.3	(82)	11

For notes, see end of table.

H

TABLE H-1 COMPOSITION OF FOODS — Continued
(For purposes of calculating, use "0" for "<1," "<.1," etc. Where a range is given, use the midpoint.)

Item No. (A)	Foods, approximate measures, units, and weight (edible part unless footnotes indicate otherwise) (B)	Grams	Water Per-cent (C)	Food energy kCal-ories (D)	Pro-tein Grams (E)	Fat Grams (F)	Carbo-hydrate Grams (G)	Calcium Milli-grams (H)	Iron Milli-grams (I)	Zinc Milli-grams (J)	Vitamin A Retinol equi-valents (K)	Thiamin Milli-grams (L)	Ribo-flavin Milli-grams (M)	Niacin Milli-grams (N)	Folacin Micro-grams (O)	Vitamin C Milli-grams (P)
	VEGETABLES AND VEGETABLE PRODUCTS—Con.															
	Corn, sweet:															
	Canned:															
	Whole kernel:—Continued															
617	Wet pack, drained solids ... 1 cup	165	76	140	4	1	33	8	.8	.8	ss58	.05	.08	1.5	64	7
	Cowpeas. See Blackeye peas. (Items 585-586).															
	Cucumber slices, ⅛ in thick (large, 2⅛-in diam.; small, 1¾-in diam.):															
618	With peel ... 6 large or 8 small slices	28	95	5	<1	<1	1	7	.3	0	7	.01	.01	.1	4	3
619	Without peel ... 6½ large or 9 small pieces	28	96	5	<1	<1	1	5	.1	0	<1	.01	.01	.1	4	3
620	Dandelion greens, cooked, drained ... 1 cup	105	90	35	2	1	7	147	1.9	[.8]	1,229	.14	.17	[1.1]	[82]	19
621	Endive, curly (including escarole), raw, small pieces. ... 1 cup	50	93	10	1	<1	2	41	.9	.4	165	.04	.07	.3	71	5
621x₁	Garlic, raw ... 1 clove	3	61	4	<1	<1	<1	1	<1	0	<1	.01	<.01	<.1	[1]	<1
621x₂	Ginger root, fresh ... 1 tsp	[5]	87	3	<1	0	<1	1	.1	[.1]	0	0			[1]	0
	Kale, cooked, drained:															
622	From raw (leaves without stems and midribs). ... 1 cup	110	88	45	5	1	7	206	1.8	(.2)	913	.11	.20	1.8	s[29]	102
623	From frozen (leaf style) ... 1 cup	130	91	40	4	1	7	157	1.3	(.2)	1,066	.08	.20	.9	(43)	49
	Lettuce, raw:															
	Butterhead, as Boston types:															
624	Head, 5-in diam ... 1 head**	220	95	25	2	<1	4	57	3.3	.7	158	.10	.10	.5	81	13
625	Leaves ... 1 outer or 2 inner or 3 heart leaves.	15	95	<1	<1	<1	<1	5	.3	<.1	15	.01	.01	<.1	6	1
	Crisphead, as Iceberg:															
626	Head, 6-in diam ... 1 head**	567	96	70	5	1	16	108	2.7	1.7	178	.32	.32	1.6	210	32
627	Wedge, ¼ of head ... 1 wedge	135	96	20	1	<1	4	27	.7	.2	45	.08	.08	.4	20	8
628	Pieces, chopped or shredded ... 1 cup	55	96	5	<1	<1	2	11	.3	.2	18	.03	.03	.2	20	3
629	Looseleaf (bunching varieties including romaine or cos), chopped or shredded pieces. ... 1 cup	55	94	10	1	<1	2	37	.8	.2	105	.03	.04	.2	98	10
	Lima beans. See Beans (items 569-570).															
630	Mushrooms, raw, sliced or chopped. ... 1 cup	70	90	20	2	<1	3	4	.6	(.9)	<1	.07	.32	2.9	16	2
631	Mustard greens, without stems and midribs, cooked, drained. ... 1 cup	140	93	30	3	1	6	193	2.5	(.3)	812	.11	.20	.8	[130]	67
632	Okra pods, 3 by ⅝ in, cooked ... 10 pods	106	91	30	2	<1	6	98	.5	[.3]	52	.14	.19	1.0	40	21
	Onions:															
	Mature:															
	Raw:															
633	Chopped ... 1 cup	170	89	65	3	<1	15	46	.9	.3	ss<1	.05	.07	.3	42	17
634	Sliced ... 1 cup	115	89	45	2	<1	10	31	.6	.2	ss<1	.03	.05	.2	23	12
635	Cooked (whole or sliced), drained. ... 1 cup	210	92	60	3	<1	14	50	.8	.2	ss<1	.06	.06	.4	27	15
636	Young green, bulb (⅜ in diam.) and white portion of top. ... 6 onions	30	88	15	<1	<1	3	12	.2	<1	<1	.02	.01	.1	11	8
637	Parsley, raw, chopped ... 1 tbsp	4	85	<1	<1	<1	<1	7	.2	(.1)	30	<.01	.01	<.1	5	6
638	Parsnips, cooked (diced or 2-in lengths). ... 1 cup	155	82	100	2	1	23	70	.9	[.4]	5	.11	.12	.2	s[37]	16

NUTRIENTS IN INDICATED QUANTITY

H

(A)	(B)	(C)	(D)	(E)	(F)	(G)	(H)	(I)	(J)	(K)	(L)	(M)	(N)	(O)	(P)
	Peas, green:														
	Canned:														
639	Whole, drained solids	1 cup	77	150	8	1	29	44	3.2	2.0	117	.15	.10	1.4	86	14
640	Strained (baby food)	1 oz (1¾ to 2 tbsp)	86	15	1	<1	3	3	.3	.1	14	.02	.03	.3	7	3
641	Frozen, cooked, drained	1 cup	82	110	8	<1	19	30	3.0	1.3	96	.43	.14	2.7	134	21
642	Peppers, hot, red, without seeds, dried (ground chili powder, added seasonings)	1 tsp	9	5	<1	<1	1	5	.3	[0]	130	<.01	.02	.2	1	<1
	Peppers, sweet (about 5 per lb, whole), stem and seeds removed:															
643	Raw	1 pod	93	15	1	<1	4	7	.5	0	31	.06	.06	.4	14	94
644	Cooked, boiled, drained	1 pod	95	15	1	<1	3	7	.4	<.1	31	.05	.05	.4	7	70
	Potatoes, cooked (see also Appendix N, Fast Foods):															
645	Baked, peeled after baking (about 2 per lb, raw)	1 potato	75	145	4	<1	33	14	1.1	.7	<1	.15	.07	2.7	14	31
	Boiled (about 3 per lb, raw):															
646	Peeled after boiling	1 potato	80	105	3	<1	23	10	.8	.4	<1	.12	.05	2.0	12	22
647	Peeled before boiling	1 potato	83	90	3	<1	20	8	.7	.4	<1	.12	.05	1.6	12	22
	French-fried, strip, 2 to 3½ in long:															
648	Prepared from raw	10 strips	45	135	2	7	18	8	.7	.1	<1	.07	.04	1.6	11	11
649	Frozen, oven heated	10 strips	53	110	2	4	17	5	.9	.2	<1	.07	.01	1.3	13	11
650	Hashed brown, prepared from frozen	1 cup	56	345	3	18	45	28	1.9	.9	<1	.11	.03	1.6	26	12
	Mashed, prepared from—															
	Raw:															
651	Milk added	1 cup	83	135	4	2	27	50	.8	.6	12	.17	.11	2.1	21	21
652	Milk and butter added	1 cup	80	195	4	9	26	50	.8	(.8)	109	.17	.11	2.1	21	19
653	Dehydrated flakes (without milk), water, milk, butter, and salt added	1 cup	79	195	4	7	30	65	.6	.8	82	.08	.08	1.9	17	11
654	Potato chips, 1¾ by 2½ in oval cross section	10 chips	2	115	1	8	10	8	.4	.2	<1	.04	.01	1.0	14	3
655	Potato salad, made with cooked salad dressing	1 cup	76	250	7	7	41	80	1.5	.6	[70]	.20	.18	2.8	17	28
656	Pumpkin, canned	1 cup	90	80	2	1	19	61	1.0	.4	1,568	.07	.12	1.5	37	12
657	Radishes, raw (prepackaged) stem ends, rootlets cut off	4 radishes	95	5	<1	<1	1	5	.2	<.1	<1	.01	.01	.1	9	5
658	Sauerkraut, canned, solids and liquid	1 cup	93	40	2	<1	9	85	1.2	1.2	12	.07	.09	.5	(7)	33
	Southern peas. See Blackeye peas (items 585-586).															
	Spinach:															
659	Raw, chopped	1 cup	91	15	2	<1	2	51	1.7	.4	446	.06	.11	.3	106	28
	Cooked, drained:															
660	From raw	1 cup	92	40	5	1	6	167	4.0	1.3	1,458	.13	.25	.9	164	50
	From frozen:															
661	Chopped	1 cup	92	45	6	1	8	232	4.3	(.6)	1,620	.14	.31	.8	(172)	39
662	Leaf	1 cup	92	45	6	1	7	200	4.8	(.6)	1,539	.15	.27	1.0	(172)	53
663	Canned, drained solids	1 cup	91	50	6	1	7	242	5.3	1.1	1,640	.04	.25	.6	119	29

For notes, see end of table.

H

TABLE H–1   COMPOSITION OF FOODS — Continued
(For purposes of calculating, use "0" for "<1," "<.1," etc. Where a range is given, use the midpoint.)

Item No. (A)	Foods, approximate measures, units, and weight (edible part unless footnotes indicate otherwise) (B)		Grams	Water Per-cent (C)	Food energy kcal-ories (D)	Pro-tein Grams (E)	Fat Grams (F)	Carbo-hydrate Grams (G)	Calcium Milli-grams (H)	Iron Milli-grams (I)	Zinc Milli-grams (J)	Vitamin A Retinol equi-valents (K)	Thiamin Milli-grams (L)	Ribo-flavin Milli-grams (M)	Niacin Milli-grams (N)	Folacin Micro-grams (O)	Vitamin C Milli-grams (P)
	VEGETABLES AND VEGETABLE PRODUCTS—Con.																
	Squash, cooked:																
664	Summer (all varieties), diced, drained	1 cup	210	96	30	2	<1	7	53	.8	.5	82	.11	.17	1.7	38	21
665	Winter (all varieties), baked, mashed	1 cup	205	81	130	4	1	32	57	1.6	.9	861	.10	.27	1.4	99	27
	Sweetpotatoes:																
	Cooked (raw, 5 by 2 in; about 2½ per lb):																
666	Baked in skin, peeled	1 potato	114	64	160	2	1	37	46	1.0	(.2)	923	.10	.08	.8	21	25
667	Boiled in skin, peeled	1 potato	151	71	170	3	1	40	48	1.1	(.2)	1,194	.14	.09	.9	27	26
668	Candied, 2½ by 2-in piece	1 piece	105	60	175	1	3	36	39	.9	.2	662	.06	.04	.4	0	11
	Canned:																
669	Solid pack (mashed)	1 cup	255	72	275	5	1	63	64	2.0	.4	1,989	.13	.10	1.5	(46)	36
670	Vacuum pack, piece 2¾ by 1 in.	1 piece	40	72	45	1	<1	10	10	.3	<1	312	.02	.02	.2	(7)	6
	Tomatoes:																
671	Raw, 2⅗-in diam. (3 per 12 oz pkg.)	1 tomato[54]	135	94	25	1	<1	6	16	.6	<1	111	.07	.05	.9	53	[55]28
672	Canned, solids and liquid	1 cup	241	94	50	2	<1	10	[55]14	1.2	.4	217	.12	.07	1.7	(66)	41
673	Tomato catsup	1 cup	273	69	290	5	1	69	60	2.2	.7	382	.25	.19	4.4	14	41
674		1 tbsp	15	69	15	<1	<1	4	3	.1	0	21	.01	.01	.2	<1	2
	Tomato juice, canned (see also item 680x, V-8 juice):																
675	Cup	1 cup	243	94	45	2	<1	10	17	2.2	.4	194	.12	.07	1.9	63	39
676	Glass (6 fl oz)	1 glass	182	94	35	2	<1	8	13	1.6	.3	146	.09	.05	1.5	47	29
676x	Tomato sauce, canned	½ cup	125	89	39	2	<1	9	14	1.1	(.3)	133	.10	.06	1.4	11	22
677	Turnips, cooked, diced	1 cup	155	94	35	1	<1	8	54	.6	[.4]	<1	.06	.08	.5	20	34
	Turnip greens, cooked, drained:																
678	From raw (leaves and stems)	1 cup	145	94	30	3	<1	5	252	1.5	2.0	827	.15	.33	.7	172	68
679	From frozen (chopped)	1 cup	165	93	40	4	<1	6	195	2.6	.7	1,139	.08	.15	.7	64	31
680	Vegetables, mixed, frozen, cooked	1 cup	182	83	115	6	1	24	46	2.4	.6	901	.22	.13	2.0	88	15
680x₁	Vegetable juice, mixed (V-8)	6 fl oz	182	94	31	2	<1	7	22	.9	[0]	127	.09	.05	1.5	29	16
680x₂	Water chestnuts, raw	4 chestnuts	58	78	46	1	0	11	2	.4	.2	0	.08	.12	.6	[13]	2
	MISCELLANEOUS ITEMS																
	Baking powders for home use:																
	Sodium aluminum sulfate:																
681	With monocalcium phosphate monohydrate	1 tsp	3	2	5	<1	<1	1	58	[0]	[0]	0	0	0	0	[0]	0
682	With monocalcium phosphate monohydrate, calcium sulfate	1 tsp	3	1	5	<1	<1	1	183	[0]	[0]	0	0	0	0	[0]	0
683	Straight phosphate	1 tsp	4	2	5	<1	<1	1	239	[0]	[0]	0	0	0	0	[0]	0
684	Low sodium	1 tsp	4	2	5	<1	<1	2	207	[0]	[0]	0	0	0	0	[0]	0
685	Barbecue sauce	1 cup	250	81	230	4	17	20	53	2.0	.3	90	.03	.03	.8	10	13
	Beverages, alcoholic:																
686	Beer	12 fl oz	360	92	150	1	0	14	18	<1	.1	[0]	.01	.11	2.2	22	[0]
	Gin, rum, vodka, whisky:																
687	80-proof	1½-fl oz jigger	42	67	95	[0]	[0]	<1	[0]	[0]	0	[0]	[0]	[0]	[0]	0	[0]

H

(A)	(B)	(C)	(D)	(E)	(F)	(G)	(H)	(I)	(J)	(K)	(L)	(M)	(N)	(O)	(P)
688	86-proof ... 1½-fl oz jigger	42	105	[0]	[0]	<1	[0]	[0]	0	[0]	[0]	[0]	[0]	0	[0]
689	90-proof ... 1½-fl oz jigger	42	110	[0]	[0]	<1	[0]	[0]	0	[0]	[0]	[0]	[0]	0	[0]
	Wines:														
690	Dessert ... 3½-fl oz glass	103	140	<1	0	8	8	[1.6]	<1	[<1]	.01	.02	[0]	2	[0]
691	Table ... 3½-fl oz glass	102	85	<1	0	4	9	.4	.1	[<1]	<.01	.01	.1	2	[0]
	Beverages, carbonated, nonalcoholic:														
692	Carbonated water, sweetened ... 12 fl oz	366	115	0	0	29	[18]	[.2]	0	0	0	0	0	[0]	0
693	Cola type ... 12 fl oz	369	145	0	0	37	[11]	[.2]	(.3)	0	0	0	0	[0]	0
694	Fruit-flavored sodas and Tom Collins mixer ... 12 fl oz	372	170	0	0	45	[15]	[.3]	<.1	0	0	0	0	[0]	0
695	Ginger ale ... 12 fl oz	366	115	0	0	29	[11]	[.2]	.1	0	0	0	0	[0]	0
695x	Mineral water, carbonated[t] ... 8 fl oz	236	[0]	0	0	[0]	33	0	[0]	[0]	[0]	[0]	[0]	[0]	[0]
696	Root beer ... 12 fl oz	370	150	0	0	39	[15]	[.2]	<.1	[0]	[0]	0	0	[0]	0
696x1	Special dietary drink, artificially sweetened ... 12 fl oz	355	0	[0]	[0]	<1	14	.5	.8	[0]	[0]	[0]	[0]	[0]	[0]
	Beverages, noncarbonated, nonalcoholic:														
696x2	Cranberry-apple juice drink ... 6 fl oz	190	135	<1	1	34	10	.2	.3	[0]	.01	.04	.1	[20]	u61
696x3	Fruit-punch drink ... 6 fl oz	190	99	<1	0	25	6	.1	.1	[0]	.04	.05	<.1	[20]	u64
696x4	Pineapple-grapefruit juice drink ... 6 fl oz	187	95	<1	<1	24	11	.6	.1	[0]	.04	.04	.5	[20]	u61
696x5	Pineapple-orange juice drink ... 6 fl oz	187	99	<1	0	24	9	.5	.1	99	.04	.04	.4	[20]	u46
696x6	Carob flour (powder)[v] ... 1 tbsp	8	14	<1	<1	7	28	(.2)	<.1	3	(<.01)	(.02)	(.1)	[0]	(0)
	Chili powder. See Peppers, hot, red (item 642).														
	Chocolate:														
697	Bitter or baking ... 1 oz	28	145	3	15	8	22	1.9	(.1)	2	.01	.07	.4	3	0
	Semisweet, see Candy, chocolate (item 539).														
697x1	Coffee, beverage prepared with 2 g of dry powder to 6 fl oz water ... 6 fl oz	180	2	(0)	(0)	(0)	w4	w.2	w0	0	0	(0)	.5	0	0
697x2	Egg roll, chicken. See item 437x1 ... 1	100	[242]	[8]	[10]	[29]	[27]	[1.0]	[.4]	[23]	[.12]	[.12]	[1.5]	[44]	[4]
	French toast. See item 437x1.														
698	Gelatin, dry ... 1 envelope	7	25	6	<1	0	[0]	[.4]	0	[0]	[0]	[0]	[0]	[0]	[4]
699	Gelatin dessert prepared with gelatin dessert powder and water ... 1 cup	240	140	4	0	34	[4]	[.2]	<.1	[0]	[.02]	[.02]	[.4]	[0]	[2]
699x	Gravy, brown, dehydrated, prepared with water (see also Appendix N, Fast Foods) ... 1 cup	261	9	<1	<1	2	7	0	0	[0]	.01	.01	.1	[0]	[0]
	Humous. See item 521x.														
	Ketchup. See items 673-674.														
	Miso. See item 522x.														
700	Mustard, prepared, yellow ... 1 tsp or individual serving pouch or cup.	5	5	<1	<1	<1	4	.1	0	[0]	[<.01]	[<.01]	[<.1]	[0]	[0]
	Olives, pickled, canned:														
701	Green ... 4 medium or 3 extra large or 2 giant[s]	16	15	<1	2	<1	8	.2	0	4	[<.01]	[<.01]	[<.1]	[0]	<1
702	Ripe, Mission ... 3 small or 2 large[ss]	10	15	<1	2	<1	9	.1	0	1	<.01	<.01	<.1	[0]	<1
	Pickles, cucumber:														
703	Dill, medium, whole, 3¾ in long, 1¼-in diam. ... 1 pickle	65	5	<1	<1	1	17	.7	.2	7	<.01	.01	<.1	<1	4
704	Fresh-pack, slices 1½-in diam, ¼ in thick. ... 2 slices	15	10	<1	<1	3	5	.3	0	2	<.01	<.01	<.1	0	1

For notes, see end of table.

H

TABLE H–1 COMPOSITION OF FOODS — Continued
(For purposes of calculating, use "0" for "<1," "<.1," etc. Where a range is given, use the midpoint.)

Item No. (A)	Foods, approximate measures, units, and weight (edible part unless footnotes indicate otherwise) (B)	Grams	Water (C) Percent	Food energy (D) kCalories	Protein (E) Grams	Fat (F) Grams	Carbohydrate (G) Grams	Calcium (H) Milligrams	Iron (I) Milligrams	Zinc (J) Milligrams	Vitamin A (K) Retinol equivalents	Thiamin (L) Milligrams	Riboflavin (M) Milligrams	Niacin (N) Milligrams	Folacin (O) Micrograms	Vitamin C (P) Milligrams
	MISCELLANEOUS ITEMS—Con.															
	Pickles, cucumber:—Continued															
705	Sweet, gherkin, small, whole, about 2½ in long, ¾-in diam. ... 1 pickle	15	61	20	<1	<1	5	2	.2	0	1	<.01	<.01	<.1	(0)	1
706	Relish, finely chopped, sweet ... 1 tbsp	15	63	20	<1	<1	5	3	.1	0	[1]	[<.01]	[<.01]	[<.1]	(0)	[1]
	Popcorn. See items 476-478.															
707	Popsicle, 3-fl oz size ... 1 popsicle	95	80	70	0	0	18	0	<.1	[0]	0	0	0	0	[0]	0
	Soups:															
	Canned, condensed:															
	Prepared with equal volume of milk:															
708	Cream of chicken ... 1 cup	245	85	180	7	10	15	172	.5	.7	[122]	.05	.27	.7	8	2
709	Cream of mushroom ... 1 cup	245	83	215	7	14	16	191	.5	.6	[50]	.05	.34	.7	10	1
710	Tomato ... 1 cup	250	84	175	7	7	23	168	.8	.3	[240]	.10	.25	1.3	21	15
	Prepared with equal volume of water:															
711	Bean with pork ... 1 cup	250	84	170	8	6	22	63	2.3	1.0	[130]	.13	.08	1.0	32	3
712	Beef broth, bouillon, consomme. ... 1 cup	240	96	30	5	0	3	<10	.5	[.5]	<1	<.01	.02	1.2	0	[0]
713	Beef noodle ... 1 cup	240	93	65	4	3	7	7	1.0	1.5	[10]	.05	.07	1.0	4	<1
714	Clam chowder, Manhattan type (with tomatoes, without milk). ... 1 cup	245	92	80	2	3	12	34	1.0	1.9	[176]	.02	.02	1.0	10	[5]
715	Cream of chicken ... 1 cup	240	92	95	3	6	8	24	.5	.6	[82]	.02	.05	.5	2	<1
716	Cream of mushroom ... 1 cup	240	90	135	2	10	10	41	.5	.6	[14]	.02	.12	.7	(4)	<1
717	Minestrone ... 1 cup	245	90	105	5	3	14	37	1.0	.7	235	.07	.05	1.0	16	[3]
718	Split pea ... 1 cup	245	85	145	9	3	21	29	1.5	1.1	44	.25	.15	1.5	2	1
719	Tomato ... 1 cup	245	91	90	2	3	16	15	.7	.2	100	.05	.05	1.2	15	12
720	Vegetable beef ... 1 cup	245	92	80	5	2	10	12	.7	3.0	270	.05	.05	1.0	12	[1]
721	Vegetarian ... 1 cup	245	92	80	2	2	13	20	1.0	.5	294	.05	.05	1.0	11	[1]
	Dehydrated:															
722	Bouillon cube, ½ in ... 1 cube	4	4	5	1	<1	<1	[<1]	.2	[0]	[0]	[.01]	[.01]	[.2]	0	[<1]
	Mixes:															
	Unprepared:															
723	Onion ... 1½-oz pkg	43	3	150	6	5	23	42	.6	.2	3	.05	.03	.3	6	6
	Prepared with water:															
724	Chicken noodle ... 1 cup	240	95	55	2	1	8	7	.2	.4	[10]	.07	.05	.5	2	<1
725	Onion ... 1 cup	240	96	35	1	1	6	10	.2	.6	<1	<.01	<.01	<.1	15	2
726	Tomato vegetable with noodles. ... 1 cup	240	93	65	1	1	12	7	.2	(.8)	48	.05	.02	.5	<1	5
	Homemade:															
726x₁	Wonton^X ... 1 cup	[250]	[90]	[268]	[22]	[12]	[16]	[33]	[3.5]	[1.7]	[135]	[.70]	[.30]	[4.6]	[30]	[5]
	Spices. See Garlic (item 621x₁), Ginger (item 621x₂), Parsley (item 637), Peppers (item 642).															
726x₂	Tea, brewed ... 1 cup	180	[178]	[0]	[0]	[0]	[0]	w4	w0	w0	[0]	[0]	[0]	[.9]	9	[0]
	Tofu. See item 528x₃.															
727	Vinegar, cider ... 1 tbsp	15	94	<1	<1	0	1	1	.1	0	[0]	[0]	[0]	[0]	[0]	[<1]
728	White sauce, medium, with enriched flour. ... 1 cup	250	73	405	10	31	22	288	.5	(.5)	[230]	.12	.43	.7	[10]	2

NUTRIENTS IN INDICATED QUANTITY

(A)	(B)	(C)	(D)	(E)	(F)	(G)	(H)	(I)	(J)	(K)	(L)	(M)	(N)	(O)	(P)	
728x	Wonton, fried .... 2 pieces	[90]	[50]	[241]	[8]	[18]	[10]	[9]	[1.4]	[.9]	[8]	[.33]	[.13]	[2.1]	[10]	[<1]
	Yeast:															
729	Baker's, dry, active .... 1 pkg	7	5	20	3	<1	3	3	1.1	.4	<1	.16	.38	2.6	Y286	<1
730	Brewer's, dry .... 1 tbsp	8	5	25	3	<1	3	[70]17	1.4	.6	<1	1.25	.34	3.0	Y313	<1

[1] Vitamin A value is largely from beta-carotene used for coloring. Riboflavin value for items 40-41 apply to products with added riboflavin.

[2] Applies to product without added vitamin A. With added vitamin A, value is 152 Retinol Equivalents (R.E.).

[3] Applies to product without vitamin A added.

[4] Applies to product with added vitamin A. Without added vitamin A, value is 6 Retinol Equivalents (R.E.).

[5] Yields 1 qt of fluid milk when reconstituted according to package directions.

[6] Applies to product with added vitamin A.

[7] Weight applies to product with label claim of 1⅓ cups equal 3.2 oz.

[8] Applies to products made from thick shake mixes and that do not contain added ice cream. Products made from milk shake mixes are higher in fat and usually contain added ice cream.

[9] Content of fat, vitamin A, and carbohydrate varies. Consult the label when precise values are needed for special diets.

[10] Applies to product made with milk containing no added vitamin A.

[11] Based on year-round average.

[12] Based on average vitamin A content of fortified margarine. Federal specifications for fortified margarine require a minimum of 15,000 International Units (I.U.) or 4,545 Retinol Equivalents (R.E.) of vitamin A per pound.

[13] Dipped in egg, milk or water, and breadcrumbs; fried in vegetable shortening.

[14] If bones are discarded, value for calcium will be greatly reduced.

[15] Dipped in egg, breadcrumbs, and flour or batter.

[16] Prepared with tuna, celery, salad dressing (mayonnaise type), pickle, onion, and egg.

[17] Outer layer of fat on the cut was removed to within approximately ½ in of the lean. Deposits of fat within the cut were not removed.

[18] Crust made with vegetable shortening and enriched flour.

[19] Made with regular margarine.

[20] Value varies widely.

[21] About one-fourth of the outer layer of fat on the cut was removed. Deposits of fat within the cut were not removed.

[22] Vegetable shortening used.

[23] Also applies to pasteurized apple cider.

[24] Applies to product without added ascorbic acid. For value of product with added ascorbic acid, refer to label.

[25] Based on product with label claim of 45% of U.S. RDA in 6 fl oz.

[26] Based on product with label claim of 100% of U.S. RDA in 6 fl oz.

[27] Weight includes peel and membranes between sections. Without these parts, the weight of the edible portion is 123 g for item 246 and 118 g for item 247.

[28] For white-fleshed varieties, value is about 2 Retinol Equivalents (R.E.) per cup; for red-fleshed varieties, 108 R.E.

[29] Weight includes seeds. Without seeds, weight of the edible portion is 57 g.

[30] Applies to product without added ascorbic acid, based on claim that 6 fl oz of reconstituted juice contain 45% or 50% of the U.S. RDA, value in milligrams is 108 or 120 for a 6-fl oz can (item 258), 36 or 40 for 1 cup of diluted juice (item 259).

[31] For products with added thiamin and riboflavin but without added ascorbic acid, values in milligrams would be 0.60 for thiamin, 0.80 for riboflavin, and trace for ascorbic acid. For products with only ascorbic acid added, value varies with the brand. Consult the label.

[32] Weight includes rind. Without rind, the weight of the edible portion is 272 g for item 271 and 149 g for item 272.

[33] Represents yellow-fleshed varieties. For white-fleshed varieties, value is 5 Retinol Equivalents (R.E.) for 1 peach, 9 R.E. for 1 cup of slices.

[34] Value represents products with added ascorbic acid. For products without added ascorbic acid, value in milligrams is 116 for a 10-oz container, 103 for 1 cup.

[35] Weight includes pits. After removal of the pits, the weight of the edible portion is 258 g for item 302, 133 g for item 303, 43 g for item 304, and 213 g for item 305.

[36] Weight includes rind and seeds. Without rind and seeds, weight of the edible portion is 426 g.

[37] Made with vegetable shortening.

[38] Applies to product made with white cornmeal. With yellow cornmeal, value is 3 Retinol Equivalents (R.E.).

[39] Applies to white varieties. For yellow varieties, value is 45 Retinol Equivalents (R.E.).

[40] Value may range from less than 1 mg to about 8 mg depending on the brand. Consult the label.

[41] Applies to product with added nutrient. Without added nutrient, value is trace.

[42] Value varies with the brand. Consult the label.

[43] Excepting angelfood cake, cakes were made from mixes containing vegetable shortening; icings, with butter.

[44] Excepting spongecake, vegetable shortening used for cake portion; butter, for icing. If butter or margarine used for cake portion, vitamin A values would be higher.

[45] Equal weights of flour, sugar, eggs, and vegetable shortening.

[46] Products are commercial unless otherwise specified.

[47] Made with enriched flour and vegetable shortening except for macaroons which do not contain flour or shortening.

[48] Icing made with butter.

H

TABLE H–1 COMPOSITION OF FOODS — Continued
(For purposes of calculating, use "0" for "<1," "<.1," etc. Where a range is given, use the midpoint.)

Item No. (A)	Foods, approximate measures, units, and weight (edible part unless footnotes indicate otherwise) (B)	Water (C) Per-cent	Food energy (D) kCal-ories	Pro-tein (E) Grams	Fat (F) Grams	Carbo-hydrate (G) Grams	Calcium (H) Milli-grams	Iron (I) Milli-grams	Zinc (J) Milli-grams	Vitamin A (K) Retinol equi-valents	Thiamin (L) Milli-grams	Ribo-flavin (M) Milli-grams	Niacin (N) Milli-grams	Folacin (O) Micro-grams	Vitamin C (P) Milli-grams
		Grams													

NUTRIENTS IN INDICATED QUANTITY

aa Applies to yellow varieties; white varieties contain only a trace.
bb Contains vegetable shortening and butter.
cc Made with corn oil.
dd Applies to product made with yellow cornmeal.
ee Made with enriched degermed cornmeal and enriched flour.
ff Product may or may not be enriched with riboflavin. Consult the label.
gg Weight includes cob. Without cob, weight is 77 g for item 612, 126 g for item 613.
hh Weight includes refuse of outer leaves and core. Without these parts, weight is 163 g.
ii Weight includes core. Without core, weight is 539 g.
jj Value based on white-fleshed varieties. For yellow-fleshed varieties, value in Retinol Equivalents (R.E.) is 7 for item 633, 5 for item 634, and 8 for item 635.
kk Weight includes cores and stem ends. Without these parts, weight is 123 g.
ll Based on year-round average. For tomatoes marketed from November through May, value is about 12 mg; from June through October, 32 mg.
mm Applies to product without calcium salts added. Value for products with calcium salts added may be as much as 63 mg for whole tomatoes, 241 mg for cut forms.
nn Weight includes pits. Without pits, weight is 13 g for item 701, 9 g for item 702.
oo Value may vary from 6 to 60 mg.
a Most of the nutrient composition of kefir was provided by product labeling and correspondence from Mathis Dairy, Decatur, Georgia.
b Nutrients estimated based on ingredients in recipe described in Agriculture Research Service, *Procedures for Calculating Nutritive Values of Home-Prepared Foods*, Agricultural Research Service Bulletin No. 62-13, Consumer Nutrition Center, Hyattsville, MD 20782, 1963.
c Values derived from label of product from EnerG Foods, Inc., P.O. Box 24723, Seattle, WA 98124.
d Values for plain, fruit, and flavored low-fat yogurt, except for water and folacin, were provided by The Dannon Company, Inc., 22-11 38th Avenue, Long Island City, NY 11101.
e Zinc content reported is for Pacific oysters (E. W. Murphy, B. W. Willis, and B. K. Watt, Provisional tables on the zinc content of foods, *Journal of the American Dietetic Association* 66, 1975: 345). Atlantic oysters are reported to have several times this amount.
f Value estimated from value for canned product from J. A. T. Pennington and H. N. Church, *Bowes and Church's Food Values of Portions Commonly Used*, 13th ed. (New York: Harper and Row, 1980).
g Iron values for white breads and rolls are based on the values for enriched corn meals, pastas, farina, and rice and represent the minimum levels of enrichment promulgated under the Federal Food, Drug and Cosmetic Act of 1955. The niacin, riboflavin, and thiamin contents of white flours and white breads and white rolls are based on the enrichment levels proposed by FDA in 1974. Riboflavin values for rice are for unenriched rice, as the levels for added riboflavin have not been approved.
h Based on white varieties. Yellow varieties contain traces of cryptoxanthine and carotene.
i The folacin in Ralston Purina, Kellogg's, and Post 40% Bran Flakes is at a level approximating 25 percent of the U.S. RDA. The folacin and zinc contents of bran flakes with raisins are assumed equal to those in fortified Kellogg's raisin bran.
j Kellogg's cornflakes are fortified with folacin. Not all brands of cornflakes are fortified.
k Values imputed by USDA, assuming a cereal such as Kix.
l Values imputed by USDA, assuming a cereal such as Corn Chex.
m Values imputed by USDA, assuming a cereal such as Cheerios.
n Based on Kellogg's product.
o Estimated weight based on frozen Sara Lee cheesecake.
p Zinc value estimated from Jiffy mix by A.W. Mahoney. Mineral contents of selected cereals and baked products, *Cereal Foods World* 27 (1982): 148.
q Dark red kidney beans may have more thiamin.
r Tofu has varying protein and water contents. Differences depend on method of preparation, type of coagulant, grade and protein content of beans. Calcium (and magnesium) contents of tofu also vary considerably, according to the coagulant used. Sea salt coagulant is high in magnesium.
s The folacin content of this food given in a literature reference was considerably higher than that recently received from USDA. The value given in brackets is an average of the two.
t Most values based on those for Perrier water; values for water, zinc, and folacin estimated.
u Vitamin C-fortified fruit drinks.
v Values in parentheses as provided in personal correspondence and by label from El Molino Mills for Cara Coa Carob powder.
w Mineral content varies with water source.
x Recipe calls for ½ lb pork and serves 4.
y The bioavailability of folacin in yeast is significantly lower than in other foods, perhaps because of the conjugase inhibitors in yeast.

APPENDIX I

Sodium and Potassium Content of Foods

Today's widespread concern about the possible overconsumption of sodium by some members of the population, and its relationship to high blood pressure, have prompted the making of this Appendix. Since potassium may contribute to normalizing blood pressure, working against sodium which may raise it (see Chapter 10), the potassium content of each food is listed next to its sodium content. The balance of the two nutrients may be of greater interest than the sodium alone.

The following table presents the same 730 foods as Appendix H, but only a brief description is given here to identify each food. The complete descriptions are in Appendix H. Occasionally, a food description differs from that of Appendix H; all differences are identified with table notes.

The potassium value for each food is taken from USDA'S Home and Garden Bulletin No. 72, *Nutritive Value of Foods*,[1] except where numbers appear in parentheses or brackets. Where Bulletin No. 72 presented a dash, we turned to other literature references[2] and adapted values

from them. When we found a potassium value for the food listed, we adjusted it for serving size, and placed the number in parentheses ( ). Where we found no value for the food listed, we adapted a value for a similar food or averaged those for several similar foods and placed the number in brackets [ ].

The sodium values are from several sources.[3] Sodium contents of foods vary widely, and the values are approximate and tentative, unlike most of those in Appendix H which are relatively precise. (See the introduction to that appendix for the methods used there.) The user of this table could round off all values below 1,000 milligrams to the nearest 25 or even 50, and could round off values above 1,000 milligrams to the nearest 100, without losing accuracy. In other words, this table is not useful for calculating a person's exact sodium intake, but can serve as a means of obtaining a rough approximation.

Many low-sodium food products are available. A few of these are identified in the table notes.

1   C. Adams and M. Richardson, *Nutritive Value of Foods, Home and Garden Bulletin No. 72* (Washington, D.C.: Government Printing Office, 1981).
2   J. A. T. Pennington and H. N. Church, *Bowes and Church's Food Values of Foods Commonly Used*, 13th ed. (New York: Harper and Row, 1980); C. F. Adams, *Nutritive Value of American Foods in Common Units, Agriculture Handbook No. 456* (Washington, D.C.: Government Printing Office, 1975).

3   U.S. Department of Agriculture, *The Sodium Content of Your Food, Home and Garden Bulletin No. 233* (Washington, D.C.: Government Printing Office, 1981); Water Quality Association, Technical paper 2/78 on *Sources of Sodium in the Diet*, available from 477 East Butterfield Road, Lombard, IL 60148; Institute of Food Technologists' Expert Panel on Food Safety and Nutrition, Dietary salt, *Food Technology*, January 1980, pp. 85-91; and Pennington and Church, 1980.

TABLE I–1 **Potassium and Sodium in Foods**

TABLE I–1 **(continued)**

FOOD AND MEASURE	POTASSIUM (mg)	SODIUM (mg)
Dairy Products		
Cheeses		
1. Blue (1 oz)	73	396
2. Camembert (1 wedge)	71	324
3. Cheddar (1 oz)	28	176[a]
4. (1 cu in)	17	108
5. (1 cup)	111	710
6. Cottage, large curd (1 cup)	190	(910)
7. Small curd (1 cup)	177	(910)
8. 2% fat (1 cup)	217	918
9. 1% fat (1 cup)	193	918
10. Dry, ½% fat (unsalted) (1 cup)	47	18
11. Cream (1 oz)	34	84
12. Mozzarella, whole (1 oz)	21	106
13. Skim (1 oz)	27	132
14. Parmesan (1 cup)	107	1,886
15. (1 tbsp)	5	94
16. (1 oz)	30	528
17. Provolone (1 oz)	39	248
18. Ricotta, whole (1 cup)	257	206
19. Skim (1 cup)	308	307
20. Romano (1 oz)	[26]	340
21. Swiss (1 oz)	31	74
22. American (process) (1 oz)	46	406[b]
23. Swiss (process) (1 oz)	61	388
24. Cheese food, American (1 oz)	79	337
25. Cheese spread, American (1 oz)	69	381
Creams		
26. Half & half (1 cup)	314	57
27. (1 tbsp)	19	6
28. Coffee (1 cup)	292	96
29. (1 tbsp)	18	6
30. Whipping, light (1 cup)	231	80
31. (1 tbsp)	15	5
32. Heavy (1 cup)	179	95
33. (1 tbsp)	11	6
34. Topping (1 cup)	88	30
35. (1 tbsp)	4	2
36. Sour cream (1 cup)	331	238
37. (1 tbsp)	17	12
38. Frozen liquid creamer (1 cup)	467	196
39. (1 tbsp)	29	12
40. Powdered creamer (1 cup)	763	188
41. (1 tsp)	16	4
42. Whipped topping, frozen (1 cup)	14	38
43. (1 tbsp)	1	2
44. Whipped topping, mix (1 cup)	121	60
45. (1 tbsp)	6	3
46. Whipped topping, pressurized (1 cup)	13	35
47. (1 tbsp)	1	2
48. Imitation sour cream (1 cup)	380	235
49. (1 tbsp)	19	12
Milks, Milk Products		
50. Whole (1 cup)	370	122[c]
51. Lowfat, 2% (1 cup)	377	122
52. Label claim normal protein (1 cup)	397	127
53. Label claim high protein (1 cup)	447	145
54. 1% fat (1 cup)	381	122
55. 1% fat normal protein (1 cup)	397	127
56. 1% fat high protein (1 cup)	444	(145)
57. Skim (1 cup)	406	128
58. Normal protein (1 cup)	418	130
59. High protein (1 cup)	446	144
60. Buttermilk (1 cup)	371	212
61. Evaporated, whole (1 cup)	764	297
62. Skim (1 cup)	845	298
63. Sweetened, condensed (1 cup)	1,136	343
64. Buttermilk, dried (1 cup)	1,910	600
65. Nonfat, instant (1 envelope)	1,552	478
66. (1 cup)	1,160	357
67. Chocolate, whole (1 cup)	417	149
68. 2% fat (1 cup)	422	150
69. 1% fat (1 cup)	426	152
70. Eggnog (1 cup)	420	138
71. Malted, chocolate (1 cup)	500	(215)
72. Natural (1 cup)	529	(215)
Ice Cream; Ice Milk		
73. Thick shake, chocolate (1 container)	672	333
74. Vanilla (1 container)	572	299
75. Ice cream, hard (½ gal)	2,052	928
76. (1 cup)	257	85
77. (3 fl oz)	96	45
78. Ice cream, soft (1 cup)	338	154
79. Hard, rich (½ gal)	1,771	864
80. (1 cup)	221	108
81. Ice milk, hard (½ gal)	2,117	(732)
82. (1 cup)	265	(89)
83. Soft (1 cup)	412	164
84. Sherbet (½ gal)	1,585	709
85. (1 cup)	198	89
Puddings, Custards		
86. Custard, baked (1 cup)	387	209

[a] 1 oz low-sodium cheddar cheese has 6 mg sodium.
[b] 1 oz low-sodium American cheese has 2 mg sodium.
[c] 1 c low-sodium milk has 5 mg sodium.

TABLE I-1 (continued)

FOOD AND MEASURE	POTASSIUM (mg)	SODIUM (mg)
87. Pudding, homemade		
chocolate (1 cup)	445	146
88. Vanilla (1 cup)	352	[251]
89. Tapioca (1 cup)	223	258
90. From mix, cooked (1 cup)	354	343
91. Instant, chocolate (1 cup)	335	820
Yogurts		
92. Yogurt, fruit flavored		
(1 container)	439	133
93. Plain (1 container)	531	159
94. Nonfat milk (1 container)	579	174
95. Whole milk (1 container)	351	107
Eggs		
96. Whole (1 egg)	65	59
97. White (1 white)	45	50
98. Yolk (1 yolk)	15	12
99. Fried (1 egg)	58	155
100. Hard cooked (1 egg)	65	61
101. Poached (1 egg)	65	[59]
102. Scrambled egg or omelet		
(1 egg)	85	164
Fats, Oils; Related Products		
103. Butter (1 stick)	29	934
104. (1 tbsp)	4	124
105. (1 pat)	1	41
106. Whipped (1 stick)	20	505
107. (1 tbsp)	2	60
108. (1 pat)	1	31
109. Shortening (1 cup)	0	0
110. (1 tbsp)	0	0
111. Lard (1 cup)	0	0
112. (1 tbsp)	0	0
113. Margarine (1 stick)	29	1,115
114. (1 tbsp)	4	138
115. (1 pat)	1	49
116. Soft (1 container)	59	1,602[d]
117. (1 tbsp)	4	98[d]
118. Whipped (1 stick)	20	490
119. (1 tbsp)	2	63
Oils		
120. Corn (1 cup)	0	0
121. (1 tbsp)	0	0
122. Olive (1 cup)	0	0
123. (1 tbsp)	0	0
124. Peanut (1 cup)	0	0
125. (1 tbsp)	0	0
126. Safflower (1 cup)	0	0
127. (1 tbsp)	0	0
128. Soybean (1 cup)	0	0
129. (1 tbsp)	0	0

[d] Value derived by averaging 9 soft margarines from Table V in J. A. T. Pennington and H. N. Church, *Bowes and Church's Food Values of Portions Commonly Used*, 13th ed. (New York: Harper and Row, 1980), p 157.

TABLE I-1 (continued)

FOOD AND MEASURE	POTASSIUM (mg)	SODIUM (mg)
130. Soybean-cottonseed (1 cup)	0	0
131. (1 tbsp)	0	0
Salad Dressings		
132. Blue cheese, regular (1 tbsp)	6	164
133. Low-kcalorie (1 tbsp)	5	177
134. French, regular (1 tbsp)	13	219
135. Low-kcalorie (1 tbsp)	13	126
136. Italian, regular (1 tbsp)	2	314
137. Low-kcalorie (1 tbsp)	2	118
138. Mayonnaise (1 tbsp)	5	84
139. Mayonnaise-type dressing,		
regular (1 tbsp)	1	88
140. Low-kcalorie (1 tbsp)	1	19
141. Tartar sauce (1 tbsp)	11	99
142. Thousand Island, regular		
(1 tbsp)	18	112
143. Low-kcalorie (1 tbsp)	17	112
144. Homemade, cooked (1 tbsp)	19	116
Fish, Shellfish, Meat, Poultry, Related Products		
145. Bluefish (3 oz)	308	87
146. Clams, raw[e] (3 oz)	200	31
147. Canned (3 oz)	119	[850]
148. Crabmeat, canned (1 cup)	149	1,350
149. Fishsticks (1 stick)	109	50
150. Haddock (3 oz)	296	150
151. Ocean perch (3 oz)	242	128
152. Oysters, raw (1 cup)	290	319[f]
153. Salmon, canned[g] (3 oz)	307	444
154. Sardines, canned (3 oz)	502	434
155. Scallops (6 scallops)	(428)	(239)[h]
156. Shad (3 oz)	320	66
157. Shrimp, canned (3 oz)	104	1,955
158. Fried (3 oz)	195	158
159. Tuna, canned (3 oz)	204	680[i]
160. Salad (1 cup)	[500][j]	[2,000][j]
Meats		
161. Bacon (2 slices)	35	250
162. Beef pot roast, regular (3 oz)	184	46
163. Lean (3 oz)	176	45
164. Ground beef, 10% fat (3 oz)	261	41
165. 21% fat (2.9 oz)	221	31
166. Beef rib roast, regular (3 oz)	189	28
167. Lean (1.8 oz)	161	24

[e] Soft clams. 3 oz hard clams have 264 mg potassium; 174 mg sodium. Potassium and sodium values from Pennington and Church, 1980.
[f] Sodium in raw oysters may be more than twice this amount, depending on preparation.
[g] Sockeye salmon. Values vary.
[h] Sodium value for steamed scallops from Pennington and Church, 1980.
[i] Sodium may be half as high, depending on brand. Low-sodium canned tuna has about 40 mg sodium in 3 oz.
[j] Rough estimates. Sodium and potassium may be much higher, depending on amounts of pickle, celery, and dressing used.

I

TABLE I-1   (continued)

FOOD AND MEASURE	POTASSIUM (mg)	SODIUM (mg)
168. Beef round roast, regular (3 oz)	279	(42)
169. Lean (2.8 oz)	268	(40)
170. Sirloin steak, regular (3 oz)	220	26
171. Lean (2 oz)	202	23
172. Braised round steak, regular (3 oz)	272	39
173. Lean (2.4 oz)	238	35
174. Corned beef, canned (3 oz)	51	803
175. Corned beef hash, canned (1 cup)	440	1,188
176. Chipped beef (2½ oz)	142	3,050
177. Beef stew (1 cup)	613	515
178. Beef pot pie (1 piece)	334	597
179. Chili, canned (1 cup)	594	1,354
180. Chop suey, homemade (1 cup)	425	1,053
181. Beef heart (3 oz)	197	88
182. Lamb chop, broiled, regular (3.1 oz)	200	47
183. Lean (2 oz)	174	42
184. Lamb leg, roasted, regular (3 oz)	241	42
185. Lean (2.5 oz)	227	40
186. Lamb shoulder roast, regular (3 oz)	206	58
187. Lean (2.3 oz)	193	54
188. Beef liver (3 oz)	323	187
189. Ham (3 oz)	199	559
190. Sliced, packaged (1 oz)	[89]	[387]
191. Canned lunchmeat (1 slice)	133	720
192. Pork chop, broiled, regular (2.7 oz)	216	[23]
193. Lean (2 oz)	192	[20]
194. Pork roast, regular (3 oz)	233	[33]
195. Lean (2.4 oz)	224	[31]
196. Pork shoulder, simmered, regular (3 oz)	158	[22]
197. Lean (2.2 oz)	146	[21]
Sausages		
198. Bologna (1 oz)	65	364
199. Braunschweiger (1 oz)	65	81
200. Brown and serve, link (1 link)	(35)	(125)
201. Deviled ham, canned (1 tbsp)	27	117
202. Frankfurter (1 frank)	121	607
203. Potted meat (1 tbsp)	[27]	[117]
204. Pork link (1 link)	35	125
205. Salami, dry (1 slice)	[49]	226
206. Cooked (1 slice)	[65]	298
207. Vienna sausage, canned (1 sausage)	[35]	152
Veal, Poultry		
208. Veal cutlet (3 oz)	258	[26]

TABLE I-1   (continued)

FOOD AND MEASURE	POTASSIUM (mg)	SODIUM (mg)
209. Veal rib roast (3 oz)	259	[41]
210. Fried chicken, breast (2.8 oz)	301	62
211. Drumstick (1.3 oz)	145	30
212. Broiled, ½ chicken (6.2 oz)	483	116
213. Canned chicken (3 oz)	117	462
214. Chicken a la king (1 cup)	404	760
215. Chicken and noodles (1 cup)	149	600
216. Chicken chow mein, canned (1 cup)	418	[718]
217. Chicken chow mein, homemade (1 cup)	473	718
218. Chicken pot pie, homemade (1 piece)	343	594
219. Roast turkey, dark (4 pieces)	338	84
220. Light (2 pieces)	349	70
221. Mixed (1 cup)	514	127
222. (3 pieces)	312	77
Fruits and Fruit Products		
223. Apple, medium (1 apple)	152	1
224. Large (1 apple)	233	2
225. Apple juice (1 cup)	250	3
226. Applesauce, sweetened (1 cup)	166	5
227. Unsweetened (1 cup)	190	5
228. Apricots, fresh (3 apricots)	301	1
229. Canned (1 cup)	604	3
230. Dried (1 cup)	1,273	34
231. Cooked, dried (1 cup)	795	18
232. Apricot nectar (1 cup)	379	1
233. Avocado, California (1 avocado)	1,303	9
234. Florida (1 avocado)	1,836	12
235. Banana (1 banana)	440	1
236. Banana flakes (1 tbsp)	92	<1
237. Blackberries (1 cup)	245	1
238. Blueberries (1 cup)	117	1
239. Sour cherries, canned (1 cup)	317	5
240. Sweet cherries, fresh (10 cherries)	129	1
241. Cranberry juice cocktail (1 cup)	25	3
242. Cranberry sauce (1 cup)	83	3
243. Dates, pitted (10 dates)	518	1
244. Chopped (1 cup)	1,153	2
245. Fruit cocktail (1 cup)	411	13
246. Grapefruit, pink or red (½ fruit)	166	2
247. White (½ fruit)	159	2
248. Canned (1 cup)	343	3
249. Grapefruit juice, pink or red (1 cup)	399	2

TABLE I–1   (continued)

FOOD AND MEASURE	POTASSIUM (mg)	SODIUM (mg)
250. White, unsweetened (1 cup)	400	10
251. Sweetened (1 cup)	405	3
252. Frozen, undiluted (6 oz)	1,250	8
253. Diluted (1 cup)	420	2
254. Dehydrated crystals mixed with water (1 cup)	412	(2)
255. Grapes, Thompson (10 grapes)	87	2
256. Tokay or Emperor (10 grapes)	99	2
257. Grape juice, canned (1 cup)	293	5
258. Frozen, undiluted (6 oz)	255	6
259. Diluted (1 cup)	85	3
260. Grape drink (1 cup)	88	3
261. Lemon (1 lemon)	102	1
262. Lemon juice, raw (1 cup)	344	2
263. Canned (1 cup)	344	2
264. Frozen (6 oz)	258	2
265. Lemonade, frozen, undiluted (6 oz)	153	4
266. Diluted (1 cup)	40	(<1)
267. Limeade, frozen, undiluted (6 oz)	129	(<1)
268. Diluted (1 cup)	32	(<1)
269. Lime juice, raw (1 cup)	256	2
270. Canned (1 cup)	256	2
271. Cantaloupe (½ melon)	682	57
272. Honeydew (1/10 melon)	374	27
273. Orange, whole (1 orange)	263	1
274. Sections (1 cup)	360	1
275. Orange juice, fresh (1 cup)	496	3
276. Canned (1 cup)	496	3
277. Frozen, undiluted (6 oz)	1,500	4
278. Diluted (1 cup)	503	3
279. Dried, mixed (1 cup)	518	2
280. Orange & grapefruit juice, frozen, undiluted (6 oz)	1,308	6
281. Diluted (1 cup)	439	(3)
282. Papaya (1 cup)	328	4
283. Peach, fresh (1 peach)	202	1
284. Slices (1 cup)	343	2
285. Canned, syrup pack (1 cup)	333	5
286. Water pack (1 cup)	334	5
287. Dried (1 cup)	1,520	26
288. Cooked (1 cup)	743	13
289. Slices, frozen (10 oz)	352	6
290. (1 cup)	310	5
291. Pear, fresh, Bartlett (1 pear)	213	3
292. Bosc (1 pear)	83	3
293. D'Anjou (1 pear)	260	4
294. Canned (1 cup)	214	3

TABLE I–1   (continued)

FOOD AND MEASURE	POTASSIUM (mg)	SODIUM (mg)
295. Pineapple, fresh (1 cup)	226	2
296. Canned (1 cup)	245	3
297. With liquid (1 slice)	101	1
298. With less liquid (1 slice)	56	1
299. Pineapple juice (1 cup)	373	(1)
300. Plums, fresh, Japanese (1 plum)	112	1
301. Prune-type (1 plum)	48	<1
302. Canned (1 cup)	367	3
303. (3 plums)	189	1
304. Prunes, dried (5 large)	298	4
305. Cooked (1 cup)	695	10
306. Prune juice (1 cup)	602	5
307. Raisins (1 cup)	1,106	39
308. (1 packet)	107	4
309. Raspberries, fresh (1 cup)	207	1
310. Frozen (10 oz)	284	3
311. Rhubarb, cooked from fresh (1 cup)	548	5
312. From frozen (1 cup)	475	8
313. Strawberries, fresh (1 cup)	244	2
314. Frozen (10 oz)	318	2
315. (16 oz)	472	5
316. Tangerine (1 tangerine)	108	2
317. Tangerine juice, canned (1 cup)	440	2
318. Watermelon (1 wedge)	426	9
Grain Products		
319. Bagel, egg (1 bagel)	41	[320]k
320. Water (1 bagel)	42	[320]k
321. Barley, raw (1 cup)	320	6
322. Biscuit, homemade (1 biscuit)	33	175
323. From mix (1 biscuit)	32	364
324. Breadcrumbs, dry (1 cup)	152l	736l
Breads		
325. Boston brown (1 slice)	131	110
326. Cracked wheat (1 loaf)	608	2,408
327. (1 slice)	34	133
328. French or Vienna (1 loaf)	408	2,633
329. French (1 slice)	32	203
330. Vienna (1 slice)	23	145
331. Italian (1 loaf)	336	2,656
332. (1 slice)	22	176
333. Raisin (1 loaf)	1,057	1,658
334. (1 slice)	58	91
335. Rye (1 loaf)	658	2,527
336. (1 slice)	36	139
337. Pumpernickel (1 loaf)	2,059	2,582
338. (1 slice)	145	182

k Rough estimate. Bagels assumed to be similar to French bread and uncoated with salt.
l 1 c salt-free breadcrumbs has 153 mg sodium and 152 mg potassium.

TABLE I–1 **(continued)**

FOOD AND MEASURE	POTASSIUM (mg)	SODIUM (mg)
339. White, soft crumb, regular loaf (1 loaf)	476	(2,309)
340. Slice (1 slice)	26	(127)[m]
341. Toasted (1 slice)	26	(130)[m]
342. Smaller slice (1 slice)	21	(102)[m]
343. Toasted (1 slice)	21	(100)[m]
344. White, soft crumb, large loaf (1 loaf)	714	(3,459)
345. Slice (1 slice)	29	(142)[m]
346. Toasted (1 slice)	29	(142)[m]
347. Smaller slice (1 slice)	25	(142)[m]
348. Toasted (1 slice)	25	(124)[m]
349. White bread cubes (1 cup)	32	(153)
350. Crumbs (1 cup)	47	(229)
351. White, firm crumb, regular loaf (1 loaf)	549	(2,309)
352. Slice (1 slice)	28	(117)[m]
353. Toasted (1 slice)	28	(102)[m]
354. White, firm crumb, large loaf (1 loaf)	1,097	(4,613)
355. Slice (1 slice)	33	(137)[m]
356. Toasted (1 slice)	33	(117)[m]
357. Whole-wheat, soft crumb (1 loaf)	1,161	(2,388)
358. Slice (1 slice)	72	(147)
359. Toasted (1 slice)	72	(126)
360. Whole-wheat, firm crumb (1 loaf)	1,238	(2,388)
361. Slice (1 slice)	68	(132)
362. Toasted (1 slice)	68	(110)
Breakfast cereals		
363. Grits, cooked, enriched (1 cup)	27	(1)[n]
364. Unenriched (1 cup)	27	(1)[n]
365. Farina, unenriched, cooked (1 cup)	25	2[o]
366. Oatmeal, cooked (1 cup)	146	1[p]
367. Wheat, rolled, cooked (1 cup)	202	(1)
368. Wheat, whole meal, cooked (1 cup)	118	519
369. Bran flakes (1 cup)	137	207
370. Raisin bran[q] (1 cup)	154	389
371. Corn flakes (1 cup)	30	245
372. Sugar coated (1 cup)	27	262
373. Corn or oat puffs (1 cup)	[44]	[285]
374. Shredded corn (1 cup)	(23)	(296)
375. Puffed oats (1 cup)	(86)	[285]

[m] 1 slice low-sodium white bread has 7 mg sodium.

[n] Regular grits. Instant grits have considerable sodium. ¼ c dry grits, for example, has about 650 mg.

[o] Regular farina. 1 c instant farina has 461 mg sodium.

[p] Regular oatmeal. 1 c instant oatmeal has about 400 mg sodium.

[q] Post's raisin bran. Others are lower in sodium; potassium varies.

TABLE I–1 **(continued)**

FOOD AND MEASURE	POTASSIUM (mg)	SODIUM (mg)
376. Puffed rice (1 cup)	15	1
377. Sugar coated (1 cup)	43	(25)
378. Wheat flakes (1 cup)	81	310
379. Puffed wheat (1 cup)	51	1
380. Sugar coated (1 cup)	63	46
381. Shredded wheat biscuit or spoon size (1 biscuit or ½ cup)	87	1
382. Wheat germ (1 tbsp)	57	<1
Buckwheat, Bulgur		
383. Buckwheat flour (1 cup)	314	1
384. Bulgur, canned (1 cup)	151	810
Cakes		
385. Angel food (1 cake)	381	(1,792)[r]
386. (1 piece)	32	(150)
387. Coffee cake (1 cake)	469	1,851
388. (1 piece)	78	310
389. Cupcakes, plain (1 cake)	21	113
390. With icing (1 cake)	42	121
391. Devil's food layer (1 cake)	1,439	2,590
392. (1 piece)	90	161
393. Devil's food cupcake (1 cake)	46	(173)
394. Gingerbread (1 cake)	1,562	1,733
395. (1 piece)	173	192
396. White (1 cake)	1,322	2,576
397. (1 piece)	82	160
398. Yellow (1 cake)	1,208	2,504
399. (1 piece)	75	156
400. Boston cream (1 cake)	734	1,538
401. (1 piece)	61	129
402. Fruitcake (1 cake)	2,250	715
403. (1 piece)	74	24
404. Sheetcake, plain (1 cake)	614	2,331
405. (1 piece)	68	258
406. Iced (1 cake)	669	2,477
407. (1 piece)	74	273
408. Pound cake (1 cake)	345	621
409. (1 piece)	20	36
410. Spongecake (1 cake)	687	1,327
411. (1 piece)	57	111
Cookies, Bars		
412. Brownies, homemade (1 brownie)	38	50
413. From mix (1 brownie)	34	78
414. Frozen (1 brownie)	44	54
415. Chocolate chip cookies (4 cookies)	56	168
416. Homemade (4 cookies)	47	138
417. Fig bars (4 bars)	111	140
418. Gingersnaps (4 snaps)	129	161
419. Macaroons (2 cookies)	176	14

[r] Sodium value calculated from sodium in ingredients of home recipe for angel food cake. Sodium in mix may be much higher; read the label.

TABLE I-1   (continued)

FOOD AND MEASURE	POTASSIUM (mg)	SODIUM (mg)
420. Oatmeal with raisins (4 cookies)	192	85
421. Plain, refrigerated dough (4 cookies)	23	264
422. Sandwich (4 cookies)	66[s]	197
423. Vanilla wafers (10 wafers)	29	102
Cornmeal		
424. Whole ground, unbolted (1 cup)	346	(1)[t]
425. Bolted (1 cup)	303	(1)[t]
426. Degermed, enriched, dry (1 cup)	166	(1)[t]
427. Cooked (1 cup)	38	(1)[t]
428. Unenriched, dry (1 cup)	166	(1)[t]
429. Cooked (1 cup)	38	(1)[t]
Crackers, Pastries, Doughnuts		
430. Graham (2 crackers)	55	94
431. Rye Wafers (2 wafers)	78	115
432. Saltines (4 crackers)	13	121
433. Danish (1 ring)	381	1,237
434. (1 pastry)	73	237
435. (1 oz)	32	102
436. Doughnuts, cake, plain (1 doughnut)	23	125
437. Raised, glazed (1 doughnut)	34	117
Macaroni		
438. Cooked, firm (1 cup)	103	1[u]
439. Tender, cold (1 cup)	64	1[u]
440. Hot (1 cup)	85	1[u]
441. Macaroni and cheese, canned (1 cup)	139	1,080
442. Homemade (1 cup)	240	1,086
Muffins, Noodles, Pancakes		
443. Muffins, homemade, blueberry (1 muffin)	46	253
444. Bran (1 muffin)	172	179
445. Corn (1 muffin)	54	192
446. Plain (1 muffin)	50	176
447. Corn, from mix (1 muffin)	44	192
448. Noodles, egg, cooked (1 cup)	70	3[u]
449. Noodles, chow mein (1 cup)	[37]	(459)
450. Pancakes, buckwheat (1 pancake)	66	125
451. Plain, home recipe (1 pancake)	33	115
452. From mix (1 pancake)	42	152

TABLE I-1   (continued)

FOOD AND MEASURE	POTASSIUM (mg)	SODIUM (mg)
Pies, Popcorn, Pretzels		
453. Apple (1 pie)	756	2,847
454. (1 piece)	108	407
455. Banana cream (1 pie)	1,847	1,365
456. (1 piece)	264	195
457. Blueberry (1 pie)	614	2,534
458. (1 piece)	88	362
459. Cherry (1 pie)	992	2,870
460. (1 piece)	142	410
461. Custard (1 pie)	1,247	2,609
462. (1 piece)	178	373
463. Lemon meringue (1 pie)	420	2,370
464. (1 piece)	60	339
465. Mince (1 pie)	1,682	4,229
466. (1 piece)	240	604
467. Peach (1 pie)	1,408	1,409
468. (1 piece)	201	201
469. Pecan (1 pie)	1,015	1,825
470. (1 piece)	145	261
471. Pumpkin (1 pie)	1,456	1,947
472. (1 piece)	208	276
473. Pie crust, homemade (1 crust)	89	1,100
474. From mix (1 crust)	179	2,603
475. Pizza (1 piece)	67	421
476. Popcorn, plain (1 cup)	[17]	[<1]
477. With oil and salt (1 cup)	[17]	[200]
478. Sugar coated (1 cup)	[17]	[<1]
479. Pretzels, twisted (1 pretzel)	21	268
480. Thin (10 pretzels)	78	1,080
481. Sticks (10 pretzels)	4	94
482. Rice, instant, hot (1 cup)	<1	450
483. Raw (1 cup)	170	11
484. Cooked (1 cup)	57	767
485. Rice, parboiled, raw (1 cup)	278	18
486. Cooked (1 cup)	75	628[v]
Rolls, Spaghetti		
487. Brown and serve (1 roll)	25	146
488. Cloverleaf or pan, commercial (1 roll)	27	193
489. Frankfurter or hamburger (1 roll)	38	292
490. Hard (1 roll)	49	313
491. Hoagie or submarine (1 roll)	122	(845)
492. Cloverleaf, homemade (1 roll)	41	98
493. Spaghetti, cooked, firm (1 cup)	103	1[u]
494. Tender (1 cup)	85	2[u]
495. With sauce, homemade (1 cup)	408	952

[s] Value in USDA table for 4 sandwich cookies was 15 mg. Value shown here is for cookies in Pennington and Church, 1980.
[t] Regular cornmeal. 1 c self-rising (degermed) cornmeal has 2,000 mg sodium.

[u] No salt added in preparation. With salt added, values are comparable to those given for rice cooked with salt (item #486).
[v] Salt added in preparation. Without salt added, 2 c cooked rice has <1 mg sodium.

TABLE I–1 (continued)

FOOD AND MEASURE	POTASSIUM (mg)	SODIUM (mg)
496. Canned (1 cup)	303	955
497. With meatballs, homemade (1 cup)	665	1,009
498. Canned (1 cup)	245	1,220
Toaster Pastries, Waffles		
499. Toaster pastry (1 pastry)	74w	218w
500. Waffle, homemade (1 waffle)	109	356
501. From mix (1 waffle)	146	515
Wheat Flours		
502. All-purpose, sifted (1 cup)	109	2
503. Unsifted (1 cup)	119	2
504. Cake, sifted (1 cup)	91	2
505. Self-rising, unsifted (1 cup)	113	1,349
506. Whole-wheat, unenriched, stirred (1 cup)	444	4
Legumes (dry), Nuts, Seeds; Related Products		
507. Almonds, chopped (1 cup)	1,005	4
508. Slivered (1 cup)	889	3
509. Great Northern beans (1 cup)	749	(13)
510. Navy beans (1 cup)	790	(13)
511. Canned beans, with frankfurters (1 cup)	668	1,374
512. With pork and tomato (1 cup)	536	1,181
513. With pork and sweet sauce (1 cup)	[637]	(969)
514. Red kidney beans (1 cup)	673	8
515. Limas, cooked from dry (1 cup)	1,163	3
516. Blackeyes, cooked from dry (1 cup)	573	[33]
517. Nuts, Brazil (1 oz)	203	<1
518. Cashew (1 cup)	650	21
519. Coconut meat, fresh (1 piece)	115	9
520. (1 cup)	205	9
521. Filberts (1 cup)	810	1
522. Lentils, cooked (1 cup)	498	[26]
523. Peanuts, roasted in oil (1 cup)	971	662
524. Peanut butter (1 tbsp)	100	19
525. Split peas, cooked (1 cup)	592	26
526. Pecans (1 cup)	712	<1
527. Seeds, pumpkin (1 cup)	1,386	[42]
528. Sunflower (1 cup)	1,334	44
529. Walnuts, black, chopped (1 cup)	575	4
530. Ground fine (1 cup)	368	2
531. English (1 cup)	540	2
Sugars and Sweets		
532. Cake icing, white, cooked (1 cup)	17	132
533. Coconut, cooked (1 cup)	277	199

TABLE I–1 (continued)

FOOD AND MEASURE	POTASSIUM (mg)	SODIUM (mg)
534. Chocolate, uncooked (1 cup)	536	165
535. Fudge, from mix (1 cup)	238	564
536. White, uncooked (1 cup)	57	160
537. Caramels, plain or chocolate (1 oz)	54	63
538. Milk chocolate (1 oz)	109	26
539. Semisweet (1 cup)	553	30
540. Chocolate-covered peanuts (1 oz)	143	17
541. Fondant (1 oz)	1	<1
542. Fudge (1 oz)	42	53
543. Gumdrops (1 oz)	1	10
544. Hard candy (1 oz)	1	9
545. Marshmallows (1 oz)	2	14
546. Cocoa powder, with dry milk (1 oz)	227	148
547. Without milk (1 oz)	142	108
548. Honey (1 tbsp)	11	1
549. Jams or preserves (1 tbsp)	18	4
550. (1 packet)	12	3
551. Jellies (1 tbsp)	14	4
552. (1 packet)	11	3
553. Syrup, chocolate, thin (1 fl oz)	106	21
554. Fudge (1 fl oz)	107	34
555. Molasses, light (1 tbsp)	183	16
556. Blackstrap (1 tbsp)	585	40
557. Sorghum (1 tbsp)	120	4
558. Table syrups (maple flavored) (1 tbsp)	1	13
559. Sugar, brown (1 cup)	757	53
560. White, granulated (1 cup)	6	1
561. (1 tbsp)	<1	<1
562. (1 packet)	<1	<1
563. Powdered, sifted (1 cup)	3	1
Vegetables and Vegetable Products		
564. Asparagus, cut, cooked from fresh (1 cup)	265	1
565. From frozen (1 cup)	396	4
566. Spears, cooked from fresh (4 spears)	110	1
567. From frozen (4 spears)	143	1
568. Canned (4 spears)	133	189
569. Lima beans, Fordhook (1 cup)	724	219
570. Baby (1 cup)	709	182
571. Green beans (snap), cooked from fresh (1 cup)	189	5
572. From frozen, cuts (1 cup)	205	1
573. French style (1 cup)	177	3
574. Canned (1 cup)	128	319
575. Yellow beans (wax), cooked from fresh (1 cup)	189	4
576. From frozen (1 cup)	221	1

w Values for potassium and sodium in toaster pastries varies with brand. Consult the label.

TABLE I-1 **(continued)**

FOOD AND MEASURE	POTASSIUM (mg)	SODIUM (mg)
577. Canned (1 cup)	128	319
578. Bean sprouts (mung), raw (1 cup)	234	5
579. Cooked (1 cup)	195	5
580. Beets, fresh cooked (2 beets)	208	43
581. (1 cup)	354	74
582. Canned, whole (1 cup)	267	378
583. Diced (1 cup)	284	401
584. Beet greens, cooked (1 cup)	481	110
585. Blackeye peas (young), cooked from fresh (1 cup)	625	(2)
586. From frozen (1 cup)	573	2
587. Broccoli, cooked from fresh (1 stalk)	481	18
588. (1 cup)	414	16
589. From frozen (1 stalk)	66	5
590. (1 cup)	392	28
591. Brussels sprouts, cooked from fresh (1 cup)	423	16
592. From frozen (1 cup)	457	22
593. Cabbage, raw, shredded (1 cup)	163	14
594. Chopped (1 cup)	210	18
595. Cooked (1 cup)	236	20
596. Cabbage, red, raw (1 cup)	188	18
597. Savoy, raw (1 cup)	188	15
598. Chinese celery cabbage, raw (1 cup)	190	17
599. White mustard cabbage, cooked (1 cup)	364	[35]
600. Carrots, raw (1 carrot)	246	34
601. (1 cup)	375	52
602. Cooked (1 cup)	344	51
603. Canned (1 cup)	186	366
604. Strained (baby food) (1 oz)	51	34
605. Cauliflower, raw (1 cup)	339	15
606. Cauliflower, cooked from fresh (1 cup)	258	11
607. From frozen (1 cup)	373	18
608. Celery (1 stalk)	136	50
609. (1 cup)	409	151
610. Collards, cooked from fresh (1 cup)	498	48
611. From frozen (1 cup)	401	27
612. Corn, cooked from fresh (1 ear)	151	<1
613. From frozen (1 ear)	291	<1
614. (1 cup)	304	<1
615. Canned, creamstyle (1 cup)	248	671[x]

FOOD AND MEASURE	POTASSIUM (mg)	SODIUM (mg)
616. Vacuum pack (1 cup)	204	577
617. Wet pack (1 cup)	160	384[x]
618. Cucumbers, with peel (6-8 slices)	45	2
619. Without peel (6-9 pieces)	45	2
620. Dandelion greens, fresh cooked (1 cup)	244	46
621. Endive (1 cup)	147	7
622. Kale, cooked from fresh (1 cup)	243	47
623. From frozen (1 cup)	251	20
624. Lettuce, butterhead (1 head)	430	16
625. (2 or 3 leaves)	40	1
626. Crisphead (1 head)	943	51
627. (1 wedge)	236	12
628. (1 cup pieces)	96	5
629. Looseleaf (1 cup)	145	5
630. Mushrooms, raw (1 cup)	290	10
631. Mustard greens, cooked from fresh (1 cup)	308	31
632. Okra, cooked from fresh (10 pods)	184	2
633. Onions, raw, chopped (1 cup)	267	17
634. Sliced (1 cup)	181	12
635. Cooked (1 cup)	231	15
636. Onions, young green (6 onions)	69	2
637. Parsley (1 tbsp)	25	2
638. Parsnips, cooked (1 cup)	587	19
639. Peas, green, canned (1 cup)	163	493[y]
640. Strained (baby food) (1 oz)	28	6
641. Cooked from frozen (1 cup)	216	184
642. Peppers, hot red, dried (1 tsp)	20	<1
643. Sweet, raw (1 pod)	157	9
644. Cooked (1 pod)	109	9
645. Potatoes, baked (1 potato)	782	5[z]
646. Boiled, then peeled (1 potato)	556	4[z]
647. Peeled, then boiled (1 potato)	385	4[z]
648. French fries, cooked from raw (10 strips)	427	15[z]
649. From frozen (10 strips)	326	15[z]
650. Hashbrowns, cooked from frozen (1 cup)	439	446[aa]

[x] 1 c low-sodium canned creamed corn has 5 mg sodium; 1 c low-sodium canned wetpack corn has 2 mg sodium.

[x] 1 c low-sodium canned creamed corn has 5 mg sodium; 1 c low-sodium canned wetpack corn has 2 mg sodium.
[y] 1 c low-sodium canned peas has 8 mg sodium.
[z] Values for sodium in potatoes assuming no added salt or seasonings containing sodium.
[aa] Salt added to hashbrowns during preparation.

TABLE I-1   **(continued)**

FOOD AND MEASURE	POTASSIUM (mg)	SODIUM (mg)
651. Mashed, cooked from raw (1 cup)	548	6
652. With milk added (1 cup)	525	63
653. From flakes (1 cup)	601	491
654. Potato chips (10 chips)	226	215
655. Potato salad (1 cup)	798	1,320
656. Pumpkin, canned (1 cup)	588	5
657. Radishes, raw (4 radishes)	58	3
658. Sauerkraut, canned (1 cup)	329	1,554
659. Spinach, raw (1 cup)	259	49
660. Spinach, cooked from fresh (1 cup)	583	94
661. From frozen (1 cup)	683	142
662. Spinach, cooked from frozen, chopped (1 cup)	688	131
663. Leaves (1 cup)	513	910[bb]
664. Squash, summer, cooked (1 cup)	296	5
665. Winter, cooked (1 cup)	945	2
666. Sweet potatoes, baked (1 potato)	342	17
667. Boiled (1 potato)	367	23
668. Candied (1 piece)	200	44
669. Canned, mashed (1 cup)	510	122
670. Vacuum pack (1 piece)	80	19
671. Tomatoes, raw (1 tomato)	300	4
672. Canned (1 cup)	523	313
673. Tomato ketchup (1 cup)	991	2,839
674. (1 tbsp)	54	156
675. Tomato juice (1 cup)	552	878[cc]
676. 1 glass (6 oz)	413	658[cc]
677. Turnips, cooked (1 cup)	291	53
678. Turnip greens, cooked from fresh (1 cup)	(246)	(17)
679. From frozen (1 cup)	246	(17)
680. Vegetables, mixed, frozen (1 cup)	348	90
Miscellaneous Items		
681. Baking powder (1 tsp)	5	405[dd]
682. With calcium sulfate (1 tsp)	(5)	(247)[dd]
683. Straight phosphate (1 tsp)	6	247[dd]
684. Low-sodium (1 tsp)	471	<1
685. Barbecue sauce (1 cup)	435	2,031
686. Beer (12 oz)	90	25
687. Whiskey, 80 proof (1½ fl oz)	1	1

y 1 c low-sodium canned peas has 8 mg sodium.
z Values for sodium in potatoes assuming no added salt or seasonings containing sodium.
aa Salt added to hashbrowns during preparation.
bb 1 c low-sodium frozen spinach leaves, cooked, have 148 mg sodium.
cc 1 c or 6-oz glass low-sodium tomato juice has about 10 mg sodium.
dd Values for sodium in baking powder vary significantly. Read the label information on individual brands.

TABLE I-1   **(continued)**

FOOD AND MEASURE	POTASSIUM (mg)	SODIUM (mg)
688. 86 proof (1½ fl oz)	1	1
689. 90 proof (1½ fl oz)	1	1
690. Wine, dessert (3½ fl oz)	77	4
691. Table (3½ fl oz)	94	5
692. Carbonated water[ee] (12 fl oz)	[0]	0
693. Colas (12 fl oz)	0	22[ff]
694. Fruit flavored soda (12 fl oz)	[0]	(25)[ff]
695. Gingerale (12 fl oz)	0	32[ff]
696. Root beer (12 fl oz)	38[gg]	29[ff]
697. Chocolate, baking (1 oz)	235	1
698. Gelatin (1 envelope)	180	8
699. Gelatin dessert, prepared (1 cup)	182	110
700. Mustard, yellow (1 tsp)	7	63
701. Olives, green (4 olives)	7	384
702. Ripe (3 olives)	2	75
703. Pickles, cucumber, dill (1 pickle)	130	928
704. Fresh pack slices (2 slices)	17	101
705. Sweet gherkins (1 pickle)	(17)	86
706. Pickle relish, sweet (1 tbsp)	[17]	107
707. Popsicle (1 popsicle)	(0)	(0)
708. Soup, made with milk, cream of chicken (1 cup)	260	1,044
709. Cream of mushroom (1 cup)	279	1,023
710. Tomato (1 cup)	418	816
711. Soup, made with water, bean with pork (1 cup)	395	1,132
712. Beef broth, bouillon, consomme (1 cup)	130	950
713. Beef noodle (1 cup)	77	782
714. Clam chowder, Manhattan (1 cup)	184	901
715. Cream of chicken (1 cup)	79	1,176
716. Cream of mushroom (1 cup)	98	955
717. Minestrone (1 cup)	314	968
718. Split pea (1 cup)	270	957
719. Tomato (1 cup)	230	760
720. Vegetable beef (1 cup)	162	990
721. Vegetarian (1 cup)	172	697
722. Bouillon cube (1 cube)	108[hh]	424
723. Soup, dry, onion (1½ oz pkg)	238	3,288

ee Tonic water.
ff Sodium content of sodas varies depending on the water source used by the manufacturer.
gg USDA value of 0 mg potassium was replaced with average of three values for rootbeer in Pennington and Church, 1980.
hh USDA value of 4 mg potassium for a beef cube was replaced with value of 108 mg found in Pennington and Church, 1980. Some sources report up to 960 mg sodium in a 4-g beef cube.

TABLE I-1   **(continued)**

FOOD AND MEASURE	POTASSIUM (mg)	SODIUM (mg)
724. Soup, dry, made with water, chicken noodle (1 cup)	19	1,047
725. Onion (1 cup)	58	841
726. Tomato vegetable with noodles (1 cup)	29	1,025
727. Vinegar cider (1 tbsp)	15	0
728. White sauce (1 cup)	348	947
729. Yeast, bakers dry active (1 pkg)	140	4
730. Brewer's dry (1 tbsp)	152	10

I

APPENDIX J

Recommended Nutrition References

CONTENTS

Books

Journals

Addresses

Specific References

People interested in nutrition often want to know where, in their own town or county, they can find reliable nutrition information. One place you are not likely to find it is the local library, where fad diet books sit side by side on the shelf with books of facts. However, wherever you live, there are several sources you can turn to:

- The Department of Health may have a nutrition expert.
- The local extension agent is often an expert.
- The food editor of your local paper may be well informed.
- The dietitian at the local hospital had to fulfill a set of qualifications before he or she became an R.D. (Registered Dietitian).
- There may be knowledgeable professors of nutrition or biochemistry at a nearby college or university.

The syndicated column on nutrition by J. Mayer and J. Dwyer, which appears in many newspapers, presents well-researched, reliable answers to current questions. The column by R. Alfin-Slater and Jelliffe is also accurate and trustworthy. In addition, you may be interested in building a nutrition library of your own. Books you can buy, journals you can subscribe to, and addresses you can write to for general information are followed by suggested readings under specific topic areas dealt with in this book's chapters.

Books

A 54-page list of references with critiques of each, *Nutrition References and Book Reviews*, is available for $2 from the Chicago Nutrition Association. (See "Addresses," below.)

This 605-page paperback ($12) has a chapter on each of 53 topics, including energy, obesity, 29 nutrients, several diseases, malnutrition, growth and its assessment, brain development, immunity, alcohol, fiber, milk intolerances, dental health, drugs, and toxins. The only major omissions seem to be nutrition and food intake and national nutrition status surveys. Watch for an update; these come out every several years:

- *Nutrition Reviews' Present Knowledge in Nutrition*, 4th ed. Washington, D.C.: Nutrition Foundation, 1976.

A scholarly volume from the *Journal of Nutrition*, five times larger than *Present Knowledge*, is:

- *Nutritional Requirements of Man, a Conspectus of Research.* New York and Washington, D.C.: Nutrition Foundation, 1980.

The *Conspectus* has major review articles on human requirements for protein, amino acids, vitamin A, calcium, zinc, vitamin C, iron, folacin, and copper.

This 1153-page volume (about $50) is a major technical reference book on nutrition topics, containing 40 encyclopedic articles on the nutrients, foods, the diet, metabolism, malnutrition, age-related needs, and nutrition in disease, with 28 appendixes:

- Goodhart, R. S., and Shils, M. E., eds. *Modern Nutrition in Health and Disease*, 6th ed. Philadelphia: Lea and Febiger, 1980.

We also recommend:

- Davidson, S., Passmore, R., Brock, J. F., and Truswell, A. S. *Human Nurition and Dietetics*, 7th ed. New York: Churchill Livingstone, 1979.

This entertaining paperback would make an excellent dis-cussion-topic source for a nutrition course; it includes arti-cles by recognized authorities on the RDA, fast foods, additives, infant nutrition, fad diets, sugar, alcohol, and most of the other topics treated in this book's Highlights:
● Hofmann, L., ed. *The Great American Nutrition Hassle*. Palo Alto, Calif.: Mayfield, 1978.

Another book that readers may wish to add to their libraries is the latest edition of *Recommended Dietary Allowances*, available from the National Academy of Sciences (see "Addresses," below).

We also recommend our own book, which explores current nutrition topics other than those treated here. The 3rd edi-tion is slated for publication in 1984:
● Hamilton, E. M. N., and Whitney, E. N., *Nutrition: Con-cepts and Controversies*, 2nd ed. St. Paul, Minn.: West, 1981.

An excellent cookbook for families wishing to prepare truly healthful meals is:
● White, A., and the Society for Nutrition Education. *The Family Health Cookbook*. New York: David McKay Com-pany, 1980.

Journals

Nutrition Today, the publication of the Nutrition Today Society, is an excellent magazine for the interested layper-son. It makes a point of raising controversial issues and providing a forum for conflicting opinions. References are seldom printed in the magazine but are available on request. Six issues per year, $12.50 ($6.25 for dietetics stu-dents), from Director of Membership Services, Nutrition Today Society. (See "Addresses," below.)

The *Journal of the American Dietetic Association*, the offi-cial publication of the ADA, contains articles of interest to dietitians and nutritionists, news of legislative action on food and nutrition, and a very useful section of abstracts of articles from many other journals of nutrition and related areas. Twelve issues per year, $24 ($12 for dietetics stu-dents), from the American Dietetic Association. (See "Addresses," below.)

Nutrition Reviews, a publication of The Nutrition Founda-tion, Inc., does much of the work for the library researcher, compiling recent evidence on current topics and present-ing extensive bibliographies. Twelve issues per year, $12

($6 for students), from the Nutrition Foundation. (See "Addresses," below.)

Nutrition and the MD is a monthly newsletter that provides up-to-date, easy to read, and practical information on nutri-tion for health care providers. It is available for $34 per year from PM, Inc. (See "Addresses," below.)

Other journals that deserve mention here are the *Journal of Nutrition, Food Technology*, the *American Journal of Clinical Nutrition*, and the *Journal of Nutrition Education*. *FDA Consumer*, a government publication with many arti-cles of interest to the consumer, is available from the Food and Drug Administration (see "Addresses," below). Many other journals of value are referred to throughout this book.

Some of this book's Highlights and the *Instructor's Man-ual's* Optional Lectures, as well as other articles of interest to consumers, are available as individual booklets. You can write for a free publication list from The Nutrition Company (address below). Many of the other organizations listed below will also provide publication lists free on request.

Addresses

U.S. Government

The U.S. Department of Agriculture (USDA) has several divisions. USDA's Food Safety and Inspection Service (FSIS) inspects and analyzes domestic and imported meat, poultry, and meat and poultry food products; establishes standards and approves recipes and labels of processed meat and poultry products; and monitors the meat and poultry industries for violations of inspection laws. To obtain publications or ask questions, write or call:
● FSIS Consumer Inquiries
USDA
Washington, DC 20250
(202) 472–4485

USDA's Agricultural Research Service (ARS) conducts research to fulfill the diverse needs of agricultural users— from farmers to consumers—in the areas of crop and animal production, protection, processing, and distribution; food safety and quality; and natural resources conservation. Write to the Information Division, ARS, USDA (same address).

USDA's Human Nutrition Information Service (HNIS) maintains USDA's Nutrient Data Bank; conducts the Nation-wide Food Consumption Survey; monitors nutrient content of the U.S. food supply; provides nutrition guidelines for education and action programs; collects and disseminates food and nutrition materials; and conducts nutrition education research. Write to:

● HNIS, USDA
Federal Center Building
Hyattsville, MD 20782

USDA's Food and Nutrition Service (FNS) administers the food stamp program; the national school lunch and school breakfast programs; the special supplemental food program for women, infants, and children (WIC); and the food distribution, child care food, summer food service, and special milk programs. Write to:

● FNS, USDA
500 12th Street SW
Washington, DC 20250

USDA's Agricultural Marketing Service (AMS) operates a variety of marketing programs and services—several of interest to consumers—that include developing grades and standards for the trading of food and other farm products and carrying out grading services on request from packers and processors; inspecting egg products for wholesomeness; administering marketing orders that aid in the marketing of milk, fruits, vegetables, and related specialty crops like nuts; and administering truth-in-seed labeling and other regulatory programs. Write to:

● Information Division, AMS, USDA
Washington, DC 20250

USDA's *Food News for Consumers*, a quarterly newsletter, is available from the Government Printing Office for $7 per year.

Other government addresses are:

● Food and Drug Administration (FDA)
5600 Fishers Lane
Rockville, MD 20852

● The Food and Nutrition Information Education Resources Center (FNIERC)
National Agriculture Library
10301 Baltimore Boulevard, Room 304
Beltsville, MD 20705
Tel: (301) 344-3719

● National Academy of Sciences/National Research Council (NAS/NRC)
2101 Constitution Avenue NW
Washington, DC 20418

● National Center for Health Statistics (NCHS)
U.S. Department of Health and Human Services (USDHHS)

● Public Health Service
3700 East–West Highway
Hyattsville, MD 20782

● U.S. Government Printing Office
The Superintendent of Documents
Washington, DC 20402

Consumer and Advocacy Groups

● Action for Children's Television (ACT)
46 Austin Street
Newtonville, MA 02160

● California Council against Health Fraud, Inc.
PO Box 1276
Loma Linda, CA 92354

● Center for Science in the Public Interest (CSPI)
1755 S Street NW
Washington, DC 20009

● Children's Foundation
1420 New York Avenue NW
Suite 800
Washington, DC 20005

● Community Nutrition Institute
1146 19th Street NW
Washington, DC 20036

● Food Research and Action Center (FRAC)
2011 I Street NW
Washington, DC 20006

Professional and Service Organizations

● American Academy of Pediatrics
PO Box 1034
Evanston, IL 60204

● American College of Nutrition
100 Manhattan Avenue #1606
Union City, NJ 07087

● American Dental Association
211 East Chicago Avenue
Chicago, IL 60611

● American Diabetes Association
2 Park Avenue
New York, NY 10016

● American Dietetic Association
430 North Michigan Avenue
Chicago, IL 60611

● American Heart Association
7320 Greenville Avenue
Dallas, TX 75231

● American Home Economics Association
2010 Massachusetts Avenue NW
Washington, DC 20036

● American Institute of Nutrition
9650 Rockville Pike
Bethesda, MD 20014

● American Medical Association
Nutrition Information Section
535 North Dearborn Street
Chicago, IL 60610

● The American National Red Cross
Food and Nutrition Consultant
National Headquarters
Washington, DC 20006

● American Public Health Association
1015 Fifteenth Street NW
Washington, DC 20005

● American Society for Clinical Nutrition
9650 Rockville Pike
Bethesda, MD 20014

● The Canadian Diabetes Association
1491 Yonge Street
Toronto, Ontario M4T 1Z5 Canada

● The Canadian Dietetic Association
123 Edward Street, Suite 601
Toronto, Ontario M5G 1E2 Canada

● The Chicago Nutrition Association
8158 Kedzie Avenue
Chicago, IL 60652

● Institute of Food Technologists
221 North La Salle Street
Chicago, IL 60601

● La Leche League International, Inc.
9616 Minneapolis Avenue
Franklin Park, IL 60131

● March of Dimes Birth Defects Foundation (National Headquarters)
1275 Mamaroneck Avenue
White Plains, NY 10605

● National Council on Alcoholism
733 Third Avenue
New York, NY 10017

● National Nutrition Consortium
1635 P Street NW, Suite 1
Washington, DC 20036

● Nutrition Company
PO Box 11102
Tallahassee, FL 32302

● Nutrition Foundation, Inc.
888 Seventeenth Street NW
Washington, DC 20036

● Nutrition Today Society
PO Box 1829
Annapolis, MD 21404

● Overeaters Anonymous (OA)
2190 190th Street
Torrance, CA 90504
(213) 320-7941

● PM, Inc. (Publisher of *Nutrition and the MD*)
14349 Victory Boulevard, #204
Van Nuys, CA 91401

● Society for Nutrition Education
1736 Franklin Street
Oakland, CA 94612

Trade Organizations

Trade organizations produce many excellent free materials on nutrition. Naturally, they also promote their own products. The student must learn to differentiate between slanted and valid information. We find the brief reviews in *Contemporary Nutrition* (General Mills), the *Dairy Council Digest*, Ross Laboratories' *Dietetic Currents*, and R. A. Seelig's reviews from the United Fresh Fruit and Vegetable Association to be generally reliable and very useful.

● ABC Corporation
1330 Avenue of the Americas
New York, NY 10019

● American Meat Institute
59 Van Buren Street
Chicago, IL 60605

● Best Foods
Consumer Service Department
Division of CPC International
Internation Plaza
Englewood Cliffs, NJ 07623

● Borden Farm Products
Division Borden Company
350 Madison Ave.
New York, NY 10017

● Campbell Soup Company
Food Service Products Division
375 Memorial Avenue
Camden, NJ 08101

● Cereal Institute
135 S. LaSalle St.
Chicago, IL 60603

J

J

● Del Monte Teaching Aids
PO Box 9075
Clinton, IA 52736

● Fleischmann's Margarines
Standard Brands, Inc.
625 Madison Avenue
New York, NY 10022

● General Foods Consumer Center
250 North Street
White Plains, NY 10625

● General Mills
PO Box 113
Minneapolis, MN 55440

● Gerber Products Company
445 State Street
Fremont, MI 49412

● H. J. Heinz
Consumer Relations
PO Box 57
Pittsburgh, PA 15230

● Hunt–Wesson Foods
Educational Services
1645 West Valencia Drive
Fullerton, CA 92634

● Kellogg Company
Department of Home Economics Services
Battle Creek, MI 49016

● McGraw–Hill Films
Care of Association Films, Inc.
600 Grand Avenue
Ridgefield, NJ 07657

● Mead Johnson Nutritionals
2404 Pennsylvania Avenue
Evansville, IN 47721

● National Commission on Egg Nutrition
205 Touvy Avenue
Park Ridge, IL 60668

● National Dairy Council
6300 North River Road
Rosemont, IL 60018–4233

● Nestle Company
Home Economics Division
100 Bloomingdale Road
White Plains, NY 10605

● Oscar Mayer Company
Consumer Service
PO Box 1409
Madison, WI 53701

● Pillsbury Company
1177 Pillsbury Building
608 Second Avenue South
Minneapolis, MN 55402

● The Potato Board
1385 South Colorado Boulevard
Suite 512
Denver, CO 80222

● Poultry and Egg National Board
8 South Michigan Avenue
Chicago, IL 60603

● Rice Council
PO Box 22802
Houston, TX 77027

● Ross Laboratories
Director of Professional Services
625 Cleveland Avenue
Columbus, OH 43216

● Sister Kenny Institute
Chicago Avenue at 27th Street
Minneapolis, MN 55407

● Soy Protein Council
1800 M Street NW
Washington, DC 20036

● Sunkist Growers
Consumer Service, Division BB
Box 7888
Valley Annex
Van Nuys, CA 91409

● VNIS (Vitamin Nutrition Information Service)
Hoffmann–LaRoche
340 Kingsland Avenue
Nutley, NJ 07110

● United Fresh Fruit and Vegetable Association
777 1st Street NW
Washington, DC 20005

● Vitamin Information Bureau
383 Madison Avenue
New York, NY 10017

● Wheat Flour Institute
309 West Jackson Boulevard
Chicago, IL 60606

Organizations Concerned with World Hunger
● Bread for the World
6411 Chillum Place NW
Washington, DC 20012

● Institute for Food and Development Policy
1885 Mission Street
San Francisco, CA 94103

● Interreligious Taskforce on U.S. Food Policy
110 Maryland Avenue NE
Washington, DC 20002

● Meals for Millions/Freedom from Hunger Foundation
1800 Olympic Boulevard
PO Drawer 680
Santa Monica, CA 90406

● Oxfam America
115 Broadway
Boston, MA 02116

● The Hunger Project
2015 Steiner Street
San Francisco, CA 94115

● Worldwatch Institute
1776 Massachusetts Avenue NW
Washington, DC 20036

United Nations

● Food and Agriculture Organization (FAO)
North American Regional Office
1325 C Street SW
Washington, DC 20025

● World Health Organization (WHO)
1211 Geneva 27
Switzerland

Specific References

Additives

Highly recommended are these discussions of all the points mentioned in the Highlights on Additives and Contaminants:

● Foster, E. M. Is there a food safety crisis? *Nutrition Today*, November/December 1982, pp. 6–13.

● Foster, E. M. How safe are our foods? *Nutrition Reviews/Supplement*, January 1982, pp. 28–34.

A good general reference on additives is the *FDA Consumer* magazine, described in full under "Food Labels."

A general review of all color additives and how the FDA regulates them:

● Damon, G. E., and Jannsen, W. F. Additives for eye appeal. *FDA Consumer*, July/August 1973, pp. 15–18.

On food-coloring agents, a recent, highly technical review is:

● Parkinson, T. M., and Brown, J. P. Metabolic fate of food colorants. *Annual Review of Nutrition* 1 (1981): 175–205.

The interesting conclusion to this article is that synthetic coloring agents have been studied more thoroughly than their natural counterparts and therefore their safety is known, while the safety of *natural* coloring agents (such as the pigments of plants) cannot be assumed on the basis of present knowledge.

The American Council on Science and Health has prepared a short report outlining its position that the Delaney Clause should be modernized. The report is available as an 11-page pamphlet, "The U.S. Food Safety Laws: Time for a Change?" from ACSH (see "Addresses," above).

A handy summary of FDA's laws and regulations is available in the 72-page paperback booklet:

● *Requirements of Laws and Regulations Enforced by the U.S. Food and Drug Administration*, U.S. Department of Health, and Human Services publication no. (FDA) 79–1042. Washington, D.C.: Government Printing Office, 1979.

The complete National Academy of Sciences' 276-page book *Report on Food Safety* became available in 1979 (write to the NAS; see "Addresses," above). The report includes case histories of saccharin, mercury, nitrites, and aflatoxin.

The review of GRAS list additives was summarized:

● Yesterday's additives = generally safe. *FDA Consumer*, March 1981, pp. 14–15.
Of the 415 GRAS substances, 305 were found to be without hazard; 68 without hazard as used; 19 without hazard as used but needing further investigation; 18 unevaluatable. Only 5 required the setting of safer usage conditions. The complete report of the select committee on GRAS substances is available for $6 from the National Technical Information Service, Springfield, VA 22161. The report includes the reassessment of all food and color additives. Ask for PB 80203789.

FDA's own report on the current uses and status of additives is a brief and clear discussion by P. Lehman. Of the 200 possible food colors, Lehman says, 31 are presently approved for use:

● Lehman, P. More than you ever thought you would know about food additives. *FDA Consumer*, April 1979 (reprint).

The issues surrounding the use of additives in foods are discussed in an interesting symposium reported in *Nutrition Reviews*, January 1980. W. J. Darby addresses the

J

question how "benefit" from additives can be quantified; V. O. Wodicka talks about risk and responsibility; and FDA's S. A. Miller discusses "the new metaphysics"—the problem of defining "zero risk."

● Risk versus benefit: The future of food safety. Underwood-Prescott Award Symposium Papers presented at Massachusetts Institute of Technology, Cambridge, Massachusetts, September 25, 1979. *Nutrition Reviews* 38 (1980): 33–64.

Three big books of food additives are available:

● *CRC Handbook: Regulatory Status of Direct Food Additives*. Boca Raton, Fl.: CRC Press, 1981.

● *Food Chemicals Codex*, 3rd ed. Washington, D.C.: National Academy Press, 1981.

● Taylor, R. J. *Food Additives*. Somerset, N.J.: Wiley, 1980.

The Nutrition Today Society (see "Addresses," above) makes available a teaching aid:

● Hall, R. L. *Additives*.

FDA also makes available a free 15-minute slide show that traces the history of color, flavor, and other additives, shows their uses, and explains FDA's regulation of them:

● *What About Food Additives?*

A new kind of "additive" is radiation, now being used by the food industry to sterilize foods for longer shelf life. Radiation does *not* leave the foods radioactive, but may create new compounds in the foods. For some pros and cons, see:

● Food irradiation—ready for a comeback. *Food Engineering*, April 1982, pp. 71–80.

Richard Wilson has written a delightful, light-hearted, and also technically sophisticated six-page demonstration of risk analysis. He compares the risks of eating a peanut-butter sandwich, walking next to a brick wall, smoking a cigarette, and others:

● Wilson, R. Analyzing the daily risks of life. *Technology Review* 81 (February 1979); reprint available from Alumni Association, Massachusetts Institute of Technology, Cambridge, MA 02139.

The fascinating subject of additives that, like BHA, accidentally turn out to help prevent toxic effects is discussed in:

● Wattenberg, L. W. Inhibitors of carcinogenesis, in *Carcinogens: Identification and Mechanisms of Action*, ed. A. C. Griffin and C. R. Shaw. New York: Raven Press, 1978. Pp. 299–316.

Alcohol

Four comprehensive papers on alcohol metabolism are the following. All four are technical, but clear and understandable. The fourth is the most detailed:

● Isselbacher, K. J. Metabolic and hepatic effects of alcohol. *New England Journal of Medicine* 296 (1977): 612–616.

● Boeker, E. A. Metabolism of ethanol. *Journal of the American Dietetic Association* 76 (1980): 550–554.

● Shaw, S., and Lieber, C. S. Nutrition and alcoholism, in *Modern Nutrition in Health and Disease*, 6th ed., ed. R. S. Goodhart, and M. E. Shils. Philadelphia: Lea and Febiger, 1980. Pp. 1220–1243.

● Eisenstein, A. B. Nutritional and metabolic effects of alcohol. *Journal of the American Dietetic Association* 81 (1982): 247–251.

For information and referrals on alcohol (not only nutrition-related), look up *Alcohol* in the telephone book, or write to the National Council on Alcoholism (see "Addresses," above). A recommended reference is:

● *Alcoholism* (pamphlet). Metropolitan Life Insurance Company (local offices in many cities).

The Nationwide Food Consumption Survey has produced some statistics on U.S. alcohol consumption. People over 14 consume an average of 1 ounce per day (probably underreported). Drinkers average 388 kcalories per day from alcohol, and receive less vitamin A and calcium in their diets than nondrinkers. For more on U.S. alcohol consumption, see:

● Windham, C. T., Wyse, B. W., and Hansen, R. G. Alcohol consumption and nutrient density of diets in the Nationwide Food Consumption Survey. *Journal of the American Dietetic Association* 82 (1983): 364–373.

For references on alcohol use in pregnancy, see "Pregnancy, Lactation, and Infancy." See also the reference by C. B. Popescu under "Food Labels."

Allergies

The *Instructor's Manual* includes an optional lecture, "Nutrition and Behavior 1: Allergies and Additives," at the end of which many useful references are listed, including cookbooks for people with food allergies.

Anorexia Nervosa

Among the most thought provoking and readable articles available on anorexia nervosa are three that appeared in the *American Journal of Nursing*, August 1980. The first is an account by an anorexic herself:

● Ciseaux, A. Anorexia nervosa: A view from the mirror. Pp. 1469–1470.

● Richardson, T. F. Anorexia nervosa: An overview. Pp. 1470–1471.

● Claggett, M. S. Anorexia nervosa: A behavioral approach. Pp. 1471–1477.

Another excellent short article by the authority H. Bruch is:
● Anorexia nervosa. *Nutrition Today*, September/October 1978, pp. 14–18.

Bruch's book is still the authoritative reference on the subject:
● Bruch, H. *The Golden Cage: The Enigma of Anorexia Nervosa.* Cambridge, Mass.: Harvard University Press, 1978.

Two excellent films on the subject are also available: *Dieting: the Danger Point,* from McGraw-Hill, and *Diet unto Death*, from ABC Learning Corporation. (See "Addresses," above.)

Three excellent articles describing therapy for and successful recover from anorexia nervosa are:
● Stordy, B. J., and coauthors. Weight gain, thermic effect of glucose and resting metabolic rate during recovery from anorexia nervosa. *American Journal of Clinical Nutrition* 30 (1977): 138–146.

● Fox., K. C., and James, N. M. Anorexia nervosa: A study of 44 strictly defined cases. *New Zealand Medical Journal* 84 (27 October 1976): 309–312.

● Lucas, A. R., Duncan, J. W., and Piens, V. The treatment of anorexia nervosa. *American Journal of Psychiatry*, September 1976, pp. 1034–1038.

Assessment of Nutrition Status
A handy desk reference for the dietitian assessing nutrition status is:
● Grant, A. *Nutritional Assessment Guidelines*, 1979. Available from Anne Grant, Box 25057, Northgate Station, Seattle, WA 98125.

A standard reference on assessment for the community nutritionist is:
● Christakis, G. *Nutritional Assessment in Health Programs*, 1973. Available from The American Public Health Association (see "Addresses," above).

For references on assessment in pregnancy, see "Pregnancy, Lactation, and Infancy."

A means of assessing expenditure in children and adults using a 3-day activity record has been validated:

● Bouchard, C., and coauthors. A method to assess energy expenditure in children and adults. *American Journal of Clinical Nutrition* 37 (1983): 461–467.

A valuable review of relative advantages and disadvantages of different methods of obtaining diet histories is:
● Stuff, J. E., and coauthors. A comparison of dietary methods in nutritional studies. *American Journal of Clinical Nutrition* 37 (1983): 300–306.

A technique that saves time is described in:
● Johnson, N. E., Nitzke, S., and VandeBerg, D. L. A reporting system for nutrient adequacy. *Home Economics Research Journal*, June 1974, pp. 210–221.

Two articles that would help the system-shopper to compare and appraise nutrient data bases and analysis systems are:
● Hoover, L. W. Computerized nutrient data bases: I. Comparison of nutrient analysis systems. *Journal of the American Dietetic Association* 82 (1983): 501–505.

● Hoover, L. W., and Perloff, B. P. Computerized nutrient data bases: II. Development of a model for appraisal of nutrient data base system capabilities. *Journal of the American Dietetic Association* 82 (1983): 506–508.

This model is available in monograph form from:
● Hoover, L. W., and Perloff, B. P. *Model for Review of Nutrient Data Base System Capabilities.* Columbia: University of Missouri-Columbia Printing Services, 1981 ($7.50).

Atherosclerosis and Diet
The American Heart Association's most recent statement on diet and heart disease reviews the evidence and reaches conclusions similar to those presented in Highlight 3:
● Rationale of the diet-heart statement of the American Heart Association. *Arteriosclerosis* 4 (1982): 177–191.

A valuable paper for physicians from the AHA is:
● *Risk Factors and Coronary Disease, a Statement for Physicians.* Dallas: American Heart Association, 1980.

See "Addresses" to write to the AHA for more on diet and heart disease.

A British review meticulously details the evidence supporting the recommendation that the general public should reduce saturated fat consumption:
● Oliver, M. F. Diet and coronary heart disease. *British Medical Bulletin* 37 (1981): 49–58.

The question whether diet is important in prevention of heart and artery disease has raised a tremendous controversy, much of it in the political arena. To find out why

J

some people think it is more a political than a physiological issue, read:

● Reader's Forum: Issues and Ideas. *Journal of Nutrition Education* 12 (1980): 186–189.

Other articles on the controversy:

● Mann, G. V. Diet-heart: End of an era. *New England Journal of Medicine* 297 (1977): 644–649.

● Ahrens, E. H. Diet and heart disease, shaping public perceptions when proof is lacking. *Arteriosclerosis* 2 (1982): 85–86.

● Nutrition Committee, American Heart Association. Diet and coronary heart disease: Another view. In *New England Journal of Medicine* 298 (1978): 1471–1473.

Some 400 pages were devoted to the controversy in:

● *Proceedings of the Conference on the Decline in Coronary Heart Disease Mortality.* Washington, D.C.: DHEW publication no. (NIH) 79–1610, May 1979.

Most of the May-June 1980 issue of *Nutrition Today* also was devoted to this controversy. The cover bore a picture of the eruption of Mount Saint Helens and suggested that the diet-heart debate was as violent as that famous volcano. An update was also published in *Nutrition and the MD*, April 1979.

Two possible food-borne causes of atherosclerosis, not treated here, are proposed in the following articles. Oster suggests that an enzyme in cow's milk (bovine xanthine oxidase) is responsible; Kummerow, that oxidation products of cholesterol and vitamin D in processed foods may be to blame:

● Oster, K. One man's meat. *Nutrition Today*, November/December 1981, p. 28.

● Kummerow, F. A. Nutrition imbalance and angiotoxins as dietary risk factors in coronary heart disease. *American Journal of Clinical Nutrition* 32 (1979): 58–83.

A concise, accurate review of the past decade's cardiovascular research is:

● Levy, R. I., and Moskowitz, J. Cardiovascular research: Decades of progress; a decade of promise. *Science* 217 (1982): 121–129.

An even-handed, readable critique of the Pritikin diet, presenting its many pros and cons, appeared in:

● The Pritikin program—claims vs. facts. *Consumer Reports*, October 1982, pp. 513–518.

The major intervention study of the late 1970s was the MRFIT (Multiple Risk Factor Intervention Trial), which was undertaken to see if reducing serum cholesterol levels, blood pressure, and smoking could reduce the risk of death from coronary heart disease in high-risk men. A two-page review, including the unexpected finding that a drug used to lower high blood pressure in the experimental subjects may have adversely affected the results, was presented in:

● Kolata, G. Heart study produces a surprise result. *Science* 218 (1982): 31–32.

The history of the MRFIT is described in:

● Zukel, W. J., Oglesby, P., and Schnaper, H. W. The multiple risk factor intervention trial (MRFIT): I. Historical perspectives. *Preventive Medicine* 10 (1981): 387–401.

To find out more about the realtionship of exercise to heart attack risk, see:

● Paffenbarger, R. S., Wing, A. L., and Hyde, R. T. Current exercise and heart attack diet. *Cardiac Rehabilitation* 10, no. 2 (1979): 1–4.

References to help health professionals and their clients devise diets for hyperlipidemia and high blood pressure include the following:

● *Planning Fat-Controlled Meals.* General Mills (see "Addresses," above).

● *Dietary Modification to Control Hyperlipidemia.* Ad Hoc Committee for Medical and Community Programs, American Heart Association, reprinted from *Circulation* 58 (1978): 381A.

● *Dietary Management of Hyperlipoproteinemia: A Handbook for Physicians and Dietitians.* DHEW publication no. (NIH) 73–110.

● *Report of the Working Group on Critical Patient Behaviors in the Dietary Management of High Blood Pressure.* DHEW publication no. (NIH) 81–2269.

● *What you should know about . . . The National Program to Control High Blood Pressure* (leaflet). DHEW publication no (NIH) 80–632.

● *High Blood Pressure Facts and Fiction* (leaflet). DHEW publication no. (NIH) 80–1218.

● *Sensible Ways to Cut Down on Sodium* (leaflet). Available from Adolph's, Ltd., Consumer Services Department, 33 Benedict Place, Greenwich, CT 06830.

● *Special Recipes for Low Sodium Diets* (booklet). General Foods (see "Addresses," above).

The NIH publications are available from the Office of Information, National Heart and Lung Institute, Bethesda, MD 20014.

See also the references under "Weight Control" for people who give up smoking.

Athlete

Women with anorexia nervosa and runners who run compulsively seem to have many psychological characteristics in common, as this interesting article points out:

● Yates, A., Leehey, K., and Shisslak, C. M. Running—an analogue of anorexia? *New England Journal of Medicine* 308 (1983): 251–255.

Weight control in athletics—sound and unsound approaches—as well as other nutrition concerns are dealt with in:

● Smith, N. J. Weight control and heat disorders in youth sports. *Journal of Adolescent Health Care* 3 (1983): 231–236.

● Lamb, D. R. Androgens and exercise. *Medicine and Science in Sports* 7 (1975): 1–5.

● Smith, N. J. Gaining and losing weight in athletics. *Journal of the American Medical Association* 236 (1976): 149–151.

A highly recommended cookbook and nutrition reference for athletes is:

● Clark, N. *The Athlete's Kitchen: A Nutrition Guide and Cookbook*. Boston: CBI, 1981 (paperback, about $10).

A study of different groups of male and female athletes (football players, wrestlers, gymnasts) revealed special nutrition concerns specific to several:

● Short, S., and Short, W. R. Four-year study of university athletes' dietary intake. *Journal of the American Dietetic Association* 82 (1983): 632–645.

Books and booklets of special interest to the athlete are:
● Katch, F. I., McArdle, W. D., and Boylan, B. R. *Getting in Shape, an Optimum Approach to Fitness and Weight Control*. Boston: Houghton-Mifflin, 1979.

● Smith, N. J. *Food for Sport*. Palo Alto, Calif.: Bull Publishing, 1976.

● Williams, M. H. *Nutritional Aspects of Human Physical and Athletic Performance*. Springfield, Ill.: Charles C. Thomas, 1976.

● *Nutrition for Athletes*, available from the American Alliance for Health, Physical Education, and Recreation, 1201 16th Street NW, Washington, DC 20036.

Four excellent articles on nutrition for the athlete appeared in *Nutrition Today*, November/December 1979:
● Hanley, D. F., Jr. Athletic training—how diet affects it. Pp. 5–9.

● Vitousek, S. H. Is more better? Pp. 10–17.

● Hursh, L. M. Practical hints about feeding athletes. Pp. 18–20.

● Hanley, D. F., Jr. Basic diet guidance for athletes. Pp. 22–23.

To get in shape physically, we suggest you use the reference by C. Bailey or F. I. Katch listed under "Weight Control," or, if running is your specialty:

● Costill, D. L. *A Scientific Approach to Distance Running*. Los Altos, Calif.: Track and Field News, 1979.

Cancer

The *Instructor's Manual* includes an optional lecture on cancer and nutrition which offers suggested references.

Carbohydrates

A compilation of 23 papers from a 1981 symposium on carbohydrates includes many on technical subjects but some of interest to the general reader, including several chapters on dietary and health aspects:

● Lineback, D. R., and Inglett, G. E., eds. *Food Carbohydrates*. Westport, Conn.: Avi, 1982 (about $45).

A major review article gives abundant information on the alternative sweeteners:

● Wang, Y. M., and Van Eys, J. Nutritional significance of fructose and sugar alcohols. In *Annual Review of Nutrition*, vol. I, ed. W. J. Darby, H. P. Broquist, and R. E. Olson. Palo Alto, Calif.: Annual Reviews, 1981. Pp. 437–475.

The *Instructor's Manual* includes an informative optional lecture: "Hypoglycemia and Nonhypoglycemia," which is also available as a separate booklet from The Nutrition Company (see "Addresses," above).

Sugar has had a major impact on human history, determining trade routes and the locations of whole cities. For the many fascinating details, turn to:

● Deevr, N. *History of Sugar*, vols. I and II. London: Chapman Hall, 1949.

The Avi handbook of sugars is available for $45:

● Pancoast, H. M., and Junk, W. R. *Handbook of Sugars*, 2nd ed. Westport, Conn.: Avi, 1980.

A film, not recommended for its accuracy, but useful for stimulating class discussion about controversies surrounding sugar, is available from Image Associates, PO Box 40106, Santa Barbara, CA 93103:

● *The Sugar Film*.

See also the references in Appendix F.

J

Children and Teenagers

The connections among malnutrition, learning, and behavior in children are clearly explained in a 33-page booklet from the National Institutes of Health:

● National Institute of Child Health and Human Development, Center for Research for Mothers and Children. *Malnutrition, Learning, and Behavior.* HHS publication no. (NIH) 76-1036. Washington, D.C.: Government Printing Office, 1976.

For people who feed children:

● Williams, J., and Smith, M. *Middle Childhood: Behavior and Development*, 2nd ed. New York: Macmillan, 1980.

In relation to the profound effect that feeding with love can have on children, E. M. Widdowson described long ago how this variable "ruined" a nutrition experiment that some investigators tried to carry out. Love and attention had a bigger effect on the children's growth than the food:

● Widdowson, E. M. Mental contentment and physical growth. *Lancet* 1 (1951): 1316–1317.

Conversely, the effect of lack of love and attention is now known to account for much of the growth and developmental failure wherever malnutrition of children is seen. A landmark article, reporting years of research, is:

● Cravioto, J. Nutrition, stimulation, mental development and learning. *Nutrition Today*, September/October 1981, pp. 4–15.

On the nutrition of children, this 205-page paperback is an authoritative, clear, understandable text, one of the best in the field:

● Pipes, P. L. *Nutrition in Infancy and Childhood.* St. Louis: Mosby, 1977.

On the prevention of adult health problems through good nutritional practices in childhood, Breslow and Somers have studied the disorders most likely to appear at every age and have suggested an agenda for screening at intervals throughout life that would detect these disorders:

● Breslow, L., and Somers, A. R. Lifetime health monitoring: A practical approach to preventive medicine. *New England Journal of Medicine* 296 (1977): 601–608.

These references also offer guidelines for screening to catch diet-related problems early in life:

● Fomon, S. J., Anderson, T. A., Stephen, H. Y. W., and Ziegler, E. E. *Nutritional Disorders of Children: Prevention, Screening, and Followup.* HHS publication no. (HSA) 76-5612. Washington, D.C.: Government Printing Office, 1976.

● Williams, C. L., and Wynder, E. L. A blind spot in preventive medicine. *Journal of the American Medical Association* 236 (1976): 2196–2197.

● Blumenthal, S., and Jesse, M. J. Prevention of atherosclerosis: A pediatric problem. *Hospital Practice*, April 1973, pp. 81–90.

A review of the recent history of the nation's child nutrition programs is presented in:
● Vaden, A. G. Child nutrition programs: past, present, future. *Professional Nutritionist*, Winter 1981, pp. 7–10.

The *School Lunch Journal* and the *School Foodservice Journal* are coming out monthly with creative new ideas about feeding children at school.

For people who feed children, this paperback encourages them to involve the children themselves in the preparation of healthful foods:
● Goodwin, M. T., and Pollen, G. *Creative Food Experiences for Children.* Washington, D.C.: Center for Science in the Public Interest, 1974. Available from Box 3099, Washington, DC 20010.

People concerned about the effects of television on children's eating habits should write to Action for Children's Television (ACT), to see what they have available. (See "Addresses," above.)

A 56-page booklet is available free from the Pennsylvania Department of Education, Division of Food Service, 8 South 13th Street, Pittsburgh, PA 15203:
● *Food with Love.*

The entire issue of *Nutrition Reviews*, February 1981, was devoted to many different aspects of adolescent nutrition.

See also "Anorexia Nervosa" and the film *Woman Child* under "Pregnancy, Lactation, and Infancy."

The *Instructor's Manual* includes two optional lectures on nutrition and behavior. These are also available as separate publications from The Nutrition Company (See "Addresses," above). Highly recommended:
● Nutrition and Behavior I: Allergies and Additives.

● Nutrition and Behavior II: Nutrient Deficiencies and Sugar.

Contaminants

Several references are available on the toxic effects of *natural* plant products. The first of these is an article, the second is a book:

● Wilson, B. J. Naturally occurring toxicants of foods. *Nutrition Reviews* 37 (1979): 305–312.

● Liener, I. E., ed. *Toxic Constituents of Plant Foodstuffs*, 2nd ed. New York: Academic Press, 1980.

A recent reevaluation of the margin of safety for mercury in seafood has reached some reassuring conclusions, which are well worth reading:

● Margolin, S. Mercury in marine seafood: The scientific medical margin of safety as a guide to the potential risk to public health. *World Review of Nutrition and Dietetics* 34 (1980): 182–265.

Lead was the subject of several articles in the October 1981 issue of *Nutrition Reviews*. The first described the interactions of nutrition and lead poisoning; the second, a typical episode of lead poisoning in a child:

● Mahaffey, K. R. Nutritional factors in lead poisoning. *Nutrition Reviews* 39 (1981): 353–362.

● Metabolism of vitamin D in lead poisoning. *Nutrition Reviews* 39 (1981): 372–373.

A thought-provoking discussion of other issues related to lead poisoning, not mentioned in Highlight 11, is:

● Wessel, M. A., and Dominski, A. Our children's daily lead. *American Scientist* 65 (1977): 294–298.

Diagnosis and treatment of lead poisoning are outlined in:
● Pincus, D., and Saccar, C. V. Lead poisoning. *American Family Physician* 19 (1979): 120–124.

Another problem related to lead and not dealt with here is the problem of detecting lead contamination in foods and using an appropriate standard. According to this important article, the standards that have been used to detect lead in foods have themselves been contaminated with lead, so that the amounts people's bodies contain may be much higher than has been thought in the past:

● Settle, D. M., and Patterson, C. C. Lead in albacore: Guide to lead pollution in Americans. *Science* 207 (1980): 1167–1176.

Lead poisoning is especially likely in low-income children because they often live in old houses near heavy traffic and are at risk for malnutrition. The WIC program, aimed at remedying nutrition problems in children under five, is an ideal program for reaching children at risk:

● Preventing lead poisoning: WIC clinics help reach children at risk. *Food and Nutrition* (a USDA publication) 10 (June 1980): 4–7.

It is recommended that you not use newspaper for grilling food because of the lead content of newsprint:

● Lao, Y. J., and Blackwell, F. O. Potential hazard from newspaper as fuel for grilling food. *Journal of Environmental Health*, January/February 1980, pp. 197–198.

Several articles of interest on food contaminants have appeared in *FDA Consumer*. The first of these expresses concern over PCB levels in fish in the waters of Colorado, Illinois, Indiana, Massachussetts, Michigan, New Jersey, New York, Ohio, Pennsylvania, and Wisconsin. The second addresses the problem of drug (for example, antibiotic) residues in the flesh of animals given feed containing drugs. The third describes FDA's priorities for reducing lead in the food supply, beginning with canned foods (solder is 98 percent lead). The fourth proposes better ways of detecting pesticides in foods:

● Level of PCB's lowered. *FDA Consumer*, September 1979, p. 3.

● Watching the food of animals that produce food. *FDA Consumer*, October 1979, pp. 15–17.

● Corwin, E. On getting the lead out of food. *FDA Consumer*, March 1982, pp. 19–21.

● Better pesticide detection proposed. *FDA Consumer*, December 1979–January 1980, pp. 26–27.

WHO (World Health Organization) has published several dozen booklets on evaluation and testing of additives, contaminants, pesticides, and the like—for example:

● *Pesticide Residues in Food*. Technical report series 592, 1976, available from WHO (see "Addresses," above).

See also the references by E. M. Foster, R. Wattenberg, and L. W. Wilson under "Additives"; also "Food Poisoning."

Cooking

The *Instructor's Manual* includes an optional lecture, "Foods in the Home," which offers tips on cooking to preserve nutrients.

Dental Health

A thorough review of the relationships between sugar and dental caries in many population groups around the world summarizes much of the evidence available as of 1982:

● Newburn, E. Sugar and dental caries—a review of human studies. *Science* 217 (1982): 418–423.

On diet and oral health, an excellent review is:
● DePaola, D. P., and Alfano, M. C. Diet and oral health. *Nutrition Today*, May/June 1977, pp. 6–11, 29–32.

Digestion and Absorption

An acquaintanceship with the GI tract lays the groundwork for an understanding of many interesting GI conditions, both trivial and serious. *Nutrition Today* offers a series of easy-to-read, colorfully illustrated articles and teaching aids on many of them. These five are by F. J. Ingelfinger:

● How to swallow and belch and cope with heartburn. *Nutrition Today*, January/February 1973. Pp. 4–13.

● *Gastrointestinal Absorption* (Teaching aid #1).

● *Gastrointestinal Malabsorption* (Teaching aid #3).

● *Gastric Function* (Teaching aid #11).

● *The Esophagus* (Teaching aid #12).

The third of these is spectacular:

● Costell, D. O., and Frank, B. B. How to treat heartburn with diet therapy. *Nutrition Today*, May/June 1971, pp. 12–21.

● Makhlouf, G. M. Function of the gallbladder. *Nutrition Today*, January/February 1982, pp. 10–15.

● Phillips, S. F., and Stephen, A. M. The structure and function of the large intestine. *Nutrition Today*, November/December 1981, pp. 4–12.

This fascinating article reveals many intimate details about the lives and activities of the cells of the small intestine described by a woman who knows them well:

● Moog, F. The lining of the small intestine. *Scientific American*, November 1981, pp. 154–176.

A teaching aid including four different slide presentations, each with an annotated syllabus, can be purchased from the Nutrition Today Society (see "Addresses," above):

● *GI Function and Dysfunction.*

The *Instructor's Manual* includes an optional lecture, "Common Digestive Problems."

Electrolytes

The *Instructor's Manual* includes an optional lecture on fluids and electrolytes that provides more detail than this book's Chapter 10.

Fats and Oils

A concise book that presents all a beginning expert might want to know about fats and oils is:

● FAO/WHO. *Dietary Fats and Oils in Human Nutrition*. Rome: FAO, 1980 (paperback, $8.50).

Two research reports on the use of sucrose polyester to lower blood cholesterol and promote weight loss in humans are:

● Mellies, M. J., and coauthors. A double blind, placebo-controlled study of sucrose polyester in hypercholesterolemic outpatients. *American Journal of Clinical Nutrition* 37 (1983): 339–346.

● Glueck, C. J., and coauthors. Sucrose polyester—substitution for dietary fats in hypocaloric diets in the treatment of familial hypercholesterolemia. *American Journal of Clinical Nutrition* 37 (1983): 347–354.

The importance of linolenic acid in the diet is reviewed by:

● Budowski, P. Review: Nutritional effects of ω3–polyunsaturated fatty acids. *Israel Journal of Medical Sciences* 17 (1980): 223–231.

An exploration into the nature and significance of dietary *trans*-fatty acids is available. Little more is known now about their cancer implications than was known at the time of the 1978 report by Enig, Munn, and Keeney, cited in the Chapter 3 footnotes; but this reference offers abundant information on the prevalence of *trans*-fatty acids in foods, their metabolism, and related subjects:

● Brisson, G. J. The enigma of the *trans* fatty acids. In *Lipids in Human Nutrition*. Englewood, N.J.: Burgess, 1981. Pp. 41–47.

Rapeseed oil is extensively used in Canada. An evaluation of its safety was presented in:

● Nolen, G. A. Biological evaluation of hydrogenated rapeseed oil. *Journal of the American Oil Chemists Society*, January 1981, pp. 31–37.

Fiber and Oxalates

A good book about fiber is:

● Inglett, G. E., and S. I. Falkehag, eds. *Dietary Fibers: Chemistry and Nutrition*. New York: Academic Press, 1979.

A book that presents the oxalate contents of many foods is:

● Ney, D. M., Hofmann, A. F., Fischer, C., and Stubblefield, N. *The Low Oxalate Diet Book*. San Diego: University of California, 1981.

For the references used in this text on fiber contents of foods, see Appendix K.

Food Choices

A set of slides on fast foods discusses their nutritional advantages and disadvantages, and suggests strategies for choosing foods:

● *Fast Food Phenomenon*. Available from Christina Stark, 3415 SW Chintimini Ave., Corvalis, OR 97330. The set is available for $36 as 48 slides or $24 as a filmstrip.

A book that explores interesting questions about human food choices is:

● Baker, L. M., ed. *The Psychobiology of Human Food Selection.* Westport, Conn.: Avi, 1982 ($27.50).

Practical pointers on buying, preparing, and cooking food can be found in:

● Peterkin, B. *Your Money's Worth in Foods.*

This 29-page booklet is available for $.60 from Home and Garden Bulletin, Government Printing Office (see "Addresses," above).

Food Composition

For the standard handbooks on food composition, see the notes in Appendix H.

Food Group Plans, Exchange Systems, Recommendations, and Dietary Guidelines

The Modified Four Food Group Plan was presented and discussed in:

● King, J. C., Cohenour, S. H., Corrucini, C. G., and Schneeman, P. Evaluation and modification of the basic four food guide. *Journal of Nutrition Education* 10 (1978): 27–29.

The Modified Four Food Group Plan includes legumes, an unfamiliar food to many people. Only about 20 of some 13,000 species are commonly eaten. Several articles in *Food Technology*, March 1981, were devoted to legumes—their nutrient contributions, the effects of their germination into sprouts ("bean sprouts"), their nutrient content when canned ("canned beans"), and related subjects.

People who want to use the exchange system for diet planning find it convenient to obtain the small booklet from the American Dietetic Association (ADA), available for under a dollar (see "Addresses," above):

● *Exchange Lists for Meal Planning.*

In conjunction with this, vegetarians will find useful:

● *Supplement to Exchange Lists for Meal Planning, Vegetarian Cookery.* The American Diabetes Association (see "Addresses," above).

A booklet that guides the vegetarian in planning diets is available for $3.00 from The Nutrition Company (see "Addresses," above).

● *Diet Planning for The Vegetarian.*

The RDA were designed for healthy, well-nourished people in the United States. A thoughtful author asks how the far-less-well-nourished people of the third world manage to get along with so much lower nutrient intakes, and what standards should be applied to them:

● Walker, A. R. P., and Walker, B. F. Recommended dietary allowances and third world populations. *American Journal of Clinical Nutrition* 34 (1981): 2319–2321.

The next article compares recommended dietary intakes and allowances around the world:

● IUNS Committee Report. Recommended dietary intakes and allowances around the world—an introduction. *Food and Nutrition Bulletin*, October 1982, pp. 34–45.

For people who want to explore in greater depth the thought processes involved in arriving at dietary guidelines broadcast for the population, the first and third of these three major references make fascinating reading:

● *Dietary Goals for the United States*, 2nd ed. U.S. Senate, Select Committee on Nutrition and Human Needs. Washington, D.C.: Government Printing Office, 1977.

● *Nutrition and Your Health, Dietary Guidelines for Americans.* Washington, D.C.: U.S. Department of Agriculture and U.S. Department of Health and Human Services, 1980.

● *Toward Healthful Diets.* Washington, D.C.: Food and Nutrition Board, National Research Council, 1980.

The controversy over whether dietary guidelines should be offered at all is described in:

● Hamilton, E. M. N., and Whitney, E. N. Controversy 3: Dietary guidelines—whose guidelines, if any, should we follow? In *Nutrition: Concepts and Controversies*, 2nd ed. St. Paul, Minn.: West, 1982. Pp. 68–73.

Food Labels

For help in reading labels, many booklets are available. One we like is available *Inside Information About the Outside of the Package*, free from Pillsbury Company (see "Addresses," above).

The best source for the general reader of the latest information on labeling laws, regulations governing additives, and all other areas under the province of the FDA is the *FDA Consumer* magazine which comes out monthly. Your library probably subscribes, or you can get a subscription of your own (see "Addresses," above).

For the exact wording of the laws relating to the food supply, and of proposals now under consideration, dig into the *Federal Register*, which arrives weekly at your library. Back issues may be found in the U.S. Government documents section.

J

The law requires that companies making alcoholic beverages should list their ingredients on labels, but they don't. For the reasons why they don't, and for an argument that they should, read:

● Popescu, C. B. Gin and tonic and ? *ACSH News and Views*, May/June 1983, pp. 6–7.

Two helpful cassettes are available from the American Dietetic Association (see "Addresses," above):

● Wyse, B., Hansen, R. G., and Sorenson, A. W. *A Practical Nutrient Density-Nutritional Quality Index for Food.*

● Robinson, M. *Food Labeling.*

Food Poisoning

The paper by Foster, listed under "Additives," includes a good perspective on food poisoning.

The *Instructor's Manual* includes an optional lecture, "Foods in the Home," that offers pointers on preventing food poisoning.

Hormones

The *Instructor's Manual* explains the body's endocrine system in full in an optional lecture, "Hormones."

Hypoglycemia

The *Instructor's Manual* includes an optional lecture, "Hypoglycemia and Nonhypoglycemia," at the end of which many informative references are listed.

Immunity

The *Instructor's Manual* includes an optional lecture that explores the relationships between nutrients and the immune system: "Nutrition and Immunity."

Metabolism

A brief and clear explanation in paperback of the ways energy flows through living things is:

● Lehninger, A. L. *Bioenergetics: The Molecular Basis of Biological Energy Transformations.* New York: W. A. Benjamin, latest edition.

A patiently detailed, meticulous description of metabolism during feasting and fasting is provided in:

● Cahill, G. F., Aoki, T. T., and Rossini, A. A. Metabolism in obesity and anorexia nervosa. In *Nutrition and the Brain*, vol. 3, ed. R. J. Wurtman and J. J. Wurtman. New York: Raven Press, 1979. Pp. 1–70.

The following beautifully written article marvels at the body's adaptations to starvation and presents fascinating speculations as to why the body "chooses" to rely on ketones (it needs a small, water–soluble derivative of fat to get across the blood-brain barrier); why it conserves glycogen except in the shock of initial fasting or in very hard exercise (it needs to save it for emergencies); how convenient it is that when the body is deprived of food its water need also diminishes; and others:

● Cahill, G. F. Starvation in man. *New England Journal of Medicine* 282 (1970): 668–675.

This article reveals that the statement that fatty acids cannot yield glucose is not quite true. There *is* one route to glucose by way of the ketone acetone (significance unknown):

● Cahill, G. F. Ketosis. *Journal of Parenteral and Enteral Nutrition* 5 (1981): 281–287.

Minerals

The principal hazards of overdosing with vitamins and minerals have been reviewed and published by the National Nutrition Consortium in a 1978 booklet, *Vitamin-Mineral Safety, Toxicity, and Misuse*, which is available from the American Dietetic Association (see "Addresses," above). The ADA also makes available two cassette tapes:

● Fletcher, D. *Trace Elements in Nutrition.*

● White, H. S. *Iron Nutrition—An Update.*

Also on iron, a 1982 review provides details of its metabolism:

● Finch, C. A., and Huebers, H. Perspectives in iron metabolism. *New England Journal of Medicine* 306 (1982): 1520–1528.

A teaching aid with slides can be ordered from the Nutrition Today Society (see "Addresses," above):

● Finch, C. A. *Iron.*

A concise and informative review of the recent information explosion about the role of zinc in nutrition is:

● Swanson, C. A., and King, J. D. Human zinc nutrition. *Journal of Nutrition Education* 11 (October–December 1979): 181–183.

An in-depth look at the implications of fluoridation is presented in:

● Richmond, V. L. Health effects associated with water fluoridation. *Journal of Nutrition Education* 11 (April–June 1979): 62–64.

The Nutrition Company (see "Addresses," above) makes available a persuasive booklet:

● *Why Should Adults Drink Milk?*

See also "Sodium and High Blood Pressure" and "Water."

Misinformation

What is a nutritionist? A superb article tells just what one can expect to find out from what kind of health professional, and offers a clear description of the credentialing of dietitians and nutritionists. The author also makes some sensible remarks about doctors:

● Carr, B. Who's got the food facts? *Health*, September 1982, pp. 43–45.

In contrast to the R.D. credential from the American Dietetic Association, a fake M.D. degree from an institution like Donsbach University is the mark of a quack. Fake degrees are described in:

● McPherrin, B. What is a nutritionist? *ACSH News and Views*, January/February 1981, pp. 4–5, 11.

Doctors have been accused of being poorly informed on nutrition issues. ACSH critizes this notion in the first of these, and a consumer defends the medical profession in the second:

● Meister, K. A. How much does your doctor know about nutrition? *ACSH News and Views*, November/December 1980, pp. 4–5.

● Stone, L. G. Get sick and send my child to college (letter to the editor). *Nutrition Today*, March/April 1981, p. 30.

A perspective on the nutrition education of doctors is offered in:

● Hamilton, E. M. N., and Whitney, E. N. Doctors, Controversy 14B in *Nutrition: Concepts and Controversies*, 2nd ed. St. Paul, Minn.: West Publishing, 1982. Pp. 485–489.

As for the question which books you can rely on, the Chicago Nutrition Association (see "Addresses," above) puts out a list of "books not recommended" as one of its many services to consumers. The list has been reprinted, with the association's permission, in Appendix A.

The American Dietetic Association has an ongoing committee on food and nutrition misinformation to answer questions about nutrition facts and rumors (see "Addresses," above).

The California Council against Health Fraud makes a lively, informative newsletter available; six issues a year, $5 for students. Ask for the *CCAHF Newsletter* (see "Addresses," above).

Among the references cited in the Highlight 1A notes is *ACSH News and Views*, a newsletter from the American Council on Science and Health. This council—composed of reputable, recognized authorities, scientists in several disciplines related to nutrition—works to provide a balanced view on consumer issues like the "denutrification" and "embalming" of foods. The council is neither pro-health foods nor pro-industry on principle, but rather looks at the evidence and reports each case on its merits. A 30-minute lecture on cassette tape ($9.50) by its president, Dr. Elizabeth Whelan, is available. Dr. Whelan's message is that the real health threats are not food additives but smoking, overeating fat, overeating generally, and lack of exercise:

● Whelan, E. The organic food rip-off. Spenco Medical Corporation, PO Box 8113, Waco, TX 76710.

The council's newsletter, *ACSH News and Views*, which comes out six times a year, is also highly recommended reading for the consumer who wants a balanced picture of nutrition and health issues (see "Addresses," above).

Many excellent publications are available on the important subject of food faddism and misinformation. A whole issue of *Nutrition Reviews* was devoted to this topic and includes a list of suggested readings to help the reader identify faddists, quacks, and promoters:

● *Nutrition Reviews/Supplement: Nutrition Misinformation and Food Faddism*, July 1974.

Dr. Deutsch has recently revised his entertaining and revealing book:

● Deutsch, R. *The New Nuts among the Berries: How Nutrition Nonsense Captured America*. Palo Alto, Calif.: Bull Publishing, 1977.

Dr. Victor Herbert's latest book is also highly recommended:

● Herbert, V., and Barrett, S. *Vitamins and "Health" Foods: The Great American Hustle*. Philadelphia: Stickley, 1981.

To see what other books are reliable references, send for the Chicago Nutrition Association's *Nutrition References and Book Reviews*, already mentioned.

The *Instructor's Manual* includes an optional lecture, "Ripoffs," that summarizes and amplifies this book's many messages on detecting nutrition misinformation.

Nutrition and the Brain

The two principal sources from which much of the information in Highlight 4 was taken are technical papers intended for the advanced student but written very clearly. The first is especially helpful about general principles and about acetylcholine; the second is a thorough review of all three systems—those involving acetylcholine, norepinephrine, and serotonin. A brief (two-page), less technical review of the same subject is provided in the third reference:

● Growdon, J. L., and Wurtman, R. J. Dietary influences on the synthesis of neurotransmitters in the brain. *Nutrition Reviews* 37 (1979): 129–136.

● Fernstrom, J. D. Effects of the diet on brain neurotransmitters. *Metabolism* 26 (1977): 207–223.

● Growdon, J. L., and Wurtman, R. J. Nutrients and neurotransmitters. *Contemporary Nutrition*, December 1979.

Nutrition and Disease

The altered nutrient needs of people with illnesses are the subject of whole textbooks for dietitians and physicians. Two of the best:

● Schneider, H. A., and Anderson, C. E., eds. *Nutritional Support of Medical Practice*, 2nd ed. Hagerstown, Md.: Lippincott, 1983.

● Barness, L. L., Coble, Y. D., MacDonald, D. I., and Christakis, G., eds. *Nutrition and Medical Practice*. Westport, Conn.: Avi, 1981.

Another we favor is our own:

● Whitney, E. N., and Cataldo, C. B. *Understanding Normal and Clinical Nutrition*. St. Paul, Minn.: West, 1983.

Nutrition and Drugs

The most authoritative (and still readable) book on the interactions of drugs with nutrients, including the vitamins, is:

● Roe, D. A. *Drug-Induced Nutritional Deficiencies*. Westport, N.Y.: Avi Publishing, 1976.

Nutritional Individuality

Three good papers on nutritional individuality are available. The first two are written in easy-to-read style for the layperson, the third is more technical and is for the professional:

● Williams, R. J. Nutritional individuality. *Human Nature*, June 1978, pp. 46–53.

● Dubos, R. The intellectual basis of nutrition science and practice. Paper presented at the NIH conference on the biomedical and behavioral basis of clinical nutrition, June 19, 1978, in Bethesda, Maryland. Reprinted in *Nutrition Today*, July/August 1979, pp. 31–34.

● Young, V. R., and Scrimshaw, N. S. Genetic and biological variability in human nutrient requirements. *American Journal of Clinical Nutrition* 32 (1979): 486–500.

Older Adults

A book that helps the reader understand the medical and social problems that develop with aging is:

● Field, M. *The Aged, the Family, and the Community*. New York: Columbia University Press, 1972.

Emphasized throughout is the need to preserve older individuals' feelings of worth and to safeguard their dignity.

The *Journal of the American Geriatrics Society* and *The Gerontologist* make good reading for the general reader.

A short article that takes a positive approach toward the nutrition problems of older people is:

● Rowe, D. Aging—a jewel in the mosaic of life. *Journal of the American Dietetic Association* 72 (1978): 478–486.

Among films and teaching aids that promote understanding of aging are:

● Pelcovits, J. Nutrition education for older Americans. *Cassette-a-Month*, February 1977. Available from the American Dietetic Association (see "Addresses," above).

● *The String Bean*, a 15- to 20-minute long film, is a hauntingly poetic masterpiece portraying an old lady's devotion to life, love, and beauty. Available from McGraw–Hill Films (see "Addresses," above).

For the provider of nutrition for the elderly, we recommend one short and one long reference. The short reference is based on the philosophy that older people should be free to choose what to eat:

● Luros, E. A rational approach to geriatric nutrition. *Dietetic Currents, Ross Timesaver* 8 (November–December 1981; 6 pages, free from Ross Labs; see "Addresses," above).

● Natow, A. B. *Geriatric Nutrition*. Boston: CBI Publishing, 1980. 332 pages, $15.95.

A chapter of Natow's book is devoted to nutrition education for the elderly, a topic not covered here. An important point she makes is that nutrition education materials need to be developed specifically for the elderly. Those prepared for younger people do not meet their needs. Indeed, the way is open for an abundance of literature and resources on nutrition for the elderly.

For help in detecting and avoiding fraudulent products and claims, see the U.S. Senate, Special Committee on Aging:

● *Frauds and Deceptions Affecting the Elderly*. Washington, D.C.: Government Printing Office, latest edition.

For help in finding all the retirement communities in your area, contact:

● Retirement, Research, and Welfare Association, Andrus Building, 215 Long Beach Boulevard, Long Beach, CA 90802.

Although originally intended for the dieter, the Weight Watchers book is useful for older people too. Many of the recipes are for one or two servings. The author has experimented with standard "down home" recipes to lower saturated fat and sugar content, thus enhancing their value for someone trying to eat in line with the *Dietary Guidelines*. Her dessert recipes using dry skimmed milk are especially recommended:

● Nidetch, J. *Weight Watchers Food Plan Diet Cookbook*. New York: The New American Library, 1982.

The *American Journal of Clinical Nutrition* devoted two entire issues—an October 1982 supplement and a November 1982 supplement—to nutrition and aging. Several articles from these issues were cited in the Chapter 15 notes, but there were many others on various body systems, individual nutrients, diet, policy, and other topics.

For the general reader, we recommend highly:

● Comfort, A. *A Good Age*. New York: Crown, 1976.

● Puner, M. *To the Good Long Life*. New York: Universe Books, 1974.

This article reviews the causes of constipation, and comments on bulking agents, stool softeners, laxatives, and other agents:

● Kallman, H. Constipation in the elderly. *American Family Physician* 27 (1983): 179–184.

Pregnancy, Lactation, and Infancy
The following paperback should be singled out for special mention:

● Worthington, B. S., Vermeersch, J., and Williams, S. R. *Nutrition in Pregnancy and Lactation*. St. Louis: Mosby, 1977.

A report, available free from the National Academy of Sciences' Food and Nutrition Board, summarizes the effects in pregnancy of tobacco, alcohol, caffeine, over-the-counter drugs, vitamin megadoses, vegetarian diets, and pica:

● Committee on Nutrition of the Mother and Preschool Child. *Alternative Dietary Practices and Nutritional Abuses in Pregnancy*, 1982. Food and Nutrition Board, 2101 Constitution Avenue, N.W., Washington, DC 20418.

For the seeker of more technical information, the *American Journal of Clinical Nutrition Supplement* published in April 1981 was devoted entirely to nutrition and nutrition assessment in pregnancy.

The person working with teenage pregnant girls should prepare by viewing this film from the March of Dimes:

● *Woman Child*.

Woman Child shows interviews with unmarried teenagers who have borne babies and makes unforgettably clear how they feel about themselves and their situations.

The entire issue of *Nutrition and the MD*, November 1980, was devoted to nutrition in pregnancy and contained many valuable pointers.

The American Council on Science and Health (ACSH) took the controversial stand in 1981 that pregnant women could drink alcohol, as long as they did so moderately. The editor of *Nutrition Today*, speaking for many authorities besides himself, angrily attacked their stand as irresponsible. His editorial, as well as the original ACSH paper, were both published in the same issue of *Nutrition Today*:

● Enloe, C. F., Jr. Thalidomide II. *Nutrition Today*, January/February 1982, pp. 16–17.

● ACSH. Alcohol use during pregnancy. *Nutrition Today*, January/February 1982, pp. 29–32.

Two other articles relevant to this debate are:

● Little, R. E. Moderate alcohol use during pregnancy and decreased infant birth weight. *American Journal of Public Health* 67 (1977): 1154–1156.

● Even moderate drinking may be hazardous to maturing fetus (medical news). *Journal of the American Medical Association* 237 (1977): 2585–2587.

An excellent ten-minute film on fetal alcohol syndrome is available from ABC (see "Addresses," above):

● *Born Drunk*.

An important film, released in 1981, demonstrates the importance of nutrition in teenage pregnancies and shows how to manage the pregnancies of preeclamptic and diabetic women. The film is available from the Society for Nutrition Education (see "Addresses," above):

● *Nutritional Management of High Risk Pregnancy*.

The authoritative reference on nutrition assessment norms for pregnant women is the National Research Council's paperback:

● *Laboratory Indices of Nutritional Status in Pregnancy*. Washington, D.C.: National Academy of Sciences, 1978.

For individualized weight-gain recommendations for underweight and overweight pregnant women, see the reference in Appendix E.

J

Many good references on breastfeeding are also available. This article presents the reasons why, in the authors' opinion, breastfeeding is best even in developed countries such as the United States and Canada:

● Jelliffe, D. B., and Jelliffe, E. F. P. "Breast is best": Modern meanings. *New England Journal of Medicine* 297 (1977): 912–915.

An outstanding, up-to-date reference for the health professional who is advising a breastfeeding mother is:

● Lawrence, R. A. *Breastfeeding: A Guide for the Medical Profession.* St. Louis: Mosby, 1980.

An international organization of women who believe in breastfeeding and who help each other with related concerns is the La Leche League. There are branches in many cities; the main office is listed in "Addresses," above. Among the league's publications are a newsletter and a manual; it also endorses the manual listed last.

● *La Leche League News* (newsletter).

● *The Womanly Art of Breastfeeding* (manual).

● Brewster, P. B. *You Can Breastfeed Your Baby . . . Even in Special Situations* (500+ pages). Emmaus, Pa.: Rodale Press, 1979.

For more information on breast milk banking, contact the local La Leche League office, or see:

● Human milk banking. *Nutrition and the MD*, March 1981.

● Williams, F. H., and Pittard, W. B., III. Human milk banking: Practical concerns for feeding premature infants. *Journal of the American Dietetic Association* 79 (1981): 565–568.

FDA Consumer published an update on drugs excreted in breast milk:

● Hecht, A. Advice on breastfeeding and drugs. *FDA Consumer*, November 1979, pp. 21–22.

If you want to learn *all* there is to know about breastfeeding, you can get a giant head start by sending for the National Academy of Sciences' 58-page booklet prepared by the Committee on Nutrition of the Mother and Preschool Child:

● *A Selected Annotated Bibliography on Breast Feeding, 1970–1977.*

Write to the Office of Publications, National Academy (see "Addresses," above).

On feeding infants, a 19-page booklet is available from the National Dairy Council (see "Addresses," above):

● *Food: From Birth to Birthday.* Publication number B205 (2), 1977.

The whole issue (all six pages) of *Nutrition and the MD*, May 1980, was devoted to infant nutrition. This resource relies extensively on the authoritative word of the American Association of Pediatrics, whose Committee on Nutrition published the following recommendations:

● Commentary on breast-feeding and infant formulas, including proposed standards for formulas. *Pediatrics* 57 (1976): 278–285.

According to a recent review, it is irresponsible to make a dogmatic statement about the timing or selection of additions of solid food to a baby's diet. This review gives the details that need to be considered:

● Nutritional adequacy of breast feeding. *Nutrition Reviews* 38 (1980): 145–147.

The USDA has published a manual giving the complete nutritional analysis of many baby foods:

● *Composition of Foods: Baby Foods—Raw, Processed, Prepared.* Agriculture Handbook no. 8–3. USDA Science and Education Administration. Washington, D.C.: Government Printing Office, 1978.

A 14-minute color film on feeding babies during their first year, excellent for showing in clinics, prenatal classes, and the like, is available from the Society for Nutrition Education (see "Addresses," above):

● *First Foods.*

This is a good paperback on infant feeding for healthy babies:

● Heslin, J. A., and Natow, A. F. *No-Nonsense Nutrition: For Your Baby's First Year.* Boston: CBI Publishing, 1978.

A booklet on nutrition for pregnant women and parents that you can consult with confidence is:

● Alfin-Slater, R. B., Aftergood, L., and Ashley, J. *Nutrition and Motherhood.* Available from PO Box 2160, 6931 Van Nuys Boulevard, Van Nuys, CA 91405.

A handy 50-page record-keeping booklet with month-by-month instructions to parents on infant feeding:

● *What Shall I Feed My Baby?* USDA. Ask for Program Aid no. 1281 (June 1981).

For the breastfeeding mother, the USDHHS makes available a short (22-page) how-to booklet:

● Breast feeding. HHS publication no. (HSA) 79–5109. Write to the Government Printing Office.

On the nutrition of infants, an excellent comprehensive reference is:

Fomon, S. J. *Infant Nutrition*, 2nd ed. Philadelphia: Saunders, 1974.

A tidy 4-page statement on the nutritional needs of infants up to a year of age was published in:
Woodruff, C. W. The science of infant nutrition and the art of infant feeding. *Journal of the American Medical Association* 240 (1978): 657–661.

A superb audiovisual aid that all clinics and doctors' offices should show to mothers-to-be is a set of about 80 slides with a cassette, prepared by the March of Dimes:
Inside My Mom.

Inside My Mom is a delightful description of pregnancy from the fetus's point of view, intended to motivate the pregnant woman to eat right. It is available from the local March of Dimes office or from the National Headquarters (see "Addresses," above). You might want to inquire what other materials they have available.

For parents who want to compare infant formulas, or who need to find alternatives to cow's milk or cow's milk formulas for their infants or children, we recommend:
Whitney, E. N., and Cataldo, C. B. Highlight 15: Choosing Formulas and Milk Substitutes, in *Understanding Normal and Clinical Nutrition*. St. Paul, Minn.: West, 1983. Pp. 559–568.

Protein

A paperback that offers a clear picture of our new and profound understanding of how genes code for enzymes, which in turn determine the structure and function of cells, tissues, and whole organisms is:
Watson, J. D. *Molecular Biology of the Gene*, 3rd ed. Menlo Park, Calif.: W. A. Benjamin, 1976.

To enhance understanding of the roles of enzymes and other proteins in the body, we recommend two optional lectures in the *Instructor's Manual*: "Nutrition and Adaptation" and "Inborn Errors."

The book edited by Pellett and Young, mentioned at the end of Appendix D, is an excellent reference on protein quality evaluation.

Sodium and High Blood Pressure

People with high blood pressure can control it with drugs and diet, and people with normal blood pressure need not bother with either. What should people with *mild* high blood pressure do? This article advances a persuasive argument in favor of "nondrug therapies," such as salt restriction, meditation, biofeedback, and exercise:

Kaplan, M. Mild hypertension: When and how to treat. *Archives of Internal Medicine* 143 (1983): 255–259.

A booklet on sodium in foods is available:
Marsh, A. C., Klippstein, R. N., and Kaplan, S. D. "The Sodium Content of Your Food," published by the USDA (booklet no. 233 in the Home and Garden Bulletin Series), available for $2 from the Government Printing Office. Mention stock number 001–000–04179–7 when ordering.

Other references on sodium in foods are mentioned in Appendix I.

For help in controlling high blood pressure:
What you should know about. . . The National Program to Control High Blood Pressure (leaflet). NIH publication no. 80–632. Bethesda, Md.: Public Health Service, National Heart, Lung, and Blood Institute, 1979.

High Blood Pressure Facts and Fiction (leaflet). NIH publication no. 80–1218. Bethesda, Md.: Public Health Service, National Heart, Lung and Blood Institute, updated.

This article outlines for professionals the general approach to hypertension management:
Moser, M. Hypertension, how therapy works. *American Journal of Nursing* 80 (1980): 937–941.

Stress and Nutrition

The "father of stress," who coined the term and spent his life studying it, is Hans Selye. A popular paperback of his, written in nontechnical language, is:
Selye, H. *The Stress of Life*, rev. ed. New York: McGraw-Hill, 1976.

A series of four excellent articles on stress appeared in the *American Journal of Nursing*. They show how the nurse can recognize and cope with stress in her very demanding job, and also how she can recognize it in patients or clients and help them to cope with it:
Smith, M. J. T., and Selye, H. Reducing the negative effects of stress. *American Journal of Nursing* 79 (November 1979): 1953–1955.

O'Flynn-Corniskey, A. J. The type A individual. *American Journal of Nursing* 79 (November 1979): 1956–1958.

Morris, C. L. Relaxation therapy in a clinic. *American Journal of Nursing* 79 (November 1979): 1958.

Richter, J. M., and Sloan, A. A relaxation technique. *American Journal of Nursing* 79 (November 1979): 1960–1964.

The article by Smith and Selye also lists the "diseases of adaptation," showing how each person has a different body system or part that may be the first to succumb to excessive stress, so that one person gets heart disease, another ulcers, another allergies, and so forth.

The standard-bearer for accuracy in vitamin claims, Dr. Victor Herbert, shows how the notion of "stress vitamins" arose and why we should not take it seriously:
● Herbert, V. The vitamin craze. *Archives of Internal Medicine* 140 (1980): 173–176.

The psychological means of managing stress are nicely described in Chapter 4 of Farquhar's delightful book, and the bibliography for that chapter suggests other good references:
● Farquhar, J. W. *The American Way of Life Need Not Be Hazardous to Your Health.* New York: Norton, 1978.

This teaching aid is a set of 13 slides designed to depict the consequences of stress. The set can be ordered from the Nutrition Today Society (see "Addresses," above):
● Selye, H. *Stress: On Just Being Sick.*

Surveys

For more information on surveys of nutrition status, see:
● *Ten-State Nutrition Survey, 1968–1970.* U.S. Department of Health and Human Services. Center for Disease Control, Atlanta, GA 30333.

● *Health and Nutrition Examination Survey (HANES) United States 1971–1973.* U.S. Department of Health and Human Services. National Center for Health Statistics, Rockville, MD 20857.

● *Nutrition Canada, National Survey,* 1973. Information Canada, Ottawa, Ontario.

● *Dietary Source Data, United States, 1971–1974,* 1979. Public Health Service. Hyattsville, MD 20782.

● *Food Consumption Profiles of White and Black Persons Aged 1–74 Years, United States, 1971–74.* HHS publication no. (PHS) 79–1658. Public Health Service, Office of Research, Statistics, 3700 East-West Highway, Hyattsville, MD 20782.

The recent Nationwide Food Consumption Survey is available from the Government Printing Office (see "Addresses," above):
● *Food Consumption: Households in the United States, Spring 1977, Nationwide Food Consumption Survey 1977–78, Report No. 1.*
Refer to publication number 001–000–04293–9. Reports for each of four regions of the United States are also available, at $8.50 each: Northeast, Report No. 2, 001–000–04294–7; North Central, Report No. 3, 001–000–04295–5; South,

Report No. 4, 001–000–04301–3; and West, Report No. 5, 001–000–04302–1.

Surveys of nutrition status have led to programs to remedy the deficiencies found. For a review, see:
● Vaden, A. G. Child nutrition programs: past, present, future. *Professional Nutritionist,* Winter 1981, pp. 7–10.

Vegetarianism

The *Instructor's Manual* includes an optional lecture, "Diet Planning for the Vegetarian," which is also available as a booklet from The Nutrition Company (see "Addresses," above), and which offers suggested references.

Vitamins

The complete terminology for the vitamins, together with their popular names and the correct chemical structures, were agreed on by the relevant scientific societies and published in:
● Nomenclature policy: Generic decriptors and trivial names for vitamins and related compounds. *Journal of Nutrition* 112 (1982): 7–14.

The hazards of overdosing with vitamins and minerals have been reviewed and described in a booklet available from the American Dietetic Association (see "Addresses," above):
● National Nutrition Consortium. *Vitamin-Mineral Safety, Toxicity, and Misuse.* The American Dietetic Association, 1978.

Douglas Ramsey, who was captured by the Vietcong in 1966 during the Vietnamese War, personally experienced severe beriberi and scurvy and lived to tell the story in a moving account:
● Seven years in captivity as Douglas K. Ramsey tells it. *Nutrition Today,* May/June 1973, pp. 14–21.

Recent research suggests that the plant pigment family of xanthophylls may be essential dietary factors for vision in primates, including humans:
● The effect of a dietary lack of xanthophyll on the eye of the monkey. *Nutrition Reviews* 38 (1980): 384–386.

The vast problem of vitamin A deficiency throughout the world is summarized in an 88-page booklet available from the World Health Organization (see "Addresses," above):
● *Vitamin A Deficiency and Xerophthalmia.* WHO/USAID Joint Meeting. Technical Report Series 590. Albany, N.Y.: Q Corporation, 1976.

The American Dietetic Association (see "Addresses," above) has made available a cassette:

● *Vitamin C.* CAM 7–78.

The entire September 1975 issue of the *Annals of the New York Academy of Sciences* (volume 258) was devoted to vitamin C; it contains 51 important articles reviewing recent research. Even the general reader might want to take this volume off the shelf and skim through it just to see how involved and extensive the work on this little vitamin really is.

The most famous and fascinating story about vitamin C is the story of how Norman Cousins, the *Saturday Review* editor, recovered from a supposedly incurable disease. Cousins researched some of the medical literature, decided that vitamin C would cure him, removed himself from the hospital, and got well with the help of vitamin C megadoses and laughter. His account of the experience is intriguing, telling how the patient's attitude, relief from stress, and faith affect healing. Highly recommended:

● Cousins, N. Anatomy of an illness (as perceived by the patient). *Nutrition Today*, May/June 1977, pp. 22–28; reprinted from the *New England Journal of Medicine* 295 (1976): 1458–1463.

The sequel, which explores further the attitudes of doctors and patients and the importance of the patient's involvement in his own cure, is also stimulating reading:

● Cousins, N. What I learned from 3,000 doctors. *Saturday Review*, February 18, 1978, pp. 12–16.

Dr. Pauling's ingenious and thought-provoking arguments in favor of taking large doses of vitamin C are presented in:

● Pauling, L. Are recommended daily allowances for vitamin C adequate? *Proceedings of the National Academy of Sciences* 71 (1974): 4442–4446.

Most of the March/April 1978 issue of *Nutrition Today* was devoted to a lively debate between Dr. Pauling and several prominent nutrition authorities. The debate brings out the major issues surrounding Dr. Pauling's new ideas about vitamin C and the differences in attitude among people attempting to assess the validity of his theories.

Dr. Pauling's latest book is:

● Pauling, L. *Vitamin C, the Common Cold and the Flu.* San Francisco: W. H. Freeman, 1976.

A thoughtful discussion of the cancer-vitamin C trials to date is provided in:

● Hodges, R. E. Vitamin C and cancer. *Nutrition Reviews* 40 (1982): 289–292.

The American Dietetic Association (see "Addresses," above) makes available a cassette:

● Herbert, V. *Megavitamin Therapy.* CAM 5–77.

Research findings on vitamin D are summarized by one of the major investigators in the area in a featured article in *Nutrition Reviews*. This would make stiff reading for the general reader, but it is recommended to anyone who wants to gain an appreciation of all the complexities. Of special interest is the new hope this research brings to renal patients, whose bone disease was untreatable until the kidney's role in vitamin D metabolism was understood:

● DeLuca, H. F. The vitamin D system in the regulation of calcium and phosphorus metabolism. *Nutrition Reviews* 37 (1979): 161–193.

Among the demonstrated ill effects of vitamin E megadoses are white blood cell damage, interference with the clotting action of vitamin K, slowing of wound healing, and damage to various body organs. The white blood cell effects are shown in:

● Prasad, J. S. Effect of vitamin E supplementation on leukocyte function. *American Journal of Clinical Nutrition* 33 (1980): 606–608.

Vitamin E therapy can be effectively used in a variety of medical situations, and these have been reviewed by:

● Horwitt, M. K. Therapeutic uses of vitamin E in medicine. *Nutrition Reviews* 38 (1980): 105–113.

The Nutrition Company (see "Addresses," above) makes available a lively discussion of how to choose vitamin-mineral supplements that includes the tables of Appendix P and the RDA table for comparison:

● *SOS—Selection of Supplements.*

See also the reference on "stress vitamins" by V. Herbert, under "Stress."

J

Water

Both of the following are classics in the literature of the history of life on earth, revealing facets of the intimate relationship between environmental water and the life of cells. Oparin's book, originally published in 1938, is available in paperback:

● Oparin, A. I. *Origin of Life.* New York: Dover, latest edition.

● Wald, G. The origin of life. *Scientific American* 190 (August 1956): 44–53; also offprint no. 47.

A teaching aid can be ordered from the Nutrition Today Society (see "Addresses," above):

● Robinson, J. *Nutrient Metabolism: Water, the Essential Nutrient.*

The following references are also informative:
● Calabrese, E. J., and Tuthill, R. W. Sources of elevated sodium levels in drinking water . . . and recommendations for reduction. *Journal of Environmental Health* 41 (1978): 151–155.

● Keller, W. D. Drinking water: A geochemical factor in human health. *Geological Society of America Bulletin* 89 (March 1978): 334–336.

● Varma, M. M., Serdahely, S. G., and Katz, H. M. Physiological effects of trace elements and chemicals in water. *Journal of Environmental Health* 39 (1976): 90–100.

California's water supply is rapidly dwindling to the point where costs will rise greatly and hard decisions will have to be made. The problem is discussed by a U.S. congressman from California in:
● Coelho, T. Water and the food supply. *Professional Nutritionist*, Spring 1981, pp. 2–3.

Weight Control

The researcher who first explained to the nutrition community how the new ideal weights were arrived at published his remarks in:
● Keys, A. Overweight, obesity, coronary heart disease and mortality. *Nutrition Reviews* 38 (1980): 297–307. This lecture was also published in *Nutrition Today*, July/August 1980, pp. 16–22.

This article reports research on the thermogenic theory of obesity. It may be that obese people have a defective sodium-potassium pump in their body cells so that they expend less energy than normal people:
● DeLuise, M., Blackburn, G. L., and Filer, J. S. Reduced activity of the red-cell sodium-potassium pump in human obesity. *New England Journal of Medicine* 303 (1980): 1017–1022.

Several articles provide insight into current research hypotheses on the control of hunger and appetite. The first relates the availability of brain fuels to food intake and body weight:
● Davis, J. D., Wirtshafter, D., Asin, K. E., and Brief, D. Sustained intracerebroventricular infusion of brain fuels reduces body weight and food intake in rats. *Science* 212 (1981): 81–83.

The second explains current thinking on how the body's fat mass may speak to the brain:
● Van Itallie, T. B., Gale, S. K., and Kissileff, H. R. Control of food intake in the regulation of depot fat: An overview. In *Advances in Modern Nutrition*, vol. 2, *Diabetes, Obesity, and Vascular Diseases*, ed. H. M. Katzen and R. J. Mahler. New York: Wiley, 1978. Pp. 427–492.

The third divulges the roles thought to be played by neurotransmitters, endogenous opiates, and other substances in the brain:
● Morley, J. E., and Levine, A. S. The central control of appetite. *Lancet* 1 (1983): 398–401.

This one concisely describes the connection of arousal with binge eating and shows how the same nervous control affects other voluntary behaviors. It concludes that the control of eating behavior is diffuse; "There *is* no special hunger center":
● Stricker, I. M. Hyperphagia. *New England Journal of Medicine* 298 (1978): 1010–1013.

These two summarize what is known about appetite control and show how many different initial stimuli merge into "a final common path":
● Castonguay, T. W., Applegate, E. A., Upton, D. E., and Stern, J. S. Hunger and appetite—old conceptions/new distinctions. *Nutrition Reviews* 41 (1983): 101–110.

● Levine, A. S., and Morley, J. E. The shortening pathways to appetite control. *Nutrition Today*, January/February 1983, pp. 6–14.

A doctor reviews for other doctors the psychological literature on obesity and suggests a screening procedure that includes a psychiatric history:
● Powers, P. S. Obesity—psychosomatic illness review, no. 2 in a series. *Psychosomatics*, October 1982, pp. 1023–1039.

The following are among the more popular behavior modification guides in paperback for the do-it-yourself dieter:
● Ferguson, J. M. *Habits, Not Diets: The Real Way to Weight Control.* Palo Alto, Calif.: Bull Publishing, 1976.

● Stuart, R. B., and Davis, B. *Slim Chance in a Fat World: Behavioral Control of Obesity.* Champaign, Ill.: Research Press, 1977.

● Nash, J. D., and Long, L. O. *Taking Charge of Your Weight and Well-Being.* Palo Alto, Calif.: Bull Publishing Company, 1978.

Weight Watchers, Inc., publishes several cookbooks, all based on the exchange system, that present sensible, nutritious, balanced meals for weight loss.

Another major reference containing voluminous recent research and scholarly reflection is:
● Stunkard, A. J., ed. *Obesity.* Philadelphia: Saunders, 1980.

The *International Journal of Obesity* began publication in 1977. Volume 1 of an even newer journal, *Appetite*, appeared in 1980.

A touching personal account by a woman who lost seventy pounds and recorded her thoughts and feelings throughout the experience:
● LeShan, E. *Winning the Losing Battle: Why I Will Never Be Fat Again*. New York: Bantam Books, 1981.

The possibility that fiber and its interplay with insulin may have an important role to play in satisfying appetite and so controlling food intake is discussed in:
● Heaton, K. W., ed. *Dietary Fibre: Current Developments of Importance to Health*. Westport, Conn.: Food and Nutrition Press, 1979.

The entire issue (six pages) of *Nutrition and the MD*, November 1979 was devoted to obesity: its causes, treatment, incidence in children, and so forth.

Metropolitan Life Insurance Company produced a film in the 1970s that has enjoyed a wide showing and has helped many people get a handle on weight control. *Song of Arthur* is available free, and makes enjoyable viewing for about twenty minutes of class time.

A thought-provoking short film shows a woman reacting to frustration and anxiety by eating a whole chocolate cake. Called *Crumb and Punishment*, the film is useful to stimulate discussion on the need for behavior change. It is available from R. L. Korschun, R.D., 7000 SW 62nd Avenue, Penthouse J, Miami, FL 33413.

A diet book that uses the exchange system—and includes exchanges for fast foods—is:
● Better Homes and Gardens' *Eat and Stay Slim*, 2nd ed. Des Moines, Iowa: Meredith, 1979.
The 1979 price was $3.95.

The *American Journal of Clinical Nutrition* published a *Supplement*, February 1980, entirely devoted to surgical and other drastic procedures for morbid obesity.

Consumer Guide put out a booklet in 1979 entitled *Diets '79*, which rated the Scarsdale Diet, the "Mayo Clinic" Diet, the Pritikin program, and many others as to whether they work, how safe they are, and how permanent their effects are. The booklet was so successful it will very likely be followed by another like it every now and then. Watch for these.

The Healthy Way to Weigh Less and *Critique of Low Carbo-* hydrate Ketogenic Weight Reduction Regimens, a pamphlet and a reprint, can be ordered from the American Medical Association (see "Addresses," above). Also from the AMA is this book for $1.00:
● *Healthy Approach to Slimming*, 1978.

The USDA makes available a handbook, useful in weight control:
● *Calories and Weight*. Washington, D.C.: Government Printing Office, 1983.

To get in shape physically, we recommend you follow the advice in one of the following (and see the references under "Athlete"):
● Bailey, C. *Fit or Fat?* Boston: Houghton Mifflin, 1977.
● Katch, F. I., McArdle, W. D., and Boylan, B. R. *Getting in Shape*. Boston: Houghton Mifflin, 1979.

The *best* diet book we've found is this paperback by the psychological director of Weight Watchers:
● Stuart, R. B. *Act Thin, Stay Thin*, rev. ed. New York: W. W. Norton (Jove edition), 1983.

People giving up smoking often develop a related nutrition problem: weight gain. The American Heart Association offers help in a booklet called *Guidelines for a Weight Control Component in a Smoking Cessation Program* and a leaflet called *Weight Control Guidance in Smoking Cessation*. (See "Addresses," above.)

A helping organization specifically designed for binge eaters, much as Alcoholics Anonymous (AA) is designed for alcohol addicts, is Overeaters Anonymous (OA). OA has many local offices around the country; its main address is listed under "Addresses," above.

The *Instructor's Manual* includes an optional lecture on the set-point theory of body weight regulation: "Set-Point."

World Hunger
The following resources provide valuable information about world hunger issues:
● *Overcoming World Hunger: The Challenge Ahead*. Report of the Presidential Commission on World Hunger. Washington, D.C.: Government Printing Office, 1980.
● Lappe, F. M., and Collins, J. *Food First: Beyond the Myth of Scarcity*. New York: Ballantine Books, 1979.
● Wortman, S., and Cummings, R. W. *To Feed This World*. Baltimore: Johns Hopkins University Press, 1978.
● Berg, A. *Malnourished People: A Policy View*. Washington, D.C.: World Bank, 1981.

J

To help people become better informed about basic data and policy making, the following references are recommended:

● *World Development Report*. The International Bank for Reconstruction and Development/The World Bank. New York: Oxford University Press. Published annually.

● *The United States and The Third World: Agenda for Action*. Overseas Development Council. New York: Praeger Publishers. Published annually.

● *North-South: A Program for Survival*. International Commission on International Development Issues. Cambridge, Mass.: MIT Press, 1980.

● *The Ending Hunger Briefing Workbook*. San Francisco: The Hunger Project, 1982.

The interrelationships between society, the environment, and the economy may be further explored in:

● Brown, L. *Building a Sustainable Society*. New York: Norton/Worldwatch Institute, 1981.

● Pimentel, D., and Pimentel, M. *Food, Energy, and Society*. New York: Wiley, 1979.

● Schumacher, E. F. *Small Is Beautiful—Economics as if People Mattered*. New York: Harper and Row, 1973.

● *The Global 2000 Report to the President: Entering the Twenty-First Century*. Council on Environmental Quality and the Department of State. Washington, D.C.: Government Printing Office, 1980.

A basic resource to help you contact the major hunger organizations lists more than 400 such organizations with their addresses:

● Worthington, L., ed. *Who's Involved With Hunger: An Organization Guide*. Washington, D.C.: World Hunger Education Service. Revised annually.

To learn how to have an impact on U.S. food policy, you may want to learn more about organizations dealing with food policy issues. Agencies especially willing to help you get the facts are listed under "Addresses," above.

J

APPENDIX   K
Dietary Fiber in Foods

Chapter 2 discussed the benefits of fiber-rich foods, made the distinction between crude fiber and dietary fiber, and concluded, tentatively, that a diet providing from 15 to 35 grams of dietary fiber a day might be beneficial and would be safe. Table K–1 shows the approximate amounts of dietary fiber in a variety of commonly eaten, fiber-rich foods. Note that most of the vegetable portions in the table are one-cup portions—twice the standard (exchange system) portion size. A one-cup portion of vegetables is not considered overly large when an objective in diet planning is to provide ample amounts of fiber. We recommend that you read the article by Southgate and coauthors from which the data of Table K–1 was derived, for an understanding of the limitations on the accuracy of the numbers in the table and for a breakdown of the fiber types into cellulose, lignin, and other sources.

TABLE K–1 **Approximate Dietary Fiber Contents of Selected Foods.**

FOOD	PORTION SIZE	DIETARY FIBER (g)
Breads and crackers		
White bread	1 slice	0.6
Whole-wheat bread	1 slice	1.8
Matzoh	1 piece	1.2
Cereals		
All-Bran	½ c	7.5
Cornflakes	¾ c	2.1
Grapenuts	1 oz	2.0
Rice Krispies	1 c	1.3
Puffed Wheat	1 c	2.2
Shredded Wheat	1 biscuit	3.1
Fruits		
Apples	1 small	2.0
Bananas	½ small	1.0
Cherries	10 large	0.8
Grapefruit	1 c	1.1
Peaches	1 medium	2.3
Pears	1 small	3.0
Plums	2 medium	1.2
Strawberries	¾ c	2.4
Legumes and Nuts		
Baked beans, canned	½ c	5.5
Peas, canned	½ c	6.0
Peanut butter	2 tbsp	2.4
Peanuts	1 tbsp	0.8
Brazil nuts	6-8 large	2.2
Vegetables		
Broccoli, cooked pieces	1 c	6.4
Brussels sprouts, cooked	1 c	4.4
Cabbage, cooked	1 c	4.1
Carrots, cooked	1 c	5.7
Cauliflower, cooked	1 c	2.3
Corn, cooked	1 c kernels	8.6
Lettuce, raw pieces	1 c	0.8
Onions, raw chopped	1 c	3.6
Peppers, green, cooked	1 c	1.5
Potatoes, cooked	1 potato	3.9
Tomatoes, canned	1 c	2.0
Tomatoes, fresh	1 tomato	1.9
Miscellaneous		
Bran, wheat	1 tbsp	4.0
Dill pickle, 3¾ × 1¼ in	1 pickle	1.0
Marmalade	1 tbsp	0.1
Strawberry jam	1 tbsp	0.2

Source: Data from *Bowes and Church's Food Values of Portions Commonly Used*, 13th ed., by J. A. T. Pennington and H. N. Church (New York: Harper and Row, 1980); D. A. T. Southgate, B. Bailey, E. Collinson, and A. F. Walker, A guide to calculating intakes of dietary fibre, *Journal of Human Nutrition* 30 (1976): 303-313, with the permission of the authors and publisher.

APPENDIX L
Exchange System

For an introduction to the use of exchange systems, see Chapter 1. The U.S. Exchange System is presented here, and the Canadian Food System is explained in Appendix M. For a complete description of the U.S. Four Food Group Plan, see Chapter 1.

The United States system divides foods into six lists—the milk, vegetable, fruit, bread, meat, and fat lists.[1] The items listed first in each group are from the standard exchange lists used in the United States. We have also listed some Chinese foods, some vegetarian foods, and some fast foods to show that the exchange system can be adapted to other uses. At the end of the section is a list of "unlimited" foods, which have negligible kcalories.

---

1   The U.S. exchange system presented here is based on material in *Exchange Lists for Meal Planning,* prepared by committees of the American Diabetes Association and the American Dietetic Association in cooperation with the National Institute of Arthritis, Metabolism, and Digestive Diseases and the National Heart and Lung Institute, National Institutes of Health, Public Health Service, U.S. Department of Health and Human Services (formerly U.S. Department of Health, Education, and Welfare).

The Chinese foods listed in these tables are reprinted from *Diabetes and Chinese Food,* ©1978, with the written permission of the Canadian Dietetic Association. We have adjusted the Canadian exchanges used in these examples so that they correspond approximately in food value to the U.S. exchanges. *Diabetes and Chinese Food* is available for a nominal charge from the Canadian Diabetes Association (address in Appendix J).

Vegetarian foods have been adapted from the *Supplement to the Exchange Lists for Meal Planning, Vegetarian Cookery,* prepared by the American Diabetes Association, Washington, D.C. area affiliate (Bethesda, Md.: The American Diabetes Association, 1978).

The fast food data are reprinted by permission from "Nutritional Analysis of Foods Served at McDonald's" (© McDonald's, 1976).

TABLE L–1 **Milk List (12 g carbohydrate, 8 g protein, 80 kcal)[a]**

AMOUNT	FOOD
Nonfat fortified milk	
1 c	Skim or nonfat milk
1 c	Buttermilk made from skim milk
1 c	Yogurt made from skim milk (plain, unflavored)
⅓ c	Powdered, nonfat dry milk, before adding liquid
½ c	Canned evaporated skim milk, before adding liquid
Low-fat fortified milk	
1 c	1% fat fortified milk (count as 1 milk and ½ fat exchange)
1 c	2% fat fortified milk (count as 1 milk and 1 fat exchange
1 c	Yogurt made from 2% fortified milk (plain, unflavored) (count as 1 milk and 1 fat exchange)
Whole milk (count as 1 milk and 2 fat exchanges)	
1 c	Whole milk
1 c	Buttermilk made from whole milk
1 c	Yogurt made from whole milk (plain, unflavored)
½ c	Canned evaporated whole milk, before adding liquid

[a] A milk exchange is a serving of food equivalent to 1 c of skim milk in its energy nutrient content. One milk exchange contains substantial amounts of carbohydrate and protein and about 80 kcal.

L

TABLE L–1   **(continued)**

AMOUNT	FOOD
Chinese foods	
1 c	Soybean milk, unsweetened
8 oz	Soybean curd (2½ × 2¾ × 2 in)
⅔ c	Soybean, cooked
Vegetarian foods	
1 c	Soy based infant formula (count as 1 milk and ½ bread exchange)
1 c	Soy milk, calcium fortified (count as 1 milk and 1 fat exchange)
1 c	Kefir (count as 1 milk and 1 fat exchange)
1 c	Goat's milk (count as 1 milk and 2 fat exchanges)
Fast foods[b]	

[b] These fast foods contain ½ milk exchange and added bread and fat: chocolate shake (3½ bread, 2 fat, 365 kcal); vanilla shake (3 bread, 1½ fat, 325 kcal); strawberry shake (3½ bread, 1½ fat, 345 kcal).

TABLE L–2   **Vegetable List**
(5 g carbohydrate, 2 g protein, 25 kcal)[a]

AMOUNT	FOOD
½ c	Asparagus
1 c	Bean sprouts (alfalfa, mung or soy)
½ c	Beets
½ c	Brussels sprouts
½ c	Cabbage
½ c	Carrots
	Carrot juice: See Fruit List
½ c	Cauliflower
½ c	Celery
½ c	Cucumbers
½ c	Dark green vegetables
½ c	Beet greens
½ c	Broccoli
½ c	Chards
½ c	Collard greens
½ c	Dandelion greens
½ c	Kale
½ c	Mustard greens
½ c	Spinach
½ c	Swiss chard
½ c	Turnip greens
½ c	Eggplant
½ c	Green pepper
½ c	Mushrooms

[a] A vegetable exchange is a serving of any vegetable that contains a moderate amount of carbohydrate, a small but significant amount of protein, and about 25 kcal.

TABLE L–2   **(continued)**

AMOUNT	FOOD
½ c	Okra
½ c	Onions
½ c	Rhubarb
½ c	Rutabaga
½ c	Sauerkraut
½ c	String beans, green or yellow
½ c	Summer squash
½ c	Tomatoes
½ c	Tomato juice
½ c	Turnips
½ c	Vegetable juice cocktail
½ c	Zucchini
Chinese foods	
1 c	Bean sprouts
½ c	Lotus root (⅓ segment)
½ c	Water chestnuts
½ c	Yam bean root

TABLE L–3   **Fruit List (10 g carbohydrate, 40 kcal)**[a]

AMOUNT	FOOD
1 small	Apple
⅓ c	Apple juice
½ c	Applesauce (unsweetened)
2 medium	Apricots, fresh
4 halves	Apricots, dried
½ small	Banana
½ c	Blackberries
½ c	Blueberries
¼ small	Cantaloupe melon
½ c	Carrot juice
10 large	Cherries
⅓ c	Cider
2	Dates
1	Fig, fresh
1	Fig, dried
1 half	Grapefruit
½ c	Grapefruit juice
12	Grapes
¼ c	Grape juice
⅛ medium	Honeydew melon
½ small	Mango

[a] A fruit exchange is a serving of fruit that contains about 10 g of carbohydrate and 40 kcal. The protein and fat content of fruit is negligible.

TABLE L-3   (continued)

AMOUNT	FOOD
1 small	Nectarine
1 small	Orange
½ c	Orange juice
¾ c	Papaya
1 medium	Peach
1 small	Pear
1 medium	Persimmon (native)
½ c	Pineapple
⅓ c	Pineapple juice
2 medium	Plums
2 medium	Prunes
¼ c	Prune juice
½ c	Raspberries
2 tbsp	Raisins
¾ c	Strawberries
1 medium	Tangerine
1 c	Watermelon

Chinese foods

1 medium	Guava, fresh
3 medium	Kumquats, fresh
4 medium	Lychee, fresh
½ small or ⅓ c	Mango
½ small or ⅓ c	Papaya
½ medium	Persimmon
⅓ medium	Pomelo

Fast foods[b]

[b] Apple and cherry pies contain 1½ exchanges of fruit but also 1 bread and 3½ fat exchanges.

TABLE L-4   **Bread–Starchy Vegetable List**
(15 g carbohydrate, 2 g protein, 70 kcal)[a]

AMOUNT	FOOD
Bread	
1 slice	White (including French and Italian)
1 slice	Whole-wheat

[a] A bread exchange is a serving of bread, cereal, or starchy vegetable that contains appreciable carbohydrate (15 g) and a small but significant amount of protein (2 g), totaling about 7() kcal.

TABLE L-4   (continued)

AMOUNT	FOOD
1 slice	Rye or pumpernickel
1 slice	Raisin
1 half	Small bagel
1 half	Small English muffin
1	Plain roll, bread
1 half	Frankfurter roll
1 half	Hamburger bun
3 tbsp	Dried bread crumbs
1 6-in	Tortilla
1¼ oz loaf	Pita (Syrian) bread

Cereal

½ c	Bran flakes
¾ c	Other ready-to-eat cereal, unsweetened
1 c	Puffed cereal, unfrosted
½ c	Cereal, cooked
½ c	Grits, cooked
½ c	White rice, millet, wild rice, or barley, cooked
⅓ c	Brown rice, cooked
½ c	Pasta, cooked (spaghetti, noodles, or macaroni)
3 c	Popcorn, popped, no fat added
2 tbsp	Cornmeal, dry
2½ tbsp	Wheat flour
3 tbsp	Buckwheat flour, dark, or rye flour
2 tbsp	Cornmeal, dry
3 tbsp	Miso
¼ c	Wheat germ
¼ c	Oats, dry
⅓ c	Wheat berries, cooked

Crackers

3	Arrowroot
2	Graham, 2½-in square
1 half	Matzoth, 4 × 6 in
20	Oyster
25	Pretzels, 3⅛ in long × ⅛ in diameter
3	Rye wafers, 2 × 3½ in
6	Saltines
4	Soda, 2½-in sq

Dried beans, peas, and lentils

½ c	Beans, peas, lentils, dried and cooked
¼ c	Baked beans, no pork, canned

TABLE L-4 (continued)

AMOUNT	FOOD

Starchy vegetables

AMOUNT	FOOD
⅓ c	Corn
1 small	Corn on cob
½ c	Lima beans
⅔ c	Parsnips
½ c	Peas, green, canned, or frozen
1 small	Potato, white
½ c	Potato, mashed
¾ c	Pumpkin
½ c	Squash (winter, acorn, or butternut)
¼ c	Yam or sweet potato

Prepared foods

AMOUNT	FOOD
1	Biscuit, 2-in diameter (count as 1 bread and 1 fat exchange)
1	Corn bread, 2 × 2 × 1 in (count as 1 bread and 1 fat exchange)
1	Corn muffin, 2-in diameter (count as 1 bread and 1 fat exchange)
5	Crackers, round butter type (count as 1 bread and 1 fat exchange)
1	Muffin, plain, small (count as 1 bread and 1 fat exchange)
8	Potatoes, french fried, 2 to 3½ in long (count as 1 bread and 1 fat exchange)
15	Potato chips or corn chips (count as 1 bread and 2 fat exchanges)
1	Pancake, 5 × ½ in (count as 1 bread and 1 fat exchange)
1	Waffle, 5 × ½ in (count as 1 bread and 1 fat exchange)

Chinese foods

AMOUNT	FOOD
1 small or ⅔ medium	Bow (Chinese steamed dough)
6	Chestnuts
1 c	Congee
¼ c	Glutinous rice, cooked
⅔ c	Gruel rice, cooked
½ c	Noodles, cooked (shrimp, thin rice, flat rice, cellophane)
2 tbsp	Rice flour or glutinous rice flour
3 small or ⅓ c	Taro
4	Wonton wrapper (5 × 5 in)

TABLE L-5 **Meat and Meat-Alternate List (7 g protein, 3 g fat + variable added fat; 55 kcal + kcalories for added fat)[a]**

AMOUNT	FOOD

Lean meat

AMOUNT	FOOD
1 oz	Beef—baby beef (very lean), chipped beef, chuck, flank steak, tenderloin, plate ribs, plate skirt steak, round (bottom, top), all cuts rump, spareribs, tripe
1 oz	Lamb—leg, rib, sirloin, loin (roast and chops), shank, shoulder
1 oz	Pork—leg (whole rump, center shank), ham, smoked (center slices)
1 oz	Veal—leg, loin, rib, shank, shoulder, cutlets
1 oz	Poultry—meat-without-skin of chicken, turkey, cornish hen, guinea hen, pheasant
1 oz	Fish—any fresh or frozen
¼ c	Canned salmon, tuna, mackerel, crab, lobster
5 (or 1 oz)	Clams, oysters, scallops, shrimp
3	Sardines, drained
1 oz	Cheese, containing less than 5% butterfat; all varieties made from skim milk
¼ c	Cottage cheese, dry and 2% butterfat
½ c	Dried beans and peas, cooked (count as 1 lean meat and 1 bread exchange)
¼ c	Baked beans, canned
¼ c	Soy flour (count as 1 lean meat and ½ bread exchange)
2 tbsp	Brewer's yeast, powder (count as 1 lean meat and ½ bread exchange)

Medium-fat meat (count as 1 lean meat and ½ fat exchange)

AMOUNT	FOOD
1 oz	Beef—ground (15% fat), corned beef (canned), rib eye, round (ground commercial)
1 oz	Pork—loin (all cuts tenderloin), shoulder arm (picnic), shoulder blade, Boston butt, Canadian bacon, boiled ham
1 oz	Liver, heart, kidney, sweetbreads (high in cholesterol)
¼ c	Cottage cheese, creamed
1 oz	Cheese—mozzarella, ricotta, farmer's cheese, Neufchatel
3 tbsp	Parmesan cheese
1	Egg (high in cholesterol)
⅓ c	Soybeans, cooked
4 oz	Soybean curd (tofu), 2½ × 2¾ × 1 in

[a] A meat exchange is a serving of protein-rich food that contains negligible carbohydrate but a significant amount of protein (7 g) and fat (3 g), roughly equivalent to the amounts in 1 oz of lean meat; contains about 55 kcal.

TABLE L-5 **(continued)**

AMOUNT	FOOD
High-fat meat (count as 1 lean meat and 1 fat exchange)	
1 oz	Beef—brisket, corned beef (brisket), ground beef (more than 20% fat), hamburger (commercial), chuck (ground commercial), roasts (rib), steaks (club and rib)
1 oz	Lamb—breast
1 oz	Pork—spare ribs, loin (back ribs), pork (ground), country-style ham, deviled ham
1 oz	Veal—breast
1 oz	Poultry—capon, duck (domestic), goose
1 oz	Cheddar-type cheeses[b]
1 slice	Cold cuts, 4½ × ⅛ in
1 small	Frankfurter
Meat Alternates	
2 tbsp	Peanut butter (count as 1 lean meat and 2½ fat exchanges)
4 tbsp	Peanuts (count as 1 lean meat, ½ bread, and 2 fat exchanges)
4 tbsp	Pumpkin or squash seeds (count as 1½ lean meat and 2 fat exchanges)
4 tbsp	Sesame or sunflower seeds (count as 1 lean meat and 2½ fat exchanges)
Chinese foods[c]	
¼ c	Canned or cooked abalone, crabmeat, eel, lobster, conch, cuttlefish, squid, octopus, fish maw, sea cucumbers, jellyfish, etc.
10 medium	River snails
2 medium	Frog legs
3 medium	Duck feet
1 medium or ½ large	Duck egg, salted
1 medium	Egg, preserved or limed
Fast foods[d]	

[b] Blue, brick, camembert, cheddar, edam, farmer's, gorgonzola, gouda, gruyere, liederkranz, limburger, mozzarella, muenster, neufchatel, parmesan (3 tbsp), ricotta, swiss.

[c] These exchanges are not separated into high-, medium-, and low-fat exchanges.

[d] Most fast-food meats are for variable numbers of exchanges and have other exchanges added: hamburger (1 high-fat meat, 2 bread, 260 kcal); cheeseburger (1½ high-fat meat, 2 bread, 306 kcal); Quarter Pounder® (3 high-fat meat, 2 bread, 420 kcal); Big Mac® (3 high-fat meat, 2½ bread, 1½ fat, 540 kcal); Quarter Pounder® with cheese (4 high-fat meat, 2 bread, 520 kcal); Egg McMuffin® (2 high-fat meat, 1½ bread, 1 fat, 350 kcal); pork sausage (1 high-fat meat, 1½ fat, 185 kcal).

TABLE L-6 **Fat List (5 g fat, 45 kcal)[a]**

AMOUNT	FOOD
Polyunsaturated fat	
1 tsp	Margarine (soft, tub, or stick)[b]
⅛	Avocado (4-in diameter)[c]
1 tsp	Oil—corn, cottonseed, safflower, soy, sunflower
1 tsp	Oil, olive[c]
1 tsp	Oil, peanut[c]
5 small	Olives[c]
10 whole	Almonds[c]
2 large whole	Pecans[c]
20 whole	Peanuts, Spanish[c]
10 whole	Peanuts, Virginia[c]
6 small	Walnuts
6 small	Nuts, other[c]
1 tsp	Tahini
1 tbsp	Hommous
1 tbsp	Pignolia nuts
Saturated fat	
1 tsp	Margarine, regular stick
1 tsp	Butter
1 tsp	Bacon fat
1 strip	Bacon, crisp
2 tbsp	Cream, light
2 tbsp	Cream, sour
1 tbsp	Cream, heavy
1 tbsp	Cream cheese
1 tbsp	French dressing[d]
1 tbsp	Italian dressing[d]
1 tsp	Lard
1 tsp	Mayonnaise[d]
2 tsp	Salad dressing, mayonnaise type[d]
¾-in cube	Salt pork
Chinese foods	
1 tsp	Sesame or chili oil
1 piece	Coconut meat, 1 × 1 × 1.2 in

[a] A fat exchange is a serving of any food that contains negligible carbohydrate and protein but appreciable fat (5 g), totaling about 45 kcal.

[b] Made with corn, cottonseed, safflower, soy, or sunflower oil only.

[c] Fat content is primarily monounsaturated.

[d] If made with corn, cottonseed, safflower, soy, or sunflower oil, can be assumed to contain polyunsaturated fat.

L

TABLE L–6   **(continued)**

AMOUNT	FOOD
2½ tsp	Coconut, grated
2 tsp	Coconut cream (no water)
1 tbsp	Sesame seeds
1-in cube	Fatty cured Chinese pork

TABLE L–7   **Unlimited Foods (negligible kcal)[a]**

AMOUNT	FOOD
	Diet kcalorie-free beverage
	Coffee
	Tea
	Bouillon without fat
	Unsweetened gelatin
	Unsweetened pickles
	Salt and pepper
	Red pepper
	Paprika
	Garlic
	Celery salt
	Parsley
	Nutmeg
	Lemon
	Mustard
	Chili powder

[a] These are "free foods" that contain negligible carbohydrate, protein, and fat and therefore negligible kcalories.

TABLE L–7   **(continued)**

AMOUNT	FOOD
	Onion salt or powder
	Horseradish
	Vinegar
	Mint
	Cinnamon
	Lime
	Raw vegetables—chicory, Chinese cabbage, endive, escarole, lettuce, parsley, radishes, watercress

Chinese foods

AMOUNT	FOOD
	Plain agar-agar
	Seasonings, spices, herbs[b] such as soy sauce, monosodium glutamate, star anise, five-spices powder
	Chinese parsley, kelp, sea girdle, laver, and seaweed hair
1 tsp	Shrimp sauce or dried shrimp
1 tsp or 2 nuts	Gingko nuts
½ block	White bean curd cheese, 1½ × ¾ × 1 in
¼ block	Red bean curd cheese, 1 × ¼ × ½ in
1 c or less	Watery vegetables, including bamboo shoots, bitter melon, bottle gourd, cabbage (celery, mustard, or spoon; fresh, pickled, spiced, salted, or salted and dried), Chinese broccoli, Chinese eggplant, fungi (black, brown, or white), snow peas, turnips (Chinese or green), watercress, winter melon, wolfberry leaves

[b] Does not include some starchy and sugar-preserved Chinese herbs.

L

APPENDIX M
The Canadian Food Guide

The Canadian food group system is similar to the U.S. exchange system, but the serving sizes and some of the foods listed are different. This food group system, as explained in the handbook *Good Health Eating Guide*, is a revision of the Canadian exchange system of meal planning.[1] A comparison of the new and old systems is presented in Table M-1. Features of the new system similar to those of the exchange system include the following:

● Foods are divided into six groups according to carbohydrate, protein, and fat content.
● Foods are interchangeable within a group.
● Most foods are eaten in measured amounts.

New features of the food group system include the following:

● An energy value is given for each food group.
● Protein foods low in fat are emphasized in the protein foods group. Protein foods containing extra fat are identified.

1   The tables in this appendix are taken from *Good Health Eating Guide* (Toronto, Ontario: Canadian Diabetes Association, 1981), and are used with the association's permission.

● The user is able to distinguish between complex and simple carbohydrates (starches and sugars).

TABLE M-1 **Canadian Food Group System Compared with Canadian Exchange System**

FOOD GROUP SYSTEM	EXCHANGE SYSTEM
1 starchy foods choice[a]	1 bread exchange
1 protein foods choice[b]	1 meat exchange
1 milk choice	1 milk exchange
1 fruits and vegetables choice	1 fruit exchange
1 fruits and vegetables choice	1 vegetable exchange (Group A)
1 fats and oils choice	1 fat exchange
Extra vegetables	1 vegetable exchange (Group B)
Extras (unmeasured)	kCalorie-free foods (List A)
Extras (small measures)	kCalorie-poor foods (List B)

[a] The word *choice* is equivalent to *exchange* or *portion* in the U.S. food systems. It refers to a weighed or measured amount of a food within a group.
[b] If protein foods high in fat are chosen, the calculations are adjusted to account for "hidden" fat.

M

TABLE M–2 **Protein Foods Group** (7 g protein, 3 g fat, 55 kcal)

FOOD	MEASURE	MASS (WEIGHT)
Cheese		
All types, made from partly skim milk, e.g. mozzarella, part-skim	1 piece, 5 cm × 2 cm × 2 cm (2″ × ¾″ × ¾″)	25 g
Cottage cheese, all types	50 mL (¼ cup)	55 g
Fish		
Anchovy (see extras)		
Canned, drained, e.g. chicken haddie, mackerel, salmon, tuna	50 mL (¼ cup)	30 g
Cod tongues/cheeks	75 mL (⅓ cup)	50 g
Fillet or Steak, e.g. Boston blue, cod, flounder, haddock, halibut, perch, pickerel, pike, salmon, shad, sole, trout, whitefish	1 piece, 6 cm × 2 cm × 2 cm (2½″ × ¾″ × ¾″)	30 g
Herring	⅓ fish	30 g
Octopus	50 mL (¼ cup)	40 g
Sardines	2 medium or 3 small	30 g
Seal, walrus	1 slice, 6 cm × 4 cm × 1 cm (2½″ × 1½″ × ½″)	25 g
Smelts	2 medium	30 g
Squid	50 mL (¼ cup)	40 g
Shellfish		
Clams, mussels, oysters, scallops, snails	3 medium	30 g
Crab, lobster, flaked	50 mL (¼ cup)	30 g
Shrimp, fresh	5 large	30 g
frozen	10 medium	30 g
canned	18 small	30 g
dry pack	50 mL (¼ cup)	30 g
Meat and poultry, e.g. beef, chicken, ham, lamb, pork, turkey, veal, wild game		
Back bacon	3 slices, thin	25 g
Chop	½ chop, with bone	35 g
Minced or ground, lean	30 mL (2 tbsps.)	25 g
Sliced, lean	1 slice, 10 cm × 5 cm × 5 mm (4″ × 2″ × ¼″)	25 g
Steak, lean	1 piece, 4 cm × 3 cm × 2 cm (1½″ × 1¼″ × ¾″)	25 g
Organ Meats		
Heart, liver	1 slice, 5 cm × 5 cm × 1 cm (2″ × 2″ × ½″)	25 g
Kidney, sweet breads, chopped	50 mL (¼ cup)	25 g
Tongue	1 slice, 8 cm × 6 cm × 5 mm (3¼″ × 2½″ × ¼″)	25 g
Tripe, 1 piece = 4 cm × 4 cm × 8 mm (1½″ × 1½″ × ⅜″)	5 pieces	50 g
Soyabean		
Bean curd or tofu, 1 block = 6 cm × 6 cm × 4 cm (2½″ × 2½″ × 1½″)	½ block	70 g

M

TABLE M–2   **(continued)**

The following choices contain extra fat, so use them less often.

FOOD	MEASURE	MASS (WEIGHT)
Cheese		
Cheese, all types made from whole milk, e.g. brick, brie, camembert, cheddar, edam, tilsit	1 piece 5 cm × 2 cm × 2 cm (2″ × ¾″ × ¾″)	25 g
Cheese, coarsely grated, e.g. cheddar	75 mL (⅓ cup)	25 g
Cheese, dry, finely grated, e.g. parmesan	45 mL (3 tbsps.)	15 g
Cheese, ricotta	50 mL (¼ cup)	55 g
Egg		
Egg, in shell, raw or cooked	1 medium	50 g
Egg, without shell, cooked or poached in water	1 medium	45 g
Egg, scrambled	50 mL (¼ cup)	55 g
Fish		
Eel	5 cm, 4 cm diameter (2″, 1½″ diameter)	50 g
Meat		
Bologna	1 slice, 5 mm, 10 cm diameter (¼″, 4″ diameter)	40 g
Canned luncheon meat	1 slice, 85 mm × 45 mm × 10 mm (3½″ × 1¾″ × ½″)	40 g
Corned beef, fresh	1 slice, 10 cm × 5 cm × 5 mm (4″ × 2″ × ¼″)	25 g
Corned beef, canned	1 slice, 75 mm × 55 mm × 5 mm (3″ × 2¼″ × ¼″)	25 g
Ground beef, medium fat	30 mL (2 tbsps.)	25 g
Meat spreads, canned	45 mL (3 tbsps.)	35 g
Pate (see fats and oils group)		
Sausage, pork, link	1 link	25 g
Sausage, garlic, Polish or knockwurst	1 slice, 1 cm, 5 cm diameter (½″, 2″ diameter)	50 g
Summer sausage or salami	1 slice, 5 mm, 10 cm diameter (¼″, 4″ diameter)	40 g
Spareribs or shortribs, with bone	10 cm × 6 cm (4″ × 2½″)	65 g
Stewing beef	1 cube, 25 mm (1″)	25 g
Wiener	½ medium	25 g
Miscellaneous		
Blood pudding	1 slice, 5 cm × 1 cm (2″ × ½″)	25 g
Peanut butter, all kinds	15 mL (1 tbsp.)	15 g

TABLE M–3   **Starchy Foods Group [15 g carbohydrate (starch), 2 g protein, 68 kcal]**

FOOD	MEASURE	MASS (WEIGHT)
Breads		
Bagel	½	25 g

M

TABLE M-3   (continued)

FOOD	MEASURE	MASS (WEIGHT)
Bread crumbs	50 mL (¼ cup)	25 g
Bread cubes	250 mL (1 cup)	25 g
Bread sticks, 11 cm × 1 cm (4½″ × ½″)	2	20 g
Brewis, cooked	50 mL (¼ cup)	45 g
English muffin, crumpet	½	25 g
Flour	40 mL (2½ tbsps.)	20 g
Hamburger bun	½	30 g
Hot dog bun	½	30 g
Kaiser roll	½	25 g
Matzoh, 15 cm (6″ square)	1	20 g
Melba toast, rectangular	4	15 g
Pita, 20 cm diameter (8″ diameter)	¼	25 g
Plain roll	1 small	25 g
Raisin bread	1 slice	25 g
Rusks	2	20 g
Rye, coarse or pumpernickel, 10 cm × 10 cm × 8 mm (4″ × 4″ × ⅜″)	½ slice	25 g
Tortilla, 15 cm (6″)	1	20 g
White (French and Italian)	1 slice	25 g
Whole wheat, cracked wheat, rye, white enriched	1 slice	25 g

Cereals

Bran flakes, 40% bran	125 mL (½ cup)	20 g
Cooked cereals, cooked	125 mL (½ cup)	125 g
dry	30 mL (2 tbsps.)	20 g
Cornmeal, cooked	125 mL (½ cup)	125 g
dry	30 mL (2 tbsps.)	20 g
Ready-to-eat unsweetened cereal	250 mL (1 cup)	20 g
Shredded wheat biscuit, rectangular or round	1	20 g
Shredded wheat bite size	125 mL (½ cup)	20 g
Wheat germ	75 mL (⅓ cup)	30 g

Cookies and biscuits

See ''Prepared Foods'' [below].

Grains

Barley, cooked	125 mL (½ cup)	120 g
dry	30 mL (2 tbsps.)	20 g
Bulgar, kasha, cooked, moist	125 mL (½ cup)	70 g
cooked, crumbly	75 mL (⅓ cup)	40 g
dry	30 mL (2 tbsps.)	20 g
Rice, cooked, loosely packed	125 mL (½ cup)	105 g
cooked, tightly packed	75 mL (⅓ cup)	70 g
Tapioca, pearl and granulated, quick cooking, dry	30 mL (2 tbsps.)	15 g

M

TABLE M-3 **(continued)**

FOOD	MEASURE	MASS (WEIGHT)
Pastas		
Macaroni, cooked	125 mL (½ cup)	70 g
Noodles, cooked	125 mL (½ cup)	80 g
Spaghetti, cooked	125 mL (½ cup)	70 g
Starchy Vegetables		
Beans and peas (dried), cooked	125 mL (½ cup)	80 g
Breadfruit	1 slice	75 g
Corn, canned, whole kernel	125 mL (½ cup)	85 g
canned, creamed	75 mL (⅓ cup)	60 g
Corn, on the cob, 13 cm, 4 cm diameter (5″, 1½″ diameter)	1 small cob	140 g
Cornstarch	30 mL (2 tbsps.)	15 g
Plantain	⅓ small	50 g
Popcorn, unbuttered, large kernel	750 mL (3 cups)	20 g
Potatoes, whipped	125 mL (½ cup)	105 g
Potatoes, whole, 13 cm, 5 cm diameter (5″, 2″ diameter)	½	95 g
Yam, sweet potatoes 13 cm, 5 cm diameter (5″, 2″ diameter)	½	75 g

Starchy Foods Group (add 1 fats and oils choice)

FOOD	MEASURE	MASS (WEIGHT)
Prepared foods		
Baking powder biscuit, 5 cm diameter (2″ diameter)	1	30 g
Cookies, plain, (e.g., digestive, oatmeal)	2	20 g
Cup cake, un-iced, 5 cm diameter (2″ diameter)	1 small	35 g
Donut, cake type, plain, 7 cm diameter (2¾″ diameter)	1	30 g
Muffin, plain, 6 cm diameter (2½″ diameter)	1 small	40 g
Pancake, homemade using 50 mL (¼ cup) batter	1 small	50 g
Potatoes, french fried, 5 cm × 9 cm (2″ × 3½″)	10	65 g
Soup, canned (prepared with equal volume of water)	250 mL (1 cup)	260 g
Waffle, homemade, using 50 mL (¼ cup) batter	1 small	35 g

TABLE M-4 **Milk Group**

TYPE OF MILK	CARBOHYDRATE	PROTEIN	FAT	ENERGY
Skim	6 g	4 g	0 g	40 calories
2%	6 g	4 g	2 g	58 calories
Whole	6 g	4 g	4 g	76 calories

FOOD	MEASURE	MASS (WEIGHT)
Milk	125 mL(½ cup)	125 g
Buttermilk	125 mL(½ cup)	125 g
Evaporated milk	50 mL(¼ cup)	50 g
Powdered milk, regular	30 mL(2 tbsps.)	15 g
instant	50 mL(¼ cup)	15 g
Unflavoured yogurt	125 mL(½ cup)	125 g

M

TABLE M-5   **Fruits and Vegetables Group [10 g carbohydrate (simple sugar), 1 g protein, 44 kcal]**

FOOD	MEASURE	MASS (WEIGHT)
Fruits (fresh, frozen without sugar, canned in water)		
Apple, raw	½ medium	75 g
raw, without skin and core	½ medium	65 g
sauce	125 mL (½ cup)	120 g
Apricot, raw	2 medium	115 g
canned, in water	4 halves, plus 30 mL (2 tbsps.) liquid	110 g
Bake-apple (cloudberries), raw	125 mL (½ cup)	120 g
Banana, 15 cm (6″), with peel	½ small	75 g
peeled	½ small	50 g
Blackberries, raw	125 mL (½ cup)	70 g
canned, in water	125 mL (½ cup), includes 30 mL (2 tbsps.) liquid	100 g
Blueberries, raw	125 mL (½ cup)	120 g
Boysenberries, raw	125 mL (½ cup)	70 g
canned, in water	125 mL (½ cup), includes 30 mL (2 tbsps.) liquid	100 g
Cantaloupe, wedge with rind, 13 cm diameter (5″ diameter)	¼	240 g
cubed or diced	250 mL (1 cup)	160 g
Cherries, raw, with pits	10	75 g
raw, without pits	10	70 g
canned, in water, with pits	75 mL (⅓ cup) includes 30 mL (2 tbsps.) liquid	90 g
canned, in water, without pits	75 mL (⅓ cup), includes 30 mL (2 tbsps.) liquid	85 g
Crabapple, raw	1 small	55 g
Cranberries, raw	250 mL (1 cup)	100 g
Figs, raw	1 medium	50 g
canned, in water	3 medium, plus 30 mL (2 tbsps.) liquid	100 g
Foxberries, raw	250 mL (1 cup)	100 g
Fruit cocktail, canned, in water	125 mL (½ cup), includes 30 mL (2 tbsps.) liquid	120 g
Fruit, mixed, cut-up	125 mL (½ cup)	120 g
Gooseberries, raw	250 mL (1 cup)	150 g
canned, in water	250 mL (1 cup), includes 30 mL (2 tbsps.) liquid	230 g
Grapefruit, raw, with rind	½ small	185 g
raw, sectioned	125 mL (½ cup)	100 g
canned, in water	125 mL (½ cup), includes 30 mL (2 tbsps.) liquid	120 g
Grapes, raw, slip skin	125 mL (½ cup)	75 g
raw, seedless	125 mL (½ cup)	75 g
canned, in water	75 mL (⅓ cup), includes 30 mL (2 tbsps.) liquid	115 g
Honeydew melon, raw, with rind	1/10	225 g
cubed or diced	250 mL (1 cup)	170 g
Guava, raw	½	50 g
Kiwi, raw, with skin	2	155 g
Kumquats, raw	3	60 g
Huckleberries, raw	125 mL (½ cup)	70 g

TABLE M–5   **(continued)**

FOOD	MEASURE	MASS (WEIGHT)
Loganberries, raw	125 mL (½ cup)	70 g
Loquats, raw	8	130 g
Lychee fruit, raw	8	120 g
Mandarin oranges, raw, with rind	1	135 g
raw, sectioned	125 mL (½ cup)	100 g
canned, in water	125 mL (½ cup), includes 30 mL (2 tbsps.) liquid	100 g
Mango, raw, without skin and seed	⅓	65 g
diced	75 mL (⅓ cup)	65 g
Nectarine	½ medium	75 g
Orange, raw, with rind	1 small	90 g
raw, sectioned	125 mL (½ cup)	90 g
Papaya, raw, with skin and seeds	¼ medium	150 g
raw, without skin and seeds	¼ medium	100 g
cubed or diced	125 mL (½ cup)	100 g
Peaches, raw with seed and skin, 6 cm (2½″) diameter	1 large	130 g
raw, sliced, diced	125 mL (½ cup)	100 g
canned, in water, halves or slices	125 mL (½ cup), includes 30 mL (2 tbsps.) liquid	120 g
Pear, raw with skin and core	½	90 g
raw, without skin and core	½	85 g
canned, in water, halves	2 halves, plus 30 mL (2 tbsps.) liquid	90 g
Persimmons, raw, native	1	30 g
raw, Japanese	¼	50 g
Pineapple, raw	1 slice, 8 cm diameter, 2 cm thick (3⅓″ diameter, ¾″ thick)	75 g
raw, diced	125 mL (½ cup)	75 g
canned, in water, sliced	2 slices, plus 15 mL (1 tbsp.) liquid	100 g
canned, in water, diced	125 mL (½ cup), includes 30 mL (2 tbsps.) liquid	100 g
canned, in juice, sliced	1 slice, plus 15 mL (1 tbsp.) liquid	55 g
canned, in juice, diced	75 mL (⅓ cup), includes 15 mL (1 tbsp.) liquid	55 g
Plums, raw, prune type	2	60 g
damson	6	65 g
Japanese	1	70 g
canned, in water	3, plus 30 mL (2 tbsps.) liquid	100 g
canned, in apple juice	2, plus 30 mL (2 tbsps.) liquid	70 g
Pomegranate, raw	½	140 g
Raspberries, raw, black or red	125 mL (½ cup)	65 g
canned, in water	125 mL (½ cup), includes 30 mL (2 tbsps.) liquid	100 g
Saskatoons (see blueberries)		
Strawberries, raw	250 mL (1 cup)	150 g
canned, in water	250 mL (1 cup), includes 30 mL (2 tbsps.) liquid	240 g
Tangelo, raw	1	205 g
Tangerine, raw	1	115 g
raw, sectioned	125 mL (½ cup)	100 g

M

TABLE M–5 **(continued)**

FOOD	MEASURE	MASS (WEIGHT)
Watermelon, raw with rind	1 wedge, 125 mm triangle, 22 mm thick (5″ triangle, 1″ thick)	310 g
cubed or diced	250 mL (1 cup)	160 g
Dried Fruit		
Apple	5 pieces	15 g
Apricot	4 halves	15 g
Banana flakes	30 mL (2 tbsps.)	15 g
Currants	30 mL (2 tbsps.)	15 g
Dates, without pits	2	15 g
Peach	1 half	15 g
Pear	1 half	15 g
Prunes, raw, with pits	2	15 g
raw, without pits	2	10 g
stewed, no liquid	2	20 g
stewed, with liquid	2, plus 15 mL (1 tbsp.) liquid	35 g
Raisins	30 mL (2 tbsps.)	15 g
Juices (no sugar added or unsweetened)		
Apricot, grape, guava, mango, prune	50 mL (¼ cup)	55 g
Apple, carrot, papaya, pear, pineapple, pomegranate	75 mL (⅓ cup)	80 g
Grapefruit, loganberry, orange, raspberry, tangelo, tangerine	125 mL (½ cup)	130 g
Tomato, tomato based mixed vegetables	250 mL (1 cup)	255 g
Vegetables (fresh, frozen, or canned)		
Artichokes, Jerusalem, mature or late season[a]	2 small	50 g
Beets, diced or sliced	125 mL (½ cup)	85 g
Carrots, diced	125 mL (½ cup)	75 g
Parsnips, mashed	125 mL (½ cup)	80 g
Peas, fresh or frozen	125 mL (½ cup)	80 g
canned	75 mL (⅓ cup)	55 g
Pumpkin, mashed	125 mL (½ cup)	45 g
Rutabagas, mashed	125 mL (½ cup)	85 g
Sauerkraut	250 mL (1 cup)	235 g
Snowpeas	10 pods	100 g
Squash, yellow or winter, mashed	125 mL (½ cup)	115 g
Succotash	75 mL (⅓ cup)	55 g
Tomatoes, canned	250 mL (1 cup)	240 g
Turnip, mashed	125 mL (½ cup)	115 g
Vegetables, mixed	125 mL (½ cup)	90 g
Water chestnuts	8 medium	50 g

[a] Jerusalem artichokes contain inulin which converts to carbohydrate during storage, in or out of ground. Jerusalem artichokes in early season (autumn) are low in carbohydrate but in late season (winter/spring) they become a Fruits and Vegetables Choice.

TABLE M–6   **Extra Vegetables Group (½ cup, 3.5 g carbohydrate, 14 kcal)**

Artichokes, globe or french	Cauliflower	Okra
Artichokes, Jerusalem, early season[a]	Celery	Onions, green or mature
	Chard	Parsley
Asparagus	Cucumber	Pepper, green or red
Bamboo shoots	Eggplant	Radish
Beans, string, green or yellow	Endive	Rhubarb
	Fiddleheads	Shallots
Bean sprouts, mung or soya	Greens: beet, collard, dandelion, mustard, turnip, etc.	Spinach
Bitter melon (balsam pear)		Sprouts: alfalfa, radish, etc.
	Kale	Tomato, raw
Bok Choy	Kohlrabi	Vegetable marrow
Broccoli	Leeks	Watercress
Brussels sprouts	Lettuce	Zucchini
Cabbage	Mushrooms	

If eaten in large amounts, the following foods must be counted as 1 fruits and vegetables choice.

Brussels sprouts, cooked, 250 mL (1 cup)	155 g
Eggplant, cooked, diced, 250 mL (1 cup)	200 g
Kohlrabi, cooked, diced, 250 mL (1 cup)	140 g
Leeks, cooked, edible parts of 4 leeks	100 g
Okra, cooked, sliced, 250 mL (1 cup)	160 g
Onion, mature, cooked, 250 mL (1 cup)	210 g
Rhubarb, cooked, no sugar added, 250 mL (1 cup)	244 g
Tomato, raw, 2 medium (6 cm or 2½″ diameter) *or* 1 large (13 cm or 5″ diameter)	270 g

[a] Jerusalem artichokes contain inulin which converts to carbohydrate during storage, in or out of ground. Jerusalem artichokes in early season (autumn) are low in carbohydrate but in late season (winter/spring) they become a Fruits and Vegetables Choice.

TABLE M–7   **Fats and Oils Group (5 g fat, 45 kcal)**

FOOD	MEASURE	MASS (WEIGHT)
Avocado pear	⅛	30 g
Bacon, side, crisp	1 slice	5 g
Butter	5 mL(1 tsp.)	5 g
Cheese spread	15 mL(1 tbsp.)	15 g
Coconut, fresh	45 mL(3 tbsps.)	15 g
dried	15 mL(1 tbsp.)	10 g
Cream, half and half (cereal) 10%	30 mL(2 tbsps.)	30 g
light (coffee) 20%	15 mL(1 tbsp.)	15 g
whipping 32-37%	15 mL(1 tbsp.)	15 g
sour 12-14%	45 mL(3 tbsps.)	35 g
Cream cheese	15 mL(1 tbsp.)	15 g

M

TABLE M-7   **(continued)**

FOOD	MEASURE	MASS (WEIGHT)
Gravy	30 mL(2 tbsps.)	30 g
Lard	5 mL(1 tsp.)	5 g
Margarine	5 mL(1 tsp.)	5 g
Nuts, shelled:		
almonds	8 nuts	20 g
Brazil nuts	2 nuts	5 g
cashews	5 nuts	10 g
filberts, hazelnuts	5 nuts	10 g
macadamia	3 nuts	5 g
peanuts	10 nuts	10 g
pecans	5 halves	5 g
pignolias, pine nuts	25 mL(5 tsps.)	10 g
pistachios, shelled	20 nuts	10 g
in shell	20 nuts	20 g
pumpkin and squash seeds	20 mL(4 tsps.)	10 g
sesame seeds	15 mL(1 tbsp.)	10 g
sunflower seeds, shelled	15 mL(1 tbsp.)	10 g
in shell	45 mL(3 tbsps.)	15 g
walnuts	4 halves	10 g
Oil, cooking and salad	5 mL	5 g
Olives, green	10	45 g
ripe	7	40 g
Pate, liverwurst, meat spreads	15 mL(1 tbsp.)	15 g
Salad dressing: blue, French, Italian, mayonnaise, thousand island	5 mL(1 tsp.)	5 g
Salt pork, raw or cooked	5 mL	5 g
Sesame oil	5 mL	5 g

TABLE M-8   **Extras (may be used without measuring)**

Beverages
Bouillon or clear broth
Bouillon from cube, powder or liquid
Coffee, clear
Consomme
Herbal teas, unsweetened
Mineral water
Soda water, club soda
Sugar-free soft drink
Tea, clear
Water

Condiments
Chow chow, unsweetened tomato pickles
Garlic
Gelatin, unsweetened
Ginger root
Horseradish, uncreamed

Lemon juice or lemon wedge
Lime juice or lime wedge
Mustard
Parsley
Pickles, unsweetened dill pickles or sour cucumber pickles
Pimentos
Soya sauce
Vinegar
Worcestershire sauce

Herbs and spices
Salt, pepper, thyme, marjoram, cinnammon, etc.

Miscellaneous
Artificial sweetener, such as cyclamate or saccharin
Baking powder, baking soda
Dulse
Flavourings and extracts, e.g. vanilla
Rennet

M

TABLE M–9   **Extras (2.5 g carbohydrate, 15 kcal, limited to amount indicated)**

Anchovy	2 fillets
Barbecue sauce	15 mL (1 tbsp.)
Bran, natural	30 mL (2 tbsps.)
Brewers yeast	5 mL (1 tsp.)
Carob powder	5 ml (1 tsp.)
Chili sauce	5 mL (1 tsp.)
Cocoa powder	5 mL (1 tsp.)
Cranberry sauce, unsweetened	15 mL (1 tbsp.)
Dietetic fruit spreads	5 mL (1 tsp.)
Ketchup	5 mL (1 tsp.)
Maraschino cherry	1 cherry
Nuts, chopped pieces	5 mL (1 tsp.)
Non-dairy coffee whitener	5 mL (1 tsp.)
Relish	5 mL (1 tsp.)
Sugar substitutes, granular	5 mL (1 tsp.) (3 to 4 packages)
Whipped topping	15 mL (1 tbsp.)
Yogurt, plain	30 mL (2 tbsps.)

M

APPENDIX N

Fast Foods

Most of the data in this table are from a publication by Ross Laboratories.[1] We appreciate their permission and that of the authors to use this information.

The numbers in brackets [ ] have been added by us. They are imputed, not laboratory-derived, values, and are tenta-tive. Most of them were arrived at by deducing the approximate composition of each food from the available nutrient composition, then turning to Appendix H to calculate estimates for the missing values.

The chief usefulness of these data is for the student conducting a Self-Study. A student who needs to know nutrient amounts in a fast food item, and who finds data missing, has to estimate values for the missing data. We thought our "educated estimates" might save trouble and improve the validity of the Self-Study results.

1   E. A. Young, E. H. Brennan, and G. L. Irving, guest eds., Update: Nutritional analysis of fast foods, *Dietetic Currents, Ross Timesaver* 8 (March/April 1981).

TABLE N-1 **Nutritional Analysis of Fast Foods**
(Dashes indicate no data available. X=Less than 2% US RDA; tr=trace.)

Food Item	Weight (g)	Energy (kcal)	Protein (g)	Fat (g)	Carbo-hydrate (g)	Calcium (mg)	Iron (mg)	Zinc (mg)	Vitamin A (RE)	Thiamin (mg)	Ribo-flavin (mg)	Niacin (mg)	Folacin (µg)	Vitamin C (mg)
ARBY'S®														
Roast Beef	140	350	22	15	32	80	3.6	[3.1]	[3]	.30	.34	5	[33]	0
Beef and Cheese	168	450	27	22	36	200	4.5	[4.0]	[103]	.38	.43	6	[35]	0
Super Roast Beef	263	620	30	28	61	100	5.4	[10.0]	[13]	.53	.43	7	[36]	0
Junior Roast Beef	74	220	12	9	21	40	1.8	[3.0]	[3]	.15	.17	3	[17]	0
Ham & Cheese	154	380	23	17	33	200	2.7	[2.4]	[100]	.75	.34	5	[35]	0
Turkey Deluxe	236	510	28	24	46	80	2.7	[3.2]	[0]	.45	.34	8	[38]	0
Club Sandwich	252	560	30	30	43	200	3.6	[4.4]	[227]	.68	.43	7	[52]	[4]

Source: Adapted from Consumer Affairs, Arby's, Inc., Atlanta, Georgia. Nutritional analysis by Technological Resources, Camden, New Jersey.

Food Item	Weight (g)	Energy (kcal)	Protein (g)	Fat (g)	Carbo-hydrate (g)	Calcium (mg)	Iron (mg)	Zinc (mg)	Vitamin A (RE)	Thiamin (mg)	Ribo-flavin (mg)	Niacin (mg)	Folacin (µg)	Vitamin C (mg)
BURGER CHEF®														
Hamburger	91	244	11	9	29	45	2.0	1.6	[34]	.17	.16	2.7	[24]	1
Cheeseburger	104	290	14	13	29	132	2.2	1.9	[81]	.18	.21	2.8	[25]	1
Double Cheeseburger	145	420	24	22	30	223	3.2	3.6	[131]	.20	.32	4.4	[26]	1
Fish Filet	179	547	21	31	46	145	2.2	1.2	[121]	.23	.22	2.7	[37]	1
Super Shef® Sandwich	252	563	29	30	44	205	4.5	4.5	[151]	.31	.40	6.0	[47]	9
Big Shef® Sandwich	186	569	23	36	38	152	3.6	3.4	[56]	.26	.31	4.7	[35]	1
TOP Shef® Sandwich	138	661	41	38	36	194	5.4	5.9	[55]	.35	.47	8.1	[35]	0
Funmeal® Feast	[269]	545	15	30	55	61	2.8	1.6	[25]	.25	.21	4.6	[41]	13
Rancher® Platter*	316	640	32	42	33	66	5.3	5.6	[350]	.29	.38	8.6	[69]	24
Mariner® Platter*	373	734	29	34	78	63	3.3	1.2	[414]	.34	.23	5.2	[104]	24
French Fries, small	68	250	2	19	20	9	0.7	<0.1	[0]	.07	.04	1.7	[15]	12
French Fries, large	85	351	3	26	28	13	0.9	<0.1	[0]	.10	.06	2.4	[19]	16
Vanilla Shake (12 oz)	336	380	13	10	60	497	0.3	1.3	[117]	.10	.66	0.5	[22]	0
Chocolate Shake (12 oz)	336	403	10	9	72	449	1.1	1.6	[88]	.16	.76	0.4	[22]	0
Hot Chocolate	[180]	198	8	8	23	271	0.7	1.1	[87]	[.10]	.39	0.3	[18]	2

* Includes salad. Source: Adapted from Burger Chef Systems, Inc., Indianapolis, Indiana. Nutritional analysis from *Handbook No. 8.* Washington: US Dept of Agriculture.

TABLE N–1 (continued)
(Dashes indicate no data available. X=Less than 2% US RDA; tr=trace.)

Food Item	Weight (g)	Energy (kcal)	Protein (g)	Fat (g)	Carbohydrate (g)	Calcium (mg)	Iron (mg)	Zinc (mg)	Vitamin A (RE)	Thiamin (mg)	Riboflavin (mg)	Niacin (mg)	Folacin (μg)	Vitamin C (mg)
CHURCH'S FRIED CHICKEN®														
White Chicken Portion	100	327	21	23	10	94	1.0	[1.2]	[48]	.10	.18	7.2	[9]	1
Dark Chicken Portion	100	305	22	21	7	15	1.3	[1.2]	[42]	.10	.27	5.3	[9]	1

Source: Adapted from Church's Fried Chicken, San Antonio, Texas. Nutritional analysis by Medallion Laboratories, Minneapolis, Minnesota.

Food Item	Weight (g)	Energy (kcal)	Protein (g)	Fat (g)	Carbohydrate (g)	Calcium (mg)	Iron (mg)	Zinc (mg)	Vitamin A (RE)	Thiamin (mg)	Riboflavin (mg)	Niacin (mg)	Folacin (μg)	Vitamin C (mg)
DAIRY QUEEN®														
Frozen Dessert	113	180	5	6	27	150	[0]	[0.4]	[30]	.09	.17	[.2]	[6]	[0]
DQ Cone, small	71	110	3	3	18	100	[0]	[0.2]	[30]	.03	.14	[.1]	[4]	[0]
DQ Cone, regular	142	230	6	7	35	200	[0]	[0.5]	[90]	.09	.26	[.3]	[8]	[0]
DQ Cone, large	213	340	10	10	52	300	[0]	[0.7]	[121]	.15	.43	[.4]	[12]	[0]
DQ Dip Cone, small	78	150	3	7	20	100	[0]	[0.2]	[30]	.03	.17	[.1]	[4]	[0]
DQ Dip Cone, regular	156	300	7	13	40	200	0.4	[0.5]	[90]	.09	.34	[.3]	[8]	[0]
DQ Dip Cone, large	234	450	10	20	58	300	0.4	[0.7]	[121]	.12	.51	[.4]	[12]	[0]
DQ Sundae, small	106	170	4	4	30	100	0.7	[0.2]	[30]	.03	.17	[.2]	[4]	[0]
DQ Sundae, regular	177	290	6	7	51	200	1.1	[0.5]	[90]	.06	.26	[.3]	[8]	[0]
DQ Sundae, large	248	400	9	9	71	300	1.8	[0.7]	[121]	.09	.43	0.4	[12]	[0]
DQ Malt, small	241	340	10	11	51	300	1.8	[0.7]	[121]	.06	.34	0.4	[12]	2
DQ Malt, regular	418	600	15	20	89	500	3.6	[1.2]	[227]	.12	.60	0.8	[21]	4
DQ Malt, large	588	840	22	28	125	600	5.4	[1.4]	[227]	.15	.85	1.2	[25]	6
DQ Float	397	330	6	8	59	200	[1.8]	[0.5]	[30]	.12	.17	[.3]	[8]	[0]
DQ Banana Split	383	540	10	15	91	350	1.8	[0.8]	[227]	.60	.60	0.8	[32]	18
DQ Parfait	284	460	10	11	81	300	1.8	[0.7]	[121]	.12	.43	0.4	[12]	[0]
DQ Freeze	397	520	11	13	89	300	[1.8]	[0.7]	[60]	.15	.34	[.6]	[12]	[0]
Mr. Misty® Freeze	411	500	10	12	87	300	[1.8]	[0.7]	[60]	.15	.34	[.5]	[12]	[0]
Mr. Misty® Float	404	440	6	8	85	200	[1.8]	[0.5]	[30]	.12	.17	[.4]	[8]	[0]
"Dilly"® Bar	85	240	4	15	22	100	0.4	[0.2]	[30]	.06	.17	[.7]	[4]	[0]
DQ Sandwich	60	140	3	4	24	60	0.4	[1.0]	[30]	.03	.14	0.4	[18]	[0]
Brazier® Cheese Dog	113	330	15	19	24	168	1.6	1.9	[81]	[.10]	.18	3.3	[25]	[0]
Brazier® Chili Dog	128	330	13	20	25	86	2.0	1.8	[50]	.15	.23	3.9	[24]	11
Brazier® Dog	99	273	11	15	23	75	1.5	1.4	[0]	.12	.15	2.6	[24]	11
Fish Sandwich	170	400	20	17	41	60	1.1	0.3	[0]	.15	.26	3.0	[37]	[0]

Food Item	Weight (g)	Energy (kcal)	Protein (g)	Fat (g)	Carbo-hydrate (g)	Calcium (mg)	Iron (mg)	Zinc (mg)	Vitamin A (RE)	Thiamin (mg)	Ribo-flavin (mg)	Niacin (mg)	Folacin (µg)	Vitamin C (mg)
Fish Sandwich w/Ch	177	440	24	21	39	150	0.4	0.3	[30]	.15	.26	3.0	[29]	[0]
Super Brazier® Dog	182	518	20	30	41	158	4.3	2.8	[0]	.42	.44	7.0	[48]	14
Super Brazier® Dog w/Ch	203	593	26	36	43	297	4.4	3.5	[30]	.43	.48	8.1	[49]	14
Super Brazier® Chili Dog	210	555	23	33	42	158	4.0	2.8	[0]	.42	.48	8.8	[48]	18
Brazier® Fries, small	71	200	2	10	25	[0]	0.4	[0]	[0]	.06	[0]	0.8	[15]	4
Brazier® Fries, large	113	320	3	16	40	[0]	0.4	0.3	[0]	.09	.03	1.2	[19]	5
Brazier® Onion Rings	85	300	6	17	33	20	0.4	0.3	[0]	.09	[0]	0.4	[7]	2

Source: Adapted from International Dairy Queen, Inc., Minneapolis, Minnesota. Nutritional analysis by Raltech Scientific Services, Inc. (formerly WARF), Madison, Wisconsin. (Nutritional analysis not applicable in the state of Texas.)

JACK IN THE BOX®

Food Item	Weight (g)	Energy (kcal)	Protein (g)	Fat (g)	Carbo-hydrate (g)	Calcium (mg)	Iron (mg)	Zinc (mg)	Vitamin A (RE)	Thiamin (mg)	Ribo-flavin (mg)	Niacin (mg)	Folacin (µg)	Vitamin C (mg)
Hamburger	97	263	13	11	29	82	2.3	1.8	[10]	.27	.18	5.6	[24]	1
Cheeseburger	109	310	16	15	28	172	2.6	2.3	[100]	.27	.21	5.4	[25]	[1]
Jumbo Jack® Hamburger	246	551	28	29	45	134	4.5	4.2	[75]	.47	.34	11.6	[47]	4
Jumbo Jack® Hamburger w/Ch	272	628	32	35	45	273	4.6	4.8	[150]	.52	.38	11.3	[49]	5
Regular Taco	83	189	8	11	15	116	1.2	1.3	[36]	.07	.08	1.8	[19]	[1]
Super Taco	146	285	12	17	20	196	1.9	2.1	[60]	.10	.12	2.8	[38]	2
Moby Jack® Sandwich	141	455	17	26	38	167	1.7	1.1	[24]	.30	.21	4.5	[30]	1
Breakfast Jack® Sandwich	121	301	18	13	28	177	2.5	1.8	[44]	.41	.47	5.1	[52]	3
French Fries	80	270	3	15	31	19	0.7	0.3	[0]	.12	.02	1.9	[14]	4
Onion Rings	85	351	5	23	32	26	1.4	0.4	[0]	.24	.12	3.1	[19]	[1]
Apple Turnover	119	411	4	24	45	11	1.4	0.2	[4]	.23	.12	2.5	[7]	[1]
Vanilla Shake*	317	317	10	6	57	349	0.2	1.0	[106]	.16	.38	0.5	[21]	[2]
Strawberry Shake*	328	323	11	7	55	371	0.6	1.1	[114]	.16	.46	0.6	[21]	[2]
Chocolate Shake*	322	325	11	7	55	348	0.7	1.1	[106]	.16	.64	0.6	[21]	[2]
Vanilla Shake	314	342	10	9	54	349	0.4	1.0	[133]	.16	.47	0.5	[21]	4
Strawberry Shake	328	380	11	10	63	351	0.3	1.0	[129]	.16	.62	0.5	[21]	[2]
Chocolate Shake	317	365	11	10	59	350	1.2	1.2	[115]	.16	.60	0.6	[21]	[2]
Ham & Cheese Omelette	174	425	21	23	32	260	4.0	2.3	[232]	.45	.70	3.0	[48]	[1]
Double Cheese Omelette	166	423	19	25	30	276	3.6	2.1	[242]	.33	.68	2.5	[48]	2
Ranchero Style Omelette	196	414	20	23	33	278	3.8	2.0	[258]	.33	.74	2.6	[48]	[1]

N

TABLE N-1 (continued)
(Dashes indicate no data available. X=Less than 2% US RDA; tr=trace.)

Food Item	Weight (g)	Energy (kcal)	Protein (g)	Fat (g)	Carbo- hydrate (g)	Calcium (mg)	Iron (mg)	Zinc (mg)	Vitamin A (RE)	Thiamin (mg)	Ribo- flavin (mg)	Niacin (mg)	Folacin (µg)	Vitamin C (mg)
French Toast	180	537	15	29	54	119	3.0	1.8	[150]	.56	.30	4.4	[36]	9
Pancakes	232	626	16	27	79	105	2.8	1.9	[100]	.63	.44	4.6	[18]	[0]
Scrambled Eggs	267	719	26	44	55	257	5.0	3.0	[210]	.69	.56	5.2	[66]	[0]

* Special formula for shakes sold in California, Arizona, Texas and Washington. Source: Adapted from Jack-in-the-Box, Foodmaker, Inc., San Diego, California. Nutritional analysis by Raltech Scientific Services, Inc. (formerly WARF), Madison, Wisconsin.

KENTUCKY FRIED CHICKEN®

Food Item	Weight (g)	Energy (kcal)	Protein (g)	Fat (g)	Carbo- hydrate (g)	Calcium (mg)	Iron (mg)	Zinc (mg)	Vitamin A (RE)	Thiamin (mg)	Ribo- flavin (mg)	Niacin (mg)	Folacin (µg)	Vitamin C (mg)
Original Recipe® Dinner*														
Wing & Rib	322	603	30	32	48	[74]	[3.5]	[3.6]	[8]	.22	.19	10.0	[51]	37
Wing & Thigh	341	661	33	38	48	[74]	[3.5]	[3.6]	[8]	.24	.27	8.4	[51]	37
Drum & Thigh	346	643	35	35	46	[74]	[3.5]	[3.6]	[8]	.25	.32	8.5	[51]	37
Extra Crispy Dinner*														
Wing & Rib	349	755	33	43	60	[74]	[3.5]	[3.6]	[8]	.31	.29	10.4	[51]	37
Wing & Thigh	371	812	36	48	58	[74]	[3.5]	[3.6]	[8]	.31	.35	10.3	[51]	37
Drum & Thigh	376	765	38	44	55	[74]	[3.5]	[3.6]	[8]	.32	.38	10.4	[51]	37
Mashed Potatoes	85	64	2	1	12	[19]	[.2]	[.2]	[0]	[0]	.02	0.8	[5]	5
Gravy	14	23	0	2	1	[0]	[0]	[0]	[0]	0	.01	0.1	[0]	[0]
Cole Slaw	91	122	1	8	13	[22]	[.2]	[.2]	[12]	[.05]	[.05]	[.3]	[30]	[42]
Rolls	21	61	2	1	11	[15]	[.4]	[.2]	[0]	.10	.04	1.0	[7]	[0]
Corn (5.5-inch ear)	135	169	5	3	31	[2]	[.5]	[.6]	[16]	.12	.07	1.2	[50]	[3]

* Includes two pieces of chicken, mashed potato and gravy, cole slaw, and roll. Source: Adapted from Kentucky Fried Chicken, Inc., Louisville, Kentucky. Nutritional analysis by Raltech Scientific Services, Inc. (formerly WARF), Madison, Wisconsin.

LONG JOHN SILVER'S®

Food Item	Weight (g)	Energy (kcal)	Protein (g)	Fat (g)	Carbo- hydrate (g)	Calcium (mg)	Iron (mg)	Zinc (mg)	Vitamin A (RE)	Thiamin (mg)	Ribo- flavin (mg)	Niacin (mg)	Folacin (µg)	Vitamin C (mg)
Fish w/Batter (2 pc)	136	366	22	22	21	[102]	[1.5]	[.8]	[56]	[.16]	[.15]	[1.9]	[26]	[1]
Fish w/Batter (3 pc)	207	549	32	32	32	[145]	[2.2]	[1.2]	[121]	[.23]	[.22]	[2.7]	[37]	[1]
Treasure Chest®	143	506	30	33	32	[82]	[2.6]	[2.3]	[32]	[.19]	[.13]	[5.2]	[35]	[18]
Chicken Planks® (4 pc)	166	457	27	23	35	[27]	[4.0]	[4.5]	[0]	[.10]	[.09]	[8.6]	[13]	[13]
Peg Legs® w/Batter (5 pc)	125	350	22	28	26	[20]	[3.0]	[3.4]	[0]	[.08]	[.07]	[6.5]	[10]	[10]
Ocean Scallops (6 pc)	120	283	11	13	30	[100]	[2.6]	[1.8]	[15]	[0]	[.03]	[1.5]	[13]	[0]
Shrimp w/Batter (6 pc)	88	268	8	13	30	[80]	[2.1]	[1.4]	[12]	[0]	[.02]	[1.2]	[10]	[0]
Breaded Oysters (6 pc)	156	441	13	19	53	[113]	[6.6]	[11.0]	[112]	[.17]	[.21]	[3.0]	[12]	[0]
Breaded Clams	142	617	18	34	61	[59]	[5.2]	[1.4]	[27]	[.08]	[.15]	[1.1]	[13]	[8]
Fish Sandwich	193	337	22	31	49	[145]	[2.2]	[1.2]	[121]	[.23]	[.22]	[2.7]	[37]	[1]

Food Item	Weight (g)	Energy (kcal)	Protein (g)	Fat (g)	Carbo-hydrate (g)	Calcium (mg)	Iron (mg)	Zinc (mg)	Vitamin A (RE)	Thiamin (mg)	Ribo-flavin (mg)	Niacin (mg)	Folacin (µg)	Vitamin C (mg)
French Fryes	85	288	4	16	33	[19]	[.7]	[.3]	[0]	[.12]	[.02]	[1.9]	[20]	[4]
Cole Slaw	113	138	1	8	16	[24]	[.2]	[.2]	[6]	[.02]	[.03]	[.2]	[14]	[23]
Corn on the Cob (1 ear)	150	176	5	4	29	[2]	[.5]	[.6]	[31]	[.09]	[.08]	[1.1]	[50]	[7]
Hushpuppies (3)	45	153	3	7	20	[6]	[.7]	[.3]	[16]	[.12]	[.03]	[.6]	[7]	[0]
Clam Chowder (8 oz)	170	107	5	3	15	[103]	[.6]	[1.1]	[73]	[.03]	[.16]	[.4]	[5]	[1]

Source: Adapted from Long John Silver's Food Shoppes, Lexington, Kentucky. Nutritional analysis by L. V. Packett, PhD. The Department of Nutrition and Food Science, University of Kentucky.

McDONALD'S®

Food Item	Weight (g)	Energy (kcal)	Protein (g)	Fat (g)	Carbo-hydrate (g)	Calcium (mg)	Iron (mg)	Zinc (mg)	Vitamin A (RE)	Thiamin (mg)	Ribo-flavin (mg)	Niacin (mg)	Folacin (µg)	Vitamin C (mg)
Egg McMuffin®	138	327	19	15	31	226	2.9	1.9	[30]	.47	.44	3.8	[55]	[0]
English Muffin, Buttered	63	186	5	5	30	117	1.5	0.5	[50]	.28	.49	2.6	[5]	1
Hotcakes w/Butter & Syrup	214	500	8	10	94	103	2.2	0.7	[75]	.26	.36	2.3	[21]	5
Sausage (Pork)	53	206	9	19	[0]	16	0.8	1.5	[0]	.27	.11	2.1	[0]	1
Scrambled Eggs	98	180	13	13	3	61	2.5	1.7	[200]	.08	.47	0.2	[33]	1
Hashbrown Potatoes	55	125	2	7	14	5	0.4	0.2	[0]	.06	[0]	0.8	[9]	4
Big Mac®	204	563	26	33	41	157	4.0	4.7	[55]	.39	.37	6.5	[37]	2
Cheeseburger	115	307	15	14	30	132	2.4	2.6	[70]	.25	.23	3.8	[25]	2
Hamburger	102	255	12	10	30	51	2.3	2.1	[25]	.25	.18	4.0	[24]	2
Quarter Pounder®	166	424	24	22	33	63	4.1	5.1	[25]	.32	.28	6.5	[33]	[0]
Quarter Pounder® w/Ch	194	524	30	31	32	219	4.3	5.7	[135]	.31	.37	7.4	[35]	3
Filet-O-Fish®	139	432	14	25	37	93	1.7	0.9	[10]	.26	.20	2.6	[37]	[0]
Regular Fries	68	220	3	12	26	9	0.6	0.3	[0]	.12	.02	2.3	[15]	13
Apple Pie	85	253	2	14	29	14	0.6	0.2	[4]	.02	.02	0.2	[7]	[0]
Cherry Pie	88	260	2	14	32	12	0.6	0.2	[10]	.03	.02	0.4	[15]	[0]
McDonaldland® Cookies	67	308	4	11	49	12	1.5	0.3	[4]	.23	.23	2.9	[5]	1
Chocolate Shake	291	383	10	9	66	320	0.8	1.4	[105]	.12	.44	0.5	[21]	[2]
Strawberry Shake	290	362	9	9	62	322	0.2	1.2	[115]	.12	.44	0.4	[21]	4
Vanilla Shake	291	352	9	8	60	329	0.2	1.2	[105]	.12	.70	0.3	[21]	3
Hot Fudge Sundae	164	310	7	11	46	215	0.6	1.0	[70]	.07	.31	1.1	[2]	3
Caramel Sundae	165	328	7	10	53	200	0.2	0.9	[85]	.07	.31	1.0	[2]	4

N

Food Item	Weight (g)	Energy (kcal)	Protein (g)	Fat (g)	Carbo- hydrate (g)	Calcium (mg)	Iron (mg)	Zinc (mg)	Vitamin A (RE)	Thiamin (mg)	Ribo- flavin (mg)	Niacin (mg)	Folacin (µg)	Vitamin C (mg)
Strawberry Sundae	164	289	7	9	46	174	0.4	0.8	[70]	.07	.30	1.0	[2]	3

Source: Adapted from McDonald's Corporation, Oak Brook, Illinois. Nutritional analysis by Raltech Scientific Services, Inc. (formerly WARF), Madison, Wisconsin.

TACO BELL®

Food Item	Weight (g)	Energy (kcal)	Protein (g)	Fat (g)	Carbo- hydrate (g)	Calcium (mg)	Iron (mg)	Zinc (mg)	Vitamin A (RE)	Thiamin (mg)	Ribo- flavin (mg)	Niacin (mg)	Folacin (µg)	Vitamin C (mg)
Bean Burrito	166	343	11	12	48	98	2.8	[2.6]	[166]	.37	.22	2.2	[51]	15
Beef Burrito	184	466	30	21	37	83	4.6	[5.7]	[168]	.30	.39	7.0	[9]	15
Beefy Tostada	184	291	19	15	21	208	3.4	[4.3]	[345]	.16	.27	3.3	[6]	13
Bellbeefer®	123	221	15	7	23	40	2.6	[2.1]	[296]	.15	.20	3.7	[24]	10
Bellbeefer® w/Ch	137	278	19	12	23	147	2.7	[2.6]	[629]	.16	.27	3.7	[26]	10
Burrito Supreme®	225	457	21	22	43	121	3.8	[3.4]	[346]	.33	.35	4.7	[66]	16
Combination Burrito	175	404	21	16	43	91	3.7	[4.1]	[167]	.34	.31	4.6	[30]	15
Enchirito®	207	454	25	21	42	259	3.8	[4.1]	[118]	.31	.37	4.7	[30]	10
Pintos 'N Cheese	158	168	11	5	21	150	2.3	[2.6]	[625]	.26	.16	0.9	[91]	9
Taco	83	186	15	8	14	120	2.5	[2.1]	[12]	.09	.16	2.9	[12]	0
Tostada	138	179	9	6	25	191	2.3	[1.2]	[315]	.18	.15	0.8	[28]	10

Sources (adapted): 1) *Menu Item Portions*, San Antonio, Texas, Taco Bell Co. July 1976. 2) Adams CF Nutritive Value of American Foods in common units in *Handbook No. 456*. Washington USDA Agricultural Research Service November 1975. 3) Church EF, Church HN (eds) *Food Values of Portions Commonly Used ed 12.* Philadelphia, JB Lippincott Co. 1975. 4) Valley Baptist Medical Center, Food Service Department *Descriptions of Mexican-American Foods*. Fort Atkinson, Wisconsin: NASCO.

WENDY'S®

Food Item	Weight (g)	Energy (kcal)	Protein (g)	Fat (g)	Carbo- hydrate (g)	Calcium (mg)	Iron (mg)	Zinc (mg)	Vitamin A (RE)	Thiamin (mg)	Ribo- flavin (mg)	Niacin (mg)	Folacin (µg)	Vitamin C (mg)
Single Hamburger	200	470	26	26	34	84	5.3	4.8	[25]	.24	.36	5.8	[48]	1
Double Hamburger	285	670	44	40	34	138	8.2	8.4	[35]	.43	.54	10.6	[72]	2
Triple Hamburger	360	850	65	51	33	104	10.7	13.5	[65]	.47	.68	14.7	[96]	2
Single w/Cheese	240	580	33	34	34	228	5.4	5.5	[65]	.38	.43	6.3	[50]	1
Double w/Cheese	325	800	50	48	41	177	10.2	10.1	[130]	.49	.75	11.4	[74]	2
Triple w/Cheese	400	1040	72	68	35	371	10.9	14.3	[145]	.80	.84	15.1	[100]	3
Chili	250	230	19	8	21	83	4.4	3.7	[120]	.22	.25	3.4	[32]	3
French Fries	120	330	5	16	41	16	1.2	0.5	[4]	.14	.07	3.0	[18]	6
Frosty	250	390	9	16	54	270	0.9	1.0	[105]	.20	.60	[0.6]	[21]	1

Source: Adapted from Wendy's International Inc., Dublin, Ohio. Nutritional analysis by Medallion Laboratories, Minneapolis, Minnesota.

Older PIZZA HUT data are invalid because of reformulation of the products.

Beverages: see Appendix H.

APPENDIX O
Recommended Nutrient Intakes

Some of the U.S. recommendations appear in the RDA table on the inside front cover. The remaining RDA are here, in Tables O–1 and O–2. The U.S. RDA used on food labels are on the inside back cover.

The Canadian recommendations are in Tables O–3 and O–4.

TABLE O–1 **Estimated Safe and Adequate Daily Dietary Intakes of Additional Selected Nutrients (United States)[a]**

| Age (years) | VITAMINS | | | TRACE ELEMENTS[b] | | |
	Vitamin K (µg)	Biotin (µg)	Pantothenic acid (mg)	Copper (mg)	Manganese (mg)	Fluoride (mg)
0-0.5	12	35	2	0.5-0.7	0.5-0.7	0.1-0.5
0.5-1	10-20	50	3	0.7-1.0	0.7-1.0	0.2-1.0
1-3	15-30	65	3	1.0-1.5	1.0-1.5	0.5-1.5
4-6	20-40	85	3-4	1.5-2.0	1.5-2.0	1.0-2.5
7-10	30-60	120	4-5	2.0-2.5	2.0-3.0	1.5-2.5
11+	50-100	100-200	4-7	2.0-3.0	2.5-5.0	1.5-2.5
Adults	70-140	100-200	4-7	2.0-3.0	2.5-5.0	1.5-4.0

[a] Because there is less information on which to base allowances, these figures are not given in the main table of the RDA and are provided here in the form of ranges of recommended intakes.
[b] Since the toxic levels for many trace elements may be only several times usual intakes, the upper levels for the trace elements given in this table should not habitually be exceeded.

TABLE O-1 **(continued)**

Age (years)	TRACE ELEMENTS[b]			ELECTROLYTES		
	Chromium (mg)	Selenium (mg)	Molybdenum (mg)	Sodium (mg)	Potassium (mg)	Chloride (mg)
0-0.5	0.01-0.04	0.01-0.04	0.03-0.06	115-350	350-925	275-700
0.5-1	0.02-0.06	0.02-0.06	0.04-0.08	250-750	425-1,275	400-1,200
1-3	0.02-0.08	0.02-0.08	0.05-0.1	325-975	550-1,650	500-1,500
4-6	0.03-0.12	0.03-0.12	0.06-0.15	450-1,350	775-2,325	700-2,100
7-10	0.05-0.2	0.05-0.2	0.1 -0.3	600-1,800	1,000-3,000	925-2,775
11+	0.05-0.2	0.05-0.2	0.15-0.5	900-2,700	1,525-4,575	1,400-4,200
Adults	0.05-0.2	0.05-0.2	0.15-0.5	1,100-3,300	1,875-5,625	1,700-5,100

[b] Since the toxic levels for many trace elements may be only several times usual intakes, the upper levels for the trace elements given in this table should not habitually be exceeded.

TABLE O-2 **Mean Heights and Weights and Recommended Energy Intakes (United States)**

AGE (years)	WEIGHT (kg)	WEIGHT (lb)	HEIGHT (cm)	HEIGHT (in)	ENERGY NEEDS[a] (kcal)	(MJ)[b]
Infants						
0.0-0.5	6	13	60	24	kg × 115 (95-145)	kg × 0.48
0.5-1.0	9	20	71	28	kg × 105 (80-135)	kg × 0.44
Children						
1-3	13	29	90	35	1,300 (900-1,800)	5.5
4-6	20	44	112	44	1,700 (1,300-2,300)	7.1
7-10	28	62	132	52	2,400 (1,650-3,300)	10.1
Males						
11-14	45	99	157	62	2,700 (2,000-3,700)	11.3
15-18	66	145	176	69	2,800 (2,100-3,900)	11.8
19-22	70	154	177	70	2,900 (2,500-3,300)	12.2
23-50	70	154	178	70	2,700 (2,300-3,100)	11.3
51-75	70	154	178	70	2,400 (2,000-2,800)	10.1
76+	70	154	178	70	2,050 (1,650-2,450)	8.6
Females						
11-14	46	101	157	62	2,200 (1,500-3,000)	9.2
15-18	55	120	163	64	2,100 (1,200-3,000)	8.8
19-22	55	120	163	64	2,100 (1,700-2,500)	8.8
23-50	55	120	163	64	2,000 (1,600-2,400)	8.4
51-75	55	120	163	64	1,800 (1,400-2,200)	7.6
76+	55	120	163	64	1,600 (1,200-2,000)	6.7
Pregnant					+300	
Lactating					+500	

[a] The energy allowances for the young adults are for men and women doing light work. The allowances for the two older age groups represent mean energy needs over these age spans, allowing for a 2 percent decrease in basal (resting) metabolic rate per decade and a reduction in activity of 200 kcal per day for men and women between 51 and 75 years, 500 kcal for men over 75 years, and 400 kcal for women over 75. The customary range of daily energy output, shown in parentheses, is based on a variation in energy needs of ± 400 kcal at any one age, emphasizing the wide range of energy intakes appropriate for any group of people. Energy allowances for children through age 18 are based on median energy intakes of children these ages followed in longitudinal growth studies. The values in parentheses are tenth and ninetieth percentiles of energy intake, to indicate the range of energy consumption among children of these ages.

[b] MJ stands for megajoules (1 MJ = 1,000 kJ).

TABLE O–3 **Recommended Nutrient Intakes for Canadians, 1983 (formerly Canadian *Dietary Standard*, 1975)**

Age	Sex	Weight (kg)	Protein (g/day)[a]	Vitamin A (RE/day)[b]	Vitamin D (µg/day)[c]	Vitamin E (mg/day)[d]
Months						
0-2	Both	4.5	11[f]	400	10	3
3-5	Both	7.0	14[f]	400	10	3
6-8	Both	8.5	16[f]	400	10	3
9-11	Both	9.5	18	400	10	3
Years						
1	Both	11	18	400	10	3
2-3	Both	14	20	400	5	4
4-6	Both	18	25	500	5	5
7-9	M	25	31	700	2.5	7
	F	25	29	700	2.5	6
10-12	M	34	38	800	2.5	8
	F	36	39	800	2.5	7
13-15	M	50	49	900	2.5	9
	F	48	43	800	2.5	7
16-18	M	62	54	1,000	2.5	10
	F	53	47	800	2.5	7
19-24	M	71	57	1,000	2.5	10
	F	58	41	800	2.5	7
25-49	M	74	57	1,000	2.5	9
	F	59	41	800	2.5	6
50-74	M	73	57	1,000	2.5	7
	F	63	41	800	2.5	6
75+	M	69	57	1,000	2.5	6
	F	64	41	800	2.5	5
Pregnancy (additonal)						
1st Trimester			15	100	2.5	2
2nd Trimester			20	100	2.5	2
3rd Trimester			25	100	2.5	2
Lactation (additional)			20	400	2.5	3

Recommended intakes of energy and of certain nutrients are not listed in this table because of the nature of the variables upon which they are based. The figures for energy are estimates of average requirements for expected patterns of activity (see Table O–4). For nutrients not shown, the following amounts are recommended: thiamin, 0.4 mg/1,000 kcal (0.48/5,000 kJ); riboflavin, 0.5 mg/1,000 kcal (0.6 mg/5,000 kJ); niacin, 7.2 NE/1,000 kcal (8.6 NE/5,000 kJ); vitamin B_6, 15 µg, as pyridoxine, per gram of protein; phosphorus, same as calcium.

Recommended intakes during periods of growth are taken as appropriate for individuals representative of the mid-point in each age group. All recommended intakes are designed to cover individual variations in essentially all of a healthy population subsisting upon a variety of common foods available in Canada. Source: *Recommended Nutrient Intakes for Canadians,* Health and Welfare Canada (Ottawa: Canadian Government Publishing Centre, 1983), Table X.1, pp. 179–180.

O

TABLE O–3 (continued)

	WATER-SOLUBLE VITAMINS			MINERALS			
Vitamin C (mg/day)	Folacin (µg/day)[e]	Vitamin B_{12} (µg/day)	Calcium (mg/day)	Magnesium (mg/day)	Iron (mg/day)	Iodine (µg/day)	Zinc (mg/day)
20	50	0.3	350	30	0.4[g]	25	2[h]
20	50	0.3	350	40	5	35	3
20	50	0.3	400	45	7	40	3
20	55	0.3	400	50	7	45	3
20	65	0.3	500	55	6	55	4
20	80	0.4	500	65	6	65	4
25	90	0.5	600	90	6	85	5
35	125	0.8	700	110	7	110	6
30	125	0.8	700	110	7	95	6
40	170	1.0	900	150	10	125	7
40	170	1.0	1,000	160	10	110	7
50	160	1.5	1,100	220	12	160	9
45	160	1.5	800	190	13	160	8
55	190	1.9	900	240	10	160	9
45	160	1.9	700	220	14	160	8
60	210	2.0	800	240	8	160	9
45	165	2.0	700	190	14	160	8
60	210	2.0	800	240	8	160	9
45	165	2.0	700	190	14[i]	160	8
60	210	2.0	800	240	8	160	9
45	165	2.0	800	190	7	160	8
60	210	2.0	800	240	8	160	9
45	165	2.0	800	190	7	160	8
0	305	1.0	500	15	6	25	0
20	305	1.0	500	20	6	25	1
20	305	1.0	500	25	6	25	2
30	120	0.5	500	80	0	50	6

[a] The primary units are grams per kilogram of body weight. The figures shown here are examples.

[b] One retinol equivalent (RE) corresponds to the biological activity of 1 µg of retinol, 6 µg of β-carotene or 12 µg of other carotenes.

[c] Expressed as cholecalciferol or ergocalciferol.

[d] Expressed as *d*-α-tocopherol equivalents, relative to which β- and γ-tocopherol and α-tocotrienol have activities of 0.5, 0.1 and 0.3 respectively.

[e] Expressed as total folate.

[f] Assumption that the protein is from breast milk or is of the same biological value as that of breast milk and that between 3 and 9 months adjustment for the quality of the protein is made.

[g] It is assumed that breast milk is the source of iron up to 2 months of age.

[h] Based on the assumption that breast milk is the source of zinc for the first 2 months.

[i] After the menopause the recommended intake is 7 mg/day.

O

TABLE O–4 **Average Energy Requirements (Canada)**

Age	Sex	Average Height (cm)	Average Weight (kg)	REQUIREMENTS[a]					
				kcal/kg[b]	MJ/kg[b]	kcal/day	MJ/day	kcal/cm	MJ/cm
Months									
0-2	Both	55	4.5	120-100	0.50-0.42	500	2.0	9	0.04
3-5	Both	63	7.0	100- 95	0.42-0.40	700	2.8	11	0.05
6-8	Both	69	8.5	95- 97	0.40-0.41	800	3.4	11.5	0.05
9-11	Both	73	9.5	97- 99	0.41	950	3.8	12.5	0.05
Years									
1	Both	82	11	101	0.42	1,100	4.8	13.5	0.06
2-3	Both	95	14	94	0.39	1,300	5.6	13.5	0.06
4-6	Both	107	18	100	0.42	1,800	7.6	17	0.07
7-9	M	126	25	88	0.37	2,200	9.2	17.5	0.07
	F	125	25	76	0.32	1,900	8.0	15	0.06
10-12	M	141	34	73	0.30	2,500	10.4	17.5	0.07
	F	143	36	61	0.25	2,200	9.2	15.5	0.06
13-15	M	159	50	57	0.24	2,800	12.0	17.5	0.07
	F	157	48	46	0.19	2,200	9.2	14	0.06
16-18	M	172	62	51	0.21	3,200	13.2	18.5	0.08
	F	160	53	40	0.17	2,100	8.8	13	0.05
19-24	M	175	71	42	0.18	3,000	12.4		
	F	160	58	36	0.15	2,100	8.8		
25-49	M	172	74	36	0.15	2,700	11.2		
	F	160	59	32	0.13	1,900	8.0		
50-74	M	170	73	31	0.13	2,300	9.6		
	F	158	63	29	0.12	1,800	7.6		
75+	M	168	69	29	0.12	2,000	8.4		
	F	155	64	23	0.10	1,500	6.0		

Source: *Recommended Nutrient Intakes for Canadians,* 1983, Table II.1, pp. 22–23.
[a] Requirements can be expected to vary within a range of ±30 percent.
[b] First and last figures are averages at the beginning and at the end of the 3-month period.

O

O

APPENDIX P
Vitamin/Mineral Supplements Compared

The following tables are useful for comparing the essential vitamin and mineral contents of supplements commonly available in the United States. Notice that blank columns have been provided for the addition of locally available products you may wish to compare with those shown here.

Not all ingredients in vitamin/mineral preparations are of proven benefit. To facilitate meaningful comparison, the table lists only the nutrients known to be needed in supplement form on occasion. Other nutrients and compounds found on the labels of these supplements are listed in the table notes.

When a supplement is needed that supplies certain particular nutrients, this table will ease the task of selecting an appropriate one. Notice, for example, that many preparations marketed for the elderly are composed largely of alcohol, with few vitamins or minerals. These are "tonics," not vitamin/mineral supplements. A tonic may be useful if the only need is for comfort and the benefit of the placebo effect, but if an elderly person needs a balanced assortment of vitamins and minerals and cannot easily take pills, it may be advisable to suggest a liquid preparation designated for infants.

Notice the very low levels of calcium present in some of these preparations. A product that supplies 20 mg of calcium provides only 2 percent of an adult's RDA for calcium and would have no significant impact on a person's calcium nutrition. For further discussion of this point, see page 389.

TABLE P-1 **Supplements for Infants and Children**

COMPANY	LEDERLE	MILES LABORATORIES	MEAD-JOHNSON	MEAD-JOHNSON	RADIANCE
PRODUCT	CENTRUM JR.	FLINSTONES PLUS IRON	POLY-VI-SOL WITH IRON (DROPS)	POLY-VI-SOL WITH IRON (CHEWABLE)	CHEWABLE FOR CHILDREN
Intended Users	*Children Over 4*	*Children 1 to 12*	*Infants*	*Children and Adults*	*Children 2 to 12*
Recommended Daily Dose	*1 tablet*	*1 tablet*	*1 ml*	*1 tablet*	*1 tablet*
Vitamins					
Vitamin A (IU)	5,000	2,500	1,500	2,500	4,000
Vitamin D (IU)	400	400	400	400	400
Vitamin E (IU)	15	15	5	15	3.4
Vitamin C (mg)	60	60	35	60	60
Thiamin (B_1) (mg)	1.5	1.05	0.5	1.05	2.0
Riboflavin (B_2) (mg)	1.7	1.2	0.6	1.2	2.4
Vitamin B_6 (mg)	2.0	1.05	0.4	1.05	2.0
Vitamin B_{12} (μg)	6.0	4.5	—	4.5	10.0
Niacin (mg)	20.0	13.5	8.0	13.5	10.0
Folacin (mg)	0.4	0.3	—	0.3	—
Minerals					
Calcium (mg)	—	—	—	—	19
Phosphorus (mg)	—	—	—	—	0.0
Iron (mg)	18	15	10	12	12
Potassium (mg)	1.6	—	—	—	4
Magnesium (mg)	25	—	—	—	22
Zinc (mg)	10	—	—	—	—
Copper (mg)	2	—	—	—	0.2
Iodine (μg)	—	—	—	—	—
Manganese (mg)	1	—	—	—	—
Cost per day*					

Radiance Chewables also contain 2 mg pantothenic acid, 10 mg biotin, 2 mg inositol, and 2 mg of a choline compound.
Neo-life Chewables also contain 10 mg pantothenic acid, 0.075 mg inositol, and 0.05 mg of a choline compound.
Williams Chewables also contain 2.5 mg pantothenic acid, and 37.5 mg biotin.
Amway Chewables also contain 5 mg pantothenic acid.
Shaklee Chewables also contain 5 mg pantothenic acid, 150 mg biotin, and 0.2 mg inositol.

P

TABLE P–1 **(continued)**

CHOCKS	NEOLIFE	J. B. WILLIAMS	UPJOHN	AMWAY NUTRILITE	SHAKLEE	OTHER
BUGS BUNNY PLUS IRON	CHEWABLE NEW-JR.	CHEWABLE POPEYE WITH MINS/IRON	UNICAP CHEWABLE	CHEWABLES	VITA-LEA CHEWABLES	
Children 1 to 12	*Children 2 and Up*	*Children*	*Children*	*Children*	*Children*	
1 tablet	*3 tablets*	*1 tablet*	*1 tablet*	*1 tablet*	*2 tablets*	
2,500	3,000	2,500	5,000	2,500	2,500	
400	300	400	400	400	200	
15	9	15	15	10	15	
60	60	60	60	40	45	
1.05	1.5	1.05	1.5	0.7	1.05	
1.2	1.5	1.2	1.7	0.8	1.2	
1.05	1.2	1.05	2.0	0.7	1.0	
4.5	3.0	4.5	6.0	3.0	4.5	
13.5	10.0	13.5	20.0	9.0	10.0	
0.3	—	0.3	0.4	0.2	0.2	
—	—	—	—	—	160	
—	—	—	—	—	125	
15	3	15	—	5	10	
—	—	40	—	—	100	
—	—	40	—	—	8	
—	—	12	—	—	1	
—	0.002	1.5	—	—	1	
—	75	105	—	—	75	
—	1	—	—	—	—	

* Since product costs varies so widely by location (and local prices have changed dramatically in the last two years), the computation of cost/day is left for the reader to complete. To compute this value, divide the total retail price by the number of doses per container. For example: XYZ vitamins are sold in bottles of 100 tablets. The recommended dose is 2 tablets per day, therefore there are 50 doses in the bottle. At $5.00 per bottle, XYZ Vitamins cost $.10 per day.

P

TABLE P-2 **Supplements for Adults**

COMPANY	LEDERLE	LEDERLE	PARKE-DAVIS	SQUIBB	MILES LAB
PRODUCT	STRESS TABS 600	CENTRUM A TO ZINC	MYADEC	THERAGRAM M	ONE-A-DAY PLUS IRON
Recommended Daily Dose	*1 tablet*	*1 tablet*	*1 tablet*	*1 tablet*	*1 tablet*
Vitamins					
Vitamin A (IU)	—	5,000	10,000	10,000	5,000
Vitamin D (IU)	—	400	400	400	400
Vitamin E (IU)	30	30	30	15	15
Vitamin C (mg)	600	90	250	200	60
Thiamin (B_1) (mg)	15.0	2.25	10.0	10.3	1.5
Riboflavin (B_2) (mg)	15.0	2.6	10.0	10.0	1.7
Vitamin B_6 (mg)	5.0	3.0	5.0	4.1	2.0
Vitamin B_{12} (μg)	12	9	6	5	6
Niacin (mg)	100	20	100	100	20
Folacin (mg)	—	0.4	0.4	—	0.4
Minerals					
Calcium (mg)	—	162	—	20	—
Phosphorus (mg)	—	125	—	—	—
Iron (mg)	—	27	20	12	18
Potassium (mg)	—	7.5	—	—	—
Magnesium (mg)	—	100	100	65	—
Zinc (mg)	—	22.5	20	1.5	00
Copper (mg)	—	3	2	2	—
Iodine (μg)	—	150	150	150	—
Manganese (mg)	—	7.5	1.25	1.0	—
Cost per day*					

Lederle Centrum A to Zinc also contains 10 mg pantothenic acid, and 45 μg biotin.
Radiance Nutri-Mega also contains 50 mg pantothenic acid, 50 μg biotin, 50 mg inositol, 50 mg PABA, 50 mg choline compound, and 80 mg lecithin.
Neo-Life Formula IV also contains 12 mg pantothenic acid, 65 mg inositol, 30 mg PABA, 30 mg lecithin, 40 mg diastase, 40 mg lipase (pancreatin), and 168 mg linoleic acid.
Origin Multivitamins also contains 20 mg pantothenic acid, 25 μg biotin, 10 mg inositol, and 20 mg of a choline compound.
Amway Nutrilite Double X also contains 10 mg pantothenic acid, 5 μg chromium, and 5 μg selenium.
J. B. Williams Vitabank also contains 18 mg pantothenic acid and 25 μg selenium.
Miles Labs One-A-Day plus Minerals also contains 10 mg pantothenic acid, 10 μg chromium, 10 μg selenium, and 10 μg molybdenum.
Lederle Stress-Tabs 600, Parke-Davis Myadec, and Squibb Theragram M also contain pantothenic acid: 20 mg, 20 mg, 18.4 mg, and 10 mg respectively.

P

TABLE P–2 (continued)

RADIANCE	NEO-LIFE	AMWAY NUTRILITE	J. B. WILLIAMS	ORIGIN	MILES LAB	OTHER
NUTRI-MEGA	FORMULA IV	DOUBLE X	VITABANK	MULTI-VITAMIN	ONE-A-DAY PLUS MINERALS	
2 tablets	*2 capsules*	*9 tablets*	*1 tablet*	*1 tablet*	*1 tablet*	
10,000	4,000	15,000	5,000	10,000	5,000	
400	400	400	400	400	400	
300	10	30	30	30	30	
300	90	500	90	250	60	
50	10	15	2.25	20	1.5	
50	10	15	2.6	20	1.7	
50	10	15	3.0	5.0	2.0	
50	10	9	9	6	6	
50	50	35	20	150	20	
0.4	0.1	0.4	0.4	0.4	0.4	
200	—	900	170	100	130	
50	—	450	130	—	100	
18	25	18	18	30	18	
30	—	—	7.5	5	5	
50	35	300	100	50	100	
15	—	15	15	7.5	15	
2	2	2	2	1	2	
150	100	150	150	150	150	
30	—	5.0	2.5	1.5	2.5	

* Since product costs varies so widely by location (and local prices have changed dramatically in the last two years), the computation of cost/day is left for the reader to complete. To compute this value, divide the total retail price by the number of doses per container. For example: XYZ vitamins are sold in bottles of 100 tablets. The recommended dose is 2 tablets per day, therefore there are 50 doses in the bottle. At $5.00 per bottle, XYZ Vitamins cost $.10 per day.

P

TABLE P–3 **Supplements and Tonics for the Elderly**

COMPANY	ROSS LABS	LEDERLE	J. B. WILLIAMS	UPJOHN	OTHER
PRODUCT	VI-DAYLIN PLUS IRON	GEVRABON	GERITOL	UNICAP SENIOR	
Recommended Daily Dose	*1 tsp*	*1 oz*	*1 oz*	*1 tablet*	
Vitamins					
Vitamin A (IU)	2,500	—	—	5,000	
Vitamin D (IU)	400	—	—	—	
Vitamin E (IU)	15	—	—	15	
Vitamin C (mg)	60	—	—	60	
Thiamin (B_1) (mg)	1.05	5.0	5.0	1.2	
Riboflavin (B_2) (mg)	1.2	2.5	5.0	1.7	
Vitamin B_6 (mg)	1.05	1.0	1.0	2.0	
Vitamin B_{12} (μg)	4.5	1.0	1.5	6.0	
Niacin (mg)	13.5	50	100	14.0	
Folacin (mg)	—	—	—	0.4	
Minerals					
Calcium (mg)	—	—	2	—	
Phosphorus (mg)	—	—	—	—	
Iron (mg)	10	15	100	10	
Potassium (mg)	—	—	—	5	
Magnesium (mg)	—	2	—	—	
Zinc (mg)	—	2	—	15	
Copper (mg)	—	—	—	2	
Iodine (μg)	—	100	—	150	
Manganese (mg)	—	2	—	1	
Alcohol (%)	0.5	18	12	—	
Cost per day*					

Lederle Gevrabon also contains 100 mg inositol and 100 mg of a choline compound.

J. B. Williams Geritol also contains 100 mg of a choline compound and 50 mg methionine.

* Since product costs varies so widely by location (and local prices have changed dramatically in the last two years), the computation of cost/day is left for the reader to complete. To compute this value, divide the total retail price by the number of doses per container. For example: XYZ vitamins are sold in bottles of 100 tablets. The recommended dose is 2 tablets per day, therefore there are 50 doses in the bottle. At $5.00 per bottle, XYZ Vitamins cost $.10 per day.

P

APPENDIX Q
Self-Studies

Self-Study 1 (Chapter 1)
Record What You Eat

Our purpose in providing these exercises is to encourage you to study your own diet. Your reaction to them may be that they are both good news and bad news. The bad news is that they will slow you down, and filling out all the forms is tedious. Like income tax returns, they have to be done carefully, with frequent checking of arithmetic and tidy handwriting, so that they will be accurate and meaningful.

The good news, however, may well outweigh the drawbacks. Most students who do these activities with thoughtful attention report that unlike income tax returns they are intriguing, informative, and often reassuring. They are also rewarding—in direct proportion to your honesty.

In this first exercise you are to make a record of your typical food intake and analyze it for the nutrients it contains. You can undertake this analysis before you have learned very much about the nutrients; having the results in front of you as you read will make the reading more meaningful. As you learn about each nutrient and ask yourself how much of the nutrient you consume, you will already have the answer in front of you, ready for interpretation and action.

1 Use three copies of Form 1* and record on them all the foods you eat for a three-day period. If, like most people, you eat differently on weekdays than on weekends, then to get a true average you should probably record for two weekdays and one weekend day—or, record your food intake for a week.

* All Self-Study forms appear at the end of Appendix Q.

As you record each food, make careful note of the measure. Estimate the amount to the nearest ounce, quarter cup, tablespoon, or other common measure. In guessing at the sizes of meat portions, it helps to know that a piece of meat the size of the palm of your hand weighs about 3 or 4 ounces. If you are unable to estimate serving sizes in cups, tablespoons, or teaspoons, try measuring out servings the size of a half-cup, tablespoon, and teaspoon onto a plate or into a bowl to see how they look. It also helps to know that a slice of cheese (like sliced American cheese) or a 1½-inch cube of cheese weighs about 1 ounce.

You may have to break down mixed dishes to their ingredients. However, many mixed dishes, including soups, are listed in the miscellaneous section at the end of Appendix H. Other mixtures are simple to analyze. A ham and cheese sandwich, for example, can be listed as 2 slices of bread, 1 tablespoon of mayonnaise, 2 ounces of ham, 1 ounce of cheese, and so on. If you can't discover all the ingredients, estimate the amounts of only the major ones, like the beef, tomatoes, and potatoes in a beef-vegetable soup.

You will, of course, make errors in estimating amounts. In calculations of this kind, errors of up to 20 percent are expected and tolerated. Still, you will have a rough approximation that will enable you to compare your nutrient intakes with the recommended ones.

Do not record any nutrient supplements you take. It will be interesting to discover whether your food choices alone deliver the nutrients you need. If they don't, you'll know better what supplement to choose.

2 Using Appendix H, calculate for each day your total intakes of kcalories, protein, fat, carbohydrate, calcium, iron, zinc, vitamin A, thiamin, riboflavin, niacin, folacin, and vitamin C (ascorbic acid). If you wish, look up fiber in Appendix K, cholesterol, linoleic acid, and other fatty acids in Appendix G, and sugar in Appendix F. (You will be given instructions in analyzing these in later Self-Studies.) If the foods you have eaten are not included in these appendixes,

read the label on the package or use your ingenuity to guess their composition, using the most similar food you can find as a guide. For example, if you ate halibut (which is not listed in Appendix H), you would not be far off in using the values for haddock or perch. If you ate cream of celery soup you might substitute the values for cream of mushroom soup. As for fast foods, their composition is given in Appendix N.

Be careful in recording the nutrient amounts in odd-size portions. For example, if you used a quarter-cup of milk, then you will have to record a fourth of the amount of every nutrient listed for a cup of milk. And note the units in which the nutrients are measured:

- Energy is measured in kcalories as explained on p. 4.
- Protein, fat, fatty acids, and carbohydrate are measured in grams (g).
- Calcium, iron, zinc, thiamin, riboflavin, niacin, vitamin C (ascorbic acid), and cholesterol are measured in milligrams (mg)—thousandths of a gram (0.001 g). Folacin is measured in micrograms (mcg or μg)—thousandths of a milligram or millionths of a gram (0.001 mg or 0.000001 g). Thus "800 mg calcium" is the same as "0.8 mg calcium," and "400 μg folacin" is the same as "0.4 mg folacin." Be sure to convert all calcium amounts to milligrams and all folacin amounts to micrograms before calculating.
- Vitamin A can be measured in international units (IU) or retinol equivalents (RE);[1] 1 RE equals 3 IU of vitamin A from animal foods or 10 IU of vitamin A from plant foods. Appendix H lists vitamin A in RE to ease comparison with the RDA, which is also in RE. (For more details, see Chapter 9.) If you eat a packaged food whose label lists vitamin A in IU, be sure to convert to RE before calculating.

If you eat a packaged food whose label lists nutrient amounts as "percent of U.S. RDA," use the table on the inside back cover to convert to grams, milligrams, micrograms, or RE. Suppose a food portion contains "25 percent of the U.S. RDA of iron," for example. The table shows that the U.S. RDA for iron is 18 milligrams. The food portion therefore contributes 25 percent of 18 milligrams, or 4.5 milligrams of iron.

3 Now total the amount of each nutrient you've consumed for each day, and transfer your totals to Form 2. Form 2 provides a convenient means of deriving and keeping on record an average intake for each nutrient.

4 As a final step, transfer your average intakes to Form 3 for future reference. For comparison, enter the intakes recommended for a person of your age and sex, using either the RDA (on the inside front cover) or the Canadian recommendations (in Appendix O), whichever you prefer. Note that no recommendations are made for intakes of fat or

carbohydrate. Guidelines for these nutrients and for others, like cholesterol and fiber, will be presented and discussed later. Succeeding Self-Studies will guide you in focusing on each of the nutrients provided by your diet.

Suspend judgment about the adequacy of your diet for the moment. You have much to learn about your individuality, the nutrients, and the recommendations before you can reach any reasonable conclusions.

5 What percentage of the kcalories you consumed comes from protein, fat, and carbohydrate? (Use Form 4 to calculate.) Is your diet in line with the U.S. *Dietary Goals* in this respect? (See Chapter 1. Remember, the *Dietary Goals* are not commandments; not everyone agrees with them.)

6 You can get an indication of whether your diet is balanced by using the Food Group Plan Scorecard (Form 5—one copy for each day). How does your diet score by these criteria?

Self–Study 2 (Chapter 2)
Examine Your Carbohydrate Intake

Having read Chapter 2, you are in a position to study your carbohydrate consumption. From the forms you filled out for Self-Study 1, answer the following questions:

1 How many grams of carbohydrate do you consume in a day?

2 How many kcalories does this represent? (Remember, 1 gram of carbohydrate contributes 4 kcalories.)

3 It is estimated that you should have 125 grams or more of carbohydrate in a day. How does your intake compare with this minimum?

4 What percentage of your total kcalories is contributed by carbohydrate (carbohydrate kcalories ÷ total kcalories × 100)?

5 How does this figure compare with the dietary goal that states that 60 percent of the kcalories in your diet should come from carbohydrate? (Note: If you are on a diet to lose weight, then this goal does not apply to you. See the exercises in Self-Study 7: Diet Planning.)

6 Another dietary goal is that no more than 10 percent of total kcalories should come from refined and other processed sugars and foods high in such sugars. To assess your intake against this standard, sort the carbohydrate-containing food items you ate into three groups:

- Foods containing complex carbohydrate (foods found on the bread and vegetable exchange lists in Appendix L or M).
- Nutritious foods containing simple carbohydrate (foods on the milk and fruit lists).
- Foods containing mostly concentrated simple carbohy-

1   One IU of vitamin A is equal to 0.344 μg of crystalline vitamin A acetate or 0.6 μg of all-*trans* beta-carotene.

drate (sugar, honey, molasses, syrup, jam, jelly, candy, cakes, doughnuts, sweet rolls, cola beverages, and so on). How many grams of carbohydrate did you consume in each of these three categories? How many kcalories (grams times 4)? What percentage of your total kcalories comes from concentrated sugars? From other simple carbohydrates? Does your concentrated sugar intake fall within the recommended maximum of 10 percent of total kcalories?

7 Estimate how many pounds of sugar (concentrated simple carbohydrate) you eat in a year (1 pound = 454 grams). How does your yearly sugar intake compare with the estimated U.S. average of about 125 pounds per person per year? (If you need additional information about the sugar in the foods you eat, look at Appendix F.)

8 Find the hidden sugar in the processed foods you buy. Refer to Appendix F, which shows how many teaspoons of sugar are in many common processed foods, or read the labels and note the position of sugar in the list of ingredients. The ingredient in the largest amount appears first. *Sugar* is not the only word to look for; be sure to count sugar's sisters as well. If different kinds of sugar appear in second, third, and fourth place on a label, then sugar is the predominant ingredient even though it isn't listed first.

9 The cereal section of a supermarket is a good place to go in pursuit of hidden sugar. (Appendix F lists about 80 cereals and shows the percentage of sucrose in each.) Make a list of the brand names of cereals in the store where you shop, and indicate if there is sugar in the list of ingredients and where in the list it is positioned. Again, be sure to count sugar by other names. It will be interesting to see how many cereals are primarily sugar products, not grain products, and how many contain no sugar.

10 Notice your own serving sizes. Many people think that the spoon they use for sugar is a teaspoon, but when it is heaped high with sugar it is more nearly two. Using your sugar spoon as you usually do, spoon ten helpings of sugar into a bowl. Now measure this sugar with a measuring spoon, using level teaspoonfuls. How many teaspoons is a spoonful of sugar as you use it?

11 Visualize your intake of concentrated sweets. Calculate this intake in grams as directed in item 6; convert to teaspoons (5 grams are about a teaspoon). Now measure into a glass or jar the same amount of sugar. People often find this a surprising experience.

12 Dentists inform us that after each exposure to sugar, the caries-causing bacteria on the teeth are maximally active for about twenty minutes, attacking the tooth enamel. The amount of sugar makes no difference; its presence alone makes this possible. Thus, 100 grams of sugar taken in ten doses is ten times worse than 100 grams of sugar taken in one dose—from the dental health point of view. What is the frequency of your exposures to sugar? What are the implications of your answer, in terms of the health of your teeth?

13 You may be interested in computing fiber intake as well. Use Tables 2–3 and 2–4 in Chapter 2 or the table in Appendix K to get a rough idea of the amount of fiber you consume. Then compare your fiber intake with the estimated 6 grams (crude fiber) provided by the typical U.S. diet in the year 1900 and with the estimated 4 grams provided today. Some authorities believe that 10 or more grams crude fiber (25 grams dietary fiber) per day is a desirable intake.

Self–Study 3 (Chapter 3) Examine Your Fat Intake

These exercises make use of the information you recorded on Forms 1 to 3.

1 How many grams of fat do you consume in a day?

2 How many kcalories does this represent? (Remember, 1 gram of fat contributes 9 kcalories.)

3 What percentage of your total kcalories is contributed by fat? (To figure this, divide fat kcalories by total kcalories, then multiply by 100, as instructed in Self-Study 1.)

4 A dietary guideline says fat should contribute not more than 30 percent of total kcalories. How does your fat intake compare with this recommendation? If it is higher, look over your food records to find out what specific foods you could cut down on or eliminate and what foods you could add to your diet to bring your total fat intake into line.

5 How much linoleic acid do you consume? (Use Appendix G.) Remembering that linoleic acid is a lipid (energy value, 9 kcalories per gram), calculate the number of kcalories it gives you. What percentage of your total kcalories comes from linoleic acid? The guideline recommends 1 to 3 percent.

6 Estimate how much cholesterol you consume daily, using Appendix G. How does your cholesterol intake compare with the suggested limit of 300 milligrams a day? If your intake is high, you might want to read Highlight 3 before arriving at any conclusions regarding the importance of this limit.

7 You may not be aware how large your meat portions are. Weigh them for a day or so to see. Then calculate how much fat you derive from meat in a day. To visualize this amount of fat, measure it from your butter or margarine dish onto a plate.

Self–Study 4 (Chapter 4) Evaluate Your Protein Intake

These exercises make use of the information you recorded on Forms 1 to 3.

Q

1 How many grams of protein do you consume in a day?

2 How many kcalories does this represent? (Remember, 1 gram of protein contributes 4 kcalories.)

3 What percentage of your total kcalories is contributed by protein?

4 The *Dietary Goals* suggest that protein should contribute about 10 to 15 percent of total kcalories. How does your protein intake compare with this recommendation? (Note: if you are on a kcalorie-restricted diet, then a higher percentage of your kcalories should come from protein. See Self-Study 7.) If your protein intake is out of line, what foods could you consume more of—or less of—to bring it into line?

5 Calculate your protein RDA (see p. 144). Is it similar to the RDA for an "average" person your age and sex as shown in the RDA Tables (inside front cover)?

6 Compare your average daily protein intake with your RDA. On the average, about what percentage of your RDA for protein are you consuming each day? If you are "average" and healthy, the RDA is probably a generous recommendation for you, and yet you are probably eating more than the recommendation. This means that you may be spending protein prices for an energy nutrient. What substitutions could you make in your day's food choices so that you would derive from carbohydrate, rather than from protein, the kcalories you need for energy?

7 How many of your protein grams are from animal, and how many from plant, foods? Assuming that the animal protein is all of high quality, no more than 20 percent of your total protein need come from this source. Should you alter the ratio of plant to animal protein in your diet? If you did, what effect would this have on the total *fat* content of your diet?

8 How is your protein intake distributed through the day? (At what times do you eat—how many grams of protein each time?) Do you have amino acids at breakfast time to help maintain your blood glucose supply from carbohydrate? At lunchtime, to replenish dwindling pools? At dinnertime, to sustain you through the evening?

9 An exercise in Self-Study 12 shows how to economize on buying protein by calculating the cost of foods per gram of protein. You might want to try that exercise now.

Self–Study 6 (Chapter 6)
Estimate Your Energy Output

The first four exercises provide a detailed method of determining your daily energy need. Exercise 1 estimates energy for basal metabolism; exercise 2, energy for muscular activities; and exercise 3, energy for the specific dynamic effect of food. Exercise 4 shows you how to put them all together to obtain your "personalized RDA" for energy.

1 First, compute the energy you need to support your basal metabolic activity. A method based on surface area has been used in previous editions of this book, but a more accurate determination can be made based on a number derived from the body weight—the "metabolic body size." The metabolic body sizes for persons of different weights are shown in Table 1. A person's metabolic body size times a factor of 70 provides an accurate estimate of basal metabolic energy needs in kcalories per day. Compute your basal metabolic energy need using Table 1.

Example: A person who weighs 110 pounds would first calculate that, because 1 kilogram is equal to 2.2 pounds, she weighs 50 kilograms (110 ÷ 2.2). Then, in Table 1, she would find her metabolic body size—18.8 kg¾. This figure times 70 provides an estimate of 1,316 kcalories per day for basal metabolic energy need.

2 Now determine the energy you need for your voluntary muscular activities. The following is an accurate method, provided that the day you select is typical. Keep a 24-hour diary of your activities. Record them on a form like Form 6.

Table 2 shows a variety of activities classified into six energy levels, depending on the extent of muscle movement involved. Look up each of your activities in the table, find the column representing its energy level, and *record the number of minutes spent on that activity in that column*. For example, if you spent 45 minutes dressing—8 of those minutes at energy level b, 23 at level c, and 12 at level d—you would put down "8" in column b, "23" in column c, and "12" in column d. Every minute of your day should be accounted for—1,440 minutes in all.

Extra energy is spent running up and down stairs. Each time you go up or down stairs, record the minutes spent in column d or e (energy levels d and e are typical of walking), but keep a separate record of the number of flights you climbed as well. Count 14 to 15 steps as one flight of stairs.

For example, suppose that during the 45 minutes you spent dressing, you went downstairs for the newspaper, came back up to lock the door, and then went down again for breakfast. You would enter all 45 minutes on the form but would also record "down twice, up once" at the bottom of the form.

After making a 24-hour record, add up the number of minutes in each column to obtain the total minutes spent at level b, the total spent at level c, and so forth. Combined, these totals should add up to 1,440 minutes.

Finally, use Form 7 to compute the total energy spent for all activities. (Notice that there is a place at the bottom of this form to calculate the extra energy spent climbing

TABLE Q–1   **Metabolic Body Size (Wt$^{3/4}$) for Body Weights from 4 to 100 Kilograms**
(An 8.8-pound infant weighs 4 kilograms; a 220-pound adult weighs 100 kilograms. Weights outside this range are available in the original reference.)

Wt (kg)	Wt¾ (kg¾)	Wt (kg)	Wt¾ (kg¾)	Wt (kg)	Wt¾ (kg¾)	Wt (kg)	Wt¾ (kg¾)
4	2.83	30	12.8	56	20.5	82	27.2
5	3.34	31	13.1	57	20.8	83	27.5
6	3.83	32	13.5	58	21.0	84	27.7
7	4.30	33	13.8	59	21.3	85	28.0
8	4.75	34	14.1	60	21.6	86	28.2
9	5.19	35	14.4	61	21.8	87	28.5
10	5.62	36	14.7	62	22.1	88	28.7
11	6.04	37	15.0	63	22.4	89	29.0
12	6.44	38	15.3	64	22.6	90	29.2
13	6.84	39	15.6	65	22.9	91	29.4
14	7.24	40	15.9	66	23.2	92	29.7
15	7.62	41	16.2	67	23.4	93	29.9
16	8.00	42	16.5	68	23.7	94	30.2
17	8.38	43	16.8	69	23.9	95	30.4
18	8.75	44	17.1	70	24.2	96	30.7
19	9.10	45	17.4	71	24.4	97	30.9
20	9.46	46	17.7	72	24.7	98	31.1
21	9.8	47	18.0	73	25.0	99	31.4
22	10.2	48	18.2	74	25.2	100	31.6
23	10.5	49	18.5	75	25.5		
24	10.8	50	18.8	76	25.8		
25	11.2	51	19.1	77	26.0		
26	11.5	52	19.4	78	26.2		
27	11.8	53	19.6	79	26.5		
28	12.2	54	19.9	80	26.7		
29	12.5	55	20.2	81	27.0		

Example: A person weighing 45 kilograms would have a metabolic body size of 17.4 kg$^{3/4}$ and would require about 1,008 (70 × 17.4) kcalories per day for basal metabolism. These data provide accurate estimates of metabolic energy needs for animals as well as people from weights of 1 gram to 1,000 kilograms. They are used by the Committee on RDA in establishing recommended energy intakes for healthy individuals.
Source: M. Kleiber, *The Fire of Life* (New York: Wiley, 1961), Chap. 10, pp. 177–216, and Appendix 24, pp. 380–385.

stairs.) By completing this form, you will arrive at an estimate of the energy you spend on muscular activity in a day.
3 Now estimate the energy you spent on the digestion and metabolism of food (SDE). If you know how many kcalories you ingested that day, use 10 percent of those kcalories. Otherwise, add the energy you used for basal metabolism and for muscular activities to obtain a subtotal. Take 10 percent of this subtotal as an estimate of the SDE.
4 Last, add all three figures—energy for BMR, energy for activities, and energy for SDE—to obtain the total energy you spent in a 24-hour period. This figure represents the best estimate you can easily obtain of the number of kcalories you need to eat each day in order to maintain your weight. It is your "personalized RDA" for energy. Keep this figure to use in Self-Study 7 on diet planning.
5 After completing exercises 1 to 4, you can classify your lifestyle as sedentary, lightly active, moderately active, or very active by the criteria described on p. 217. A sedentary person, for example, spends 50 percent as much energy on muscular activities as on BMR. What percentage do you spend?

Example: Ms. R's basal metabolic rate is 1,200 kcalories per day, and she uses 600 kcalories per day for muscular activities. Since 600 is 50 percent of 1,200, her lifestyle is classed as sedentary.
6 The preceding five exercises dealt with kcalorie output. Now learn to estimate your kcalorie input, using the exchange system. Consult the record of the foods you ate on a typical day (from Self-Study 1), translate each food into an exchange, and record it on Form 8. Refer to Appendix L for the U.S., or Appendix M for the Canadian, exchange system. For foods not specifically listed there, use your judgment as to where they fit best in the system.

Q

After recording all your foods on Form 8 and classifying each into an exchange grouping, gather together all the milk exchanges and enter them on Form 9. Do the same for the vegetable exchanges, the fruit exchanges, and the others. Then use a single kcalorie value for each exchange (see the box on p. 212) to estimate the total kcalories you consumed that day.

How closely does your kcalorie estimate agree with the calculated amount you arrived at in Self-Study 1? If there is a big discrepancy, how do you account for it? In view of your finding here, would a greater familiarity with the exchange system be useful to you in the future? If so, practice using it some more by repeating this exercise, using the second and third days' records of Self-Study 1.

Self–Study 7 (Chapter 7) Practice Diet Planning

Diets can be planned using the exchange system to gain weight, lose weight, or stay the same. For practice in the use of this convenient system, try planning two diets, one for weight maintenance or gain, the other for weight loss. Use your own "personalized RDA for energy," derived in Self-Study 6, as a baseline for planning.

Diet for Weight Maintenance or Gain

1 Set your daily kcalorie level. If you choose to maintain weight, it should be equal to your "personalized RDA." If you wish to gain weight, it should be at least 500 kcalories above that (see Self-Study 6).

2 Decide on the proportions in which protein, fat, and carbohydrate kcalories will be represented in the diet. A suggested ratio is about 10 to 15 percent of the kcalories from protein, not more than 30 percent from fat, and the rest from carbohydrate. Given the daily kcalorie level you chose, how many kcalories will you allot to each nutrient?

3 Translate these kcalorie amounts into grams. (Remember, 1 gram of protein or carbohydrate = 4 kcalories; 1 gram of fat = 9 kcalories.) Enter these gram amounts and your intended kcalorie total at the top of Form 10.

4 Now decide how many exchanges of milk, vegetables, and fruit you'd like to have each day; enter these numbers in the form; and compute the number of grams of carbohydrate, protein, and fat they will deliver (don't compute kcalories yet). See p. 16 or Appendix L or M for the exchange system values. (Caution: Use pencil. You'll want to change these numbers several times before you finalize your plan.)

Only one more set of foods—the bread exchanges—contribute any carbohydrate to the diet. Select the number of

TABLE Q–2 Energy Levels and Their Energy Cost

Energy Level	Type of Activity	Energy Cost (kcal/kg/min)[a]	
		Woman	Man
a	Sleep or lying still, relaxed[b]	0.000	0.000
b	Sitting or standing still (includes activities like sewing, writing, eating)	0.001–0.007	0.003–0.012
c	Very light activity (like driving a car, walking slowly on level ground)	0.009–0.016	0.014–0.022
d	Light exercise (sweeping, eating, walking normally carrying books)	0.018–0.035	0.023–0.040
e	Moderate exercise (fast walking, dancing, bicycling, cleaning vigorously, moving furniture)	0.036–0.053	0.042–0.060
f	Heavy exercise (fast dancing, fast uphill walking, hitting tennis ball, swimming, gymnastics)	0.055	0.062

[a] Measured in kilocalories per kilogram per minute above basal energy.
[b] For purposes of this exercise, these are assumed to be at the basal level of energy.
Source: Adapted from J. V. G. A. Durnin and R. Passmore, *Energy, Work and Leisure* (London: Heinemann Educational Books, 1976).

bread exchanges that will bring your total carbohydrate intake close to the amount you want. Adjust the numbers of these four exchanges until they seem reasonable to you.

Suggestions: Diets for adults should include two to three milk exchanges daily, two or more vegetable exchanges, and at least two and preferably more fruit exchanges. The number of bread exchanges is variable, but the bread list includes many nutritious foods containing complex carbohydrates. It is not unusual for women's diets to include four to six bread exchanges and for men's to include twice as many or even more. High kcalorie diets can have many more of all of these carbohydrate-containing exchanges.

If you have a special fondness for sugar or sugar-containing foods, add a line to Form 10 under Bread, and allow yourself some "sugar exchanges" (see p. 63). At the end of this step, you should have a carbohydrate gram total within about 10 percent of the number you planned in step 3.

5 Subtotal the protein grams delivered by these four types of foods. Only one more list of foods—the meat exchanges—will contribute any protein to the diet. Select the number

of meat exchanges you need to bring your total protein intake close to what you planned in step 3.

Note: The recommended intake of carbohydrate is high compared with what many people are used to. Planners often find that once they have completed step 4 of this procedure they have almost used up their protein allowance and must therefore drastically limit their consumption of meat exchanges. If it works out this way for you, you have two choices. You can accept the dictates of this pattern and resolve to limit your intake of meats and meat substitutes accordingly. Or you can increase the number of protein grams you will allow yourself (step 3) and reduce carbohydrate and/or fat to keep the kcalorie level within bounds.

At the end of this step, you should have a protein gram total that agrees (within 10 percent) with your plan of step 3.

6 Subtotal the fat grams delivered by these five categories of foods. Now use the fat exchanges to bring your total fat intake up to the level planned in step 3.

7 Fill in the kcalorie amounts contributed by the exchanges you have selected, and check to see that the total agrees (within 10 percent) with the kcalorie level you set in step 1. The completed form now indicates the total exchanges of each type that you will consume on each day of your diet.

8 Distribute the exchanges you have selected into a meal pattern like that on Form 11. You may want to plan four to six meals a day or to have only one snack; if so, or if you have other preferences, make your own form.

9 Finally, to see how your diet plan might work out on an actual day, make a sample menu. Look over the exchange lists and choose foods you would like to eat that fit the pattern you worked out in step 8. For example:

My meal pattern for breakfast specifies:
1 fruit exchange.
2 bread exchanges.
1 milk exchange.
1 sugar exchange.
1 fat exchange.
So I might choose:
½ c orange juice.
¾ oz dry cereal and 1 slice bread, toasted.
½ c milk on the cereal and ½ c milk in a glass.
1 tsp sugar on the cereal.
1 pat margarine on the toast.

Diet for Weight Loss

1 Set your daily kcalorie level. If you wish to lose a pound a week, set it 500 kcalories per day below your "personalized RDA." You could set it higher or lower than this, but on no account should you set it below 1,000 kcalories per day unless your height is below average (see pp. 218–219).

2 Decide on the proportions in which protein, fat, and carbohydrate kcalories will be represented in the diet. A suggested ratio is that offered in Chapter 7, Table 7–3: about 33 percent of the kcalories from each energy nutrient.

3 Translate these kcalorie amounts into grams, as in the previous diet plan, and enter them and your kcalorie level into Form 10.

4 Now, using pencil on Form 10, decide on the number of carbohydrate-containing exchanges you'll have, as in step 4 of the first plan. Try to include two milk, two vegetable, and at least two fruit exchanges, and make up the rest of your carbohydrate intake with bread exchanges. Allow no sugar unless you really can't do without it. At the end of this step you should have a carbohydrate gram total within about 10 percent of the number you planned in step 3.

5 Now subtotal the protein grams you have so far, and bring your total protein intake up to the level of your plan by adding meat exchanges. At the end of this step, you should have a protein gram total that agrees (within 10 percent) with your plan of step 3.

6 Now subtotal the fat grams you have so far, and add fat exchanges to bring your total fat intake up to the level planned in step 3.

7 Fill in the kcalorie amounts contributed by the exchanges you have selected, and check to see that the total agrees (within 10 percent) with the kcalorie level you set in step 1.

8 Distribute the exchanges into a meal pattern, using Form 11 or your own form based on your own preferences.

9 Make a day's sample menus, as in step 9 of the first plan.

Self–Study 8 (Chapter 8) Evaluate Your Intakes of B Vitamins and Vitamin C

Several of these exercises make use of the information you recorded on Forms 1 to 3.

1 Look up and record your recommended intake of thiamin (from the RDA tables on the inside front cover or from the Canadian *Dietary Standard* in Appendix O). Also record your actual intake, from the average derived on Form 2 (Self-Study 1). What percentage of your recommended intake did you consume? Was this enough? What foods contribute the greatest amount of thiamin to your diet? If you consumed more than the recommendation, was this too much? Why or why not? In what ways would you change your diet to improve your thiamin intake?

2 Repeat exercise 1 using riboflavin as the subject.

3 Estimate your niacin intake using the method outlined

Q

on p. 283. Did you consume enough niacin preformed in foods to meet your recommended intake? If not, did you consume enough extra protein to bring your intake up to the recommendation? What do you suppose are the limitations on this means of estimating niacin intake?

4 Find alternative sources of riboflavin for the person who doesn't drink milk. Many people avoid milk products because of allergy, lactose intolerance, or personal preference. How can these people meet their riboflavin needs without drinking milk? Plan a day's menus around the favorite foods of the U.S. South (pork, fish, chicken, greens, corn bread, hominy grits, and sweet potatoes) to provide adequacy for thiamin and riboflavin. Be sure not to exceed the appropriate kcalorie level. Is it necessary to eat *enriched* corn bread and grits in order to get enough of these nutrients? Show your calculations.

Alternatively, plan a day's menus around your own favorite foods (if you avoid milk) or around the favorite foods of a friend of yours who dislikes milk. Is it necessary for you or your friend to eat *enriched* or *whole-grain* breads or cereals in order to get enough riboflavin? Show your calculations.

5 Explode some of the myths surrounding the vitamins. Go to a health food store and interview the owner or salesperson about the virtues of the products being sold there. Jot down these claims and the evidence cited to substantiate them. Which claims would you be inclined to believe on the basis of the evidence? Which are examples of the kinds of misinformation we have cautioned you about?

6 Record your recommended intake of folacin and compare it with your actual intake from Self-Study 1. Which are your best food sources of folacin? Remembering that folacin is destroyed by processing and cooking, do you have ample raw, whole-food sources of folacin? The food contents of folacin and the folacin RDA are approximate, so even if your folacin intake appears low, you may not have a physiological deficiency. Still, it is worthwhile to know how your intake compares with the recommendation, and to take steps to increase it if it seems low.

7 Look up and record your recommended intake of vitamin C. Also record a possible maximum intake (suggestion: 250 milligrams). Now record your actual intake from Self-Study 1. Was it within this range? What foods contribute the greatest amount of vitamin C to your diet? If you consumed less than the minimum or more than the maximum, in what ways could you change your diet to improve it in this respect?

8 Suppose a person dislikes fruits but likes vegetables. Find a substitute for fruit sources of vitamin C. How much of a serving of greens would she have to consume daily to meet her recommended intake for vitamin C? How many servings of potatoes would meet the recommended intake? Cabbage is a favorite vegetable of the Chinese. How much cabbage must a person eat to consume the recommended intake of vitamin C? Mexicans eat citrus fruits infrequently but use green bell peppers and tomatoes daily. Can they meet their vitamin C needs this way?

9 Return to the health food store and ask about the virtues of vitamin C supplements. Jot down the claims and the evidence cited to substantiate them. Which claims are you inclined to believe? Which seem false? Why?

Self–Study 9 (Chapter 9) Evaluate Your Intakes of Vitamins A, D, E, and K

These exercises make use of the information you recorded in Self-Study 1.

1 Look up and record your recommended intake of vitamin A. Note that this recommendation is stated in RE units.

2 What percentage of your recommended intake of vitamin A did you consume? Was this enough? What foods contribute the greatest amount of vitamin A to your diet? What percentage of your intake comes from plant foods? If you consumed more than the recommendation, was this too much? Why or why not? In what ways would you change your diet to improve it in this respect?

3 Tables of food composition do not show vitamins D, E, and K, but you can guess at the adequacy of your intake. For vitamin D, answer the following questions. Do you drink fortified milk (read the label)? Eat eggs? Fortified breakfast cereal? Liver? Are you in the sun frequently? (Remember, though, that excessive exposure to sun can cause skin cancer in susceptible individuals.)

4 For vitamin E, consider the foods you ate in 24 hours. Vitamin E often accompanies linoleic acid in foods. Did you consume enough linoleic acid? (The recommendation is 1 to 3 percent of total kcalories from linoleic acid, as specified in Self-Study 3).

5 For vitamin K, does your diet include 2 cups of milk or the equivalent in milk products every day? Does it include leafy vegetables frequently (every other day)? Do you take antibiotics regularly (which inhibit the production of vitamin K by your intestinal bacteria)?

6 Return to the health food store and ask some more questions, this time about the fat-soluble vitamins. Does the salesperson try to alert you to the risks of overdosing with these vitamins?

Self–Study 10 (Chapter 10) Evaluate Your Intakes of Major Minerals

1 Look up and record your recommended intake of calcium. Also record your actual intake, from the average derived on Form 2 (Self-Study 1). What percentage of your recommended intake did you consume? Was this enough? What foods contribute the greatest amount of calcium to your diet? If you consumed more than the recommendation, was this too much? Why or why not? In what ways would you change your diet to improve it in this respect? Remember that, although greens are high in calcium, the calcium is unavailable.

2 Estimate your sodium intake, using Appendix I. A dietary goal quoted in Chapter 10 is to restrict added salt intake to 5 grams per day or less. This means 2 grams (2,000 milligrams) of sodium in the added salt. (By "added salt," we mean salt added in processing or by you in cooking or at the table. It is assumed that foods you eat already contain about 3 grams of naturally occurring salt. So in calculating, count only the sodium you find in processed foods and in the salt shaker.)

Is your salt intake ample by this standard? Excessive? Should you consider making any changes, and if so, what kind?

Some authorities feel that the dietary goal for sodium should not apply to everyone but only to those who have a hereditary tendency toward heart disease, especially hypertension. Are these conditions characteristic of your family? The quiz in Highlight 3 gives you a means of estimating your risk of heart disease. The higher your score on that quiz, the more critical your sodium intake probably is.

3 Find alternative calcium sources for someone who doesn't drink milk. Plan a day's menus around this person's favorite foods.

Self–Study 11 (Chapter 11) Evaluate Your Intakes of Trace Minerals

1 Look up and record your recommended intake of iron. Also record your actual intake. What percentage of your recommended intake did you consume? Was this enough?

2 Which of the foods you eat supply the most iron? Rank your top five iron contributors. How many were meats? Legumes? Greens? Did any of them fall outside these classes? If so, what were they? How much of a contribution does enriched or whole-grain bread or cereal make to your iron intake? Are there refined bread/cereal products in your diet, such as pastries, that you could replace with enriched or whole-grain products to increase your iron intake?

3 Compute your iron absorption from a meal of your choosing. Three factors go into the calculation—first, how much of the iron in the meal was heme and how much was nonheme iron; second, how much vitamin C was in the meal; and third, how much total meat, fish, and poultry (MFP) was consumed. Here's how it works.[2] First, answer these six questions:

(1) How much iron was from animal tissues (MFP)? _____ mg

(2) Forty percent of this is heme iron. _____ mg heme iron

(3) How much iron was from other sources? _____ mg

(4) This, plus 60 percent of (1), is nonheme iron. _____ mg nonheme iron.

(5) How much vitamin C was in the meal? Less than 25 mg is low; 25 to 75 mg is medium; more than 75 mg is high.

(6) How much MFP was in the meal? Less than 1 oz lean MFP is low; more than 3 oz is high.

Now you're ready to calculate. You absorbed:

23 percent of the heme iron (2). _____ mg heme iron absorbed

Now, take your best score from (5) and (6). If either C or MFP was high, the availability of your nonheme iron was high. If neither was high but either was medium, the availability of your nonheme iron was medium. If both were low, your nonheme iron had poor availability. You absorbed:

High availability: 8 percent of the nonheme iron.

Medium availability: 5 percent.

Poor availability: 3 percent. _____ mg nonheme iron absorbed

Add the two together:

_____ mg heme iron absorbed.

_____ mg nonheme iron absorbed.

Total = _____ mg iron absorbed.

The RDA assumes you will absorb 10 percent of the iron you ingest. Thus, if you are a man of any age or a woman over 50 years old (RDA 10 milligrams), you need to absorb 1 milligram per day; if a woman 11 to 50 years old (RDA 18 milligrams), 1.8 milligrams.

---

2   Based on the method of E. R. Monsen and coauthors, Estimation of available dietary iron, *American Journal of Clinical Nutrition* 31 (1978): 134–141. Moderate iron stores assumed.

a need to learn more about individual foods
contributions of iron to the diet, look up some of
owing in Appendix H: different kinds of liver; differ-
green, leafy vegetables; various breads and cereals (do
enriched breads have more or less iron than whole-grain
breads, or are they about the same?); nuts and legumes;
dried fruits; molasses and other sugar sources. Pay particular attention to the foods you eat. Then plan several days'
menus you would enjoy that provide your recommended
intake.

5 Are you in an area of the country where the soil is iodine-
poor? If so, do you use iodized salt?

6 Record your recommended zinc intake and the amount
you actually consumed. What percentage of your recommended intake did you obtain from your diet? Which were
your best food sources? What guidelines do you need to
follow to be sure of obtaining enough zinc from the foods
you eat?

7 Is the water in your county fluoridated? (Call the County
Health Department.) If not, how do you and your family
ensure that your intakes of fluoride are optimal?

8 Review your three-day food record (Self-Study 1) and
separate the foods you ate into two categories: predominantly natural, unprocessed foods like those on the
exchange lists and highly processed foods, such as TV dinners, pastries, and instant gravies. Beside each food, record
its kcalorie value. How many total kcalories did you consume in three days? Of these, what percentage came from
highly processed foods? In light of the discussion of trace
elements in Chapter 11, what implications do you suppose
this estimate has for the nutritional adequacy of your diet?

Self–Study 12
(Chapter and Highlight 12)
Use Nutrient Density to
Help Assess Food Choices

1 Highlight 12 described food labels and the need for consumers to know how nutritious are the foods they buy. The
concept of nutrient density helps people estimate the nutritional value of foods. Using this concept, you can decide
which of your favorite foods are the most nutritious.

Pick a food, any food you are curious about, and follow
this procedure, using Form 12 to record the information:
a. Record your recommended kcalorie intake and your recommended intakes for protein, vitamins, and minerals from
the inside front cover or from Appendix O. (Self-Study 6
directed you to calculate how much energy you need for a
typical day. You may use this personalized calculation in

place of your recommended kcalorie intake if you feel it is
more accurate.)
b. Look up in Appendix H the number of kcalories and the
amounts of protein, vitamins, and minerals provided by a
serving of the food you are interested in, and list these
numbers under your recommended intakes.
c. Determine what percentage of your recommended
intake for kcalories a serving of the food provides. This will
be your *comparison number*.
d. Determine what percentage of your recommended
intake for each nutrient a serving of the food provides.
e. Divide each percentage derived for the nutrients by the
comparison number to give each nutrient a score.
f. The food might be considered nutritious if it receives a
score greater than 1 for each of four nutrients or greater
than 2 for each of two. By this standard, how nutritious is
the food you selected? Repeat this procedure several times
to study a variety of the foods in your diet.

2 An alternative way to visualize the nutrient density of a
food is to graph its energy and nutrient contributions
against your energy and nutrient RDA. For example, suppose your RDA were as follows: Energy, 2,500 kcalories;
protein, 56 grams; vitamins and minerals as in the U.S. RDA
table (inside back cover). You would draw on graph paper
a set of tall bars representing 100 percent of those RDA (see
Figure Q–1). Then you would look up the food in Appendix H, find its kcalorie and nutrient contributions, and compute each as a percentage of your RDA.

Home-made spaghetti with tomato sauce and cheese is
used here as an example. A cup provides 260 kcalories, or
about 10 percent of your 2,500-kcalorie RDA, so you would
color in 10 percent of the energy bar. The food contributes
9 grams of protein, or about 16 percent of your 56-gram
RDA, so you would color in about 16 percent of the protein
bar. Then you would proceed across the graph, representing every nutrient as a percentage of your RDA.

Now, compare the heights of the *nutrient* bars with that
of the *energy* bar. Almost all are as tall or taller, showing
that, in general, the food's contribution of nutrients (relative to your need) is as great as or greater than its contribution of energy (relative to your need).
a. Do this exercise for a person on a weight-loss diet whose
energy allowance is only 1,300 kcalories a day. Would the
spaghetti dish be of appropriate nutrient density for such a
person? Why or why not?
b. Do this exercise for a food you like to eat. Does its
nutrient density appear favorable on the graph?

3 Review your food records (Self-Study 1) and list from
them the foods that made the major contributions to your
kcalorie intakes on the days you studied. Jot down by each
food your reason for choosing it:

● Personal preference (I like it).
● Habit or tradition (It's familiar; I always eat it).

- Social pressure (It was offered; I couldn't refuse).
- Familiarity (It's a family food).
- Availability (I was hungry and it was the only food offered).
- Convenience (I was too rushed to prepare anything else).
- Economy (It was a food I could afford).
- Nutritional value (I thought it was good for me).
- Other (explain).

From what you know now, you can make a good guess about the nutritive value of each of these foods. In some cases you will find that a food chosen primarily because it tastes good to you is also nutritious—a happy surprise. In others, you may find that a food you thought was nutritious is not especially noteworthy in this sense. Such insights can help guide you toward food selections that meet your needs for pleasure as well as for good nutrition.

4 Having completed all the exercises to this point, you are in a position to decide whether you really need your vitamin-mineral supplement or other supplements. For each nutrient you've studied, compare your RDA, the amount you consume, and the amount contributed by your supplement. Does the supplement make up for a deficit in your intake, or is it an unnecessary extra? Perhaps, with the appropriate food choices, you can dispense with it.

5 You may want to know if the U.S. RDA used on labels is similar to your own RDA, so that the label information applies to you. Jot down your RDA for each nutrient from the inside front cover, and the U.S. RDA from the inside back cover. Compare them. Which of your RDA are out of line with the U.S. RDA? (For example, a food that contains only 50 percent of the U.S. RDA for iron would contain almost 100 percent of a man's iron RDA.)

6 Test the "ballpark estimate" versus the calculation method of assessing a person's nutrient intakes. Start with the information on a three-day dietary record—your own or someone else's. First, use the exchange system values of Chapters 1 and 7 and the tables in Chapters 8 to 11 to estimate the person's intakes of kcalories, protein, calcium, iron, zinc, vitamin A, thiamin, riboflavin, folacin, and vitamin C. Then use the calculation method: look up every food in Appendix H. Record the time each method takes you. In terms of improved accuracy from calculating instead of estimating, is the extra time worth spending? The answer will vary from one person to the next, depending on the foods in the record and on your skill in using the tables.

7 For the food shopper interested in economizing: protein food is one of the most costly items in the food budget. To cut down on food costs, calculate the cost per gram of the protein delivered by various foods. Form 13 will help in making these comparisons. You might wish to enter your own food choices in the spaces at the top.

FIGURE 1   **Nutrient density of home-made spaghetti with tomato sauce and cheese for a person with the nutrient needs shown. (Item 495 in Appendix H. Note that vitamin A is expressed in RE.)** TH12-2

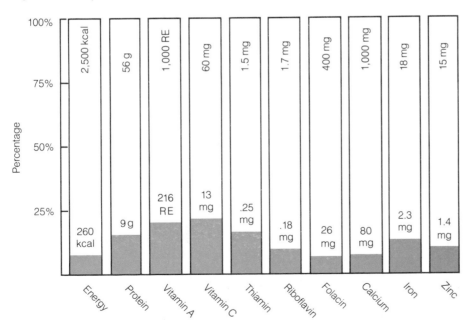

Q

FORM 1   **Nutrient Intakes (Use One Form for Each Day)**

Food	Approximate Measure or Weight	Energy[a] (kcal)	Protein[b] (g)	Fat[b] (g)	Carbo- hydrate[b] (g)	Calcium[a] (mg)	Iron[c] (mg)	Zinc[b] (mg)	Vitamin A[a] (RE)	Thiamin[c] (mg)	Riboflavin[c] (mg)	Niacin[b] (mg)	Folacin[a] (μg)	Vitamin C[b] (mg)
Total														

[a] Compute these values to the nearest whole number.
[b] Compute these values to one decimal place.
[c] Compute these values to two decimal places.

FORM 2 **Average Daily Energy and Nutrient Intakes**

Day	Energy (kcal)	Protein (g)	Fat (g)	Carbo-hydrate (g)	Calcium (mg)	Iron (mg)	Zinc (mg)	Vitamin A (RE)	Thiamin (mg)	Riboflavin (mg)	Niacin (mg)	Folacin (µg)	Vitamin C (mg)
1													
2													
3													
Total													
Average daily intake (divide total by 3)													

FORM 3 **Comparison with a Standard Intake**

Day	Energy (kcal)	Protein (g)	Fat (g)	Carbo-hydrate (g)	Calcium (mg)	Iron (mg)	Zinc (mg)	Vitamin A (RE)	Thiamin (mg)	Riboflavin (mg)	Niacin (mg)	Folacin (µg)	Vitamin C (mg)
Average daily intake (from Form 2)													
Standard[a]													
Intake as percentage of standard[b]													

[a] Taken from RDA tables (inside front cover) or *Recommended Nutrient Intakes for Canadians* (Appendix O).
[b] For example, if your intake of protein was 50 g and the standard for a person your age and sex was 46 g, then you consumed (50 ÷ 46) × 100, or 109 percent of the standard.

Q

FORM 4 **Percentage of kCalories from Protein, Fat, and Carbohydrate**

From Form 3:

Protein: _____ g/day × 4 kcal/g = (P) _____ kcal/day

Fat: _____ g/day × 9 kcal/g = (F) _____ kcal/day

Carbohydrate: _____ g/day × 4 kcal/g = (C) _____ kcal/day

Total kcal/day = (T) _____ kcal/day

Percentage of kcalories from protein:

$$\frac{(P)}{(T)} \times 100 = \text{\_\_\_\_\_ \% of total kcalories}$$

Percentage of kcalories from fat:

$$\frac{(F)}{(T)} \times 100 = \text{\_\_\_\_\_ \% of total kcalories}$$

Percentage of kcalories from carbohydrate:

$$\frac{(C)}{(T)} \times 100 = \text{\_\_\_\_\_ \% of total kcalories}$$

Note: The three percentages can total 99, 100, or 101, depending on the way in which figures were rounded off earlier.

FORM 5 **Food Selection Scorecard**

FOOD GROUP AND RECOMMENDED INTAKE	YOUR INTAKE FROM GROUP (SPECIFY FOOD AND AMOUNT)	YOUR SCORE
Fruits and vegetables—4 or more portions (½ cup cooked edible portion or 3-4 oz, 100 g, raw); at least 1 raw daily		
1 portion vitamin A–rich dark green or deep orange fruit or vegetable (any food with more than your RDA) = 10 points (no more than 10 points allowed)		
1 portion vitamin C–rich fruit or vegetable (any food with more than your RDA) = 10 points (no more than 10 points allowed)		
Other fruits and vegetables, incuding potatoes = 2.5 each		
Subtotal (no more than 25 points allowed)		
Breads and cereals—4 or more portions of whole-grain or enriched (1 oz dry-weight cereal or 1-oz slice bread or equivalent grain product)		
1 portion cereal or 2 bread equivalents = 10 points (no more than 10 points allowed)		
Other bread equivalents = 5 points each		
Subtotal (no more than 25 points allowed)		
Milk and milk products—2 or more portions (8 oz fluid milk; calcium equivalents are 1⅓ oz hard cheese, 1⅓ c cottage cheese, 1 pint ice milk or ice cream)		
One portion = 12.5 points		
Subtotal (no more than 25 points allowed)		

Q

FORM 5   (continued)

FOOD GROUP AND RECOMMENDED INTAKE	YOUR INTAKE FROM GROUP (SPECIFY FOOD AND AMOUNT)	YOUR SCORE

Meat and meat substitutes—2 or more portions of meat (2–3 oz of cooked lean meat, fish, poultry; protein equivalents are 2 eggs, 2 oz hard cheese, or ½ c cottage cheese) and 2 portions legumes or nuts (¾ c cooked legumes, 4 tbsp peanut butter, 1 oz nuts or sunflower seeds); count cheese either in milk group or in meat group, not both

2 portions meat = 12.5 points

2 portions legumes = 12.5 points

    Subtotal (no more than 25 points allowed)

    Grand total (no more than 100 points)

The above are foundation foods. Additional foods are those that do not fit into the above groupings but add flavor, interest, variety, and (often) kcalories. List those eaten:

_____   _____   _____
_____   _____   _____
_____   _____   _____

FORM 6   **Minutes Spent at Each Energy Level**

CLOCK TIME	TOTAL MINUTES	ACTIVITY	ENERGY LEVEL[a]					
			a	*b*	*c*	*d*	*e*	*f*
7:00 – 7:45	45	Dressing		8	23	14		
7:45 – 8:15	30	Eating	26	4				
8:15 – 9:00	45	Biking to school			4	25	16	

(Stairs: up   *I*
            down   *II*   )

Total

[a] See Table 6–2 for an explanation of these levels.

FORM 7 **Energy Cost for Muscular Activities (Exclusive of Basal Metabolism and the Effect of Food)**

ENERGY LEVEL	TOTAL MINUTES SPENT		ENERGY COST PER MINUTE (KCAL/KG/MIN)			TOTAL ENERGY COST PER KG (KCAL/KG)
			Women	*Men*		
a		×	0.000	0.000	=	0.000
b		×	0.001–0.007	0.003–0.012	=	
c		×	0.009–0.016	0.014–0.022	=	
d		×	0.018–0.035	0.023–0.040	=	
e		×	0.036–0.053	0.042–0.060	=	
f		×	0.055	0.062		
Subtotal	1,440					

Extra energy spent on stairs:

Flights down		×	0.012		=
Flights up		×	0.036		=

Total kcal/kg/24 hours

Now multiply by body weight (kg) to arrive at total energy spent on activities for the day: × ___ kg

= ___ kcal/day

FORM 8 **Foods Eaten in One Day Translated into Exchanges**

FOOD I ATE	PORTION OR AMOUNT	EXCHANGE LIST	NUMBER OF EXCHANGES
Banana	1 medium	fruit	2

FORM 9 **kCalories Consumed in One Day Based on Exchanges**

EXCHANGE LIST	TOTAL EXCHANGES	× KCAL/EXCHANGE =	ENERGY (KCAL)
Milk[a]		× 80 =	
Vegetables		× 25 =	
Fruit		× 40 =	
Bread		× 70 =	
Meat[b]		× 55 =	
Fat		× 45 =	
Sugar, tsp.		× 20 =	
		Total:	kcal

[a] If you used whole milk, add 2 fats for each cup of milk you drank. If you used low-fat milk, add 1 fat for each cup.

[b] If you used high-fat meat, add 1 fat for each ounce of meat. If you used medium-fat meat, add ½ fat for each ounce.

FORM 10 **Diet Planning by Exchange Groups** TH7-2

		Amounts to be Delivered[b]			
		Carbohydrate	Protein	Fat	Energy[c]
Exchange List	*Number of Exchanges[a]*	——— g	——— g	——— g	——— kcal
Milk					
Vegetable					
Fruit					
Bread					
Meat					
Fat					
	Total actually delivered				

[a] From steps 4, 5, 6.

[b] From step 3.

[c] From step 7.

Q

FORM 11   **Meal Patterns** TH7-3

EXCHANGE LIST	TOTAL EXCHANGES TO BE CONSUMED DAILY[a]	EXCHANGES CONSUMED AT EACH MEAL				
		BREAKFAST	LUNCH	SNACK	DINNER	SNACK
Milk						
Vegetable						
Fruit						
Bread						
Meat						
Fat						

[a] From Form 10, column 2.

FORM 12   **Nutrient Density of a Food**

Food chosen for analysis _____

	Energy (kcal)	Protein (g)	Calcium (mg)	Iron (mg)	Zinc (mg)	Vitamin A (RE)	Thiamin (mg)	Riboflavin[a] (mg)	Folacin (μg)	Vitamin C (mg)
① Your recommended intake										
② Amount provided by one serving of the food										
Percentage of recommended intake provided by one serving	③ Comparison number	④								④
⑤ Nutrition score										

⑥   Is the food nutritious? _____

[a] A complete calculation would include niacin, but we have omitted it because of the difficulty in estimating niacin derived from tryptophan (see Chapter 8).

FORM 13   **Calculating the Relative Costs of Protein**

	REGULAR HAMBURGER	LOW-FAT MILK	PLAIN CORNFLAKES	PEANUT BUTTER	EGGS	CANNED PORK AND BEANS
Grams protein per measure	23 g / 3 oz			4 g / 1 tbsp		
Amount of food to provide 10 g protein						
Cost of unit amount of food						
Cost of amount of food to provide 10 g protein						
Cost of 1 g protein						

Q

Index

Numbers in **bold face** refer to pages where definitions or major discussions appear. Numbers in *italics* refer to illustrations, diagrams, or chemical structures. A number followed by a "t" (e.g., 354t) refers to a table. Letters A, B, C, etc., refer to Appendixes. The letters IM refer to the *Instructor's Manual*.

A

AAP (address), J
Absorption, **155–182**, J
 see also nutrient names
Abuse. *See* Alcohol, Drug, Sugar
Acetaldehyde, 306–307
Acetate/acetic acid, *89*, 196–197
Acetone, **206**
Acetyl CoA, 101, 196–197, *200, 202,* 204–205
Acetylcholine, **152**
Acid, **89**, 135, 374, B
 ash diet, **378**
 -base balance, 135–136, 308, 377–379
 former, 378t
 gastric, 161
 group, **89**, *124*
 indigestion, 161
 see also Acidosis, Amino acid, Fatty acid
Acidosis, **136–137**
Acne (and vitamin A), 331
ACSH News and Views, A, J
ACT (address), J
ACTH, *186*
Active site (of enzyme), 271
Active transport, 172
Activity (physical). *See* Exercise
ADA (address), J
Adaptation, 205, 206, 208, IM
Addiction, **265**; *see also* Alcohol, Sugar
Additives, 35–36, 95, **397–408, 398, 399,** IM
 incidental/indirect/intentional, 369, **398,** 439, 446
 on labels, 483
 salt and sugar as, 75–76, 382, 485–486
 suggested references, J

see also Contaminants
Addresses (for nutrition information), J
Adenosine diphosphate. *See* ATP
Adenosine triphosphate. *See* ATP
Adequacy (of diet). *See* Diet planning
ADH (antidiuretic hormone), *186,* **311, 369**
ADH (enzyme). *See* Alcohol dehydrogenase
Adipose cell, 86; *see also* Fat (in body)
Adolescence (Adolescent, Teenager), 234, **533–545,** O
 alcohol and drug use, 539–541
 diet planning for, 535–536
 pregnancy in, 538–539
 suggested references, J
 see also Acne, Anorexia nervosa, Growth, RDA
ADP. *See* ATP
Adrenal gland, 51, 152, *186*
Adrenaline, **51**
Adrenocorticotropin, *186*
Advertising (food), 83, 528–529
Aerobic, **224**; *see also* Exercise
Aging. *See* Older adults
Agriculture (and world hunger), 357–359
AHA. *See* American Heart Association
AHEA (address), J
AIN (address), J
Alanine, 124, C
Alarm reaction (of stress), *186*
Albumin, 136, 422, 423, 457t, **458,** E
Alcohol, 4, *54,* **305–313,** J
 abuse and malnutrition, 142
 addiction (inherited), 540
 consumption and HDL, 120
 dehydrogenase, **305–307**

diet planning and, 30, 255, 472
effects on nutrients, 280, 283, 288, 309, 330, 540, 561
kcalories in, 255t
metabolism of, 305–310, *307*
quiz (alcoholism), IM
suggested references, J
see also Adolescence, Fetal alcohol syndrome, Older adults, Pregnancy, Sugar
Aldehyde, **95**
Aldosterone, *186,* 369, 380
Alimentary canal, **157–165**
Alkaline ash diet, **378**
Alkaline phosphatase, **338**
Alkalosis, 136, **137**
Allergy(ies), 516, IM
 breast milk and, 502, 503
 milk, 59, *391*
 suggested reference, J
Alpha cell, 51
Alpha-tocopherol, C
Alternative sweeteners. *See* Sweeteners
AMA (address), J
Amenorrhea, 223
American Heart Association (AHA), 118
Amino acid(s), **123–146,** *124,* C
 absorption of, 164–175
 chemical structure of, *124,* C
 coenzymes and, 273
 energy source, 200
 essential, **131**
 limiting, **131**
 metabolism of, 194, 199, *200,* 201, *202,* 297, 309
 niacin synthesis from 283
 sulfur containing, 394
 supplementation, 167, 423
 transport system, 169

214